Brain Computations and Connectivity

Brain Computations and Connectivity

Edmund T. Rolls

Oxford Centre for Computational Neuroscience
Oxford
England

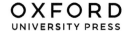

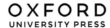

Great Clarendon Street, Oxford, OX2 6DP,
United Kingdom

Oxford University Press is a department of the University of Oxford.
It furthers the University's objective of excellence in research, scholarship,
and education by publishing worldwide. Oxford is a registered trade mark of
Oxford University Press in the UK and in certain other countries

© Edmund T. Rolls 2023

The moral rights of the author have been asserted

Some rights reserved. No part of this publication may be reproduced, stored in
a retrieval system, or transmitted, in any form or by any means, for commercial purposes,
without the prior permission in writing of Oxford University Press, or as expressly
permitted by law, by licence or under terms agreed with the appropriate
reprographics rights organization.

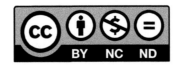

This is an open access publication, available online and distributed under the terms of a
Creative Commons Attribution – Non Commercial – No Derivatives 4.0
International licence (CC BY-NC-ND 4.0), a copy of which is available at
http://creativecommons.org/licenses/by-nc-nd/4.0/.

Enquiries concerning reproduction outside the scope of this licence
should be sent to the Rights Department, Oxford University Press, at the address above

Published in the United States of America by Oxford University Press
198 Madison Avenue, New York, NY 10016, United States of America

British Library Cataloguing in Publication Data

Data available

Library of Congress Control Number: 2023940370

ISBN 978–0–19–888791–1

DOI: 10.1093/oso/9780198887911.001.0001

Printed and bound by
CPI Group (UK) Ltd, Croydon, CR0 4YY

Links to third party websites are provided by Oxford in good faith and
for information only. Oxford disclaims any responsibility for the materials
contained in any third party website referenced in this work.

Preface

This book, *Brain Computations and Connectivity* is an update to Rolls *Brain Computations: What and How* published by Oxford University Press in 2021. A key part of this updated version of *Brain Computations: What and How* is the addition of much new evidence that has emerged since 2021 on the connectivity of the human brain, which by analysing the effective or causal connectivity between 360 cortical regions, enriches our understanding of information processing streams in the human cerebral cortex. Knowing how one cortical region connects to other cortical regions helps to provide a deeper understanding of how each stage in a processing stream contributes to the computations being performed, as each processing stream is now becoming better defined.

The addition in *Brain Computations and Connectivity* of much new evidence on the connectivity of the human brain is leading to better understanding of what is computed in different human brain regions, which in turn has implications for how the computations are performed. The added emphasis in this book on the organisation, connectivity, and functions of 360 cortical regions in the human brain increases the application of new approaches taken to understanding how the brain works that are described in this book, by making the evidence very relevant to the human brain, and thereby to those who are interested in disorders of the human brain, including neurologists and psychiatrists, as well as to all those interested in understanding how the human brain works in health and disease. The enables the computational approaches to understanding brain function described in this book to be combined with and made highly relevant to understanding human brain function. It is hoped that these developments in understanding human brain function by including analysis of the connectivity of the 360 cortical regions in the Human Connectome Project Multimodal Parcellation (HCP-MMP) atlas (Glasser et al., 2016a; Huang et al., 2022) as described here will provide a foundation for future research that by using the HCP-MMP can be related to the connectivity and functions of these 360 cortical regions in the human brain that are described in this book. The title of this book, *Brain Computations and Connectivity*, refers to the importance of this type of connectivity in understanding what and how the brain computes.

Another feature of this book is that it adopts what was described as a 'grand unifying approach' in a review in the journal *Brain* (Manohar, 2022) of *Brain Computations: What and How* (Rolls, 2021b) in that it takes a biologically plausible approach to how the brain computes, rather than invoking the artificial intelligence approach of deep learning to try to account for brain computation. The approach to how the brain computes in this book is biologically plausible in that it utilises primarily local synaptic modification rules to set up the synaptic connections between neurons, and unsupervised learning, yet considers how far this can take us in understanding how the brain operates. This approach is quite different to the deep learning approach used now in much machine learning and AI, which backpropagates an error backwards through the network to correct every synaptic weight in all preceding layers of the network, but there is no connectivity in the brain for that. Moreover, the learning in the brain is largely unsupervised, whereas deep learning approaches typically require a supervisor for each output neuron, which in turn requires what must be computed for each output neuron to be specified by the designer of the deep network. The point is developed (in Chapter 19) that machine learning might benefit from understanding some of the unsupervised approaches used by the brain to solve complex problems, including navigation, attention, semantics, and even syntax. The title of this book, *Brain Computations and Connectivity*, also refers to this concept that the actual connectivity at the local level of neurons and synapses that is found in the brain is important in understanding what and how it computes.

My aim in making this book Open Access is to make the scholarship and ideas in this book easily available to colleagues, in the interests of better understanding the human brain in health and disease. This book can be cited as Rolls, E. T. (2023) *Brain Computations and Connectivity*, Oxford University Press, Oxford. The book can be downloaded from https://www.oxcns.org or from the Oxford University Press website. An advantage of publication of this book as a .pdf is that it contains extensive hyperlinks, enabling readers to quickly cross-refer to other parts of the book or to citations. With the .pdf, figures can also be expanded to show details.

Many scientists, and many others, are interested in how the brain works. In order to understand this, we need to know **what** computations are performed by different brain systems; and **how** they are computed by each of these systems.

The aim of this book is to elucidate what is computed in different brain systems; and to describe current computational approaches and models of how each of these brain systems computes.

To understand how our brains work, it is essential to know **what** is computed in each part of the brain. That can be addressed by utilising evidence relevant to computation from many areas of neuroscience. Knowledge of the connections between different brain regions is important, for this shows that the brain is organised as systems, with whole series of brain regions devoted for example to visual processing. That provides a foundation for examining the computation performed by each brain region, by comparing what is represented in a brain regions with what is represented in the preceding and following brain regions, using techniques of for example neurophysiology and functional neuroimaging. The ways in which effective connectivity is now available for 360 cortical regions are introduced in Chapter 1, with the results of these new analyses found throughout this book. Neurophysiology at the single neuron level is needed because this is the level at which information is transmitted between the computing elements of the brain, the neurons. Evidence from the effects of brain damage, including that available from neuropsychology, is needed to help understand what different parts of the system do, and indeed what each part is necessary for. Functional neuroimaging is useful to indicate where in the human brain different processes take place, and to show which functions can be dissociated from each other. So for each brain system, evidence on what is computed at each stage, and what the system as a whole computes, is essential.

To understand how our brains work, it is also essential to know **how** each part of the brain computes. That requires a knowledge of what is computed by each part of the brain, but it also requires knowledge of the network properties of each brain region. This involves knowledge of the connectivity between the neurons in each part of the brain, and knowledge of the synaptic and biophysical properties of the neurons. It also requires knowledge of the theory of what can be computed by networks with defined connectivity.

There are at least three key goals of the approaches described here. One is to understand ourselves better, and how we work and think. A second is to be better able to treat the system when it has problems, for example in mental illnesses. Medical applications are a very important aim of the type of research described here. A third, is to be able to emulate the operation of parts of our brains, which some in the field of artificial intelligence (AI) would like to do to produce useful computers that incorporate some of the principles of computation utilised by the brain. All of these goals require, and cannot get off the ground, without a firm foundation in what is computed by brain systems, and theories and models of how it is computed. To understand the operation of the whole brain, it is necessary to show how the different brain systems operate together: but a necessary foundation for this is to know what is computed in each brain system, and the connectivity between the different regions involved.

Part of the enterprise here is to stimulate new theories and models of how parts of the brain work. The evidence on what is computed in different brain systems had advanced rapidly in the last 50 years, and provides a reasonable foundation for the enterprise, though there is much that remains to be learned. Theories of how the computation is performed are less advanced, but progress is being made, and current models are described in this book for many brain systems, in the expectation that before further advances are made, knowledge of the considerable current evidence on how the brain computes provides a useful starting point, especially as current theories do take into account the limitations that are likely to be imposed by the neural architectures present in our brains. In this book, the focus is on biologically plausible algorithms for brain computation, rather than for example deep learning which does not appear to be how the brain learns and computes (Sections B.12 and B.14).

The simplest way to delineate **brain computation** is to examine what information is represented at each stage of processing, and how this is different from stage to stage. For example in the primary visual cortex (V1), neurons respond to simple stimuli such as bars or edges or gratings and have small receptive fields. Little can be read off from the firing rates about for example whose face is represented from a small number of neurons in V1. On the other hand, after four or five stages of processing, in the inferior temporal visual cortex, information can be read from the firing rates of neurons about whose face is being viewed, and indeed there is remarkable invariance with respect to the position, size, contrast and even in some cases view of the face. That is a major computation, and indicates what can be achieved by biological neuronal network computation.

These approaches can only be taken to understand brain function because there is considerable localization of function in the brain, quite unlike a digital computer. One fundamental reason for localization of function in the brain is that this minimizes the total length of the connections between neurons, and thus brain size. Another is that it simplifies the genetic information that has to be provided in order to build the brain, because the connectivity instructions can refer considerably to local connections. These points are developed in my book *Cerebral Cortex: Principles of Operation* (Rolls, 2016b).

That brings me to what is different about the present book and *Cerebral Cortex: Principles of Operation* (Rolls, 2016b). *Cerebral Cortex: Principles of Operation* took on the enormous task of making progress with understanding how the major part of our brains, the cerebral cortex, works, by understanding its principles of operation. The present book builds on that approach, and uses it as background, but has the different aim of taking each of our brain systems, and describing *what* they compute, and then what is known about *how* each system computes. The issue of how they compute relies for many brain systems on how the cortex operates, so *Cerebral Cortex: Principles of Operation* provides an important complement to the present book.

With its focus on what and how each brain system computes, a field that includes computational neuroscience, this book is distinct from the many excellent books on neuroscience that describe much evidence about brain structure and function, but do not aim to provide an understanding of how the brain works at the computational level. This book aims to forge an understanding of how some key brain systems may operate at the computational level, so that we can understand how the brain actually performs some of its complex and necessarily computational functions in memory, perception, attention, decision-making, cognitive functions, and actions.

Indeed, as one of the key aims of this book is to describe **what computations** are performed by different brain systems, I have chosen to include in this book some of the key actual discoveries in neuroscience that I believe help to define what computations are performed in different brain systems. Part of the aim of citing the original pioneering discoveries is to show how conceptual advances have been made in our understanding of what is computed in each region of our brains, for understanding the key discoveries provides a foundation for further advances.

That makes this book very different from many of the textbooks of neuroscience (such as *Principles of Neural Science* (Kandel et al., 2021)), and some of the textbooks of theoretical neuroscience that describe principles of operation of neurons or of networks of neurons (Dayan and Abbott, 2001; Hertz et al., 1991; Gerstner et al., 2014), but not in general what is computed in different brain systems, and how it is computed. Further, there are likely to be great developments in our understanding of *how* the brain computes, and this book is intended to set out a framework for new developments, by providing an analysis of what is computed by different brain systems, and providing some current approaches to how these computations may be performed. I believe that this book, and its predecessor *Brain Computations: What and How*, is pioneering in what I propose is the necessary approach to understanding brain function, understanding 'What' is computed by each brain region, and 'How' it is computed.

A test of whether one's understanding is correct is to simulate the processing on a computer, and to show whether the simulation can perform the tasks performed by the brain, and whether the simulation has similar properties to the real brain. This approach to neural computation leads to a precise definition of how the computation is performed, and to precise and quantitative tests of the theories produced. How memory systems in the brain work is a paradigm example of this approach, because memory-like operations which involve altered functionality as a result of synaptic modification are at the heart of how many computations in the brain are performed. It happens that attention and decision-making can be understood in terms of interactions between and fundamental operations in memory systems in the cortex, and therefore it is natural to address these areas of cognitive neuroscience in this book. The same fundamental concepts based on the operation of neuronal circuitry can be applied to all these functions, as is shown in this book.

One of the distinctive properties of this book is that it links the neural computation approach not only firmly to neuronal neurophysiology, which provides much of the primary data about how the brain operates, but also to psychophysical studies (for example of attention); to neuropsychological studies of patients with brain damage; and to functional magnetic resonance imaging (fMRI) (and other neuroimaging) approaches. The empirical evidence that is brought to bear is largely from non-human primates and from humans, because of the considerable similarity of their cortical systems, and the major differences in their systems-level computational organization from that of rodents, as set out in Section 19.10.

Another feature of the book is that it aims to describe the principles of operation of the brain, and in doing that, frequently refers to the original research in which those principles were discovered. Another feature of the book is that I have also chosen to make each Chapter relatively understandable on its own, which may involve some information also present in other parts of the book, so that readers with an interest in one part of the brain can benefit by reading the relevant chapters, rather than necessarily having to read the whole book.

The overall aims of the book are developed further, and the plan of the book is described, in Chapter 1. Appendix B describes the fundamental operation of key networks of the type that are likely to be the building blocks of brain function. Appendix C describes quantitative, information theoretic, approaches to how information is represented in the brain, which is an essential framework for understanding what is computed in a brain system, and how it is computed. Appendix D describes Matlab software that has been made available with this book to provide simple demonstrations of the operation of some key neuronal networks related to cortical function; to show how the information represented by neurons can be measured; and to provide a tutorial version of the VisNet program for invariant visual object recognition described in Chapter 2. The neural networks programs are also provided in Python. The programs are available at https://www.oxcns.org.

Part of the material described in the book reflects work performed in collaboration with many colleagues, whose tremendous contributions are warmly appreciated. The contributions of many will be evident from the references cited in the text. Especial appreciation is due to Alessandro Treves, Gustavo Deco, Sylvia Wirth, and Simon M. Stringer, who have contributed greatly in always interesting and fruitful research collaborations on computational and related aspects of brain function, and to many neurophysiology and functional neuroimaging colleagues who have contributed to the empirical discoveries that provide the foundation to which the computational neuroscience must always be closely linked, and whose names are cited throughout the text. Charl Ning (University of Warwick) is thanked for help with translating the Matlab neural network programs described in Appendix D into Python. Dr Patrick Mills and Imogen Kruse are thanked for very helpful comments on an earlier version of this book. Much of the work described would not have been possible without financial support from a number of sources, particularly the Medical Research Council of the UK, the Human Frontier Science Program, the Wellcome Trust, and the James S. McDonnell Foundation. I am also grateful to many colleagues who I have consulted while writing this book. The Gatsby Foundation is thanked for a grant towards the cost of making this book Open Access. The book was typeset by the author using LaTeX and WinEdt.

Updates to and .pdfs of many of the publications cited in this book are available at https://www.oxcns.org. Updates and corrections to the text and notes are also available at https://www.oxcns.org.

I dedicate this work to the overlapping group: my family, friends, and colleagues – in salutem praesentium, in memoriam absentium.

Contents

1 Introduction — 1
  1.1 What and how the brain computes: introduction — 1
  1.2 What and how the brain computes: plan of the book — 3
  1.3 Neurons — 5
  1.4 Neurons in a network — 6
  1.5 Synaptic modification — 8
  1.6 Long-term potentiation and long-term depression — 10
      1.6.1 Long-Term Potentiation — 10
      1.6.2 Long-Term Depression — 13
      1.6.3 Spike Timing-Dependent Plasticity — 14
  1.7 Information encoding by neurons, and distributed representations — 15
      1.7.1 Definitions — 16
      1.7.2 Advantages of sparse distributed encoding — 17
  1.8 Neuronal network approaches versus connectionism — 18
  1.9 Introduction to three neuronal network architectures — 19
  1.10 Systems-level analysis of brain function — 22
  1.11 Brodmann areas — 22
  1.12 Human Connectome Project Multi-Modal Parcellation atlas of the human cortex — 27
  1.13 Connectivity of the human brain — 36
      1.13.1 Connections analyzed with diffusion tractography — 37
      1.13.2 Functional connectivity — 37
      1.13.3 Effective connectivity — 37
  1.14 The fine structure of the cerebral neocortex — 39
      1.14.1 The fine structure and connectivity of the neocortex — 39
      1.14.2 Excitatory cells and connections — 40
      1.14.3 Inhibitory cells and connections — 41
      1.14.4 Quantitative aspects of cortical architecture — 44
      1.14.5 Functional pathways through the cortical layers — 46
      1.14.6 The scale of lateral excitatory and inhibitory effects, and modules — 51

2 The ventral visual system — 53
  2.1 Introduction and overview — 53
      2.1.1 Introduction — 53
      2.1.2 Overview of what is computed in the ventral visual system — 53
      2.1.3 Overview of how computations are performed in the ventral visual system — 57
      2.1.4 What is computed in the ventral visual system is unimodal, and is related to other 'what' systems after the inferior temporal visual cortex — 58
  2.2 What: V1 – primary visual cortex — 60
  2.3 What: V2 and V4 – intermediate processing areas in the ventral visual system — 61
  2.4 What: Invariant representations of faces and objects in the inferior temporal visual cortex — 62
      2.4.1 Reward value is not represented in the primate ventral visual system — 62
      2.4.2 Translation invariant representations — 63
      2.4.3 Reduced translation invariance in natural scenes — 64

	2.4.4	Size and spatial frequency invariance	67
	2.4.5	Combinations of features in the correct spatial configuration	67
	2.4.6	A view-invariant representation	69
	2.4.7	Learning in the inferior temporal cortex	71
	2.4.8	A sparse distributed representation is what is computed in the ventral visual system	74
	2.4.9	Face expression, gesture, and view	80
	2.4.10	Specialized regions in the temporal cortical visual areas	80
2.5		The connectivity of the ventral visual pathways in humans	85
	2.5.1	A Ventrolateral Visual Cortical Stream to the inferior temporal visual cortex for object and face representations	86
	2.5.2	A Visual Cortical Stream to the cortex in the inferior bank of the superior temporal sulcus involved in semantic representations	89
	2.5.3	A Visual Cortical Stream to the cortex in the superior bank of the superior temporal sulcus involved in multimodal semantic representations including visual motion, auditory, somatosensory and social information	89
2.6		How the computations are performed: approaches to invariant object recognition	92
	2.6.1	Feature spaces	93
	2.6.2	Structural descriptions and syntactic pattern recognition	94
	2.6.3	Template matching and the alignment approach	96
	2.6.4	Invertible networks that can reconstruct their inputs	97
	2.6.5	Deep learning	98
	2.6.6	Feature hierarchies	98
2.7		Hypotheses about how the computations are performed in a feature hierarchy approach	104
2.8		VisNet: a model of how the computations are performed in the ventral visual system	107
	2.8.1	The architecture of VisNet	108
	2.8.2	Initial experiments with VisNet	117
	2.8.3	The optimal parameters for the temporal trace used in the learning rule	124
	2.8.4	Different forms of the trace learning rule, and error correction	126
	2.8.5	The issue of feature binding, and a solution	134
	2.8.6	Operation in a cluttered environment	147
	2.8.7	Learning 3D transforms	154
	2.8.8	Capacity of the architecture, and an attractor implementation	159
	2.8.9	Vision in natural scenes – effects of background versus attention	162
	2.8.10	The representation of multiple objects in a scene	170
	2.8.11	Learning invariant representations using spatial continuity	172
	2.8.12	Lighting invariance	173
	2.8.13	Deformation-invariant object recognition	175
	2.8.14	Learning invariant representations of scenes and places	176
	2.8.15	Finding and recognising objects in natural scenes	178
	2.8.16	Non-accidental properties, and transform invariant object recognition	181
2.9		Further approaches to invariant object recognition	183
	2.9.1	Other types of slow learning	183
	2.9.2	HMAX	183
	2.9.3	Minimal recognizable configurations	188
	2.9.4	Hierarchical convolutional deep neural networks	189
	2.9.5	Sigma-Pi synapses	190
	2.9.6	A principal dimensions approach to coding in the inferior temporal visual cortex	190
2.10		Visuo-spatial scratchpad memory, and change blindness	192
2.11		Processes involved in object identification	194
2.12		Top-down attentional modulation is implemented by biased competition	195
2.13		Highlights on how the computations are performed in the ventral visual system	198

3 The dorsal visual system   201

3.1		Introduction, and overview of the dorsal cortical visual stream	201

3.2		Global motion in the dorsal visual system	202
3.3		Invariant object-based motion in the dorsal visual system	204
3.4		What is computed in the dorsal visual system: visual coordinate transforms	206
	3.4.1	The transform from retinal to head-based coordinates	207
	3.4.2	The transform from head-based to allocentric bearing coordinates	208
	3.4.3	A transform from allocentric bearing coordinates to allocentric spatial view coordinates	209
3.5		How visual coordinate transforms are computed in the dorsal visual system	211
	3.5.1	Gain modulation	211
	3.5.2	Mechanisms of gain modulation using a trace learning rule	211
	3.5.3	Gain modulation by eye position to produce a head-centered representation in Layer 1 of VisNetCT	213
	3.5.4	Gain modulation by head direction to produce an allocentric bearing to a landmark in Layer 2 of VisNetCT	214
	3.5.5	Gain modulation by place to produce an allocentric spatial view representation in Layer 3 of VisNetCT	215
	3.5.6	The utility of the coordinate transforms in the dorsal visual system	216
3.6		The human Dorsal Visual Cortical Stream	217
	3.6.1	Dorsal stream visual division regions	217
	3.6.2	MT+ complex regions (FST, LO1, LO2, LO3, MST, MT, PH, V3CD and V4t)	218
	3.6.3	Intraparietal sulcus posterior parietal cortex, regions (AIP, LIPd, LIPv, MIP, VIP; with IP0, IP1 and IP2)	219
	3.6.4	Area 7 regions	220

4 The taste and flavor system — 221

4.1		Introduction and overview	221
	4.1.1	Introduction	221
	4.1.2	Overview of what is computed in the taste and flavor system	221
	4.1.3	Overview of how computations are performed in the taste and flavor system	223
4.2		Taste and related pathways: what is computed	223
	4.2.1	Hierarchically organised anatomical pathways	223
	4.2.2	Taste neuronal tuning become more selective through the taste hierarchy	226
	4.2.3	The primary, insular, taste cortex represents what taste is present and its intensity	228
	4.2.4	The secondary, orbitofrontal, taste cortex, and its representation of the reward value and pleasantness of taste	229
	4.2.5	Sensory-specific satiety is computed in the orbitofrontal cortex	231
	4.2.6	Oral texture is represented in the primary and secondary taste cortex: viscosity and fat texture	234
	4.2.7	Vision and olfaction converge using associative learning with taste to represent flavor in the secondary but not primary taste cortex	236
	4.2.8	Top-down attention and cognition can modulate taste and flavor representations in the taste cortical areas	238
	4.2.9	The tertiary taste cortex in the anterior cingulate cortex provides the rewards for action-reward outcome learning	240
	4.2.10	Taste, oral texture and flavor provide the rewards for eating, and the gut provides satiety signals	241
4.3		Taste and related pathways: how the computations are performed	245
	4.3.1	Increased selectivity of taste and flavor neurons through the hierarchy by competitive learning and convergence	245
	4.3.2	Pattern association learning of associations of visual and olfactory stimuli with taste	245
	4.3.3	Rule-based reversal of visual to taste associations in the orbitofrontal cortex	246
	4.3.4	Sensory-specific satiety is implemented by adaptation of synapses onto orbitofrontal cortex neurons	246
	4.3.5	Top-down cognitive and attentional modulation is implemented by biased activation	247

5 The olfactory system — 251

5.1 Introduction 251
  5.1.1 Overview of what is computed in the olfactory system 251
  5.1.2 Overview of how the computations are performed in the olfactory system 252
5.2 What is computed in the olfactory system 253
  5.2.1 1000 gene-encoded olfactory receptor types, and 1000 corresponding glomerulus types in the olfactory bulb 253
  5.2.2 The primary olfactory, pyriform, cortex: olfactory feature combinations are what is represented 255
  5.2.3 Orbitofrontal cortex: olfactory neuronal response selectivity 256
  5.2.4 Orbitofrontal cortex: olfactory to taste convergence 257
  5.2.5 Orbitofrontal cortex: olfactory to taste association learning and reversal 257
  5.2.6 Orbitofrontal cortex: olfactory reward value is represented 259
  5.2.7 Cognitive influences on olfactory representations in the orbitofrontal cortex 260
5.3 How computations are performed in the olfactory system 262
  5.3.1 Olfactory receptors, and the olfactory bulb 262
  5.3.2 Olfactory (pyriform) cortex 263
  5.3.3 Orbitofrontal cortex 267

6 The somatosensory system 268

6.1 What is computed in the somatosensory system 268
  6.1.1 The receptors and periphery 268
  6.1.2 The anterior somatosensory cortex, areas 1, 2, 3a, and 3b, in the anterior parietal cortex 268
  6.1.3 The ventral somatosensory stream: areas S2 and PV, in the lateral parietal cortex 269
  6.1.4 The dorsal somatosensory stream to area 5 and then 7b, in the posterior parietal cortex 270
  6.1.5 Somatosensory representations in the insula 272
  6.1.6 Somatosensory and temperature inputs to the orbitofrontal cortex, affective value, pleasant touch, and pain 272
  6.1.7 Decision-making in the somatosensory system 276
  6.1.8 Somatosensory cortical regions and connectivity in humans 278
6.2 How computations are performed in the somatosensory system 284
  6.2.1 Hierarchical computation in the somatosensory system 284
  6.2.2 Computations for pleasant touch and pain 284
  6.2.3 The mechanisms for somatosensory decision-making 285

7 The auditory system 286

7.1 Introduction, and overview of computations in the auditory system 286
7.2 Auditory Localization 287
7.3 Ventral and dorsal cortical auditory pathways 290
7.4 The ventral cortical auditory stream 291
7.5 The dorsal cortical auditory stream 293
7.6 Auditory cortical regions and connectivity in humans 293
  7.6.1 Early Auditory cortical regions 294
  7.6.2 Ventral auditory cortical streams 294
  7.6.3 Dorsal auditory cortical streams 295
  7.6.4 Other auditory system cortical connectivities 297
7.7 How the computations are performed in the auditory system 298

8 The temporal cortex 299

8.1 Introduction and overview 299
8.2 Middle temporal gyrus and face expression and gesture 299
8.3 Semantic representations in the temporal lobe neocortex 301
  8.3.1 Neurophysiology of the medial temporal lobe, including concept cells 301

		8.3.2	Neuropsychology	303

	8.3.2	Neuropsychology	303
	8.3.3	Functional neuroimaging	303
	8.3.4	Brain stimulation	304
8.4	Connectivity and functions of the human temporal lobe regions related to semantics		305
	8.4.1	Group 1 semantic regions that include regions in the ventral bank of the Superior Temporal Sulcus	306
	8.4.2	Group 3 semantic regions that include regions in the dorsal bank of the Superior Temporal Sulcus	309
8.5	The mechanisms for semantic learning in the human anterior temporal lobe		311

9 The hippocampus, memory, and spatial function — 313

9.1	Introduction and overview		313
	9.1.1	Overview of what is computed by the hippocampal system	313
	9.1.2	Overview of how the computations are performed by the hippocampal system	315
9.2	What is computed in the hippocampus		316
	9.2.1	Systems-level anatomy	316
	9.2.2	Evidence from the effects of damage to the hippocampus	319
	9.2.3	Episodic memories need to be recalled from the hippocampus, and can be used to help build neocortical semantic memories	321
	9.2.4	Systems-level neurophysiology of the primate including human hippocampus	324
	9.2.5	Spatial view cells in primates including humans, and foveal vision	342
	9.2.6	Head direction cells in the presubiculum	344
	9.2.7	Perirhinal cortex, recognition memory, and long-term familiarity memory	346
	9.2.8	Connectivity of the human hippocampal system	353
9.3	How computations are performed in the hippocampal system		364
	9.3.1	Historical development of the theory of the hippocampus	364
	9.3.2	Hippocampal circuitry	366
	9.3.3	Medial entorhinal cortex, spatial processing streams, and grid cells	369
	9.3.4	Lateral entorhinal cortex, object processing streams, and the generation of time cells in the hippocampus	372
	9.3.5	CA3 as an autoassociation memory	378
	9.3.6	Dentate granule cells	397
	9.3.7	CA1 cells	400
	9.3.8	Backprojections to the neocortex, memory recall, and consolidation	405
	9.3.9	Backprojections to the neocortex – quantitative aspects	409
	9.3.10	Simulations of hippocampal operation	413
	9.3.11	The learning of spatial view and place cell representations	414
	9.3.12	Linking the inferior temporal visual cortex to spatial view and place cells	416
	9.3.13	A scientific theory of the art of memory: scientia artis memoriae	418
	9.3.14	How navigation is performed	419
	9.3.15	Navigational computations using neuron types found in primates including humans	423
9.4	Tests of the theory of hippocampal cortex operation		432
	9.4.1	Dentate gyrus (DG) subregion of the hippocampus	432
	9.4.2	CA3 subregion of the hippocampus	435
	9.4.3	CA1 subregion of the hippocampus	442
9.5	Comparison of spatial processing and computations in primates including humans vs rodents		445
	9.5.1	Similarities and differences between the spatial representations in primates and rodents	445
	9.5.2	Hippocampal computational similarities and differences between primates and rodents	447
9.6	Synthesis: the hippocampus: memory, navigation, or both?		450
9.7	Comparison with other theories of hippocampal function		454

10 The parietal cortex, spatial functions, and navigation — 459

- 10.1 Introduction and overview — 459
  - 10.1.1 Overview of what is computed in the parietal cortex — 459
  - 10.1.2 Overview of how the computations are performed in the parietal cortex — 460
- 10.2 Inferior parietal cortex somatosensory stream, PF regions — 460
- 10.3 Intraparietal sulcus posterior parietal cortex, regions AIP, LIPd, LIPv, MIP, VIP, IP0, IP1, and IP2 — 464
- 10.4 Posterior superior parietal cortex, regions 7AL, 7Am, 7PC, 7PL, and 7Pm — 466
- 10.5 Inferior parietal cortex, visual regions PFm, PGi, PGs and PGp — 467
  - 10.5.1 Region PGi — 469
  - 10.5.2 Region PGs — 470
  - 10.5.3 Region PFm — 470
  - 10.5.4 Region PGp — 471
- 10.6 Navigation: What computations are performed in the parietal and related cortex — 473
- 10.7 How the computations are performed in the parietal cortex — 474

11 The orbitofrontal cortex, amygdala, reward value, emotion, and decision-making — 475

- 11.1 Introduction and overview — 475
  - 11.1.1 Introduction — 475
  - 11.1.2 Overview of what is computed in the orbitofrontal cortex — 475
  - 11.1.3 Overview of how the computations are performed by the orbitofrontal cortex — 478
- 11.2 The topology and connections of the orbitofrontal cortex — 479
  - 11.2.1 Inputs to the orbitofrontal cortex — 480
  - 11.2.2 Outputs of the orbitofrontal cortex — 482
- 11.3 What is computed in the orbitofrontal cortex — 483
  - 11.3.1 The orbitofrontal cortex represents reward value — 483
  - 11.3.2 Neuroeconomic value is represented in the orbitofrontal cortex — 490
  - 11.3.3 A representation of face and voice expression and other socially relevant stimuli in the orbitofrontal cortex — 492
  - 11.3.4 Negative reward prediction error neurons in the orbitofrontal cortex — 495
  - 11.3.5 The human medial orbitofrontal cortex represents rewards, and the lateral orbitofrontal cortex non-reward and punishers — 500
  - 11.3.6 Decision-making in the orbitofrontal / ventromedial prefrontal cortex — 502
  - 11.3.7 The ventromedial prefrontal cortex and memory — 504
  - 11.3.8 The orbitofrontal cortex and emotion — 506
  - 11.3.9 Emotional orbitofrontal vs rational routes to action — 508
  - 11.3.10 The connectivity of the human orbitofrontal cortex, and its relation to function — 521
  - 11.3.11 Mental problems associated with the orbitofrontal cortex — 528
- 11.4 What is computed in the amygdala for emotion — 529
  - 11.4.1 Overview of the functions of the amygdala in emotion — 529
  - 11.4.2 The amygdala and the associative processes involved in emotion-related learning — 530
  - 11.4.3 Connections of the amygdala — 531
  - 11.4.4 Effects of amygdala lesions — 532
  - 11.4.5 Amygdala lesions in primates — 532
  - 11.4.6 Amygdala lesions in rats — 534
  - 11.4.7 Neuronal activity in the primate amygdala to reinforcing stimuli — 535
  - 11.4.8 Neuronal responses in the amygdala to faces — 536
  - 11.4.9 Evidence from humans — 538
  - 11.4.10 Connectivity of the human amygdala — 539
- 11.5 How the computations are performed in the orbitofrontal cortex — 544
  - 11.5.1 Decision-making in attractor networks in the brain — 544
  - 11.5.2 Analyses of reward-related decision-making mechanisms in the orbitofrontal cortex — 549
  - 11.5.3 A model for reversal learning in the orbitofrontal cortex — 554

		11.5.4	A theory and model of non-reward neural mechanisms in the orbitofrontal cortex	559

	11.6	Highlights: the special computational roles of the orbitofrontal cortex	560

12 The cingulate cortex — 564

- 12.1 Introduction to and overview of the cingulate cortex — 564
  - 12.1.1 Introduction — 564
  - 12.1.2 Overview of what is computed in the cingulate cortex — 565
  - 12.1.3 Overview of how the computations are performed by the cingulate cortex — 567
- 12.2 Anterior cingulate cortex — 568
  - 12.2.1 Anterior cingulate cortex anatomy and connections in primates — 568
  - 12.2.2 Anterior cingulate cortex: A framework — 569
  - 12.2.3 Anterior cingulate cortex and action-outcome representations — 571
  - 12.2.4 Anterior cingulate cortex lesion effects — 572
  - 12.2.5 Anterior cingulate cortex and ventromedial prefrontal cortex connectivity and functions in humans — 572
  - 12.2.6 Pregenual anterior cingulate representations of reward value, and supracallosal anterior cingulate representations of punishers and non-reward — 575
  - 12.2.7 The human supracallosal anterior cingulate cortex, dACC, and action-outcome learning — 578
  - 12.2.8 Reward value outputs from the orbitofrontal and pregenual anterior cortex, and vmPFC, to the hippocampal memory system — 579
  - 12.2.9 The pregenual anterior cingulate cortex has connectivity with the septal cholinergic system that is involved in memory consolidation — 579
  - 12.2.10 Reward value outputs from the orbitofrontal and pregenual anterior cortex, and vmPFC, to the hippocampal system to provide the goals for navigation — 580
  - 12.2.11 Subgenual cingulate cortex — 581
- 12.3 Posterior cingulate cortex — 581
  - 12.3.1 Introduction and overview — 581
  - 12.3.2 Postero-ventral posterior cingulate and medial parietal regions 31pd, 31pv, d23ab, v23ab and 7m, and their relation to episodic memory — 582
  - 12.3.3 Antero-dorsal Posterior Cingulate Division regions 23d, 31a, PCV; and RSC, POS2, and POS1; and their relation to navigation and executive function — 584
  - 12.3.4 Dorsal Visual Transitional area and ProStriate region: the retrosplenial scene area — 587
- 12.4 Mid-cingulate cortex, the cingulate motor area, and action–outcome learning — 588
- 12.5 How the computations are performed by the cingulate cortex — 589
  - 12.5.1 The anterior cingulate cortex and emotion — 589
  - 12.5.2 Action-outcome learning in the supracallosal anterior cingulate cortex (dACC) — 590
  - 12.5.3 Connectivity of the posterior cingulate cortex with the hippocampal memory system — 592
- 12.6 Synthesis and conclusions — 593

13 The prefrontal cortex — 596

- 13.1 Introduction and overview — 596
- 13.2 Divisions of the lateral prefrontal cortex — 600
  - 13.2.1 The dorsolateral prefrontal cortex — 600
  - 13.2.2 The caudal prefrontal cortex — 603
  - 13.2.3 The ventrolateral prefrontal cortex — 603
- 13.3 The connectivity and computational organisation of the human prefrontal cortex — 603
  - 13.3.1 Inferior frontal gyrus — 604
  - 13.3.2 Dorsolateral prefrontal cortex division — 606
- 13.4 The lateral prefrontal cortex and top-down attention — 609
- 13.5 The frontal pole cortex — 612

13.6		How the computations are performed in the prefrontal cortex	613
	13.6.1	Cortical short-term memory systems and attractor networks	613
	13.6.2	Prefrontal cortex short-term memory networks, and their relation to perceptual networks	615
	13.6.3	Mapping from one representation to another in short-term memory	620
	13.6.4	The mechanisms of top-down attention	621
	13.6.5	Computational necessity for a separate, prefrontal cortex, short-term memory system	622
	13.6.6	Synaptic modification is needed to set up but not to reuse short-term memory systems	623
	13.6.7	Sequence memory	623
	13.6.8	Working memory, and planning	623

14 Language and syntax in the brain — 624

14.1		Introduction and overview	624
	14.1.1	Introduction	624
	14.1.2	Overview	624
14.2		What is computed in different brain systems to implement language	626
	14.2.1	The Wernicke-Lichtheim-Geschwind hypothesis	626
	14.2.2	The dual-stream hypothesis of speech comprehension	627
	14.2.3	Reading requires different brain systems to hearing speech	627
	14.2.4	Semantic representations	629
	14.2.5	Syntactic processing	630
	14.2.6	The parietal cortex: supramarginal and angular gyri	631
14.3		Cortical regions for language and their connectivity in humans	631
	14.3.1	A semantic system that includes the inferior bank of the superior temporal sulcus including object representations	632
	14.3.2	A semantic system that includes the superior bank of the superior temporal sulcus including visual motion, auditory, somatosensory and social information	634
	14.3.3	Multimodal semantic representations	635
	14.3.4	Broca's area and related regions (TGv 44 45 47l SFL 55b)	637
14.4		Hypotheses about how semantic representations are computed	640
14.5		A neurodynamical hypothesis about how syntax is computed	641
	14.5.1	Binding by synchrony?	641
	14.5.2	Syntax using a place code	642
	14.5.3	Temporal trajectories through a state space of attractors	642
	14.5.4	Hypotheses about the implementation of language in the cerebral cortex	643
	14.5.5	Tests of the hypotheses – a model	646
	14.5.6	Tests of the hypotheses – findings with the model	651
	14.5.7	Evaluation of the hypotheses	654
	14.5.8	Further approaches	658

15 The motor cortical areas — 660

15.1		Introduction and overview	660
15.2		What is computed in different cortical motor-related areas	661
	15.2.1	Ventral parietal and ventral premotor cortex F4	661
	15.2.2	Superior parietal areas with activity related to reaching	661
	15.2.3	Inferior parietal areas with activity related to grasping, and ventral premotor cortex F5	662
15.3		The mirror neuron system	662
15.4		How the computations are performed in motor cortical and related areas	664

16 The basal ganglia — 665

16.1		Introduction and overview	665
16.2		Systems-level architecture of the basal ganglia	666

16.3	What computations are performed by the basal ganglia?		669
	16.3.1	Effects of striatal lesions	669
	16.3.2	Neuronal activity in different parts of the striatum	670
16.4	How do the basal ganglia perform their computations?		683
	16.4.1	Interaction between neurons and selection of output	683
	16.4.2	Convergence within the basal ganglia, useful for stimulus-response habit learning	686
	16.4.3	Dopamine as a reward prediction error signal for reinforcement learning in the striatum	688
16.5	Comparison of computations for selection in the basal ganglia and cerebral cortex		692

17 Cerebellar cortex   695

17.1	Introduction		695
17.2	Architecture of the cerebellum		697
	17.2.1	The connections of the parallel fibres onto the Purkinje cells	697
	17.2.2	The climbing fibre input to the Purkinje cell	698
	17.2.3	The mossy fibre to granule cell connectivity	698
17.3	Modifiable synapses of parallel fibres onto Purkinje cell dendrites		700
17.4	The cerebellar cortex as a perceptron		701
17.5	Cognitive functions of the cerebellum		702
	17.5.1	Anatomical connections from most neocortical regions	702
	17.5.2	Functional connectivity of different cortical systems with different parts of the cerebellum	703
	17.5.3	Activation of different cerebellar cortical regions in different tasks	703
	17.5.4	Damage to different parts of the cerebellum can produce different cognitive, emotional, and motor impairments	703
	17.5.5	Neocortical–cerebellar cortical computations for cognition	703
17.6	Highlights: differences between cerebral and cerebellar cortex microcircuitry		707

18 Cortical attractor dynamics and connectivity, stochasticity, psychiatric disorders, and aging   709

18.1	Introduction and overview		709
	18.1.1	Introduction	709
	18.1.2	Overview	709
18.2	The noisy cortex		711
	18.2.1	Reasons why the brain is inherently noisy and stochastic	711
	18.2.2	Attractor networks, energy landscapes, and stochastic neurodynamics	714
	18.2.3	A multistable system with noise	719
	18.2.4	Stochastic dynamics and the stability of short-term memory	721
	18.2.5	Stochastic dynamics in decision-making, and the evolutionary utility of probabilistic choice	725
	18.2.6	Selection between conscious vs unconscious decision-making, and free will	726
	18.2.7	Stochastic dynamics and creative thought	728
	18.2.8	Stochastic dynamics and unpredictable behavior	729
18.3	Attractor dynamics and schizophrenia		729
	18.3.1	Introduction	729
	18.3.2	A dynamical systems hypothesis of the symptoms of schizophrenia	730
	18.3.3	Reduced functional connectivity of some brain regions in schizophrenia	733
	18.3.4	Beyond the disconnectivity hypothesis of schizophrenia: reduced forward but not backward connectivity	734
18.4	Attractor dynamics and obsessive-compulsive disorder		738
	18.4.1	Introduction	738
	18.4.2	A hypothesis about obsessive-compulsive disorder	739
	18.4.3	Glutamate and increased depth of the basins of attraction	741
18.5	Depression and attractor dynamics		742

		18.5.1	Introduction	742
		18.5.2	A non-reward attractor theory of depression	743
		18.5.3	The orbitofrontal cortex, and the theory of depression	745
		18.5.4	Altered connectivity of the orbitofrontal cortex in depression	746
		18.5.5	Activations of the orbitofrontal cortex related to depression	751
		18.5.6	Implications, and possible treatments, and subtypes of depression	753
		18.5.7	Mania and bipolar disorder	756
	18.6	Attractor stochastic dynamics, aging, and memory		758
		18.6.1	NMDA receptor hypofunction	758
		18.6.2	Dopamine and norepinephrine	760
		18.6.3	Impaired synaptic modification	760
		18.6.4	Cholinergic function and memory	761
	18.7	High blood pressure, reduced hippocampal functional connectivity, and impaired memory		766
	18.8	Brain development, and structural differences in the brain		766

19 Computations by different types of brain, and by artificial neural systems 768

	19.1	Introduction and overview		768
	19.2	Computations that combine different computational systems in the brain to produce behavior		769
	19.3	Brain computation compared to computation on a digital computer		769
	19.4	Brain computation compared with artificial deep learning networks		775
	19.5	Reinforcement Learning		778
	19.6	Levels of explanation, and the mind-brain problem		780
		19.6.1	A levels of explanation theory of causality, and the relation between the mind and the brain	780
		19.6.2	Downward or Upward Causality?	782
		19.6.3	Consciousness - a Higher Order Syntactic Thought theory	784
		19.6.4	Levels of explanation, and levels of investigation	785
	19.7	Biologically plausible computation in the brain: a grand unifying theory?		787
	19.8	Brain-Inspired Intelligence		791
	19.9	Brain-Inspired Medicine		792
		19.9.1	Computational psychiatry and neurology	792
		19.9.2	Reward systems in the brain, and their application to understanding food intake control and obesity	793
		19.9.3	Multiple Routes to Action	796
	19.10	Primates including humans have different brain organisation than rodents		796
		19.10.1	The visual system	796
		19.10.2	The taste system	797
		19.10.3	The olfactory system	798
		19.10.4	The somatosensory system	798
		19.10.5	The auditory system	799
		19.10.6	The hippocampal system, memory, and navigation	799
		19.10.7	The orbitofrontal cortex and amygdala	800
		19.10.8	The cingulate cortex	801
		19.10.9	The motor system	802
		19.10.10	Language	802

A Introduction to linear algebra for neural networks 803

	A.1	Vectors		803
		A.1.1	The inner or dot product of two vectors	803
		A.1.2	The length of a vector	805
		A.1.3	Normalizing the length of a vector	805

		A.1.4	The angle between two vectors: the normalized dot product	805

- A.1.4   The angle between two vectors: the normalized dot product   805
- A.1.5   The outer product of two vectors   806
- A.1.6   Linear and non-linear systems   807
- A.1.7   Linear combinations, linear independence, and linear separability   808
- A.2   Application to understanding simple neural networks   809
  - A.2.1   Capability and limitations of single-layer networks   810
  - A.2.2   Non-linear networks: neurons with non-linear activation functions   812
  - A.2.3   Non-linear networks: neurons with non-linear activations   813

B   Neuronal network models   815

- B.1   Introduction   815
- B.2   Pattern association memory   815
  - B.2.1   Architecture and operation   816
  - B.2.2   A simple model   818
  - B.2.3   The vector interpretation   821
  - B.2.4   Properties   822
  - B.2.5   Prototype extraction, extraction of central tendency, and noise reduction   825
  - B.2.6   Speed   825
  - B.2.7   Local learning rule   826
  - B.2.8   Implications of different types of coding for storage in pattern associators   831
- B.3   Autoassociation or attractor memory   832
  - B.3.1   Architecture and operation   832
  - B.3.2   Introduction to the analysis of the operation of autoassociation networks   834
  - B.3.3   Properties   836
  - B.3.4   Diluted connectivity and the storage capacity of attractor networks   843
  - B.3.5   Use of autoassociation networks in the brain   854
- B.4   Competitive networks, including self-organizing maps   855
  - B.4.1   Function   855
  - B.4.2   Architecture and algorithm   856
  - B.4.3   Properties   857
  - B.4.4   Utility of competitive networks in information processing by the brain   862
  - B.4.5   Guidance of competitive learning   864
  - B.4.6   Topographic map formation   866
  - B.4.7   Invariance learning by competitive networks   870
  - B.4.8   Radial Basis Function networks   871
  - B.4.9   Further details of the algorithms used in competitive networks   873
- B.5   Continuous attractor networks   876
  - B.5.1   Introduction   876
  - B.5.2   The generic model of a continuous attractor network   878
  - B.5.3   Learning the synaptic strengths in a continuous attractor network   879
  - B.5.4   The capacity of a continuous attractor network: multiple charts   881
  - B.5.5   Continuous attractor models: path integration   882
  - B.5.6   Stabilization of the activity packet within a continuous attractor network   884
  - B.5.7   Continuous attractor networks in two or more dimensions   886
  - B.5.8   Mixed continuous and discrete attractor networks   887
- B.6   Network dynamics: the integrate-and-fire approach   888
  - B.6.1   From discrete to continuous time   888
  - B.6.2   Continuous dynamics with discontinuities   889
  - B.6.3   An integrate-and-fire implementation   893
  - B.6.4   The speed of processing of attractor networks   894
  - B.6.5   The speed of processing of a four-layer hierarchical network   897
  - B.6.6   Spike response model   900
- B.7   Network dynamics: introduction to the mean-field approach   901
- B.8   Mean-field based neurodynamics   902
  - B.8.1   Population activity   903
  - B.8.2   The mean-field approach used in a model of decision-making   905
  - B.8.3   The model parameters used in the mean-field analyses of decision-making   907
  - B.8.4   A basic computational module based on biased competition   908

	B.8.5	Multimodular neurodynamical architectures	909
B.9		Interacting attractor networks	911
B.10		Sequence memory implemented by adaptation in an attractor network	915
B.11		Error correction networks	915
	B.11.1	Architecture and general description	916
	B.11.2	Generic algorithm for a one-layer error correction network	916
	B.11.3	Capability and limitations of single-layer error-correcting networks	917
	B.11.4	Properties	920
B.12		Error backpropagation multilayer networks	922
	B.12.1	Introduction	922
	B.12.2	Architecture and algorithm	923
	B.12.3	Properties of multilayer networks trained by error backpropagation	927
B.13		Deep learning using stochastic gradient descent	928
B.14		Deep convolutional networks	928
B.15		Contrastive Hebbian learning: the Boltzmann machine	930
B.16		Deep Belief Networks	931
B.17		Reinforcement learning	932
	B.17.1	Associative reward–penalty algorithm of Barto and Sutton	933
	B.17.2	Reward prediction error or delta rule learning, and classical conditioning	934
	B.17.3	Temporal Difference (TD) learning	935
B.18		Learning in the neocortex	938
B.19		Forgetting in cortical associative neural networks, and memory reconsolidation	940
B.20		Genes and self-organization build neural networks in the cortex	945
	B.20.1	Introduction	945
	B.20.2	Hypotheses about the genes that build cortical neural networks	946
	B.20.3	Genetic selection of neuronal network parameters	950
	B.20.4	Simulation of the evolution of neural networks using a genetic algorithm	952
	B.20.5	Evaluation of the gene-based evolution of single-layer networks	961
	B.20.6	The gene-based evolution of multi-layer cortical systems	964
	B.20.7	Summary	965
B.21		Highlights	965

C Neuronal encoding, and information theory — 967

C.1		Information theory	968
	C.1.1	The information conveyed by definite statements	968
	C.1.2	Information conveyed by probabilistic statements	969
	C.1.3	Information sources, information channels, and information measures	970
	C.1.4	The information carried by a neuronal response and its averages	971
	C.1.5	The information conveyed by continuous variables	974
C.2		The information carried by neuronal responses	976
	C.2.1	The limited sampling problem	976
	C.2.2	Correction procedures for limited sampling	977
	C.2.3	The information from multiple cells: decoding procedures	978
	C.2.4	Information in the correlations between cells: a decoding approach	982
	C.2.5	Information in the correlations between cells: second derivative approach	987
C.3		Neuronal encoding results	990
	C.3.1	The sparseness of the distributed encoding used by the brain	991
	C.3.2	The information from single neurons	1002
	C.3.3	The information from single neurons: temporal codes versus rate codes	1005
	C.3.4	The information from single neurons: the speed of information transfer	1008
	C.3.5	The information from multiple cells: independence versus redundancy	1019
	C.3.6	Should one neuron be as discriminative as the whole organism?	1023
	C.3.7	The information from multiple cells: the effects of cross-correlations	1025
	C.3.8	Conclusions on cortical neuronal encoding	1029

	C.4	Information theory terms – a short glossary	1033
	C.5	Highlights	1034

D Simulation software for neuronal networks, and information analysis of neuronal encoding   1035

	D.1	Introduction	1035
	D.2	Autoassociation or attractor networks	1036
	D.2.1	Running the simulation	1036
	D.2.2	Exercises	1038
	D.3	Pattern association networks	1038
	D.3.1	Running the simulation	1038
	D.3.2	Exercises	1040
	D.4	Competitive networks and Self-Organizing Maps	1041
	D.4.1	Running the simulation	1041
	D.4.2	Exercises	1042
	D.5	Further developments	1043
	D.6	Matlab code for a tutorial version of VisNet	1043
	D.7	Matlab code for information analysis of neuronal encoding	1044
	D.8	Matlab code to illustrate the use of spatial view cells in navigation	1044
	D.9	The Automated Anatomical Labelling Atlas 3, AAL3	1044
	D.10	The extended Human Connectome Project extended atlas, HCPex	1044
	D.11	Highlights	1044

Bibliography   1045

Index   1139

C.4 Information theory terms – a short glossary
C.5 Exercises

D. **Simulation software for neuronal networks, and information analysis of neuronal circuits**

Bibliography

Index

1 Introduction

1.1 What and how the brain computes: introduction

The subject of this book is how the brain works. In order to understand this, it is essential to know **what** is computed by different brain systems; and **how** the computations are performed. The aim of this book is to elucidate what is computed in different brain systems; and to describe current computational approaches and models of how each of these brain systems computes. Understanding the brain in this way has enormous potential for understanding ourselves better in health and in disease. Potential applications of this understanding are to the treatment of the brain in disease; and to artificial intelligence which will benefit from knowledge of how the brain performs many of its extraordinarily impressive functions. This book is pioneering in taking this approach to brain function: to consider **what** is computed by many of our brain systems; and **how** it is computed.

To understand how our brains work, it is essential to know **what** is computed in each part of the brain. That can be addressed by utilising evidence relevant to computation from many areas of neuroscience. Knowledge of the connections between different brain areas is important, for this shows that the brain is organised as systems, with whole series of brain areas devoted for example to visual processing. That provides a foundation for examining the computation performed by each brain area, by comparing what is represented in a brain area with what is represented in the preceding and following brain areas, using techniques of for example neurophysiology and functional neuroimaging. Neurophysiology at the single neuron level is needed because this is the level at which information is transmitted between the computing elements of the brain, the neurons. Evidence from the effects of brain damage, including that available from neuropsychology, is needed to help understand what different parts of the system do, and indeed what each part is necessary for. Functional neuroimaging is useful to indicate where in the human brain different processes take place, and to show which functions can be dissociated from each other. So for each brain system, evidence on what is computed at each stage, and what the system as a whole computes, is essential.

To understand how our brains work, it is also essential to know **how** each part of the brain computes. That requires a knowledge of what is represented and computed by the neurons in each part of the brain, but it also requires knowledge of the network properties of each brain region. This involves knowledge of the connectivity between the neurons in each part of the brain, and knowledge of the synaptic and biophysical properties of the neurons. It also requires knowledge of the theory of what can be computed by networks with defined connectivity.

There are at least three key goals of the approaches described here. One is to understand ourselves better, and how we work and think. A second is to be better able to treat the system when it has problems, for example in mental illnesses. Medical applications are a very important aim of the type of research described here. A third goal, is to be able to emulate and learn from the operation of parts of our brains, which some in the field of artificial intelligence (AI) would like to do to produce more useful computers and machines. All of these goals require, and cannot get off the ground, without a firm foundation in what is computed by brain systems, and theories and models of how it is computed. To understand the operation of the whole brain, it is necessary to show how the different brain systems operate together: but a necessary foundation for this is to know what is computed in each brain system.

Part of the enterprise here is to stimulate new theories and models of how parts of the brain work. The evidence on what is computed in different brain systems has advanced rapidly in the last 50 years, and provides a reasonable foundation for the enterprise, though there is much that remains to be learned. Theories of how the computation is performed are less advanced, but progress is being made, and current models are described in this book for many brain systems. Before further advances are made, knowledge of the considerable current evidence on how the brain computes provides a useful stating point, especially as current theories do take into account the limitations that are likely to be imposed by the neural architectures present in our brains.

The simplest way to define **brain computation** is to examine what information is represented at each stage of processing, and how this is different from stage to stage. For example in the primary visual cortex (V1), neurons respond to simple stimuli such as bars or edges or gratings and have small receptive fields. Little can be read off about for example whose face is represented from the firing rates of a small number of neurons in V1. On the other hand, after four or five stages of processing, in the inferior temporal visual cortex, information can be read from the firing rates of neurons about whose face is being viewed, and indeed there is remarkable invariance with respect to the position, size, contrast and even in some cases view of the face. That is a major computation, and indicates what can be achieved by biological neuronal network computation.

These approaches can only be taken to understand brain function because there is considerable localization of function in the brain, quite unlike a digital computer. One fundamental reason for localization of function in the brain is that this minimizes the total length of the connections between neurons, and thus brain size. Another is that it simplifies the genetic information that has to be provided in order to build the brain, because the connectivity instructions can refer considerably to local connections. These points are developed in my book *Cerebral Cortex: Principles of Operation* (Rolls, 2016b).

That brings me to what is different about the present book and *Cerebral Cortex: Principles of Operation* (Rolls, 2016b). The previous book took on the enormous task of making progress with understanding how the major part of our brains, the cerebral cortex, works, by understanding its principles of operation. The present book builds on that approach, and uses it as background, but has the different aim of taking each of our brain systems, and describing *what* they compute, and then what is known about *how* each system computes. The issue of how they compute relies for many brain systems on how the cortex operates, so *Cerebral Cortex: Principles of Operation* provides an important complement to the present book.

One of the distinctive properties of this book is that it links the neural computation approach not only firmly to neuronal neurophysiology, which provides much of the primary data about how the brain operates, but also to psychophysical studies (for example of attention); to neuropsychological studies of patients with brain damage; and to functional magnetic resonance imaging (fMRI) (and other neuroimaging) approaches. The empirical evidence that is brought to bear is largely from non-human primates and from humans, because of the considerable similarity of their cortical systems, and the overall aims to understand the human brain, and the disorders that arise after brain damage.

In selecting the research findings on 'what' is computed in different brain systems and on 'how' it is computed, to include in this book, I have selected pioneering research that has helped to identify key computational principles involved for different brain systems. Discoveries that have laid the foundation for our understanding as research has developed are emphasized. That has meant that much excellent neuroscience research could not be included in this book: but the aim of the book instead is to identify computational principles of operation of brain systems, providing some of the key research discoveries that have helped to identify those principles. I hope that future research will extend this aim further.

1.2 What and how the brain computes: plan of the book

In the rest of Chapter 1, I introduce some of the background for understanding brain computation, such as how single neurons operate, how some of the essential features of this can be captured by simple formalisms, and some of the biological background to what it can be taken happens in the nervous system, such as synaptic modification based on information available locally at each synapse.

Each of the following Chapters has parts concerned with **what** is computed in a brain system, followed with parts concerned with **how** it is computed.

Chapters 2–7 consider the main sensory processing systems of the brain: the ventral visual system with its functions in invariant object recognition (2); the dorsal visual system involved in spatial visual processing, actions in space, and the spatial coordinate transforms that are needed (3); the taste system (4); the olfactory system (5); the somatosensory system (6); and the auditory system (7).

Chapter 8 considers the functions of the temporal lobe, including its functions in semantic representations.

Chapter 9 considers the functions of the hippocampus, which combines neocortical 'what', 'where' and reward information to implement episodic memory, and its later recall back to the neocortex which is implicated in memory consolidation.

Chapter 10 considers the functions of the parietal cortex, which receives much input from the dorsal processing streams concerned with the location of stimuli and actions in space – the 'where and action' processing stream, and which is also involved in navigation.

Chapter 11 describes the functions of the orbitofrontal cortex and amygdala, which compute reward value from inputs received from the ventral processing streams, and are therefore central to understanding the implementation in the brain of emotion and reward-related decision-making. Chapter 12 shows how the anterior cingulate cortex has functions related to the initiation of goal-directed action given its inputs from the orbitofrontal cortex about reward value and its connections with the mid-cingulate motor parts of the cingulate; and how the posterior cingulate cortex has major connections that link 'what' and 'where' neocortical systems with the hippocampus, making it an important component of the episodic memory system, and perhaps with connected cortical regions involved in navigation.

Chapter 13 describes the prefrontal cortex, which provides off-line short-term and working memory, and the associated functions of planning and top-down attention.

Chapter 14 describes brain systems involved in language and syntax.

Chapter 15 describes motor cortical areas. Chapter 16 describes the basal ganglia, and Chapter 17 the cerebellum, which are both involved in motor function, but which are now also implicated in emotional, social, and cognitive functions.

Chapter 18 describes factors that influence the dynamics and stability of cortical systems, and how these are different in some mental disorders including Schizophrenia, Obsessive-Compulsive Disorder and Depression.

Chapter 19 describes how the functions of each of these systems provide a foundation for understanding functions implemented by the whole brain, including many types of complex and useful behaviors. This Chapter also compares computations in the brain with those performed in digital computers including with machine learning algorithms. This is intended to be a useful guide for engineers and artificial intelligence experts who may wish to learn from how computations are performed in the brain, and how to emulate the computations performed by the brain. This Chapter also compares the systems-level organisation of computations in rodent brains with those in primate including human brains, and provides evidence that there are many differences in the systems-level computations between rodent and primate including human brains, which is why this book focusses on computations in primate including human brains.

The Appendices are updated somewhat from those in *Cerebral Cortex: Principles of Operation* (Rolls, 2016b), and are provided in this book for those who do not have access to *Cerebral Cortex*. Appendix A provides an introduction to the linear algebra that is useful background for the description of the fundamental operation of key networks found in the brain. Appendix B describes the fundamental operation of key networks of the type that are likely to be the building blocks of brain function. Appendix C shows how information theory can be applied to analyze what is represented by populations of neurons and thus to understand brain function. Appendix D describes Matlab software that has been made available with this book to provide simple demonstrations of the operation of some key neuronal networks related to cortical function; to show how the information represented by neurons can be measured; and to provide a tutorial version of the VisNet program for invariant visual object recognition described in Chapter 2. The neural networks programs are also provided in Python. The programs are available at https://www.oxcns.org.

I start the rest of Chapter 1 with some history showing how recently it is that our understanding of the (computational) principles of operation of the brain and cerebral cortex has started to develop.

Before the 1960s there were many and important discoveries about the phenomenology of the cortex, for example that damage in one part would affect vision, and in another part movement, with electrical stimulation often producing the opposite effect. The principles may help us to understand these phenomena, but the phenomena provide limited evidence about how the cortex works, apart from the very important principle of localization of function (see Rolls (2016b)), and the important principle of hierarchical organization (Hughlings Jackson, 1878; Swash, 1989) (see Rolls (2016b)) which has been supported by increasing evidence on the connections between different cortical areas, which is a fundamental building block for understanding brain computations.

In the 1960s David Hubel and Torsten Wiesel made important discoveries about the stimuli that activate primary visual cortex neurons, showing that they respond to bar-like or edge-like visual stimuli (Hubel and Wiesel, 1962, 1968, 1977), instead of the small circular receptive fields in the preceding stage the lateral geniculate nucleus neurons. This led them to suggest the elements of a model of how this might come about, by cortical neurons that respond to elongated lines of lateral geniculate neurons (Fig. 2.5). This led to the concept that hierarchical organization over a series of cortical areas might at each stage form combinations of the features represented in the previous cortical area, in what might be termed feature combination neurons.

However, before 1970 there were few ideas about how the cerebral cortex operates computationally.

David Marr was a pioneer who helped to open the way to an understanding of how the details of cortical anatomy and connectivity help to develop quantitative theories of how cortical areas may compute, including the cerebellar cortex (Marr, 1969), the neocortex (Marr, 1970), and the hippocampal cortex (Marr, 1971). Marr was hampered by some lack in detail of the available anatomical knowledge, and did not for example hypothesize that the hippocampal CA3 network was an autoassociation memory. He attempted to test his theory of the cerebellum with Sir John (Jack) Eccles by stimulating the climbing fibres in the cerebellum while providing an input from the parallel fibres to a Purkinje cell, but the experiment did not succeed, partly because of a lack of physiological knowledge about the firing rates of climbing fibres, which are low, rarely more than 10 spikes/s, whereas they had stimulated at much higher frequencies. Perhaps in part because David Marr was ahead of the experimental techniques available at the time to test his theories of network operations of cortical systems, he focussed in his later work on more conceptual rather that neural network based approaches, which he applied to understanding vision. This also had only limited success at least in understanding invariant object recognition (Marr, 1982), again related to the lack of available experimental data (Rolls, 2011c).

Very stimulating advances in thinking about cortical function were made in books by Abeles (1991), Braitenberg and Schüz (1991) and Creutzfeldt (1995), but many advances have been made since those books (Rolls, 2016b).

Theories of operation are essential to understanding the brain - e.g. collective computation in attractor networks, and emergent properties. It cannot be done just by molecular biology, though that provides useful tools, and potentially ways to ameliorate brain dysfunction.

I emphasize that to understand brain including cortical function, and processes such as memory, perception, attention, and decision-making in the brain, we are dealing with large-scale computational systems with interactions between the parts, and that this understanding requires analysis at the computational and global level of the operation of many neurons to perform together a useful function. Understanding at the molecular level is important for helping to understand how these large-scale computational processes are implemented in the brain, but will not by itself give any account of what computations are performed to implement these cognitive functions. Instead, understanding cognitive functions such as object recognition, memory recall, attention, and decision-making requires single neuron data to be closely linked to computational models of how the interactions between large numbers of neurons and many networks of neurons allow these cognitive problems to be solved. The single neuron level is important in this approach, for the single neurons can be thought of as the computational units of the system, and is the level at which the information is exchanged by the spiking activity between the computational elements of the brain. The single neuron level is therefore, because it provides the level at which information is communicated between the computing elements of the brain, the fundamental level of information processing, and the level at which the information can be read out (by recording the spiking neuronal activity) in order to understand what information is being represented and processed in each cortical area.

1.3 Neurons in the brain, and their representation in neuronal networks

Neurons in the vertebrate brain typically have, extending from the cell body, large dendrites that receive inputs from other neurons through connections called synapses. The synapses operate by chemical transmission. When a synaptic terminal receives an all-or-nothing action potential from the neuron of which it is a terminal, it releases a transmitter that crosses the synaptic cleft and produces either depolarization or hyperpolarization in the postsynaptic neuron, by opening particular ion channels. (A textbook such as Kandel, Koester, Mack and Siegelbaum (2021) gives further information on this process.) Summation of a number of such depolarizations or excitatory inputs within the time constant of the receiving neuron, which is typically 15–25 ms, produces sufficient depolarization that the neuron fires an action potential. There are often 5,000–20,000 inputs per neuron. Examples of cortical neurons are

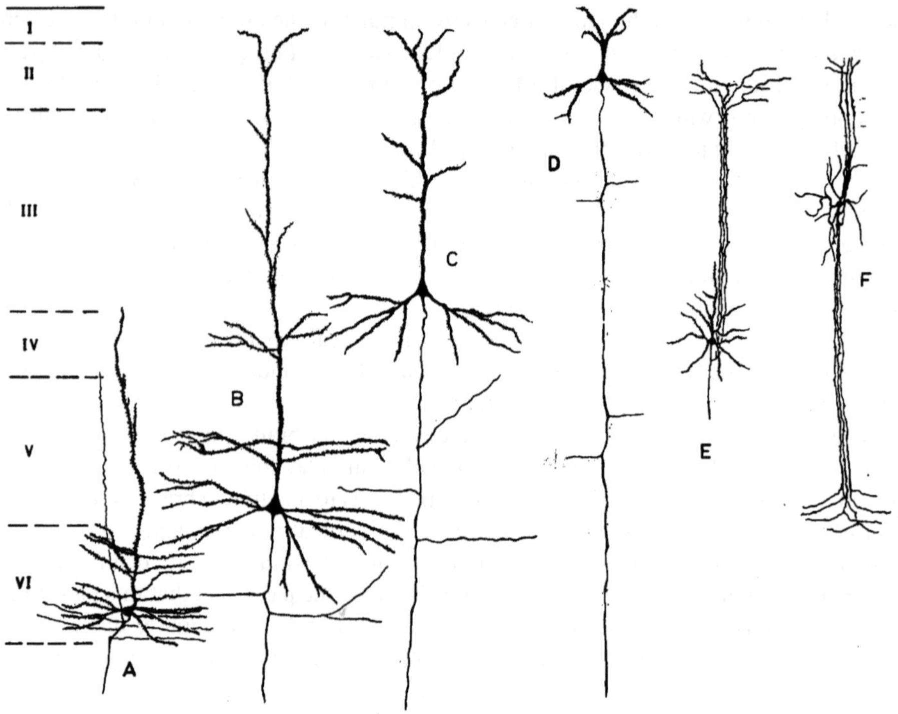

Fig. 1.1 Examples of neurons found in the brain. Cell types in the cerebral neocortex are shown. The different laminae of the cortex are designated I–VI, with I at the surface. Cells A–D are pyramidal cells in the different layers. Cell E is a spiny stellate cell, and F is a double bouquet cell.) (From Edward G. Jones and Alan Peters; Cerebral Cortex, Functional Properties of Cortical Cells volume 2, published 1984 [Springer Science + Business Media New York], reproduced with permission of SNCSC. Figure 1.1 is copyright protected and excluded from the open access license.)

shown in Figs. 1.1, 1.12, 1.13, and 9.20, further examples are shown in Shepherd (2004), and schematic drawings are shown in Shepherd and Grillner (2010). Once firing is initiated in the cell body (or axon initial segment of the cell body), the action potential is conducted in an all-or-nothing way to reach the synaptic terminals of the neuron, whence it may affect other neurons. Any inputs the neuron receives that cause it to become hyperpolarized make it less likely to fire (because the membrane potential is moved away from the critical threshold at which an action potential is initiated), and are described as inhibitory. The neuron can thus be thought of in a simple way as a computational element that sums its inputs within its time constant and, whenever this sum, minus any inhibitory effects, exceeds a threshold, produces an action potential that propagates to all of its output synaptic terminals. This simple idea is incorporated in many neuronal network models using a formalism of a type described in the next section.

1.4 A formalism for approaching the operation of single neurons in a network

Let us consider a neuron i as shown in Fig. 1.2, which receives inputs from axons that we label j through synapses of strength w_{ij}. The first subscript (i) refers to the output neuron that receives synaptic inputs, and the second subscript (j) to the particular input. j counts from 1 to C, where C is the number of synapses or connections received. The firing rate of the ith neuron is denoted as y_i, and that of the jth input to the neuron as x_j. To express the

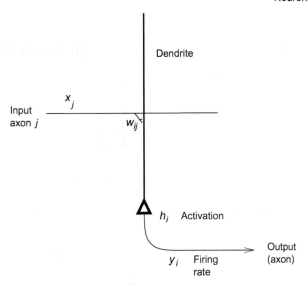

Fig. 1.2 Notation used to describe an individual neuron in a network model. By convention, we generally represent the dendrite as thick, and vertically oriented (as this is the normal way that neuroscientists view cortical pyramidal cells under the microscope); and the axon as thin. The cell body or soma is indicated between them by the triangle, as many cortical neurons have a pyramidal shape. The firing rate we also call the activity of the neuron.

idea that the neuron makes a simple linear summation of the inputs it receives, we can write the activation of neuron i, denoted h_i, as

$$h_i = \sum_j x_j w_{ij} \tag{1.1}$$

where $\sum_j$ indicates that the sum is over the C input axons (or connections) indexed by j to each neuron. The multiplicative form here indicates that activation should be produced by an axon only if it is firing, and depending on the strength of the synapse w_{ij} from input axon j onto the dendrite of the receiving neuron i. Equation 1.1 indicates that the strength of the activation reflects how fast the axon j is firing (that is x_j), and how strong the synapse w_{ij} is. The sum of all such activations expresses the idea that summation (of synaptic currents in real neurons) occurs along the length of the dendrite, to produce activation at the cell body, where the activation h_i is converted into firing y_i. This conversion can be expressed as

$$y_i = f(h_i) \tag{1.2}$$

which indicates that the firing rate is a function (f) of the postsynaptic activation. The function is called the activation function in this case. The function at its simplest could be linear, so that the firing rate would be proportional to the activation (see Fig. 1.3a). Real neurons have thresholds, with firing occurring only if the activation is above the threshold. A threshold linear activation function is shown in Fig. 1.3b. This has been useful in formal analysis of the properties of neural networks. Neurons also have firing rates that become saturated at a maximum rate, and we could express this as the sigmoid activation function shown in Fig. 1.3c. Another simple activation function, used in some models of neural networks, is the binary threshold function (Fig. 1.3d), which indicates that if the activation is below threshold, there is no firing, and that if the activation is above threshold, the neuron fires maximally. Some non-linearity in the activation function is an advantage, for it enables many useful computations to be performed in neuronal networks, including removing interfering effects of similar memories, and enabling neurons to perform logical operations, such as firing only if several inputs are present simultaneously.

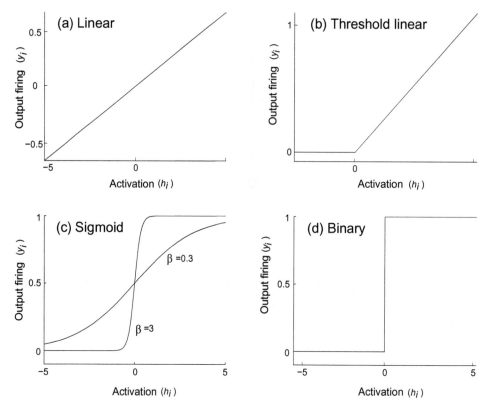

Fig. 1.3 Different types of activation function. The activation function relates the output activity (or firing rate), y_i, of the neuron (i) to its activation, h_i. (a) Linear. (b) Threshold linear. (c) Sigmoid. [One mathematical exemplar of this class of activation function is $y_i = 1/(1 + \exp(-2\beta h_i))$.] The output of this function, also sometimes known as the logistic function, is 0 for an input of $-\infty$, 0.5 for 0, and 1 for $+\infty$. The function incorporates a threshold at the lower end, followed by a linear portion, and then an asymptotic approach to the maximum value at the top end of the function. The parameter β controls the steepness of the almost linear part of the function round $h_i = 0$. If β is small, the output goes smoothly and slowly from 0 to 1 as h_i goes from $-\infty$ to $+\infty$. If β is large, the curve is very steep, and approximates a binary threshold activation function. (d) Binary threshold.

A property implied by Equation 1.1 is that the postsynaptic membrane is electrically short, and so summates its inputs irrespective of where on the dendrite the input is received. In real neurons, the transduction of current into firing frequency (the analogue of the transfer function of Equation 1.2) is generally studied not with synaptic inputs but by applying a steady current through an electrode into the soma. Examples of the resulting curves, which illustrate the additional phenomenon of firing rate adaptation, are shown in Fig. 1.4.

1.5 Synaptic modification

For a neuronal network to perform useful computation, that is to produce a given output when it receives a particular input, the synaptic weights must be set up appropriately. This is often performed by synaptic modification occurring during learning.

A simple learning rule that was originally presaged by Donald Hebb (1949) proposes that synapses increase in strength when there is conjunctive presynaptic and postsynaptic activity. The Hebb rule can be expressed more formally as follows

$$\delta w_{ij} = \alpha y_i x_j \tag{1.3}$$

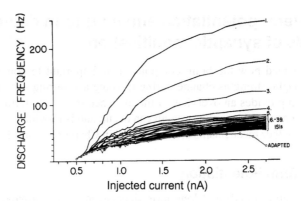

Fig. 1.4 Activation function of a hippocampal CA1 neuron. Frequency – current plot (the closest experimental analogue of the activation function) for a CA1 pyramidal cell. The firing frequency (in Hz) in response to the injection of 1.5 s long, rectangular depolarizing current pulses has been plotted against the strength of the current pulses (in nA) (abscissa). The first 39 interspike intervals (ISIs) are plotted as instantaneous frequency (1 / ISI), together with the average frequency of the adapted firing during the last part of the current injection (circles and broken line). The plot indicates a current threshold at approximately 0.5 nA, a linear range with a tendency to saturate, for the initial instantaneous rate, above approximately 200 Hz, and the phenomenon of adaptation, which is not reproduced in simple non-dynamical models (see further Appendix A5 of Rolls and Treves 1998). (Reproduced from Lanthorn, T., Storm, J. and Andersen, P. (1984) Current-to-frequency transduction in CA1 hippocampal pyramidal cells: Slow prepotentials dominate the primary range firing. *Experimental Brain Research* 53: 431–443, Copyright © Springer-Verlag.)

where δw_{ij} is the change of the synaptic weight w_{ij} which results from the simultaneous (or conjunctive) presence of presynaptic firing x_j and postsynaptic firing y_i (or strong depolarization), and α is a learning rate constant that specifies how much the synapses alter on any one pairing. The presynaptic and postsynaptic activity must be present approximately simultaneously (to within perhaps 100–500 ms in the real brain).

The Hebb rule is expressed in this multiplicative form to reflect the idea that both presynaptic and postsynaptic activity must be present for the synapses to increase in strength. The multiplicative form also reflects the idea that strong pre- and postsynaptic firing will produce a larger change of synaptic weight than smaller firing rates. The Hebb rule thus captures what is typically found in studies of associative Long-Term Potentiation (LTP) in the brain, described in Section 1.6.

One useful property of large neurons in the brain, such as cortical pyramidal cells, is that with their short electrical length, the postsynaptic term, y_i, is available on much of the dendrite of a cell. The implication of this is that once sufficient postsynaptic activation has been produced, any active presynaptic terminal on the neuron will show synaptic strengthening. This enables associations between coactive inputs, or correlated activity in input axons, to be learned by neurons using this simple associative learning rule.

If, in contrast, a group of coactive axons made synapses close together on a small dendrite, then the local depolarization might be intense, and only these synapses would modify onto the dendrite. (A single distant active synapse might not modify in this type of neuron, because of the long electrotonic length of the dendrite.) The computation in this case is described as Sigma-Pi ($\Sigma\Pi$), to indicate that there is a local product computed during learning; this allows a particular set of locally active synapses to modify together, and then the output of the neuron can reflect the sum of such local multiplications (see Rumelhart and McClelland (1986), Koch (1999)). Sigma-Pi neurons are not used in most of the networks described in this book. There has been some work on how such neurons, if present in the brain, might utilize this functionality in the computation of invariant representations (Mel et al., 1998; Mel and Fiser, 2000) (see Section 2.9).

1.6 Long-term potentiation and long-term depression as models of synaptic modification

In order to understand how the brain computes, it is important to consider the rules that describe how synaptic strengths change during learning and during self-organization of the brain. This section provides an overview of the evidence from long-term potentiation about how associative changes in synaptic strength can occur, and is provided as background reference information. Other mechanisms are considered in Chapters 16 and 17.

1.6.1 Long-Term Potentiation

Long-term potentiation (LTP) and long-term depression (LTD) provide useful models of some of the synaptic modifications that occur in the brain. The synaptic changes found appear to be synapse-specific, and to depend on information available locally at the synapse. LTP and LTD may thus provide a good model of the biological synaptic modifications involved in real neuronal network operations in the brain. Some of the properties of LTP and LTD are described next, together with evidence that implicates them in learning in at least some brain systems. Even if they turn out not to be the basis for the synaptic modifications that occur during learning, they have many of the properties that would be needed by some of the synaptic modification systems used by the brain.

Long-term potentiation is a use-dependent and sustained increase in synaptic strength that can be induced by brief periods of synaptic stimulation (Bliss and Collingridge, 2013; Takeuchi, Duszkiewicz and Morris, 2014; Bliss and Collingridge, 2019; Moser, Moser and Siegelbaum, 2021). It is usually measured as a sustained increase in the amplitude of electrically evoked responses in specific neural pathways following brief trains of high-frequency stimulation. For example, high frequency stimulation of the Schaffer collateral inputs from the CA3 hippocampal cells to the CA1 cells results in a larger response recorded from the CA1 cells to single test pulse stimulation of the pathway. LTP is long-lasting, in that its effect can be measured for hours in hippocampal slices, and in chronic in vivo experiments in some cases it may last for months. LTP becomes evident rapidly, typically in less than 1 minute. LTP is in some brain systems associative. This is illustrated in Fig. 1.5c, in which a weak input to a group of cells (e.g. the commissural input to CA1) does not show LTP unless it is given at the same time as (i.e. associatively with) another input (which could be weak or strong) to the cells. The associativity arises because it is only when sufficient activation of the postsynaptic neuron to exceed the threshold of NMDA receptors (see below) is produced that any learning can occur. The two weak inputs summate to produce sufficient depolarization to exceed the threshold. This associative property is shown very clearly in experiments in which LTP of an input to a single cell only occurs if the cell membrane is depolarized by passing current through it at the same time as the input arrives at the cell. The depolarization alone, or the input alone, is not sufficient to produce the LTP, and the LTP is thus associative. Moreover, in that the presynaptic input and the postsynaptic depolarization must occur at about the same time (within approximately 500 ms), the LTP requires temporal contiguity. LTP is also synapse-specific, in that, for example, an inactive input to a cell does not show LTP even if the cell is strongly activated by other inputs (Fig. 1.5b, input B).

These spatiotemporal properties of long term potentiation can be understood in terms of actions of the inputs on the postsynaptic cell, which in the hippocampus has two classes of receptor, NMDA (N-methyl-D-aspartate) and AMPA (alpha-amino-3-hydroxy-5-methyl-isoxasole-4-propionic acid), activated by the glutamate released by the presynaptic terminals. The NMDA receptor channels are normally blocked by Mg^{2+}, but when the cell is strongly depolarized by strong tetanic stimulation of the type necessary to induce LTP, the Mg^{2+} block

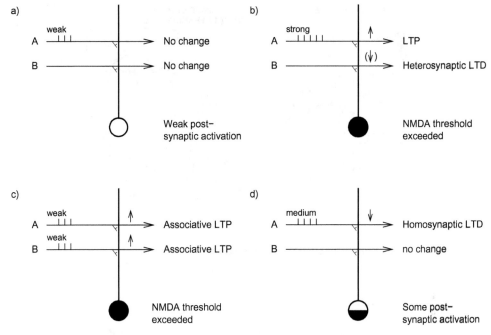

Fig. 1.5 Schematic illustration of synaptic modification rules as revealed by long-term potentiation (LTP) and long-term depression (LTD). The activation of the postsynaptic neuron is indicated by the extent to which its soma is black. There are two sets of inputs to the neuron: A and B. (a) A weak input (indicated by three spikes) on the set A of input axons produces little postsynaptic activation, and there is no change in synaptic strength. (b) A strong input (indicated by five spikes) on the set A of input axons produces strong postsynaptic activation, and the active synapses increase in strength. This is LTP. It is homosynaptic in that the synapses that increase in strength are the same as those through which the neuron is activated. LTP is synapse-specific, in that the inactive axons, B, do not show LTP. They either do not change in strength, or they may weaken. The weakening is called heterosynaptic LTD, because the synapses that weaken are other than those through which the neuron is activated (hetero- is Greek for other). (c) Two weak inputs present simultaneously on A and B summate to produce strong postsynaptic activation, and both sets of active synapses show LTP. (d) Intermediate strength firing on A produces some activation, but not strong activation, of the postsynaptic neuron. The active synapses become weaker. This is homosynaptic LTD, in that the synapses that weaken are the same as those through which the neuron is activated (homo- is Greek for same).

is removed, and Ca^{2+} entering via the NMDA receptor channels triggers events that lead to the potentiated synaptic transmission (see Fig. 1.6 (Horowitz and Horwitz, 2019)). Part of the evidence for this is that NMDA antagonists such as AP5 (D-2-amino-5-phosphonopentanoate) block LTP. Further, if the postsynaptic membrane is voltage clamped to prevent depolarization by a strong input, then LTP does not occur. The voltage-dependence of the NMDA receptor channels introduces a threshold and thus a non-linearity that contributes to a number of the phenomena of some types of LTP, such as cooperativity (many small inputs together produce sufficient depolarization to allow the NMDA receptors to operate); associativity (a weak input alone will not produce sufficient depolarization of the postsynaptic cell to enable the NMDA receptors to be activated, but the depolarization will be sufficient if there is also a strong input); and temporal contiguity between the different inputs that show LTP (in that if inputs occur non-conjunctively, the depolarization shows insufficient summation to reach the required level, or some of the inputs may arrive when the depolarization has decayed). Once the LTP has become established (which can be within one minute of the strong input to the cell), the LTP is expressed through the AMPA receptors, in that the NMDA receptor antagonist AP5 blocks only the establishment of LTP, and not its subsequent expression (Bliss and Collingridge, 2013; Siegelbaum and Kandel, 2013).

There are a number of possibilities about what change is triggered by the entry of Ca^{2+} to the postsynaptic cell to mediate LTP. One possibility is that somehow a messenger (such as

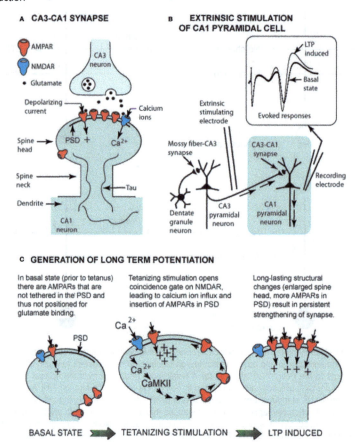

Fig. 1.6 The mechanism of induction of Long-Term Potentiation (LTP) for the CA3 to CA1 synapses in the hippocampus. (A) CA3-CA1 synaptic structure showing glutamate receptors (AMPA receptors AMPARs and an NMDA receptor NMDAR) linked to the post-synaptic density (PSD), a multiprotein assembly that orients receptors to face the presynaptic CA3 terminal. Tau is a structural protein. (B) Electrical circuit for recording CA1 pyramidal neuron-evoked responses. The insert shows the evoked response prior to a tetanizing (high frequency) stimulation (basal state), and an enhanced response following the tetanizing stimulation (LTP-induced). (C) Change in spine head shape before and after the tetanizing stimulation. The latter induces a rapid (within seconds) increase in spine head size, allowing insertion of AMPARs into the PSD. Within minutes, the spine head has slightly shrunken to a long lasting (hours) form with additional AMPARs in the PSD (LTP-induced). In more detail, during normal, low-frequency synaptic transmission glutamate released from the terminals of CA3 Schaffer collateral axons acts on both NMDA and AMPA receptors in the postsynaptic membrane of dendritic spines (the site of excitatory input) of CA1 neurons. Sodium and K^+ flow through the AMPA receptors but not through the NMDA receptors because their pore is blocked by Mg^{2+} at negative membrane potentials. During a high-frequency tetanus the large depolarization of the postsynaptic membrane (caused by strong activation of the AMPA receptors) relieves the Mg^{2+} blockade of the NMDA receptors, allowing Ca^{2+}, Na^+, and K^+ to flow through these channels. The resulting increase of Ca^{2+} in the dendritic spine triggers calcium-dependent kinases–calcium/calmodulin-dependent kinase (CaMKII), leading to induction of LTP. (From Horowitz,J.M. and Horwitz,B.A. 2019. Extreme neuroplasticity of hippocampal CA1 pyramidal neurons in hibernating mammalian species. Frontiers in Neuroanatomy 13:9. doi: 10.3389/fnana.2019.00009.)

NO) reaches the presynaptic terminals from the postsynaptic membrane and, if the terminals are active, causes them to release more transmitter in future whenever they are activated by an action potential. Consistent with this possibility is the observation that, after LTP has been induced, more transmitter appears to be released from the presynaptic endings. Another possibility is that the postsynaptic membrane changes just where Ca^{2+} has entered, so that AMPA receptors become more responsive to glutamate released in future. Consistent with this possibility is the observation that after LTP, the postsynaptic cell may respond more to locally applied glutamate (using a microiontophoretic technique).

The rule that underlies associative LTP is thus that synapses connecting two neurons become stronger if there is conjunctive presynaptic and (strong) postsynaptic activity. This learning rule for synaptic modification is sometimes called the Hebb rule, after Donald Hebb of McGill University who drew attention to this possibility, and its potential importance in learning (Hebb, 1949).

In that LTP is long-lasting, develops rapidly, is synapse-specific, and is in some cases associative, it is of interest as a potential synaptic mechanism underlying some forms of memory. Evidence linking it directly to some forms of learning comes from experiments in which it has been shown that the drug AP5 infused so that it reaches the hippocampus to block NMDA receptors blocks spatial learning mediated by the hippocampus (Morris, 1989; Martin, Grimwood and Morris, 2000; Takeuchi, Duszkiewicz and Morris, 2014). The task learned by the rats was to find the location relative to cues in a room of a platform submerged in an opaque liquid (milk). Interestingly, if the rats had already learned where the platform was, then the NMDA infusion did not block performance of the task. This is a close parallel to LTP, in that the learning, but not the subsequent expression of what had been learned, was blocked by the NMDA antagonist AP5. Although there is still some uncertainty about the experimental evidence that links LTP to learning (Martin, Grimwood and Morris, 2000; Lynch, 2004; Takeuchi, Duszkiewicz and Morris, 2014), there is a need for a synapse-specific modifiability of synaptic strengths on neurons if neuronal networks are to learn. If LTP is not always an exact model of the synaptic modification that occurs during learning, then something with many of the properties of LTP is nevertheless needed, and is likely to be present in the brain given the functions known to be implemented in many brain regions.

In another model of the role of LTP in memory, Davis (2000) has studied the role of the amygdala in learning associations to fear-inducing stimuli. He has shown that blockade of NMDA synapses in the amygdala interferes with this type of learning, consistent with the idea that LTP also provides a useful model of this type of learning. NMDA receptors in the amygdala are also involved in the extinction of conditioned fear responses (Davis, 2011).

1.6.2 Long-Term Depression

Long-Term Depression (LTD) can also occur. It can in principle be associative or non-associative. In associative LTD, the alteration of synaptic strength depends on the pre- and postsynaptic activities. There are two types. Heterosynaptic LTD occurs when the postsynaptic neuron is strongly activated, and there is low presynaptic activity (see Fig. 1.5b input B, and Table B.1 on page 828). Heterosynaptic LTD is so-called because the synapse that weakens is other than (hetero-) the one through which the postsynaptic neuron is activated. Heterosynaptic LTD is important in associative neuronal networks, and in competitive neuronal networks (see Appendix B). In competitive neural networks it would be helpful if the degree of heterosynaptic LTD depended on the existing strength of the synapse, and there is some evidence that this may be the case (see Appendix B). Homosynaptic LTD occurs when the presynaptic neuron is strongly active, and the postsynaptic neuron has some, but low, activity (see Fig. 1.5d and Table B.1). Homosynaptic LTD is so-called because the synapse that weakens is the same as (homo-) the one that is active. Heterosynaptic and homosynaptic LTD are found in the neocortex (Artola and Singer, 1993; Singer, 1995; Frégnac, 1996) and hippocampus (Christie, 1996), and in many cases are dependent on activation of NMDA receptors (Fazeli and Collingridge, 1996; Bliss and Collingridge, 2013). LTD in the cerebellum is evident as weakening of active parallel fibre to Purkinje cell synapses when the climbing fibre connecting to a Purkinje cell is active (Ito, 1984, 1989, 1993b,a, 2006, 2010).

Neuromodulators such as dopamine and acetylcholine can influence LTP and LTD (Bazzari and Parri, 2019; Fremaux and Gerstner, 2015). The ways in which dopamine acts to modulate learning are described in Chapter 16, and the importance of cholinergic modulation in human memory consolidation (Rolls, 2022b) is described in Chapter 9.

1.6.3 Spike Timing-Dependent Plasticity

An interesting time-dependence of LTP and LTD has been observed, with LTP occurring especially when the presynaptic spikes precede by a few ms the post-synaptic activation, and LTD occurring when the pre-synaptic spikes follow the post-synaptic activation by a few milliseconds (ms) (Markram, Lübke, Frotscher and Sakmann, 1997; Bi and Poo, 1998, 2001; Senn, Markram and Tsodyks, 2001; Dan and Poo, 2004, 2006; Markram, Gerstner and Sjöström, 2012; Fremaux and Gerstner, 2015). This is referred to as spike timing-dependent plasticity, STDP. This type of temporally asymmetric Hebbian learning rule, demonstrated in the hippocampus and neocortex, can induce associations over time, and not just between simultaneous events. Networks of neurons with such synapses can learn sequences (Minai and Levy, 1993), enabling them to predict the future state of the postsynaptic neuron based on past experience (Abbott and Blum, 1996) (see further Koch (1999), Markram, Pikus, Gupta and Tsodyks (1998) and Abbott and Nelson (2000)). This mechanism, because of its apparent time-specificity for periods in the range of ms or tens of ms, could also encourage neurons to learn to respond to temporally synchronous pre-synaptic firing (Gerstner, Kreiter, Markram and Herz, 1997; Gutig and Sompolinsky, 2006), and indeed to decrease the synaptic strengths from neurons that fire at random times with respect to the synchronized group. This mechanism might also play a role in the normalization of the strength of synaptic connection strengths onto a neuron. A version of STDP learning that adjusts the eligibility of synapses for learning provides a more explicit way for controlling the strength of the synaptic weights onto a neuron (El Boustani, Yger, Fregnac and Destexhe, 2012). Further, there is accumulating evidence (Sjöström, Turrigiano and Nelson, 2001) that a more realistic description of the protocols for inducing LTP and LTD probably requires a combination of dependence on spike timing – to take into account the effects of the backpropagating action potential – and dependence on the sub-threshold depolarization of the postsynaptic neuron. However these spike timing-dependent synaptic modifications may be evident primarily at low firing rates rather than those that often occur in the brain (Sjöström, Turrigiano and Nelson, 2001), and may not be especially reproducible in the cerebral neocortex (Fregnac et al., 2010), though interest in STDP, especially from theoretical perspectives, continues (Feldman, 2012, 2009; Fremaux and Gerstner, 2015). Neuromodulators such as dopamine and acetylcholine may also modulate STDP, and modelling approaches show how a delayed modulator such as a reward signal could influence STDP if there is a STDP eligibility trace that lasts until the reward is received (Fremaux and Gerstner, 2015).

However, under the somewhat steady-state conditions of the firing of neurons in the higher parts of the ventral visual system on the 10 ms timescale that are observed not only when single stimuli are presented for 500 ms (see Fig. 2.16), but also when macaques have found a search target and are looking at it (in the experiments described in Sections 2.4.3 and 2.8.9.1), the average of the presynaptic and postsynaptic rates are likely to be the important determinants of synaptic modification. Part of the reason for this is that correlations between the firing of simultaneously recorded inferior temporal cortex neurons are not common, and if present are not very strong or typically restricted to a short time window in the order of 10 ms (Rolls and Treves, 2011; Rolls, 2016b). This point is also made in the context that each neuron has thousands of inputs, several tens of which are normally likely to be active when a cell is firing above its spontaneous firing rate and is strongly depolarized. This may make it unlikely statistically that there will be a strong correlation between a particular presynaptic spike and postsynaptic firing, and thus that STDP is a main determinant of synaptic strength under these natural conditions.

Synaptic modification for learning is considered further by Rolls (2016b), and some of the implications of different types of synaptic modification are considered in Appendix B.

1.7 Information encoding by neurons, and distributed representations

Most neurons in the cortex respond selectively to different stimuli, and the firing rate increases with the intensity of the stimulus. One example comes from the taste system, where some neurons are tuned to respond best to sweet, others to salt, others to sour, others to bitter, and others to umami (Chapter 4). Their firing rates increase as the intensity of the stimulus increases (in this case, the concentration of the tastant). In the primary visual cortex, some neurons respond to a stimulus at the fovea, and other neurons to a stimulus at a particular retinal position with respect to the fovea. Thus which neurons are active carries or encodes the information. This is called **place coding**, or (firing) **rate** encoding (as it is the number of action potential spikes that is important, and not the detailed timing of the spikes as with temporal encoding). This is also sometimes referred to as **labelled line encoding**, or grandmother cell encoding, if the neurons are very selective, which they are not usually. Indeed, the information is usually distributed across a population of neurons that are each somewhat differently tuned to a small proportion of a stimulus set. This is called distributed encoding, and is considered soon. The term 'place coding' probably has its origin in cortical maps, where the stimuli to which a neuron responds depends on the place of the neuron in the map. However, often in the cortex the coding is in high dimensional spaces that do not map easily into a 2D map, but the concept that the stimulus is encoded by which neurons are active still holds very firmly, as described in Appendix C, and we can use the term place coding. We will refer to this type of encoding as place coding or rate coding.

In some parts of the brain, the firing frequency of neurons encodes what the stimulus is, and this happens in the peripheral parts of the auditory system, where some neurons can follow the frequency of auditory stimuli up to about 1,000 Hz (Chapter 7). This is a type of **temporal encoding**, in which timing information can be important. The temporal information in this firing can be important in auditory localisation; but it is notable that the brain recodes this at the first central synapse in the brain into a place code / rate code, in which the particular neurons that are active encode the sound frequency (Chapter 7), because temporal encoding is difficult to maintain accurately when time delays and transmission time differences depend on factors such as the exact diameter of nerve fibres. It is presumably because of the difficulty of maintaining accurate timing in the brain that we have such large transmission lines in the dorsal 'magnocellular' visual system, for if the conduction time is fast (as it is with magnocellular neurons), then any absolute differences in transmission times can be minimised. This may be important when motion is being computed in the dorsal visual system. Thus in general temporal encoding is used as little as possible in the brain; and when the time of arrival is important, the brain uses large metabolic resources by employing magnocellular neurons. It has also been argued by some that the timing of spikes within a spike train carries information, but that hypothesis is shown in Appendix C not to apply in several brain systems (Tovee, Rolls, Treves and Bellis, 1993; Rolls, Franco, Aggelopoulos and Jerez, 2006b). At its simplest, such temporal encoding might involve different latencies of neuronal responses for different stimuli, but wherever that has been tested (apart as mentioned in the auditory system), the amount of information encoded by the latencies is small compared to that in the firing rates of neurons; and the information from the latency is redundant with respect to the rate information, i.e. the latency adds nothing useful to the encoding by firing rate using a place code (Appendix C) (Tovee, Rolls, Treves and Bellis, 1993; Rolls, Franco, Aggelopoulos and Jerez, 2006b; Verhagen, Baker, Vasan, Pieribone and Rolls, 2023).

In the remainder of this section, we consider place / rate coding, and the advantages of using sparse distributed place / rate coding for the representation of information in the brain, and for use in brain computations.

When considering the operation of many neuronal networks in the brain, it is found that many useful properties arise if each input to the network (arriving on the axons as the vector of input firing rates **x**) is encoded in the activity of an ensemble or population of the axons or input lines (distributed encoding), and is not signalled by the activity of a single input, which is called local encoding. We start off with some definitions, and then highlight some of the differences, and summarize some evidence that shows the type of encoding used in some brain regions. Then in Appendix B (e.g. Table B.2), I show how many of the useful properties of the neuronal networks described depend on distributed encoding. Evidence on the encoding actually found in visual cortical areas is described in Chapters 2 and 3, in Appendix C, and by Rolls and Treves (2011).

1.7.1 Definitions

All of the following apply to what is termed above 'place coding'.

A *local representation* is one in which all the information that a particular stimulus or event occurred is provided by the activity of one of the neurons. In a famous example, a single neuron might be active only if one's grandmother was being seen. An implication is that most neurons in the brain regions where objects or events are represented would fire only very rarely. A problem with this type of encoding is that a new neuron would be needed for every object or event that has to be represented. There are many other disadvantages of this type of encoding, many of which will become apparent in this book. Moreover, there is evidence that objects are represented in the brain by a different type of encoding (sparse distributed encoding, Appendix C; and Rolls and Treves (2011)).

A *fully distributed representation* is one in which all the information that a particular stimulus or event occurred is provided by the activity of the full set of neurons. If the neurons are binary (e.g. either active or not), the most distributed encoding is when half the neurons are active for any one stimulus or event.

A *sparse distributed representation* is a distributed representation in which a small proportion of the neurons is active at any one time. In a sparse representation with binary neurons, less than half of the neurons are active for any one stimulus or event. For binary neurons, we can use as a measure of the sparseness the proportion of neurons in the active state. For neurons with real, continuously variable, values of firing rates, the sparseness a^p of the representation provided by the population can be measured, by extending the binary notion of the proportion of neurons that are firing, as

$$a^p = \frac{(\sum_{i=1}^{N} y_i/N)^2}{\sum_{i=1}^{N} y_i^2/N} \tag{1.4}$$

where y_i is the firing rate of the ith neuron in the set of N neurons (Treves and Rolls, 1991). This is referred to as the population sparseness, and measures of sparseness including that for a single neuron are considered in detail in Section C.3.1 and by Rolls (2016b). A low value of the sparseness a^p indicates that few neurons are firing for any one stimulus.

Coarse coding utilizes overlaps of receptive fields, and can compute positions in the input space using differences between the firing levels of coactive cells (e.g. color-tuned cones in the retina). The representation implied is very distributed. Fine coding (in which, for example, a neuron may be 'tuned' to the exact orientation and position of a stimulus) implies more sparse coding.

1.7.2 Advantages of sparse distributed encoding

One advantage of distributed encoding is that the similarity between two representations can be reflected by the correlation between the two patterns of activity that represent the different stimuli. We have already introduced the idea that the input to a neuron is represented by the activity of its set of input axons x_j, where j indexes the axons, numbered from $j = 1, C$ (see Fig. 1.2 and Equation 1.1). Now the set of activities of the input axons is a vector (a vector is an ordered set of numbers; Appendix A provides a summary of some of the concepts involved). We can denote as $\mathbf{x}^1$ the vector of axonal activity that represents stimulus 1, and $\mathbf{x}^2$ the vector that represents stimulus 2. Then the similarity between the two vectors, and thus the two stimuli, is reflected by the correlation between the two vectors. The correlation will be high if the activity of each axon in the two representations is similar; and will become more and more different as the activity of more and more of the axons differs in the two representations. Thus the similarity of two inputs can be represented in a graded or continuous way if (this type of) distributed encoding is used. This enables generalization to similar stimuli, or to incomplete versions of a stimulus (if it is, for example, partly seen or partly remembered), to occur. With a local representation, either one stimulus or another is represented, each by its own neuron firing, and similarities between different stimuli are not encoded.

Another advantage of distributed encoding is that the number of different stimuli that can be represented by a set of C components (e.g. the activity of C axons) can be very large. A simple example is provided by the binary encoding of an 8-element vector. One component can code for which of two stimuli has been seen, 2 components (or bits in a computer byte) for 4 stimuli, 3 components for 8 stimuli, 8 components for 256 stimuli, etc. That is, the number of stimuli increases exponentially with the number of components (or, in this case, axons) in the representation. (In this simple binary illustrative case, the number of stimuli that can be encoded is 2^C.) Put the other way round, even if a neuron has only a limited number of inputs (e.g. a few thousand), it can nevertheless receive a great deal of information about which stimulus was present. This ability of a neuron with a limited number of inputs to receive information about which of potentially very many input events is present is probably one factor that makes computation by the brain possible. With local encoding, the number of stimuli that can be encoded increases only linearly with the number C of axons or components (because a different component is needed to represent each new stimulus). (In our example, only 8 stimuli could be represented by 8 axons.)

In the real brain, there is now good evidence that in a number of brain systems, including the high-order visual and olfactory cortices, and the hippocampus, distributed encoding with the above two properties, of representing similarity, and of exponentially increasing encoding capacity as the number of neurons in the representation increases, is found (Rolls and Tovee, 1995b; Abbott, Rolls and Tovee, 1996; Rolls, Treves and Tovee, 1997b; Rolls, Treves, Robertson, Georges-François and Panzeri, 1998b; Rolls, Franco, Aggelopoulos and Reece, 2003b; Rolls, Aggelopoulos, Franco and Treves, 2004; Franco, Rolls, Aggelopoulos and Treves, 2004; Aggelopoulos, Franco and Rolls, 2005; Rolls, Franco, Aggelopoulos and Jerez, 2006b; Rolls and Treves, 2011; Rolls, 2016b) (Appendix C). For example, in the primate inferior temporal visual cortex, the number of faces or objects that can be represented increases approximately exponentially with the number of neurons in the population (Rolls and Treves, 2011; Rolls, 2016b). If we consider instead the information about which stimulus is seen, we see that this rises approximately linearly with the number of neurons in the representation (Fig. 2.18). This corresponds to an exponential rise in the number of stimuli encoded, because information is a log measure (see Fig. 2.19 and Rolls (2016b)). A similar result has been found for the encoding of position in space by the primate hippocampus (Rolls, Treves, Robertson, Georges-François and Panzeri, 1998b).

It is particularly important that the information can be read from the ensemble of neurons using a simple measure of the similarity of vectors, the correlation (or dot product, see Appendix B) between two vectors (e.g. Fig. 2.18). The importance of this is that it is essentially vector similarity operations that characterize the operation of many neuronal networks (see Appendix B). The neurophysiological results show that both the ability to reflect similarity by vector correlation, and the utilization of exponential coding capacity, are properties of real neuronal networks found in the brain.

To emphasize one of the points being made here, although the binary encoding used in the 8-bit vector described above has optimal capacity for binary encoding, it is not optimal for vector similarity operations. For example, the two very similar numbers 127 and 128 are represented by 01111111 and 10000000 with binary encoding, yet the correlation or bit overlap of these vectors is 0. The brain, in contrast, uses a code that has the attractive property of exponentially increasing capacity with the number of neurons in the representation, though it is different from the simple binary encoding of numbers used in computers; and at the same time the brain codes stimuli in such a way that the code can be read off with simple dot product or correlation-related decoding, which is what is specified for the elementary neuronal network operation shown in Equation 1.2 (see Section 1.7).

1.8 Neuronal network approaches versus connectionism

The approach taken in this book is to introduce how real neuronal networks in the brain may compute, and thus to achieve a fundamental and realistic basis for understanding brain function. This may be contrasted with connectionism, which aims to understand cognitive function by analysing processing in neuron-like computing systems (Rumelhart and McClelland, 1986; McLeod, Plunkett and Rolls, 1998). Connectionist systems are neuron-like in that they analyze computation in systems with large numbers of computing elements in which the information which governs how the network computes is stored in the connection strengths between the nodes (or "neurons") in the network. However, in many connectionist models the individual units or nodes are not intended to model individual neurons, and the variables that are used in the simulations are not intended to correspond to quantities that can be measured in the real brain. Moreover, connectionist approaches use learning rules in which the synaptic modification (the strength of the connections between the nodes) is determined by algorithms that require information that is not local to the synapse, that is, evident in the pre- and post-synaptic firing rates (see further Appendix B). Instead, in many connectionist systems, information about how to modify synaptic strengths is propagated backwards from the output of the network to affect neurons hidden deep within the network (see Section B.12). Because it is not clear that this is biologically plausible, we have instead in this text concentrated on introducing neuronal network architectures which are more biologically plausible, and which use a local learning rule. Connectionist approaches (see for example McClelland and Rumelhart (1986), McLeod, Plunkett and Rolls (1998)) are very valuable, for they show what can be achieved computationally with networks in which the connection strength determines the computation that the network achieves with quite simple computing elements. However, as models of brain function, many connectionist networks achieve almost too much, by solving problems with a carefully limited number of "neurons" or nodes, which contributes to the ability of such networks to generalize successfully over the problem space. Connectionist schemes thus make an important start to understanding how complex computations (such as language) could be implemented in brain-like systems. In doing this, connectionist models often use simplified representations of the inputs and outputs, which are often crucial to the way in which the problem is solved. In addition, they may use learning algorithms that are really too powerful for the brain to perform, and therefore they can be taken only as a guide to how cognitive functions might be implemented by neuronal networks in the brain. In this book, we focus on more biologically plausible neuronal networks.

1.9 Introduction to three neuronal network architectures

With neurons of the type outlined in Section 1.4, and an associative learning rule of the type described in Section 1.5, three neuronal network architectures arise that appear to be used in many different brain regions. The three architectures will be described in Appendix B, and a brief introduction is provided here.

In the first architecture (see Fig. 1.7a and b), pattern associations can be learned. The output neurons are driven by an unconditioned stimulus (for example the taste of food). A conditioned stimulus (for example the sight of food) reaches the output neurons by associatively modifiable synapses w_{ij}. If the conditioned stimulus is paired during learning with activation of the output neurons produced by the unconditioned stimulus, then later, after learning, due to the associative synaptic modification, the conditioned stimulus alone will produce the same output as the unconditioned stimulus. **Pattern association networks** are described in Section B.2.

In the second architecture, an **autoassociation or attractor network**, the output neurons have recurrent associatively modifiable synaptic connections w_{ij} to other neurons in the network (see Fig. 1.7c). When an external input causes the output neurons to fire, then associative links are formed through the modifiable synapses that connect the set of neurons that is active. Later, if only a fraction of the original input pattern is presented, then the associative synaptic connections or weights allow the whole of the memory to be retrieved. This is called completion. Because the components of the pattern are associated with each other as a result of the associatively modifiable recurrent connections, this is called an autoassociative memory. It is believed to be used in the cortex for many purposes, including short-term memory; episodic memory, in which the parts of a memory of an episode are associated together; and helping to define the response properties of cortical neurons, which have collaterals between themselves within a limited region. Autoassociation or attractor networks are described in Section B.3.

In the third architecture, a **competitive network**, the main input to the output neurons is received through associatively modifiable synapses w_{ij} (see Fig. 1.7d). Because of the initial values of the synaptic strengths, or because every axon does not contact every output neuron, different patterns tend to activate different output neurons. When one pattern is being presented, the most strongly activated neurons tend via lateral inhibition to inhibit the other neurons. For this reason the network is called competitive. During the presentation of that pattern, associative modification of the active axons onto the active postsynaptic neuron takes place. Later, that or similar patterns will have a greater chance of activating that neuron or set of neurons. Other neurons learn to respond to other input patterns. In this way, a network is built that can categorize patterns, placing similar patterns into the same category. This is useful as a preprocessor for sensory information, self-organizes to produce feature analyzers, and finds uses in many other parts of the brain too. Competitive networks are described in

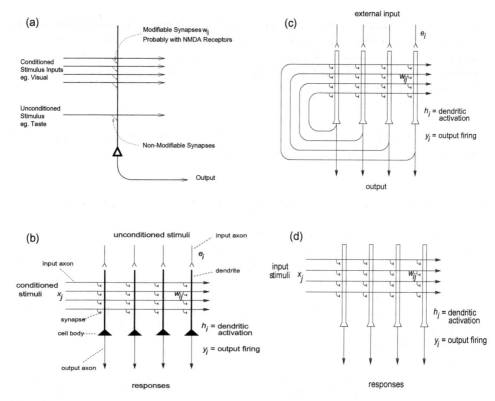

Fig. 1.7 Three network architectures that use local learning rules: (a) pattern association network introduced with a single output neuron; (b) pattern association network; (c) autoassociation network; (d) competitive network. Cortical pyramidal cell bodies are represented by triangular shapes, and the dendrites of each cell are shown above, with the axons shown below. The negative feedback inhibitory neurons are not shown.

Section B.4, and, importantly, perform unsupervised learning in that there is no teacher specifying how each neuron should respond. Instead, the categories are learned from the statistics present in the inputs.

Competitive networks enable new representations in the brain to be formed, by learning to respond to different combinations of inputs. The inputs are sometimes referred to as features. An example in vision might be that a common co-occurrence of two input features, such as a horizontal and vertical line, might enable a 'T' junction to be learned. Combinations of just a few features (termed low order combinations) need to be learned at any one stage, otherwise there would be a combinatorial explosion in the number of feature analyzers needed (Feldman, 1985). The building of feature analyzers using competitive learning is a key aspect of the operation of hierarchical networks, as described in Chapter 2.

All three architectures require inhibitory interneurons, which receive inputs from the principal neurons in the network (usually the pyramidal cells shown in Fig. 1.7) and implement feedback inhibition by connections to the pyramidal cells. The inhibition is usually implemented by GABA neurons, and maintains a small proportion of the pyramidal cells active.

These are three fundamental building blocks for neural architectures in the cortex. They are often used in combination with each other. Because they are some of the building blocks of some of the architectures found in the cerebral cortex, they are described in Appendix B.

These three architectures illustrate some of the important types of learning that can be implemented in Neural Networks, as described in more detail in Appendix B. First, competitive learning is an example of **unsupervised learning**, in that the system self-organizes based on the statistics of the inputs being received, without an external teacher to guide its learning. This is used in the model of invariant visual object recognition, VisNet, described in Chapter 2. This type of learning must be very common in the brain, in that there is often no external teacher to help the system self-organise, let alone an external teacher for every neuron. Unsupervised learning is relatively little used in the machine learning community at present, and there are likely to be important lessons learned from how unsupervised learning is used in the brain.

Pattern association learning is an example of **supervised learning**, in that each output neuron has an external input that specifies the output that each neuron should produce. This external input is e_i in Fig. 1.7b. In the pattern association networks shown in Fig. 1.7b the inputs x_j learn to produce the required outputs just by associative synaptic modification, and this type of learning is common in the brain. In machine learning, the learning rule may be much more powerful, and may involve calculating an error between the output that is required for each neuron, and the actual output that is being produced by the inputs x_j. A one-layer network with such error correction learning is referred to as a one-layer error correction network or one-layer perceptron, and is described in Section B.11. The brain does in general not have the architecture required for this type of learning, as there is no separate teacher for each neuron to specify what its firing should be for every input, and no way to compare the actual firing with the target firing to compute an error to correct the appropriate synaptic weight. The only part of the brain where the architecture might be suitable is the cerebellum, where there is a single climbing fibre for each Purkinje cell, as described in Chapter 17. The error correction type of learning can be implemented in machine learning in a multilayer network, in which inputs are applied to the bottom layer of the network, and every neuron in the output layer has a teacher. In the backpropagation of error algorithm described in Section B.12, the error is backpropagated though all the layers of the network to calculate the error that should be used to correct the firing of every neuron in all the hidden layers not connected to the input or output. This is a non-local type of synaptic modification, and could not easily be implemented in the cortex, partly because there is no teacher for each neuron, and partly because of the implausibility of computing the backpropagated errors through every layer, although attempts have been made (O'Reilly and Munakata, 2000; Guerguiev et al., 2017). Although deep learning trained by error backpropagation is used widely for classifying inputs in machine learning, there is no clear evidence yet that it is or could be implemented in the cortex. The brain may solve similar problems, but in other ways, with one example being invariant visual object recognition as described in Chapter 2.

A third type of learning is **reinforcement learning**, in which there is a single reward signal for the whole network, as described in Sections B.17 and 19.5. This type of learning may be implemented in the brain for the slow learning of stimulus-response habits in the basal ganglia, using dopamine to provide a reward prediction error signal as described in Section 16.4.3.

A fourth learning system is that exemplified by the autoassociation network system illustrated in Fig. 1.7c and described in Section B.3. This is a network that stores information and can retrieve it using a partial cue, and can maintain it using the positive feedback implemented by the recurrent collateral connections. This type of network plays key roles in episodic memory (Chapter 9), short-term memory and attention, and planning (Chapter 13), semantic memory (Chapter 8), and indeed in cortical computation (Rolls, 2016b). This is key to understanding brain function, but is little used in machine learning as other mechanisms can be used in digital computers.

1.10 Systems-level analysis of brain function

To understand the computations in the brain, it is essential to understand the systems-level organization of the brain, in order to understand how the networks in each region provide a particular computational function as part of an overall computational scheme. These systems-level processing streams are described in the different Chapters of this book. The description is based primarily on studies in non-human primates, for they have well-developed cortical areas that in many cases correspond to those found in humans, and it has been possible to analyze their connectivity and their functions by recording the activity of neurons in them.

Some of the processing streams involved in sensory and related memory and emotional functions are shown in Fig. 1.8. Some of these regions are shown in the drawings of the primate brain in Figs. 2.3, 2.1, and 3.1.

The hippocampus receives inputs from both the 'what' and the 'where' visual systems (Figs. 1.8 and 2.3, and Chapter 9). By rapidly learning associations between conjunctive inputs in these systems, it is able to form memories of particular events occurring in particular places at particular times. To do this, it needs to store whatever is being represented in each of many cortical areas at a given time, and later to recall the whole memory from a part of it. The types of network it contains that are involved in this memory function are described in Chapter 9.

The dorsolateral parts of the prefrontal cortex receive inputs from dorsal stream processing pathways, and the ventrolateral parts from the ventral stream processing pathways, as shown in Figs. 2.4, 2.3 and 3.1. These lateral prefrontal cortical areas, including Brodmann area (BA) 46, provide short-term memory functions, providing the basis for functions such as top-down attention, short-term memory, working memory, and planning (Chapter 13). These lateral prefrontal cortex areas can be thought of as providing processing that need not be dominated by perceptual processing, as must the posterior visual and parietal lobe spatial areas if incoming stimuli are to be perceived, but can instead be devoted to processing recent information that may no longer be present in perceptual areas.

The orbitofrontal cortex, areas BA 11, 12 and 13 (Figs. 1.8, 11.2, 2.3 and 3.1), receives information from the 'what' systems for vision, taste, olfaction, touch, and audition), forms multimodal representations, and computes reward value. It is therefore of fundamental importance for emotional, motivational, and social behavior (see Chapter 11).

1.11 Brodmann areas

A very brief outline of some of the connections and functions of different Brodmann areas (Brodmann, 1909, 1925) is provided here, intended mainly for those who are not familiar with them. Brodmann used cytoarchitecture of the cortex studied with a microscope to distinguish different areas, but because function reflects the architecture, different Brodmann areas also to a considerable extent have different functions. Some of these areas are shown by the numbers in Figs. 1.9, 2.3, 2.1, and 3.1. However, a more modern parcellation of the cortex based on function as well as structure produced by the Human Connectome Project and used for the connectivity studies described in this book is described in Section 1.12 and illustrated in Figs. 1.10 and 1.11.

Brodmann areas:
Areas 3, 1 & 2 – Primary somatosensory cortex (in the postcentral gyrus). This is numbered rostral to caudal as 3,1,2. This region is associated with the sense and localization of touch, temperature, vibration, and pain. There is a map or homunculus of different parts of the body.

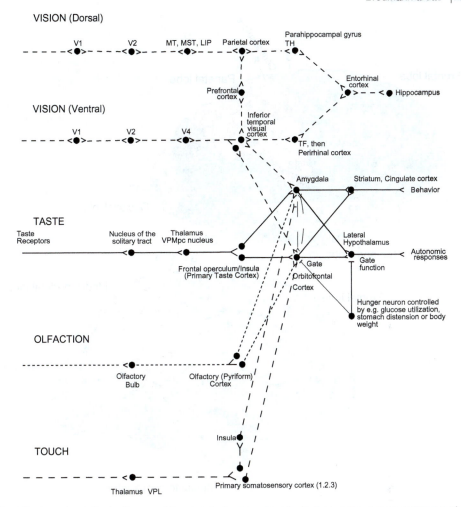

Fig. 1.8 The pathways involved in some different cortical systems described in the text. Forward connections start from early cortical areas on the left. To emphasise that backprojections are important in many memory systems, they are made explicit in the synaptic terminals drawn in the upper part of the diagram, but are a property of most of the connections shown. The top pathway, also shown in Fig. 3.1, shows the connections in the 'dorsal or where visual pathway' from V1 to V2, MT, MST, 7a etc, with some connections reaching the dorsolateral prefrontal cortex and frontal eye fields. The second pathway, also shown in Fig. 2.1, shows the connections in the 'ventral or what visual pathway' from V1 to V2, V4, the inferior temporal visual cortex, etc., with some connections reaching the amygdala and orbitofrontal cortex. The two systems project via the parahippocampal gyrus and perirhinal cortex respectively to the hippocampus, and both systems have projections to the dorsolateral prefrontal cortex. The taste pathways project after the primary taste cortex to the orbitofrontal cortex and amygdala. The olfactory pathways project from the primary olfactory, pyriform, cortex to the orbitofrontal cortex and amygdala. The bottom pathway shows the connections from the primary somatosensory cortex, areas 1, 2 and 3, to the mid-insula, orbitofrontal cortex, and amygdala. Somatosensory areas 1, 2 and 3 also project via area 5 in the parietal cortex, to area 7b.

A lesion in this area may cause agraphesthesia, asterognosia, loss of vibration, proprioception and fine touch, and potentially hemineglect if the non-dominant hemisphere is affected. (Chapter 6).

Area 4 – Primary motor cortex (in the precentral gyrus). This is the area responsible for executing fine motor movements, which includes contralateral finger/hand/wrist or orofacial movements, learned motor sequences, breathing control, and voluntary blinking. There is a motor map in area 4, which approximately corresponds to the map in the primary somatosensory cortex. A lesion in this area may cause paralysis of the contralateral side of the body, including facial palsy, arm or leg monoparesis, and hemiparesis. (Chapter 15.)

24 | Introduction

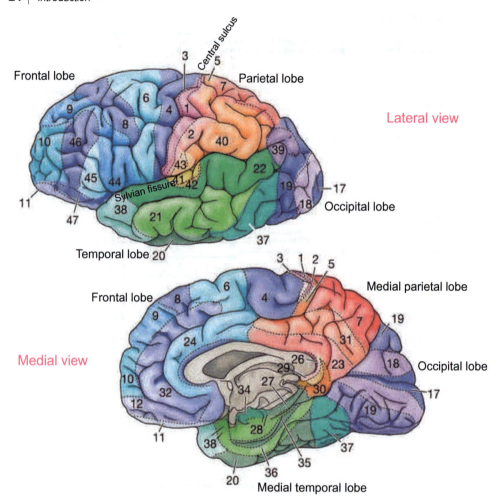

Fig. 1.9 Brodmann areas. Upper left: lateral view of the human brain. The front of the brain is on the left. Lower right: Medial view of the human brain. The front of the brain is on the left. (Modified from Purves,D., Augustine,G.J., Fitzpatrick,D. et al., editors (2019) Neuroscience. International Edition. © Oxford University Press: Oxford.)

Area 5 – Somatosensory association cortex. Brodmann area 5 is part of the superior parietal cortex, and is a secondary somatosensory area that receives inputs from the primary somatosensory cortex, and projects to parietal area 7b. A lesion in the left superior parietal lobe may cause ideomotor apraxia, which is the loss of ability to produce purposeful, skilled movements as a result of brain pathology not due to physical weakness, paralysis, lack of coordination or sensory loss. Astereognosis (also known as tactile agnosia) is also possible, which would lead to loss of ability to recognize objects by feeling or handling them. (Chapter 6.)

Area 6 – Premotor and Supplementary Motor Cortex (Secondary Motor Cortex). This projects to motor cortex area 4, and can be thought of as a higher order motor cortical area. This region is critical for the sensory guidance of movement and control of proximal and trunk muscles, and contributes to the planning of complex and coordinated motor movements. A lesion here may affect sensory guidance of movement and control of proximal and trunk muscles. Damage to the lateral premotor area 6 may result in kinetic apraxia (which would appear as coarse or unrefined movements that no longer have the appearance of being practiced over time). (Chapter 15.)

Area 7 – 7b: Somatosensory Association Cortex in the anterior part of the superior parietal lobule on the lateral surface. 7a: Visuospatial association cortex in the posterior part of the superior parietal lobule on the lateral surface. The precuneus medially is involved in spatial function including the sense of self (Scott et al., 2005). (Chapter 6.)

Area 8 – A higher order motor cortical area, which projects to area 6. Area 8 includes the frontal eye fields, which are involved in making saccades based on information in short-term memory (Goldberg and Walker, 2013). (Chapter 15.)

Area 9 – is in the dorsolateral/anterior prefrontal cortex (DLPFC). This region is a high order cortical area responsible for motor planning, organization, and regulation, and sustaining attention and working memory. The DLPFC projects to areas such as Area 8. The DLPFC plays an important role in working memory, and hence is important in planning. Area 46 is a part of the dorsolateral prefrontal cortex around and within the principal sulcus, and is involved in spatial working memory (dorsally), and object working memory (ventrally) (Chapter 13.)

Area 10 – Anterior prefrontal cortex (most rostral part of superior and middle frontal gyri). This region is involved in strategic processes of memory retrieval and executive functions (such as reasoning, task flexibility, problem solving, planning, execution, working memory, processing emotional stimuli, inferential reasoning, decision making, calculation of numerical processes, etc.). (Chapter 13.) The ventral medial prefrontal cortex area 10m and the anterior and medial parts of the orbitofrontal cortex are sometimes referred to as the ventromedial prefrontal cortex. (Chapter 11.)

Area 11 – Medial Orbitofrontal cortex, anterior part. (Figs. 11.2 and 11.3. Chapter 11)

Area 12 – Lateral orbitofrontal cortex. (Figs. 11.2 and 11.3. Chapter 11)

Area 13 – Medial orbitofrontal cortex, posterior part (Ongur et al., 2003; Carmichael and Price, 1994; Ongur and Price, 2000; Rolls, 2019e; Rolls et al., 2023c). Areas 11–13 are illustrated in Figs. 11.2 and 11.3, and are involved in reward value, non-reward, and emotion (Rolls, 2019e). (Chapter 11.)

Areas 14–16 Insular cortex. The anterior part contains the taste cortex, and below is visceral / autonomic cortex (Rolls, 2016c). More posteriorly, there are somatotopically organised somatosensory representations. (Chapter 6.)

Area 17 – Primary visual cortex (V1). The primary visual cortex is located in the occipital lobe at the back of the brain, and contains a well-defined map of the visual field. Depending on where and how damage and lesions occur to this region, partial or complete cortical blindness can result; for example, if the upper bank of the calcarine sulcus is damaged, then the lower bank of the visual field is affected. Patients with damage to the striate cortex may show blindsight, in which they deny seeing objects, but can often guess better than chance (Weiskrantz, 1998). (Chapter 2.)

Area 18 – Secondary visual cortex (V2). (Chapter 2.)

Area 19 – Associative visual cortex (V3,V4,V5). (Chapters 2 and 3.)

Area 20 – Inferior temporal gyrus. Includes parts of the inferior temporal visual cortex, which includes area 21 in macaques. (Chapter 2.)

Area 21 – Middle temporal gyrus and part of inferior frontal gyrus. In humans, parts of the middle temporal gyrus may correspond to parts of the cortex in the macaque cortex in the superior temporal sulcus. It contains face expression cells, and is implicated also in humans in theory of mind and autism (Cheng, Rolls, Gu, Zhang and Feng, 2015). (Chapter 2.)

Area 22 – Auditory association cortex (in the Superior Temporal Gyrus, of which the caudal part is usually considered to be within Wernicke's area which is involved in language comprehension). (Chapter 7.)

Area 23 – Ventral posterior cingulate cortex (Rolls, 2019c). (Figs. 12.2 and 12.1). (Chapter 12.)

Area 24 – Part of anterior cingulate cortex and mid-cingulate cortex (Rolls, 2019c; Rolls et

al., 2023c). (Figs. 12.2 and 12.1). (Chapter 12.)
Area 25 – Subgenual cingulate cortex (involved in autonomic function) (Rolls, 2019c). (Figs. 12.2 and 12.1. Chapter 12.)
Area 26 – Ectosplenial portion of the retrosplenial region of the cerebral cortex (Rolls, 2019c; Rolls et al., 2023i). (Figs. 9.1 and 12.1. Chapters 10 and 12.)
Area 27 – Part of the parahippocampal gyrus that may correspond to the presubiculum. (Chapter 9.)
Area 28 – Entorhinal cortex. The gateway to and from the hippocampus (Fig. 9.1). The medial entorhinal cortex contains grid (place) cells in rodents, and grid (spatial view) cells in primates. (Chapter 9.)
Area 29 – Retrosplenial cingulate cortex. Processes spatial information, with connections with the hippocampus. (Figs. 12.2 and 12.1). (Chapter 12.)
Area 30 – Retrosplenial cingulate cortex (Rolls, 2019c; Rolls et al., 2023i). (Figs. 12.2 and 12.1). (Chapter 12.)
Area 31 – Dorsal posterior cingulate cortex (Rolls, 2019c; Rolls et al., 2023i). (Figs. 12.2 and 12.1). (Chapter 12.)
Area 32 – Part of anterior cingulate cortex (Rolls, 2019c). (Figs. 12.2 and 12.1). (Chapter 12.)
Area 33 – Part of anterior cingulate cortex (Rolls, 2019c; Rolls et al., 2023c). (Figs. 12.2 and 12.1). (Chapter 12.)
Area 34 – Part of the parahippocampal gyrus (Fig. 9.1). (Chapter 9.)
Area 35 – Perirhinal cortex (in the rhinal sulcus) (Fig. 9.1). Connects visual and other ventral stream cortical areas to and from the entorhinal cortex and thus hippocampus. (Chapter 9.)
Area 36 – Also perirhinal cortex (in the rhinal sulcus). (Chapter 9.)
Area 37 – Fusiform gyrus. This region is involved in face, object, and scene representation. It receives from earlier cortical visual areas. (Chapter 2.)
Area 38 – Temporopolar area (most rostral part of the superior and middle temporal gyri). Involved in semantic representations. (Chapters 8 and 14).
Area 39 – Angular gyrus. In the inferior parietal lobule. May be involved in contributions of the dorsal stream to semantic processing. (Sections 14.2.6 and Chapter 14.)
Area 40 – Supramarginal gyrus, in the inferior parietal lobule, is involved in phonological word processing in the left hemisphere of right-handed people. A lesion here causes language disorders characterized by fluent speech paraphasias where words are jumbled and nonsensical sentences are spoken. (Sections 14.2.6 and Chapter 14.)
Areas 41 and 42 – Auditory cortex. (Chapter 7).
Area 43 – Primary gustatory cortex in the anterior insula. (Chapter 4).
Areas 44–45 Area 44 (inferior frontal gyrus pars opercularis) and area 45 (inferior frontal gyrus pars triangularis) are together often known as Broca's area in the dominant hemisphere. This region is associated with the praxis of speech (motor speech programming). This includes being able to put together the binding elements of language, selecting information among competing sources, sequencing motor/expressive elements, cognitive control mechanisms for syntactic processing of sentences, and construction of complex sentences and speech patterns. Lesions in this area cause Broca's aphasia: a deficit in the ability to speak and produce the proper words/sounds, even though the person maintains the ability to comprehend language. (Chapter 14.)
Area 45 – Inferior frontal gyrus pars triangularis, and part of Broca's area. (Chapter 14.)
Area 46 – Dorsolateral prefrontal cortex. Area 46 is a part of the dorsolateral prefrontal cortex around and within the principal sulcus, and is involved in spatial working memory (dorsally), and object working memory (ventrally). (Chapter 13.)
Area 47 – Inferior frontal gyrus, pars orbitalis. Often termed 12/47, the lateral orbitofrontal

cortex. (Chapter 11.)
Area 48 – Retrosubicular area (a small part of the medial surface of the temporal lobe).
Area 49 – Parasubicular area in a rodent.
Area 52 – Parainsular area (at the junction of the temporal lobe and the insula).

One atlas that we have found useful for research purposes is the automated anatomical labelling atlas AAL2 and AAL3, which includes detailed divisions of the orbitofrontal cortex (Rolls et al., 2015a, 2020d) (Section D.9).

1.12 Human Connectome Project Multi-Modal Parcellation atlas of the human cortex

The Human Connectome Project multimodal parcellation atlas (HCP-MMP) provides a very useful parcellation of human cerebral cortical areas (Glasser et al., 2016b,a). The atlas is multimodal in that each region is defined by a combination of four criteria, architecture (T1w/T2w myelin content and cortical thickness maps which can be identified with MRI), resting-state functional connectivity, and task-based fMRI activation in seven tasks, using a 3T MRI scanner (Glasser et al., 2016a). The HCP-MMP v1.0 atlas includes 180 cortical areas in each hemisphere, based on analyses in 210 participants. The areas defined include many areas that are of interest because of evidence on their functions, such as parieto-temporal cortex areas LIP, VIP, MT, MST, and occipital areas including V1, V2, V3, V4 etc. The boundaries of each cortical region are defined using this approach based on a combination of the multimodal evidence obtained in all of these ways. This potentially makes this atlas able to discriminate more reliably between different cortical regions with potentially different functions and connectivity than any other atlas based on evidence from a single modality.

Given the usefulness of the parcellation provided in the HCP-MMP atlas (Glasser et al., 2016a), we have provided an extended version of the atlas, HCPex, that extends it with 66 subcortical areas, provides it in volumetric form useful for many types of neuroimaging software (e.g. SPM (Friston et al., 2006) https://www.fil.ion.ucl.ac.uk/spm/ and FSL (Jenkinson et al., 2012; Smith et al., 2004) https://fsl.fmrib.ox.ac.uk), and by providing a reordered version with an option to revert to the original order (Huang et al., 2022). The order of cortical regions defined in HCPex and shown in Tables 1.1–1.6 is used throughout this book. We note that this atlas helps in the analysis of brain structure and function, for many of the cortical areas defined in the HCP-MMP / HCPex atlas are known about functionally, many can be related to corresponding regions in macaques in which much detailed neurophysiology is available, and the atlas helps new investigations of the brain to be related to the known functions of those anatomically defined brain areas.

We note that surface-based registration such as that provided by the HCP-MMP leads to better spatial localization of cortical areas than volumetric methods (Coalson et al., 2018; Glasser et al., 2016b) such as those commonly used and made available in neuroimaging software such as SPM and FSL. However, given that much neuroimaging analysis is performed with software such as SPM and FSL, and that volumetric analysis enables subcortical areas to be easily included straightforwardly in the atlas which is an aim of HCPex, we have provided HCPex which is in volumetric space (Huang, Rolls, Feng and Lin, 2022). At the same time, where better localization is required than may be provided with HCPex, we appreciate and recommend the use of the surface-based version HCP-MMP v1.0 (Glasser et al., 2016a), for the reasons set out by Coalson et al. (2018). In fact, for most of the effective connectivity analyses described in this book, the cortical connectivity was measured with the surface-based parcellation, and the connectivity with subcortical areas was measured with HCPex. We

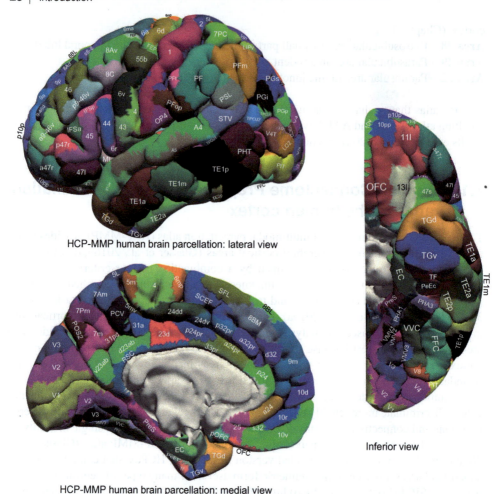

Fig. 1.10 Anatomical regions in the Human Connectome Project Multimodal Parcellation atlas (HCP-MMP) of the human cortical regions. Cortical regions are shown as defined in the HCP-MMP atlas (Glasser et al., 2016a), and in its extended version HCPex (Huang, Rolls et al. (2022)). The regions are shown on images of the human brain without the sulci expanded to show which cortical HCP-MMP regions are normally visible, for comparison with Fig. 1.11. Abbreviations are provided in Tables 1.1–1.6.

further note that an advantage of the HCP-MMP / HCPex atlas is that the effective connectivity, functional connectivity, and connections measured with diffusion tractography have been measured and described between all 360 cortical regions, and this provides a rich foundation for future studies of the functions and computations of the human cerebral cortex (Rolls et al., 2022a,b, 2023e,h,c,f,i,d,b,a). This is likely to be facilitated when a corresponding atlas for macaques now in development becomes available. These papers also relate the connectivities of each of these HCP-MMP regions to the functions of these cortical regions.

Cortical regions defined in the HCP-MMP / HCPex atlas are shown in Figs. 1.10 and 1.11, with a list of the cortical regions in Tables 1.1–1.6 and of the subcortical regions in HCPex in Table 1.7. Coronal slices to further help visualization of the locations in the brain of these cortical regions are provided by Huang, Rolls, Feng and Lin (2022). Descriptions of most of these cortical regions including their connectivity and functions are provided in the different Chapters of this book. Short summaries of some of the key Divisions in the HCP-MMP and HCPex atlases (Glasser et al., 2016a; Huang et al., 2022) are provided next with reference to Tables 1.1–1.6.

Human Connectome Project Multi-Modal Parcellation atlas of the human cortex | 29

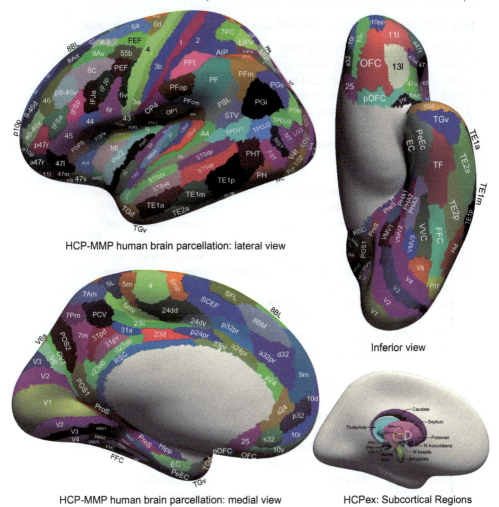

Fig. 1.11 Anatomical regions in the Human Connectome Project Multimodal Parcellation atlas HCP-MMP of the human cortical regions. Cortical Regions are shown as defined in the HCP-MMP atlas (Glasser et al., 2016a), and in its extended version HCPex which includes the thalamus and the other subcortical areas shown (Huang, Rolls et al. (2022)). The regions are shown on images of the human brain with the sulci expanded to show all cortical HCP-MMP regions, for comparison with Fig. 1.12. Abbreviations are provided in Tables 1.1–1.6.

The main visual processing cortical regions are in the Primary Visual, Early Visual, Dorsal Visual Stream, Ventral Visual Stream, and MT+ Complex Divisions in Table 1.1, and in the Lateral Temporal Division in Table 1.3, and their connectivity and functions are described in Chapters 2 and 3, and by Rolls et al. (2023e).

The main somatosensory and motor cortical regions are in the SomatoSensory, ParaCentral and MidCingulate, Premotor, and Posterior Opercular Divisions in Table 1.2, and in the Insula / Frontal Opercular Division in Table 1.3, and their connectivity and functions are described in Chapters 6 and 15, and by Rolls et al. (2023f). Regions 23c, 24dd and 24dv are the midcingulate premotor cortex described by Vogt (2016) and Rolls et al. (2023i).

The main auditory cortical regions are in the Early Auditory, and Auditory Association Divisions in Table 1.2, and their connectivity and functions are described in Chapter 7 and by Rolls et al. (2023h). However some of the regions in the 'Auditory Association' Division are in fact multimodal, include visual and auditory responsiveness to social stimuli, and are also

Table 1.1 Cortical regions in the HCP-MMP atlas in the order used in the HCPex atlas

ID (L, R)	Region	Region Long Name	Cortical Division
1, 181	V1	Primary Visual Cortex	Primary Visual
2, 182	V2	Second Visual Area	Early Visual
3, 183	V3	Third Visual Area	Early Visual
4, 184	V4	Fourth Visual Area	Early Visual
5, 185	IPS1	IntraParietal Sulcus Area 1	Dorsal Stream Visual
6, 186	V3A Area	V3A	Dorsal Stream Visual
7, 187	V3B Area	V3B	Dorsal Stream Visual
8, 188	V6	Sixth Visual Area	Dorsal Stream Visual
9, 189	V6A	Area V6A	Dorsal Stream Visual
10, 190	V7	Seventh Visual Area	Dorsal Stream Visual
11, 191	FFC	Fusiform Face Complex	Ventral Stream Visual
12, 192	PIT	Posterior InferoTemporal complex	Ventral Stream Visual
13, 193	V8	Eighth Visual Area	Ventral Stream Visual
14, 194	VMV1	VentroMedial Visual Area 1	Ventral Stream Visual
15, 195	VMV2	VentroMedial Visual Area 2	Ventral Stream Visual
16, 196	VMV3	VentroMedial Visual Area 3	Ventral Stream Visual
17, 197	VVC	Ventral Visual Complex	Ventral Stream Visual
18, 198	FST	Area FST	MT+ Complex
19, 199	LO1	Area Lateral Occipital 1	MT+ Complex
20, 200	LO2	Area Lateral Occipital 2	MT+ Complex
21, 201	LO3	Area Lateral Occipital 3	MT+ Complex
22, 202	MST	Medial Superior Temporal Area	MT+ Complex
23, 203	MT	Middle Temporal Area	MT+ Complex
24, 204	PH	Area PH	MT+ Complex
25, 205	V3CD	Area V3CD	MT+ Complex
26, 206	V4t	Area V4t	MT+ Complex

involved in semantic representations for language, as described in Chapters 8, 2 and 14.5, and by Rolls et al. (2022b), Rolls et al. (2023e), and Pitcher and Ungerleider (2021).

Table 1.2 Cortical regions in the HCP-MMP atlas in the order used in the HCPex atlas

ID (L, R)	Region	Region Long Name	Cortical Division
27, 207	1	Area 1	SomaSens Motor
28, 208	2	Area 2	SomaSens Motor
29, 209	3a	Area 3a	SomaSens Motor
30, 210	3b	Primary Sensory Cortex	SomaSens Motor
31, 211	4	Primary Motor Cortex	SomaSens Motor
32, 212	23c	Area 23c	ParaCentral MidCing
33, 213	24dd	Dorsal Area 24d	ParaCentral MidCing
34, 214	24dv	Ventral Area 24d	ParaCentral MidCing
35, 215	5L	Area 5L	ParaCentral MidCing
36, 216	5m	Area 5m	ParaCentral MidCing
37, 217	5mv	Area 5m ventral	ParaCentral MidCing
38, 218	6ma	Area 6m anterior	ParaCentral MidCing
39, 219	6mp	Area 6mp	ParaCentral MidCing
40, 220	SCEF	Supplementary and Cingulate Eye Field	ParaCentral MidCing
41, 221	55b	Area 55b	Premotor
42, 222	6a	Area 6 anterior	Premotor
43, 223	6d	Dorsal area 6	Premotor
44, 224	6r	Rostral Area 6	Premotor
45, 225	6v	Ventral Area 6	Premotor
46, 226	FEF	Frontal Eye Fields	Premotor
47, 227	PEF	Premotor Eye Field	Premotor
48, 228	43	Area 43	Posterior Opercular
49, 229	FOP1	Frontal Opercular Area 1	Posterior Opercular
50, 230	OP1	Area OP1-SII	Posterior Opercular
51, 231	OP2-3	Area OP2-3-VS	Posterior Opercular
52, 232	OP4	Area OP4-PV	Posterior Opercular
53, 233	52	Area 52	Early Auditory
54, 234	A1	Primary Auditory Cortex	Early Auditory
55, 235	LBelt	Lateral Belt Complex	Early Auditory
56, 236	MBelt	Medial Belt Complex	Early Auditory
57, 237	PBelt	ParaBelt Complex	Early Auditory
58, 238	PFcm	Area PFcm	Early Auditory
59, 239	RI	RetroInsular Cortex	Early Auditory
60, 240	A4	Auditory 4 Complex	Auditory Association
61, 241	A5	Auditory 5 Complex	Auditory Association
62, 242	STGa	Area STGa	Auditory Association
63, 243	STSda	Area STSd anterior	Auditory Association
64, 244	STSdp	Area STSd posterior	Auditory Association
65, 245	STSva	Area STSv anterior	Auditory Association
66, 246	STSvp	Area STSv posterior	Auditory Association
67, 247	TA2	Area TA2	Auditory Association

Table 1.3 Cortical regions in the HCP-MMP atlas in the order used in the HCPex atlas

ID (L, R)	Region	Region Long Name	Cortical Division
68, 248	AAIC	Anterior Agranular Insula Complex	Insula FrontalOperc
69, 249	AVI	Anterior Ventral Insular Area	Insula FrontalOperc
70, 250	FOP2	Frontal Opercular Area 2	Insula FrontalOperc
71, 251	FOP3	Frontal Opercular Area 3	Insula FrontalOperc
72, 252	FOP4	Frontal Opercular Area 4	Insula FrontalOperc
73, 253	FOP5	Area Frontal Opercular 5	Insula FrontalOperc
74, 254	Ig	Insular Granular Complex	Insula FrontalOperc
75, 255	MI	Middle Insular Area	Insula FrontalOperc
76, 256	PI	Para-Insular Area	Insula FrontalOperc
77, 257	Pir	Piriform Cortex	Insula FrontalOperc
78, 258	PoI1	Area Posterior Insular 1	Insula FrontalOperc
79, 259	PoI2	Posterior Insular Area 2	Insula FrontalOperc
80, 260	H	Hippocampus	Medial Temporal
81, 261	PreS	PreSubiculum	Medial Temporal
82, 262	EC	Entorhinal Cortex	Medial Temporal
83, 263	PeEc	Perirhinal Ectorhinal Cortex	Medial Temporal
84, 264	TF	Area TF	Medial Temporal
85, 265	PHA1	ParaHippocampal Area 1	Medial Temporal
86, 266	PHA2	ParaHippocampal Area 2	Medial Temporal
87, 267	PHA3	ParaHippocampal Area 3	Medial Temporal
88, 268	PHT	Area PHT	Lateral Temporal
89, 269	TE1a	Area TE1 anterior	Lateral Temporal
90, 270	TE1m	Area TE1 Middle	Lateral Temporal
91, 271	TE1p	Area TE1 posterior	Lateral Temporal
92, 272	TE2a	Area TE2 anterior	Lateral Temporal
93, 273	TE2p	Area TE2 posterior	Lateral Temporal
94, 274	TGd	Area TG dorsal	Lateral Temporal
95, 275	TGv	Area TG Ventral	Lateral Temporal
96, 276	PSL	PeriSylvian Language Area	TPO
97, 277	STV	Superior Temporal Visual Area	TPO
98, 278	TPOJ1	Area TemporoParietoOccipital Junction 1	TPO
99, 279	TPOJ2	Area TemporoParietoOccipital Junction 2	TPO
100, 280	TPOJ3	Area TemporoParietoOccipital Junction 3	TPO

The hippocampal memory system is in the Medial Temporal Division in Table 1.3, with its closely related regions in the Posterior Cingulate Division shown in Table 1.4. Their connectivity and functions are described in Chapters 9 and 10, and by Rolls et al. (2022a), Rolls et al. (2023i), Rolls et al. (2023d), Rolls (2023c), and Rolls (2022b).

The human language-related cortical regions are in the Temporo-Parietal-Occipital TPO Division in Table 1.3, and regions 44, 45 and 47l (Broca's area) in Table 1.6. Their connectivity and functions are described in Chapter 14, and by Rolls et al. (2022b).

Table 1.4 Cortical regions in the HCP-MMP atlas in the order used in the HCPex atlas

ID (L, R)	Region	Region Long Name	Cortical Division
101, 281	7AL	Lateral Area 7A Superior Parietal	
102, 282	7Am	Medial Area 7A	Superior Parietal
103, 283	7PC	Area 7PC	Superior Parietal
104, 284	7PI	Lateral Area 7P	Superior Parietal
105, 285	7Pm	Medial Area 7P	Superior Parietal
106, 286	AIP	Anterior IntraParietal Area	Superior Parietal
107, 287	LIPd	Area Lateral IntraParietal dorsal	Superior Parietal
108, 288	LIPv	Area Lateral IntraParietal ventral	Superior Parietal
109, 289	MIP	Medial IntraParietal Area	Superior Parietal
110, 290	VIP	Ventral IntraParietal Complex	Superior Parietal
111, 291	IP0	Area IntraParietal 0	Inferior Parietal
112, 292	IP1	Area IntraParietal 1	Inferior Parietal
113, 293	IP2	Area IntraParietal 2	Inferior Parietal
114, 294	PF	Area PF Complex	Inferior Parietal
115, 295	PFm	Area PFm Complex	Inferior Parietal
116, 296	PFop	Area PF Opercular	Inferior Parietal
117, 297	PFt	Area PFt	Inferior Parietal
118, 298	PGi	Area PGi	Inferior Parietal
119, 299	PGp	Area PGp	Inferior Parietal
120, 300	PGs	Area PGs	Inferior Parietal
121, 301	23d	Area 23d	Posterior Cingulate
122, 302	31a	Area 31a	Posterior Cingulate
123, 303	31pd	Area 31pd	Posterior Cingulate
124, 304	31pv	Area 31p ventral	Posterior Cingulate
125, 305	7m	Area 7m	Posterior Cingulate
126, 306	d23ab	Area dorsal 23 a+b	Posterior Cingulate
127, 307	DVT	Dorsal Transitional Visual Area	Posterior Cingulate
128, 308	PCV	PreCuneus Visual Area	Posterior Cingulate
129, 309	POS1	Parieto-Occipital Sulcus Area 1	Posterior Cingulate
130, 310	POS2	Parieto-Occipital Sulcus Area 2	Posterior Cingulate
131, 311	ProS	ProStriate Area	Posterior Cingulate
132, 312	RSC	RetroSplenial Complex	Posterior Cingulate
133, 313	v23ab	Area ventral 23 a+b	Posterior Cingulate

The parietal cortex regions involved in visuo-spatial and related multimodal functions are in the Superior Parietal and Inferior Parietal Divisions in Table 1.4, and their connectivity and functions are described in Chapter 10, and by Rolls et al. (2023d).

Table 1.5 Cortical regions in the HCP-MMP atlas in the order used in the HCPex atlas

ID (L, R)	Region	Region Long Name	Cortical Division
134, 314	10r	Area 10r	AntCing MedPFC
135, 315	10v	Area 10v	AntCing MedPFC
136, 316	25	Area 25	AntCing MedPFC
137, 317	33pr	Area 33 prime	AntCing MedPFC
138, 318	8BM	Area 8BM	AntCing MedPFC
139, 319	9m	Area 9 Middle	AntCing MedPFC
140, 320	a24	Area a24	AntCing MedPFC
141, 321	a24pr	Anterior 24 prime	AntCing MedPFC
142, 322	a32pr	Area anterior 32 prime	AntCing MedPFC
143, 323	d32	Area dorsal 32	AntCing MedPFC
144, 324	p24	Area posterior 24	AntCing MedPFC
145, 325	p24pr	Area Posterior 24 prime	AntCing MedPFC
146, 326	p32	Area p32	AntCing MedPFC
147, 327	p32pr	Area p32 prime	AntCing MedPFC
148, 328	pOFC	Posterior OFC Complex	AntCing MedPFC
149, 329	s32	Area s32	AntCing MedPFC
150, 330	10d	Area 10d	OrbPolaFrontal
151, 331	10pp	Polar 10p	OrbPolarFrontal
152, 332	11l	Area 11l	OrbPolarFrontal
153, 333	13l	Area 13l	OrbPolarFrontal
154, 334	47m	Area 47m	OrbPolarFrontal
155, 335	47s	Area 47s	OrbPolarFrontal
156, 336	a10p	Area anterior 10p	OrbPolarFrontal
157, 337	OFC	Orbital Frontal Complex	OrbPolarFrontal
158, 338	p10p	Area posterior 10p	OrbPolarFrontal

The orbitofrontal cortex and ventromedial prefrontal cortex regions involved in reward valuation and emotion, and the anterior cingulate cortex involved in linking reward to action in action-outcome learning, are in the Orbitofrontal and Polar Frontal, and Anterior Cingulate and Medial Prefrontal Cortex Divisions in Table 1.5, and their connectivity and functions are described in Chapters 11 and 12, and by Rolls et al. (2023c) and Rolls et al. (2023b).

Table 1.6 Cortical regions in the HCP-MMP atlas in the order used in the HCPex atlas

ID (L, R)	Region	Region Long Name	Cortical Division
159, 339	44	Area 44	Inferior Frontal
160, 340	45	Area 45	Inferior Frontal
161, 341	47l	Area 47l (47 lateral)	Inferior Frontal
162, 342	a47r	Area anterior 47r	Inferior Frontal
163, 343	IFJa	Area IFJa	Inferior Frontal
164, 344	IFJp	Area IFJp	Inferior Frontal
165, 345	IFSa	Area IFSa	Inferior Frontal
166, 346	IFSp	Area IFSp	Inferior Frontal
167, 347	p47r	Area posterior 47r	Inferior Frontal
168, 348	46	Area 46	Dorsolateral Prefrontal
169, 349	8Ad	Area 8Ad	Dorsolateral Prefrontal
170, 350	8Av	Area 8Av	Dorsolateral Prefrontal
171, 351	8BL	Area 8B Lateral	Dorsolateral Prefrontal
172, 352	8C	Area 8C	Dorsolateral Prefrontal
173, 353	9-46d	Area 9-46d	Dorsolateral Prefrontal
174, 354	9a	Area 9 anterior	Dorsolateral Prefrontal
175, 355	9p	Area 9 Posterior	Dorsolateral Prefrontal
176, 356	a9-46v	Area anterior 9-46v	Dorsolateral Prefrontal
177, 357	i6-8	Inferior 6-8 Transitional Area	Dorsolateral Prefrontal
178, 358	p9-46v	Area posterior 9-46v	Dorsolateral Prefrontal
179, 359	s6-8	Superior 6-8 Transitional Area	Dorsolateral Prefrontal
180, 360	SFL	Superior Frontal Language Area	Dorsolateral Prefrontal

The prefrontal cortex cortical regions involved in short-term memory, working memory, planning, and attention are in the Inferior Frontal, and Dorsolateral Prefrontal Cortex Divisions in Table 1.6, and their connectivity and functions are described in Chapter 13, and by Rolls et al. (2023f) and Rolls et al. (2023a).

Table 1.7 Subcortical regions in the HCPex atlas

ID (L, R)	Region	Region Long Name	Cortical Division
361, 394	AV	Thalamus: Anteroventral Nucleus	
362, 395	CeM	Thalamus: Central medial	
363, 396	CL	Thalamus: Central lateral	
364, 397	CM	Thalamus: Centralmedian	
365, 398	LD	Thalamus: Laterodorsal	
366, 399	LGN	Thalamus: Lateral Geniculate	
367, 400	LP	Thalamus: Lateral Posterior	
368, 401	L-Sg	Thalamus: Limitans Suprageniculate	
369, 402	MDl	Thalamus: Mediodorsolateral parvocellular	
370, 403	MDm	Thalamus: Mediodorsomedial magnocellular	
371, 404	MGN	Thalamus: Medial Geniculate	
372, 405	MV(Re)	Thalamus: Reuniens	
373, 406	Pf	Thalamus: Parafascicular	
374, 407	PuA	Thalamus: Pulvinar anterior	
375, 408	PuI	Thalamus: Pulvinar inferior	
376, 409	PuL	Thalamus: Pulvinar lateral	
377, 410	PuM	Thalamus: Pulvinar medial	
378, 411	VA	Thalamus: Ventral Anterior	
379, 412	VLa	Thalamus: Ventral Lateral Anterior	
380, 413	VLp	Thalamus: Ventral Lateral Posterior	
381, 414	VPL	Thalamus: Ventral posterolateral	
382, 415	Putam	Putamen	
383, 416	Caud	Caudate	
384, 417	NAc	Nucleus Accumbens	
385, 418	Gpe	Globus pallidus externalis	
386, 419	Gpi	Globus pallidus internalis	
387, 420	Amyg	Amygdala	
388, 421	SNpc	Substantia nigra pars compacta	
389, 422	SNpr	Substantia nigra pars reticulata	
390, 423	VTA	Ventral tegmental area	
391, 424	MB	Mammillary bodies	
392, 425	Septum	Septal nuclei	
393, 426	Nb	Nucleus basalis	

The subcortical regions involved in many functions that are in the HCPex atlas (Huang, Rolls, Feng and Lin, 2022) are listed in Table 1.7, and their connectivity and functions are described in Chapter 16 and elsewhere (Rolls et al., 2023b,c; Rolls, 2022b).

1.13 Connectivity of the human brain

To understand what computations are performed by each brain region, and how they are performed, it is very helpful to know the connectivity of different brain regions. The inputs to a brain region for example influence what computations it can perform, and the regions to which it is connected help to define what functions its computations are used for. Brief descriptions of some methods that are used to investigate the connectivity of the human brain are described next.

1.13.1 Connections analyzed with diffusion tractography

Diffusion tractography uses MRI to measure the diffusion of water in the human brain, and this tends to occur along fibre tracts, so provides some evidence about connections in the brain (Catani and Thiebaut de Schotten, 2008; Lerch et al., 2017; Maier-Hein et al., 2017; Jeurissen et al., 2019).

Diffusion tractography can provide evidence about fibre pathways linking different brain regions. Diffusion tractography shows only direct connections, so comparison with effective connectivity (described below) can help to suggest which effective connectivities may be mediated directly or trans-synaptically. Diffusion tractography does not provide evidence about the direction of connections. The term 'connections' is appropriate for use for diffusion tractography, for it provides evidence about anatomical connections.

Diffusion tractography as a method for following connections and measuring their strength is supported by comparisons made in macaques between diffusion tractography and conventional anatomical methods with tracers (van den Heuvel et al., 2015; Donahue et al., 2016).

The methods used in the application of diffusion tractography in the investigations included in this book are described by Huang, Rolls, Hsu, Feng and Lin (2021). Diffusion tractography cannot follow fibres where they become unmyelinated within the cortex, and that is one of its limitations. Another is that it does not work well for long connections across the midline of the human brain (Huang et al., 2021).

1.13.2 Functional connectivity

Functional connectivity is measured by the Pearson correlation between the BOLD (Blood Oxygenation-Level Dependent) fMRI signal in each pair of brain regions, and can provide evidence that may relate to interactions between brain regions, while providing no evidence about causal direction-specific effects. A high functional connectivity may in this scenario thus reflect strong physiological interactions between areas, and provides a different type of evidence to effective connectivity described next. Functional connectivity measured between cortical regions typically ranges continuously between 0.9 and -0.3, so a threshold such as 0.4 is often utilised to view the stronger functional connectivities. No subtraction of the global signal was used in the investigations described here, because this produces many apparently negative functional connectivities that are difficult to interpret, as described in the Supplementary Material of Cheng, Rolls, Qiu, Liu, Tang, Huang, Wang, Zhang, Lin, Zheng, Pu, Tsai, Yang, Lin, Wang, Xie and Feng (2016a).

1.13.3 Effective connectivity

Effective connectivity measures the effect of one brain region on another, and utilizes differences detected at different times in the signals in each connected pair of brain regions to infer effects of one brain region on another. One such approach is dynamic causal modelling, but it applies most easily to activation studies, and is typically limited to measuring the effective connectivity between just a few brain areas (Valdes-Sosa et al., 2011; Bajaj et al., 2016; Friston, 2009), though there have been moves to extend it to resting state studies and more brain areas (Razi et al., 2017; Frassle et al., 2017).

The method used here (Rolls et al., 2023e,h,c, 2022a, 2023i,f,d, 2022b, 2023b) was developed from a Hopf algorithm to enable measurement of effective connectivity between many brain areas, described by Deco et al. (2019). A principle is that the functional connectivity is measured at time t and time $t + tau$, where tau is typically 2 s to take into account the time within which a change in the BOLD signal can occur, and then the effective connectivity model is trained by error correction until it can generate the functional connectivity matrices at time t and time $t + tau$. Full details of the algorithm and its validation are provided elsewhere (Rolls et al., 2022a), and a short description is provided next. The directionality described in these papers has been investigated and validated with analyses using magnetoencephalography (MEG), which operates on a much faster time scale of ms (Rolls et al., 2023a).

To infer the effective connectivity, we use a whole-brain model that allows us to simulate the BOLD activity across all brain regions and time. We use the so-called Hopf computational model, which integrates the dynamics of Stuart-Landau oscillators, expressing the activity of each brain region coupled together by the strength of the connectivity in each direction between every pair of brain regions (Deco et al., 2017b). The local dynamics of each brain area (node) is given by Stuart-Landau oscillators which expresses the normal form of a supercritical Hopf bifurcation, describing the transition from noisy to oscillatory dynamics (Kuznetsov, 2013). It has been shown that the Hopf whole-brain model successfully simulates empirical electrophysiology (Freyer et al., 2011, 2012), MagnetoEncephalography (Deco et al., 2017a) and fMRI (Deco et al., 2017b; Kringelbach et al., 2015; Kringelbach and Deco, 2020). The Hopf whole-brain model can be expressed mathematically as follows:

$$\frac{dx_i}{dt} = \overbrace{[a_i - x_i^2 - y_i^2]x_i - \omega_i y_i}^{Local\,Dynamics} + \overbrace{G\Sigma_{j=1}^{N} C_{ij}(x_j - x_i)}^{Coupling} + \overbrace{\beta\eta_i(t)}^{Gaussian\,Noise} \quad (1.5)$$

$$\frac{dy_i}{dt} = \overbrace{[a_i - x_i^2 - y_i^2]y_i + \omega_i x_i}^{Local\,Dynamics} + \overbrace{G\Sigma_{j=1}^{N} C_{ij}(y_j - y_i)}^{Coupling} + \overbrace{\beta\eta_i(t)}^{Gaussian\,Noise} \quad (1.6)$$

Equations 1.5 and 1.6 describe the coupling of Stuart-Landau oscillators through an effective connectivity matrix C. The $x_i(t)$ term represents the simulated BOLD signal data of brain area i. The values of $y_i(t)$ are relevant to the dynamics of the system but are not part of the information read out from the system. In these equations, $\eta_i(t)$ provides additive Gaussian noise with standard deviation β. The Stuart-Landau oscillators for each brain area i express a Hopf normal form that has a supercritical bifurcation at $a_i = 0$, so that if $a_i > 0$ the system has a stable limit cycle with frequency with frequency $f_i = \omega_i/2$ (where ω_i is the angular velocity); and when $a_i < 0$ the system has a stable fixed point representing a low activity noisy state. The intrinsic frequency f_i of each Stuart-Landau oscillator corresponding to a brain area i is in the 0.008–0.08 Hz band (i=1, ..., 360 cortical regions). The intrinsic frequencies are fitted from the data, provided here by the averaged peak frequency of the narrowband BOLD signals of each brain region. The coupling term representing the input received in node i from every other node j, is weighted by the corresponding effective connectivity C_{ij}. The coupling is the canonical diffusive coupling, which approximates the simplest (linear) part of a general coupling function. G denotes the global coupling weight, scaling equally the total input received in each brain area. While the oscillators are weakly coupled, the periodic orbit of the uncoupled oscillators is preserved.

The effective connectivity matrix can be derived by optimizing the conductivity of each existing anatomical connection as specified by the Structural Connectivity matrix (measured with tractography (Huang et al., 2021)) in order to fit the empirical functional connectivity (FC) pairs and the lagged FC^{tau} pairs. By this, we are able to infer a non-symmetric Effective Connectivity matrix (see Gilson et al. (2016)). Note that FC^{tau}, i.e. the lagged functional connectivity between pairs, lagged at tau s, breaks the symmetry and thus is fundamental for our purpose. Specifically, we compute the distance between the model FC simulated from the current estimate of the effective connectivity and the empirical data FC^{emp}, as well as the simulated model FC^{tau} and empirical data FC^{tauemp} and adjust each effective connection (entry in the effective connectivity matrix) separately with a gradient-descent approach. The model is run repeatedly with the updated effective connectivity until the fit converges towards a stable value.

We can start with the anatomical connectivity obtained with probabilistic tractography from diffusion MRI (which might help the algorithm by utilising as a constraint connections known to be absent in the brain); or with a C matrix initialized to zero (which has a potential advantage that it is not influenced by possible errors in the diffusion tractography). The latter is implemented in our research for the reason given, but in practice the algorithm produced similar results with either method (Rolls et al., 2022a). The following procedure is used to update each entry C_{ij} in the effective connectivity matrix

$$C_{ij} = C_{ij} + \epsilon((FC_{ij}^{\text{emp}} - FC_{ij}) + (FC_{ij}^{\text{tauemp}} - FC_{ij}^{\text{tau}})) \qquad (1.7)$$

where ϵ is a learning rate constant, and i and j are the (brain region) nodes. For the implementation, tau was set to 2 s. The maximum effective connectivity was set to a value of 0.2, and was found between V1 and V2.

1.14 Introduction to the fine structure of the cerebral neocortex

An important part of the approach to understanding how the cerebral cortex could implement its computational processes is to take into account as much as possible its fine structure and connectivity, as these provide important indicators of and constraints on how it computes. An introductory description is provided in this section (1.14), and a description that considers the operational / computational principles of neocortex, and compares them to pyriform cortex and hippocampal cortex, is provided by Rolls (2016b). A comparison of the network architecture and computations of the neocortex, cerebellum, and basal ganglia is provided in Section 17.5.5.

1.14.1 The fine structure and connectivity of the neocortex

The neocortex comprises most areas of the cerebral cortex apart from the hippocampal cortex and pyriform cortex, and most of the cortical regions shown in Figs. 1.9, 1.10 and 1.11. Different areas of the neocortex can be distinguished by the appearance of the cells (cytoarchitecture) and fibres or axons (myeloarchitecture), but nevertheless, the basic organization of the different neocortical areas has many similarities, and it is this basic organization that is considered here. Useful sources for more detailed descriptions of neocortical structure and function are the books in the series 'Cerebral Cortex' edited by Jones and Peters (Jones and Peters (1984) and Peters and Jones (1984)) and many other resources (Douglas, Markram and Martin, 2004; Shepherd, 2004; Shepherd and Grillner, 2010; da Costa and Martin, 2010; Harris and Mrsic-Flogel, 2013; Kubota, 2014; Harris and Shepherd, 2015; Shepherd and Rowe, 2017). The detailed understanding of the cell types and their patterns of connections is now benefitting from molecular markers (Harris and Shepherd, 2015; Bernard et al., 2012). Approaches to quantitative aspects of the connectivity are provided by Braitenberg and Schüz (1991), Braitenberg and Schüz (1998), Abeles (1991), and by Rolls (2016b). Some of the connections described in Sections 1.14.2 and 1.14.3 are shown schematically in Figs. 1.15 and 1.16. Further analysis of some of the computationally most relevant aspects of neocortical circuitry (see Fig. 1.17) are provided by Rolls (2016b).

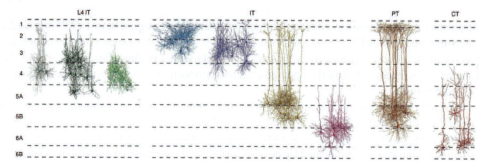

Fig. 1.12 Dendritic morphology of excitatory neurons in S1 whisker barrel cortex. L4 IT shows the three morphological classes of L4 intratelencephalic (IT) neurons: pyramidal, star pyramidal and spiny stellate cells. Under IT are other intratelencephalic neurons of L2, L3, 5A/B and 6. PT shows pyramidal tract neurons of L5B. CT shows corticothalamic neurons of L6. (Adapted with permission from Marcel Oberlaender, Christiaan P.J. de Kock, Randy M. Bruno, Alejandro Ramirez, Hanno S. Meyer, Vincent J. Dercksen, Moritz Helmstaedter and Bert Sakmann (2012) Cell type-specific three-dimensional structure of thalamocortical circuits in a column of rat vibrissal cortex. *Cerebral Cortex* 22: 2375–2391. © Oxford University Press.)

1.14.2 Excitatory cells and connections

Some of the cell types found in the neocortex are shown in Fig. 1.1. Cells A–D are pyramidal cells. The dendrites (shown thick in Fig. 1.1) are covered in spines, which receive the excitatory synaptic inputs to the cell. Pyramidal cells with cell bodies in different laminae of the cortex (shown in Fig. 1.1 as I–VI) not only have different distributions of their dendrites, but also different distributions of their axons (shown thin in Fig. 1.1), which connect both within that cortical area and to other brain regions outside that cortical area (see labelling at the bottom of Fig. 1.15). Further examples of cell types, from S1 (somatosensory) rat whisker barrel cortex, are shown in Fig. 1.12 (Harris and Shepherd, 2015).

The main information-bearing afferents to a cortical area have many terminals in layer 4. (By these afferents, we mean primarily those from the thalamus; or for higher cortical regions from the preceding cortical region. We do not mean the cortico-cortical backprojections; nor the subcortical cholinergic, noradrenergic, dopaminergic, and serotonergic inputs, which are numerically minor, although they are important in setting cortical cell thresholds, excitability, and adaptation, see for example Douglas, Markram and Martin (2004).) In primary sensory cortical areas only, there are spiny stellate cells in a rather expanded layer 4, and the thalamic terminals synapse onto these cells (Lund, 1984; Martin, 1984; Douglas and Martin, 1990; Douglas, Markram and Martin, 2004; Levitt, Lund and Yoshioka, 1996; da Costa and Martin, 2013; Harris and Shepherd, 2015). (Primary sensory cortical areas receive their inputs from the primary sensory thalamic nucleus for a sensory modality. An example is the primate striate cortex which receives inputs from the lateral geniculate nucleus, which in turn receives inputs from the retinal ganglion cells. Spiny stellate cells are so-called because they have radially arranged, star-like, dendrites. Their axons usually terminate within the cortical area in which they are located.) Each thalamic axon makes 1,000–10,000 synapses, not more than several (or at most 10) of which are onto any one spiny stellate cell. In addition to these afferent terminals, there are some terminals of the thalamic afferents onto pyramidal cells with cell bodies in layers 6 and 3 (Martin, 1984) (and terminals onto inhibitory interneurons such as basket cells, which thus provide for a feedforward inhibition) (see Fig. 1.13). Even in layer 4, the thalamic axons provide less than 20% of the synapses. The number of thalamo-cortical connections received by a cortical cell is relatively low, in the range 18–191 (da Costa and Martin, 2013). The spiny stellate neurons in layer 4 have axons which terminate in layers 3 and 2, at least partly on dendrites of pyramidal cells with cell bodies in layers 3 and 2. (These synapses are of Type I, that is are asymmetrical and are on spines, so that they are excitatory. Their transmitter is glutamate.) These layer 3 and 2 pyramidal cells provide the onward cortico-cortical projection with axons which project into layer 4 of the next cortical area. For example, layer 3 and 2 pyramidal cells in the primary visual (striate) cortex of the macaque monkey project into the second visual area (V2), layer 4.

In non-primary sensory areas, important information-bearing afferents from a preceding cortical area terminate in layer 4, but there are no or few spiny stellate cells in this layer (Lund, 1984; Levitt, Lund and Yoshioka, 1996). Layer 4 still looks 'granular' (due to the presence of many small cells), but these cells are typically small pyramidal cells (Lund, 1984). (It may be noted here that spiny stellate cells and small pyramidal cells are similar in many ways, with a few main differences including the absence of a major apical dendrite in a spiny stellate which accounts for its non-pyramidal, star-shaped, appearance; and for many spiny stellate cells, the absence of an axon that projects outside its cortical area.) The terminals presumably make synapses with these small pyramidal cells, and also presumably with the dendrites of cells from other layers, including the basal dendrites of deep layer 3 pyramidal cells (see Fig. 1.15).

The axons of the *superficial (layer 2 and 3) pyramidal cells* have collaterals and terminals in layer 5 (see Fig. 1.15), and synapses are made with the dendrites of the layer 5 pyramidal cells (Martin, 1984). The axons also typically project out of that cortical area, and on to the next cortical area in sequence, where they terminate in layer 4, forming the forward cortico-cortical projection. It is also from these pyramidal cells in some sensory regions that are high in the hierarchy that projections to the amygdala arise (Amaral, Price, Pitkanen and Carmichael, 1992).

The axons of the *layer 5 pyramidal cells* have many collaterals in layer 6 (see Fig. 1.1), where synapses could be made with the layer 6 pyramidal cells (based on indirect evidence, see Fig. 13 of Martin (1984)), and axons of these cells typically leave the cortex to project to subcortical sites (such as the striatum), or back to the preceding cortical area to terminate in layer 1. It is remarkable that there are as many of these backprojections as there are forward connections between two sequential cortical areas. The possible computational significance of this connectivity is considered in Chapter 9.

The *layer 6 pyramidal cells* have prolific dendritic arborizations in layer 4 (see Fig. 1.1), and some receive synapses from thalamic afferents (Martin, 1984) (but see Shepherd and Yamawaki (2021)), and also presumably from pyramidal cells in other cortical layers. The axons of these cells form backprojections to the thalamic nucleus which projects into that cortical area, and also axons of cells in layer 6 contribute to the backprojections to layer 1 of the preceding cortical area (see Jones and Peters (1984) and Peters and Jones (1984); see Figs. 1.1 and 1.15). Layer 6 pyramidal cells also project to layer 4, where thalamic afferents terminate. Layer 6 is thus closely related to the thalamus.

Although the pyramidal and spiny stellate cells form the great majority of neocortical neurons with excitatory outputs, there are in addition several further cell types (see Peters and Jones (1984), Chapter 4). Bipolar cells are found in layers 3 and 5, and are characterized by having two dendritic systems, one ascending and the other descending, which, together with the axon distribution, are confined to a narrow vertical column often less than 50 μm in diameter (Peters, 1984a). Bipolar cells form asymmetrical (presumed excitatory) synapses with pyramidal cells, and may serve to emphasize activity within a narrow vertical column.

1.14.3 Inhibitory cells and connections

There are a number of types of neocortical inhibitory neurons. All are described as smooth in that they have few spines, and use GABA (gamma-amino-butyric acid) as a transmitter. (In older terminology they were called Type II.) A number of types of inhibitory neuron

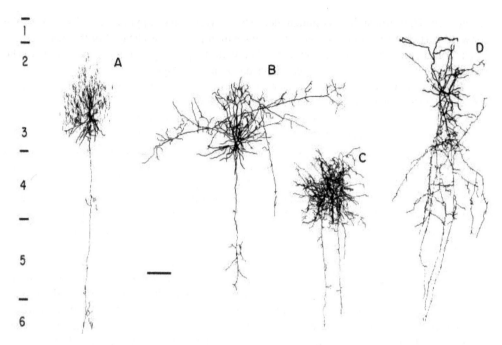

Fig. 1.13 Smooth (inhibitory) cells from cat visual cortex. (A) Chandelier or axoaxonic cell. (B) Large basket cell of layer 3. Basket cells, present in layers 3–6, have few spines on their dendrites so that they are described as smooth, and have an axon which participates in the formation of weaves of preterminal axons which surround the cell bodies of pyramidal cells and form synapses directly onto the cell body. (C) Small basket or clutch cell of layer 3. The major portion of the axonal arbor is confined to layer 4. (D) Double bouquet cell. The axon collaterals run vertically. The cortical layers are as indicated. Bar = 100 μm. (Adapted from Rodney Douglas, Henry Markram and Kevin Martin (2004) Neocortex. In Gordon M. Shepherd (ed), *The Synaptic Organization of the Brain* 5e, pp. 499–558. © Oxford University Press.)

can be distinguished, best by their axonal distributions (Szentagothai, 1978; Peters and Regidor, 1981; Douglas, Markram and Martin, 2004; Douglas and Martin, 2004; Shepherd and Grillner, 2010; Harris and Mrsic-Flogel, 2013). One type is the *basket cell*, present in layers 3–6, which has few spines on its dendrites so that it is described as smooth, and has an axon that participates in the formation of weaves of preterminal axons which surround the cell bodies of pyramidal cells and form synapses directly onto the cell body, but also onto the dendritic spines (Somogyi, Kisvarday, Martin and Whitteridge, 1983) (Fig. 1.13). Basket cells comprise 5–7% of the total cortical cell population, compared with approximately 72% for pyramidal cells (Sloper and Powell, 1979b,a). Basket cells receive synapses from the main extrinsic afferents to the neocortex, including thalamic afferents (Fig. 1.13), so that they must contribute to a feedforward type of inhibition of pyramidal cells. The inhibition is feedforward in that the input signal activates the basket cells and the pyramidal cells by independent routes, so that the basket cells can produce inhibition of pyramidal cells that does not depend on whether the pyramidal cells have already fired. Feedforward inhibition of this type not only enhances stability of the system by damping the responsiveness of the pyramidal cell simultaneously with a large new input, but can also be conceived of as a mechanism which normalizes the magnitude of the input vector received by each small region of neocortex (see further Appendix B). In fact, the feedforward inhibitory mechanism allows the pyramidal cells to be set at the appropriate sensitivity for the input they are about to receive. Basket cells can also be polysynaptically activated by an afferent volley in the thalamo-cortical projection (Martin, 1984), so that they may receive inputs from pyramidal cells, and thus participate in feedback inhibition of pyramidal cells.

The transmitter used by the basket cells is gamma-amino-butyric acid (GABA), which

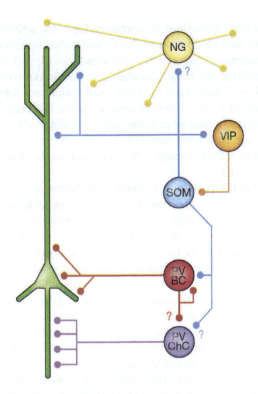

Fig. 1.14 Classes of neocortical inhibitory interneuron.
Parvalbumin-expressing interneurons (PVs) are capable of firing rapidly and with high temporal precision. They consist of two main subgroups: basket cells (BCs) that target the soma and proximal dendrites of principal cells (typically pyramidal cells shown in green), and chandelier cells (ChCs) that target the axon initial segment. PV cells receive strong excitatory inputs from thalamus and cortex, as well as inhibition from other PVs. A key role of these cells is to stabilize the activity of cortical networks using negative feedback: their absence leads to epileptiform activity, whereas more moderate chronic dysfunction of these cells has been implicated in diseases such as schizophrenia.
Somatostatin-expressing interneurons (SOMs) consist largely of Martinotti cells that target the tuft dendrites of principal cells, as well as inhibiting other interneurons. Consistent with their targeting of dendritic tufts, these cells have been implicated in behavior-dependent control of dendritic integration, as well as in more general lateral inhibition. Connections from principal cells to SOMs show facilitating synapses. In contrast to PVs, SOMs receive the majority of their input from local principal cells but little inhibition or thalamic drive.
5HT3A-receptor-expressing interneurons are the most numerous interneuron of the superficial layers. They contain two prominent subgroups: neurogliaform cells (NGs), which are thought to release GABA by volume transmission; and cells that express vasoactive intestinal peptide (VIP) and preferentially target SOMs. Putative 5HT3A-receptor-expressing cells have been implicated in the control of cortical circuits by higher-order cortex and the thalamus. (Reproduced from Harris,K.D. and Mrsic-Flogel,T.D. (2013) Cortical connectivity and sensory coding. Nature 503: 51–58, Copyright © Springer Nature Limited.)

opens chloride channels in the postsynaptic membrane. Because the reversal potential for Cl^- is approximately -10 mV relative to rest, opening the Cl^- channels does produce an inhibitory postsynaptic potential (IPSP), which results in some hyperpolarization, especially in the dendrites. This is a subtractive effect, hence it is a linear type of inhibition (Douglas and Martin, 1990; Douglas, Markram and Martin, 2004). However, a major effect of the opening of the Cl^- channels in the cell body is that this decreases the membrane resistance, thus producing a shunting effect. The importance of shunting is that it decreases the magnitude of excitatory postsynaptic potentials (EPSPs) (cf. Andersen, Dingledine, Gjerstad, Langmoen and Laursen (1980) for hippocampal pyramidal cells), so that the effect of shunting is to produce division (i.e. a multiplicative reduction) of the excitatory inputs received by the cell, and not just to act by subtraction (see further Bloomfield (1974), Martin (1984), Douglas and

Martin (1990)). Thus, when modelling the normalization of the activity of cortical pyramidal cells, it is common to include division in the normalization function (cf. Appendix B). It is notable that the dendrites of basket cells can extend laterally 0.5 mm or more (primarily within the layer in which the cell body is located), and that the axons can also extend laterally from the cell body 0.5–1.5 mm. Thus the basket cells produce a form of lateral inhibition which is quite spatially extensive. There is some evidence that each basket cell may make 4–5 synapses with a given pyramidal cell, that each pyramidal cell may receive from 10–30 basket cells, and that each basket cell may inhibit approximately 300 pyramidal cells (Martin, 1984; Douglas and Martin, 1990; Douglas, Markram and Martin, 2004). The basket cells are sometimes called clutch cells.

A second type of GABA-containing inhibitory interneuron is the *axoaxonic (or 'chandelier') cell*, named because it synapses onto the initial segment of the axon of pyramidal cells. The pyramidal cells receiving this type of inhibition are almost all in layers 2 and 3, and much less in the deep cortical layers. One effect that axoaxonic cells probably produce is thus prevention of outputs from layer 2 and 3 pyramidal cells reaching the pyramidal cells in the deep layers, or from reaching the next cortical area. Up to five axoaxonic cells converge onto a pyramidal cell, and each axoaxonic cell may project to several hundred pyramidal cells scattered in a region that may be several hundred microns in length (Martin, 1984; Peters, 1984b). This implies that axoaxonic cells provide a rather simple device for preventing runaway overactivity of pyramidal cells, but little is known yet about the afferents to axoaxonic cells, so that the functions of these neurons are very incompletely understood.

A third type of (usually smooth and inhibitory) cell is the *double bouquet cell*, which has primarily vertically organized axons. These cells have their cell bodies in layer 2 or 3, and have an axon traversing layers 2–5, usually in a tight bundle consisting of varicose, radially oriented collaterals often confined to a narrow vertical column 50 μm in diameter (Somogyi and Cowey, 1984). Double bouquet cells receive symmetrical, type II (presumed inhibitory) synapses, and also make type II synapses, perhaps onto the apical dendrites of pyramidal cells, so that these neurons may serve, by this double inhibitory effect, to emphasize activity within a narrow vertical column.

An overview of neocortical inhibitory neurons is shown in Fig. 1.14.

1.14.4 Quantitative aspects of cortical architecture

Some quantitative aspects of cortical architecture are described, because, although only preliminary data are available, they are crucial for developing an understanding of how the neocortex could work. Further evidence is provided by Braitenberg and Schüz (1991), and by Abeles (1991). Typical values, many of them after Abeles (1991), are shown in Table 1.8. The figures given are for a rather generalized case, and indicate the order of magnitude. The number of synapses per neuron (20,000) is an estimate for monkeys; those for humans may be closer to 40,000, and for the mouse, closer to 8,000. The number of 18,000 excitatory synapses made by a pyramidal cell is set to match the number of excitatory synapses received by pyramidal cells, for the great majority of cortical excitatory synapses are made from axons of cortical, principally pyramidal, cells.

Microanatomical studies show that pyramidal cells rarely make more than one connection with any other pyramidal cell, even when they are adjacent in the same area of the cerebral cortex. An interesting calculation takes the number of local connections made by a pyramidal cell within the approximately 1 mm of its local axonal arborization (say 9,000), and the number of pyramidal cells with dendrites in the same region, and suggests that the probability that a pyramidal cell makes a synapse with its neighbour is low, approximately 0.1 (Braitenberg and Schüz, 1991; Abeles, 1991) (see further Hill et al. (2012) and Markram et al.

Table 1.8 Typical quantitative estimates for neocortex reflecting estimates in macaques. (Some of the information in this Table is adapted from M. Abeles, *Corticonics, Neural Circuits of the Cerebral Cortex*, p. 59, Table 1.5.4, Copyright © 1991, Cambridge University Press. Human data from Bethlehem et al. (2022)).

Neuronal density	20,000–40,000/mm^3
Neuronal composition:	
Pyramidal	75%
Spiny stellate	10%
Inhibitory neurons, for example smooth stellate, chandelier	15%
Synaptic density	8×10^8/mm^3
Numbers of synapses on pyramidal cells:	
Excitatory synapses from remote sources onto each neuron	9,000
Excitatory synapses from local sources onto each neuron	9,000
Inhibitory synapses onto each neuron	2,000
Pyramidal cell dendritic length	10 mm
Number of synapses made by axons of pyramidal cells	18,000
Number of synapses on inhibitory neurons	2,000
Number of synapses made by inhibitory neurons	300
Dendritic length density	400 m/mm^3
Axonal length density	3,200 m/mm^3
Typical cortical thickness	2 mm (3 mm in humans)
Cortical area	
human	150,000 mm^2
macaque (assuming 2 mm for cortical thickness)	30,000 mm^2
rat (assuming 2 mm for cortical thickness)	300 mm^2

(2015)). This fits with the estimate from simultaneous recording of nearby pyramidal cells using spike-triggered averaging to monitor time-locked EPSPs (Abeles, 1991; Thomson and Deuchars, 1994).

Now the implication of the pyramidal cell to pyramidal cell connectivity just described is that within a cortical area of perhaps 1 mm^2, the region within which typical pyramidal cells have dendritic trees and their local axonal arborization, there is a probability of excitatory-to-excitatory cell connection of 0.1. Moreover, this population of mutually interconnected neurons is served by 'its own' population of inhibitory interneurons (which have a spatial receiving and sending zone in the order of 1 mm^2), enabling local threshold setting and optimization of the set of neurons with 'high' (0.1) connection probability in that region. Such an architecture is effectively recurrent or re-entrant. It may be expected to show some of the properties of recurrent networks, including the fast dynamics described in Appendix B. Such fast dynamics may be facilitated by the fact that cortical neurons in the awake behaving monkey generally have a low spontaneous rate of firing of a few spikes/s (personal observations; see for example Rolls and Tovee (1995b), Rolls, Treves, Tovee and Panzeri (1997d), and Franco, Rolls, Aggelopoulos and Jerez (2007)), which means that even any small additional input may produce some spikes sooner than would otherwise have occurred, because some of the neurons may be very close to a threshold for firing. It might also show some of the autoassociative retrieval of information typical of autoassociation networks, if the synapses between the nearby pyramidal cells have the appropriate (Hebbian) modifiability. In this context, the value of 0.1 for the probability of a connection between nearby neocortical pyramidal cells is of interest, for the connection probability between hippocampal CA3 pyramidal is approximately 0.02–0.04, and this is thought to be sufficient to sustain associative retrieval (see

Appendix B, Rolls and Treves (1998), and Rolls (2012b)). The role of this diluted connectivity of the recurrent excitatory synapses between nearby neocortical pyramidal cells and between hippocampal CA3 cells as underlying a principle of operation of the cerebral cortex is considered by Rolls (2016b).

In the neocortex, each 1 mm^2 region within which there is a relatively high density of recurrent collateral connections between pyramidal cells probably overlaps somewhat continuously with the next. This raises the issue of modules in the cortex, described by many authors as regions of the order of 1 mm^2 (with different authors giving different sizes), in which there are vertically oriented columns of neurons that may share some property (for example, responding to the same orientation of a visual stimulus), and that may be anatomically marked (for example (Powell, 1981; Mountcastle, 1984; Douglas et al., 1996; da Costa and Martin, 2010)). The anatomy just described, with the local connections between nearby (1 mm) pyramidal cells, and the local inhibitory neurons, may provide a network basis for starting to understand the columnar architecture of the neocortex, for it implies that local recurrent connectivity on this scale implementing local re-entrancy is a feature of cortical computation. We can note that the neocortex could not be a single, global, autoassociation network, because the number of memories that could be stored in an autoassociation network, rather than increasing with the number of neurons in the network, is limited by the number of recurrent connections per neuron, which is in the order of 10,000 (see Table 1.8), or less, depending on the species, as pointed out by O'Kane and Treves (1992). This would be an impossibly small capacity for the whole cortex. It is suggested that instead a principle of cortical design is that it does have in part local connectivity, so that each part can have its own processing and storage, which may be triggered by other modules, but is a distinct operation from that which occurs simultaneously in other modules Rolls (2016b).

An interesting parallel between the hippocampus and any small patch of neocortex is the allocation of a set of many small excitatory (usually non-pyramidal, spiny stellate or granular) cells at the input side. In the neocortex this is layer 4, in the hippocampus the dentate gyrus Rolls (2016b). In both cases, these cells receive the feedforward inputs and relay them to a population of pyramidal cells (in layers 2–3 of the neocortex and in the CA3 field of the hippocampus) which have extensive recurrent collateral connections. In both cases, the pyramidal cells receive inputs both as relayed by the preprocessing array and directly. Such analogies might indicate that the functional roles of neocortical layer 4 cells and of dentate granule cells could be partially the same Rolls (2016b).

The short-range high density of connectivity may also contribute to the formation of cortical topographic maps, as described in Section B.4.6. This may help to ensure that different parameters of the input space are represented in a nearly continuous fashion across the cortex, to the extent that the reduction in dimensionality allows it; or when preserving strict continuity is not possible, to produce the clustering of cells with similar response properties, as illustrated for example by color 'blobs' in striate cortex, or by the local clustering of face cells in the temporal cortical visual areas (Rolls, 2007e, 2008b, 2011d, 2012d).

1.14.5 Functional pathways through the cortical layers

Because of the complexity of the circuitry of the cerebral cortex, some of which is summarized in Figs. 1.15, 1.16 and 1.17, there are only preliminary indications available now of how information is processed through cortical layers and between cortical areas (da Costa and Martin, 2010; Harris and Mrsic-Flogel, 2013; Harris and Shepherd, 2015; Rolls, 2016b). For the following description, reference should be made to Figs. 1.15, 1.16 and 1.17.

In primary sensory cortical areas, the main extrinsic 'forward' input is from the thalamus, and ends in layer 4, where synapses are formed onto spiny stellate cells. These in turn project

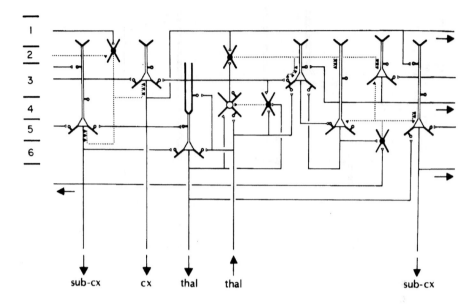

Fig. 1.15 Basic circuit for visual cortex. Excitatory neurons, which are spiny and use glutamate as a transmitter, and include the pyramidal and spiny stellate cells, are indicated by open somata; their axons are indicated by solid lines, and their synaptic boutons by open symbols. Inhibitory (smooth, GABAergic) neurons are indicated by black (filled) somata; their axons are indicated by dotted lines, and their synaptic boutons by solid symbols. thal, thalamus; cx, cortex; sub-cx, subcortex. Cortical layers 1–6 are as indicated. (Adapted from Rodney Douglas, Henry Markram and Kevin Martin (2004) Neocortex. In Gordon M. Shepherd (ed), *The Synaptic Organization of the Brain* 5e, pp. 499–558. © Oxford University Press.)

heavily onto pyramidal cells in layers 3 and 2, which in turn send projections forward to the next cortical area. The situation is made more complex than this by the fact that the thalamic afferents also synapse onto the basal dendrites in or close to the layer 2 pyramidal cells, as well as onto layer 6 pyramidal cells and inhibitory interneurons. Given that the functional implications of this particular architecture are not fully clear, it would be of interest to examine the strength of the functional links between thalamic afferents and different classes of cortical cell using cross-correlation techniques, to determine which neurons are strongly activated by thalamic afferents with monosynaptic or polysynaptic delays. Given that this is technically difficult, an alternative approach has been to use electrical stimulation of the thalamic afferents to classify cortical neurons as mono- or poly-synaptically driven, then to examine the response properties of the neuron to physiological (visual) inputs, and finally to fill the cell with horseradish peroxidase so that its full structure can be studied (see for example Martin (1984)). Using these techniques, it has been shown in the cat visual cortex that spiny stellate cells can indeed be driven monosynaptically by thalamic afferents to the cortex. Further, many of these neurons have S-type receptive fields, that is they have distinct on and off regions of the receptive field, and respond with orientation tuning to elongated visual stimuli (Martin, 1984) (see Rolls and Deco (2002)). Further, consistent with the anatomy just described, pyramidal cells in the deep part of layer 3, and in layer 6, could also be monosynaptically activated by thalamic afferents, and had S-type receptive fields (Martin, 1984). Also consistent with the anatomy just described, pyramidal cells in layer 2 were di- (or poly-) synaptically activated by stimulation of the afferents from the thalamus, but also had S-type receptive fields.

In contrast to these 'core' thalamo-cortical inputs to primary sensory cortical areas which

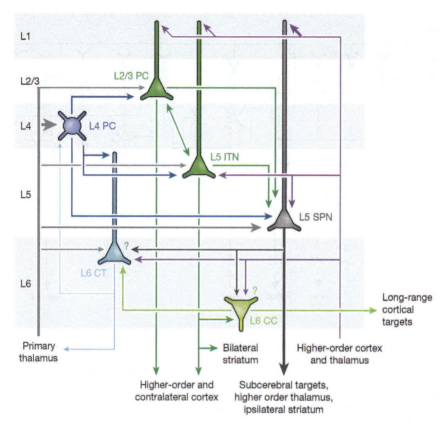

Fig. 1.16 Canonical connectivity of cortical principal cells. Line thickness represents the strength of a pathway. Sensory information arrives from primary thalamus into all cortical layers, but most densely into L4 and the L5–L6 border. Contextual inputs from higher-order cortex and thalamus most densely target L1, L5 and L6, but avoid L4.
L4 principal cells comprise two morphological classes, pyramidal and spiny stellate cells. L4 principal cells project to all layers, but most strongly L2/3. However they receive little intracolumnar input in return.
L2/3 principal cells send outputs L5, and to the next cortical area in the hierarchy L4.
Upper L5 (L5A) 'Intratelencephalic neurons' project locally upward to L2/3 and to the striatum and send backprojections to the preceding cortical area in the hierarchy. They show firing rate adaptation.
Lower L5 (L5B) 'Subcerebral projection neurons' (SPNs) are larger cells with prominent dendritic tufts in L1. They project to subcerebral motor centres for example via the pyramidal tract, and send collaterals to the striatum and higher-order thalamus with large, strong 'driver' synapses. They show little adaptation, and may fire in bursts.
L6 Corticocortical cells (CCs) have small dendritic trees, and long-range horizontal axons.
L6 Corticothalamic cells (CTs) send projections to the thalamus which, unlike those of L5 SPNs, are weak, and target the reticular and specific thalamic nuclei. Corticothalamic cells also project to cortical layer 4, where they strongly target interneurons, as well as hyperpolarizing principal cells via group II mGluRs (metabotropic glutamate receptors). Consistent with this connectivity, optogenetic stimulation of L6 in vivo suppresses cortical activity, suggesting a role of this layer in gain control or translaminar inhibition. (Reproduced from Harris,K.D. and Mrsic-Flogel,T.D. (2013). Cortical connectivity and sensory coding. Nature 503: 51–58. Copyright © Springer Nature.)

carry the main input to such cortical areas, 'matrix' thalamo-cortical connections from higher-order thalamic nuclei project to non-primary cortical areas, further up in the hierarchy (Harris and Shepherd, 2015). In higher cortical areas, the main inputs that drive the cortex come instead from the preceding cortical area in a hierarchy, and not from the 'matrix' thalamic nucleus (Harris and Shepherd, 2015; Shepherd and Yamawaki, 2021).

Inputs could reach the layer 5 pyramidal cells from the pyramidal cells in layers 2 and 3, the axons of which ramify extensively in layer 5, in which the layer 5 pyramidal cells have widespread basal dendrites (see Fig. 1.1), and also perhaps from thalamic afferents. Many layer 5 pyramidal cells are di- or trisynaptically activated by stimulation of the thalamic afferents, consistent with them receiving inputs from monosynaptically activated deep layer 3 pyramidal cells, or from disynaptically activated pyramidal cells in layer 2 and upper layer 3 (Martin, 1984). Upper L5 (L5A) 'Intratelencephalic neurons' project locally upward to L2/3 and to the striatum and send backprojections to the preceding cortical area in the hierarchy. They show firing rate adaptation (i.e. their firing rates gradually decrease over short time periods). Lower L5 (L5B) 'Subcerebral projection neurons' (SPNs) are larger cells with prominent dendritic tufts in L1. They project to subcerebral motor centres for example via the pyramidal tract, and send collaterals to the striatum and higher-order thalamus with large, strong 'driver' synapses (Harris and Mrsic-Flogel, 2013; Harris and Shepherd, 2015). They may also provide some cortico-cortical backprojections, which terminate in superficial layers of the cerebral cortex, including layer 1 (see Rolls (2016b)). They show little adaptation, and may fire in bursts. These neurons may have a less sparse representation than those in L2/3, with this representation being useful for high information transmission. (In contrast, the more sparse representation in L2/L3 pyramidal cells may be useful when information is being stored in the recurrent collaterals, for this maximizes the number of patterns that can be stored and correctly retrieved. This may be one reason why the cerebral neocortex has superficial pyramidal cell layers (L2/L3) which are separate from the deep pyramidal cell layers (L5/L6) (see further Rolls (2016b) and Rolls and Mills (2017)).

L6 Corticocortical cells (CCs) have small dendritic trees, and long-range horizontal axons. L6 Corticothalamic cells (CTs) send projections to the thalamus which, unlike those of L5 Subcerebral projection neurons (typically pyramidal tract neurons), are weak, and target the reticular nucleus, and a particular thalamic nucleus which then sends thalamo-cortical connections back to the cortical region that connects to that part of the thalamus. Some of these are pyramidal tract neurons. One type of thalamo-cortical neuron described as 'matrix' type (found typically in thalamic regions that project to non-primary sensory / association cortical areas (Harris and Shepherd, 2015)) sends connections to L2/3 and L5A pyramidal cells, which then connect to cortico-thalamic cells (Shepherd and Yamawaki, 2021). This thus forms a loop with excitatory synapses throughout, so control by inhibitory neurons is needed, but the CT influence on thalamic cells is weak, so this may not be a strong positive feedback loop (Shepherd and Yamawaki, 2021). Corticothalamic cells have low conduction speed, so their effect is slow. Matrix type thalamocortical cells also project to cortical layer 1 (Harris and Shepherd, 2015). Corticothalamic cells also project to cortical layer 4, where they strongly target interneurons, as well as hyperpolarizing principal cells via group II mGluRs. Consistent with this connectivity, optogenetic stimulation of L6 in vivo suppresses cortical activity, suggesting a role of this layer in gain control or translaminar inhibition (Harris and Mrsic-Flogel, 2013). The cortico-thalamic connections involving CT cells may accordingly be for some type of control function, rather than performing any new computation (by which I mean for example autoassociation, pattern association, or competitive learning). In many types of behavior, CT cells are rather silent, so their function is a mystery (Harris and Shepherd, 2015; Shepherd and Yamawaki, 2021).

What Fig. 1.16 does not bring out is what I consider to be the key anatomical and computational feature of the cortex, excitatory connections between pyramidal cells implemented by the recurrent collateral connections (Rolls, 2016b, 2021c). These are shown for neocortex in the canonical neocortical circuit of Rolls (2016b) (Fig. 1.17). The recurrent collateral connections are associatively modifiable. The concept is that this anatomy and physiology provides for what computationally are attractor networks (Section B.3), which provide the neocortex with its key computational properties of implementing a local short-term memory that can be implemented by ongoing firing, providing the basis for planning; and semantic networks, which enable attributes of individual objects or people to be associated with the individual. In neocortex, the anatomical evidence suggests that there are separate attractor networks in

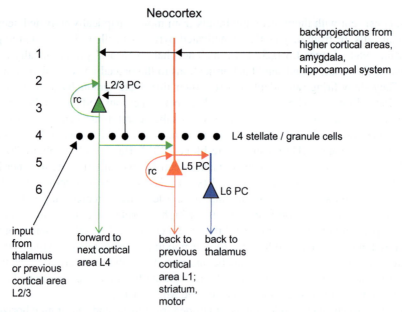

Fig. 1.17 Functional canonical microcircuit of the neocortex (see text). The cortical layers are numbered 1–6, with layer 1 at the surface of the cortex, and layer 6 adjacent to the white matter consisting of axonal connections to other brain areas. Recurrent collateral connections (rc) are shown as a loop back to a particular population of cells, of which just one neuron is shown in this and Figs. 5.7 and 9.22. In primates the feedforward projection neurons are concentrated in L3B; and the main feedback projection neurons are in L6 and Lower L5 (L5B), but some L2 and L3A neurons do send backprojections (Markov et al 2014b). Some L6 cortico-thalamic neurons send a projection to L4 (see text). (From Rolls, E. T. (2016) Cerebral Cortex: Principles of Operation. Oxford University Press: Oxford.)

the superficial layers (2 and 3), and in the deep layers (layer 5) (Rolls, 2016b). These may be specialised for somewhat different functions, with the superficial attractor networks involved in the main feedforward computations from area to area of the cerebral cortex; and the deep layer specialized for outputs to motor and related structures such as the striatum, and for backprojections to the preceding cortical area (Rolls and Mills, 2017), consistent with what is shown in Fig. 1.17.

A key feature of the neocortical recurrent collateral system is that it is local, extending just several mm from any given neuron. This provides a basis for separate attractor networks in nearby cortical regions spaced only several mm apart, and this is necessary to provide for high memory capacity of the whole neocortex, made possible by the partial independence of the local attractors. Without this relative independence of nearby attractors, the total memory capacity of the cortex would be determined by the leading term of the number of recurrent collateral synapses onto any one neuron, as described in Section B.3 (O'Kane and Treves, 1992). Because the recurrent collaterals are local, the total memory capacity of the cortex is the number of memories that could be stored in any one local attractor network (of order 10,000, if the number C of recurrent collaterals onto each pyramidal cell is 10,000), multiplied by the number of local attractor networks in the cortex, divided by a factor of 2–3 due to interference between nearby attractors with some overlap of anatomical connectivity as one moves across the cortical sheet (Roudi and Treves, 2006, 2008). If the human neocortical surface area is of order 1,900 cm^2, and each local neocortical attractor has a diameter of 3 mm (and thus an area of approximately 7 mm^2), then the number of independent attractor networks would be approximately 27,000, each with a memory capacity of at least several thousand items. The locality of the recurrent collaterals in the neocortex also means that it tends to support topological maps (Section B.4.6), with this locality of neocortical processing in turn contributing to the convergence from area to area as one moves up a cortical hierarchy (Rolls, 2016b).

This fundamental aspect of neocortical architecture and principle of operation, its locality, is in complete contrast to the hippocampus as described in Chapter 9 in which the CA3 cells provide a single attractor network so that any item can be associated with any other item to form an episodic memory (Fig. 9.22); and with the olfactory pyriform cortex as described in Section 5.3.2 (see Fig. 5.7) in which there is no topology in the input space of odors as represented in the glomeruli of the olfactory bulb, so that associations may need to be found throughout the olfactory space. The locality of the dense recurrent collateral excitatory connections between pyramidal cells is a fundamental principle of the evolution and operation of the neocortex.

Further consideration of how computations are performed by cortical circuitry are provided in Section B.18, and by Rolls (2016b), Rolls and Mills (2017), and Rolls (2021c).

Studies on the function of inhibitory pathways in the cortex are also beginning. The fact that basket cells often receive strong thalamic inputs, and that they terminate on pyramidal cell bodies where part of their action is to shunt the membrane, suggests that they act in part as a feedforward inhibitory system that normalizes the thalamic influence on pyramidal cells by dividing their response in proportion to the average of the thalamic input received (see Appendix B). The smaller and numerous smooth (or sparsely spiny) non-pyramidal cells that are inhibitory may receive inputs from pyramidal cells as well as inhibit them, so that these neurons could perform the very important function of recurrent or feedback inhibition (see Appendix B). It is only feedback inhibition that can take into account not only the inputs received by an area of cortex, but also the effects that these inputs have, once multiplied by the synaptic weight vector on each neuron, so that recurrent inhibition is necessary for competition and contrast enhancement (see Appendix B).

Another way in which the role of inhibition in the cortex can be analyzed is by applying a drug such as bicuculline using iontophoresis (which blocks GABA receptors to a single neuron), while examining the response properties of the neuron (see Sillito (1984)). With this technique, it has been shown that in the visual cortex of the cat, layer 4 simple cells lose their orientation and directional selectivity. Similar effects are observed in some complex cells, but the selectivity of other complex cells may be less affected by blocking the effect of endogenously released GABA in this way (Sillito, 1984). One possible reason for this is that the inputs to complex cells must often synapse onto the dendrites far from the cell body, and distant synapses will probably be unaffected by the GABA receptor blocker released near the cell body. The experiments reveal that inhibition is very important for the normal selectivity of many visual cortex neurons for orientation and the direction of movement. Many of the cells displayed almost no orientation selectivity without inhibition. This implies that not only is the inhibition important for maintaining the neuron on an appropriate part of its activation function, but also that lateral inhibition between neurons is important because it allows the responses of a single neuron (which need not be markedly biased by its excitatory input) to have its responsiveness set by the activity of neighbouring neurons (see Appendix B).

1.14.6 The scale of lateral excitatory and inhibitory effects, and the concept of modules

The forward cortico-cortical afferents to a cortical area sometimes have a columnar pattern to their distribution, with the column width 200–300 μm in diameter (see Eccles (1984)). Similarly, individual thalamo-cortical axons often end in patches in layer 4 which are 200–300 μm in diameter (Martin, 1984). The dendrites of spiny stellate cells are in the region of 500 μm in diameter, and their axons can distribute in patches 200–300 μm across, separated by distances of up to 1 mm (Martin, 1984). The dendrites of layer 2 and 3 pyramidal cells can be approximately 300 μm in diameter, but after this the relatively narrow column appears to become less important, for the axons of the superficial pyramidal cells can distribute over 1 mm or more, both in layers 2 and 3, and in layer 5 (Martin, 1984). Other neurons that may contribute to the maintenance of processing in relatively narrow columns are the double bouquet cells, which because they receive inhibitory inputs, and themselves produce inhibition, all within a column perhaps 50 μm across (see above), would tend to enhance local excitation. The bipolar cells, which form excitatory synapses with pyramidal cells, may also serve to emphasize activity within a narrow vertical column approximately 50 μm across. These two mechanisms for enhancing local excitation operate against a much broader-ranging set of lateral inhibitory processes, and could it is suggested have the effect of increasing contrast between the firing rates of pyramidal cells 50 μm apart, and thus be very important in competitive interactions between pyramidal cells. Indeed, the lateral inhibitory effects are broader than the excitatory effects described so far, in that for example the axons of basket cells spread laterally 500 μm or more (see above) (although those of the small, smooth non-pyramidal cells are closer to 300 μm – see Peters and Saint Marie (1984)). Such short-range local excitatory interactions with longer range inhibition not only provide for contrast enhancement and for competitive interactions, but also can result in the formation of maps in which neurons with similar responses are grouped together and neurons with dissimilar response are more widely separated (see Appendix B). Thus these local interactions are consistent with the possibilities that cortical pyramidal cells form a competitive network (see Appendix B and below), and that cortical maps are formed at least partly as a result of local interactions of this kind in a competitive network (see Section B.4.6).

The type of genetic specification that could provide the fundamental connectivity rules between cortical areas, which would then self-organize the details of the exact synaptic connectivity, have been considered by Rolls and Stringer (2000). They compared the connectivity of different cortical areas, thereby suggested a set of rules that the genes might be specifying, and then simulated using genetic algorithms the selection of the appropriate rules for solving particular types of computational problem, including pattern association memory, autoassociation memory, and competitive learning (see Rolls (2016b) and Section B.20). Although molecular studies are making progress in studying categories of cortical neurons based on their genetic signature (Zeisel et al., 2018), these approaches have not yet focussed on the key question of the few genes that specify the connections of each cortical area that enable the classes of neuron in one cortical area to recognise the classes of neuron in other cortical areas with which they should make connections (Rolls and Stringer, 2000).

In contrast to the relatively localized terminal distributions of forward cortico-cortical and thalamo-cortical afferents, the cortico-cortical backward projections that end in layer 1 have a much wider horizontal distribution, of up to several millimetres (mm). It is suggested that this enables the backward-projecting neurons to search over a larger number of pyramidal cells in the preceding cortical area for activity that is conjunctive with their own (Rolls, 2016b, 2021c).

2 The ventral visual system

2.1 Introduction and overview

2.1.1 Introduction

Information in the *'ventral or what'* visual cortical processing stream projects after the primary visual cortex, area V1, to the secondary visual cortex (V2), and then via area V4 to the posterior and then to the anterior inferior temporal visual cortex (see Figs. 1.8, 2.1, and 2.3). The ventral visual system performs invariant visual object recognition, that is, it encodes objects by the level of the anterior inferior temporal cortex, and the representation is relatively invariant with respect to where for example the object is on the retina, its size, and even for some neurons its view. That makes the output of this system ideal as an input to memory systems and for systems that learn the reward value of visual stimuli, for if the output system learns something about the object when one transform is shown (e.g. one view), then the learning automatically generalizes to other transforms. That is a key computation performed by this system. We start with overviews: first about what is computed, and then about how it is computed.

2.1.2 Overview of what is computed in the ventral visual system

What is computed in the ventral visual system is described in Sections 2.1.4 to 2.4 with an overview here.

1. The primate retina has a fovea with closely packed cones and ganglion cells that provide for high visual acuity at the fovea (Rolls and Cowey, 1970). This shapes the computations performed in the ventral visual system, and indeed in systems such as the hippocampus and orbitofrontal cortex that receive from the ventral visual system. Object recognition of typically one or a very few objects is performed primarily with the high resolution fovea when an object is being fixated. This greatly simplifies visual object recognition, because the whole scene does not have to be processed simultaneously, as occurs in some artificial vision systems. The extrafoveal retina is used more to attract attention, so that the eyes move to foveate the stimulus in order to identify it. Foveal vision thus requires mechanisms to saccade to fixate on objects, and to track moving objects to keep them on the fovea, and these mechanisms are implemented in the dorsal visual system and superior colliculus.
2. The retina provides a pixel-based representation in retinal coordinates, which has no transform invariances, and moreover which changes greatly whenever an object moves even a small amount on the retina, and when the eyes move even a little. That means that a major computation is needed in the ventral visual system, to produce a transform-invariant representation of objects, faces, etc that can be read off easily by other brain systems.
3. The retinal pixel-level representation is passed by the lateral geniculate nucleus of the thalamus, which provides some further lateral inhibition to that already implemented between the retinal ganglion cells for high-pass spatial frequency filtering, useful for contrast enhancement of boundaries and contrast equalization over different parts of retinal space.

54 | The ventral visual system

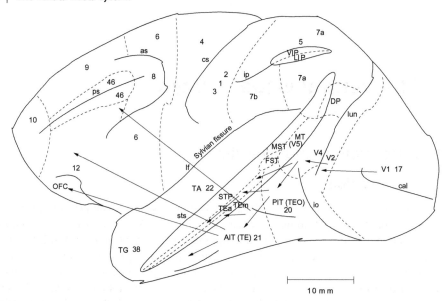

Fig. 2.1 Lateral view of the macaque brain showing the connections in the 'ventral or what visual pathway' from V1 to V2, V4, the inferior temporal visual cortex, etc., with some connections reaching the amygdala and orbitofrontal cortex. as, arcuate sulcus; cal, calcarine sulcus; cs, central sulcus; lf, lateral (or Sylvian) fissure; lun, lunate sulcus; ps, principal sulcus; io, inferior occipital sulcus; ip, intraparietal sulcus (which has been opened to reveal some of the areas it contains); sts, superior temporal sulcus (which has been opened to reveal some of the areas it contains). AIT, anterior inferior temporal cortex; FST, visual motion processing area; LIP, lateral intraparietal area; MST, visual motion processing area; MT, visual motion processing area (also called V5); OFC, orbitofrontal cortex; PIT, posterior inferior temporal cortex; STP, superior temporal plane; TA, architectonic area including auditory association cortex; TE, architectonic area including high order visual association cortex, and some of its subareas TEa and TEm; TG, architectonic area in the temporal pole; V1–V4, visual areas 1–4; VIP, ventral intraparietal area; TEO, architectonic area including posterior visual association cortex. The numbers refer to architectonic areas, and have the following approximate functional equivalence: 1, 2, 3, somatosensory cortex (posterior to the central sulcus); 4, motor cortex; 5, superior parietal lobule; 7a, inferior parietal lobule, visual part; 7b, inferior parietal lobule, somatosensory part; 6, lateral premotor cortex; 8, frontal eye field; 12, inferior convexity prefrontal cortex; 46, dorsolateral prefrontal cortex.

4. The primary visual cortex converts the circular centre-surround receptive field representation received from the lateral geniculate nucleus into a massively expanded new representation in which the receptive fields are elongated so that the neurons respond to bars or edges with a given orientation and size / spatial frequency. The expansion of neuron numbers helps to decorrelate the representation provided across neurons of retinal inputs, which in turn helps in the process of forming neurons that respond to low-order combinations of features (such as a horizontal and vertical edge that join) at subsequent levels of visual processing. Binocular neurons are formed.

5. V2 neurons have larger receptive fields (typically 2 deg) than those in V1 (typically 1 deg), and V4 neurons have large receptive fields (typically 4 deg). Neurons in V2 and V4 respond to more complex shapes than those in V1. Some respond to visual texture, and some respond to both shape and texture, which may be useful for segregating objects from their background. V2 and V4 neurons are often tuned to stereoscopic depth, and/or to color.

6. Posterior inferior temporal visual cortex neurons (BA 20, TEO) have larger receptive fields, but are still not very translation invariant, in that small eye movements to a different position result in different sets of neurons being active.

7. Rolls and colleagues discovered many of the key properties of anterior inferior temporal (AIT) visual cortex neurons, as described in this Chapter and summarized elsewhere (Rolls, 2021d). These macaque anterior inferior temporal cortex neurons have large re-

ceptive fields often with a diameter of 70 degrees when an object is seen against a blank background. This means that their responses do not depend on completely precise fixation of an object, and indeed, their response can be translation (shift) invariant over tens of degrees. Their responses can be relatively selective for objects or faces: by which I mean that they can be selective for some and not other objects, or some but not other faces. Their responses to objects are often quite invariant with respect to changes of not only position, but also of object size, spatial frequency, contrast, and even in some cases of the view of an object or face. In other cases, the neurons are view-specific, encoding for example a view of the right but not the left profile of a particular person.

8. The responses of AIT neurons thus provide a basis for object and face recognition, and indeed which object or face was presented can be read out from the responses of small numbers of these selective neurons, as shown by information theoretic analyses (Appendix C). Moreover, their responses are relatively uncorrelated with each other, so that over tens of neurons the information from a population of these neurons increases approximately linearly. Put another way, the number of objects or faces that can be encoded by these neurons increases approximately exponentially with the number of neurons (as information is a logarithmic measure) (with populations of tens of neurons). The tuning of these neurons is sparse distributed, with the distributed property allowing useful generalization, and the sparseness providing high capacity in terms of the number of objects that can be encoded. Each neuron has an approximately exponential probability distribution of firing rates, with most objects producing low firing rates, and high firing rates to a few objects or faces. The code can be read out by dot (or inner) product decoding, which is highly biologically plausible, because receiving neurons then only need to sum the firing rates of their inputs weighted by their synaptic strengths to correctly decode the stimulus. Most of the information is present in the firing rates, with a little in the response latencies, and rather little in any stimulus-dependent cross-correlations between the firing of different neurons.

9. The response fields of AIT neurons shrink to a few degrees in complex visual scenes. This enables neurons to be selective for an object being fixated, so that information can be passed to brain regions such as the hippocampus and orbitofrontal cortex that enable the learning that is implemented in these brain regions to be selective for the object being fixated, which is what is needed biologically, and not for the whole scene. AIT neurons in such crowded scenes even have some asymmetry around the fovea, so that different neurons can encode not only what object is present, but where it is relative to the fovea if it is close to the fovea.

10. The responses of AIT neurons, and thereby V4 neurons by backprojections, can also be influenced by top-down attention. For example, if a stimulus at one position in a receptive field is relevant to a task, the response to a stimulus in that position can be enhanced relative to a stimulus in another part of the receptive field. Similar top-down attention can also operate for objects. These effects can be modelled by top-down biased competition using cortico-cortical backprojections. The origins of these top-down influences include the prefrontal cortex.

11. There is some evidence that IT neurons can modify their responses over the first few presentations of objects or faces to learn how to best categorize the new objects or faces, without disrupting existing representations.

12. In primates, the reward vs punishment value of stimuli are not represented in the inferior temporal visual cortex, as shown by visual discrimination reversal experiments, and by devaluation experiments in which the reward value is reduced to zero by feeding to satiety. The reward value of visual stimuli is learned in the orbitofrontal cortex and amygdala. This

clear separation of reward value from perceptual representations is a key feature of the organisation of primate perceptual systems, and ensures that we do not go blind to objects when their reward value is decreased to zero; and that we can learn about for example the location of objects even when their reward value is currently zero.

13. In addition to this inferior temporal cortex system, in which we are speaking primarily about the cortex that forms the inferior temporal gyrus (area 21, TE), there is also a whole set of visual areas in the cortex in the superior temporal sulcus (STS), running from posterior to anterior, Many of these neurons require movement in order to respond, but are nevertheless often object or face selective. Such neurons may respond for example to a head turning towards the viewer, or for other neurons away from the viewer. These neurons may be useful for encoding gesture with social significance, for some of these neurons may respond to the head turning away from the viewer, or to the eyes closing, both of which indicate breaking of social contact, and which co-occur so could arise by learned association. Some of these neurons code in object-based coordinates, in that they may respond to a head performing ventral flexion with respect to the body, independently of whether the head is the correct way up or inverted (which of course reverses the optic flow but not the object-based description). These neurons provide very clear evidence for object-based descriptions of objects in the temporal lobe cortical visual areas.

14. Some temporal lobe neurons, especially in the cortex in the STS or close to this, encode face expression, and some of these respond to face gesture (movement), such as lip-smacking, which is an affiliative / social gesture in macaques.

15. Although processing in the temporal cortical visual areas is primarily unimodal (visual) as far as AIT, there are neurons in the cortex in the STS that respond to auditory stimuli, including the sounds of macaque vocalizations and humans speaking (Baylis et al., 1987). It is likely that some neurons in these areas in macaques learn to respond by association to corresponding visual and auditory stimuli, such as the sight and sound of a macaque lip-smacking, and single neurons with auditory as well as visual responses have now been described in macaques (Khandhadia et al., 2021). In humans in temporal lobe areas, such multimodal neurons have been recorded, and have been termed 'concept cells' (Quian Quiroga, 2012), and neurons with some similar properties are found in macaques (Rolls, 2023d).

16. Although much of what we know about what is computed in the ventral visual stream can be best established by neuronal recording in macaques, the results of fMRI investigations in humans, in which the activity of tens of thousands of neurons is averaged, is at least consistent. The point here is that because the code used by these neurons is often independent, the details of what is being computed can be most clearly established by recording the activity of neurons and populations of neurons, with some of the examples provided above and in the rest of this Chapter providing evidence on the richness of what is represented.

17. In humans, effective connectivity analyses and the use of the Human Connectome Project HCP-MMP atlas show how the ventral visual stream visual pathways connect via the fusiform face cortex FFC to the inferior temporal visual cortex, and then via the lateral parahippocampal gyrus TF to provide 'what' inputs to the hippocampal ventral visual system (Rolls et al., 2023e) (Section 2.5). The inferior temporal cortex in humans has connectivity to the semantic systems in the banks of the superior temporal sulcus that extend up into the inferior parietal cortex region PGi (Section 2.5.2).

Many of these neurophysiological discoveries were made by Rolls and colleagues, and are described below and elsewhere (Rolls, 1984, 2000a, 2011d, 2012d, 2016b, 2021d), where citations are provided. These discoveries have been confirmed and extended, for example

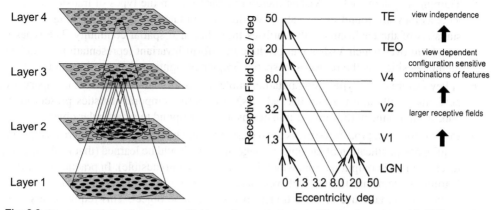

Fig. 2.2 Convergence in the visual system. Right – as it occurs in the brain. V1, visual cortex area V1; TEO, posterior inferior temporal cortex; TE, anterior inferior temporal cortex (IT). Left – as implemented in VisNet, a model of invariant visual object recognition. Convergence through the network is designed to provide fourth layer neurons with information from across the entire input retina, by providing an increase of receptive field size of 2.5 times at each stage. Layer 1 of the model corresponds to V2 in the brain.

by showing that the clustering of face cells appears as face patches with fMRI (Freiwald, Tsao and Livingstone, 2009; Rust and DiCarlo, 2010; Freiwald, 2020; Tsao, 2014; Freedman, 2015; Aparicio, Issa and DiCarlo, 2016; Arcaro and Livingstone, 2021).

2.1.3 Overview of how computations are performed in the ventral visual system

How the computations are performed in the ventral visual system is described in Sections 2.6–2.9 with an overview here.

1. Invariant visual object recognition is implemented in the ventral visual system using only about 5 stages of hierarchical processing, V1, V2, V4, posterior inferior temporal cortex, and anterior inferior temporal cortex. This allows approximately 15 ms of processing time for each stage. That is just sufficient for processes implemented by recurrent collaterals such as attractor network computations to be involved.

2. Although there are as many backprojections as forward projections between each pair of stages of the hierarchy, these are used for memory recall and top-down attention, and probably not for backpropagation of error learning, which is prima facie biologically implausible.

3. A biologically plausible form of learning to categorize new stimuli is competitive learning, and this is at present the most plausible candidate mechanism for how object and face representations are learned over successive stages of the hierarchy, with convergence from stage to stage consistent with the increase of receptive field size from stage to stage (Fig. 2.2).

4. Because different views of an object can be quite different, a mechanism is needed to associate together different transforms of the same object. An associative synaptic learning rule that incorporates a short-term trace of previous neuronal activity is proposed in the VisNet model to enable these associations to be learned, utilising the property of the natural world that temporally close visual stimuli are statistically likely to be different transforms of the same object (Rolls, 1992a, 2012d, 2016b, 2021d). Systems (such as HMAX) without this 'slow learning' capability fail in this key aspect of visual object recognition, transform-invariant representations of objects.

5. Training a system such as VisNet therefore benefits from the types of transforms of objects as they are found in the natural world, to facilitate this type of learning about the statistics of the environment that utilises time, but also spatial continuity. The types of transform over which VisNet can produce transform-invariant representations of objects include position on the retina, size, spatial frequency, lighting, deformation, and view.
6. A key feature of the type of computation implemented in VisNet is that it is unsupervised, performed without a teacher. Instead, VisNet uses the temporal statistics present in the natural environment to learn the transforms that correspond to a particular object or face.
7. In contrast, AI approaches such as deep learning using backpropagation of errors typically require prespecification of the object categories that should be learned (that is, the use of a teacher for each output neuron, which is biologically implausible). In practice these deep learning systems are trained with very large numbers of exemplars of a class, typically without systematic use of close transforms of the same object. This requires very large numbers of training trials. Deep learning networks may have up to 100 layers, again biologically implausible. Moreover, little is learned from these deep learning models about how the brain solves complex problems such as invariant visual object and face recognition, because deep convolutional learning does not use biological constraints such as local learning rules, and when mappings from images to categories are found, clear computational principles of how the mapping is achieved are largely not understood (Plebe and Grasso, 2019). VisNet is the most biologically plausible approach to how computations in the ventral visual system for invariant object and face recognition are performed using unsupervised 'slow', memory trace-based, learning (Rolls, 2021d).
8. Other proposals such as feature spaces are too simple to implement object recognition for the reasons give above, though features such as texture, and color may be usefully combined with shape information to help invariant visual object recognition in a VisNet-like system. Object-based systems that utilise connections between parts also seem implausible, because of the requirement of powerful syntax to describe how all the parts are joined together.
9. VisNet implements a feature hierarchy approach to object recognition. Feature hierarchy networks are biologically plausible in that they can be implemented with local synaptic learning rules (needing only the activity in the pre-synaptic and post-synaptic neurons), implemented in competitive networks (described in Section B.4). They are evolutionarily economical in that the same type of competitive network can be utilised in each stage of the hierarchy, without the need for evolution to optimise many different types of network and the genetic specification for them; and in that they can be used in every sensory system.
10. Invariant visual object recognition is one of the major and difficult computations performed by the primate (including of course human) brain, and developments in this field of current or new approaches will be important.

2.1.4 What is computed in the ventral visual system is unimodal, and is related to other 'what' systems after the inferior temporal visual cortex

The ventral visual system systems-level organization is illustrated in Figs. 1.8, 2.1, 2.3, and 2.4, and these Figures show that anatomically the ventral visual system receives inputs from the retina, and not from other modalities (such as taste or smell). The unimodal nature of the processing is also shown by the fact that neurons in the inferior temporal cortex respond primarily to visual stimuli, and not to taste or olfactory stimuli, etc. (Rolls, 2000a; Baylis, Rolls and Leonard, 1987; Rolls, 2012d, 2016b). The computation that must be performed along

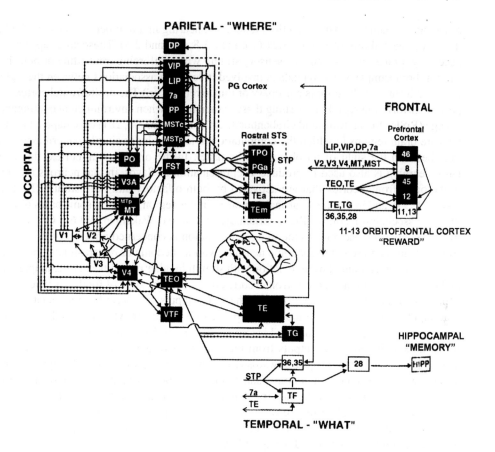

Fig. 2.3 Visual processing pathways in monkeys. Solid lines indicate connections arising from both central and peripheral visual field representations; dotted lines indicate connections restricted to peripheral visual field representations. Shaded boxes in the 'ventral (lower) or what' stream indicate visual areas related primarily to object vision; shaded boxes in the 'dorsal or where' stream indicate areas related primarily to spatial vision; and white boxes indicate areas not clearly allied with only one stream. Abbreviations: DP, dorsal prelunate area; FST, fundus of the superior temporal area; HIPP, hippocampus; LIP, lateral intraparietal area; MSTc, medial superior temporal area, central visual field representation; MSTp, medial superior temporal area, peripheral visual field representation; MT, middle temporal area; MTp, middle temporal area, peripheral visual field representation; PO, parieto-occipital area; PP, posterior parietal sulcal zone; STP, superior temporal polysensory area; V1, primary visual cortex; V2, visual area 2; V3, visual area 3; V3A, visual area 3, part A; V4, visual area 4; and VIP, ventral intraparietal area. Inferior parietal area 7a; prefrontal areas 8, 11 to 13, 45 and 46 are from Brodmann (1925). Inferior temporal areas TE and TEO, parahippocampal area TF, temporal pole area TG, and inferior parietal area PG are from Von Bonin and Bailey (1947). Rostral superior temporal sulcal (STS) areas are from Seltzer and Pandya (1978) and VTF is the visually responsive portion of area TF (Boussaoud, Desimone and Ungerleider 1991). Area 46 in the dorsolateral prefrontal cortex is involved in short-term memory. (Modified from Ungerleider, L. G. (1995) Functional brain imaging studies of cortical mechanisms for memory. Science 270: 769–775. Copyright © The American Association for the Advancement of Science.)

this stream is primarily to build a representation of objects that shows invariance. After this processing, the visual representation is interfaced to other sensory systems in areas in which simple associations must be learned between stimuli in different modalities (see Chapters 9 and 11). The representation must thus be in a form in which the simple generalization properties of associative networks can be useful. Given that the association is about what object is present (and not where it is on the retina), the representation computed in sensory systems must be in a form that allows the simple correlations computed by associative networks to reflect similarities between objects, and not between their positions on the retina.

The ventral visual stream converges with other 'what' and mainly unimodal information processing streams for taste, olfaction, touch, and hearing in a number of areas, particularly the amygdala and orbitofrontal cortex (see Figs. 1.8, 2.1, and 2.3). These areas appear to be necessary for learning to associate sensory stimuli with reinforcing (rewarding or punishing) stimuli. For example, the amygdala is involved in learning associations between the sight of food and its taste. (The taste is a primary or innate reinforcer.) The orbitofrontal cortex is especially involved in rapidly relearning these associations, when environmental contingencies change (Rolls, 2014a; Rolls and Grabenhorst, 2008; Rolls, 2000d, 2019e) (Chapter 11). They thus are brain regions in which the computation at least includes simple pattern association (e.g. between the sight of an object and its taste). In the orbitofrontal cortex, this association learning is also used to produce a representation of flavor, in that neurons are found in the orbitofrontal cortex that are activated by both olfactory and taste stimuli (Rolls and Baylis, 1994), and in that the neuronal responses in this region reflect in some cases olfactory to taste association learning (Rolls, Critchley, Mason and Wakeman, 1996b; Critchley and Rolls, 1996b). In these regions too, the representation is concerned not only with what sensory stimulus is present, but for some neurons, with its hedonic or reward-related properties, which are often computed by association with stimuli in other modalities. For example, many of the visual neurons in the orbitofrontal cortex respond to the sight of food only when hunger is present. This probably occurs because the visual inputs here have been associated with a taste input to this region, with the taste response only occurring when the food is rewarding because hunger is present (Chapter 11) (Rolls, 2014a, 2015d; Rolls and Grabenhorst, 2008; Rolls, 2000d, 2016b). The outputs from these associative memory systems, the amygdala and orbitofrontal cortex, project onwards (Fig. 1.8) to structures such as the hypothalamus, through which they control autonomic and endocrine responses such as salivation and insulin release to the sight of food; to the cingulate cortex for actions to be learned to lead to the reward outcomes signalled by the orbitofrontal cortex (Rolls, 2019c) (Chapter 12); and to the striatum, including the ventral striatum, through which behavioral responses to learned reinforcing stimuli are produced (Chapter 16).

What is computed in the ventral visual system can best be appreciated by considering the properties of anterior inferior temporal cortex (AIT) neurons, as this can be considered as the end of the primate ventral visual system, and this is described in Section 2.4. The next two sections provide some background on the stages of visual processing that lead to the inferior temporal visual cortex.

2.2 What: V1 – primary visual cortex

In V1, concentric center-antagonistic surround receptive fields (RF) become a minority, while orientation selectivity emerges, as discovered by Hubel and Wiesel (1962) and illustrated in Fig. 2.5. Second, many neurons become selective for motion direction. Third, many cells have 'complex' RFs, that is, they respond to both light increments and decrements in their RFs, compared to 'simple' cells which do not. Fourth, most cells become driven by both eyes and many are tuned to stereoscopic depth. Fifth, V1 cells become more selective for spatial frequency. In addition, some cells show double color opponency (Vanni, Hokkanen, Werner and Angelucci, 2020). The receptive field diameters are typically 1–2 degrees in the foveal region. A Difference of Gaussian function fits the centre-surround organization (Vanni et al., 2020), but an alternative formulation which fits essentially as well is that the receptive fields of simple cells can be modelled by 2D-Gabor functions (Daugman, 1988) as described in Section 2.8.1.4. Further descriptions of V1 are provided in Kandel et al. (2021), and in Chapter 2 of Rolls and Deco (2002).

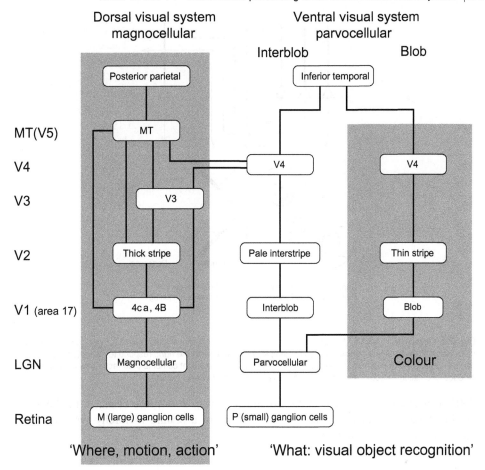

Fig. 2.4 A schematic diagram of the visual pathways from the retina to visual cortical areas. LGN, lateral geniculate nucleus; V1, primary visual cortex; V2, V3, V4, and MT, other visual cortical areas; M, magnocellular; P, parvocellular.

2.3 What: V2 and V4 – intermediate processing areas in the ventral visual system

In V2, latencies of early neuronal responses are approximately 60–70 ms, compared to 30–50 ms in V1 (Vanni et al., 2020). Many V2 cells assign contrast edges to particular objects, that is, encode border ownership (Vanni et al., 2020). This may be useful for separating objects from their background.

Some neurons in V4 code jointly for object shape and for object texture/color (Pasupathy et al., 2019; Kim et al., 2019), while others code for these separately. The combination of shape with texture may facilitate the segmentation of objects from their background. the corresponding area in humans is V4 and the lateral occipital cortex (LOC).

The size of the receptive fields in V4 is intermediate between that of V1 and the inferior temporal visual cortex, and has a diameter in degrees of approximately 1.0 + 0.625 x receptive field eccentricity (and is thus approximately 4 degrees at 5 degrees of eccentricity, the edge of the fovea) (Kim et al., 2019). Because the receptive fields are larger in V4 than V1, V4 neurons can respond to extended combinations of features in the correct relative positions to form for example curves or corners (Roe et al., 2012; Jiang et al., 2021).

Some neurons in V2 and V4 respond to end-stopped lines, to tongues flanked by inhibitory subregions, to combinations of lines, or to combinations of colors (Rolls and Deco,

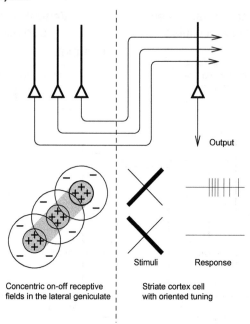

Fig. 2.5 Receptive fields in the lateral geniculate have concentric on-centre off-surround (or vice versa) receptive fields (left). Neurons in the striate cortex, such as the simple cell illustrated on the right, respond to elongated lines or edges at certain orientations. A suggestion that the lateral geniculate neurons might combine their responses in the way shown to produce orientation-selective simple cells was made by Hubel and Wiesel (1962).

2002; Hegde and Van Essen, 2000; Ito and Komatsu, 2004; Roe et al., 2012; Jiang et al., 2021)). *What* is computed here is useful as part of a feature hierarchy system for object recognition, as described below.

2.4 What: Invariant representations of faces and objects in the inferior temporal visual cortex

2.4.1 Reward value is not represented in the primate ventral visual system

The representation in the inferior temporal cortex is independent of whether the object is associated with reward or punishment, that is the representation is about objects per se (Rolls, Judge and Sanghera, 1977; Rolls, Aggelopoulos and Zheng, 2003a). This was shown in visual discrimination reversal experiments in which inferior temporal cortex neurons respond to an object independently of its association with reward vs punishment value, as illustrated in Fig. 2.6. It was also shown that IT neurons do not alter their responses after the reward value of a food-related visual stimulus is reduced to zero, by feeding to satiety (Rolls et al., 1977). Importantly, this is in contrast to what happens one synapse further on, in the orbitofrontal cortex, in the same test situations (Thorpe, Rolls and Maddison, 1983; Rolls, Critchley, Mason and Wakeman, 1996b; Critchley and Rolls, 1996a). As noted above, this clear separation of perceptual representations in the inferior temporal visual cortex from reward value (see Chapter 11) is a key feature of the organisation of primate perceptual systems (it is found in the taste and olfactory systems too, see Chapters 4 and 5), and ensures that we do not go blind to objects when their reward value is decreased to zero; and that we can learn about for example the location of objects even when their reward value is currently zero.

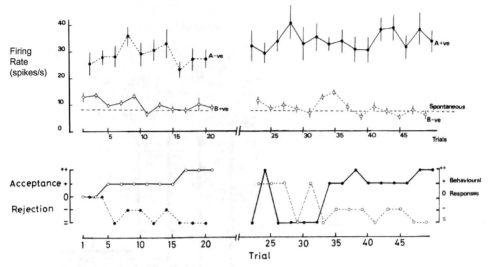

Fig. 2.6 Examples of the responses of a neuron in the inferior temporal visual cortex, showing that its responses (firing rate in spikes/s, upper panel) do not reverse when the reward association of the visual stimuli reverses. For the first 21 trials of the visual discrimination task, visual stimulus A was aversive (–ve, because if the monkey licked he obtained saline), and visual stimulus B was associated with reward (+ve, because if the monkey licked when he saw this stimulus, he obtained fruit juice). The neuron responded more to stimulus A than to stimulus B. After trial 21, the contingencies reversed (so that A was now +ve, and B –ve). The monkey learned the reversal correctly by about trial 35 (lower panel). However, the inferior temporal cortex neuron did not reverse when the reinforcement contingency reversed – it continued to respond to stimulus A after the reversal, even though the stimulus was now +ve. Thus this, and other inferior temporal cortex neurons, respond to the physical aspects of visual stimuli, and not to the stimuli based on their reinforcement association or the reinforcement contingency. (Reprinted from E. T. Rolls, S. J. Judge, and M. K. Sanghera (1977) Activity of neurones in the inferotemporal cortex of the alert monkey. Brain Research 130: 229–238. Copyright © Elsevier Ltd.)

2.4.2 Translation invariant representations

There is convergence from each small part of a region to the succeeding region (or layer in the hierarchy) in such a way that the receptive field sizes of neurons (for example 1 degree near the fovea in V1) become larger by a factor of approximately 2.5 with each succeeding stage (see Fig. 2.2). [The typical parafoveal receptive field sizes found would not be inconsistent with the calculated approximations of, for example, 8 degrees in V4, 20 degrees in TEO, and 50 degrees in anterior inferior temporal cortex (Boussaoud et al., 1991) (see Fig. 2.2).] Such zones of convergence would overlap continuously with each other (Fig. 2.2). This convergent connectivity provides part of the basis for the fact that many neurons in the temporal cortical visual areas respond to a stimulus relatively independently of where it is in their receptive field, and moreover maintain their stimulus selectivity when the stimulus appears in different parts of their large visual receptive field (Gross, Desimone, Albright and Schwartz, 1985; Tovee, Rolls and Azzopardi, 1994; Rolls, Aggelopoulos and Zheng, 2003a). This is called translation or shift invariance. In addition to having topologically appropriate connections, it is necessary for the connections to have the appropriate synaptic weights to perform the mapping of each set of features, or object, to the same set of neurons in IT. How this could be achieved is addressed in the computational neuroscience models described later in this Chapter and elsewhere (Wallis and Rolls, 1997; Rolls and Deco, 2002; Rolls and Stringer, 2006b; Stringer, Perry, Rolls and Proske, 2006; Rolls, 2012d, 2016b, 2021d).

64 | The ventral visual system

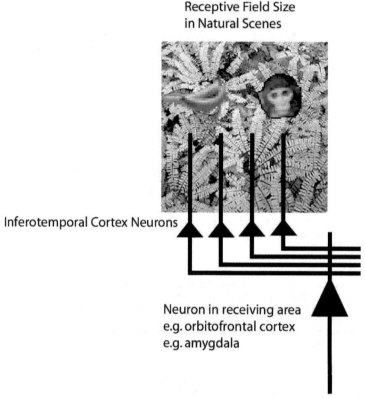

Fig. 2.7 Objects shown in a natural scene, in which the task was to search for and touch one of the stimuli. The objects in the task as run were smaller. The diagram shows that if the receptive fields of inferior temporal cortex neurons are large in natural scenes with multiple objects (in this scene, bananas and a face), then any receiving neuron in structures such as the orbitofrontal cortex and amygdala would receive information from many stimuli in the field of view, and would not be able to provide evidence about each of the stimuli separately.

2.4.3 Reduced translation invariance in natural scenes, and the selection of a rewarded object

Until recently, research on translation invariance considered the case in which there is only one object in the visual field. What happens in a cluttered, natural, environment? Do all objects that can activate an inferior temporal neuron do so whenever they are anywhere within the large receptive fields of inferior temporal neurons? If so, the output of the visual system might be confusing for structures that receive inputs from the temporal cortical visual areas. If one of the objects in the visual field was associated with reward, and another with punishment, would the output of the inferior temporal visual cortex to reward / emotion-related brain systems be an amalgam of both stimuli? If so, how would we be able to choose between the stimuli, and have an emotional response to one but not perhaps the other, and select one for action and not the other (see Fig. 2.7)?

In an investigation of this, it was found that even if an effective face was present in the parafovea, an IT neuron represented correctly (by a low firing rate) a non-effective face at the fovea (Rolls and Tovee, 1995a). This provides evidence that in situations with more than one stimulus present, IT neurons still represent what is at the fovea. This makes the interface to action simpler, in that what is at the fovea can be interpreted (e.g. by an associative memory) partly independently of the surroundings, and choices and actions can be directed if appropriate to what is at the fovea (cf. Ballard (1993)). These findings are a step towards understanding how the visual system functions in a normal environment (see also Gallant,

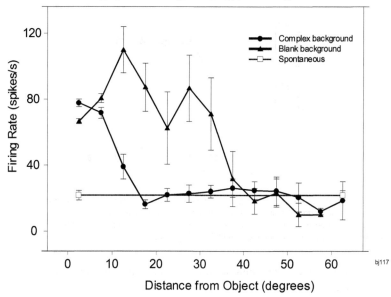

Fig. 2.8 Firing of a temporal cortex cell to an effective visual stimulus presented either in a blank background or in a natural scene, as a function of the angle in degrees at which the monkey was fixating away from the effective stimulus. The task was to search for and touch the stimulus. (After Rolls, E. T., Aggelopoulos,N.C. and Zheng,F. 2003 The receptive fields of inferior temporal cortex neurons in natural scenes. Journal of Neuroscience 23: 339–348.)

Connor and Van-Essen (1998), Stringer and Rolls (2000), Sheinberg and Logothetis (2001), and Rolls and Deco (2006)).

To investigate further how information is passed from the inferior temporal cortex (IT) to other brain regions to enable stimuli to be selected from natural scenes for action, Rolls, Aggelopoulos and Zheng (2003a) analyzed the responses of single and simultaneously recorded IT neurons to stimuli presented in complex natural backgrounds. In one situation, a visual fixation task was performed in which the monkey fixated at different distances from the effective stimulus. In another situation the monkey had to search for two objects on a screen, and a touch of one object was rewarded with juice, and of another object was punished with saline (see Fig. 2.7 for a schematic overview, and Fig. 2.69 on page 162 for the actual display). In both situations neuronal responses to the effective stimuli for the neurons were compared when the objects were presented in the natural scene or on a plain background. It was found that the overall response of the neuron to objects was sometimes somewhat reduced when they were presented in natural scenes, though the selectivity of the neurons remained. However, the main finding was that the magnitudes of the responses of the neurons typically became much less in the real scene the further the monkey fixated in the scene away from the object (see Figs. 2.8 and 2.70, and Section 2.8.9.1).

It is proposed that this reduced translation invariance in natural scenes helps an unambiguous representation of an object that may be the target for action to be passed to the brain regions that receive from the primate inferior temporal visual cortex. It helps with the binding problem, by reducing in natural scenes the effective receptive field of inferior temporal cortex neurons to approximately the size of an object in the scene. The computational utility and basis for this is considered in Section 2.8.9 and by Rolls and Deco (2002), Trappenberg, Rolls and Stringer (2002), Deco and Rolls (2004), Aggelopoulos and Rolls (2005), and Rolls and Deco (2006), and includes an advantage for what is at the fovea because of the large cortical

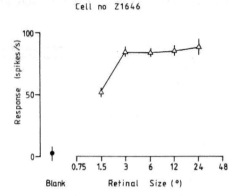

Fig. 2.9 Typical response of an inferior temporal cortex face-selective neuron to faces of different sizes. The size subtended at the retina in degrees is shown. (From Rolls,E.T. and Baylis,G.C. (1986) Size and contrast have only small effects on the responses to faces of neurons in the cortex of the superior temporal sulcus of the monkey. Experimental Brain Research 65: 38–48. Copyright © Springer Nature.)

magnification of the fovea, and shunting interactions between representations weighted by how far they are from the fovea.

These discoveries indicate that the principle of *what* is computed in the ventral visual system is to provide strong weight to whatever is close to the fovea in natural environments. This principle of operation is very important in interfacing the visual system to action systems, because the effective stimulus in making inferior temporal cortex neurons fire is in natural scenes usually on or close to the fovea. This means that the spatial coordinates of where the object is in the scene do not have to be represented in the inferior temporal visual cortex, nor passed from it to the action selection system, as the latter can assume that the object making IT neurons fire is close to the fovea in natural scenes. Thus the position in visual space being fixated provides part of the interface between sensory representations of objects and their coordinates as targets for actions in the world. The small receptive fields that include the fovea of IT neurons in natural scenes make this possible. After this, local, egocentric, processing implemented in the dorsal visual processing stream using e.g. stereodisparity may be used to guide action towards objects being fixated (Rolls and Deco, 2002; Rolls, 2016b) (see Section 3.4).

The reduced receptive field size in complex natural scenes also enables emotions to be selective to just what is being fixated, because this is the information that is transmitted by the firing of IT neurons to structures such as the orbitofrontal cortex and amygdala that are involved in emotion as described in Chapter 11.

Another principle of what is computed is that the whole scene is not processed simultaneously by the ventral visual system, as that greatly simplifies the process of object recognition. Successive fixations to different parts of the scene then enable a representation of a whole scene to be built up, over time, and to be held effectively in memory.

Interestingly, although the size of the receptive fields of inferior temporal cortex neurons become reduced in natural scenes so that neurons in IT respond primarily to the object being fixated, there is nevertheless frequently some asymmetry in the receptive fields (see Section 2.8.10 and Fig. 2.74). This provides a partial solution to how multiple objects and their position close to the fovea in a scene can be captured with a single glance (Aggelopoulos and Rolls, 2005), and is another principle of *what* is computed in the ventral visual system.

2.4.4 Size and spatial frequency invariance

It was discovered that some neurons in the inferior temporal visual cortex and cortex in the anterior part of the superior temporal sulcus (IT/STS) respond relatively independently of the size of an effective face stimulus, with a mean size invariance (to a half maximal response) of 12 times (3.5 octaves) (Rolls and Baylis, 1986). An example of the responses of an inferior temporal cortex face-selective neuron to faces of different sizes is shown in Fig. 2.9. This is not a property of a simple single-layer network (see Fig. 2.26), nor of neurons in V1, which respond best to small stimuli, with a typical size-invariance of 1.5 octaves. Also, the neurons typically continued to respond to a face when the information in it had been reduced from 3D to a 2D representation in grey on a monitor, with a response that was on average 0.5 of that to a real face.

Another transform over which recognition is relatively invariant is spatial frequency. For example, a face can be identified when it is blurred (when it contains only low spatial frequencies), and when it is high-pass spatial frequency filtered (when it looks like a line drawing). If the face images to which these neurons respond are low-pass filtered in the spatial frequency domain (so that they are blurred), then many of the neurons still respond when the images contain frequencies only up to 8 cycles per face. Similarly, the neurons still respond to high-pass filtered images (with only high spatial frequency edge information) when frequencies down to only 8 cycles per face are included (Rolls, Baylis and Leonard, 1985). Face recognition shows similar invariance with respect to spatial frequency (see Rolls, Baylis and Leonard (1985)). Further analysis of these neurons with narrow (octave) bandpass spatial frequency filtered face stimuli shows that the responses of these neurons to an unfiltered face can not be predicted from a linear combination of their responses to the narrow band stimuli (Rolls, Baylis and Hasselmo, 1987). This lack of linearity of these neurons, and their responsiveness to a wide range of spatial frequencies (see also their broad critical band masking (Rolls, 2008b)), indicate that in at least this part of the primate visual system recognition does not occur using Fourier analysis of the spatial frequency components of images.

The utility of *what* is computed in this representation for memory systems in the brain is that the output of the visual system will represent an object invariantly with respect to position on the retina, size, etc, and this simplifies the functionality required of the (multiple) memory systems, which need then to simply associate the object representation with reward (orbitofrontal cortex and amygdala), associate it with position in the environment (hippocampus), recognise it as familiar (perirhinal cortex), associate it with a motor response in a habit memory (basal ganglia), etc. (Rolls, 2007d, 2016b, 2012d, 2014a). The associations can be relatively simple, involving for example Hebbian associativity (see chapters throughout this book, and Appendix B).

It has been discovered that some neurons in the temporal cortical visual areas actually represent the absolute size of objects such as faces independently of viewing distance (Rolls and Baylis, 1986). This could be called neurophysiological size constancy. The utility of *what* is computed by this small population of neurons is that the absolute size of an object is a useful feature to use as an input to neurons that perform object recognition. Faces only come in certain sizes.

2.4.5 Combinations of features in the correct spatial configuration

Many neurons in this processing stream respond to combinations of features (including objects), but not to single features presented alone, and the features must have the correct spatial arrangement. This has been shown, for example, with faces, for which it was discovered by masking out or presenting parts of the face (for example eyes, mouth, or hair) in isolation, or by jumbling the features in faces, that some cells in the cortex in IT/STS respond only if two

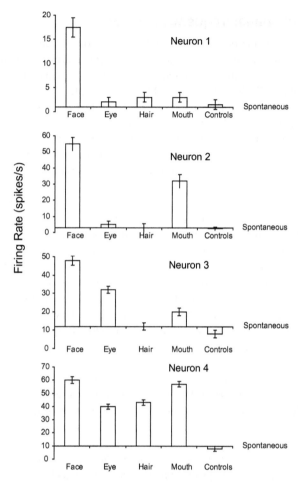

Fig. 2.10 Responses of four temporal cortex neurons to whole faces and to parts of faces. The mean firing rate ± sem are shown. The responses are shown as changes from the spontaneous firing rate of each neuron. Some neurons respond to one or several parts of faces presented alone. Other neurons (of which the top one is an example) respond only to the combination of the parts (and only if they are in the correct spatial configuration with respect to each other as shown by Rolls et al 1994b). The control stimuli were non-face objects. (After Perrett,D.I., Rolls, E. T. and Caan,W. (1982) Visual neurons responsive to faces in the monkey temporal cortex. Experimental Brain Research 47: 329–342.)

or more features are present, and are in the correct spatial arrangement (Perrett, Rolls and Caan, 1982; Rolls, Tovee, Purcell, Stewart and Azzopardi, 1994b). Fig. 2.10 shows examples of four neurons, the top one of which responds only if all the features are present, and the others of which respond not only to the full face, but also to one or more features. Corresponding evidence has been found for non-face cells. For example, Tanaka et al. (1990) showed that some posterior inferior temporal cortex neurons might only respond to the combination of an edge and a small circle if they were in the correct spatial relationship to each other.

Evidence consistent with the suggestion that neurons are responding to combinations of a few variables represented at the preceding stage of cortical processing is that some neurons in V2 and V4 respond to end-stopped lines, to tongues flanked by inhibitory subregions, to combinations of lines, or to combinations of colors (see Rolls and Deco (2002), Hegde and Van Essen (2000) and Ito and Komatsu (2004)). Neurons that respond to combinations of features but not to single features contained in those combinations indicate that the system is non-linear (Elliffe, Rolls and Stringer, 2002).

The fact that some temporal cortex neurons respond to objects or faces consisting of a set of features only if the whole combination of features is present and they are in the correct spatial arrangement with respect to each other (not jumbled) is part of the evidence that some inferior temporal cortex neurons are tuned to respond to objects or faces, and are part of a feature hierarchy system as described in Section 2.6.6.

If a task requires in addition to the normal representation of objects by the inferior temporal cortex, the ability to discriminate between stimuli composed of highly overlapping feature conjunctions in a low-dimensional feature space, then the perirhinal cortex may contribute to this type of discrimination, as described in Section 9.2.7.

2.4.6 A view-invariant representation

For recognizing and learning about objects (including faces), it is important that an output of the visual system should be not only translation- and size-invariant, but also relatively view-invariant. In an investigation of whether there are such neurons, we discovered that some temporal cortical neurons reliably responded differently to the faces of two different individuals independently of viewing angle (Hasselmo, Rolls, Baylis and Nalwa, 1989b) (see example in Fig. 2.11 upper), although in most cases (16/18 neurons) the response was not perfectly view-independent. Mixed together in the same cortical regions there are neurons with view-dependent responses (Hasselmo, Rolls, Baylis and Nalwa, 1989b; Rolls and Tovee, 1995b; Chang and Tsao, 2017) (see example in Fig. 2.11 lower)). Such neurons might respond, for example, to a view of a profile of a monkey but not to a full-face view of the same monkey (Perrett, Smith, Potter, Mistlin, Head, Milner and Jeeves, 1985b; Hasselmo, Rolls, Baylis and Nalwa, 1989b).

These discoveries of view-dependent, partially view-independent, and view-independent representations in the same cortical regions are consistent with the hypothesis discussed below that view-independent representations are being built in these regions by associating together the outputs of neurons that have different view-dependent responses to the same individual. These findings also provide evidence that one output of the visual system includes representations of what is being seen, in a view-independent way that would be useful for object recognition and for learning associations about objects; and that another output is a view-based representation that would be useful in social interactions to determine whether another individual is looking at one, and for selecting details of motor responses, for which the orientation of the object with respect to the viewer is required (Rolls and Deco, 2002; Rolls, 2016b).

Further evidence that some neurons in the temporal cortical visual areas have object-based rather than view-based responses comes from a study of a population of neurons that responds to moving faces (Hasselmo, Rolls, Baylis and Nalwa, 1989b). For example, four neurons responded vigorously to a head undergoing ventral flexion, irrespective of whether the view of the head was full face, of either profile, or even of the back of the head. These different views could only be specified as equivalent in object-based coordinates. Further, the movement specificity was maintained across inversion, with neurons responding for example to ventral flexion of the head irrespective of whether the head was upright or inverted (see example in Fig. 2.12). In this procedure, retinally encoded or viewer-centered movement vectors are reversed, but the object-based description remains the same.

Also consistent with object-based encoding is the discovery of a small number of neurons that respond to images of faces of a given absolute size, irrespective of the retinal image size or distance (Rolls and Baylis, 1986).

Neurons with view invariant responses to objects seen naturally in their home cages by macaques have also been discovered (Booth and Rolls, 1998). The stimuli were presented for 0.5 s on a color video monitor while the monkey performed a visual fixation task. The

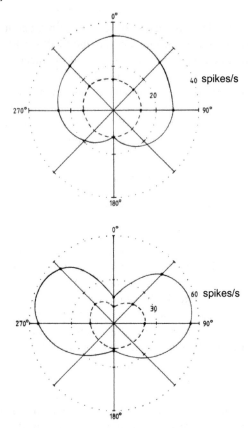

Fig. 2.11 Upper: View invariant response of an inferior temporal cortex neuron to two faces. In the polar response plot, 0° is the front of the face, and 90° the right profile. The firing rate in spikes/s is shown by the distance from the centre of the plot. The responses to two different faces are shown by the solid and dashed lines. The neuron discriminated between the faces, apart from the view of the back of the head. Lower: View dependent response of an inferior temporal cortex neuron to two faces. The neuron responded best to the left and right profiles. Some neurons respond to only one of the profiles, and this neuron had a small preference for the left profile. (After Hasselmo,M.E., Rolls, E. T., Baylis,G.C. and Nalwa,V. (1989) Object-centered encoding by face-selective neurons in the cortex in the superior temporal sulcus of the monkey. Experimental Brain Research 75: 417–429.)

stimuli were images of 10 real plastic objects that had been in the monkey's cage for several weeks, to enable him to build view invariant representations of the objects. Control stimuli were views of objects that had never been seen as real objects. The neurons analyzed were in the TE cortex in and close to the ventral lip of the anterior part of the superior temporal sulcus. Many neurons were found that responded to some views of some objects. However, for a smaller number of neurons, the responses occurred only to a subset of the objects (using ensemble encoding), irrespective of the viewing angle. Moreover, the firing of a neuron on any one trial, taken at random and irrespective of the particular view of any one object, provided information about which object had been seen, and this information increased approximately linearly with the number of neurons in the sample (see Fig. 2.13). This is strong quantitative evidence that some neurons in the inferior temporal cortex provide an invariant representation of objects. Moreover, the results of Booth and Rolls (1998) show that the information is available in the firing rates, and has all the desirable properties of distributed representations described above, including exponentially high coding capacity, and rapid speed of readout of the information.

Further evidence consistent with these findings is that some studies have shown that the responses of some visual neurons in the inferior temporal cortex do not depend on the pres-

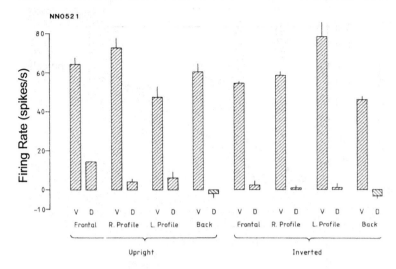

Fig. 2.12 Object-centred encoding: Neuron responding to ventral flexion (V) of the head independently of view even when the head was inverted. Ventral flexion is tilting the head from the full frontal view forwards to face down at 45 degrees. Dorsal flexion is tilting the head until it is looking 45 degrees up. The response is shown as a change in firing rate in spikes/s ± sem from the spontaneous firing rate. (After Hasselmo,M.E., Rolls, E. T., Baylis,G.C. and Nalwa,V. (1989) Object-centered encoding by face-selective neurons in the cortex in the superior temporal sulcus of the monkey. Experimental Brain Research 75: 417–429.)

ence or absence of critical features for maximal activation (Perrett, Rolls and Caan, 1982; Tanaka, 1993, 1996). For example, the responses of neuron 4 in Fig. 2.10 responded to several of the features in a face when these features were presented alone (Perrett, Rolls and Caan, 1982). In another example, Mikami, Nakamura and Kubota (1994) showed that some TE cells respond to partial views of the same laboratory instrument(s), even when these partial views contain different features. Such functionality is important for object recognition when part of an object is occluded, by for example another object. In a different approach, Logothetis, Pauls, Bulthoff and Poggio (1994) have reported that in monkeys extensively trained (over thousands of trials) to treat different views of computer generated wire-frame 'objects' as the same, a small population of neurons in the inferior temporal cortex did respond to different views of the same wire-frame object (see also Logothetis and Sheinberg (1996)). However, extensive training is not necessary for invariant representations to be formed, and indeed no explicit training in invariant object recognition was given in the experiment by Booth and Rolls (1998), as Rolls' hypothesis (1992a) is that view invariant representations can be learned by associating together the different views of objects as they are moved and inspected naturally in a period that may be in the order of a few seconds. Evidence for this is described in Section 2.4.7.

2.4.7 Learning of new representations in the temporal cortical visual areas

To investigate the idea that visual experience might guide the formation of the responsiveness of neurons so that they provide an economical and ensemble-encoded representation of items actually present in the environment, the responses of inferior temporal cortex face-selective neurons have been analyzed while a set of new faces were shown. Some of the neurons studied in this way altered the relative degree to which they responded to the different members of the set of novel faces over the first few (1–2) presentations of the set (Rolls, Baylis, Hasselmo and Nalwa, 1989a) (see examples in Fig. 2.14). If in a different experiment a single novel face

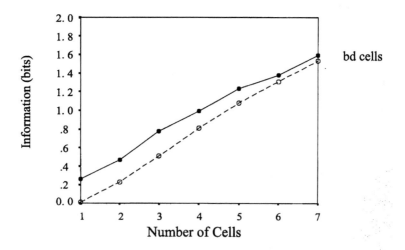

Fig. 2.13 View-independent object encoding: information in a population of different numbers of inferior temporal cortex cells available from a single trial, in which one view was shown, about which of 10 objects each with 4 different views in the stimulus set had been seen. The solid symbols show the information decoded with a Bayesian probability estimator algorithm, and the open symbols with dot product decoding. (After Booth,M.C.A. and Rolls, E. T. (1998) View-invariant representations of familiar objects by neurons in the inferior temporal visual cortex. Cerebral Cortex 8: 510–523.)

was introduced when the responses of a neuron to a set of familiar faces were being recorded, the responses to the set of familiar faces were not disrupted, while the responses to the novel face became stable within a few presentations. Alteration of the tuning of individual neurons in this way may result in a good discrimination over the population as a whole of the faces known to the monkey. This evidence is consistent with the categorization being performed by self-organizing competitive neuronal networks, as described in Section B.4. Consistent findings have been described more recently (Freedman, 2015).

Further evidence that these neurons can learn new representations very rapidly comes from an experiment in which binarized black and white (two-tone) images of faces that blended with the background were used (see Fig. 2.15, left). These did not activate face-selective neurons. Full grey-scale images of the same photographs were then shown for ten 0.5 s presentations (Fig. 2.15, middle). In a number of cases, if the neuron happened to be responsive to that face, when the binarized version of the same face was shown next (Fig. 2.15, right), the neurons responded to it (Tovee, Rolls and Ramachandran, 1996). This is a direct parallel to the same phenomenon that is observed psychophysically, and provides dramatic evidence that these neurons are influenced by only a very few seconds (in this case 5 s) of experience with a visual stimulus (Tovee et al., 1996). We have shown a neural correlate of this effect using similar stimuli and a similar paradigm in a PET (positron emission tomography) neuroimaging study in humans, with a region showing an effect of the learning found for faces in the right temporal lobe, and for objects in the left temporal lobe (Dolan, Fink, Rolls, Booth, Holmes, Frackowiak and Friston, 1997).

The discovery that inferior temporal visual cortex neurons can learn rapidly in an unsupervised way to categorise new objects or faces (Rolls, Baylis, Hasselmo and Nalwa, 1989a) has been confirmed, with size invariance requiring temporal contiguity (Li and DiCarlo, 2010) as predicted by the VisNet model of memory trace rule dependent learning and related psychophysics (Perry, Rolls and Stringer, 2006), and it has been confirmed that reward is not necessary for this type of self-organising learning of invariant representations (Li and DiCarlo, 2012). The psychophysical discovery of the importance in humans of associations over time

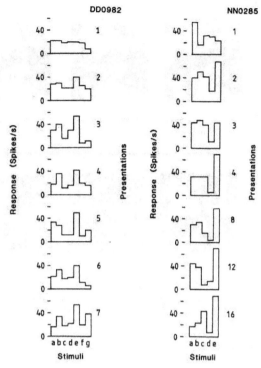

Fig. 2.14 Learning in the responses of inferior temporal cortex neurons. Results for two face-selective neurons are shown. On presentation 1 a set of 7 completely novel faces was shown when recording from neuron DD0982. The firing rates elicited on 1-sec presentations of each stimulus (a-g) are shown. After the first presentation, the set of stimuli was repeated in random sequence for a total of 7 iterations. After the first two presentations, the relative responses of the neuron to the different stimuli settled down to a fairly reliable response profile to the set of stimuli (as shown by statistical analysis). NN0285 – data from a similar experiment with another neuron, and another completely new set of face stimuli. (After Rolls, E. T., Baylis,G.C. Hasselmo,M.E. and Nalwa,V. (1989) The effect of learning on the face-selective responses of neurons in the cortex in the superior temporal sulcus of the monkey. Experimental Brain Research 76: 153–164.)

for helping to build invariant object representations (Perry, Rolls and Stringer, 2006) has been confirmed in further psychophysical investigations in humans (Jia, Hong and DiCarlo, 2021).

Such rapid learning of representations of new objects appears to be a major type of learning in which the temporal cortical areas are involved. Ways in which this learning could occur are considered later in this Chapter. In addition, some of these neurons may be involved in a short term memory for whether a particular familiar visual stimulus (such as a face) has been seen recently. The evidence for this is that some of these neurons respond differently to recently seen stimuli in visual memory tasks (Baylis and Rolls, 1987; Miller and Desimone, 1994; Xiang and Brown, 1998). In the inferior temporal visual cortex proper, neurons respond more to novel than to familiar stimuli, but treat the stimuli as novel if one or more other stimuli intervene between the first (novel) and second (familiar) presentations of a particular stimulus (Baylis and Rolls, 1987). More ventrally, in what is in or close to the perirhinal cortex, these memory spans may hold for several intervening stimuli in the same task (Xiang and Brown, 1998) (see Section 9.2.7). Some neurons in these areas respond more when a sample stimulus reappears in a delayed match to sample task with intervening stimuli (Miller and Desimone, 1994), and the basis for this using a short term memory implemented in the prefrontal cortex is described in Section 13.6.1. Neurons in the more ventral (perirhinal) cortical area respond

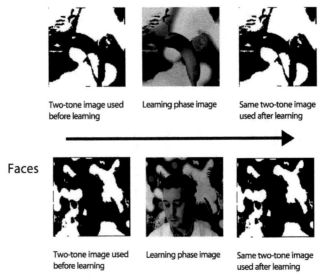

Fig. 2.15 Images of the type used to investigate rapid learning in the neurophysiological experiments of Tovee, Rolls and Ramachandran (1996) and the PET imaging study of Dolan, Fink, Rolls et al. (1997). When the black and white (two-tone) images at the left are shown, the objects or faces are not generally recognized. After the full grey scale images (middle) have been shown for a few seconds, humans and inferior temporal cortex neurons respond to the faces or objects in the black and white images (right).

during the delay in a match to sample task with a delay between the sample stimulus and the to-be-matched stimulus (Miyashita, 1993; Renart, Parga and Rolls, 2000) (see Section 9.2.7).

2.4.8 A sparse distributed representation is what is computed in the ventral visual system

An important question for understanding brain function is whether a particular object (or face) is represented in the brain by the firing of one or a few gnostic (or 'grandmother') cells (see Barlow (1972)), or whether instead the firing of a group or ensemble of cells each with somewhat different responsiveness provides the representation. We tested this experimentally, and discovered that *what* is computed in the ventral visual system is a sparse distributed representation of objects and faces of a type that can easily be read by neurons in the next brain areas, as described next. Advantages of distributed codes include generalization and graceful degradation (fault tolerance), and a potentially very high capacity in the number of stimuli that can be represented (that is exponential growth of capacity with the number of neurons in the representation) (see Appendix B, Rolls and Treves (1998), Rolls (2016b), and Rolls and Treves (2011)). If the ensemble encoding is sparse, this provides a good input to an associative memory, for then large numbers of stimuli can be stored (see Appendix B, Chapters 2 and 3 of Rolls and Treves (1998), and Rolls (2016b)). A quantitative analysis of information encoding by inferior temporal cortex neurons and by neurons in other brain areas is provided in Appendix B.

We discovered that in the inferior temporal visual cortex and cortex in the anterior part of the superior temporal sulcus (IT/STS), responses of a group of neurons, but not of a single neuron, provide evidence about which face was shown. We showed, for example, that these neurons typically respond with a graded set of firing rates to different faces, with firing rates from 120 spikes/s to the most effective face, to no response at all to a number of the least effective faces (Baylis, Rolls and Leonard, 1985; Rolls and Tovee, 1995b; Rolls, 2016b). In

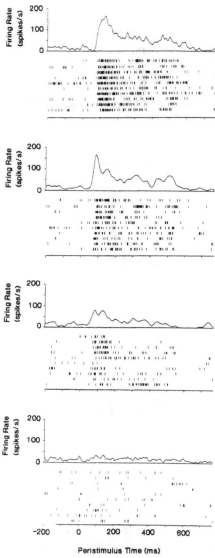

Fig. 2.16 Peristimulus time histograms and rastergrams showing the responses on different trials (originally in random order) of a face-selective neuron in the inferior temporal visual cortex to four different faces. (In the rastergrams each vertical line represents one spike from the neuron, and each row is a separate trial. Each block of the Figure is for a different face.) (Reproduced from M. J. Tovee, E. T. Rolls, A. Treves, and R. P. Bellis. (1993) Information encoding and the responses of single neurons in the primate temporal visual cortex. Journal of Neurophysiology 70: 640–654. © The American Physiological Society.)

fact, the firing rate probability distribution of a single neuron to a set of stimuli is approximately exponential (Rolls and Tovee, 1995b; Treves, Panzeri, Rolls, Booth and Wakeman, 1999; Rolls, 2016b; Baddeley, Abbott, Booth, Sengpiel, Freeman, Wakeman and Rolls, 1997; Franco, Rolls, Aggelopoulos and Jerez, 2007). To provide examples, Fig. 2.16 shows typical firing rate changes of a single neuron on different trials to each of several different faces. This makes it clear that from the firing rate on any one trial, information is available about which stimulus was shown, and that the firing rate is graded, with a different firing rate response of the neuron to each stimulus.

The distributed nature of the encoding typical for neurons in the inferior temporal visual cortex is illustrated in Fig. 2.17, which shows that temporal cortical neurons typically re-

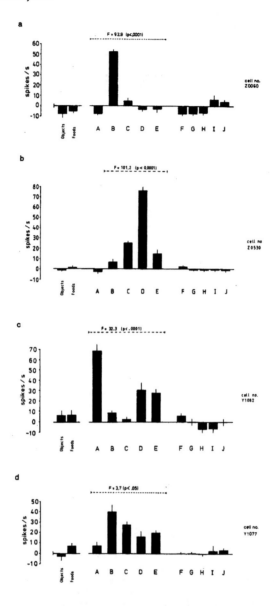

Fig. 2.17 Responses of four different temporal cortex visual neurons to a set of five faces (A–E), and, for comparison, to a wide range of non-face objects and foods. F–J are non-face stimuli. The means and standard errors of the responses computed over 8–10 trials are shown. (Reprinted from G.C. Baylis, E.T. Rolls, C.M. Leonard. (1985) Selectivity between faces in the responses of a population of neurons in the cortex in the superior temporal sulcus of the monkey. Brain Research 342: 91–102. Copyright © Elsevier Ltd.)

sponded to several members of a set of five faces, with each neuron having a different profile of responses to each face (Baylis, Rolls and Leonard, 1985). It would be difficult for most of these single cells to tell which of even five faces, let alone which of hundreds of faces, had been seen. Yet across a population of such neurons, much information about the particular face that has been seen is provided, as shown below.

The single neuron selectivity or sparseness a^s of the activity of inferior temporal cortex neurons was 0.65 over a set of 68 stimuli including 23 faces and 45 non-face natural scenes, and a measure called the response sparseness a_r^s of the representation, in which the spon-

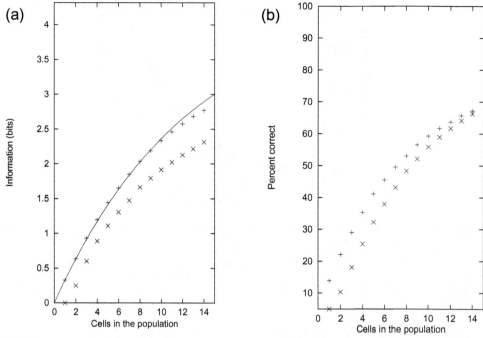

Fig. 2.18 (a) The values for the average information available in the responses of different numbers of inferior temporal visual cortex neurons on each trial, about which one of a set of 20 face stimuli has been shown. The decoding method was Dot Product (DP, ×) or Probability Estimation (PE, +). The full line indicates the amount of information expected from populations of increasing size, when assuming random correlations within the constraint given by the ceiling (the information in the stimulus set, I = 4.32 bits). (b) The percent correct for the corresponding data to those shown in (a). The measurement period was 500 ms. (After Rolls, E. T., Treves, A. and Tovee, M.J. (1997) The representational capacity of the distributed encoding of information provided by populations of neurons in the primate temporal visual cortex. Experimental Brain Research 114: 149–162.)

taneous rate was subtracted from the firing rate to each stimulus so that the responses of the neuron were being assessed, was 0.38 across the same set of stimuli (Rolls and Tovee, 1995b). [For the definition of sparseness see Section C.3.1, and Appendix B. For binary neurons (firing for example either at a high rate or not at all), the single neuron sparseness is the proportion of stimuli that a single neuron responds to. These definitions, and what is found in cortical neuronal representations, are described further elsewhere (Franco, Rolls, Aggelopoulos and Jerez, 2007; Rolls and Treves, 2011; Rolls, 2016b).]

It has been possible to apply information theory (see Appendix C) to show that each neuron conveys on average approximately 0.4 bits of information about which face in a set of 20 faces has been seen (Tovee and Rolls, 1995; Tovee, Rolls, Treves and Bellis, 1993; Rolls, Treves, Tovee and Panzeri, 1997d). If a neuron responded to only one of the faces in the set of 20, then it could convey (if noiseless) 4.6 bits of (stimulus-specific) information about one of the faces (when that face was shown). If, at the other extreme, it responded to half the faces in the set, it would convey 1 bit of information about which face had been seen on any one trial. In fact, the average maximum (stimulus-specific) information about the best stimulus was 1.8 bits of information. This provides good evidence not only that the representation is distributed, but also that it is a sufficiently reliable representation that useful information can be obtained from it.

An important discovery is that when the information available from a population of neurons about which of 20 faces has been seen is considered, the information increases approximately linearly as the number of neurons in the population increases from 1 to 14 (Rolls,

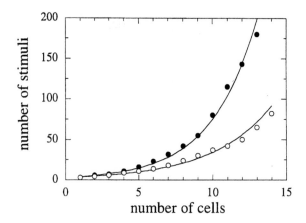

Fig. 2.19 The number of stimuli (in this case from a set of 20 faces) that are encoded in the responses of different numbers of neurons in the temporal lobe visual cortex, based on the results shown in Fig. 2.18. The solid circles are the result of the raw calculation, and the open circles correspond to the cross-validated case. (After Rolls, E. T., Treves,A. and Tovee,M.J. (1997) The representational capacity of the distributed encoding of information provided by populations of neurons in the primate temporal visual cortex. Experimental Brain Research 114: 149–162; and Abbott,L.F., Rolls, E. T. and Tovee,M.J. (1996) Representational capacity of face coding in monkeys. Cerebral Cortex 6: 498–505.)

Treves and Tovee, 1997b; Abbott, Rolls and Tovee, 1996) (see Fig. 2.18 and Section C.3.5). Remembering that the information in bits is a logarithmic measure, this shows that the representational capacity of this population of cells increases exponentially (see Fig. 2.19). This is the case both when an optimal, probability estimation, form of decoding of the activity of the neuronal population is used, and also when the neurally plausible dot product type of decoding is used (Fig. 2.18). (The dot product decoding assumes that what reads out the information from the population activity vector is a neuron or a set of neurons that operates just by forming the dot product of the input population vector and its synaptic weight vector – see Rolls, Treves and Tovee (1997b), and Appendix B.) By simulation of further neurons and further stimuli, we have shown that the capacity grows very impressively, approximately as shown in Fig. 2.19 (Abbott, Rolls and Tovee, 1996). The result has been replicated with simultaneously recorded neurons (Rolls, Franco, Aggelopoulos and Reece, 2003b; Rolls, Aggelopoulos, Franco and Treves, 2004; Rolls, 2016b). This result is exactly what would be hoped for from a distributed representation. This result is not what would be expected for local encoding, for which the number of stimuli that could be encoded would increase linearly with the number of cells. (Even if the grandmother cells were noisy, adding more replicates to increase reliability would not lead to more than a linear increase in the number of stimuli that can be encoded as a function of the number of cells.) Moreover, the encoding in the inferior temporal visual cortex about objects remains based on the spike count from each neuron, and not on the relative time of firing of each neuron or stimulus-dependent synchronization, when analyzed with simultaneous single neuron recording (Rolls, Franco, Aggelopoulos and Reece, 2003b; Rolls, Aggelopoulos, Franco and Treves, 2004; Franco, Rolls, Aggelopoulos and Treves, 2004) even in natural scenes when an attentional task is being performed (Aggelopoulos, Franco and Rolls, 2005). Further, we discovered that much of the information is available in short times of e.g. 20 or 50 ms (Tovee and Rolls, 1995; Rolls, Franco, Aggelopoulos and Jerez, 2006b), so that the receiving neuron does not need to integrate over a long time period to estimate a firing rate.

These findings, provided more fully and with equations in Appendix C, provide very firm evidence that the encoding built at the end of the visual system is distributed, and that part of the power of this representation is that by receiving inputs from relatively small numbers

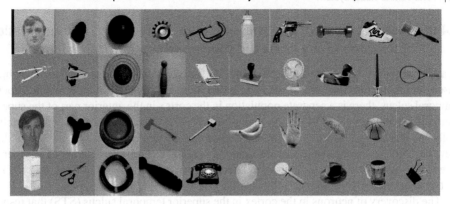

Fig. 2.20 Some examples of the objects and faces encoded by anterior inferior temporal cortex neurons (see text, and further examples in Fig. C.7).

of such neurons, neurons at the next stage of processing (for example in memory structures such as the hippocampus, amygdala, and orbitofrontal cortex) would obtain information about which of a very great number of objects or faces had been shown (Rolls and Treves, 2011).

In this sense, the inferior temporal visual cortex provides a representation of objects and faces, in which information about which object or face is shown is made explicit in the firing of the neurons in such a way that the information can be read off very simply by memory systems such as the orbitofrontal cortex, amygdala, and perirhinal cortex / hippocampal systems. The information can be read off using dot product decoding, that is by using a synaptically weighted sum of inputs from inferior temporal cortex neurons (see further Rolls (2016b) and Section 9.2.7). Examples of some of the types of objects and faces that are encoded in this way by anterior inferior temporal cortex neurons are shown in Fig. 2.20.

This representational capacity of neuronal populations has fundamental implications for the connectivity of the brain, for it shows that neurons need not have hundreds of thousands or millions of inputs to have available to them information about what is represented in another population of cells, but that instead the real numbers of perhaps 8,000–10,000 synapses per neuron would be adequate for them to receive considerable information from the several different sources between which this set of synapses is allocated.

It may be noted that it is unlikely that there are further processing areas beyond those described where ensemble coding changes into grandmother cell encoding. Anatomically, there does not appear to be a whole further set of visual processing areas present in the brain; and outputs from the temporal lobe visual areas such as those described are taken directly to limbic and related regions such as the amygdala and orbitofrontal cortex, and via the perirhinal and entorhinal cortex to the hippocampus (see Chapter 9, Rolls (2000a), Rolls (2016b), and Rolls (2011d)). Indeed, tracing this pathway onwards, we have found a population of neurons with face-selective responses in the amygdala, and in the majority of these neurons, different responses occur to different faces, with ensemble (not local) coding still being present (Leonard, Rolls, Wilson and Baylis, 1985). The amygdala, in turn, projects to another structure that may be important in other behavioral responses to faces, the ventral striatum, and comparable neurons have also been found in the ventral striatum (Williams, Rolls, Leonard and Stern, 1993). We have also recorded from face-responding neurons in the part of the orbitofrontal cortex that receives from the IT/STS cortex, and discovered that the encoding there is also not local but is distributed (Rolls, Critchley, Browning and Inoue, 2006a).

2.4.9 Face expression, gesture, and view represented in a population of neurons in the cortex in the superior temporal sulcus

In addition to the population of neurons that code for face identity, which tend to have object-based representations and are in areas TEa and TEm on the ventral bank of the superior temporal sulcus, there is a separate population in the cortex in the anterior part of the superior temporal sulcus (e.g. area TPO) that conveys information about facial expression (Hasselmo, Rolls and Baylis, 1989a) (see e.g. Fig. 2.21). Some of the neurons in this region tend to have view-based representations (so that information is conveyed for example about whether the face is looking at one, or is looking away), and might respond to moving faces, and to facial gesture (Hasselmo, Rolls, Baylis and Nalwa, 1989b).

The discovery of neurons in the cortex in the superior temporal sulcus (STS) that respond to face expression, face and head movement, and social signals such as breaking eye contact by closing the eyes or by turning the head to break eye contact (Baylis, Rolls and Leonard, 1987; Hasselmo, Rolls and Baylis, 1989a; Hasselmo, Rolls, Baylis and Nalwa, 1989b) led to the proposal that these cortical regions are involved in social behavior. That proposal has now been accepted (Pitcher and Ungerleider, 2021). The discoveries also led to the proposal that this visual cortical stream involved a combination of information from the ventral and dorsal visual streams (Hasselmo, Rolls and Baylis, 1989a; Hasselmo, Rolls, Baylis and Nalwa, 1989b), and that also has been accepted (Pitcher and Ungerleider, 2021). The connectivity that underlies this convergence in humans (Rolls et al., 2023e) is described in Section 2.5. This STS system has been proposed to be the source of the inputs to neurons in the primate orbitofrontal cortex that have similar responses to socially relevant face expression and gesture (Rolls, Critchley, Browning and Inoue, 2006a). These neurons in the orbitofrontal cortex are likely to be important in social and emotional responses to faces, in that face and voice expression processing is impaired by damage to the human orbitofrontal cortex (Hornak, Rolls and Wade, 1996; Hornak, Bramham, Rolls, Morris, O'Doherty, Bullock and Polkey, 2003). Impairments of processing in this STS visual stream have been implicated in autism by the lower functional connectivity of these STS cortical regions in people with autism spectrum disorder (Cheng, Rolls, Gu, Zhang and Feng, 2015; Cheng, Rolls, Zhang, Sheng, Ma, Wan, Luo and Feng, 2016b; Rolls, Zhou, Cheng, Gilson, Deco and Feng, 2020f).

Thus information in cortical areas that project to the amygdala and orbitofrontal cortex includes information about face identity, and about face expression and gesture (Rolls, Critchley, Browning and Inoue, 2006a; Leonard, Rolls, Wilson and Baylis, 1985; Rolls, 2011d). Both types of information are important in social and emotional responses to other primates (including humans), which must be based on who the individual is as well as on the face expression or gesture being made (Rolls, 2014a). One output from the amygdala for this information is probably via the ventral striatum, for a small population of neurons has been found in the ventral striatum with responses selective for faces (Rolls and Williams, 1987a; Williams, Rolls, Leonard and Stern, 1993).

2.4.10 Specialized regions in the temporal cortical visual areas

As we have just seen, some neurons respond to face identity, and others to face expression (Hasselmo, Rolls and Baylis, 1989a; Rolls, 2011d, 2014a). The neurons responsive to expression were found primarily in the cortex in the superior temporal sulcus, while the neurons responsive to identity were found in the inferior temporal gyrus. In more detail, the face-selective neurons described in this book are found mainly between 7 mm and 3 mm posterior to the sphenoid reference, which in a 3–4 kg macaque corresponds to approximately 11 to 15 mm anterior to the interaural plane (Baylis, Rolls and Leonard, 1987; Rolls, 2007e,c, 2011d,

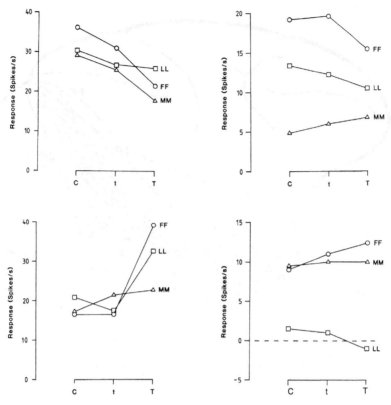

Fig. 2.21 There is a population of neurons in the cortex in the superior temporal sulcus (STS) with responses tuned to respond differently to different face expressions. The cells in the two left panels did not discriminate between individuals (faces MM, FF, and LL), but did discriminate between different expressions on the faces of those individuals (C, calm expression; t, mild threat; T, strong threat). In contrast, the cells in the right two panels responded differently to different individuals, and did not discriminate between different expressions. The neurons that discriminated between expressions were found mainly in the cortex in the fundus of the superior temporal sulcus; the neurons that discriminated between identity were in contrast found mainly in the cortex in the lateral part of the ventral lip of the superior temporal sulcus (areas TEa and TEm). (Reproduced with permission from Michael E. Hasselmo, Edmund T. Rolls and Gordon C. Baylis (1989) The role of expression and identity in the face-selective responses of neurons in the temporal visual cortex of the monkey. Copyright © 1989 Elsevier Ltd.)

2012d). The 'middle face patch' of Tsao, Freiwald, Tootell and Livingstone (2006) was at A6, which is probably part of the posterior inferior temporal cortex. In the anterior inferior temporal cortex areas we have investigated, there are separate regions specialized for face identity in areas TEa and TEm on the ventral lip of the superior temporal sulcus and the adjacent gyrus, and for face expression and movement in the cortex deep in the superior temporal sulcus (Hasselmo, Rolls and Baylis, 1989a; Baylis, Rolls and Leonard, 1987; Rolls, 2007e, 2011d, 2012d) (see Sections 2.4.9 and 2.4.10).

A further way in which some of these neurons in the cortex in the superior temporal sulcus may be involved in social interactions is that some of them respond to gestures, for example to a face undergoing ventral flexion (i.e. the head bending at the neck forwards and down) (Perrett, Smith, Potter, Mistlin, Head, Milner and Jeeves, 1985b; Hasselmo, Rolls, Baylis and Nalwa, 1989b). The interpretation of these neurons as being useful for social interactions is that in some cases these neurons respond not only to ventral head flexion, but also to the eyes lowering and the eyelids closing (Hasselmo, Rolls, Baylis and Nalwa, 1989b). These movements (turning the head away, breaking eye contact, and eyelid lowering) often occur

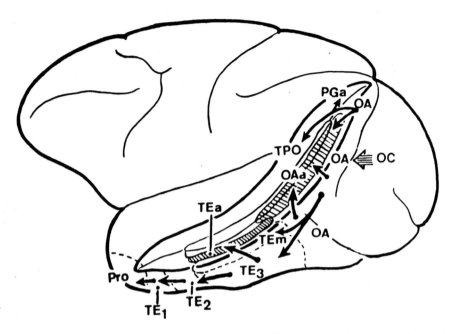

Fig. 2.22 Lateral view of the macaque brain (left hemisphere) showing the different architectonic areas (e.g. TEm, TEa) in and bordering the anterior part of the superior temporal sulcus (STS) of the macaque (see text). The STS has been drawn opened to reveal to reveal the cortical areas inside it, and is circumscribed by a thick line. (From Seltzer,B. and Pandya,D.N. (1978) Afferent cortical connections and architectonics of the superior temporal sulcus and surrounding cortex in the rhesus monkey. Brain Research 149: 1–24. Copyright © Elsevier Ltd.)

together when a monkey is breaking social contact with another, and neurons that respond to these components could be built by associative synaptic modification. It is also important when decoding facial expression to retain some information about the direction of the head relative to the observer, for this is very important in determining whether a threat is being made in your direction. The presence of view–dependent, head and body gesture (Hasselmo, Rolls, Baylis and Nalwa, 1989b), and eye gaze (Perrett, Smith, Potter, Mistlin, Head, Milner and Jeeves, 1985b), representations in some of these cortical regions where face expression is represented is consistent with this requirement. In contrast, the TE areas (more ventral, mainly in the macaque inferior temporal gyrus), in which neurons tuned to face identity (Hasselmo, Rolls and Baylis, 1989a) and with view–independent responses (Hasselmo, Rolls, Baylis and Nalwa, 1989b) are more likely to be found, may be more related to an object–based representation of identity. Of course, for appropriate social and emotional responses, both types of subsystem would be important, for it is necessary to know both the direction of a social gesture, and the identity of the individual, in order to make the correct social or emotional response (Rolls, 2014a).

Further evidence for specialization of function in the different architectonically defined areas of the temporal cortex (Seltzer and Pandya, 1978) (see Fig. 2.22) was found by Baylis, Rolls and Leonard (1987). Areas TPO, PGa and IPa are multimodal, with neurons that respond to visual, auditory and/or somatosensory inputs. The more ventral areas in the inferior temporal gyrus (areas TE3, TE2, TE1, TEa and TEm) are primarily unimodal visual areas. Areas in the cortex in the anterior and dorsal part of the superior temporal sulcus (e.g. TPO, IPa and IPg) have neurons specialized for the analysis of moving visual stimuli. Neurons responsive primarily to faces are found more frequently in areas TPO, TEa and TEm, where they comprise approximately 20% of the visual neurons responsive to stationary stimuli, in contrast to the other temporal cortical areas in which they comprise 4–10%. The stimuli that activate other cells in these TE regions include simple visual patterns such as gratings, and combinations of simple stimulus features (Gross, Desimone, Albright and Schwartz, 1985; Baylis, Rolls and Leonard, 1987; Tanaka, Saito, Fukada and Moriya, 1990). If patches are identified by fMRI, the proportion of neurons tuned to for example faces may be high (Tsao, Freiwald, Tootell and Livingstone, 2006; Freiwald, Tsao and Livingstone, 2009; Tsao, 2014; Freiwald, 2020; Arcaro and Livingstone, 2021). Due to the fact that face-selective neurons have a wide distribution (Baylis, Rolls and Leonard, 1987), and also occur in different patches (Tsao et al., 2006; Tsao, 2014), it might be expected that only large lesions, or lesions that interrupt outputs of these visual areas, would produce readily apparent face-processing deficits.

Another specialization is that areas TEa and TEm, which receive inter alia from the cortex in the intraparietal sulcus, have neurons that are tuned to binocular disparity, so that information derived from stereopsis about the 3D structure of objects is represented in the inferior temporal cortical visual areas (Janssen, Vogels and Orban, 1999, 2000). Interestingly, these neurons respond only when the black and white regions in the two eyes are correlated (that is, when a white patch in one eye corresponds to a white patch in the other eye) (Janssen et al., 2003). This corresponds to what we see perceptually and consciously. In contrast, in V1, MT and MST, depth-tuned neurons can respond to anticorrelated depth images, that is where white in one eye corresponds to black in the other (Parker, Cumming and Dodd, 2000; DeAngelis, Cumming and Newsome, 2000; Parker, 2007), and this may be suitable for eye movement control, but much less for shape and object discrimination and identification. It may be expected that other depth cues, such as perspective, surface shading, and occlusion, affect the response properties of some neurons in inferior temporal cortex visual areas. Binocular disparity, and information from these other depth cues, may be used to compute the absolute size of objects, which is represented independently of the distance of the object for a small proportion of inferior temporal cortex neurons (Rolls and Baylis, 1986). Knowing the absolute size of an object is useful evidence to include in the identification of an object. Although cues from binocular disparity can thus drive some temporal cortex visual neurons, and there is a small proportion of inferior temporal neurons that respond better to real faces and objects than to 2D representations on a monitor, it is found that the majority of TE neurons respond as well or almost as well to 2D images on a video monitor as to real faces or objects (Perrett, Rolls and Caan, 1982). Moreover, the tuning of inferior temporal cortex neurons to images of faces or objects on a video monitor is similar to that to real objects (personal observations of E. T. Rolls).

Neuroimaging data in humans, while not being able to address the details of what is encoded in a brain area or of how it is encoded, does provide evidence consistent with the neurophysiology that there are different face processing systems in the human brain, and different processing subsystems for faces, objects, moving objects, scenes, and agents performing actions (Spiridon, Fischl and Kanwisher, 2006; Grill-Spector and Malach, 2004; Epstein and Kanwisher, 1998; Morin, Hadj-Bouziane, Stokes, Ungerleider and Bell, 2015; Nasr, Liu, Devaney, Yue, Rajimehr, Ungerleider and Tootell, 2011; Weiner and Grill-Spector, 2015; Deen, Koldewyn, Kanwisher and Saxe, 2015; Pitcher, Ianni and Ungerleider, 2019; Zhang, Japee, Stacy, Flessert and Ungerleider, 2020; Haxby, Gobbini and Nastase, 2020; Pitcher and Ungerleider, 2021). For example, Kanwisher, McDermott and Chun (1997) and Ishai, Ungerleider, Martin, Schouten and Haxby (1999) have shown activation by faces of an area in the fusiform gyrus; Hoffman and Haxby (2000) have shown that distinct areas are activated by eye gaze and face identity; Dolan, Fink, Rolls, Booth, Holmes, Frackowiak and Friston (1997) have shown that a fusiform gyrus area becomes activated after humans learn to identify faces in complex scenes; and the amygdala (Morris, Fritch, Perrett, Rowland, Young, Calder and Dolan, 1996) and orbitofrontal cortex (Blair, Morris, Frith, Perrett and Dolan, 1999; Rolls,

2014a) may become activated particularly by certain face expressions. Cortical regions in humans that respond to faces, body parts, objects, scenes (Pitcher et al., 2019; Vogels, 2022) and word form (Vinckier et al., 2007; Dehaene and Cohen, 2011) and the connectivity between them (Rolls et al., 2023e) are considered further in Section 2.5. Consistent with the neurophysiology described below and by Baylis, Rolls and Leonard (1987), human fMRI studies are able to detect small patches of non-face and other types of responsiveness in areas that appeared to respond primarily to one category such as faces (Grill-Spector, Sayres and Ress, 2006; Haxby, 2006).

Different inferior temporal cortex neurons in macaques not only provide different types of information about different aspects of faces, as described above, but also respond differently to different *categories* of visual stimuli, with for example some neurons conveying information primarily about faces, and others about objects (Rolls and Tovee, 1995b; Rolls, Treves, Tovee and Panzeri, 1997d; Booth and Rolls, 1998; Rolls and Treves, 2011; Rolls, 2012d, 2016b). In fact, when recording in the inferior temporal cortex, one finds small clustered groups of neurons, with neurons within a cluster responding to somewhat similar attributes of stimuli, and different clusters responding to different categories or types of visual stimuli. For example, within the set of neurons responding to moving faces, there are some neuronal clusters that respond to for example ventral and dorsal flexion of the head on the body; others that respond to axial rotation of the head; others that respond to the sight of mouth movements; and others that respond to the gaze direction in a face being viewed (Hasselmo, Rolls, Baylis and Nalwa, 1989b; Perrett, Smith, Potter, Mistlin, Head, Milner and Jeeves, 1985b). The parts of the body to which neurons in the cortex in the superior temporal sulcus respond include not only to heads, moving for example with respect to the body (Hasselmo, Rolls, Baylis and Nalwa, 1989b) (e.g. Fig. 2.12), but also to body parts, and to images of bodies walking (Perrett, Smith, Mistlin, Chitty, Head, Potter, Broennimann, Milner and Jeeves, 1985a; Pitcher, Ianni and Ungerleider, 2019; Vogels, 2022), both of which may be important in social behavior.

Within the domain of objects, some neuronal clusters respond based on the shapes of the object (e.g. responding to elongated and not round objects), others respond based on the texture of the object being viewed, and others are sensitive to what the object is doing (Hasselmo, Rolls, Baylis and Nalwa, 1989b; Perrett, Smith, Mistlin, Chitty, Head, Potter, Broennimann, Milner and Jeeves, 1985a). Within a cluster, each neuron is tuned differently, and may combine at least partly with information predominant in other clusters, so that at least some of the neurons in a cluster can become quite selective between different objects, with the preference for individual objects showing the usual exponential firing rate distribution (Rolls, 2016b). Using optical imaging in macaques, Tanaka and colleagues (Tanaka, 1996) have seen comparable evidence for different localized clusters of neuronal activation produced by different types or categories of stimuli.

The principle that Rolls proposes underlies this local clustering is the representation of the high dimensional space of objects and their features into a two-dimensional cortical sheet using the local self-organizing mapping principles described in Section B.4.6 and illustrated in a Matlab program described in Appendix D. In this situation, these principles produce maps that have many fractures, but nevertheless include local clusters of similar neurons. Exactly this clustering can be produced in the model of visual object recognition, VisNet, described in Section 2.8 by replacing the lateral inhibition filter shown in Fig. 2.29 with a difference of Gaussians filter of the type illustrated in Fig. B.21. Such a difference of Gaussians filter would reflect the effects of short range excitatory (recurrent collateral) connections between cortical pyramidal cells, and slightly longer range inhibition produced through inhibitory interneurons. These local clusters minimize the wiring length between neurons, if the computations involve exchange of information within neurons of a similar general type, as will usually be the case (see Section B.4.6). Minimizing wiring length is crucial in keeping brain size relatively low (see Section B.4.6). Another useful property of such self-organizing maps is that they encourage distributed representations in which semi-continuous similarity functions are mapped. This is potentially useful in building representations that then generalize usefully when new stimuli are shown between representations that are already set up continuously in the map.

Another fundamental contribution and key aspect of neocortical design facilitated by the short-range recurrent excitatory connections is that the attractors that are formed are local. This is fundamentally important, for if the neocortex had long-range connectivity, it would tend to be able to form only as many attractor states as there are connections per neocortical neuron, which would be a severe limit on cortical memory capacity (O'Kane and Treves, 1992) (see further Sections 1.14.4, B.9, Rolls (2016b), and Spalla et al. (2021)).

It is consistent with this general conceptual background that Kreiman, Koch and Fried (2000) and others ((De Falco et al., 2016; Ison et al., 2015; Quian Quiroga, 2012) see Fried, Rutishauser, Cerf and Kreiman (2014) and Rolls (2015c)) have described some neurons in the human temporal lobe that seem to respond to categories of object or to concepts of people. This is consistent with the principles just described, although in humans backprojections from language or other cognitive areas concerned for example with tool use might also influence the categories represented in high order cortical areas, as described in Section B.4.5, and by Farah, Meyer and McMullen (1996), Farah (2000) and Rolls (2016b). In fact, neurons recorded in the macaque inferior temporal visual cortex predict by a weighted sum the recognition of objects by human observers (Majaj, Hong, Solomon and DiCarlo, 2015), providing evidence that what has been discovered in the inferior temporal cortex is relevant to understanding human visual object recognition. Moreover, this also indicates that inferior temporal cortex neurons provide a useful goal for what the models of object recognition described in Section 2.6 must account for, in order to provide a basis for understanding human visual object recognition.

2.5 The connectivity of the ventral visual pathways in humans

It is now possible to consider how the ventral stream visual pathways are organised in humans by considering the connectivity between ventral stream visual regions in the human brain. This approach builds on the Human Connectome Project Multimodal Parcellation atlas (HCP-MMP) (Glasser et al., 2016a; Huang et al., 2022) introduced in Section 1.12, and measures diffusion tractography, functional connectivity, and effective connectivity as described in Sections 1.13.1 - 1.13.3. The connectivities described here were measured in 171 participants imaged at 7T in the Human Connectome Project (Glasser et al., 2016b). By using this high resolution atlas, and by measuring effective connectivity between the regions defined in it to help identify the flow of information, and adding what has been discovered from neurophysiology in macaques and from activation studies in humans, a framework is provided for understanding *what* computations are performed at different stages of processing in the human brain, and that in turn has implications for *how* the computations are performed. Several visual streams have been identified in humans (Rolls et al., 2023e), and are described next.

2.5.1 A Ventrolateral Visual Cortical Stream to the inferior temporal visual cortex for object and face representations

The Ventrolateral Visual Cortical Stream is characterized by effective connectivities that lead towards the inferior temporal visual cortex. After a progression from V1 > V2 > V3 > V4 (where > indicates the general progression but does not exclude some connectivity that is more than between strictly adjacent levels in the hierarchy), V4 (and to some extent V3) have effective connectivity to HCP-MMP ventral visual division regions such as PIT (a posterior inferior temporal cortex region identified in humans) and V8. PIT, and to some extent V8, then have connectivity to FFC, the 'fusiform face cortex' (Fig. 2.23), which is in the fusiform gyrus in which scenes are represented medially (Sulpizio et al., 2020), then objects and faces, and next moving laterally, words in a visual word form area (Dehaene and Cohen, 2011). This can be considered as a series of representations each at a different spatial scale of size from medial to lateral. FFC in turn has connectivity to posterior inferior temporal cortex regions TE2p and PH (and PH also connects to TE2p). PH and TE2p project to PHT, which in turn projects to TE1p, and to an anterior inferior temporal cortex region TE2a. The posterior inferior temporal cortex regions TE1p and TE2p project to anterior inferior temporal cortex regions TE2a, TE1m and TE1a (Fig. 2.23).

TE1a then projects anteriorly to temporal pole region TGd which is involved in semantic representations for language (Rolls et al., 2022b) (Chapter 8). Other regions related to language, temporo-parieto-occipital regions TPOJ1, TPOJ2 and TPOJ3 (Rolls et al., 2022b), also receive effective connectivity from ventrolateral visual cortical stream regions including the FFC, providing a route for face and word form inputs to reach language-related regions (Figs. 2.24 and 2.25). We therefore have a route through the ventrolateral visual stream as shown schematically in Fig. 2.23 which can now be shown to reach human language-related cortical regions. This ventrolateral cortical visual stream also provides 'what' visual outputs (Rolls et al., 2023e) to the orbitofrontal cortex / vmPFC reward/punishment emotion-related system (Rolls et al., 2023c); to the hippocampal memory system as a 'what' component of episodic memory (Rolls et al., 2022a); and to the prefrontal cortex for short-term memory and planning (Rolls et al., 2023f); and to the cortex in the superior temporal sulcus (STS) involved in multimodal representations relevant to social behavior and to semantics, which is described next.

These findings are supported by tract-tracing studies in macaques (Kravitz et al., 2013, 2011), though more cortical regions are distinguished in the human brain, and the advantage of studying the connectivity in humans with a parcellation such as the HCP-multimodal parcellation (Glasser et al., 2016a; Huang et al., 2022) is that we are now dealing with identifiable systems in humans that other studies (fMRI, lesion etc) in humans can directly relate to by reference to the HCP-multimodal parcellation, and that the connectivity in humans relates to the strength of connections in both directions between every pair of cortical regions, not only to whether anatomical connections can be traced.

Key discoveries that we made with neuronal recordings in macaques as described in Section 2.4 about this ventrolateral visual cortical stream leading to the anterior inferior temporal visual cortex (IT) are that IT neurons code for objects and not their reward value (Rolls et al., 1977); that some neurons code for faces (Perrett et al., 1979, 1982); that IT neurons use sparse distributed encoding for face identity (Baylis, Rolls and Leonard, 1985; Rolls, Treves, Tovee and Panzeri, 1997d) with relatively independent information provided by populations of neurons (Treves, Panzeri, Rolls, Booth and Wakeman, 1999; Rolls, Treves and Tovee, 1997b; Rolls and Treves, 2011); that feature combinations in the correct spatial position encode faces and objects (Perrett, Rolls and Caan, 1982; Desimone, Albright, Gross and Bruce, 1984); and that IT neurons have representations of objects that are invariant with respect to

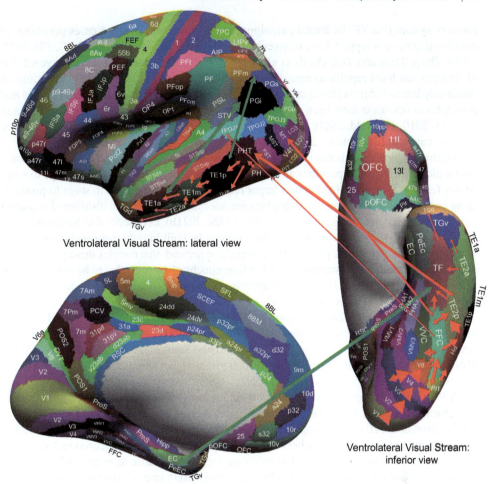

Fig. 2.23 Effective connectivity of the Ventrolateral Visual Cortical Stream which reaches inferior temporal cortex TE regions in which objects and faces are represented: schematic overview. A green arrow shows how the Ventrolateral Visual Stream provides 'what' input to the hippocampal memory system via parahippocampal gyrus TF to perirhinal PeEc connectivity from FFC, PH, TE1p, TE2a and TE2p. The Ventrolateral Visual Stream also provides input to the semantic language system via TGd. The Ventrolateral Visual Stream also has connectivity to the inferior parietal visual area PFm, PGs and PGi as indicated by 2 green arrows. The widths of the lines and the size of the arrowheads indicate the magnitude and direction of the effective connectivity. (From Rolls,E.T., Deco,G., Huang,C-C. and Feng,J. (2023) Multiple cortical visual streams in humans. Cerebral Cortex 33: 3319-3349. doi: 10.1093/cercor/bhac276. Copyright © Oxford University Press.)

transforms including retinal position (Tovee, Rolls and Azzopardi, 1994; Gross, Desimone, Albright and Schwartz, 1985), size and contrast (Rolls and Baylis, 1986), spatial frequency (Rolls et al., 1985, 1987), and in some cases to view (Booth and Rolls, 1998; Hasselmo, Rolls, Baylis and Nalwa, 1989b). For natural vision, we discovered in complex natural scenes that IT neurons respond primarily to the object being fixated (Sheinberg and Logothetis, 2001; Rolls et al., 2003a; Aggelopoulos and Rolls, 2005) by reducing their receptive field size (Rolls et al., 2003a) which simplifies the interpretation of the output of IT by structures such as the orbitofrontal cortex which implements object-reward association learning (Rolls, Critchley, Mason and Wakeman, 1996b; Thorpe, Rolls and Maddison, 1983; Rolls, 2019e,f) and the hippocampal system which implements object-scene location learning (Rolls, Xiang and Franco, 2005c; Rolls and Xiang, 2006; Rolls, 2023c). The 'what' information to the hippocampal memory system (via TF the lateral parahippocampal cortex and in some cases perirhinal or entorhinal cortex) is tapped from this ventrolateral object/face system from FFC, PH, PHT, TE2p, TE1p, TE2a and TGd (Rolls et al., 2023e) (Fig. 2.23). Moreover, we discovered that IT neurons can learn rapidly to represent new objects without disturbing representations of previously learned objects (Rolls et al., 1989b). Results consistent with these discoveries and principles of operation have been reported (Freiwald, Tsao and Livingstone, 2009; Rust and DiCarlo, 2010; Freiwald, 2020; Tsao, 2014; Freedman, 2015; Aparicio, Issa and DiCarlo, 2016; Arcaro and Livingstone, 2021).

The hierarchical organisation of the connectivity of the Ventrolateral Visual Stream shown schematically in Fig. 2.23 provides an architecture that with convergence from stage to stage allows features to be combined across larger receptive fields from stage to stage to produce, using competitive learning, neurons that become specialised with sparse distributed encoding to represent different objects and faces (Rolls, 1992a, 2021b), as described in Sections 2.6.6–2.13. Invariances such as position, size and view can be built into the neuronal responses by using a local synaptic learning rule in the competitive network that enables these properties of objects, which tend to be invariant over short time epochs of 1 - several s, to be learned by the neurons (Rolls, 1992a, 2021b). This unsupervised self-organising learning system with only local synaptic learning rules has been built into a model, VisNet, that shows how this learning can take place (Rolls, 1992a; Wallis and Rolls, 1997; Rolls, 2021d,b; Stringer et al., 2007b; Perry et al., 2006; Stringer and Rolls, 2002; Elliffe et al., 2002). A similar approach has been developed by others (Franzius et al., 2007; Wiskott and Sejnowski, 2002; Wyss et al., 2006). This biologically plausible approach to invariant visual object recognition is described in the rest of this Chapter.

A very different approach to object recognition using deep convolutional networks (Rajalingham et al., 2018; Yamins et al., 2014; Cadieu et al., 2014; Yamins and DiCarlo, 2016; Rajalingham et al., 2018) is biologically implausible, because in the brain there is no teacher for each output neuron, and errors between the firing rate of each output neuron and a putative teacher's instruction cannot be used to calculate for every synapse at every earlier stage of the hierarchy and then backpropagated back to correct every one of those synaptic strengths (Rolls, 2021b,d) (see Sections B.12 B.14 and 2.9.4). Further, top-down processes such as memory recall (Treves and Rolls, 1994; Rolls and Treves, 1994; Rolls, 2021b) and top-down attention (Deco and Rolls, 2005a, 2004; Rolls, 2021b) can be implemented biologically plausibly by the cortico-cortical backprojection effective connectivities found in the real brain (Fig. 2.23), and that associative memory recall / top-down attention functionality is likely to be inconsistent with error backpropagation. Moreover most of the deep learning approaches to vision utilise convolutional deep learning (see Sections 2.9.4, 19.4, and B.14), with the convolution part also being biologically implausible. Comparing neurons recorded in the brain with the units found in deep learning algorithms tuned to produce neurons that resemble those in the brain (Cadieu, Hong, Yamins, Pinto, Ardila, Solomon, Majaj and DiCarlo, 2014; Yamins, Hong, Cadieu, Solomon, Seibert and DiCarlo, 2014; Yamins and DiCarlo, 2016; Rajalingham, Issa, Bashivan, Kar, Schmidt and DiCarlo, 2018; Jia, Hong and DiCarlo, 2021; Zhuang, Yan, Nayebi, Schrimpf, Frank, DiCarlo and Yamins, 2021) seems like a poorly founded exercise, for two reasons. First, the solutions found by deep convolution networks and other machine learning algorithms for image to category mapping may be very different to those found in a system such as the brain that uses only local learning rules and is restricted to only 4–5 layers in the hierarchy. Second, it is difficult to know what can be learned about how primate including human vision works computationally from deep learning and related machine learning algorithms, given that the understanding of exactly how these machine learning algorithms reach their mapping is almost un-understood, apart from the recipe that makes them work (Plebe and Grasso, 2019; Bowers et al., 2023).

2.5.2 A Visual Cortical Stream to the cortex in the inferior bank of the superior temporal sulcus involved in semantic representations

One output of the Ventrolateral Visual Cortical Stream for object and face information is to the cortex in the inferior parts of the Superior Temporal Sulcus (STS), regions STSva and STSvp (Rolls et al., 2022b). These inferior cortical regions in the STS have been identified by a community analysis as part of a ventral temporal lobe semantic system involved in language (Rolls et al., 2022b). The visual inputs to regions STSva and STSvp in this ventral STS semantic system are described here. The visual inputs to these inferior STS regions STSva and STSvp are shown in Fig. 2.24, and come from inferior temporal visual cortex (TE1a, TE1m and TE2a), temporal pole (TGd and TGv), and parietal PGi. Other connectivities shown with green arrows in Fig. 2.24 are with the memory-related parts of the posterior cingulate cortex (31pd and 31pv) (Rolls et al., 2023i); and from the ventromedial prefrontal cortex (vmPFC, in particular 10v and 10r) (Rolls et al., 2023c). STSva and STSvp have connectivity directed towards Broca's area 44 and 45, and related areas (47s, 47l), and to the Superior Frontal Language region SFL (Rolls et al., 2022b). This 'inferior STS cortex semantic network', for which the visual input is described here, is described in more detail for the same participants elsewhere (Rolls et al., 2022b) (see Chapter 8).

This inferior (/ventral) STS cortex network that includes STSva and STSvp is considered to be separate from the superior (/dorsal) STS cortex network described below that includes STSda and STSdp because these regions fall into different semantic connectivity networks as shown by a community analysis (Rolls et al., 2022b). The inferior network is likely to be more involved in invariant object and face identity representations for static visual stimuli of the type represented in the inferior temporal visual cortex, whereas the superior (/dorsal) regions are more likely to be involved in responses to face expression and visual motion including that which can be combined with auditory stimuli such as the sight and sound of a vocalization (Baylis, Rolls and Leonard, 1987; Hasselmo, Rolls, Baylis and Nalwa, 1989b; Hasselmo, Rolls and Baylis, 1989a; Rolls, 2021b; Rolls, Deco, Huang and Feng, 2022b; Rolls, Rauschecker, Deco, Huang and Feng, 2023h) (see Section 2.4).

2.5.3 A Visual Cortical Stream to the cortex in the superior bank of the superior temporal sulcus involved in multimodal semantic representations including visual motion, auditory, somatosensory and social information

In the superior bank of the cortex in the Superior Temporal Sulcus (STS), regions STSda and STSdp have been identified by a community analysis as part of a superior temporal lobe semantic system involved in language (Rolls et al., 2022b). The visual inputs to regions STSda and STSdp in this superior STS semantic system are described here. Visual inputs reach STSdp from PGi (Rolls et al., 2023e) (Fig. 2.25), and provide a route for moving visual stimuli / objects analyzed in the parietal cortex to reach STS regions (Rolls et al., 2023d). Visual inputs also reach STSdp from the Superior Temporal Visual (STV) region which receives from both MT and FFC (Fig. 2.25), and which as described below could contribute to the neuronal activity in the cortex in the STS which has been shown to respond to moving heads, faces and objects in macaques (Hasselmo et al., 1989b,a). STSda and STSdp also have connectivity from STSva and STSvp which have strong connectivity with the Ventrolateral Visual Stream (Figs. 2.23 and 2.25). STSda and STSdp also receive auditory effective connectivity from A5 (Fig. 2.25) (Rolls et al., 2023h). STSdp has connectivity directed towards Broca's area 44 and 45, and related areas (47l), and to the PeriSylvian Language region PSL and to the Superior Frontal Language region SFL (Rolls et al., 2022b).

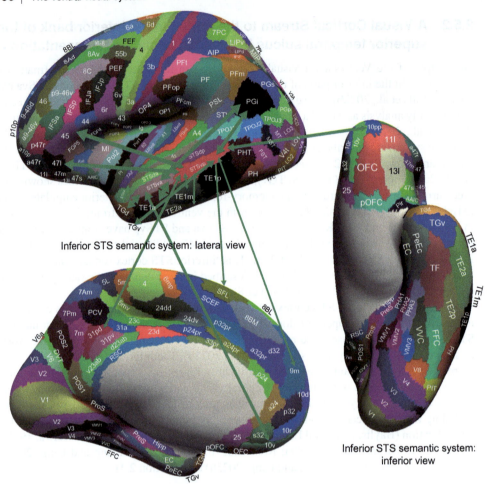

Fig. 2.24 Inferior bank of the STS cortex semantic system in STSva and STSvp: schematic overview. An output of the Ventrolateral Visual System for object and face information is to the cortex in the inferior parts of the Superior Temporal Sulcus, STSva and STSvp. The visual inputs to these inferior STS cortex regions are shown with green arrows, and come from TE1a, TE1m, TE2a, TGd, TGv, and PGi. Other connectivities are with the memory-related parts of the posterior cingulate cortex (31pd and 31pv); and from the vmPFC (10v and 10r). STSva and STSvp have connectivity directed towards Broca's area 44 and 45, and related areas (47s), and to the Superior Frontal Language region (SFL). (From Rolls,E.T., Deco,G., Huang,C-C. and Feng,J. (2023) Multiple cortical visual streams in humans. Cerebral Cortex 33: 3319-3349. doi: 10.1093/cercor/bhac276. Copyright © Oxford University Press.)

This 'superior STS cortex semantic system' thus enables multimodal representations including visual, auditory, and probably also somatosensory via PGi, to gain access to the language system. This is a major output of cortical visual processing for use in language, described in more detail elsewhere (Rolls et al., 2022b). There is also a link via TF to the hippocampal memory system (Fig. 2.25) (Rolls et al., 2022a).

Discoveries in macaques provide an indication for what is represented in these STS regions. It was discovered that single neurons in the macaque STS respond to face expression and also to face and head movement to encode the social relevance of stimuli (Hasselmo, Rolls, Baylis and Nalwa, 1989b; Hasselmo, Rolls and Baylis, 1989a). For example, a neuron might respond to closing of the eyes, or to turning of the head away from facing the viewer, both of which break social contact (Hasselmo et al., 1989b,a). Some neurons respond to the direction of gaze (Perrett et al., 1987). It was found that many of the neurons in the STS respond only or

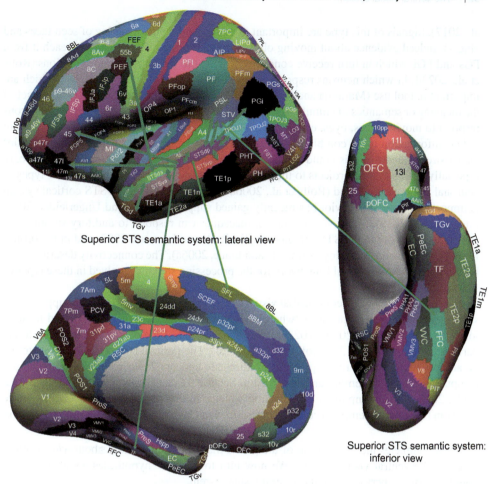

Fig. 2.25 Superior bank of the STS semantic system in STSda and STSdp: schematic overview. Visual inputs for moving visual stimuli / objects reach STSdp from PGi. Visual inputs also reach STSdp from the Superior Temporal Visual area which receives from FFC. STSda and STSdp also have connectivity from STSva and STSvp which have strong connectivity with the Ventrolateral Visual Stream (Fig. 2.23). STSda and STSdp also receive auditory effective connectivity from A5. STSdp has connectivity directed towards Broca's area 44 and 45, and related areas (47l), and to the PeriSylvian Language region PSL and to the Superior Frontal Language region SFL. (From Rolls,E.T., Deco,G., Huang,C-C. and Feng,J. (2023) Multiple cortical visual streams in humans. Cerebral Cortex 33: 3319-3349. doi: 10.1093/cercor/bhac276. Copyright © Oxford University Press.)

much better to moving faces or objects (Hasselmo et al., 1989a), whereas in the anterior inferior temporal cortex neurons were discovered that respond well to static visual stimuli, and are tuned for face identity (Perrett, Rolls and Caan, 1982; Rolls, 1984, 2000a; Rolls and Treves, 2011; Rolls, Treves, Tovee and Panzeri, 1997d; Rolls, Treves and Tovee, 1997b; Hasselmo, Rolls and Baylis, 1989a). It has been proposed that PGi, with its inputs from PGs which has connectivity with superior parietal and intraparietal regions that encode visual motion, is part of this processing stream for socially relevant face-related information (Rolls et al., 2023d). Consistent with this, the effective connectivity is stronger from PGi to STS regions (Rolls et al., 2023e). In humans, representations of this type could provide part of the basis for the development of systems to interpret the significance of such stimuli, including theory of mind. Consistent with this proposal, activations in the temporo-parietal junction region are related to theory of mind (DiNicola et al., 2020; Buckner and DiNicola, 2019; Schurz et al., 2017). Signals of this type are important in understanding the meaning of seen faces and objects. Indeed evidence about moving objects present in the STS cortex may reach it from PGs and PGi, which in turn receive connectivity from the intraparietal sulcus regions (Rolls et al., 2023d) in which neurons respond to visual motion and to grasping objects which are important in tool use (Maravita and Romano, 2018), which is another fundamental aspect of the meaning or semantics of stimuli. We proposed that the cortex in the STS in which neurons respond to moving faces, eyes, etc and to changing facial expression enables ventral stream 'what' information to be combined with dorsal stream motion information to form a third visual stream, and that this could be useful for social functions (Hasselmo et al., 1989b,a), especially as this system projects to the orbitofrontal cortex / vmPFC where similar types of neuronal response are found (Rolls et al., 2006a). The concept that this STS cortical system is important in social behavior has recently gained support (Pitcher and Ungerleider, 2021; Pitcher et al., 2019). Moreover, neurons in macaques can respond to auditory stimuli such as vocalisation both in the STS regions (Baylis, Rolls and Leonard, 1987) and in the orbitofrontal cortex (Rolls, Critchley, Browning and Inoue, 2006a). The connectivity described here helps to provide a functional framework for the processing streams involved in these types of function.

The connectivity of a ventromedial visual cortical stream leading to the parahippocampal scene area and hippocampus as a 'where' input for episodic memory is described in Section 9.2.8.1 (Rolls et al., 2023e, 2022a; Rolls, 2023c), and of the dorsal visual stream to the parietal cortex in Section 3.6 (Rolls et al., 2023e,d). The parietal cortex visual inputs to the parahippocampal scene area to provide for idiothetic update of 'where' inputs to the hippocampus for episodic memory are described in Section 9.2.8.2 (Rolls et al., 2023e,d, 2022a; Rolls, 2023c). Visual inputs to the semantic systems in the ventral and dorsal banks of the cortex in the superior temporal sulcus are described in Chapter 8 (Rolls et al., 2023e, 2022b).

That completes the elaboration of the points made in Section 2.1.2 about *what* is computed in the ventral visual system. We now turn to consider hypotheses about *how* these computations are performed in the ventral visual system.

2.6 How the computations are performed: approaches to invariant object recognition

Given that a key computation performed in the ventral visual system is invariant visual object recognition, we now consider several approaches to **how** this computation is performed in the brain. In this section, a number of approaches are briefly reviewed. Then we turn to the most biologically plausible approach so far, a feature hierarchy system, and then in Section 2.8 we consider developments of this that enable the object recognition to be transform invariant, in the VisNet model.

We start by emphasizing that generalization to different positions, sizes, views etc. of an object is not a simple property of one-layer neural networks. Although neural networks do generalize well, the type of generalization they show naturally is to vectors which have a high dot product or correlation with what they have already learned. To make this clear, Fig. 2.26 is a reminder that the activation h_i of each neuron is computed as

$$h_i = \sum_j x_j w_{ij} \qquad (2.1)$$

where the sum is over the C input axons, indexed by j. Now consider translation (or shift) of

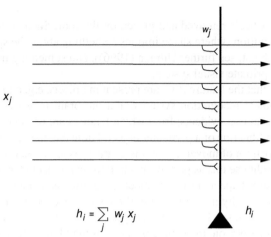

Fig. 2.26 A neuron that computes a dot product of the input pattern with its synaptic weight vector generalizes well to other patterns based on their similarity measured in terms of dot product or correlation, but shows no translation (or size, etc.) invariance.

the input pattern vector by one position. The dot product will now drop to a low level, and the neuron will not respond, even though it is the same pattern, just shifted by one location. This makes the point that special processes are needed to compute invariant representations. Network approaches to such invariant pattern recognition are described in this chapter, and the nature of the problem to be solved is described further in Section B.4.7 and Fig. B.24 on page 871. Once an invariant representation has been computed by a sensory system, it is in a form that is suitable for presentation to a pattern association or autoassociation neural network (see Appendix B). This is key to understanding computationally how the inferior temporal visual cortex interfaces to be associated with reward value in the orbitofrontal cortex, and how IT interace to the episodic memory system in the hippocampus.

A number of different computational approaches that have been taken both in artificial vision systems and as suggestions for how the brain performs invariant object recognition are described in the following parts of this section (2.6). This places in context the approach that appears to be taken in the brain and that forms the basis for VisNet described in Section 2.8.

2.6.1 Feature spaces

One very simple possibility for performing object classification is based on feature spaces, which amount to lists of the features that are present in a particular object. The features might consist of textures, colors, areas, ratios of length to width, etc. The spatial arrangement of the features is not taken into account. If n different properties are used to characterize an object, each viewed object is represented by a set of n real numbers. It then becomes possible to represent an object by a point R^n in an n-dimensional space (where R is the resolution of the real numbers used). Such schemes have been investigated (Tou and Gonzalez, 1974; Gibson, 1950, 1979; Bolles and Cain, 1982; Mundy and Zisserman, 1992; Selfridge, 1959; Mel, 1997), but, because the relative positions of the different parts are not implemented in the object recognition scheme, are not sensitive to spatial jumbling of the features. For example, if the features consisted of nose, mouth, and eyes, such a system would respond to faces with jumbled arrangements of the eyes, nose, and mouth, which does not match human vision, nor the responses of macaque inferior temporal cortex neurons, which are sensitive to the spatial arrangement of the features in a face (Rolls, Tovee, Purcell, Stewart and Azzopardi, 1994b). Similarly, such an object recognition system might not distinguish a normal car from a car with the back wheels removed and placed on the roof. Such systems do not therefore perform shape recognition (where shape implies something about the spatial arrangement of features within an object, see further Ullman (1996)), and something more is needed, and is implemented in the primate visual system.

However, I note that the features that are present in objects, e.g. a furry texture, are useful to incorporate in object recognition systems, and the brain may well use, and the model VisNet in principle can use, evidence from which features are present in an object as part of the evidence for identification of a particular object. I note that the features might consist also of for example the pattern of movement that is characteristic of a particular object (such as a buzzing fly), and might use this as part of the input to final object identification.

The capacity to use shape in invariant object recognition is fundamental to primate vision, but may not be used or fully implemented in the visual systems of some other animals with less developed visual systems. For example, pigeons may correctly identify pictures containing people, a particular person, trees, pigeons etc, but may fail to distinguish a figure from a scrambled version of a figure (Herrnstein, 1984; Cerella, 1986). Thus their object recognition may be based more on a collection of parts than on a direct comparison of complete figures in which the relative positions of the parts are important. Even if the details of the conclusions reached from that research are revised (Wasserman, Kirkpatrick-Steger and Biederman, 1998), it nevertheless does appear that at least some birds may use computationally simpler methods than those needed for invariant shape recognition. For example, it may be that when some birds are trained to discriminate between images in a large set of pictures, they tend to rely on some chance detail of each picture (such as a spot appearing by mistake on the picture), rather than on recognition of the shapes of the object in the picture (Watanabe, Lea and Dittrich, 1993).

2.6.2 Structural descriptions and syntactic pattern recognition

A second approach to object recognition is to decompose the object or image into parts, and to then produce a structural description of the relations between the parts. The underlying assumption is that it is easier to capture object invariances at a level where parts have been identified. This is the type of scheme for which Marr and Nishihara (1978) and Marr (1982) opted. The particular scheme (Binford, 1981) they adopted consists of generalized cones, series of which can be linked together to form structural descriptions of some, especially animate, stimuli (see Fig. 2.27). Such schemes assume that there is a 3D internal model (structural description) of each object. Perception of the object consists of parsing or segmenting the scene into objects, and then into parts, then producing a structural description of the object, and then testing whether this structural description matches that of any known object stored in the system. Other examples of structural description schemes include those of Winston (1975), Sutherland (1968), and Milner (1974). The relations in the structural description may need to be quite complicated, for example 'connected together', 'inside of', 'larger than' etc.

Perhaps the most developed model of this type is the recognition by components (RBC) model of Biederman (1987), implemented in a computational model by Hummel and Biederman (1992). His small set (less than 50) of primitive parts named 'geons' include simple 3D shapes such as boxes, cylinders and wedges. Objects are described by a syntactically linked list of the relations between each of the geons of which they are composed. Describing a table in this way (as a flat top supported by three or four legs) seems quite economical. The emphasis more recently has been on the non-accidental properties of objects, which are maintained when objects transform (Kim and Biederman, 2012). Other schemes use 2D surface patches as their primitives (Dane and Bajcsy, 1982; Brady, Ponce, Yuille and Asada, 1985; Faugeras

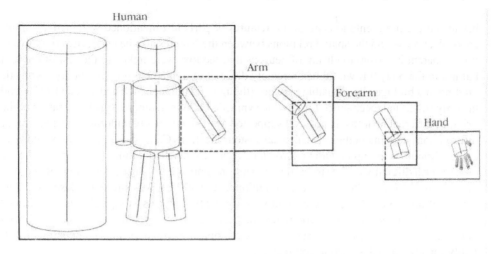

Fig. 2.27 A 3D structural description of an object based on generalized cone parts. Each box corresponds to a 3D model, with its model axis on the left side of the box and the arrangement of its component axes on the right. In addition, some component axes have 3D models associated with them, as indicated by the way the boxes overlap. (Reproduced from Marr, D. and Nishihara, H.K. (1978) Representation and recognition of the spatial organization of three dimensional structure. Proceedings of the Royal Society of London B 200: 269–294. © Royal Society.)

and Hebert, 1986; Faugeras, 1993). When 3D objects are being recognized, the implication is that the structural description is a 3D description. This is in contrast to feature hierarchical systems, in which recognition of a 3D object from any view might be accomplished by storing a set of associated 2D views (see below, Section 2.6.6).

There are a number of difficulties with schemes based on structural descriptions, some general, and some with particular reference to the potential difficulty of their implementation in the brain. First, it is not always easy to decompose the object into its separate parts, which must be performed before the structural description can be produced. For example, it may be difficult to produce a structural description of a cat curled up asleep from separately identifiable parts. Identification of each of the parts is also frequently very difficult when 3D objects are seen from different viewing angles, as key parts may be invisible, occluded, or highly distorted. This is particularly likely to be difficult in 3D shape perception. It appears that being committed to producing a correct description of the parts before other processes can operate is making too strong a commitment early on in the recognition process.

A second difficulty is that many objects or animals that can be correctly recognized have rather similar structural descriptions. For example, the structural descriptions of many four-legged animals are rather similar. Rather more than a structural description seems necessary to identify many objects and animals.

A third difficulty, which applies especially to biological systems, is the difficulty of implementing the syntax needed to hold the structural description as a 3D model of the object, of producing a syntactic structural description on the fly (in real time, and with potentially great flexibility of the possible arrangement of the parts), and of matching the syntactic description of the object in the image to all the stored representations in order to find a match. An example of a structural description for a limb might be body > thigh > shin > foot > toes. In this description > means 'is linked to', and this link must be between the correct pair of descriptors. If we had just a set of parts, without the syntactic or relational linking, then there would be no way of knowing whether the toes are attached to the foot or to the body. In fact, worse than this, there would be no evidence about what was related to what, just a set of parts. Such syntactical relations are difficult to implement in neuronal networks, because if the representations of all the features or parts just mentioned were active simultaneously, how would the spatial relations between the features also be encoded? (How would it be apparent just from the firing of neurons that the toes were linked to the rest of the foot but not to the body?) It would be extremely difficult to implement this 'on the fly' syntactic binding in a biologically plausible network (though cf. Hummel and Biederman (1992)), and the only suggested mechanism for flexible syntactic binding, temporal synchronization of the firing of different neurons, is not well supported as a quantitatively important mechanism for information encoding in the ventral visual system (Sections C.2.5 and C.3.7), and would have major difficulties in implementing correct, relational, syntactic binding (see Section 2.8.5.1).

A fourth difficulty of the structural description approach is that segmentation into objects must occur effectively before object recognition, so that the linked structural description list can be of one object. Given the difficulty of segmenting objects in typical natural cluttered scenes (Ullman, 1996), and the compounding problem of overlap of parts of objects by other objects, segmentation as a first necessary stage of object recognition adds another major difficulty for structural description approaches.

A fifth difficulty is that metric information, such as the relative size of the parts that are linked syntactically, needs to be specified in the structural description (Stankiewicz and Hummel, 1994), which complicates the parts that have to be syntactically linked.

It is because of these difficulties that even in artificial vision systems implemented on computers, where almost unlimited syntactic binding can easily be implemented, the structural description approach to object recognition has not yet succeeded in producing a scheme which actually works in more than an environment in which the types of objects are limited, and the world is far from the natural world, consisting for example of 2D scenes (Mundy and Zisserman, 1992).

Although object recognition in the brain is unlikely to be based on the structural description approach, for the reasons given above, and the fact that the evidence described in this chapter supports a feature hierarchy rather than the structural description implementation in the brain, it is certainly the case that humans can provide verbal, syntactic, descriptions of objects in terms of the relations of their parts, and that this is often a useful type of description. Humans may therefore it is suggested supplement a feature hierarchical object recognition system built into their ventral visual system with the additional ability to use the type of syntax that is necessary for language to provide another level of description of objects. This is of course useful in, for example, engineering applications.

2.6.3 Template matching and the alignment approach

Another approach to object recognition is template matching, comparing the image on the retina with a stored image or picture of an object. This is conceptually simple, but there are in practice major problems. One major problem is how to align the image on the retina with the stored images, so that all possible images on the retina can be compared with the stored template or templates of each object.

The basic idea of the alignment approach (Ullman, 1996) is to compensate for the transformations separating the viewed object and the corresponding stored model, and then compare them. For example, the image and the stored model may be similar, except for a difference in size. Scaling one of them will remove this discrepancy and improve the match between them. For a 2D world, the possible transforms are translation (shift), scaling, and rotation. Given for example an input letter of the alphabet to recognize, the system might, after segmentation (itself a very difficult process if performed independently of (prior to) object recognition), compensate for translation by computing the centre of mass of the object, and shifting the character to a 'canonical location'. Scale might be compensated for by calculating the convex hull (the smallest envelope surrounding the object), and then scaling the image. Of course how the shift and scaling would be accomplished is itself a difficult point – easy to perform on a computer using matrix multiplication as in simple computer graphics, but not the sort of computation that could be performed easily or accurately by any biologically plausible network. Compensating for rotation is even more difficult (Ullman, 1996). All this has to happen before the segmented canonical representation of the object is compared to the stored object templates with the same canonical representation. The system of course becomes vastly more complicated when the recognition must be performed of 3D objects seen in a 3D world, for now the particular view of an object after segmentation must be placed into a canonical form, regardless of which view, or how much of any view, may be seen in a natural scene with occluding contours. However, this process is helped, at least in computers that can perform high precision matrix multiplication, by the fact that (for many continuous transforms such as 3D rotation, translation, and scaling) all the possible views of an object transforming in 3D space can be expressed as the linear combination of other views of the same object (see Chapter 5 of Ullman (1996); Koenderink and van Doorn (1991); and Koenderink (1990)).

This alignment approach is the main theme of the book by Ullman (1996), and there are a number of computer implementations (Lowe, 1985; Grimson, 1990; Huttenlocher and Ullman, 1990; Shashua, 1995). However, as noted above, it seems unlikely that the brain is able to perform the high precision calculations needed to perform the transforms required to align any view of a 3D object with some canonical template representation. For this reason, and because the approach also relies on segmentation of the object in the scene before the template alignment algorithms can start, and because key features may need to be correctly identified to be used in the alignment (Edelman, 1999), this approach is not considered further here.

However, it is certainly the case that humans are very sensitive to precise feature configurations (Ullman et al., 2016).

We may note here in passing that some animals with a less computationally developed visual system appear to attempt to solve the alignment problem by actively moving their heads or eyes to see what template fits, rather than starting with an image on the eye and attempting to transform it into canonical coordinates. This 'active vision' approach used for example by some invertebrates has been described by Land (1999) and Land and Collett (1997).

2.6.4 Invertible networks that can reconstruct their inputs

Hinton, Dayan, Frey and Neal (1995) and Hinton and Ghahramani (1997) (see Section B.15) have argued that cortical computation is invertible, so that for example the forward transform of visual information from V1 to higher areas loses no information, and there can be a backward transform from the higher areas to V1. A comparison of the reconstructed representation in V1 with the actual image from the world might in principle be used to correct all the synaptic weights between the two (in both the forward and the reverse directions), in such a way that there are no errors in the transform. This suggested reconstruction scheme would seem to involve non-local synaptic weight correction (though see Section B.15 for a suggested, although still biologically implausible, neural implementation), or other biologically implausible operations. The scheme also does not seem to provide an account for why or how the responses of inferior temporal cortex neurons become the way they are (providing information about which object is seen relatively independently of position on the retina, size, or view). The whole forward transform performed in the brain seems to lose much of the information about the size, position and view of the object, as it is evidence about which object is present invariant of its size, view, etc. that is useful to the stages of processing about objects that follow. Because of these difficulties, and because the backprojections are needed for processes such as recall (see Rolls (2016b) and Section 9.3.8), this invertible network approach is not considered further in this book.

In the context of recall, if the visual system were to perform a reconstruction in V1 of a visual scene from what is represented in the inferior temporal visual cortex, then it might be supposed that remembered visual scenes might be as information-rich (and subjectively as full of rich detail) as seeing the real thing. This is not the case for most humans, and indeed this point suggests that at least what reaches consciousness from the inferior temporal visual cortex (which is activated during the recall of visual memories) is the identity of the object (as made explicit in the firing rate of the neurons), and not the low-level details of the exact place, size, and view of the object in the recalled scene, even though, according to the reconstruction argument, that information should be present in the inferior temporal visual cortex.

Another difficulty is that if the backprojections are used for top-down attention and recall, as seems to be the case (Rolls, 2016b), then associative modifiability of the top-down backprojections is appropriate, and may not be compatible with invertible networks.

2.6.5 Deep learning

Another approach, from the machine learning area, is that of deep convolutional networks (LeCun, Kavukcuoglu and Farabet, 2010; LeCun, Bengio and Hinton, 2015), which are described in Sections B.14 and 2.9.4. Convolutional networks are a biologically-inspired trainable architecture that can learn invariant features. Each stage in a ConvNet is composed of a filter bank, some non-linearities, and feature pooling layers. With multiple stages, a ConvNet can learn multi-level hierarchies of features (LeCun et al., 2010, 2015). Non-linearities that include rectification and local contrast normalization are important in such systems (Jarrett et al., 2009) (and are of course properties of VisNet).

Convolutional networks are very biologically implausible, in that each unit (or 'neuron') receives from only typically a 3 x 3 or 2 x 2 unit patch of the preceding area; by using lateral weight copying within a layer; by having up to 140 or more layers stacked on top of each other in the hierarchy; by using the non-biologically plausible backpropagation of error training algorithm; and by using a teacher for every neuron in the output layer. Interestingly, unlike VisNet, there is no attempt in general to teach the network transform invariance by presenting images with spatial continuity, and no attempt to take advantage of the statistics of the world to help it learn which transforms are probably of the same object by capitalising on temporal continuity (Rolls, 2021d). Further, convolutional networks cannot explain the sensitivity of humans to precise feature configurations (Ullman et al., 2016). Although the computations involved are very different, comparisons of neurons in the brain with the neurons found in deep learning networks have been made (Yamins and DiCarlo, 2016; Rajalingham, Issa, Bashivan, Kar, Schmidt and DiCarlo, 2018), and are evaluated in Section 2.9.4.

2.6.6 Feature hierarchies and 2D view-based object recognition

The hierarchical organisation of the ventral visual system is illustrated in Fig. 2.2. This lends itself as a suitable framework for a *feature hierarchy* approach to 2D shape and object encoding and recognition, which is illustrated in Fig. 2.28.

2.6.6.1 The feature hierarchy approach to object recognition

In the feature hierarchy approach, the system starts with some low-level description of the visual scene, in terms for example of oriented straight line segments of the type that are rep-

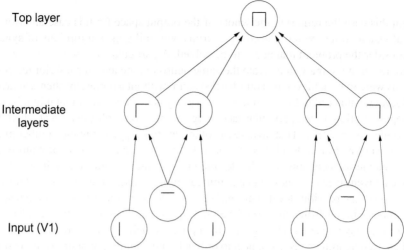

Fig. 2.28 The feature hierarchy approach to object recognition. The inputs may be neurons tuned to oriented straight line segments. In early intermediate levels neurons respond to a combination of these inputs in the correct spatial position with respect to each other. In further intermediate levels, of which there may be several, neurons respond with some invariance to the feature combinations represented early, and form higher order feature combinations. Finally, in the top level, neurons respond to combinations of what is represented in the preceding intermediate level, and thus provide evidence about objects in a position (and scale and even view) invariant way. Convergence through the network is designed to provide top level neurons with information from across the entire input retina, as part of the solution to translation invariance, and other types of invariance are treated similarly.

resented in the responses of primary visual cortex (V1) neurons (Hubel and Wiesel, 1962; Miller, 2016) (Fig. 2.5), and then builds, in repeated hierarchical levels, features based on what is represented in previous levels. A feature may thus be defined as a combination of what is represented in the previous level. For example, after V1, features might consist of combinations of straight lines, which might represent longer curved lines (Zucker, Dobbins and Iverson, 1989), or terminated lines (in fact represented in V1 as end-stopped cells), corners, 'T' junctions which are characteristic of obscuring edges, and (at least in humans) the arrow and 'Y' vertices that are characteristic properties of human environments such as the corners of a building or room. Evidence that such feature combination neurons are present in V2 is that some neurons respond to combinations of line elements that join at different angles (Hegde and Van Essen, 2000; Ito and Komatsu, 2004). (An example of this might be a neuron responding to a 'V' shape at a particular orientation.) As one ascends the hierarchy, neurons might respond to more complex trigger features (such as two parts of a complex figure in the correct spatial arrangement with respect to each other, as shown by Tanaka (1996) for V4 and posterior inferior temporal cortex neurons). In the (anterior) inferior temporal visual cortex, we showed that some face-selective neurons respond to combinations of features such as eyes, mouth, and hair, but not to these components presented individually, or in a configuration with the parts rearranged (Perrett, Rolls and Caan, 1982; Rolls, Tovee, Purcell, Stewart and Azzopardi, 1994b), and this is captured by hierarchical competitive networks (Robinson and Rolls, 2015). Further on, neurons might respond to combinations of several such intermediate-level feature combination neurons, and thus come to respond systematically differently to different objects, and thus to convey information about which object is present. This approach received neurophysiological support early on from the results of Hubel and Wiesel (1962; 1968) in the cat and monkey, and much of the data described in Chapter 5 of Rolls and Deco (2002) (available at https://www.oxcns.org as a .pdf) are consistent with this scheme.

One advantage of feature hierarchy systems is that they can map the whole of an input space (in this case the retina) to the whole of the output space (in this case anterior inferior temporal visual cortex) without needing neurons with millions and millions of synaptic inputs. Consider the problem that needs to be solved. A particular face seen over a wide range of positions on the retina will activate the same neuron in the anterior inferior temporal cortex. If this were to be achieved in a one-level system, without a hierarchy, then a neuron in the second level would need to have connections to every neuron in level 1 that might be involved in the representation of that particular face image at every possible position at which the face might be placed on level 1. That involves a combinatorial explosion in the number of connections that every neuron in level 2 would need to the enormous numbers of neurons in level 1. Instead, a hierarchical approach divides the problem into several stages, in which any one neuron at a given stage responds to just a limited set of combinations of neuronal firing over a small region of the previous level. This enables a single neuron in the top level to respond to a combination of inputs from any part of the input space, as illustrated in Fig. 2.2. Moreover, if the neurons at any one level self-organize by a process such as competitive learning (Section B.4), then each neuron needs to connect to only a limited number of neurons in the preceding level (e.g. 10,000), and the competition helps to ensure that different neurons within a local cortical region within which lateral inhibition operates through the inhibitory interneurons learn to respond to different combinations of features in the input space. Moreover, not every combination of inputs needs to be encoded by neurons, but only those that occur during self-organization given the statistics of the world. For example, natural image statistics reflect the presence of structure in the input space, in for example edges in a scene, so that not every possible combination of pixels in the input space need to be encoded, for vision in a world with natural image statistics.

A second advantage is that the feature analyzers can be built out of the rather simple competitive networks described in Section B.4 that use a local learning rule, and have no external teacher, so that they are rather biologically plausible. Another advantage is that, once trained at lower levels on sets of features common to most objects, the system can then learn new objects quickly using only its higher levels (Elliffe, Rolls and Stringer, 2002).

A related third advantage is that, if implemented with competitive nets as in the case of VisNet (see Section 2.8), then neurons are allocated by self-organization to represent just the features present in the natural statistics of real images (cf. Field (1994)), and not every possible feature that could be constructed by random combinations of pixels on the retina.

A related fourth advantage of feature hierarchy networks is that because they can utilize competitive networks, they can still produce a good estimate of what is in the image under non-ideal conditions, when only parts of objects are visible because for example of occlusion by other objects, etc. The reasons for this are that competitive networks assess the evidence for the presence of certain 'features' to which they are tuned using a dot product operation on their inputs, so that they are inherently tolerant of missing input evidence; and reach a state that reflects the best hypothesis or hypotheses (with soft competition) given the whole set of inputs, because there are competitive interactions between the different neurons (see Section B.4).

A fifth advantage of a feature hierarchy system is that, as shown in Section 2.8.6, the system does not need to perform segmentation into objects as part of pre-processing, nor does it need to be able to identify parts of an object, and can also operate in cluttered scenes in which the object may be partially obscured. The reason for this is that once trained on objects, the system then operates somewhat like an associative memory, mapping the image properties forward onto whatever it has learned about before, and then by competition selecting just the most likely output to be activated. Indeed, the feature hierarchy approach provides a mechanism by which processing at the object recognition level could feed back using back-projections to early cortical areas to provide top-down guidance to assist segmentation Rolls

(2016b). Although backprojections are not built into VisNet2 (Rolls and Milward, 2000), they have been added when attentional top-down processing must be incorporated (Deco and Rolls, 2004).

A sixth advantage of feature hierarchy systems is that they can naturally utilize features in the images of objects that are not strictly part of a shape description scheme, such as the fact that different objects have different textures, colors etc. Feature hierarchy systems, because they utilize whatever is represented at earlier stages in forming feature combination neurons at the next stage, naturally incorporate such 'feature list' evidence into their analysis, and have the advantages of that approach (see Section 2.6.1 and also Mel (1997)). Indeed, the feature space approach can utilize a hybrid representation, some of whose dimensions may be discrete and defined in structural terms, while other dimensions may be continuous and defined in terms of metric details (Biederman, 1987), and others may be concerned with non-shape properties such as texture and color (cf. Edelman (1999)).

A seventh advantage of feature hierarchy systems is that they do not need to utilize 'on the fly' or run-time arbitrary binding of features. Instead, the spatial syntax is effectively hardwired into the system when it is trained, in that the feature combination neurons have learned to respond to their set of features when they are in a given spatial arrangement on the retina.

An eighth advantage of feature hierarchy systems is that they can self-organize (given the right functional architecture, trace synaptic learning rule, and the temporal statistics of the normal visual input from the world), with no need for an external teacher to specify for each output neuron what it must respond to. The need for a teacher is a major argument against the biological plausibility of deep learning approaches such as convolution nets to visual object recognition (see Sections 2.6.5 and 2.9.4). In a feature hierarchy network the correct, object, representation can self-organize itself given rather economically specified genetic rules for building the network (Rolls and Stringer, 2000). Artificial neuronal network approaches to invariant object recognition could have major benefits if they could self-organize like the brain without pre-specification of what should be learned, and indeed what each output neuron should learn (see Sections 2.6.5 and 2.9.4).

Ninth, hierarchical visual systems may recognize 3D objects based on a limited set of 2D views of objects, and the same architectural rules just stated and implemented in VisNet will correctly associate together the different views of an object. It is part of the concept, and consistent with neurophysiological data (Tanaka, 1996), that the neurons in the upper levels will generalize correctly within a view (see Section 2.8.7).

Tenth, another advantage of cortical feature hierarchy systems is that they can operate fast, in approximately 20 ms per level (see Sections B.4 and B.6.5).

Eleventh, although hierarchical cortical systems so far have been described in a feed-forward mode of operation, they are completely compatible with backprojections, again connected mainly between adjacent levels, to implement top-down effects of attention and cognition, and to implement memory recall (Rolls, 2016b). The connectivity requirements in terms of the number of input and output connections of each neuron are met best by having backprojection connections mainly between adjacent levels of the backprojection hierarchy. As described by Rolls (2016b), the backprojections must not dominate the bottom-up (feedforward) connections, and therefore are relatively weak, which is facilitated by their termination in layer 1 of the cortex, well away from the cell body, and where the effects can be shunted if there are strong bottom-up inputs.

Twelfth, hierarchical cortical systems are also consistent with local recurrent collateral connections within a small region within a level of the hierarchy, to implement memory and constraint satisfaction functions as described by Rolls (2016b).

Thirteenth, some artificial neural networks are invertible (Hinton et al., 1995; Hinton and

Ghahramani, 1997), and operate by minimizing an error between an input representation and a reconstructed input representation based on a forward pass to the top of the hierarchy, and a backward pass down the hierarchy. There are a number of reasons why this seems implausible for cortical architecture. One is that information appears to be lost in the forward pass in the neocortex, for example in computing position and view invariant representations at the top of the network, for use in subsequent stages of processing. That makes it unlikely that what is represented at the top of a cortical network could be used to reconstruct the input. Another problem is how an error-correction synaptic modification rule might be computed and applied to the appropriate synapses of the neurons at every stage of the cortical architecture. A third difficulty is that if the backprojections are used for top-down attention and recall, as seems to be the case (Rolls, 2016b), then associative modifiability of the top-down backprojections is appropriate, and may not be compatible with invertible networks.

Fourteenth, feature hierarchies are biologically plausible, and evolutionarily economical. They are biologically plausible in that they can be implemented with local synaptic learning rules (needing only the activity in the pre-synaptic and post-synaptic neurons), in competitive networks (described in Section B.4). They are evolutionarily economical in that the same type of competitive network can be utilised in each stage of the hierarchy, without the need for evolution to optimise many different types of network and the genetic specification for them; and can be used in every sensory system.

A number of problems need to be solved for such feature hierarchy systems to provide a useful model of, for example, object recognition in the primate visual system.

First, some way needs to be found to keep the number of feature combination neurons realistic at each stage, without undergoing a combinatorial explosion. If a separate feature combination neuron was needed to code for every possible combination of n types of feature each with a resolution of 2 levels (binary encoding) in the preceding stage, then 2^n neurons would be needed. The suggestion that is made in Section 2.7 is that by forming neurons that respond to low-order combinations of features (neurons that respond to a combination of only say 2–4 features from the preceding stage), the number of actual feature analyzing neurons can be kept within reasonable numbers. By reasonable I mean the number of neurons actually found at any one stage of the visual system, which, for V4 might be in the order of 60×10^6 neurons (assuming a volume for macaque V4 of approximately 2,000 mm^3, and a cell density of 20,000–40,000 neurons per mm^3, see Table 1.8). This is certainly a large number; but the fact that a large number of neurons is present at each stage of the primate visual system is in fact consistent with the hypothesis that feature combination neurons are part of the way in which the brain solves object recognition.

Another factor that also helps to keep the number of neurons under control is the statistics of the visual world, which contain great redundancies. The world is not random, and indeed the statistics of natural images are such that many regularities are present (Field, 1994), and not every possible combination of pixels on the retina needs to be separately encoded.

A third factor that helps to keep the number of connections required onto each neuron under control is that in a multilevel hierarchy each neuron can be set up to receive connections from only a small region of the preceding level. Thus an individual neuron does not need to have connections from all the neurons in the preceding level. Over multiple levels, the required convergence can be produced so that the same neurons in the top level can be activated by an image of an effective object anywhere on the retina (see Fig. 2.2).

A second problem of feature hierarchy approaches is how to map all the different possible images of an individual object through to the same set of neurons in the top level by modifying the synaptic connections (see Fig. 2.2). The solution discussed in Sections 2.7, 2.8.1.1 and 2.8.4 is the use of a synaptic modification rule with a short-term memory trace of the previous activity of the neuron, to enable it to learn to respond to the now transformed version of what was seen very recently, which, given the statistics of looking at the visual world, will probably be an input from the same object.

A third problem of feature hierarchy approaches is how they can learn in just a few seconds of inspection of an object to recognize it in different transforms, for example in different positions on the retina in which it may never have been presented during training. A solution to this problem is provided in Section 2.8.5, in which it is shown that this can be a natural property of feature hierarchy object recognition systems, if they are trained first for all locations on the intermediate level feature combinations of which new objects will simply be a new combination, and therefore require learning only in the upper levels of the hierarchy.

A fourth potential problem of feature hierarchy systems is that when solving translation invariance they need to respond to the same local spatial arrangement of features (which are needed to specify the object), but to ignore the global position of the whole object. It is shown in Section 2.8.5 that feature hierarchy systems can solve this problem by forming feature combination neurons at an early stage of processing (e.g. V1 or V2 in the brain) that respond with high spatial precision to the local arrangement of features. Such neurons would respond differently for example to L, +, and T if they receive inputs from two line-responding neurons. It is shown in Section 2.8.5 that at later levels of the hierarchy, where some of the intermediate level feature combination neurons are starting to show translation invariance, then correct object recognition may still occur because only one object contains just those sets of intermediate level neurons in which the spatial representation of the features is inherent in the encoding.

After the immediately following description of early models of a feature hierarchy approach implemented in the Cognitron and Neocognitron, we turn in Section 2.7 to hypotheses of *how* the key computations could be performed in the ventral visual system. These are developed in the context of a feature hierarchy approach to invariant visual object recognition. Then in Section 2.8, the VisNet model of *how* these computations are implemented in the ventral visual system is described.

2.6.6.2 The Cognitron and Neocognitron

An early computational model of a hierarchical feature-based approach to object recognition, joining other early discussions of this approach (Selfridge, 1959; Sutherland, 1968; Barlow, 1972; Milner, 1974), was proposed by Fukushima (1975; 1980; 1989; 1989; 1991). His model used two types of cell within each layer to approach the problem of invariant representations. In each layer, a set of 'simple cells', with defined position, orientation, etc. sensitivity for the stimuli to which they responded, was followed by a set of 'complex cells', which generalized a little over position, orientation, etc. This simple cell – complex cell pairing within each layer provided some invariance. When a neuron in the network using competitive learning with its stimulus set, which was typically letters on a 16×16 pixel array, learned that a particular feature combination had occurred, that type of feature analyzer was replicated in a non-local manner throughout the layer, to provide further translation invariance. Invariant representations were thus learned by using a convolution (and this was the forerunner of deep convolutional networks (Section B.14), but is biologically implausible). This is this very different to VisNet. Up to eight layers were used. The network could learn to differentiate letters, even with some translation, scaling, or distortion. Although internally it is organized and learns very differently to VisNet, it is an independent example of the fact that useful invariant pattern recognition can be performed by multilayer hierarchical networks. A major biological implausibility of the system is that once one neuron within a layer learned, other similar neurons were set up throughout the layer by a non-local process. A second biological limitation was that no learning rule or self-organizing process was specified as to how the complex cells can provide translation invariant representations of simple cell responses – this was simply handwired. Solutions to both these issues are provided by VisNet.

2.7 Hypotheses about how the computations are performed in a feature hierarchy approach to for invariant object recognition

The neurophysiological findings described in Section 2.4, and wider considerations on the possible computational properties of the cerebral cortex (Rolls, 1990b, 1989f, 1992a, 1994a, 1995a, 1997c, 2000a; Rolls and Treves, 1998; Rolls and Deco, 2002; Rolls, 2016b), led to the following outline working hypotheses on object recognition by visual cortical mechanisms (see Rolls (1992a) which is a paper delivered to the Royal Society on 8-9 July 1991, Rolls (2012d), and Rolls (2021d)). The principles underlying the processing of faces and other objects may be similar, but more neurons may become allocated to represent different aspects of faces because of the need to recognize the faces of many different individuals, that is to identify many individuals within the category faces.

Cortical visual processing for object recognition is considered to be organized as a set of hierarchically connected cortical regions consisting at least of V1, V2, V4, posterior inferior temporal cortex (TEO), inferior temporal cortex (e.g. TE3, TEa and TEm), and anterior temporal cortical areas (e.g. TE2 and TE1) (in macaques). (This stream of processing has many connections with a set of cortical areas in the anterior part of the superior temporal sulcus, including area TPO.) There is convergence from each small part of a region to the succeeding region (or layer in the hierarchy) in such a way that the receptive field sizes of neurons (e.g. 1 degree near the fovea in V1) become larger by a factor of approximately 2.5 with each succeeding stage (and the typical parafoveal receptive field sizes found would not be inconsistent with the calculated approximations of e.g. 8 degrees in V4, 20 degrees in TEO, and 50 degrees in the inferior temporal cortex (Boussaoud, Desimone and Ungerleider, 1991)) (see Fig. 2.2 on page 57). Such zones of convergence would overlap continuously with each other (see Fig. 2.2). This connectivity would be part of the architecture by which translation invariant representations are computed.

Each layer is considered to act partly as a set of local self-organizing competitive neuronal networks with overlapping inputs. (The region within which competition would be implemented would depend on the spatial properties of inhibitory interneurons, and might operate over distances of 1–2 mm in the cortex.) These competitive nets operate by a single set of forward inputs leading to (typically non-linear, e.g. sigmoid) activation of output neurons; of competition between the output neurons mediated by a set of feedback inhibitory interneurons which receive from many of the principal (in the cortex, pyramidal) cells in the net and project back (via inhibitory interneurons) to many of the principal cells and serve to decrease the firing rates of the less active neurons relative to the rates of the more active neurons; and then of synaptic modification by a modified Hebb rule, such that synapses to strongly activated output neurons from active input axons strengthen, and from inactive input axons weaken (see Section B.4). A biologically plausible form of this learning rule that operates well in such networks is

$$\delta w_{ij} = \alpha y_i (x_j - w_{ij}) \tag{2.2}$$

where α is a learning rate constant, and x_j and w_{ij} are in appropriate units (see Section B.4). Such competitive networks operate to detect correlations between the activity of the input neurons, and to allocate output neurons to respond to each cluster of such correlated inputs. These networks thus act as categorizers. In relation to visual information processing, they would remove redundancy from the input representation, and would develop low entropy representations of the information (cf. Barlow (1985), Barlow, Kaushal and Mitchison (1989)). Such competitive nets are biologically plausible, in that they utilize Hebb-modifiable forward excitatory connections, with competitive inhibition mediated by cortical inhibitory neurons. The competitive scheme I suggest would not result in the formation of 'winner-take-all' or 'grandmother' cells, but would instead result in a small ensemble of active neurons representing each input with a sparse distributed representation (Rolls, 1990b, 1989f; Rolls and Treves, 1998; Rolls, 2012d) (see Section B.4). The scheme has the advantages that the output neurons learn better to distribute themselves between the input patterns (cf. Bennett (1990)), and that the sparse representations formed have utility in maximizing the number of memories that can be stored when, towards the end of the visual system, the visual representation of objects is interfaced to associative memory (Rolls, 1990b, 1989f; Rolls and Treves, 1998)[1].

Translation invariance would be computed in such a system by utilizing competitive learning to detect regularities in inputs when real objects are translated in the physical world. The hypothesis is that because objects have continuous properties in space and time in the world, an object at one place on the retina might activate feature analyzers at the next stage of cortical processing, and when the object was translated to a nearby position, because this would occur in a short period (e.g. 0.5 s), the membrane of the postsynaptic neuron would still be in its 'Hebb-modifiable' state (caused for example by calcium entry as a result of the voltage-dependent activation of NMDA receptors), and the presynaptic afferents activated with the object in its new position would thus become strengthened on the still-activated postsynaptic neuron. It is suggested that the short temporal window (e.g. 0.5 s) of Hebb-modifiability helps neurons to learn the statistics of objects moving and more generally transforming in the physical world, and at the same time to form different representations of different feature combinations or objects, as these are physically discontinuous and present less regular correlations to the visual system (Rolls, 1992a, 2021d). Földiák (1991) has proposed computing an average activation of the postsynaptic neuron to assist with the same problem. One idea here is that the temporal properties of the biologically implemented synaptic learning mechanism are such that it is well suited to detecting the relevant continuities in the world of real objects (Rolls, 1992a, 2021d). Another suggestion (Rolls, 1992a, 2021d) is that a memory trace for what has been seen in the last 300 ms appears to be implemented by a mechanism as simple as continued firing of inferior temporal neurons after the stimulus has disappeared, as has been found in masking experiments (Rolls and Tovee, 1994; Rolls, Tovee, Purcell, Stewart and Azzopardi, 1994b; Rolls, Tovee and Panzeri, 1999b; Rolls, 2003, 2016b).

I also proposed (Rolls, 1992a) that other invariances, for example size, spatial frequency, and rotation invariance, could be learned by a comparable process. (Early processing in V1 that enables different neurons to represent inputs at different spatial scales would allow combinations of the outputs of such neurons to be formed at later stages. Scale invariance would then result from detecting at a later stage which neurons are almost conjunctively active as the size of an object alters.) It is proposed that this process takes place at each stage of the

---

[1] In that each neuron has graded responses centred about an optimal input, the proposal has some of the advantages with respect to hypersurface reconstruction described by Poggio and Girosi (1990a). However, the system I propose learns differently, in that instead of using perhaps non-biologically plausible algorithms to optimally locate the centres of the receptive fields of the neurons, the neurons use graded competition to spread themselves throughout the input space, depending on the statistics of the inputs received, and perhaps with some guidance from backprojections (see below). In addition, the competitive nets I propose use as a distance function the dot product between the input vector to a neuron and its synaptic weight vector, whereas radial basis function networks use a Gaussian measure of distance (see Section B.4.8). Both systems benefit from the finite width of the response region of each neuron which tapers from a maximum, and is important for enabling the system to generalize smoothly from the examples with which it has learned (cf. Poggio and Girosi (1990b), Poggio and Girosi (1990a)), to help the system to respond for example with the correct invariances as described below.

multiple-layer cortical processing hierarchy, so that invariances are learned first over small regions of space, and then over successively larger regions. This limits the size of the connection space within which correlations must be sought.

Increasing complexity of representations could also be built in such a multiple layer hierarchy by similar mechanisms. At each stage or layer the self-organizing competitive nets would result in combinations of inputs becoming the effective stimuli for neurons. In order to avoid the combinatorial explosion, it is proposed, following Feldman (1985), that low-order combinations of inputs would be what is learned by each neuron. (Each input would not be represented by activity in a single input axon, but instead by activity in a set of active input axons.) Evidence consistent with this suggestion that neurons are responding to combinations of a few variables represented at the preceding stage of cortical processing is that some neurons in V1 respond to combinations of bars or edges (see Section 2.5 of Rolls and Deco (2002); Sillito et al. (1995); and Shevelev et al. (1995)); V2 and V4 respond to end-stopped lines, to angles formed by a combination of lines, to acute curvature, to tongues flanked by inhibitory subregions, and to combinations of colors (Hegde and Van Essen, 2000; Rolls and Deco, 2002; Ito and Komatsu, 2004; Carlson et al., 2011; Kourtzi and Connor, 2011; Roe et al., 2012; Nandy et al., 2013; Kim et al., 2019; Jiang et al., 2021); in posterior inferior temporal cortex to stimuli which may require two or more simple features to be present (Tanaka, Saito, Fukada and Moriya, 1990); and in the temporal cortical face processing areas to images that require the presence of several features in a face (such as eyes, hair, and mouth) in order to respond (Perrett, Rolls and Caan, 1982; Yamane, Kaji and Kawano, 1988) (see Chapter 5 of Rolls and Deco (2002), Rolls (2007e), Rolls (2016b), Rolls (2011d), and Fig. 2.10). (Precursor cells to face-responsive neurons might, it is suggested, respond to combinations of the outputs of the neurons in V1 that are activated by faces, and might be found in areas such as V4.)

It is an important part of this proposal that some local spatial information would be inherent in the features that were being combined. For example, cells might not respond to the combination of an edge and a small circle unless they were in the correct spatial relation to each other. (This is in fact consistent with the data of Tanaka, Saito, Fukada and Moriya (1990), and with our data on face neurons, in that some faces neurons require the face features to be in the correct spatial configuration, and not jumbled (Rolls, Tovee, Purcell, Stewart and Azzopardi, 1994b).) The local spatial information in the features being combined would ensure that the representation at the next level would contain some information about the (local) arrangement of features. Further low-order combinations of such neurons at the next stage would include sufficient local spatial information so that an arbitrary spatial arrangement of the same features would not activate the same neuron, and this is the proposed, and limited, solution that this mechanism would provide for the feature binding problem (Elliffe, Rolls and Stringer, 2002). By this stage of processing a view-dependent representation of objects suitable for view-dependent processes such as behavioral responses to face expression and gesture would be available.

It is also proposed that view-independent representations could be formed by the same type of computation, operating to combine a limited set of views of objects (Rolls, 1992a, 2021d). The plausibility of providing view-independent recognition of objects by combining a set of different views of objects has been proposed by a number of investigators (Koenderink and Van Doorn, 1979; Poggio and Edelman, 1990; Logothetis, Pauls, Bulthoff and Poggio, 1994; Ullman, 1996). Consistent with the suggestion that the view-independent representations are formed by combining view-dependent representations in the primate visual system, is the fact that in the temporal cortical areas, neurons with view-independent representations of faces are present in the same cortical areas as neurons with view-dependent representations (from which the view-independent neurons could receive inputs) (Hasselmo,

Rolls, Baylis and Nalwa, 1989b; Perrett, Smith, Potter, Mistlin, Head, Milner and Jeeves, 1985b; Booth and Rolls, 1998). This solution to 'object-based' representations is very different from that traditionally proposed for artificial vision systems, in which the coordinates in 3D space of objects are stored in a database, and general-purpose algorithms operate on these to perform transforms such as translation, rotation, and scale change in 3D space (e.g. Marr (1982)). In the present, much more limited but more biologically plausible scheme, the representation would be suitable for recognition of an object, and for linking associative memories to objects, but would be less good for making actions in 3D space to particular parts of, or inside, objects, as the 3D coordinates of each part of the object would not be explicitly available. It is therefore proposed that visual fixation is used to locate in foveal vision part of an object to which movements must be made, and that local disparity and other measurements of depth then provide sufficient information for the motor system to make actions relative to the small part of space in which a local, view-dependent, representation of depth would be provided (using computations of the type described in Section 3.4 and by Rolls (2020b)).

The computational processes proposed above operate by an unsupervised learning mechanism, which utilizes statistical regularities in the physical environment to enable representations to be built (Rolls, 2021d). In some cases it may be advantageous to utilize some form of mild teaching input to the visual system, to enable it to learn for example that rather similar visual inputs have very different consequences in the world, so that different representations of them should be built. In other cases, it might be helpful to bring representations together, if they have identical consequences, in order to use storage capacity efficiently. It is proposed elsewhere (Rolls, 1990b, 1989f; Rolls and Treves, 1998; Rolls, 2016b) (as described in Section B.4.5) that the backprojections from each adjacent cortical region in the hierarchy (and from the amygdala and hippocampus to higher regions of the visual system) play such a role by providing guidance to the competitive networks suggested above to be important in each cortical area. This guidance, and also the capability for recall, are it is suggested implemented by Hebb-modifiable connections from the backprojecting neurons to the principal (pyramidal) neurons of the competitive networks in the preceding stages (Rolls, 1990b, 1989f; Rolls and Treves, 1998; Rolls, 2016b) (see Section B.4).

The computational processes outlined above use sparse distributed coding with relatively finely tuned neurons with a graded response region centred about an optimal response achieved when the input stimulus matches the synaptic weight vector on a neuron. The distributed nature of the coding but with fine tuning would help to limit the combinatorial explosion, to keep the number of neurons within the biological range. The graded response region would be crucial in enabling the system to generalize correctly to solve for example the invariances. However, such a system would need many neurons, each with considerable learning capacity, to solve visual perception in this way. This is fully consistent with the large number of neurons in the visual system, and with the large number of, probably modifiable, synapses on each neuron (e.g. 10,000). Further, the fact that many neurons are tuned in different ways to faces is consistent with the fact that in such a computational system, many neurons would need to be sensitive (in different ways) to faces, in order to allow recognition of many individual faces when all share a number of common properties.

2.8 VisNet: a model of how the computations are performed in the ventral visual system

The feature hierarchy approach to invariant object recognition was introduced in Sections 2.6.6 and 2.7, and advantages and disadvantages of it were discussed. Hypotheses about how object recognition could be implemented in the brain that are consistent with much of the neurophysiology discussed in Section 2.4 and elsewhere (Rolls and Deco, 2002; Rolls, 2007e, 2016b, 2011d, 2012d) were set out in Section 2.7. These hypotheses effectively incorporate a feature hierarchy system while encompassing much of the neurophysiological evidence. In this Section (2.8), we consider the computational issues that arise in such feature hierarchy systems, and in the brain systems that implement visual object recognition. The issues are considered with the help of a particular model, VisNet, which requires precise specification of the hypotheses, and at the same time enables them to be explored and tested numerically and quantitatively. However, we emphasize that the issues to be covered in Section 2.8 are key and major computational issues for architectures of this feature hierarchical type (Rolls and Stringer, 2006b), and are very relevant to understanding how any mechanism for invariant object recognition is implemented in the cerebral cortex.

*It is worth emphasising that each of the investigations described in this section (2.8) with VisNet address issues that need to be accounted for by any theory and model of **how** the computations are performed in the ventral visual system.*

A feature of the research with VisNet is that most of the investigations have been performed to account for particular neurophysiological findings, and the results obtained with VisNet have then been compared with the neuronal responses found in the cerebral cortex, in particular in the inferior temporal visual cortex (Rolls, 2012d; Rolls and Webb, 2014; Webb and Rolls, 2014; Robinson and Rolls, 2015; Rolls and Mills, 2018; Rolls, 2021d).

VisNet is a model of invariant object recognition based on Rolls' (1992a) hypotheses (Section 2.7). It is a computer simulation that allows hypotheses to be tested and developed about how multilayer hierarchical networks of the type proposed to be implemented in the visual cortical pathways operate (Rolls, 2016b, 2012d, 2021d). The architecture captures a number of aspects of the architecture of the visual cortical pathways, and is described next. The model of course, as with all models, requires precise specification of what is to be implemented, and at the same time involves specified simplifications of the real architecture, as investigations of the fundamental aspects of the information processing being performed are more tractable in a simplified and at the same time quantitatively specified model. First the architecture of the model is described, and this is followed by descriptions of key issues in such multilayer feature hierarchical models, such as the issue of feature binding, the optimal form of training rule for the whole system to self-organize, the operation of the network in natural environments and when objects are partly occluded, how outputs about individual objects can be read out from the network, and the capacity of the system.

A version of VisNet written entirely in Matlab for simplicity is made available in connection with the publication of this book (Rolls, 2023a) at https://www.oxcns.org (see Appendix D). Although it is not the full version of VisNet with which the research described next has been performed which is written in C, and will not perform identically to the full version, the Matlab version may be useful for tutorial use to help make explicit how the computations are performed in this example of a network that can learn invariant representations with unsupervised learning.

2.8.1 The architecture of VisNet

Fundamental elements of Rolls' (1992a) theory for how cortical networks might implement invariant object recognition are described in Section 2.7. They provide the basis for the design of VisNet, and can be summarized as:

- A series of competitive networks, organized in hierarchical layers, exhibiting mutual inhibition over a short range within each layer. These networks allow combinations of features or inputs occurring in a given spatial arrangement to be learned by neurons, ensuring that higher order spatial properties of the input stimuli are represented in the network.

- A convergent series of connections from a localized population of cells in preceding layers to each cell of the following layer, thus allowing the receptive field size of cells to increase through the visual processing areas or layers.
- A modified Hebb-like learning rule incorporating a temporal trace of each cell's previous activity, which, it is suggested, will enable the neurons to learn transform invariances.

The first two elements of Rolls' theory are used to constrain the general architecture of a network model, VisNet, of the processes just described that is intended to learn invariant representations of objects. The simulation results described in this chapter using VisNet show that invariant representations can be learned by the architecture. It is moreover shown that successful learning depends crucially on the use of the modified Hebb rule. The general architecture simulated in VisNet, and the way in which it allows natural images to be used as stimuli, has been chosen to enable some comparisons of neuronal responses in the network and in the brain to similar stimuli to be made.

2.8.1.1 The memory trace learning rule

The synaptic learning rule implemented in the VisNet simulations utilizes the spatio-temporal constraints placed upon the behavior of 'real-world' objects to learn about natural object transformations. By presenting consistent sequences of transforming objects the cells in the network can learn to respond to the same object through all of its naturally transformed states, as described by Földiák (1991), Rolls (1992a), Wallis, Rolls and Földiák (1993), Wallis and Rolls (1997) and Rolls (2021d). The learning rule incorporates a decaying trace of previous cell activity and is henceforth referred to simply as the 'trace' learning rule. The learning paradigm described here is intended in principle to enable learning of any of the transforms tolerated by inferior temporal cortex neurons, including position, size, view, lighting, and spatial frequency (Rolls, 1992a, 1994a, 1995a, 1997c, 2000a; Rolls and Deco, 2002; Rolls, 2007e,c, 2008b, 2016b, 2012d; Rolls and Webb, 2014; Webb and Rolls, 2014; Robinson and Rolls, 2015; Rolls and Mills, 2018; Rolls, 2021d).

To clarify the reasoning behind this point, consider the situation in which a single neuron is strongly activated by a stimulus forming part of a real world object. The trace of this neuron's activation will then gradually decay over a time period in the order of 0.5 s. If, during this limited time window, the net is presented with a transformed version of the original stimulus then not only will the initially active afferent synapses modify onto the neuron, but so also will the synapses activated by the transformed version of this stimulus. In this way the cell will learn to respond to either appearance of the original stimulus. Making such associations works in practice because it is very likely that within short time periods different aspects of the same object will be being inspected. The cell will not, however, tend to make spurious links across stimuli that are part of different objects because of the unlikelihood in the real world of one object consistently following another.

Various biological bases for this temporal trace have been advanced:

- The persistent firing of neurons for as long as 100–400 ms observed after presentations of stimuli for 16 ms (Rolls and Tovee, 1994) could provide a time window within which to associate subsequent images. Maintained activity may potentially be implemented by recurrent connections between as well as within cortical areas (Rolls and Treves, 1998; Rolls, 2016b) (see Section 13.6.1)[2].

---

[2]The prolonged firing of inferior temporal cortex neurons during memory delay periods of several seconds, and associative links reported to develop between stimuli presented several seconds apart (Miyashita, 1988) are on too long a time scale to be immediately relevant to the present theory. In fact, associations between visual events occurring several seconds apart would, under *normal* environmental conditions, be detrimental to the operation of a

- The binding period of glutamate in the NMDA channels, which may last for 100 ms or more, may implement a trace rule by producing a narrow time window over which the *average* activity at each presynaptic site affects learning (Rolls, 1992a; Rhodes, 1992; Földiák, 1991; Spruston, Jonas and Sakmann, 1995; Hestrin, Sah and Nicoll, 1990).
- Chemicals such as nitric oxide may be released during high neural activity and gradually decay in concentration over a short time window during which learning could be enhanced (Földiák, 1991; Montague, Gally and Edelman, 1991).

The trace update rule used in the baseline simulations of VisNet (Wallis and Rolls, 1997) is equivalent to both Foldiak's used in the context of translation invariance and to the earlier rule of Sutton and Barto (1981) explored in the context of modelling the temporal properties of classical conditioning, and can be summarized as follows:

$$\delta w_j = \alpha \bar{y}^\tau x_j \qquad (2.3)$$

where

$$\bar{y}^\tau = (1-\eta) y^\tau + \eta \bar{y}^{\tau-1} \qquad (2.4)$$

and

- x_j: j^{th} input to the neuron.
- $\bar{y}^\tau$: Trace value of the output of the neuron at time step τ.
- w_j: Synaptic weight between j^{th} input and the neuron.
- y: Output from the neuron.
- α: Learning rate. Annealed between unity and zero.
- η: Trace value. The optimal value varies with presentation sequence length.

To bound the growth of each neuron's synaptic weight vector, $\mathbf{w}_i$ for the ith neuron, its length is explicitly normalized (a method similarly employed by von der Malsburg (1973) which is commonly used in competitive networks, see Section B.4). An alternative, more biologically relevant implementation, using a local weight bounding operation which utilizes a form of heterosynaptic long-term depression (see Section 1.6), has in part been explored using a version of the Oja (1982) rule (see Wallis and Rolls (1997)).

Learning for layer 1 of VisNet (corresponding to V2) uses purely Hebbian training, without a temporal trace (Rolls and Milward, 2000). The reason for this is that it is essential to form feature combination neurons that respond for example to combinations of edges before any invariance learning is introduced, because the spatial structure of objects can only be specified if the relative positions of features is defined by feature combination neurons.

2.8.1.2 The network implemented in VisNet

The network itself is designed as a series of hierarchical, convergent, competitive networks, in accordance with the hypotheses advanced above. The actual network consists of a series of four layers, constructed such that the convergence of information from the most disparate parts of the network's input layer can potentially influence firing in a single neuron in the final layer – see Fig. 2.2. This corresponds to the scheme described by many researchers (Van Essen et al., 1992; Rolls, 1992a, for example) as present in the primate visual system – see Fig. 2.2. The forward connections to a cell in one layer are derived from a topologically related and confined region of the preceding layer. The choice of whether a connection between neurons in adjacent layers exists or not is based upon a Gaussian distribution of connection probabilities which roll off radially from the focal point of connections for each neuron. (A

---

network of the type described here, because they would probably arise from different objects. In contrast, the system described benefits from associations between visual events which occur close in time (typically within 1 s), as they are likely to be from the same object.

minor extra constraint precludes the repeated connection of any pair of cells.) In particular, the forward connections to a cell in one layer come from a small region of the preceding layer defined by the radius in Table 2.1 which will contain approximately 67% of the connections from the preceding layer. Table 2.1 shows the dimensions for VisNetL, the system we have been using since 2008, which is a (16x) larger version of the version of VisNet than used in most of our earlier investigations, which utilized 32x32 neurons per layer.

Table 2.1 VisNet dimensions. Dimensions shows the number of neurons in each of the 4 layers. # Connections shows the number of synaptic connections onto each neuron. Radius shows the radius of the connectivity from the previous layer of a single neuron (see text).

	Dimensions	# Connections	Radius
Layer 4	128x128	100	48
Layer 3	128x128	100	36
Layer 2	128x128	100	24
Layer 1	128x128	272	24
Input layer	256x256x32	–	–

Figure 2.2 shows the general convergent network architecture used. Localization and limitation of connectivity in the network is intended to mimic cortical connectivity, partially because of the clear retention of retinal topology through regions of visual cortex. This architecture also encourages the gradual combination of features from layer to layer which has relevance to the binding problem, as described in Section 2.8.5[3].

2.8.1.3 Competition and lateral inhibition

In order to act as a competitive network some form of mutual inhibition is required within each layer, which should help to ensure that all stimuli presented are evenly represented by the neurons in each layer. This is implemented in VisNet by a form of lateral inhibition. The idea behind the lateral inhibition, apart from this being a property of cortical architecture in the brain, was to prevent too many neurons that received inputs from a similar part of the preceding layer responding to the same activity patterns. The purpose of the lateral inhibition was to ensure that different receiving neurons coded for different inputs. This is important in reducing redundancy (see Section B.4). The lateral inhibition is conceived as operating within a radius that was similar to that of the region within which a neuron received converging inputs from the preceding layer (because activity in one zone of topologically organized

---

[3] Modelling topological constraints in connectivity leads to an issue concerning neurons at the edges of the network layers. In principle these neurons may either receive no input from beyond the edge of the preceding layer, or have their connections repeatedly sample neurons at the edge of the previous layer. In practice either solution is liable to introduce artificial weighting on the few active inputs at the edge and hence cause the edge to have unwanted influence over the development of the network as a whole. In the real brain such edge-effects would be naturally smoothed by the transition of the locus of cellular input from the fovea to the lower acuity periphery of the visual field. However, it poses a problem here because we are in effect only simulating the small high acuity foveal portion of the visual field in our simulations. As an alternative to the former solutions Wallis and Rolls (1997) elected to form the connections into a toroid, such that connections wrap back onto the network from opposite sides. This wrapping happens at all four layers of the network, and in the way an image on the 'retina' is mapped to the input filters. This solution has the advantage of making all of the boundaries effectively invisible to the network. Further, this procedure does not itself introduce problems into evaluation of the network for the problems set, as many of the critical comparisons in VisNet involve comparisons between a network with the same architecture trained with the trace rule, or with the Hebb rule, or not trained at all. In practice, it is shown below that only the network trained with the trace rule solves the problem of forming invariant representations.

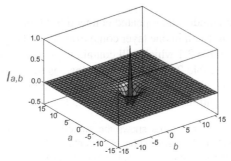

Fig. 2.29 Contrast-enhancing filter, which has the effect of local lateral inhibition. The parameters δ and σ in Equation 2.5 modify the amount and extent of inhibition respectively.

processing within a layer should not inhibit processing in another zone in the same layer, concerned perhaps with another part of the image)[4].

The lateral inhibition and contrast enhancement just described is actually implemented in VisNet2 (Rolls and Milward, 2000) in two stages, to produce filtering of the type illustrated in Fig. 2.29. This lateral inhibition is implemented by convolving the activation of the neurons in a layer with a spatial filter, I, where δ controls the contrast and σ controls the width, and a and b index the distance away from the centre of the filter

$$I_{a,b} = \begin{cases} -\delta e^{-\frac{a^2+b^2}{\sigma^2}} & \text{if } a \neq 0 \text{ or } b \neq 0, \\ 1 - \sum_{a \neq 0, b \neq 0} I_{a,b} & \text{if } a = 0 \text{ and } b = 0. \end{cases} \quad (2.5)$$

This is a filter that leaves the average activity unchanged. A modified version of this filter designed as a difference of Gaussians with the same inhibition but shorter range local excitation is being tested to investigate whether the self-organizing maps that this promotes (Section B.4.6) help the system to provide some continuity in the representations formed. The concept is that this may help the system to code efficiently for large numbers of untrained stimuli that fall between trained stimuli in similarity space.

The second stage involves contrast enhancement. In VisNet (Wallis and Rolls, 1997), this was implemented by raising the neuronal activations to a fixed power and normalizing the resulting firing within a layer to have an average firing rate equal to 1.0. In VisNet2 (Rolls and Milward, 2000) and in subsequent simulations a more biologically plausible form of the activation function, a sigmoid, is used:

$$y = f^{\text{sigmoid}}(r) = \frac{1}{1 + e^{-2\beta(r-\alpha)}} \quad (2.6)$$

where r is the activation (or firing rate) of the neuron after the lateral inhibition, y is the firing rate after the contrast enhancement produced by the activation function, and β is the slope or gain and α is the threshold or bias of the activation function. The sigmoid bounds the firing rate between 0 and 1 so global normalization is not required. The slope and threshold are held constant within each layer. The slope is constant throughout training, whereas the threshold

---

[4] Although the extent of the lateral inhibition actually investigated by Wallis and Rolls (1997) in VisNet operated over adjacent pixels, the lateral inhibition introduced by Rolls and Milward (2000) in what they named VisNet2 and which has been used in subsequent simulations operates over a larger region, set within a layer to approximately half of the radius of convergence from the preceding layer. Indeed, Rolls and Milward (2000) showed in a problem in which invariant representations over 49 locations were being used with a 17 face test set, that the best performance was with intermediate range lateral inhibition, using the parameters for σ shown in Table 2.3. These values of σ set the lateral inhibition radius within a layer to be approximately half that of the spread of the excitatory connections from the preceding layer.

is used to control the sparseness of firing rates within each layer. The (population) sparseness of the firing within a layer is defined (Rolls and Treves, 1998) as:

$$a = \frac{(\sum_i y_i/n)^2}{\sum_i y_i^2/n} \qquad (2.7)$$

where n is the number of neurons in the layer. To set the sparseness to a given value, e.g. 5%, the threshold is set to the value of the 95th percentile point of the activations within the layer. (Unless otherwise stated here, the neurons used the sigmoid activation function as just described.)

In most simulations with VisNet2 and later (Rolls, 2021d), the sigmoid activation function was used with parameters (selected after a number of optimization runs) similar to those shown in Table 2.2.

Table 2.2 Sigmoid parameters and sparseness in the tutorial version of VisNet (Section D.6)

Layer	1	2	3	4
Sparseness	0.01	0.01	0.01	0.01
Slope β	10	10	10	10

In addition, the lateral inhibition parameters normally used in VisNet2 simulations are similar to those shown in Table 2.3 but scaled to reflect the size of the network.

Table 2.3 Lateral inhibition parameters for the 25-location runs in the 32x32 version of VisNet used by Rolls and Milward (2000).

Layer	1	2	3	4
Radius, σ	1.38	2.7	4.0	6.0
Contrast, δ	1.5	1.5	1.6	1.4

2.8.1.4 The input to VisNet

VisNet is provided with a set of input filters which can be applied to an image to produce inputs to the network that correspond to those provided by simple cells in visual cortical area 1 (V1). The purpose of this is to enable within VisNet the more complicated response properties of cells between V1 and the inferior temporal cortex (IT) to be investigated, using as inputs natural stimuli such as those that could be applied to the retina of the real visual system. This is to facilitate comparisons between the activity of neurons in VisNet and those in the real visual system, to the same stimuli. In VisNet no attempt is made to train the response properties of simple cells, but instead we start with a defined series of filters to perform fixed feature extraction to a level equivalent to that of simple cells in V1, as have other researchers in the field (Hummel and Biederman, 1992; Buhmann, Lange, von der Malsburg, Vorbrüggen and Würtz, 1991; Fukushima, 1980), because we wish to simulate the more complicated response properties of cells between V1 and the inferior temporal cortex (IT). In many papers before 2012 we used difference of Gaussian filters, but more recently we have used Gabor filters to simulate V1 similar to those described and used by Deco and Rolls (2004).

The Gabor filters are described next. Following Daugman (1988) the receptive fields of the simple cell-like input neurons are modelled by 2D-Gabor functions. The Gabor receptive fields have five degrees of freedom given essentially by the product of an elliptical Gaussian and a complex plane wave. The first two degrees of freedom are the 2D-locations of the receptive field's centre; the third is the size of the receptive field; the fourth is the orientation of the boundaries separating excitatory and inhibitory regions; and the fifth is the symmetry. This fifth degree of freedom is given in the standard Gabor transform by the real and imaginary part, i.e by the phase of the complex function representing it, whereas in a biological context this can be done by combining pairs of neurons with even and odd receptive fields. This design is supported by the experimental work of Pollen and Ronner (1981), who found simple cells in quadrature-phase pairs. Even more, Daugman (1988) proposed that an ensemble of simple cells is best modelled as a family of 2D-Gabor wavelets sampling the frequency domain in a log-polar manner as a function of eccentricity. Experimental neurophysiological evidence constrains the relation between the free parameters that define a 2D-Gabor receptive field (De Valois and De Valois, 1988). There are three constraints fixing the relation between the width, height, orientation, and spatial frequency (Lee, 1996). The first constraint posits that the aspect ratio of the elliptical Gaussian envelope is 2:1. The second constraint postulates that the plane wave tends to have its propagating direction along the short axis of the elliptical Gaussian. The third constraint assumes that the half-amplitude bandwidth of the frequency response is about 1 to 1.5 octaves along the optimal orientation. Further, we assume that the mean is zero in order to have an admissible wavelet basis (Lee, 1996).

In more detail, the Gabor filters are constructed as follows (Deco and Rolls, 2004). We consider a pixelized grey-scale image given by a $N \times N$ matrix $\Gamma_{ij}^{\text{orig}}$. The subindices ij denote the spatial position of the pixel. Each pixel value is given a grey level brightness value coded in a scale between 0 (black) and 255 (white). The first step in the preprocessing consists of removing the DC component of the image (i.e. the mean value of the grey-scale intensity of the pixels). (The equivalent in the brain is the low-pass filtering performed by the retinal ganglion cells and lateral geniculate cells. The visual representation in the LGN is essentially a contrast invariant pixel representation of the image, i.e. each neuron encodes the relative brightness value at one location in visual space referred to the mean value of the image brightness.) We denote this contrast-invariant LGN representation by the $N \times N$ matrix Γ_{ij} defined by the Equation

$$\Gamma_{ij} = \Gamma_{ij}^{\text{orig}} - \frac{1}{N^2} \sum_{i=1}^{N} \sum_{j=1}^{N} \Gamma_{ij}^{\text{orig}}. \tag{2.8}$$

Feedforward connections to a layer of V1 neurons perform the extraction of simple features like bars at different locations, orientations and sizes. Realistic receptive fields for V1 neurons that extract these simple features can be represented by 2D-Gabor wavelets. Lee (1996) derived a family of discretized 2D-Gabor wavelets that satisfy the wavelet theory and the neurophysiological constraints for simple cells mentioned above. They are given by an expression of the form

$$G_{pqkl}(x, y) = a^{-k} \Psi_{\Theta_l}(a^{-k}(x - 2p), a^{-k}(y - 2q)) \tag{2.9}$$

where

$$\Psi_{\Theta_l} = \Psi(x \cos(l\Theta_0) + y \sin(l\Theta_0), -x \sin(l\Theta_0) + y \cos(l\Theta_0)), \tag{2.10}$$

and the mother wavelet is given by

$$\Psi(x, y) = \frac{1}{\sqrt{2\pi}} e^{-\frac{1}{8}(4x^2 + y^2)} [e^{i\kappa x} - e^{-\frac{\kappa^2}{2}}]. \tag{2.11}$$

In the above equations $\Theta_0 = \pi/L$ denotes the step size of each angular rotation; l the index of rotation corresponding to the preferred orientation $\Theta_l = l\pi/L$; k denotes the octave;

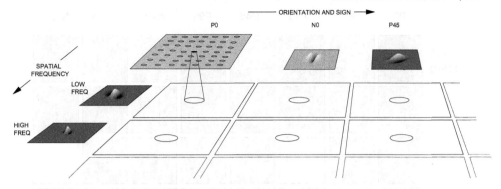

Fig. 2.30 The filter sampling paradigm. Here each square represents the retinal image presented to the network after being filtered by a difference of gaussian filter of the appropriate orientation sign and frequency. The circles represent the consistent retinotopic coordinates used to provide input to a layer 1 cell. The filters double in spatial frequency towards the reader. Left to right the orientation tuning increases from $0°$ in steps of $45°$, with segregated pairs of positive (P) and negative (N) filter responses. (Reprinted from Wallis,G. and Rolls, E. T. (1997) Invariant face and object recognition in the visual system. Progress in Neurobiology 51: 167–194. Copyright © Elsevier Ltd.)

and the indices pq the position of the receptive field centre at $c_x = p$ and $c_y = q$. In this form, the receptive fields at all levels cover the spatial domain in the same way, i.e. by always overlapping the receptive fields in the same fashion. In the model we use $a = 2$, $b = 1$ and $\kappa = \pi$ corresponding to a spatial frequency bandwidth of one octave. We used symmetric filters with the angular spacing between the different orientations set to 45 degrees; and with 4 filter frequencies spaced one octave apart starting with 0.5 cycles per pixel, and with the sampling from the spatial frequencies set as shown in Table 2.4. Each individual filter is tuned to spatial frequency (0.0625 to 0.5 cycles / pixel over four octaves); orientation ($0°$ to $135°$ in steps of $45°$); and sign (± 1) (Rolls, 2021d).

Table 2.4 VisNet layer 1 connectivity. The frequency is in cycles per pixel

Frequency	0.5	0.25	0.125	0.0625
# Connections	201	50	13	8

Of the 272 layer 1 connections, the number for each group is as shown in Table 2.4.

Cells of layer 1 of VisNet receive a topologically consistent, localized, random selection of the filter responses in the input layer, under the constraint that each cell samples every filter spatial frequency and receives a constant number of inputs. Figure 2.30 shows pictorially the general filter sampling paradigm, and Fig. 2.31 the typical connectivity to a layer 1 cell from the filters of the input layer. The blank squares indicate that no connection exists between the layer 1 cell chosen and the filters of that particular orientation, sign, and spatial frequency.

2.8.1.5 Measures for network performance

A neuron can be said to have learnt an invariant representation if it discriminates one set of stimuli from another set, across all transformations. For example, a neuron's response is translation invariant if its response to one set of stimuli irrespective of presentation is consistently higher than for all other stimuli irrespective of presentation location. Note that we state 'set of stimuli' since neurons in the inferior temporal cortex are not generally selective for a single stimulus but rather a subpopulation of stimuli (Baylis, Rolls and Leonard, 1985; Abbott, Rolls and Tovee, 1996; Rolls, Treves and Tovee, 1997b; Rolls and Treves, 1998; Rolls and Deco, 2002; Rolls, 2007e; Franco, Rolls, Aggelopoulos and Jerez, 2007; Rolls and Treves, 2011) (see Appendix C). The measure of network performance used in VisNet1 (Wallis and Rolls, 1997), the 'Fisher metric' (referred to in some figure labels as the Discrim-

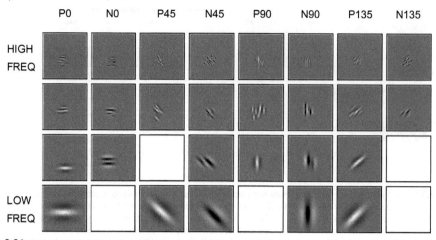

Fig. 2.31 Typical connectivity before training between a single cell in the first layer of the network and the input layer, represented by plotting the receptive fields of every input layer cell connected to the particular layer 1 cell. Separate input layer cells have activity that represents a positive (P) or negative (N) output from the bank of filters which have different orientations in degrees (the columns) and different spatial frequencies (the rows). Here the overall receptive field of the layer 1 cell is centred just below the centre-point of the retina. The connection scheme allows for relatively fewer connections to lower frequency cells than to high frequency cells in order to cover a similar region of the input at each frequency. A blank square indicates that there is no connection to the layer 1 neuron from an input neuron with that particular filter type. (After Wallis,G. and Rolls, E. T. (1997) Invariant face and object recognition in the visual system. Progress in Neurobiology 51: 167–194. Copyright © Elsevier Ltd.)

ination Factor), reflects how well a neuron discriminates between stimuli, compared to how well it discriminates between different locations (or more generally the images used rather than the objects, each of which is represented by a set of images, over which invariant stimulus or object representations must be learned). The Fisher measure is very similar to taking the ratio of the two F values in a two-way ANOVA, where one factor is the stimulus shown, and the other factor is the position in which a stimulus is shown. The measure takes a value greater than 1.0 if a neuron has more different responses to the stimuli than to the locations. That is, values greater than 1 indicate invariant representations when this measure is used in the following figures. Further details of how the measure is calculated are given by Wallis and Rolls (1997).

Measures of network performance based on information theory and similar to those used in the analysis of the firing of real neurons in the brain (see Appendix C) were introduced by Rolls and Milward (2000) for VisNet2, and are used in later papers (Rolls, 2021d). A single cell information measure was introduced which is the maximum amount of information the cell has about any one stimulus / object independently of which transform (e.g. position on the retina) is shown. Because the competitive algorithm used in VisNet tends to produce local representations (in which single cells become tuned to one stimulus or object), this information measure can approach $\log_2 N_S$ bits, where N_S is the number of different stimuli. Indeed, it is an advantage of this measure that it has a defined maximal value, which enables how well the network is performing to be quantified. Rolls and Milward (2000) showed that the Fisher and single cell information measures were highly correlated, and given the advantage just noted of the information measure, it was adopted in Rolls and Milward (2000) and subsequent papers. Rolls and Milward (2000) also introduced a multiple cell information measure, which has the advantage that it provides a measure of whether all stimuli are encoded by different neurons in the network. Again, a high value of this measure indicates good performance.

For completeness, further specification is provided next of the two information theoretic measures, which are described in detail by Rolls and Milward (2000) (see Appendix C for introduction of the concepts, and Appendix D for availability of a Matlab version of the code). The measures assess the extent to which either a single cell, or a population of cells, responds to the same stimulus invariantly with respect to its location, yet responds differently to different stimuli. The measures effectively show what one learns about which stimulus was presented from a single presentation of the stimulus at any randomly chosen location. Results for top (4th) layer cells are shown. High information measures thus show that cells fire similarly to the different transforms of a given stimulus (object), and differently to the other stimuli. The single cell stimulus-specific information, $I(s, R)$, is the amount of information the set of responses, R, has about a specific stimulus, s (see Rolls, Treves, Tovee and Panzeri (1997d) and Rolls and Milward (2000)). $I(s, R)$ is given by

$$I(s, R) = \sum_{r \in R} P(r|s) \log_2 \frac{P(r|s)}{P(r)} \qquad (2.12)$$

where r is an individual response from the set of responses R of the neuron. For each cell the performance measure used was the maximum amount of information a cell conveyed about any one stimulus. This (rather than the mutual information, $I(S, R)$ where S is the whole set of stimuli s), is appropriate for a competitive network in which the cells tend to become tuned to one stimulus[5].

If all the output cells of VisNet learned to respond to the same stimulus, then the information about the set of stimuli S would be very poor, and would not reach its maximal value of $\log_2$ of the number of stimuli (in bits). The second measure that is used here is the information provided by a set of cells about the stimulus set, using the procedures described by Rolls, Treves and Tovee (1997b) and Rolls and Milward (2000). The multiple cell information is the mutual information between the whole set of stimuli S and of responses R calculated using a decoding procedure in which the stimulus s' that gave rise to the particular firing rate response vector on each trial is estimated. (The decoding step is needed because the high dimensionality of the response space would lead to an inaccurate estimate of the information if the responses were used directly, as described by Rolls, Treves and Tovee (1997b) and Rolls and Treves (1998).) A probability table is then constructed of the real stimuli s and the decoded stimuli s'. From this probability table, the mutual information between the set of actual stimuli S and the decoded estimates S' is calculated as

$$I(S, S') = \sum_{s,s'} P(s, s') \log_2 \frac{P(s, s')}{P(s)P(s')} \qquad (2.13)$$

This was calculated for the subset of cells which had as single cells the most information about which stimulus was shown. In particular, in Rolls and Milward (2000) and subsequent papers, the multiple cell information was calculated from the first five cells for each stimulus that had maximal single cell information about that stimulus, that is from a population of 35 cells if there were seven stimuli (each of which might have been shown in for example 9 or 25 positions on the retina, or other types of transform).

2.8.2 Initial experiments with VisNet

Having established a network model, Wallis and Rolls (1997) (following a first report by Wallis, Rolls and Földiák (1993)) described four experiments in which the theory of how invariant representations could be formed was tested using a variety of stimuli undergoing a number of

---

[5] $I(s, R)$ has also been termed the stimulus-specific surprise, see DeWeese and Meister (1999). Its average across stimuli is the mutual information $I(S, R)$.

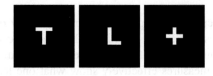

Fig. 2.32 The three stimuli used in the first two VisNet experiments. (After Wallis,G. and Rolls, E. T. (1997) Invariant face and object recognition in the visual system. Progress in Neurobiology 51: 167–194. Copyright © Elsevier Ltd.)

natural transformations. In each case the network produced neurons in the final layer whose responses were largely invariant across a transformation and highly discriminating between stimuli or sets of stimuli.

2.8.2.1 'T','L' and '+' as stimuli: learning translation invariance

One of the classical properties of inferior temporal cortex face cells is their invariant response to face stimuli translated across the visual field (Tovee, Rolls and Azzopardi, 1994). In this first experiment, the learning of translation invariant representations by VisNet was investigated.

In order to test the network a set of three stimuli, based upon probable 3D edge cues – consisting of a 'T', 'L' and '+' shape – was constructed[6]. The actual stimuli used are shown in Fig. 2.32. These stimuli were chosen partly because of their significance as form cues, but on a more practical note because they each contain the same fundamental features – namely a horizontal bar conjoined with a vertical bar. In practice this means that the oriented simple cell filters of the input layer cannot distinguish these stimuli on the basis of which features are present. As a consequence of this, the representation of the stimuli received by the network is non-orthogonal and hence considerably more difficult to classify than was the case in earlier experiments involving the trace rule (Földiák, 1991). The expectation is that layer 1 neurons would learn to respond to spatially selective combinations of the basic features thereby helping to distinguish these non-orthogonal stimuli. The trajectory followed by each stimulus consisted of sweeping left to right horizontally across three locations in the top row, and then sweeping back, right to left across the middle row, before returning to the right hand side across the bottom row – tracing out a 'Z' shape path across the retina. Unless stated otherwise this pattern of nine presentation locations was adopted in all image translation experiments described by Wallis and Rolls (1997).

Training was carried out by permutatively presenting all stimuli in each location a total of 800 times. The sequence described above was followed for each stimulus, with the sequence start point and direction of sweep being chosen at random for each of the 800 training trials.

Figures 2.33 and 2.34 show the response after training of a first layer neuron selective for the 'T' stimulus. The weighted sum of all filter inputs reveals the combination of horizontally and vertically tuned filters in identifying the stimulus. In this case many connections to the lower frequency filters have been reduced to zero by the learning process, except at the relevant orientations. This contrasts strongly with the random wiring present before training, as seen previously in Fig. 2.31. It is important that neurons at early stages of feature hierarchy networks respond to combinations of features in defined relative spatial positions, before invariance is built into the system, as this is part of the way that the binding problem is solved, as described in more detail in Section 2.8.5 and by Elliffe, Rolls and Stringer (2002). The feature combination tuning is illustrated by the VisNet layer 1 neuron shown in Figs. 2.33 and 2.34.

Likewise, Fig. 2.35 depicts two neural responses, but now from the two intermediate layers of the network, taken from the top 30 most highly invariant cells, not merely the top

---

[6]Chakravarty (1979) described the application of these shapes as cues for the 3D interpretation of edge junctions, and Tanaka et al. (1991) have demonstrated the existence of cells responsive to such stimuli in IT.

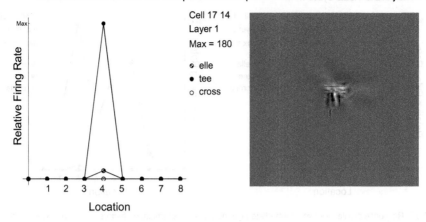

Fig. 2.33 The left graph shows the response of a VisNet layer 1 neuron to the three training stimuli for the nine training locations. Alongside this are the results of summating all the filter inputs to the neuron. The discrimination factor for this cell was 1.04.

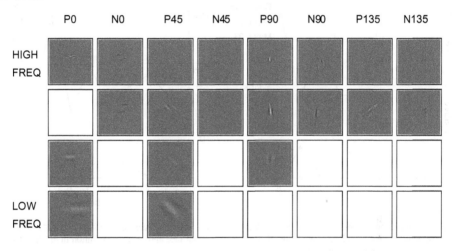

Fig. 2.34 The same cell as in the previous figure and the same input reconstruction results but separated into four rows of differing spatial frequency, and eight columns representing the four filter tuning orientations in positive and negative complementary pairs.

two or three. The gradual increase in the discrimination indicates that the tolerance to shifts of the preferred stimulus gradually builds up through the layers.

The results for layer 4 neurons are illustrated in Fig. 2.36. By this stage translation-invariant, stimulus-identifying, cells have emerged. The response profiles confirm the high level of neural selectivity for a particular stimulus irrespective of location.

Figure 2.37 contrasts the measure of invariance, or discrimination factor, achieved by cells in the four layers, averaged over five separate runs of the network. Translation invariance clearly increases through the layers, with a considerable increase in translation invariance between layers 3 and 4. This sudden increase may well be a result of the geometry of the network, which enables cells in layer 4 to receive inputs from any part of the input layer.

Having established that invariant cells have emerged in the final layer, we now consider the role of the trace rule, by assessing the network tested under two new conditions. Firstly, the performance of the network was measured before learning occurs, that is with its initially random connection weights. Secondly, the network was trained with η in the trace rule set to 0, which causes learning to proceed in a traceless, standard Hebbian, fashion. (Hebbian learning is purely associative, as shown for example in Equation B.29.)

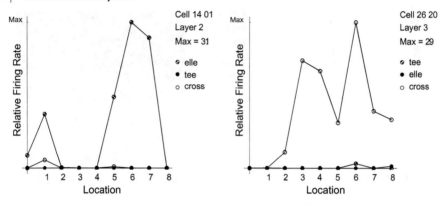

Fig. 2.35 Response profiles for two intermediate layer neurons – discrimination factors 1.34 and 1.64 – in the L, T, and + experiment. (After Wallis,G. and Rolls, E. T. (1997) Invariant face and object recognition in the visual system. Progress in Neurobiology 51: 167–194. Copyright © Elsevier Ltd.)

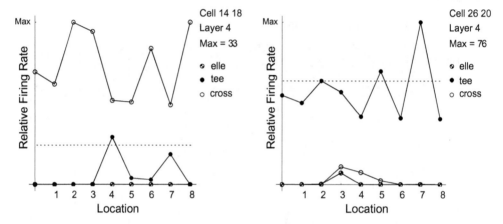

Fig. 2.36 Response profiles for two fourth layer VisNet neurons – discrimination factors 4.07 and 3.62 – in the L, T, and + experiment. (After Wallis,G. and Rolls, E. T. (1997) Invariant face and object recognition in the visual system. Progress in Neurobiology 51: 167–194.)

Figure 2.38 shows the results under the three training conditions. The results show that the trace rule is the decisive factor in establishing the invariant responses in the layer 4 neurons. It is interesting to note that the Hebbian learning results are actually *worse* than those achieved by chance in the untrained net. In general, with Hebbian learning, the most highly discriminating cells barely rate higher than 1. This value of discrimination corresponds to the case in which a cell responds to only one stimulus and in only one location. The poor performance with the Hebb rule comes as a direct consequence of the presentation paradigm being employed. If we consider an image as representing a vector in multidimensional space, a particular image in the top left-hand corner of the input retina will tend to look more like any other image in that same location than the same image presented elsewhere. A simple competitive network using just Hebbian learning will thus tend to categorize images by *where* they are rather than what they are – the exact opposite of what the net was intended to learn. This comparison thus indicates that a small memory trace acting in the standard Hebbian learning paradigm can radically alter the normal vector averaging, image classification, performed by a Hebbian-based competitive network.

One question that emerges about the representation in the final layer of the network relates to how evenly the network divides up its resources to represent the learnt stimuli. It is conceivable that one stimulus stands out among the set of stimuli by containing very distinc-

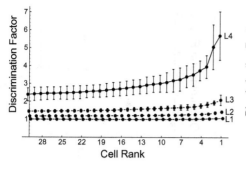
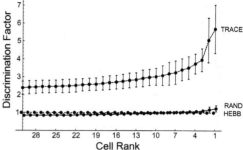

Fig. 2.37 Variation in VisNet neural discrimination factors as a measure of performance for the top 30 most highly discriminating cells through the four layers of the network, averaged over five runs of the network in the L, T, and + experiment. (After Wallis,G. and Rolls, E. T. (1997) Invariant face and object recognition in the visual system. Progress in Neurobiology 51: 167–194.)

Fig. 2.38 Variation in neural discrimination factors as a measure of performance for the top 30 most highly discriminating cells in the fourth layer for the three training regimes, averaged over five runs of the network. (After Wallis,G. and Rolls, E. T. (1997) Invariant face and object recognition in the visual system. Progress in Neurobiology 51: 167–194. Copyright © Elsevier Ltd.)

tive features which would make it easier to categorize. This may produce an unrepresentative number of neurons with high discrimination factors which are in fact all responding to the same stimulus. It is important that at least some cells code for (or provide information about) each of the stimuli. As a simple check on this, the preferred stimulus of each cell was found and the associated measure of discrimination added to a total for each stimulus. This measure in practice never varied by more than a factor of 1.3:1 for all stimuli. The multiple cell information measure used in some later figures addresses the same issue, with similar results.

2.8.2.2 'T','L', and '+' as stimuli: Optimal network parameters

The second series of investigations described by Wallis and Rolls (1997) using the 'T','L' and '+' stimuli, centred upon finding optimal parameters for elements of the network, such as the optimal trace time constant η, which controls the relative effect of previous activities on current learning as described above. The network performance was gauged using a single 800 epoch training run of the network with the median discrimination factor (with the upper and lower quartile values) for the top sixteen cells of the fourth layer being displayed at each parameter value.

Figure 2.39 displays the effect of varying the value of η for the nine standard presentation locations. The optimal value of η might conceivably change with the alteration of the number of training locations, and indeed one might predict that it would be smaller if the number of presentation locations was reduced. To confirm this, network performance was also measured for presentation sweeps over only five locations. Figure 2.40 shows the results of this experiment, which confirm the expected shift in the general profile of the curve towards shorter time constant values. Of course, the optimal value of η derived is in effect a compromise between optimal values for the three layers in which the trace operates. Since neurons in each layer have different effective receptive field sizes, one would expect each layer's neurons to be exposed to different portions of the full sweep of a particular stimulus. This would in turn suggest that the optimal value of η will grow through the layers.

2.8.2.3 Faces as stimuli: translation invariance

The aim of the next set of experiments described by Wallis and Rolls (1997) was to start to address the issues of how the network operates when invariant representations must be learned for a larger number of stimuli, and whether the network can learn when much more complicated, real biological stimuli (faces) are used. The set of face images used appears in Fig. 2.41. In practice, to equalize luminance the D.C. component of the images was removed.

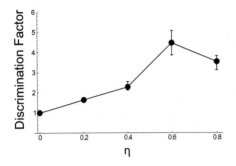
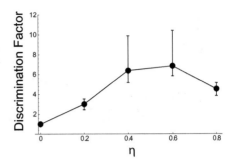

Fig. 2.39 Variation in VisNet network performance as a function of the trace rule parameter η in neurons of layers 2 to 4 – over nine locations in the L, T and + experiment. (After Wallis,G. and Rolls, E. T. (1997) Invariant face and object recognition in the visual system. Progress in Neurobiology 51: 167–194.)

Fig. 2.40 Variation in network performance as a function of the trace rule parameter η in neurons of layers 2 to 4 – over five presentation locations in the L, T and + experiment. (After Wallis,G. and Rolls, E. T. (1997) Invariant face and object recognition in the visual system. Progress in Neurobiology 51: 167–194. Copyright © Elsevier Ltd.)

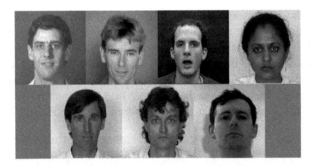

Fig. 2.41 Seven faces used as stimuli in the face translation experiment. (After Wallis,G. and Rolls, E. T. (1997) Invariant face and object recognition in the visual system. Progress in Neurobiology 51: 167–194. Copyright © Elsevier Ltd.)

In addition, so as to minimize the effect of cast shadows, an oval Hamming window was applied to the face image which also served to remove any hard edges of the image relative to the plain background upon which they were set.

The results of training in the translation invariance paradigm with 7 faces each in 9 locations are shown in Figs. 2.42, 2.43 and 2.44. The network produces neurons with high discrimination factors, and this only occurs if it is trained with the trace rule. Some layer 4 neurons showed a somewhat distributed representation, as illustrated in the examples of layer 4 neurons shown in Fig. 2.42. The more recent Matlab version of VisNet available from 2022 (Section D.6) would obtain perfect performance on this type of problem, with layer 4 neurons responding to only one object or face with complete invariance, that is a high response to one face invariantly of the transform, with no response to any other face or object.

In order to check that there was an invariant representation in layer 4 of VisNet that could be read by a receiving population of neurons, a fifth layer was added to the net which fully sampled the fourth layer cells. This layer was in turn trained in a supervised manner using gradient descent or with a Hebbian associative learning rule. Wallis and Rolls (1997) showed that the object classification performed by the layer 5 network was better if the network had been trained with the trace rule than when it was untrained or was trained with a Hebb rule.

2.8.2.4 Faces as stimuli: view invariance

Given that the network had been shown to be able to operate usefully with a more difficult translation invariance problem, we next addressed the question of whether the network can

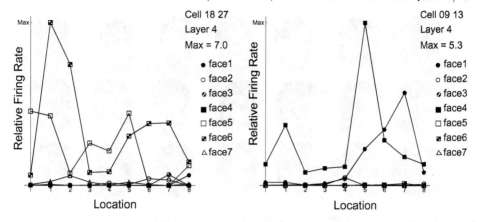

Fig. 2.42 Response profiles for two VisNet neurons in the fourth layer – discrimination factors 2.64 and 2.10. The net was trained on 7 faces each in 9 locations. (After Wallis,G. and Rolls, E. T. (1997) Invariant face and object recognition in the visual system. Progress in Neurobiology 51: 167–194.)

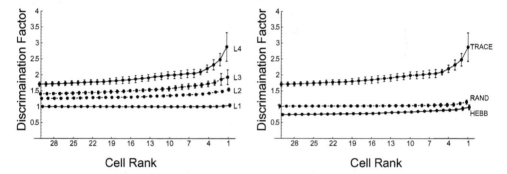

Fig. 2.43 Variation in VisNet network performance for the top 30 most highly discriminating neurons through the four layers of the network, averaged over five runs of the network. The net was trained on 7 faces each in 9 locations. (After Wallis,G. and Rolls, E. T. (1997) Invariant face and object recognition in the visual system. Progress in Neurobiology 51: 167–194.)

Fig. 2.44 Variation in network performance for the top 30 most highly discriminating cells in the fourth layer for the three training regimes, averaged over five runs of the network. The net was trained on 7 faces each in 9 locations. (After Wallis,G. and Rolls, E. T. (1997) Invariant face and object recognition in the visual system. Progress in Neurobiology 51: 167–194. Copyright © Elsevier Ltd.)

solve other types of transform invariance, as we had intended. The next experiment addressed this question, by training the network on the problem of 3D stimulus rotation, which produces non-isomorphic transforms, to determine whether the network can build a view-invariant categorization of the stimuli (Wallis and Rolls, 1997). The trace rule learning paradigm should, in conjunction with the architecture described here, prove capable of learning any of the transforms tolerated by IT neurons, so long as each stimulus is presented in short sequences during which the transformation occurs and can be learned. This experiment continued with the use of faces but now presented them centrally in the retina in a sequence of different views of a face. The images used are shown in Fig. 2.45. The faces were again smoothed at the edges to erase the harsh image boundaries, and the D.C. term was removed. During the 800 epochs of learning, each stimulus was chosen at random, and a sequence of preset views of it was shown, rotating the face either to the left or to the right.

Although the actual number of images being presented is smaller, some 21 views in all, there is good reason to think that this problem may be harder to solve than the previous translation experiments. This is simply due to the fact that all 21 views exactly overlap with

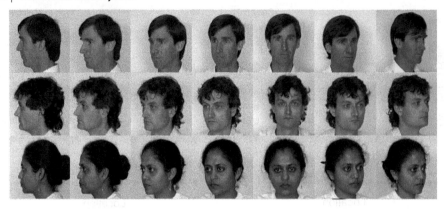

Fig. 2.45 Three faces in seven different views used as stimuli in an experiment in view-invariant recognition by VisNet. (After Wallis,G. and Rolls, E. T. (1997) Invariant face and object recognition in the visual system. Progress in Neurobiology 51: 167–194. Copyright © Elsevier Ltd.)

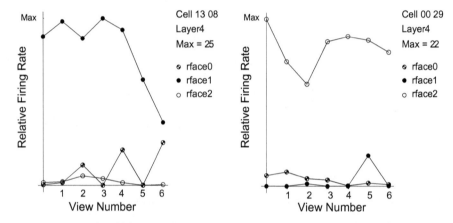

Fig. 2.46 Response profiles for cells in the last two layers of the VisNet network – discrimination factors 11.12 and 12.40 – in the experiment with seven different views of each of three faces. (After Wallis,G. and Rolls, E. T. (1997) Invariant face and object recognition in the visual system. Progress in Neurobiology 51: 167–194. Copyright © Elsevier Ltd.)

one another. The net was indeed able to solve the invariance problem, with examples of invariant layer 4 neuron response profiles appearing in Fig. 2.46.

Figure 2.47 confirms the improvement in invariant stimulus representation found through the layers, and that layer 4 provides a considerable improvement in performance over the previous layers. Figure 2.48 shows the Hebb trained and untrained nets performing equally poorly, whilst the trace trained net shows good invariance across the entire 30 cells selected.

2.8.3 The optimal parameters for the temporal trace used in the learning rule

The trace used in VisNet enables successive features that, based on the natural statistics of the visual input, are likely to be from the same object or feature complex to be associated together. For good performance, the temporal trace needs to be sufficiently long that it covers the period in which features seen by a particular neuron in the hierarchy are likely to come from the same object. On the other hand, the trace should not be so long that it produces associations between features that are parts of different objects, seen when for example the eyes move to another object. One possibility is to reset the trace during saccades between different objects. If explicit trace resetting is not implemented, then the trace should, to opti-

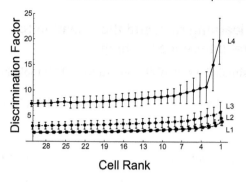

Fig. 2.47 Variation in VisNet network performance for the top 30 most highly discriminating cells through the four layers of the network, averaged over five runs of the network in the experiment with seven different views of each of three faces. (After Wallis,G. and Rolls, E. T. (1997) Invariant face and object recognition in the visual system. Progress in Neurobiology 51: 167–194.)

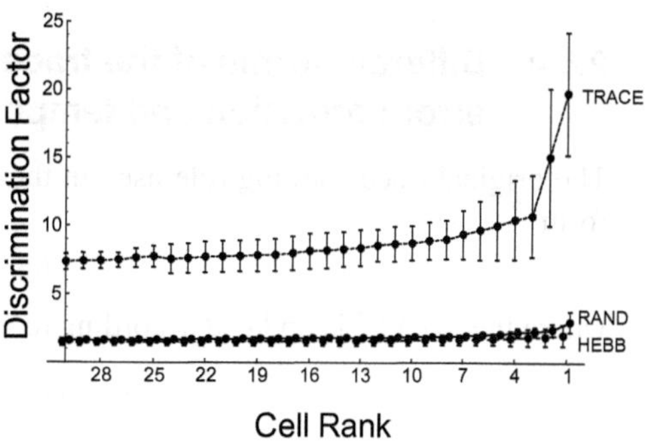

Fig. 2.48 Variation in VisNet network performance for the top 30 most highly discriminating cells in the fourth layer for the three training regimes, averaged over five runs of the network in the experiment with seven different views of each of three faces. (After Wallis,G. and Rolls, E. T. (1997) Invariant face and object recognition in the visual system. Progress in Neurobiology 51: 167–194. Copyright © Elsevier Ltd.)

mize the compromise implied by the above, lead to strong associations between temporally close stimuli, and increasingly weaker associations between temporally more distant stimuli. In fact, the trace implemented in VisNet has an exponential decay, and it has been shown that this form is optimal in the situation where the exact duration over which the same object is being viewed varies, and where the natural statistics of the visual input happen also to show a decreasing probability that the same object is being viewed as the time period in question increases (Wallis and Baddeley, 1997). Moreover, as is made evident in Figs. 2.40 and 2.39, performance can be enhanced if the duration of the trace does at the same time approximately match the period over which the input stimuli are likely to come from the same object or feature complex. Nevertheless, good performance can be obtained in conditions under which the trace rule allows associations to be formed only between successive items in the visual stream (Rolls and Milward, 2000; Rolls and Stringer, 2001a).

It is also the case that the optimal value of η in the trace rule is likely to be different for different layers of VisNet, and for cortical processing in the 'what' visual stream. For early layers of the system, small movements of the eyes might lead to different feature combinations providing the input to cells (which at early stages have small receptive fields), and a short duration of the trace would be optimal. However, these small eye movements might be around the same object, and later layers of the architecture would benefit from being able to associate together their inputs over longer times, in order to learn about the larger scale properties that characterize individual objects, including for example different views of objects observed as an object turns or is turned. Thus the suggestion is made that the temporal trace could be effectively longer at later stages (e.g. inferior temporal visual cortex) compared to early stages (e.g. V4 and posterior inferior temporal cortex) of processing in the visual system. In addition, as will be shown in Section 2.8.5, it is important to form feature combinations with high spatial precision before invariance learning supported by a temporal trace starts, in order that the feature combinations and not the individual features have invariant representations. This leads to the suggestion that the trace rule should either not operate, or be short, at early stages of cortical visual processing such as V1. This is reflected in the operation of VisNet2, which does not use a temporal trace in layer 1 (Rolls and Milward, 2000).

2.8.4 Different forms of the trace learning rule, and their relation to error correction and temporal difference learning

The original trace learning rule used in the simulations of Wallis and Rolls (1997) took the form

$$\delta w_j = \alpha \bar{y}^\tau x_j^\tau \qquad (2.14)$$

where the trace $\bar{y}^\tau$ is updated according to

$$\bar{y}^\tau = (1 - \eta)y^\tau + \eta \bar{y}^{\tau-1}. \qquad (2.15)$$

The parameter $\eta \in [0, 1]$ controls the relative contributions to the trace $\bar{y}^\tau$ from the instantaneous firing rate y^τ and the trace at the previous time step $\bar{y}^{\tau-1}$, where for $\eta = 0$ we have $\bar{y}^\tau = y^\tau$ and equation 2.14 becomes the standard Hebb rule

$$\delta w_j = \alpha y^\tau x_j^\tau. \qquad (2.16)$$

At the start of a series of investigations of different forms of the trace learning rule, Rolls and Milward (2000) demonstrated that VisNet's performance could be greatly enhanced with a modified Hebbian learning rule that incorporated a trace of activity from the preceding time steps, with no contribution from the activity being produced by the stimulus at the current time step. This rule took the form

$$\delta w_j = \alpha \bar{y}^{\tau-1} x_j^\tau. \qquad (2.17)$$

The trace shown in Equation 2.17 is in the postsynaptic term, and similar effects were found if the trace was in the presynaptic term, or in both the pre- and the postsynaptic terms. The crucial difference from the earlier rule (see Equation 2.14) was that the trace should be calculated up to only the preceding timestep, with no contribution to the trace from the firing on the current trial to the current stimulus. How might this be understood?

One way to understand this is to note that the trace rule is trying to set up the synaptic weight on trial τ based on whether the neuron, based on its previous history, is responding to that stimulus (in other transforms, e.g. position). Use of the trace rule at $\tau - 1$ does this, that is it takes into account the firing of the neuron on previous trials, with no contribution from the firing being produced by the stimulus on the current trial. On the other hand, use of the trace at time τ in the update takes into account the current firing of the neuron to the stimulus in that particular position, which is not a good estimate of whether that neuron should be allocated to invariantly represent that stimulus. Effectively, using the trace at time τ introduces a Hebbian element into the update, which tends to build position-encoded analyzers, rather than stimulus-encoded analyzers. (The argument has been phrased for a system learning translation invariance, but applies to the learning of all types of invariance.) A particular advantage of using the trace at $\tau - 1$ is that the trace will then on different occasions (due to the randomness in the location sequences used) reflect previous histories with different sets of positions, enabling the learning of the neuron to be based on evidence from the stimulus present in many different positions. Using a term from the current firing in the trace (i.e. the trace calculated at time τ) results in this desirable effect always having an undesirable element from the current firing of the neuron to the stimulus in its current position (or any other transform).

2.8.4.1 The modified Hebbian trace rule and its relation to error correction

The rule of Equation 2.17 corrects the weights using a postsynaptic trace obtained from the previous firing (produced by other transforms of the same stimulus), with no contribution to the trace from the current postsynaptic firing (produced by the current transform of the stimulus). Indeed, insofar as the current firing y^τ is not the same as $\overline{y}^{\tau-1}$, this difference can be thought of as an error. This leads to a conceptualization of using the difference between the current firing and the preceding trace as an error correction term, as noted in the context of modelling the temporal properties of classical conditioning by Sutton and Barto (1981), and developed next in the context of invariance learning (see Rolls and Stringer (2001a)).

First, we re-express the rule of Equation 2.17 in an alternative form as follows. Suppose we are at timestep τ and have just calculated a neuronal firing rate y^τ and the corresponding trace $\overline{y}^\tau$ from the trace update Equation 2.15. If we assume $\eta \in (0, 1)$, then rearranging Equation 2.15 gives

$$\overline{y}^{\tau-1} = \frac{1}{\eta}(\overline{y}^\tau - (1-\eta)y^\tau), \tag{2.18}$$

and substituting Equation 2.18 into Equation 2.17 gives

$$\delta w_j = \alpha \frac{1}{\eta}(\overline{y}^\tau - (1-\eta)y^\tau)x_j^\tau$$
$$= \alpha \frac{1-\eta}{\eta}(\frac{1}{1-\eta}\overline{y}^\tau - y^\tau)x_j^\tau$$
$$= \hat{\alpha}(\hat{\beta}\overline{y}^\tau - y^\tau)x_j^\tau \tag{2.19}$$

where $\hat{\alpha} = \alpha \frac{1-\eta}{\eta}$ and $\hat{\beta} = \frac{1}{1-\eta}$. The modified Hebbian trace learning rule (2.17) is thus equivalent to Equation 2.19 which is in the general form of an error correction rule (Hertz, Krogh and Palmer, 1991). That is, rule (2.19) involves the subtraction of the current firing rate y^τ from a target value, in this case $\hat{\beta}\overline{y}^\tau$.

Although above we have referred to rule (2.17) as a modified Hebbian rule, I note that it is only associative in the sense of associating *previous* cell firing with the current cell inputs. In the next section we continue to explore the error correction paradigm, examining five alternative examples of this sort of learning rule.

2.8.4.2 Five forms of error correction learning rule

Error correction learning rules are derived from gradient descent minimization (Hertz, Krogh and Palmer, 1991), and continually compare the current neuronal output to a target value t and adjust the synaptic weights according to the following Equation at a particular timestep τ

$$\delta w_j = \alpha(t - y^\tau)x_j^\tau. \tag{2.20}$$

In this usual form of gradient descent by error correction, the target t is fixed. However, in keeping with our aim of encouraging neurons to respond similarly to images that occur close together in time it seems reasonable to set the target at a particular timestep, t^τ, to be some function of cell activity occurring close in time, because encouraging neurons to respond to temporal classes will tend to make them respond to the different variants of a given stimulus (Földiák, 1991; Rolls, 1992a; Wallis and Rolls, 1997). For this reason, Rolls and Stringer (2001a) explored a range of error correction rules where the targets t^τ are based on the trace of neuronal activity calculated according to Equation 2.15. I note that although the target is not a fixed value as in standard error correction learning, nevertheless the new learning rules perform gradient descent on each timestep, as elaborated below. Although the target may be varying early on in learning, as learning proceeds the target is expected to become more and more constant, as neurons settle to respond invariantly to particular stimuli. The first set of five error correction rules we discuss are as follows.

$$\delta w_j = \alpha(\beta\overline{y}^{\tau-1} - y^\tau)x_j^\tau, \tag{2.21}$$

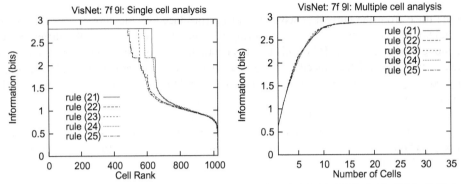

Fig. 2.49 Numerical results for VisNet with the five error correction rules (2.21), (2.22), (2.23), (2.24), (2.25) (with positive clipping of synaptic weights) trained on 7 faces in 9 locations. On the left are single cell information measures, and on the right are multiple cell information measures. (After Rolls, E. T. and Stringer,S.M. (2001) Invariant object recognition in the visual system with error correction and temporal difference learning. Network: Computation in Neural Systems 12: 111–129.)

$$\delta w_j = \alpha(\beta y^{\tau-1} - y^\tau)x_j^\tau, \qquad (2.22)$$

$$\delta w_j = \alpha(\beta \overline{y}^\tau - y^\tau)x_j^\tau, \qquad (2.23)$$

$$\delta w_j = \alpha(\beta \overline{y}^{\tau+1} - y^\tau)x_j^\tau, \qquad (2.24)$$

$$\delta w_j = \alpha(\beta y^{\tau+1} - y^\tau)x_j^\tau, \qquad (2.25)$$

where updates (2.21), (2.22) and (2.23) are performed at timestep τ, and updates (2.24) and (2.25) are performed at timestep $\tau + 1$. (The reason for adopting this convention is that the basic form of the error correction rule (2.20) is kept, with the five different rules simply replacing the term t.) It may be readily seen that Equations (2.22) and (2.25) are special cases of Equations (2.21) and (2.24) respectively, with $\eta = 0$.

These rules are all similar except for their targets t^τ, which are all functions of a temporally nearby value of cell activity. In particular, rule (2.23) is directly related to rule (2.19), but is more general in that the parameter $\hat{\beta} = \frac{1}{1-\eta}$ is replaced by an unconstrained parameter β. In addition, we also note that rule (2.21) is closely related to a rule developed in Peng, Sha, Gan and Wei (1998) for view invariance learning. The above five error correction rules are biologically plausible in that the targets t^τ are all local cell variables (see Appendix B and Rolls and Treves (1998)). In particular, rule (2.23) uses the trace $\overline{y}^\tau$ from the current time level τ, and rules (2.22) and (2.25) do not need exponential trace values $\overline{y}$, instead relying only on the instantaneous firing rates at the current and immediately preceding timesteps. However, all five error correction rules involve decrementing of synaptic weights according to an error which is calculated by subtracting the current activity from a target.

Numerical results with the error correction rules trained on 7 faces in 9 locations are presented in Fig. 2.49. For all the results shown the synaptic weights were clipped to be positive during the simulation, because it is important to test that decrementing synaptic weights purely within the positive interval $w \in [0, \infty]$ will provide significantly enhanced performance. That is, it is important to show that error correction rules do not necessarily require possibly biologically implausible modifiable negative weights. For each of the rules (2.21), (2.22), (2.23), (2.24), (2.25), the parameter β has been individually optimized to the following respective values: 4.9, 2.2, 2.2, 3.8, 2.2. On the left and right are results with the single and multiple cell information measures, respectively. Comparing Fig. 2.49 with Fig. 2.50 shows that all five error correction rules offer considerably improved performance over both the standard trace rule (2.14) and rule (2.17). From the left-hand side of Fig. 2.49 it can be seen that rule (2.21) performs best, and this is probably due to two reasons. Firstly, rule (2.21)

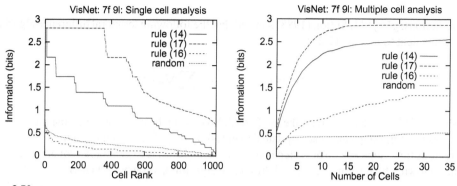

Fig. 2.50 Numerical results for VisNet with the standard trace rule (2.14), learning rule (2.17), the Hebb rule (2.16), and random weights, trained on 7 faces in 9 locations: single cell information measure (left), multiple cell information measure (right). (After Rolls, E. T. and Stringer,S.M. (2001) Invariant object recognition in the visual system with error correction and temporal difference learning. Network: Computation in Neural Systems 12: 111–129.)

incorporates an exponential trace $\overline{y}^{\tau-1}$ in its target t^τ, and we would expect this to help neurons to learn more quickly to respond invariantly to a class of inputs that occur close together in time. Hence, setting $\eta = 0$ as in rule (2.22) results in reduced performance. Secondly, unlike rules (2.23) and (2.24), rule (2.21) does not contain any component of y^τ in its target. If we examine rules (2.23), (2.24), we see that their respective targets $\beta\overline{y}^\tau$, $\beta\overline{y}^{\tau+1}$ contain significant components of y^τ.

2.8.4.3 Relationship to temporal difference learning

Rolls and Stringer (2001a) not only considered the relationship of rule (2.17) to error correction, but also considered how the error correction rules shown in Equations (2.21), (2.22), (2.23), (2.24) and (2.25) are related to temporal difference learning (Sutton, 1988; Sutton and Barto, 1998). Sutton (1988) described temporal difference methods in the context of prediction learning. These methods are a class of incremental learning techniques that can learn to predict final outcomes through comparison of successive predictions from the preceding time steps (Section B.17.3). This is in contrast to traditional supervised learning, which involves the comparison of predictions only with the final outcome. Consider a series of multistep prediction problems in which for each problem there is a sequence of observation vectors, $\mathbf{x}^1$, $\mathbf{x}^2$, ..., $\mathbf{x}^m$, at successive timesteps, followed by a final scalar outcome z. For each sequence of observations temporal difference methods form a sequence of predictions y^1, y^2, ..., y^m, each of which is a prediction of z. These predictions are based on the observation vectors $\mathbf{x}^\tau$ and a vector of modifiable weights $\mathbf{w}$; i.e. the prediction at time step τ is given by $y^\tau(\mathbf{x}^\tau, \mathbf{w})$, and for a linear dependency the prediction is given by $y^\tau = \mathbf{w}^T\mathbf{x}^\tau$. (Note here that $\mathbf{w}^T$ is the transpose of the weight vector $\mathbf{w}$.) The problem of prediction is to calculate the weight vector $\mathbf{w}$ such that the predictions y^τ are good estimates of the outcome z.

The supervised learning approach to the prediction problem is to form pairs of observation vectors $\mathbf{x}^\tau$ and outcome z for all time steps, and compute an update to the weights according to the gradient descent equation

$$\delta\mathbf{w} = \alpha(z - y^\tau)\nabla_\mathbf{w} y^\tau \qquad (2.26)$$

where α is a learning rate parameter and $\nabla_\mathbf{w}$ indicates the gradient with respect to the weight vector $\mathbf{w}$. However, this learning procedure requires all calculation to be done at the end of the sequence, once z is known. To remedy this, it is possible to replace method (2.26) with a temporal difference algorithm that is mathematically equivalent but allows the computational workload to be spread out over the entire sequence of observations. Temporal difference methods are a particular approach to updating the weights based on the values of successive predictions, y^τ, $y^{\tau+1}$. Sutton (1988) showed that the following temporal difference algorithm is equivalent to method (2.26)

$$\delta \mathbf{w} = \alpha (y^{\tau+1} - y^\tau) \sum_{k=1}^{\tau} \nabla_\mathbf{w} y^k, \qquad (2.27)$$

where $y^{m+1} \equiv z$. However, unlike method (2.26) this can be computed incrementally at each successive time step since each update depends only on $y^{\tau+1}$, y^τ and the sum of $\nabla_\mathbf{w} y^k$ over previous time steps k. The next step taken in Sutton (1988) is to generalize equation (2.27) to the following final form of temporal difference algorithm, known as 'TD(λ)'

$$\delta \mathbf{w} = \alpha (y^{\tau+1} - y^\tau) \sum_{k=1}^{\tau} \lambda^{\tau-k} \nabla_\mathbf{w} y^k \qquad (2.28)$$

where $\lambda \in [0, 1]$ is an adjustable parameter that controls the weighting on the vectors $\nabla_\mathbf{w} y^k$. Equation (2.28) represents a much broader class of learning rules than the more usual gradient descent-based rule (2.27), which is in fact the special case TD(1).

A further special case of Equation (2.28) is for $\lambda = 0$, i.e. TD(0), as follows

$$\delta \mathbf{w} = \alpha (y^{\tau+1} - y^\tau) \nabla_\mathbf{w} y^\tau. \qquad (2.29)$$

But for problems where y^τ is a linear function of $\mathbf{x}^\tau$ and $\mathbf{w}$, we have $\nabla_\mathbf{w} y^\tau = \mathbf{x}^\tau$, and so Equation (2.29) becomes

$$\delta \mathbf{w} = \alpha (y^{\tau+1} - y^\tau) \mathbf{x}^\tau. \qquad (2.30)$$

If we assume the prediction process is being performed by a neuron with a vector of inputs $\mathbf{x}^\tau$, synaptic weight vector $\mathbf{w}$, and output $y^\tau = \mathbf{w}^T \mathbf{x}^\tau$, then we see that the TD(0) algorithm (2.30) is identical to the error correction rule (2.25) with $\beta = 1$. In understanding this comparison with temporal difference learning, it may be useful to note that the firing at the end of a sequence of the transformed exemplars of a stimulus is effectively the temporal difference target z. This establishes a link to temporal difference learning (described further in Section B.17.3). Further, I note that from learning epoch to learning epoch, the target z for a given neuron will gradually settle down to be more and more fixed as learning proceeds.

We now explore in more detail the relation between the error correction rules described above and temporal difference learning. For each sequence of observations with a single outcome the temporal difference method (2.30), when viewed as an error correction rule, is attempting to adapt the weights such that $y^{\tau+1} = y^\tau$ for all successive pairs of time steps – the same general idea underlying the error correction rules (2.21), (2.22), (2.23), (2.24), (2.25). Furthermore, in Sutton and Barto (1998), where temporal difference methods are applied to reinforcement learning, the TD(λ) approach is again further generalized by replacing the target $y^{\tau+1}$ by any weighted average of predictions y from arbitrary future timesteps, e.g. $t^\tau = \frac{1}{2} y^{\tau+3} + \frac{1}{2} y^{\tau+7}$, including an exponentially weighted average extending forward in time. So a more general form of the temporal difference algorithm has the form

$$\delta \mathbf{w} = \alpha (t^\tau - y^\tau) \mathbf{x}^\tau, \qquad (2.31)$$

where here the target t^τ is an arbitrary weighted average of the predictions y over future timesteps. Of course, with standard temporal difference methods the target t^τ is always an average over *future* timesteps $k = \tau + 1, \tau + 2$, etc. But in the five error correction rules this is only true for the last exemplar (2.25). This is because with the problem of prediction, for example, the ultimate target of the predictions $y^1, ..., y^m$ is a final outcome $y^{m+1} \equiv z$.

However, this restriction does not apply to our particular application of neurons trained to respond to temporal classes of inputs within VisNet. Here we only wish to set the firing rates $y^1,...,y^m$ to the same value, not some final given value z. However, the more general error correction rules clearly have a close relationship to standard temporal difference algorithms. For example, it can be seen that Equation (2.22) with $\beta = 1$ is in some sense a temporal mirror image of Equation (2.30), particularly if the updates δw_j are added to the weights w_j only at the end of a sequence. That is, rule (2.22) will attempt to set $y^1,...,y^m$ to an *initial* value $y^0 \equiv z$. This relationship to temporal difference algorithms allowed us to begin to exploit established temporal difference analyses to investigate the convergence properties of the error correction methods (Rolls and Stringer, 2001a).

Although the main aim of Rolls and Stringer (2001a) in relating error correction rules to temporal difference learning was to begin to exploit established temporal difference analyses, they observed that the most general form of temporal difference learning, TD(λ), in fact suggests an interesting generalization to the existing error correction learning rules for which we currently have $\lambda = 0$. Assuming $y^\tau = \mathbf{w}^T\mathbf{x}^\tau$ and $\nabla_\mathbf{w} y^\tau = \mathbf{x}^\tau$, the general Equation (2.28) for TD(λ) becomes

$$\delta \mathbf{w} = \alpha(y^{\tau+1} - y^\tau)\sum_{k=1}^{\tau} \lambda^{\tau-k}\mathbf{x}^k \qquad (2.32)$$

where the term $\sum_{k=1}^{\tau} \lambda^{\tau-k}\mathbf{x}^k$ is a weighted sum of the vectors $\mathbf{x}^k$. This suggests generalizing the original five error correction rules (2.21), (2.22), (2.23), (2.24), (2.25) by replacing the term x_j^τ by a weighted sum $\hat{x}_j^\tau = \sum_{k=1}^{\tau} \lambda^{\tau-k}x_j^k$ with $\lambda \in [0,1]$. In Sutton (1988) $\hat{x}_j^\tau$ is calculated according to

$$\hat{x}_j^\tau = x_j^\tau + \lambda \hat{x}_j^{\tau-1} \qquad (2.33)$$

with $\hat{x}_j^0 \equiv 0$. This gives the following five temporal difference-inspired error correction rules

$$\delta w_j = \alpha(\beta \overline{y}^{\tau-1} - y^\tau)\hat{x}_j^\tau, \qquad (2.34)$$

$$\delta w_j = \alpha(\beta y^{\tau-1} - y^\tau)\hat{x}_j^\tau, \qquad (2.35)$$

$$\delta w_j = \alpha(\beta \overline{y}^\tau - y^\tau)\hat{x}_j^\tau, \qquad (2.36)$$

$$\delta w_j = \alpha(\beta \overline{y}^{\tau+1} - y^\tau)\hat{x}_j^\tau, \qquad (2.37)$$

$$\delta w_j = \alpha(\beta y^{\tau+1} - y^\tau)\hat{x}_j^\tau, \qquad (2.38)$$

where it may be readily seen that Equations (2.35) and (2.38) are special cases of equations (2.34) and (2.37) respectively, with $\eta = 0$. As with the trace $\overline{y}^\tau$, the term $\hat{x}_j^\tau$ is reset to zero when a new stimulus is presented. These five rules can be related to the more general TD(λ) algorithm, but continue to be biologically plausible using only local cell variables. Setting $\lambda = 0$ in rules (2.34), (2.35), (2.36), (2.37), (2.38), gives us back the original error correction rules (2.21), (2.22), (2.23), (2.24), (2.25) which may now be related to TD(0).

Numerical results with error correction rules (2.34), (2.35), (2.36), (2.37), (2.38), and $\hat{x}_j^\tau$ calculated according to equation (2.33) with $\lambda = 1$, with positive clipping of weights, trained on 7 faces in 9 locations are presented in Fig. 2.51. For each of the rules (2.34), (2.35), (2.36), (2.37), (2.38), the parameter β has been individually optimized to the following respective values: 1.7, 1.8, 1.5, 1.6, 1.8. On the left and right are results with the single and multiple cell information measures, respectively. Comparing these five temporal difference-inspired rules it can be seen that the best performance is obtained with rule (2.38) where many more cells reach the maximum level of performance possible with respect to the single cell information measure. In fact, this rule offered the best such results. This may well be due to the fact that

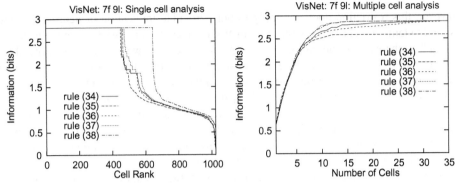

Fig. 2.51 Numerical results for VisNet with the five temporal difference-inspired error correction rules (2.34), (2.35), (2.36), (2.37), (2.38), and $\hat{x}_j^\tau$ calculated according to Equation (2.33) (with positive clipping of synaptic weights) trained on 7 faces in 9 locations. On the left are single cell information measures, and on the right are multiple cell information measures. (After Rolls, E. T. and Stringer, S.M. (2001) Invariant object recognition in the visual system with error correction and temporal difference learning. Network: Computation in Neural Systems 12: 111–129.)

this rule may be directly compared to the standard TD(1) learning rule, which itself may be related to classical supervised learning for which there are well known optimality results, as discussed further by Rolls and Stringer (2001a).

From the simulations described by Rolls and Stringer (2001a) it appears that the form of optimization described above associated with TD(1) rather than TD(0) leads to better performance within VisNet. Comparing Figs. 2.49 and 2.51 shows that the TD(1)-like rule (2.38) with $\lambda = 1.0$ and $\beta = 1.8$ gives considerably superior results to the TD(0)-like rule (2.25) with $\beta = 2.2$. In fact, the former of these two rules provided the best single cell information results in these studies. It is hypothesized that these results are related to the fact that only a finite set of image sequences is presented to VisNet, and so the type of optimization performed by TD(1) for repeated presentations of a finite data set is more appropriate for this problem than the form of optimization performed by TD(0).

2.8.4.4 Evaluation of the different training rules

In terms of biological plausibility, I note the following. First, all the learning rules investigated by Rolls and Stringer (2001a) are local learning rules, and in this sense are biologically plausible (see Appendix B). (The rules are local in that the terms used to modify the synaptic weights are potentially available in the pre- and post-synaptic elements.)

Second I note that all the rules do require some evidence of the activity on one or more previous stimulus presentations to be available when the synaptic weights are updated. Some of the rules, e.g. learning rule (2.23), use the trace $\overline{y}^\tau$ from the current time level, while rules (2.22) and (2.25) do not need to use an exponential trace of the neuronal firing rate, but only the instantaneous firing rates y at two successive time steps. It is known that synaptic plasticity does involve a combination of separate processes each with potentially differing time courses (Koch, 1999), and these different processes could contribute to trace rule learning. Another mechanism suggested for implementing a trace of previous neuronal activity is the continuing firing for often 300 ms produced by a short (16 ms) presentation of a visual stimulus (Rolls and Tovee, 1994) that is suggested to be implemented by local cortical recurrent attractor networks (Rolls and Treves, 1998; Rolls, 2016b) (Section 13.6).

Third, I note that in utilizing the trace in the targets t^τ, the error correction (or temporal difference inspired) rules perform a comparison of the instantaneous firing y^τ with a temporally nearby value of the activity, and this comparison involves a subtraction. The subtraction provides an error, which is then used to increase or decrease the synaptic weights. This is a somewhat different operation from long-term depression (LTD) as well as long term potentiation (LTP), which are *associative* changes which depend on the pre- and post-synaptic activity. However, it is interesting to note that an error correction rule which appears to involve a subtraction of current firing from a target might be implemented by a combination of an associative process operating with the trace, and an anti-Hebbian process operating to remove the effects of the current firing. For example, the synaptic updates $\delta w_j = \alpha(t^\tau - y^\tau)x_j^\tau$ can be decomposed into two separate associative processes $\alpha t^\tau x_j^\tau$ and $-\alpha y^\tau x_j^\tau$, that may occur independently. (The target, t^τ, could in this case be just the trace of previous neural activity from the preceding trials, excluding any contribution from the current firing.) Another way to implement an error correction rule using associative synaptic modification would be to force the post-synaptic neuron to respond to the error term. Although this has been postulated to be an effect that could be implemented by the climbing fibre system in the cerebellum (Ito, 1989, 1984, 2013) (Chapter 17), there is no similar system known for the neocortex, and it is not clear how this particular implementation of error correction might operate in the neocortex.

In Section 2.8.4.2 we describe five learning rules as error correction rules. We now discuss an interesting difference of these error correction rules from error correction rules as conventionally applied. It is usual to derive the general form of error correction learning rule from gradient descent minimization in the following way (Hertz, Krogh and Palmer, 1991). Consider the idealized situation of a single neuron with a number of inputs x_j and output $y = \sum_j w_j x_j$, where w_j are the synaptic weights. We assume that there are a number of input patterns and that for the kth input pattern, $\mathbf{x}^k = [x_1^k, x_2^k, ...]^T$, the output y^k has a target value t^k. Hence an error measure or cost function can be defined as

$$e(\mathbf{w}) = \frac{1}{2}\sum_k (t^k - y^k)^2 = \frac{1}{2}\sum_k (t^k - \sum_j w_j x_j^k)^2. \quad (2.39)$$

This cost function is a function of the input patterns $\mathbf{x}^k$ and the synaptic weight vector $\mathbf{w} = [w_1, w_2, ...]^T$. With a fixed set of input patterns, we can reduce the error measure by employing a gradient descent algorithm to calculate an improved set of synaptic weights. Gradient descent achieves this by moving downhill on the error surface defined in $\mathbf{w}$ space using the update

$$\delta w_j = -\alpha \frac{\partial e}{\partial w_j} = \alpha \sum_k (t^k - y^k) x_j^k. \quad (2.40)$$

If we update the weights after each pattern k, then the update takes the form of an error correction rule

$$\delta w_j = \alpha(t^k - y^k)x_j^k, \quad (2.41)$$

which is also commonly referred to as the delta rule or Widrow–Hoff rule (see Widrow and Hoff (1960) and Widrow and Stearns (1985)). Error correction rules continually compare the neuronal output with its pre-specified target value and adjust the synaptic weights accordingly. In contrast, the way Rolls and Stringer (2001a) introduced of utilizing error correction is to specify the target as the activity trace based on the firing rate at nearby timesteps. Now the actual firing at those nearby time steps is not a pre-determined fixed target, but instead depends on how the network has actually evolved. This effectively means the cost function $e(\mathbf{w})$ that is being minimized changes from timestep to timestep. Nevertheless, the concept of calculating an error, and using the magnitude and direction of the error to update the synaptic weights, is the similarity Rolls and Stringer (2001a) made to gradient descent learning.

To conclude this evaluation, the error correction and temporal difference rules explored by Rolls and Stringer (2001a) provide interesting approaches to help understand invariant pattern recognition learning. Although we do not know whether the full power of these rules is expressed in the brain, we provided suggestions about how they might be implemented. At the same time, I note that the original trace rule used by Földiák (1991), Rolls (1992a), Wallis, Rolls and Földiák (1993), and Wallis and Rolls (1997) is a simple associative rule, is therefore biologically very plausible, and, while not as powerful as many of the other rules introduced by Rolls and Stringer (2001a), can nevertheless solve the same class of problem. Rolls and Stringer (2001a) also emphasized that although they demonstrated how a number of new error correction and temporal difference rules might play a role in the context of view invariant object recognition, they may also operate elsewhere where it is important for neurons to learn to respond similarly to temporal classes of inputs that tend to occur close together in time.

2.8.5 The issue of feature binding, and a solution

In this section we investigate two key issues that arise in hierarchical layered network architectures, such as VisNet, other examples of which have been described and analyzed by Fukushima (1980), Ackley, Hinton and Sejnowski (1985), Rosenblatt (1961), Riesenhuber and Poggio (1999b) and Serre, Oliva and Poggio (2007b) (see also Section 2.9.2). One issue is whether the network can discriminate between stimuli that are composed of the same basic alphabet of features. The second issue is whether such network architectures can find solutions to the spatial binding problem. These issues are addressed next and by Elliffe, Rolls and Stringer (2002).

The first issue investigated is whether a hierarchical layered network architecture of the type exemplified by VisNet can discriminate stimuli that are composed of a limited set of features and where the different stimuli include cases where the feature sets are subsets and supersets of those in the other stimuli. A question is whether if the network has learned representations of both the parts and the wholes, will the network identify that the whole is present when it is shown, and not just that one or more parts is present? (In many investigations with VisNet, complex stimuli (such as faces) were used where each stimulus might contain unique features not present in the other stimuli.) To address this issue, Elliffe, Rolls and Stringer (2002) used stimuli that are composed from a set of four features which are designed so that each feature is spatially separate from the other features, and no unique combination of firing caused for example by overlap of horizontal and vertical filter outputs in the input representation distinguishes any one stimulus from the others. The results described in Section 2.8.5.4 show that VisNet can indeed learn correct invariant representations of stimuli that do consist of feature sets where individual features do not overlap spatially with each other and where the stimuli can be composed of sets of features which are supersets or subsets of those in other stimuli. Fukushima and Miyake (1982) did not address this crucial issue where different stimuli might be composed of subsets or supersets of the same set of features, although they did show that stimuli with partly overlapping features could be discriminated by the Neocognitron.

In Section 2.8.5.6 we address the spatial binding problem in architectures such as VisNet. This computational problem that needs to be addressed in hierarchical networks such as the primate visual system and VisNet is how representations of features can be (e.g. translation) invariant, yet can specify stimuli or objects in which the features must be specified in the correct spatial arrangement. This is the feature binding problem, discussed for example by von der Malsburg (1990), and arising in the context of hierarchical layered systems (Ackley, Hinton and Sejnowski, 1985; Fukushima, 1980; Rosenblatt, 1961). The issue is whether or not features are bound into the correct combinations in the correct relative spatial positions, or if alternative combinations of known features or the same features in different relative spatial positions would elicit the same responses. All this has to be achieved while at the same time producing position invariant recognition of the whole combination of features, that is, the object. This is a major computational issue that needs to be solved for memory systems in the brain to operate correctly. This can be achieved by what is effectively a learning process that builds into the system a set of neurons in the hierarchical network that enables the recognition process to operate correctly with the appropriate position, size, view etc. invariances.

2.8.5.1 Syntactic binding of separate neuronal ensembles by synchronization

The problem of syntactic binding of neuronal representations, in which some features must be bound together to form one object, and other simultaneously active features must be bound together to represent another object, has been addressed by von der Malsburg (see von der Malsburg (1990)). He has proposed that this could be performed by temporal synchronization of those neurons that were temporarily part of one representation in a different time slot from other neurons that were temporarily part of another representation. The idea is attractive in allowing arbitrary relinking of features in different combinations. Singer, Engel, Konig, and colleagues (Singer, Gray, Engel, Konig, Artola and Brocher, 1990; Engel, Konig, Kreiter, Schillen and Singer, 1992; Singer and Gray, 1995; Singer, 1999; Fries, 2015; Uran, Peter, Lazar, Barnes, Klon-Lipok, Shapcott, Roese, Fries, Singer and Vinck, 2022), and others (Abeles, 1991) have obtained some evidence that when features must be bound, synchronization of neuronal populations can occur (but see Shadlen and Movshon (1999)), and this has been modelled (Hummel and Biederman, 1992).

Synchronization to implement syntactic binding has a number of disadvantages and limitations (see also Rolls (2016b), and Riesenhuber and Poggio (1999a). The greatest computational problem is that synchronization does not by itself define the spatial relations between the features being bound, so is not just as a binding mechanism adequate for shape recognition. For example, temporal binding might enable features 1, 2 and 3, which might define one stimulus to be bound together and kept separate from for example another stimulus consisting of features 2, 3 and 4, but would require a further temporal binding (leading in the end potentially to a combinatorial explosion) to indicate the relative spatial positions of the 1, 2 and 3 in the 123 stimulus, so that it can be discriminated from e.g. 312.

A second problem with the synchronization approach to the spatial binding of features is that, when stimulus-dependent temporal synchronization has been rigourously tested with information theoretic approaches, it has so far been found that most of the information available is in the number of spikes, with rather little, less than 5% of the total information, in stimulus-dependent synchronization (Aggelopoulos, Franco and Rolls, 2005; Franco, Rolls, Aggelopoulos and Treves, 2004; Rolls, Aggelopoulos, Franco and Treves, 2004) (see Section C.3.7). For example, Aggelopoulos, Franco and Rolls (2005) showed that when macaques used object-based attention to search for one of two objects to touch in a complex natural scene, between 99% and 94% of the information was present in the firing rates of inferior temporal cortex neurons, and less that 5% in any stimulus-dependent synchrony that was present between the simultaneously recorded inferior temporal cortex neurons. The implication of these results is that any stimulus-dependent synchrony that is present is not quantitatively important as measured by information theoretic analyses under natural scene conditions when feature binding, segmentation of objects from the background, and attention are required (Rolls and Treves, 2011). This has been found for the inferior temporal cortex, a brain region where features are put together to form representations of objects (Rolls and Deco, 2002), and where attention has strong effects, at least in scenes with blank backgrounds (Rolls, Aggelopoulos and Zheng, 2003a). It would of course also be of interest to test the same hypothesis in earlier visual areas, such as V4, with quantitative, information theoretic, techniques. However, it is found that stimulus-dependent correlations between the firing of neurons far from increasing the information available from a population of neurons, in fact typically limits the amount of information that can be extracted from a neuronal population (Panzeri et al., 2022), providing further evidence against the binding by neuronal temporal synchronisation hypothesis.

In connection with rate codes, it should be noted that a rate code implies using the number of spikes that arrive in a given time, and that this time can be very short, as little as 20–50 ms, for very useful amounts of information to be made available from a population of neurons (Tovee, Rolls, Treves and Bellis, 1993; Rolls and Tovee, 1994; Rolls, Tovee, Purcell, Stewart and Azzopardi, 1994b; Tovee and Rolls, 1995; Rolls, Tovee and Panzeri, 1999b; Rolls, 2003; Rolls, Franco, Aggelopoulos and Jerez, 2006b) (see Section C.3.4).

A third problem with the 'Communication Through Coherence' hypothesis (Fries, 2015; Uran et al., 2022) whereby synchrony of oscillations between coupled cortical areas enhances communication between those areas is that in a formal model of coupled attractor networks, the strength of the coupling between the networks that was sufficient for information transfer was far lower than that required to force oscillations in each of the two networks to become coherent, that is, phase coupled (Rolls, Webb and Deco, 2012). Our investigation provides evidence that gamma oscillations can arise in strongly activated networks with high firing rates, and that communication between networks can occur perfectly well at much lower connectivities between the networks that is required for coherence. Our evidence is for *'Communication Before Coherence'* (Rolls, Webb and Deco, 2012). It could be that these phenomena of gamma oscillations and coherence arise as spandrels–as effects of over-stimulation of neuronal populations that do not serve a useful computational function (Rolls, 2016b).

In the context of VisNet, and how the real visual system may operate to implement object recognition, the use of synchronization does not appear to match the way in which the visual system is organized. For example, von der Malsburg's argument would indicate that, using only a two-layer network, synchronization could provide the necessary feature linking to perform object recognition with relatively few neurons, because they can be reused again and again, linked differently for different objects. In contrast, the primate uses a considerable part of its cortex, perhaps 50% in monkeys, for visual processing, with therefore what could be in the order of 6×10^8 neurons and 6×10^{12} synapses involved (estimating from the values given in Table 1.8), so that the solution adopted by the real visual system may be one that relies on many neurons with simpler processing than arbitrary syntax implemented by synchronous firing of separate assemblies suggests. On the other hand, a solution such as that investigated by VisNet, which forms low-order combinations of what is represented in previous layers, is very demanding in terms of the number of neurons required, and this matches what is found in the primate visual system.

2.8.5.2 Sigma-Pi neurons

Another approach to a binding mechanism is to group spatial features based on local mechanisms that might operate for closely adjacent synapses on a dendrite (in what is a Sigma-Pi type of neuron, see Sections 2.9 and A.2.3) (Finkel and Edelman, 1987; Mel, Ruderman and Archie, 1998; Mel, Schiller and Poirazi, 2017). A problem for such architectures is how to force one particular neuron to respond to the same feature combination invariantly with respect to all the ways in which that feature combination might occur in a scene.

2.8.5.3 Binding of features and their relative spatial position by feature combination neurons

The approach to the spatial binding problem that is proposed for VisNet is that individual neurons at an early stage of processing are set up (by learning without a temporal trace learning rule) to respond to low order combinations of input features occurring in a given relative

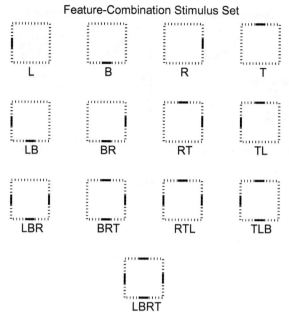

Fig. 2.52 Demonstration that VisNet can form separate representations of stimuli that are subsets or supersets of each other. All members of the full object set are shown, using a dotted line to represent the central 32×32 square on which the individual features are positioned, with the features themselves shown as dark line segments. Nomenclature is by acronym of the features present. (After Elliffe,M.C.M., Rolls, E. T. and Stringer,S.M. (2002) Invariant recognition of feature combinations in the visual system. Biological Cybernetics 86: 59–71. Copyright © Springer Nature.)

spatial arrangement and position on the retina (Rolls, 1992a, 1994a, 1995a; Wallis and Rolls, 1997; Rolls and Treves, 1998; Elliffe, Rolls and Stringer, 2002; Rolls and Deco, 2002; Rolls, 2016b) (cf. Feldman (1985)). (By low order combinations of input features we mean combinations of a few input features. By forming neurons that respond to combinations of a few features in the correct spatial arrangement the advantages of the scheme for syntactic binding are obtained, yet without the combinatorial explosion that would result if the feature combination neurons responded to combinations of many input features so producing potentially very specifically tuned neurons which very rarely responded.) Then invariant representations are developed in the next layer from these feature combination neurons which already contain evidence on the local spatial arrangement of features. Finally, in later layers, only one stimulus would be specified by the particular set of low order feature combination neurons present, even though each feature combination neuron would itself be somewhat invariant. The overall design of the scheme is shown in Fig. 2.28. Evidence that many neurons in V1 respond to combinations of spatial features with the correct spatial configuration is now starting to appear (see Section 2.7), and neurons that respond to feature combinations (such as two lines with a defined angle between them, and overall orientation) are found in V2 (Hegde and Van Essen, 2000; Ito and Komatsu, 2004). The tuning of a VisNet layer 1 neuron to a combination of features in the correct relative spatial position is illustrated in Figs. 2.33 and 2.34.

2.8.5.4 Discrimination between stimuli with super- and sub-set feature combinations

Some investigations with VisNet (Wallis and Rolls, 1997) have involved groups of stimuli that might be identified by some unique feature common to all transformations of a particular stimulus. This might allow VisNet to solve the problem of transform invariance by simply learning to respond to a unique feature present in each stimulus. For example, even in the

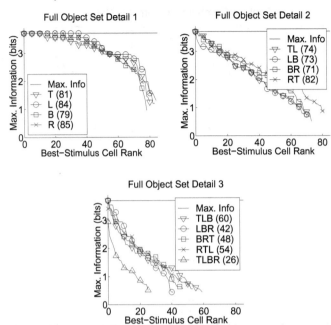

Fig. 2.53 Demonstration that VisNet can form separate representations of stimuli that are subsets or supersets of each other. Performance of VisNet on the full set of stimuli shown in Fig. 2.52. Separate graphs showing the information available about the stimulus for cells tuned to respond best to each of the stimuli are shown. The number of cells responding best to each of the stimuli is indicated in parentheses. The information values are shown for the different cells ranked according to how much information about that stimulus they encode. Separate graphs are shown for cells tuned to stimuli consisting of single features, pairs of features, and triples of features as well as the quadruple feature stimulus TLBR. (After Elliffe,M.C.M., Rolls, E. T. and Stringer,S.M. (2002) Invariant recognition of feature combinations in the visual system. Biological Cybernetics 86: 59–71. Copyright © Springer Nature.)

case where VisNet was trained on invariant discrimination of T, L, and +, the representation of the T stimulus at the spatial filter level inputs to VisNet might contain unique patterns of filter outputs where the horizontal and vertical parts of the T join. The unique filter outputs thus formed might distinguish the T from for example the L.

Elliffe, Rolls and Stringer (2002) tested whether VisNet is able to form transform invariant cells with stimuli that are specially composed from a common alphabet of features, with no stimulus containing any firing in the spatial filter inputs to VisNet not present in at least one of the other stimuli. The limited alphabet enables the set of stimuli to consist of feature sets which are subsets or supersets of those in the other stimuli.

For these experiments the common pool of stimulus features chosen was a set of two horizontal and two vertical 8×1 bars, each aligned with the sides of a 32×32 square. The stimuli can be constructed by arbitrary combination of these base level features. I note that effectively the stimulus set consists of four features, a top bar (T), a bottom bar (B), a left bar (L), and a right bar (R). Figure 2.52 shows the complete set used, containing every possible image feature combination.

To train the network a stimulus was presented in a randomized sequence of nine locations in a square grid across the 128×128 input retina. The central location of the square grid was in the centre of the 'retina', and the eight other locations were offset 8 pixels horizontally and/or vertically from this. Two different learning rules were used, 'Hebbian' (2.16), and 'trace' (2.17), and also an untrained condition with random weights. As in earlier work (Wallis and Rolls, 1997; Rolls and Milward, 2000) only the trace rule led to any cells with invariant responses, and the results shown here are for networks trained with the trace rule for layers 2–4.

The results with VisNet trained on the set of stimuli shown in Fig. 2.52 with the trace rule are as follows. Firstly, it was found that single neurons in the top layer learned to differentiate between the stimuli in that the responses of individual neurons were maximal for one of the stimuli and had no response to any of the other stimuli invariantly with respect to location. Secondly, to assess how well every stimulus was encoded for in this way, Fig. 2.53 shows the information available about each of the stimuli consisting of feature singles, feature pairs, feature triples, and the quadruple-feature stimulus 'TLBR'. The single cell information available from the 26–85 cells with best tuning to each of the stimuli is shown. The cells in general conveyed translation invariant information about the stimulus to which they responded, with indeed cells which perfectly discriminated one of the stimuli from all others over every testing position (for all stimuli except 'RTL' and 'TLBR').

The results presented show clearly that the VisNet paradigm can accommodate networks that can perform invariant discrimination of objects which have a subset–superset relationship. The result has important consequences for feature binding and for discriminating stimuli for other stimuli which may be supersets of the first stimulus. For example, a VisNet cell which responds invariantly to feature combination TL can genuinely signal the presence of exactly that combination, and will not necessarily be activated by T alone, or by TLB. The basis for this separation by competitive networks of stimuli that are subsets and supersets of each other is described in Section B.4, by Rolls (2016b), and by Rolls and Treves (1998, Section 4.3.6).

2.8.5.5 Feature binding and re-use of feature combinations at different levels of a hierarchical network

A key property of a feature hierarchy object recognition system is that it may be possible at intermediate layers of the network to form feature combination neurons that can be useful for a number of different objects in each of which a particular feature combination may be present. If this is a property of encoding in the ventral visual system, this would help the capacity in terms of the number of objects that can be encoded to be high, because feature combination neurons in the intermediate layers could be used for many different objects, with orthogonal representations of whole objects only made explicit in neuronal firing at a late or the last stage of processing. Rolls and Mills (2018) tested the hypothesis that this could be implemented by the relatively simple and biologically plausible architecture of VisNet by training VisNet to identify separately every single feature and feature combinations of an object by its final layer (4); and then examining whether in VisNet's intermediate layers (2 and 3) single neurons typically responded to features or low-order feature combinations that were components of several whole objects represented orthogonally in layer 4. The underlying overall hypothesis here is that at any layer of VisNet neurons need only learn low-order feature combinations; and that if this is repeated over several layers, then by the last layer neurons will become object selective (Rolls, 1992a, 2012d, 2016b). This overcomes any need at all for neurons to respond to high order feature combinations at any one layer, which would be biologically implausible as it would require so many neurons. At the same time, this feature-hierarchy approach would enable neurons in the final layer or layers to respond as if they were sensitive to a high order combination of features, that is, to be quite object selective (though using a sparse distributed representation), as has been found for neurons in the inferior temporal visual cortex (Rolls and Tovee, 1995b; Rolls et al., 1997d; Booth and Rolls, 1998; Franco et al., 2007; Rolls et al., 1997b; Rolls, 2012d, 2016b).

This was tested by training VisNet on the set of 13 objects shown in Fig. 2.54 (Rolls and Mills, 2018). Single neurons in layer 4 coded for each of the objects separately, as expected. In Layer 3 the neurons were a little less selective for separate objects, and might respond best to one object, but might also have good responses to one or more other objects. In layers 2

140 | The ventral visual system

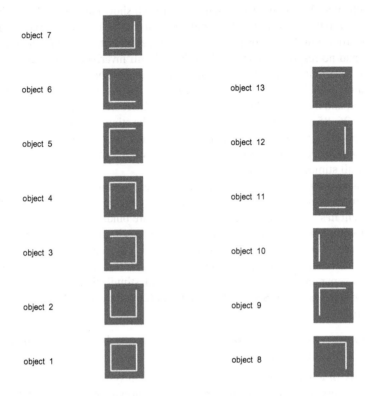

Fig. 2.54 Encoding of information in intermediate layers of VisNet. Stimuli used to investigate coding of feature combinations in intermediate layers of VisNet. Every feature or feature combination with adjacent features was a different object to be learned as a different object by VisNet. (After Rolls, E. T. and Mills, W.P.C. (2018) Non-accidental properties, metric invariance, and encoding by neurons in a model of ventral stream visual object recognition, VisNet. Neurobiology of Learning and Memory 152: 20–31. Copyright © Elsevier Inc.)

and 1 of Visnet, some neurons might respond best to one object, but might also have good responses to one or several other objects. For example, some of these intermediate layer neurons responded to features (such as a top edge) or feature combinations that are a component of several different objects.

This thus demonstrates the important principle in VisNet as a hierarchical unsupervised network approach to computations in the ventral visual system, that representations in intermediate layers can be used for several different objects represented as different objects in the top layer of the hierarchy (layer 4 in VisNet). The distributed tuning of neurons in intermediate layers enables the capacity, the number of objects that can be represented, to be high (Rolls and Mills, 2018; Rolls, 2021d).

2.8.5.6 Feature binding in a hierarchical network with invariant representations of local feature combinations

In this section we consider the ability of output layer neurons to learn new stimuli if the lower layers are trained solely through exposure to simpler feature combinations from which the new stimuli are composed. A key question we address is how invariant representations of low order feature combinations in the early layers of the visual system are able to uniquely specify the correct spatial arrangement of features in the overall stimulus and contribute to preventing false recognition errors in the output layer.

The problem, and its proposed solution, can be treated as follows. Consider an object

1234 made from the features 1, 2, 3 and 4. The invariant low order feature combinations might represent 12, 23, and 34. Then if neurons at the next layer respond to combinations of the activity of these neurons, the only neurons in the next layer that would respond would be those tuned to 1234, not to for example 3412, which is distinguished from 1234 by the input of a pair neuron responding to 41 rather than to 23. The argument (Rolls, 1992a) is that low-order spatial feature combination neurons in the early stage contain sufficient spatial information so that a particular combination of those low-order feature combination neurons specifies a unique object, even if the relative positions of the low-order feature combination neurons are not known, because they are somewhat invariant.

The architecture of VisNet is intended to solve this problem partly by allowing high spatial precision combinations of input features to be formed in layer 1. The actual input features in VisNet are, as described above, the output of oriented spatial-frequency tuned filters, and the combinations of these formed in layer 1 might thus be thought of in a simple way as for example a T or an L or for that matter a Y. Then in layer 2, application of the trace rule might enable neurons to respond to a T with limited spatial invariance (limited to the size of the region of layer 1 from which layer 2 cells receive their input). Then an 'object' such as H might be formed at a higher layer because of a conjunction of two Ts in the same small region.

To show that VisNet can actually solve this problem, Elliffe, Rolls and Stringer (2002) performed the experiments described next. They trained the first two layers of VisNet with feature pair combinations, forming representations of feature pairs with some translation invariance in layer 2. Then they used feature triples as input stimuli, allowed no more learning in layers 1 and 2, and then investigated whether layers 3 and 4 could be trained to produce invariant representations of the triples where the triples could only be distinguished if the local spatial arrangement of the features within the triple had effectively to be encoded in order to distinguish the different triples. For this experiment, they needed stimuli that could be specified in terms of a set of different features (they chose vertical (1), diagonal (2), and horizontal (3) bars) each capable of being shown at a set of different relative spatial positions (designated A, B and C), as shown in Fig. 2.55. The stimuli are thus defined in terms of what features are present and their precise spatial arrangement with respect to each other. The length of the horizontal and vertical feature bars shown in Fig. 2.55 is 8 pixels. To train the network a stimulus (that is a pair or triple feature combination) is presented in a randomized sequence of nine locations in a square grid across the 128×128 input retina. The central location of the square grid is in the centre of the 'retina', and the eight other locations are offset 8 pixels horizontally and/or vertically from this. We refer to the two and three feature stimuli as 'pairs' and 'triples', respectively. Individual stimuli are denoted by three numbers which refer to the individual features present in positions A, B and C, respectively. For example, a stimulus with positions A and C containing a vertical and diagonal bar, respectively, would be referred to as stimulus 102, where the 0 denotes no feature present in position B. In total there are 18 pairs (120, 130, 210, 230, 310, 320, 012, 013, 021, 023, 031, 032, 102, 103, 201, 203, 301, 302) and 6 triples (123, 132, 213, 231, 312, 321). This nomenclature not only defines which features are present within objects, but also the spatial relationships of their component features. Then the computational problem can be illustrated by considering the triple 123. If invariant representations are formed of single features, then there would be no way that neurons higher in the hierarchy could distinguish the object 123 from 213 or any other arrangement of the three features. An approach to this problem (see e.g. Rolls (1992a)) is to form early on in the processing neurons that respond to overlapping combinations of features in the correct spatial arrangement, and then to develop invariant representations in the next layer from these neurons which already contain evidence on the local spatial arrangement of features. An example might be that with the object 123, the invariant feature pairs would

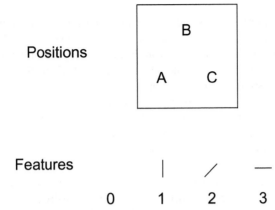

Fig. 2.55 VisNet layer 4 neurons can generalize to transforms never previously seen of stimuli. Feature combinations for experiments of Section 2.8.5.6: there are 3 features denoted by 1, 2 and 3 (including a blank space 0) that can be placed in any of 3 positions A, B, and C. Individual stimuli are denoted by three consecutive numbers which refer to the individual features present in positions A, B and C respectively. In the experiments in Section 2.8.5.6, layers 1 and 2 were trained on stimuli consisting of pairs of the features, and layers 3 and 4 were trained on stimuli consisting of triples. Then the network was tested to show whether layer 4 neurons would distinguish between triples, even though the first two layers had only been trained on pairs. In addition, the network was tested to show whether individual cells in layer 4 could distinguish between triples even in locations where the triples were not presented during training. (After Elliffe,M.C.M., Rolls, E. T. and Stringer,S.M. (2002) Invariant recognition of feature combinations in the visual system. Biological Cybernetics 86: 59–71. Copyright © Springer Nature)

Table 2.5 The different training regimes used in VisNet experiments 1–4 of Section 2.8.5.6. In the no training condition the synaptic weights were left in their initial untrained random values.

	Layers 1, 2	Layers 3, 4
Experiment 1	trained on pairs	trained on triples
Experiment 2	no training	no training
Experiment 3	no training	trained on triples
Experiment 4	trained on triples	trained on triples

represent 120, 023, and 103. Then if neurons at the next layer correspond to combinations of these neurons, the only next layer neurons that would respond would be those tuned to 123, not to for example 213. The argument is that the low-order spatial feature combination neurons in the early stage contain sufficient spatial information so that a particular combination of those low-order feature combination neurons specifies a unique object, even if the relative positions of the low-order feature combination neurons are not known because these neurons are somewhat translation invariant (cf. also Fukushima (1988)).

The stimuli used in the experiments of Elliffe, Rolls and Stringer (2002) were constructed from pre-processed component features as discussed in Section 2.8.5.4. That is, base stimuli containing a single feature were constructed and filtered, and then the pairs and triples were constructed by merging these pre-processed single feature images. In the first experiment layers 1 and 2 of VisNet were trained with the 18 feature pairs, each stimulus being presented in sequences of 9 locations across the input. This led to the formation of neurons that responded to the feature pairs with some translation invariance in layer 2. Then they trained layers 3 and 4 on the 6 feature triples in the same 9 locations, while allowing no more learning in layers 1 and 2, and examined whether the output layer of VisNet had developed transform invariant neurons to the 6 triples. The idea was to test whether layers 3 and 4 could be trained to produce invariant representations of the triples where the triples could only be distinguished if the local spatial arrangement of the features within the triple had effectively

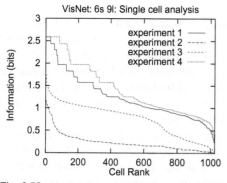 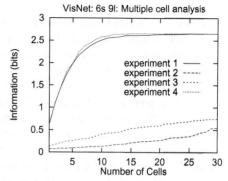

Fig. 2.56 VisNet layer 4 neurons can generalize to transforms never previously seen of stimuli. Numerical results for experiments 1–4 as described in Table 2.5, with the trace learning rule (2.17). On the left are single cell information measures, and on the right are multiple cell information measures. (After Elliffe,M.C.M., Rolls, E. T. and Stringer,S.M. (2002) Invariant recognition of feature combinations in the visual system. Biological Cybernetics 86: 59–71. Copyright © Springer Nature.)

to be encoded in order to distinguish the different triples. The results from this experiment were compared and contrasted with results from three other experiments which involved different training regimes for layers 1,2 and layers 3,4. All four experiments are summarized in Table 2.5. Experiment 2 involved no training in layers 1,2 and 3,4, with the synaptic weights left unchanged from their initial random values. These results are included as a baseline performance with which to compare results from the other experiments 1, 3 and 4. The model parameters used in these experiments were as described by Rolls and Milward (2000) and Rolls and Stringer (2001a).

In Fig. 2.56 we present numerical results for the four experiments listed in Table 2.5. On the left are the single cell information measures for all top (4th) layer neurons ranked in order of their invariance to the triples, while on the right are multiple cell information measures. To help to interpret these results we can compute the maximum single cell information measure according to

$$\text{Maximum single cell information} = \log_2(\text{Number of triples}), \qquad (2.42)$$

where the number of triples is 6. This gives a maximum single cell information measure of 2.6 bits for these test cases. First, comparing the results for experiment 1 with the baseline performance of experiment 2 (no training) demonstrates that even with the first two layers trained to form invariant responses to the pairs, and then only layers 3 and 4 trained on feature triples, layer 4 is indeed capable of developing translation invariant neurons that can discriminate effectively between the 6 different feature triples. Indeed, from the single cell information measures it can be seen that a number of cells have reached the maximum level of performance in experiment 1. In addition, the multiple cell information analysis presented in Fig. 2.56 shows that all the stimuli could be discriminated from each other by the firing of a number of cells. Analysis of the response profiles of individual cells showed that a fourth layer cell could respond to one of the triple feature stimuli and have no response to any other of the triple feature stimuli invariantly with respect to location.

A comparison of the results from experiment 1 with those from experiment 3 (see Table 2.5 and Fig. 2.56) reveals that training the first two layers to develop neurons that respond invariantly to the pairs (performed in experiment 1) actually leads to improved invariance of 4th layer neurons to the triples, as compared with when the first two layers are left untrained (experiment 3).

Two conclusions follow from these results (Elliffe, Rolls and Stringer, 2002). First, a hierarchical network that seeks to produce invariant representations in the way used by VisNet can solve the feature binding problem. In particular, when feature pairs in layer 2 with some translation invariance are used as the input to later layers, these later layers can nevertheless build invariant representations of objects where all the individual features in the stimulus must occur in the correct spatial position relative to each other. This is possible because the feature combination neurons formed in the first layer (which could be trained just with a Hebb rule) do respond to combinations of input features in the correct spatial configuration, partly because of the limited size of their receptive fields (see e.g. Fig. 2.31).

The second conclusion is that even though early layers can in this case only respond to small feature subsets, these provide, with no further training of layers 1 and 2, an adequate basis for learning to discriminate in layers 3 and 4 stimuli consisting of combinations of larger numbers of features. Indeed, comparing results from experiment 1 with experiment 4 (in which all layers were trained on triples, see Table 2.5) demonstrates that training the lower layer neurons to develop invariant responses to the pairs offers almost as good performance as training all layers on the triples (see Fig. 2.56).

2.8.5.7 Stimulus generalization to new locations

Another important aspect of the architecture of VisNet is that it need not be trained with every stimulus in every possible location. Indeed, part of the hypothesis (Rolls, 1992a) is that training early layers (e.g. 1–3) with a wide range of visual stimuli will set up feature analyzers in these early layers which are appropriate later on with no further training of early layers for new objects. For example, presentation of a new object might result in large numbers of low order feature combination neurons in early layers of VisNet being active, but the particular set of feature combination neurons active would be different for the new object. The later layers of the network (in VisNet, layer 4) would then learn this new set of active layer 3 neurons as encoding the new object. However, if the new object was then shown in a new location, the same set of layer 3 neurons would be active because they respond with spatial invariance to feature combinations, and given that the layer 3 to 4 connections had already been set up by the new object, the correct layer 4 neurons would be activated by the new object in its new untrained location, and without any further training.

To test this hypothesis, Elliffe, Rolls and Stringer (2002) repeated the general procedure of experiment 1 of Section 2.8.5.6, training layers 1 and 2 with feature pairs, but then instead trained layers 3 and 4 on the triples in only 7 of the original 9 locations. The crucial test was to determine whether VisNet could form top layer neurons that responded invariantly to the 6 triples when presented over all nine locations, not just the seven locations at which the triples had been presented during training. The results are presented in Fig. 2.57, with single cell information measures on the left and multiple cell information measures on the right. VisNet is still able to develop some fourth layer neurons with perfect invariance, that is which have invariant responses over all nine location, as shown by the single cell information analysis. The response profiles of individual fourth layer cells showed that they can continue to discriminate between the triples even in the two locations where the triples were not presented during training. In addition, the multiple cell analysis shown in Fig. 2.57 demonstrates that a small population of cells was able to discriminate between all of the stimuli irrespective of location, even though for two of the test locations the triples had not been trained at those particular locations during the training of layers 3 and 4.

2.8.5.8 Discussion of feature binding in hierarchical layered networks

Elliffe, Rolls and Stringer (2002) thus first showed (see Section 2.8.5.4) that hierarchical feature detecting neural networks can learn to respond differently to stimuli that consist of unique combinations of non-unique input features, and that this extends to stimuli that are direct subsets or supersets of the features present in other stimuli.

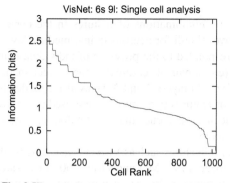
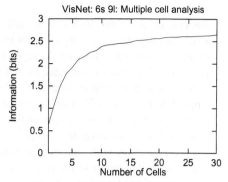

Fig. 2.57 VisNet layer 4 neurons can generalize to transforms never previously seen of stimuli. Generalization to new locations: numerical results for a repeat of experiment 1 of Section 2.8.5.6 with the triples presented at only 7 of the original 9 locations during training, and with the trace learning rule (2.17). On the left are single cell information measures, and on the right are multiple cell information measures. (After Elliffe,M.C.M., Rolls, E. T. and Stringer,S.M. (2002) Invariant recognition of feature combinations in the visual system. Biological Cybernetics 86: 59–71. Copyright © Springer Nature.)

Second, Elliffe, Rolls and Stringer (2002) investigated (see Section 2.8.5.6) the hypothesis that hierarchical layered networks can produce identification of unique stimuli even when the feature combination neurons used to define the stimuli are themselves partly translation invariant. The stimulus identification should work correctly because feature combination neurons in which the spatial features are bound together with high spatial precision are formed in the first layer. Then at later layers when neurons with some translation invariance are formed, the neurons nevertheless contain information about the relative spatial position of the original features. There is only then one object which will be consistent with the set of active neurons at earlier layers, which though somewhat translation invariant as combination neurons, reflect in the activity of each neuron information about the original spatial position of the features. I note that the trace rule training used in early layers (1 and 2) in Experiments 1 and 4 would set up partly invariant feature combination neurons, and yet the late layers (3 and 4) were able to produce during training neurons in layer 4 that responded to stimuli that consisted of unique spatial arrangements of lower order feature combinations. Moreover, and very interestingly, Elliffe, Rolls and Stringer (2002) were able to demonstrate that VisNet layer 4 neurons would respond correctly to visual stimuli at untrained locations, provided that the feature subsets had been trained in early layers of the network at all locations, and that the whole stimulus had been trained at some locations in the later layers of the network.

The results described by Elliffe, Rolls and Stringer (2002) thus provide one solution to the feature binding problem. The solution that has been shown to work in the model is that in a multilayer competitive network, feature combination neurons that encode the spatial arrangement of the bound features are formed at intermediate layers of the network. Then neurons at later layers of the network which respond to combinations of active intermediate layer neurons do contain sufficient evidence about the local spatial arrangement of the features to identify stimuli because the local spatial arrangement is encoded by the intermediate layer neurons. The information required to solve the visual feature binding problem thus becomes encoded by self-organization into what become hard-wired properties of the network. In this sense, feature binding is not solved at run time by the necessity to instantaneously set up arbitrary syntactic links between sets of co-active neurons. The computational solution proposed to the superset/subset aspect of the binding problem will apply in principle to other multilayer competitive networks, although the issues considered here have not been explicitly addressed in architectures such as the Neocognitron (Fukushima and Miyake, 1982).

Consistent with these hypotheses about how VisNet operates to achieve, by layer 4, position-invariant responses to stimuli defined by combinations of features in the correct spatial arrangement, investigations of the effective stimuli for neurons in intermediate layers of VisNet showed as follows. In layer 1, cells responded to the presence of individual features, or to low order combinations of features (e.g. a pair of features) in the correct spatial arrangement at a small number of nearby locations. In layers 2 and 3, neurons responded to single features or to higher order combinations of features (e.g. stimuli composed of feature triples) in more locations. These findings provide direct evidence that VisNet does operate as described above to solve the feature binding problem.

A further issue with hierarchical multilayer architectures such as VisNet is that false binding errors might occur in the following way (Mozer, 1991; Mel and Fiser, 2000). Consider the output of one layer in such a network in which there is information only about which pairs are present. How then could a neuron in the next layer discriminate between the whole stimulus (such as the triple 123 in the above experiment) and what could be considered a more distributed stimulus or multiple different stimuli composed of the separated subparts of that stimulus (e.g. the pairs 120, 023, 103 occurring in 3 of the 9 training locations in the above experiment)? The problem here is to distinguish a single object from multiple other objects containing the same component combinations (e.g. pairs). We proposed that part of the solution to this general problem in real visual systems is implemented through lateral inhibition between neurons in individual layers, and that this mechanism, implemented in VisNet, acts to reduce the possibility of false recognition errors in the following two ways.

First, consider the situation in which neurons in layer N have learned to represent low order feature combinations with location invariance, and where a neuron n in layer $N+1$ has learned to respond to a particular set Ω of these feature combinations. The problem is that neuron n receives the same input from layer N as long as the same set Ω of feature combinations is present, and cannot distinguish between different spatial arrangements of these feature combinations. The question is how can neuron n respond only to a particular favoured spatial arrangement Ψ of the feature combinations contained within the set Ω. We suggest that as the favoured spatial arrangement Ψ is altered by rearranging the spatial relationships of the component feature combinations, the new feature combinations that are formed in new locations will stimulate additional neurons nearby in layer $N+1$, and these will tend to inhibit the firing of neuron n. Thus, lateral inhibition within a layer will have the effect of making neurons more selective, ensuring neuron n responds only to a single spatial arrangement Ψ from the set of feature combinations Ω, and hence reducing the possibility of false recognition.

The second way in which lateral inhibition may help to reduce binding errors is through limiting the sparseness of neuronal firing rates within layers. In our discussion above the spurious stimuli we suggested that might lead to false recognition of triples were obtained from splitting up the component feature combinations (pairs) so that they occurred in separate training locations. However, this would lead to an increase in the number of features present in the complete stimulus; triples contain 3 features while their spurious counterparts would contain 6 features (resulting from 3 separate pairs). For this simple example, the increase in the number of features is not dramatic, but if we consider, say, stimuli composed of 4 features where the component feature combinations represented by lower layers might be triples, then to form spurious stimuli we need to use 12 features (resulting from 4 triples occurring in separate locations). But if the lower layers also represented all possible pairs then the number of features required in the spurious stimuli would increase further. In fact, as the size of the stimulus increases in terms of the number of features, and as the size of the component feature combinations represented by the lower layers increases, there is a combinatorial explosion in terms of the number of features required as we attempt to construct spurious stimuli to trigger false recognition. And the construction of such spurious stimuli will then be prevented through setting a limit on the sparseness of firing rates within layers, which will in turn set a limit on the number of features that can be represented. Lateral inhibition is likely to contribute in both these ways to the performance of VisNet when the stimuli consist of subsets and supersets of each other, as described in Section 2.8.5.4.

Another way in which the problem of multiple objects is addressed is by limiting the size of the receptive fields of inferior temporal cortex neurons so that neurons in IT respond primarily to the object being fixated, but with nevertheless some asymmetry in the receptive fields (see Section 2.8.10). Multiple objects are then 'seen' by virtue of being added to a visuo-spatial scratchpad, as addressed in Section 2.10.

A related issue that arises in this class of network is whether forming neurons that respond to feature combinations in the way described here leads to a combinatorial explosion in the number of neurons required. The solution to this issue that is proposed is to form only low-order combinations of features at any one stage of the network (Rolls (1992a); cf. Feldman (1985)). Using low-order combinations limits the number of neurons required, yet enables the type of computation that relies on feature combination neurons that is analyzed here to still be performed. The actual number of neurons required depends also on the redundancies present in the statistics of real-world images. Even given these factors, it is likely that a large number of neurons would be required if the ventral visual system performs the computation of invariant representations in the manner captured by the hypotheses implemented in VisNet. Consistent with this, a considerable part of the non-human primate brain is devoted to visual information processing. The fact that large numbers of neurons and a multilayer organization are present in the primate ventral visual system is actually thus consistent with the type of model of visual information processing described here.

2.8.6 Operation in a cluttered environment

In this section I consider how hierarchical layered networks of the type exemplified by Vis-Net operate in cluttered environments. Although there has been much work involving object recognition in cluttered environments with artificial vision systems, many such systems typically rely on some form of explicit segmentation followed by search and template matching procedure (see Ullman (1996) for a general review). In natural environments, objects may not only appear against cluttered (natural) backgrounds, but also the object may be partially occluded. Biological nervous systems operate in quite a different manner to those artificial vision systems that rely on search and template matching, and the way in which biological systems cope with cluttered environments and partial occlusion is likely to be quite different also.

One of the factors that will influence the performance of the type of architecture considered here, hierarchically organized series of competitive networks, which form one class of approaches to biologically relevant networks for invariant object recognition (Fukushima, 1980; Rolls, 1992a; Wallis and Rolls, 1997; Poggio and Edelman, 1990; Rolls and Treves, 1998; Rolls, 2016b, 2012d, 2021d), is how lateral inhibition and competition are managed within a layer. Even if an object is not obscured, the effect of a cluttered background will be to fire additional neurons, which will in turn to some extent compete with and inhibit those neurons that are specifically tuned to respond to the desired object. Moreover, where the clutter is adjacent to part of the object, the feature analysing neurons activated against a blank background might be different from those activated against a cluttered background, if there is no explicit segmentation process. We consider these issues next, following investigations of Stringer and Rolls (2000).

148 | The ventral visual system

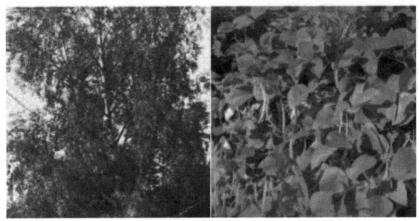

Fig. 2.58 Cluttered backgrounds used in VisNet simulations: backgrounds 1 and 2 are on the left and right respectively. (After Stringer,S.M. and Rolls, E. T. (2000) Position invariant recognition in the visual system with cluttered environments. Neural Networks 13: 305–315. Copyright © Elsevier Ltd.)

2.8.6.1 VisNet simulations with stimuli in cluttered backgrounds

In this section I show that recognition of objects learned previously against a blank background is hardly affected by the presence of a natural cluttered background. I go on to consider what happens when VisNet is set the task of learning new stimuli presented against cluttered backgrounds.

The images used for training and testing VisNet in the simulations described next performed by Stringer and Rolls (2000) were specially constructed. There were 7 face stimuli approximately 64 pixels in height constructed without backgrounds from those shown in Fig. 2.41. In addition there were 3 possible backgrounds: a blank background (greyscale 127, where the range is 0–255), and two cluttered backgrounds as shown in Fig. 2.58 which are 128×128 pixels in size. Each image presented to VisNet's 128×128 input retina was composed of a single face stimulus positioned at one of 9 locations on either a blank or cluttered background. The cluttered background was intended to be like the background against which an object might be viewed in a natural scene. If a background is used in an experiment described here, the same background is always used, and it is always in the same position, with stimuli moved to different positions on it. The 9 stimulus locations are arranged in a square grid across the background, where the grid spacings are 32 pixels horizontally or vertically. Before images were presented to VisNet's input layer they were pre-processed by the standard set of input filters which accord with the general tuning profiles of simple cells in V1 (Hawken and Parker, 1987); full details are given in Rolls and Milward (2000). To train the network a sequence of images is presented to VisNet's retina that corresponds to a single stimulus occurring in a randomized sequence of the 9 locations across a background. At each presentation the activation of individual neurons is calculated, then their firing rates are calculated, and then the synaptic weights are updated. After a stimulus has been presented in all the training locations, a new stimulus is chosen at random and the process repeated. The presentation of all the stimuli across all locations constitutes 1 epoch of training. In this manner the network is trained one layer at a time starting with layer 1 and finishing with layer 4. In the investigations described in this subsection, the numbers of training epochs for layers 1–4 were 50, 100, 100 and 75 respectively.

In this experiment (see Stringer and Rolls (2000), experiment 2), VisNet was trained with the 7 face stimuli presented on a blank background, but tested with the faces presented on each of the 2 cluttered backgrounds. Figure 2.59 shows results for experiment 2, with single and multiple cell information measures on the left and right respectively. It can be seen that

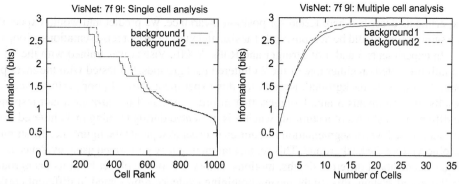

Fig. 2.59 VisNet can recognise stimuli against a cluttered background. Numerical results for experiment 2, with the 7 faces presented on a blank background during training and a cluttered background during testing. On the left are single cell information measures, and on the right are multiple cell information measures. (After Stringer,S.M. and Rolls, E. T. (2000) Position invariant recognition in the visual system with cluttered environments. Neural Networks 13: 305–315. Copyright © Elsevier Ltd.)

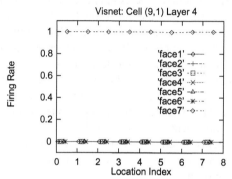

Fig. 2.60 VisNet can recognise stimuli against a cluttered background. Response profiles of a top layer neuron to the 7 faces from experiment 2 of Stringer and Rolls (2000), with the faces presented against cluttered background 1 during testing. (After Stringer,S.M. and Rolls, E. T. (2000) Position invariant recognition in the visual system with cluttered environments. Neural Networks 13: 305–315. Copyright © Elsevier Ltd.)

a number of cells have reached the maximum possible single cell information measure of 2.8 bits ($\log_2$ of the number of stimuli) for this test case, and that the multiple cell information measures also reach the 2.8 bits indicating perfect performance. Compared to performance when shown against a blank background, there was very little deterioration in performance when testing with the faces presented on either of the two cluttered backgrounds. This is an interesting result to compare with many artificial vision systems that would need to carry out computationally intensive serial searching and template matching procedures in order to achieve such results. In contrast, the VisNet neural network architecture is able to perform such recognition relatively quickly through a simple feedforward computation. Further results from this experiment are presented in Fig. 2.60 where we show the response profiles of a 4th layer neuron to the 7 faces presented on cluttered background 1 during testing. It can be seen that this neuron achieves excellent invariant responses to the 7 faces even with the faces presented on a cluttered background. The response profiles are independent of location but differentiate between the faces in that the responses are maximal for only one of the faces and minimal for all other faces.

This is an interesting and important result, for it shows that after learning, special mechanisms for segmentation and for attention are not needed in order for neurons already tuned by previous learning to the stimuli to be activated correctly in the output layer. Although the experiments described here tested for position invariance, we predict and would expect that the same results would be demonstrable for size and view invariant representations of objects.

In experiments 3 and 4 of Stringer and Rolls (2000), VisNet was trained with the 7 face stimuli presented on either one of the 2 cluttered backgrounds, but tested with the faces presented on a blank background. Results for this experiment showed poor performance. The results of experiments 3 and 4 suggest that in order for a cell to *learn* invariant responses to different transforms of a stimulus when it is presented during training in a cluttered background, some form of segmentation is required in order to separate the figure (i.e. the stimulus or object) from the background. This segmentation might be performed using evidence in the visual scene about different depths, motions, colors, etc. of the object from its background. In the visual system, this might mean combining evidence represented in different cortical areas, and might be performed by cross-connections between cortical areas to enable such evidence to help separate the representations of objects from their backgrounds in the form-representing cortical areas.

Another mechanism that helps the operation of architectures such as VisNet and the primate visual system to learn about new objects in cluttered scenes is that the receptive fields of inferior temporal cortex neurons become much smaller when objects are seen against natural backgrounds (Sections 2.8.9.1 and 2.8.9). This will help greatly to learn about new objects that are being fixated, by reducing responsiveness to other features elsewhere in the scene.

Another mechanism that might help the learning of new objects in a natural scene is attention. An attentional mechanism might highlight the current stimulus being attended to and suppress the effects of background noise, providing a training representation of the object more like that which would be produced when it is presented against a blank background. The mechanisms that could implement such attentional processes are described in Chapter 13. If such attentional mechanisms do contribute to the development of view invariance, then it follows that cells in the temporal cortex may only develop transform invariant responses to objects to which attention is directed.

Part of the reason for the poor performance in experiments 3 and 4 was probably that the stimuli were always presented against the same fixed background (for technical reasons), and thus the neurons learned about the background rather than the stimuli. Part of the difficulty that hierarchical multilayer competitive networks have with learning in cluttered environments may more generally be that without explicit segmentation of the stimulus from its background, at least some of the features that should be formed to encode the stimuli are not formed properly, because the neurons learn to respond to combinations of inputs which come partly from the stimulus, and partly from the background. To investigate this, Stringer and Rolls (2000) performed experiment 5 in which layers 1–3 were pretrained with stimuli to ensure that good feature combination neurons for stimuli were available, and then allowed learning in only layer 4 when stimuli were presented in the cluttered backgrounds. Layer 4 was then trained in the usual way with the 7 faces presented against a cluttered background. The results for this experiment are shown in Fig. 2.61, with single and multiple cell information measures on the left and right respectively. It was found that prior random exposure to the face stimuli led to much improved performance. Indeed, it can be seen that a number of cells have reached the maximum possible single cell information measure of 2.8 bits for this test case, although the multiple cell information measures do not quite reach the 2.8 bits that would indicate perfect performance for the complete face set.

These results demonstrate that the problem of developing position invariant neurons to stimuli occurring against cluttered backgrounds may be ameliorated by the prior existence of stimulus-tuned feature-detecting neurons in the early layers of the visual system, and that these feature-detecting neurons may be set up through previous exposure to the relevant class of objects. When tested in cluttered environments, the background clutter may of course

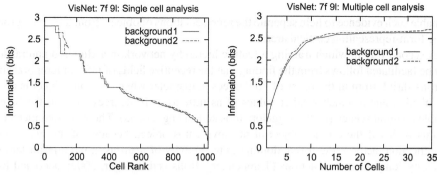

Fig. 2.61 VisNet can recognise stimuli against a cluttered background. Numerical results for experiment 5 of Stringer and Rolls (2000). In this experiment VisNet is first exposed to a completely random sequence of faces in different positions against a blank background during which layers 1–3 are allowed to learn. This builds general feature detecting neurons in the lower layers that are tuned to the face stimuli, but cannot develop view invariance since there is no temporal structure to the order in which different views of different faces occur. Then layer 4 is trained in the usual way with the 7 faces presented against a cluttered background, where the images are now presented such that different views of the same face occur close together in time. On the left are single cell information measures, and on the right are multiple cell information measures. (After Stringer,S.M. and Rolls, E. T. (2000) Position invariant recognition in the visual system with cluttered environments. Neural Networks 13: 305–315. Copyright © Elsevier Ltd.)

activate some other neurons in the output layer, but at least the neurons that have learned to respond to the trained stimuli are activated. The result of this activity is sufficient for the activity in the output layer to be useful, in the sense that it can be read off correctly by a pattern associator connected to the output layer. Indeed, Stringer and Rolls (2000) tested this by connecting a pattern associator to layer 4 of VisNet. The pattern associator had seven neurons, one for each face, and 1,024 inputs, one from each neuron in layer 4 of VisNet. The pattern associator learned when trained with a simple associative Hebb rule (equation 2.16 on page 126) to activate the correct output neuron whenever one of the faces was shown in any position in the uncluttered environment. This ability was shown to be dependent on invariant neurons for each stimulus in the output layer of VisNet, for the pattern associator could not be taught the task if VisNet had not been previously trained with a trace learning rule to produce invariant representations. Then it was shown that exactly the correct neuron was activated when any of the faces was shown in any position with the cluttered background. This readoff by a pattern associator is exactly what we hypothesize takes place in the brain, in that the inferior temporal visual cortex (where neurons with invariant responses are found) projects to structures such as the orbitofrontal cortex and amygdala, where associations between the invariant visual representations and stimuli such as taste and touch are learned (Rolls and Treves, 1998; Rolls, 1999a, 2014a, 2019f,e) (see Chapter 11). Thus testing whether the output of an architecture such as VisNet can be used effectively by a pattern associator is a very biologically relevant way to evaluate the performance of this class of architecture.

2.8.6.2 Learning invariant representations of an object with multiple objects in the scene and with cluttered backgrounds

The results of the experiments just described suggest that in order for a neuron to *learn* invariant responses to different transforms of a stimulus when it is presented during training in a cluttered background, some form of segmentation is required in order to separate the figure (i.e. the stimulus or object) from the background. This segmentation might be performed using evidence in the visual scene about different depths, motions, colors, etc. of the object from its background. In the visual system, this might mean combining evidence represented in different cortical areas, and might be performed by cross-connections between cortical areas to enable such evidence to help separate the representations of objects from their backgrounds in the form-representing cortical areas.

A second way in which training a feature hierarchy network in a cluttered natural scene may be facilitated follows from the finding that the receptive fields of inferior temporal cortex neurons shrink from in the order of 70 degrees in diameter when only one object is present in a blank scene to much smaller values of as little as 5–10 degrees close to the fovea in complex natural scenes (Rolls, Aggelopoulos and Zheng, 2003a). The proposed mechanism for this is that if there is an object at the fovea, this object, because of the high cortical magnification factor at the fovea, dominates the activity of neurons in the inferior temporal cortex by competitive interactions (Trappenberg, Rolls and Stringer, 2002; Deco and Rolls, 2004) (see Section 2.8.9). This allows primarily the object at the fovea to be represented in the inferior temporal cortex, and, it is proposed, for learning to be about this object, and not about the other objects in a whole scene.

Third, top-down spatial attention (Deco and Rolls, 2004, 2005b; Rolls and Deco, 2006; Rolls, 2008f, 2016b) (see Section 2.12) could bias the competition towards a region of visual space where the object to be learned is located.

Fourth, if object 1 is presented during training with different objects present on different trials, then the competitive networks that are part of VisNet will learn to represent each object separately, because the features that are part of each object will be much more strongly associated together, than are those features with the other features present in the different objects seen on some trials during training (Stringer and Rolls, 2008; Stringer, Rolls and Tromans, 2007b). It is a natural property of competitive networks that input features that co-occur very frequently together are allocated output neurons to represent the pattern as a result of the learning. Input features that do not co-occur frequently, may not have output neurons allocated to them. This principle may help feature hierarchy systems to learn representations of individual objects, even when other objects with some of the same features are present in the visual scene, but with different other objects on different trials. With this fundamental and interesting property of competitive networks, it has now become possible for VisNet to self-organize invariant representations of individual objects, even though each object is always presented during training with at least one other object present in the scene (Stringer and Rolls, 2008; Stringer, Rolls and Tromans, 2007b).

2.8.6.3 VisNet simulations with partially occluded stimuli

In this section I examine the recognition of partially occluded stimuli. Many artificial vision systems that perform object recognition typically search for specific markers in stimuli, and hence their performance may become fragile if key parts of a stimulus are occluded. However, in contrast it us demonstrated that the model of invariance learning in the brain discussed here can continue to offer robust performance with this kind of problem, and that the model is able to correctly identify stimuli with considerable flexibility about what part of a stimulus is visible.

In these simulations (Stringer and Rolls, 2000), training and testing was performed with a blank background to avoid confounding the two separate problems of occlusion and background clutter. In object recognition tasks, artificial vision systems may typically rely on being able to locate a small number of key markers on a stimulus in order to be able to identify it. This approach can become fragile when a number of these markers become obscured. In contrast, biological vision systems may generalize or complete from a partial input as a result of the use of distributed representations in neural networks, and this could lead to greater robustness in situations of partial occlusion.

In this experiment (6 of Stringer and Rolls (2000)), the network was first trained with the 7 face stimuli without occlusion, but during testing there were two options: either (i) the top

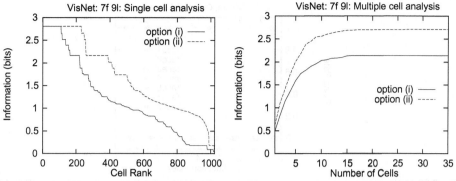

Fig. 2.62 VisNet can recognise correctly even when part of the object or face is occluded. Numerical results for experiment 6 of Stringer and Rolls, 2000, with the 7 faces presented on a blank background during both training and testing. Training was performed with the whole face. However, during testing there are two options: either (i) the top half of all the faces are occluded, or (ii) the bottom half of all the faces are occluded. On the left are single cell information measures, and on the right are multiple cell information measures. (After Stringer,S.M. and Rolls, E. T. (2000) Position invariant recognition in the visual system with cluttered environments. Neural Networks 13: 305–315. Copyright © Elsevier Ltd.)

halves of all the faces were occluded, or (ii) the bottom halves of all the faces were occluded. Since VisNet was tested with either the top or bottom half of the stimuli no stimulus features were common to the two test options. This ensures that if performance is good with both options, the performance cannot be based on the use of a single feature to identify a stimulus. Results for this experiment are shown in Fig. 2.62, with single and multiple cell information measures on the left and right respectively. When compared with the performance without occlusion (Stringer and Rolls, 2000), Fig. 2.62 shows that there is only a modest drop in performance in the single cell information measures when the stimuli are partially occluded.

For both options (i) and (ii), even with partially occluded stimuli, a number of cells continue to respond maximally to one preferred stimulus in all locations, while responding minimally to all other stimuli. However, comparing results from options (i) and (ii) shows that the network performance is better when the bottom half of the faces is occluded. This is consistent with psychological results showing that face recognition is performed more easily when the top halves of faces are visible rather than the bottom halves (see Bruce (1988)). The top half of a face will generally contain salient features, e.g. eyes and hair, that are particularly helpful for recognition of the individual, and it is interesting that these simulations appear to further demonstrate this point. Furthermore, the multiple cell information measures confirm that performance is better with the upper half of the face visible (option (ii)) than the lower half (option (i)). When the top halves of the faces are occluded the multiple cell information measure asymptotes to a suboptimal value reflecting the difficulty of discriminating between these more difficult images. Further results from experiment 6 are presented in Fig. 2.63 where we show the response profiles of a 4th layer neuron to the 7 faces, with the bottom half of all the faces occluded during testing. It can be seen that this neuron continues to respond invariantly to the 7 faces, responding maximally to one of the faces but minimally for all other faces.

Thus this model of the ventral visual system offers robust performance with this kind of problem, and the model is able to correctly identify stimuli with considerable flexibility about what part of a stimulus is visible, because it is effectively using distributed representations and associative processing (Stringer and Rolls, 2000).

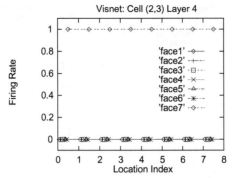

Fig. 2.63 VisNet can recognise correctly even when part of the object or face is occluded. Response profiles of a top layer neuron to the 7 faces from experiment 6 of Stringer and Rolls (2000), with the bottom half of all the faces occluded during testing. (After Stringer,S.M. and Rolls, E. T. (2000) Position invariant recognition in the visual system with cluttered environments. Neural Networks 13: 305–315. Copyright © Elsevier Ltd.)

2.8.7 Learning 3D transforms

In this section investigations of Stringer and Rolls (2002) are described that show that trace learning can in the VisNet architecture solve the problem of in-depth rotation invariant object recognition by developing representations of the transforms which features undergo when they are on the surfaces of 3D objects. Moreover, it is shown that having learned how features on 3D objects transform as the object is rotated in depth, the network can correctly recognize novel 3D variations within a generic view of an object which is composed of previously learned feature combinations.

Rolls' hypothesis of how object recognition could be implemented in the brain postulates that trace rule learning helps invariant representations to form in two ways (Rolls, 1992a, 1994a, 1995a, 2000a, 2016b, 2012d, 2021d). The first process enables associations to be learned between different generic 3D views of an object where there are different qualitative shape descriptors. One example of this would be the front and back views of an object, which might have very different shape descriptors. Another example is provided by considering how the shape descriptors typical of 3D shapes, such as Y vertices, arrow vertices, cusps, and ellipse shapes, alter when most 3D objects are rotated in 3 dimensions. At some point in the 3D rotation, there is a catastrophic rearrangement of the shape descriptors as a new generic view can be seen (Koenderink, 1990). An example of a catastrophic change to a new generic view is when a cup being viewed from slightly below is rotated so that one can see inside the cup from slightly above. The bottom surface disappears, the top surface of the cup changes from a cusp to an ellipse, and the inside of the cup with a whole set of new features comes into view. The second process is that within a generic view, as the object is rotated in depth, there will be no catastrophic changes in the qualitative 3D shape descriptors, but instead the quantitative values of the shape descriptors alter. For example, while the cup is being rotated within a generic view seen from somewhat below, the curvature of the cusp forming the top boundary will alter, but the qualitative shape descriptor will remain a cusp. Trace learning could help with both processes. That is, trace learning could help to associate together qualitatively different sets of shape descriptors that occur close together in time, and describe for example the generically different views of a cup. Trace learning could also help with the second process, and learn to associate together the different quantitative values of shape descriptors that typically occur when objects are rotated within a generic view.

There is evidence that some neurons in the inferior temporal cortex may show the two types of 3D invariance. First, Booth and Rolls (1998) showed that some inferior temporal cortex neurons can respond to different generic views of familiar 3D objects. Second, some neurons do generalize across quantitative changes in the values of 3D shape descriptors while faces (Hasselmo, Rolls, Baylis and Nalwa, 1989b) and objects (Tanaka, 1996; Logothetis, Pauls and Poggio, 1995) are rotated within generic views. Indeed, Logothetis, Pauls and Poggio (1995) showed that a few inferior temporal cortex neurons can generalize to novel (untrained) values of the quantitative shape descriptors typical of within-generic view object rotation.

In addition to the qualitative shape descriptor changes that occur catastrophically between different generic views of an object, and the quantitative changes of 3D shape descriptors that occur within a generic view, there is a third type of transform that must be learned for correct invariant recognition of 3D objects as they rotate in depth. This third type of transform is that which occurs to the surface features on a 3D object as it transforms in depth. The main aim here is to consider mechanisms that could enable neurons to learn this third type of transform, that is how to generalize correctly over the changes in the surface markings on 3D objects that are typically encountered as 3D objects rotate within a generic view. Examples of the types of perspectival transforms investigated are shown in Fig. 2.64. Surface markings on the sphere that consist of combinations of three features in different spatial arrangements undergo characteristic transforms as the sphere is rotated from 0 degrees towards −60 degrees and +60 degrees. We investigated whether the class of architecture exemplified by VisNet, and the trace learning rule, can learn about the transforms that surface features of 3D objects typically undergo during 3D rotation in such a way that the network generalizes across the change of the quantitative values of the surface features produced by the rotation, and yet still discriminates between the different objects (in this case spheres). In the cases being considered, each object is identified by surface markings that consist of a different spatial arrangement of the same three features (a horizontal, vertical, and diagonal line, which become arcs on the surface of the object).

It has been suggested that the finding that neurons may offer some degree of 3D rotation invariance after training with a single view (or limited set of views) represents a challenge for existing trace learning models, because these models assume that an initial exposure is required during learning to every transformation of the object to be recognized (Riesenhuber and Poggio, 1998). Stringer and Rolls (2002) showed as described here that this is not the case, and that such models can generalize to novel within-generic views of an object provided that the characteristic changes that the features show as objects are rotated have been learned previously for the sets of features when they are present in different objects.

Elliffe, Rolls and Stringer (2002) demonstrated for a 2D system how the existence of translation invariant representations of low order feature combinations in the early layers of the visual system could allow correct stimulus identification in the output layer even when the stimulus was presented in a novel location where the stimulus had not previously occurred during learning. The proposal was that the low-order spatial feature combination neurons in the early stages contain sufficient spatial information so that a particular combination of those low-order feature combination neurons specifies a unique object, even if the relative positions of the low-order feature combination neurons are not known because these neurons are somewhat translation invariant (see Section 2.8.5.6). Stringer and Rolls (2002) extended this analysis to feature combinations on 3D objects, and indeed in their simulations described in this section therefore used surface markings for the 3D objects that consisted of triples of features.

The images used for training and testing VisNet were specially constructed for the purpose of demonstrating how the trace learning paradigm might be further developed to give rise to neurons that are able to respond invariantly to novel within-generic view perspectives of an object, obtained by rotations in-depth up to 30 degrees from any perspectives encountered during learning. The stimuli take the form of the surface feature combinations of 3-dimensional rotating spheres, with each image presented to VisNet's retina being a 2-

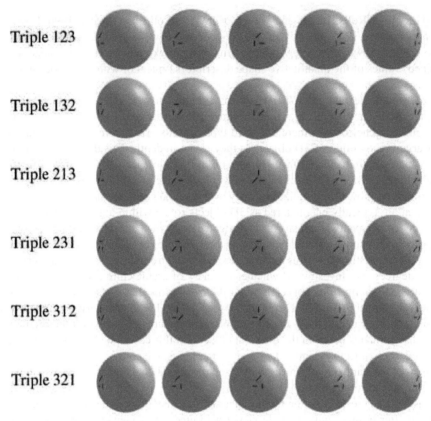

Fig. 2.64 VisNet can learn 3D perspectival transforms of features. Representations of the 6 visual stimuli with 3 surface features (triples) presented to VisNet during the simulations described in Section 2.8.7. Each stimulus is a sphere that is uniquely identified by a unique combination of three surface features (a vertical, diagonal and horizontal arc), which occur in 3 relative positions A, B, and C. Each row shows one of the stimuli rotated through the 5 different rotational views in which the stimulus is presented to VisNet. From left to right the rotational views shown are: (i) −60 degrees, (ii) −30 degrees, (iii) 0 degrees (central position), (iv) +30 degrees, and (v) +60 degrees. (After Stringer, S.M. and Rolls, E. T. (2002) Invariant object recognition in the visual system with novel views of 3D objects. Neural Computation 14: 2585–2596. Copyright © Elsevier Ltd.)

dimensional projection of the surface features of one of the spheres. Each stimulus is uniquely identified by two or three surface features, where the surface features are (1) vertical, (2) diagonal, and (3) horizontal arcs, and where each feature may be centred at three different spatial positions, designated A, B, and C, as shown in Fig. 2.64. The stimuli are thus defined in terms of what features are present and their precise spatial arrangement with respect to each other. We refer to the two and three feature stimuli as 'pairs' and 'triples', respectively. Individual stimuli are denoted by three numbers which refer to the individual features present in positions A, B and C, respectively. For example, a stimulus with positions A and C containing a vertical and diagonal bar, respectively, would be referred to as stimulus 102, where the 0 denotes no feature present in position B. In total there are 18 pairs (120, 130, 210, 230, 310, 320, 012, 013, 021, 023, 031, 032, 102, 103, 201, 203, 301, 302) and 6 triples (123, 132, 213, 231, 312, 321).

To train the network each stimulus was presented to VisNet in a randomized sequence of five orientations with respect to VisNet's input retina, where the different orientations are obtained from successive in-depth rotations of the stimulus through 30 degrees. That is, each stimulus was presented to VisNet's retina from the following rotational views: (i) −60°, (ii) −30°, (iii) 0° (central position with surface features facing directly towards VisNet's retina), (iv) 30°, (v) 60°. Figure 2.64 shows representations of the 6 visual stimuli with 3 surface features (triples) presented to VisNet during the simulations. (For the actual simulations described here, the surface features and their deformations were what VisNet was trained and tested with, and the remaining blank surface of each sphere was set to the same greyscale as the background.) Each row shows one of the stimuli rotated through the 5 different rotational views in which the stimulus is presented to VisNet. At each presentation the activation of individual neurons is calculated, then the neuronal firing rates are calculated, and then the synaptic weights are updated. Each time a stimulus has been presented in all the training orientations, a new stimulus is chosen at random and the process repeated. The presentation of all the stimuli through all 5 orientations constitutes 1 epoch of training. In this manner the network was trained one layer at a time starting with layer 1 and finishing with layer 4. In the investigations described here, the numbers of training epochs for layers 1–4 were 50, 100, 100 and 75, respectively.

In experiment 1, VisNet was trained in two stages. In the first stage, the 18 feature pairs were used as input stimuli, with each stimulus being presented to VisNet's retina in sequences of five orientations as described above. However, during this stage, learning was only allowed to take place in layers 1 and 2. This led to the formation of neurons which responded to the feature pairs with some rotation invariance in layer 2. In the second stage, we used the 6 feature triples as stimuli, with learning only allowed in layers 3 and 4. However, during this second training stage, the triples were only presented to VisNet's input retina in the first 4 orientations (i)–(iv). After the two stages of training were completed, Stringer and Rolls (2002) examined whether the output layer of VisNet had formed top layer neurons that responded invariantly to the 6 triples when presented in all 5 orientations, not just the 4 in which the triples had been presented during training. To provide baseline results for comparison, the results from experiment 1 were compared with results from experiment 2 which involved no training in layers 1,2 and 3,4, with the synaptic weights left unchanged from their initial random values.

In Fig. 2.65 numerical results are given for the experiments described. On the left are the single cell information measures for all top (4th) layer neurons ranked in order of their invariance to the triples, while on the right are multiple cell information measures. To help to interpret these results we can compute the maximum single cell information measure according to

$$\text{Maximum single cell information} = \log_2(\text{Number of triples}), \qquad (2.43)$$

where the number of triples is 6. This gives a maximum single cell information measure of 2.6 bits for these test cases. The information results from the experiment demonstrate that even with the triples presented to the network in only four of the five orientations during training, layer 4 is indeed capable of developing rotation invariant neurons that can discriminate effectively between the 6 different feature triples in all 5 orientations, that is with correct recognition from all five perspectives. In addition, the multiple cell information for the experiment reaches the maximal level of 2.6 bits, indicating that the network as a whole is capable of perfect discrimination between the 6 triples in any of the 5 orientations. These results may be compared with the very poor baseline performance from the control experiment, where no learning was allowed before testing. Further results from experiment 1 are presented in Fig. 2.66 where we show the response profiles of a top layer neuron to the 6 triples. It can be seen that this neuron has achieved excellent invariant responses to the 6 triples: the response profiles are independent of orientation, but differentiate between triples in that the responses are maximal for triple 132 and minimal for all other triples. In particular, the cell responses are maximal for triple 132 presented in all 5 of the orientations.

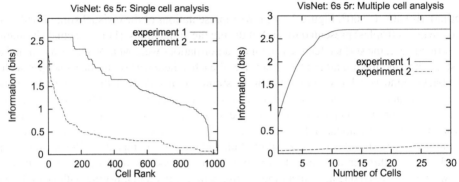

Fig. 2.65 VisNet can learn 3D perspectival transforms of features. Numerical results for experiments 1 and 2: on the left are single cell information measures, and on the right are multiple cell information measures. (After Stringer,S.M. and Rolls, E. T. (2002) Invariant object recognition in the visual system with novel views of 3D objects. Neural Computation 14: 2585–2596. Copyright © Elsevier Ltd.)

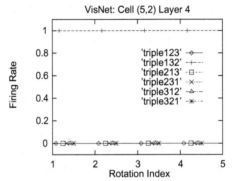

Fig. 2.66 VisNet can learn 3D perspectival transforms of features. Numerical results for experiment 1: response profiles of a top layer neuron to the 6 triples in all 5 orientations. (After Stringer,S.M. and Rolls, E. T. (2002) Invariant object recognition in the visual system with novel views of 3D objects. Neural Computation 14: 2585–2596. Copyright © Elsevier Ltd.)

Stringer and Rolls (2002) also performed a control experiment to show that the network really had learned invariant representations specific to the kinds of 3D deformations undergone by the surface features as the objects rotated in-depth. In the control experiment the network was trained on 'spheres' with non-deformed surface features; and then as predicted the network failed to operate correctly when it was tested with objects with the features present in the transformed way that they appear on the surface of a real 3D object.

Stringer and Rolls (2002) were thus able to show how trace learning can form neurons that can respond invariantly to novel rotational within-generic view perspectives of an object, obtained by within-generic view 3D rotations up to 30 degrees from any view encountered during learning. They were able to show in addition that this could occur for a novel view of an object which was not an interpolation from previously shown views. This was possible given that the low order feature combination sets from which an object was composed had been learned about in early layers of VisNet previously. The within-generic view transform invariant object recognition described was achieved through the development of true 3-dimensional representations of objects based on 3-dimensional features and feature combinations, which, unlike 2-dimensional feature combinations, are invariant under moderate in-depth rotations of the object. Thus, in a sense, these rotation invariant representations encode a form of 3-dimensional knowledge with which to interpret the visual input from the real world, that is able provide a basis for robust rotation invariant object recognition with novel perspectives. The particular finding in the work described here was that VisNet can learn how the surface features on 3D objects transform as the object is rotated in depth, and can use knowledge of the characteristics of the transforms to perform 3D object recognition. The knowledge embodied in the network is knowledge of the 3D properties of objects, and in this sense assists the recognition of 3D objects seen from different views.

The process investigated by Stringer and Rolls (2002) will only allow invariant object recognition over moderate 3D object rotations, since rotating an object through a large angle may lead to a catastrophic change in the appearance of the object that requires the new qualitative 3D shape descriptors to be associated with those of the former view. In that case, invariant object recognition must rely on the first process referred to at the start of this Section (2.8.7) in order to associate together the different generic views of an object to produce view invariant object identification. For that process, association of a few cardinal or generic views is likely to be sufficient (Koenderink, 1990). The process described in this section of learning how surface features transform is likely to make a major contribution to the within-generic view transform invariance of object identification and recognition.

Further investigation of how VisNet can learn to recognise objects despite catastrophic changes in view during 3D object rotation is described in Section 2.9.2 (Robinson and Rolls, 2015).

Poggio and colleagues (Leibo, Liao, Anselmi, Freiwald and Poggio, 2017) have further evidence that the type of learning rule used in VisNet, i.e. Hebbian associative learning combined with a mechanism to maintain the synaptic weight vector at a constant length, exemplified by the Oja rule (Oja, 1982; Wallis and Rolls, 1997) (Section B.4.9.2), is useful to account for the properties of some neurons recorded in the inferior temporal visual cortex. Although in our recordings many neurons responded differently to a right and left profile of a face, they refer to some neurons that respond to both the left and right profile of a face, similar to the type of neuron illustrated in the lower part of Fig. 2.11 (Hasselmo, Rolls, Baylis and Nalwa, 1989b). They show that this type of learning rule is particularly well suited to learning this type of responsiveness (Leibo et al., 2017), providing further support for the VisNet approach to invariant visual object and face learning in the brain which uses a learning rule of this type.

2.8.8 Capacity of the architecture, and incorporation of a trace rule into a recurrent architecture with object attractors

One issue that has not been considered extensively so far is the capacity of hierarchical feedforward networks of the type exemplified by VisNet that are used for invariant object recognition. One approach to this issue is to note that VisNet operates in the general mode of a competitive network, and that the number of different stimuli that can be categorized by a competitive network is in the order of the number of neurons in the output layer, as described in Section B.4. Given that the successive layers of the real visual system (V1, V2, V4, posterior inferior temporal cortex, anterior inferior temporal cortex) are of the same order of magnitude[7], VisNet is designed to work with the same number of neurons in each successive layer. The hypothesis is that because of redundancies in the visual world, each layer of the system by its convergence and competitive categorization can capture sufficient of the statistics of the visual input at each stage to enable correct specification of the properties of the world that specify objects. For example, V1 does not compute all possible combinations of a few lateral geniculate inputs, but instead represents linear series of geniculate inputs to form edge-like and bar-like feature analyzers, which are the dominant arrangement of pixels found

---

[7]Of course the details are worth understanding further. V1 is for example somewhat larger than earlier layers, but on the other hand serves the dorsal as well as the ventral stream of visual cortical processing.

at the small scale in natural visual scenes. Thus the properties of the visual world at this stage can be captured by a small proportion of the total number of combinations that would be needed if the visual world were random. Similarly, at a later stage of processing, just a subset of all possible combinations of line or edge analyzers would be needed, partly because some combinations are much more frequent in the visual world, and partly because the coding because of convergence means that what is represented is for a larger area of visual space (that is, the receptive fields of the neurons are larger), which also leads to economy and limits what otherwise would be a combinatorial need for feature analyzers at later layers. The hypothesis thus is that the effects of redundancies in the input space of stimuli that result from the statistical properties of natural images (Field, 1987), together with the convergent architecture with competitive learning at each stage, produces a system that can perform invariant object recognition for large numbers of objects. Large in this case could be within one or two orders of magnitude of the number of neurons in any one layer of the network (or cortical area in the brain). The extent to which this can be realized can be explored with simulations of the type implemented in VisNet, in which the network can be trained with natural images which therefore reflect fully the natural statistics of the stimuli presented to the real brain.

Another approach to the issue of the capacity of networks that use trace-learning to associate together different instances (e.g. views) of the same object is to reformulate the issue in the context of autoassociation (attractor) networks, where analytic approaches to the storage capacity of the network are well developed (see Section B.3, Amit (1989), and Rolls (2016b)). This approach to the storage capacity of attractor networks that associate together different instantiations of an object to form invariant representations has been developed by Parga and Rolls (1998) and Elliffe, Rolls, Parga and Renart (2000), and is described next.

In this approach, the storage capacity of a *recurrent* network which performs for example view invariant recognition of objects by associating together different views of the same object which tend to occur close together in time, was studied (Parga and Rolls, 1998; Elliffe, Rolls, Parga and Renart, 2000). The architecture with which the invariance is computed is a little different to that described earlier. In the model of Rolls ((1992a), (1994a), (1995a), Wallis and Rolls (1997), Rolls and Milward (2000), and Rolls and Stringer (2006b)), the postsynaptic memory trace enabled different afferents from the preceding stage to modify onto the same postsynaptic neuron (see Fig. 2.67). In that model there were no recurrent connections between the neurons, although such connections were one way in which it was postulated the memory trace might be implemented, by simply keeping the representation of one view or aspect active until the next view appeared. Then an association would occur between representations that were active close together in time (within e.g. 100–300 ms).

In the model developed by Parga and Rolls (1998) and Elliffe, Rolls, Parga and Renart (2000), there is a set of inputs with fixed synaptic weights to a network. The network itself is a recurrent network, with a trace rule incorporated in the recurrent collaterals (see Fig. 2.68). When different views of the same object are presented close together in time, the recurrent collaterals learn using the trace rule that the different views are of the same object. After learning, presentation of any of the views will cause the network to settle into an attractor that represents all the views of the object, that is which is a view invariant representation of an object.

We envisage a set of neuronal operations which set up a synaptic weight matrix in the recurrent collaterals by associating together because of their closeness in time the different views of the same object.

Parga and Rolls (1998) and Elliffe, Rolls, Parga and Renart (2000) were able to show that the number of objects P_o that can be stored is approximately

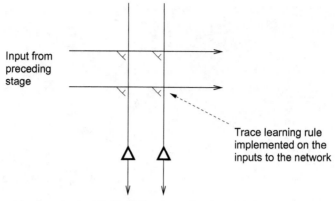

Fig. 2.67 The learning scheme implemented in VisNet. A trace learning rule is implemented in the feedforward inputs to a competitive network. (After Parga,N. and Rolls, E. T. (1998) Transform invariant recognition by association in a recurrent network. Neural Computation 10: 1507–1525. © Massachusetts Institute of Technology.)

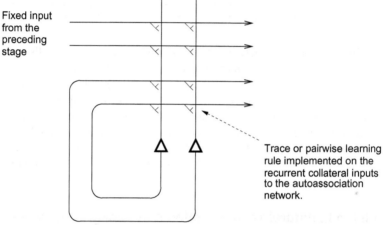

Fig. 2.68 The learning scheme considered by Parga and Rolls (1998) and Elliffe, Rolls, Parga and Renart (2000). There are inputs to the network from the preceding stage via unmodifiable synapses, and a trace or pairwise associative learning rule is implemented in the recurrent collateral synapses of an autoassociative memory to associate together the different exemplars (e.g. views) of the same object. (After Parga,N. and Rolls, E. T. (1998) Transform invariant recognition by association in a recurrent network. Neural Computation 10: 1507–1525. © Massachusetts Institute of Technology.)

$$P_o = \frac{k\,C}{s} \tag{2.44}$$

where C is the number of synapses on each neuron devoted to the recurrent collaterals from other neurons in the network, s is the number of views of each object, and k is a factor that is in the region of 0.07–0.09 (Parga and Rolls, 1998). There is a heavy cost to be paid for large numbers of views s, and the approach of using the recurrent collaterals as an attractor network to perform transform invariant object recognition has not been pursued further. However, the recurrent collaterals could be useful to help to store categories of objects learned by using VisNet-like mechanisms. The object recurrent attractor would help to 'clean up' a somewhat ambiguous image into one or another object category, and indeed evidence for this has been found (Akrami et al., 2009).

It is useful to contrast the different nature of the invariant object recognition problem studied here, and the paired associate learning task studied by Miyashita and colleagues (Miyashita and Chang, 1988; Fujimichi, Naya, Koyano, Takeda, Takeuchi and Miyashita, 2010; Miyashita, 2019). In the invariant object recognition case no particular learning pro-

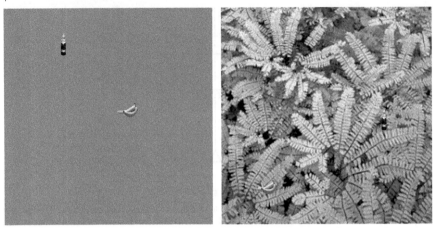

Fig. 2.69 The visual search task. The monkey had to search for and touch an object (in this case a banana) when shown in a complex natural scene, or when shown on a plain background. In each case a second object is present (a bottle) which the monkey must not touch. The stimuli are shown to scale. The screen subtended 70 deg × 55 deg. (After Rolls, E. T., Aggelopoulos,N.C., and Zheng,F. (2003) The receptive fields of inferior temporal cortex neurons in natural scenes. Journal of Neuroscience 23: 339–348. © by The Society for Neuroscience.)

tocol is required to produce an activity of the inferior temporal cortex cells responsible for invariant object recognition that is maintained for 300 ms. The learning can occur rapidly, and the learning occurs between stimuli (e.g. different views) which occur with no intervening delay. In the paired associate task, which had the aim of providing a model of semantic memory, the monkeys must learn to associate together two stimuli that are separated in time (by a number of seconds), and this type of learning can take weeks to train. During the delay period the sustained activity is rather low in the experiments, and thus the representation of the first stimulus that remains is weak, and can only poorly be associated with the second stimulus.

2.8.9 Vision in natural scenes – effects of background versus attention

Object-based attention refers to attention to an object. For example, in a visual search task the object might be specified as what should be searched for, and its location must be found. In spatial attention, a particular location in a scene is pre-cued, and the object at that location may need to be identified. Here we consider some of the neurophysiology of object selection and attention in the context of a feature hierarchy approach to invariant object recognition. The computational mechanisms of attention, including top-down biased competition, are described in Chapter 13.

2.8.9.1 Neurophysiology of object selection in the inferior temporal visual cortex

Much of the neurophysiology, psychophysics, and modelling of attention has been with a small number, typically two, of objects in an otherwise blank scene. In this Section, I consider how attention operates in complex natural scenes, and in particular describe how the inferior temporal visual cortex operates to enable the selection of an object in a complex natural scene (see also Rolls and Deco (2006)). The inferior temporal visual cortex contains distributed and invariant representations of objects and faces (Rolls, 2000a; Booth and Rolls, 1998; Rolls, Treves and Tovee, 1997b; Rolls and Tovee, 1995b; Tovee, Rolls and Azzopardi, 1994; Hasselmo, Rolls and Baylis, 1989a; Rolls and Baylis, 1986; Rolls, 2007e,f,c, 2011d, 2012d, 2016b).

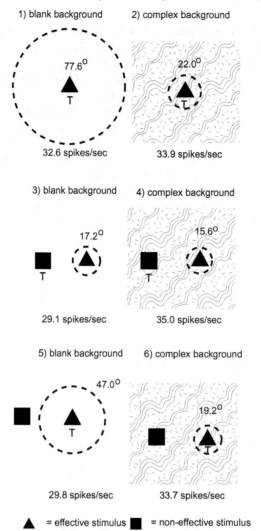

Fig. 2.70 Receptive field sizes of inferior temporal cortex neurons shrink in complex natural scenes. Summary of the receptive field sizes of inferior temporal cortex neurons to a 5 degree effective stimulus presented in either a blank background (blank screen) or in a natural scene (complex background). The stimulus that was a target for action in the different experimental conditions is marked by T. When the target stimulus was touched, a reward was obtained. The mean receptive field diameter of the population of neurons analyzed, and the mean firing rate in spikes/s, is shown. The stimuli subtended 5 deg × 3.5 deg at the retina, and occurred on each trial in a random position in the 70 deg × 55 deg screen. The dashed circle is proportional to the receptive field size. Top row: responses with one visual stimulus in a blank (left) or complex (right) background. Middle row: responses with two stimuli, when the effective stimulus was not the target of the visual search. Bottom row: responses with two stimuli, when the effective stimulus was the target of the visual search. (After Rolls, E. T., Aggelopoulos,N.C., and Zheng,F. (2003) The receptive fields of inferior temporal cortex neurons in natural scenes. Journal of Neuroscience 23: 339–348. © by The Society for Neuroscience.)

To investigate how attention operates in complex natural scenes, and how information is passed from the inferior temporal cortex (IT) to other brain regions to enable stimuli to be selected from natural scenes for action, Rolls, Aggelopoulos and Zheng (2003a) analyzed the responses of inferior temporal cortex neurons to stimuli presented in complex natural backgrounds. The monkey had to search for two objects on a screen, and a touch of one object was rewarded with juice, and of another object was punished with saline (see Fig. 2.7 for a schematic illustration and Fig. 2.69 for a version of the display with examples of the stimuli shown to scale). Neuronal responses to the effective stimuli for the neurons were compared when the objects were presented in the natural scene or on a plain background. It was found that the overall response of the neuron to objects was hardly reduced when they were presented in natural scenes, and the selectivity of the neurons remained. However, the main finding was that the magnitudes of the responses of the neurons typically became much less in the real scene the further the monkey fixated in the scene away from the object (see Fig. 2.8). A small receptive field size has also been found in inferior temporal cortex neurons when monkeys have been trained to discriminate closely spaced small visual stimuli (DiCarlo and Maunsell, 2003).

It is proposed that this reduced translation invariance in natural scenes helps an unambiguous representation of an object which may be the target for action to be passed to the brain regions that receive from the primate inferior temporal visual cortex. It helps with the binding problem, by reducing in natural scenes the effective receptive field of at least some inferior temporal cortex neurons to approximately the size of an object in the scene.

It is also found that in natural scenes, the effect of object-based attention on the response properties of inferior temporal cortex neurons is relatively small, as illustrated in Fig. 2.70 (Rolls, Aggelopoulos and Zheng, 2003a).

2.8.9.2 Attention in natural scenes – a computational account

The results summarized in Fig. 2.70 for 5 degree stimuli show that the receptive fields were large (77.6 degrees) with a single stimulus in a blank background (top left), and were greatly reduced in size (to 22.0 degrees) when presented in a complex natural scene (top right). The results also show that there was little difference in receptive field size or firing rate in the complex background when the effective stimulus was selected for action (bottom right, 19.2 degrees), and when it was not (middle right, 15.6 degrees) (Rolls, Aggelopoulos and Zheng, 2003a). (For comparison, the effects of attention against a blank background were much larger, with the receptive field increasing from 17.2 degrees to 47.0 degrees as a result of object-based attention, as shown in Fig. 2.70, left middle and bottom.)

Trappenberg, Rolls and Stringer (2002) have suggested what underlying mechanisms could account for these findings, and simulated a model to test the ideas. The model utilizes an attractor network representing the inferior temporal visual cortex (implemented by the recurrent connections between inferior temporal cortex neurons), and a neural input layer with several retinotopically organized modules representing the visual scene in an earlier visual cortical area such as V4 (see Fig. 2.71). The attractor network aspect of the model produces the property that the receptive fields of IT neurons can be large in blank scenes by enabling a weak input in the periphery of the visual field to act as a retrieval cue for the object attractor. On the other hand, when the object is shown in a complex background, the object closest to the fovea tends to act as the retrieval cue for the attractor, because the fovea is given increased weight in activating the IT module because the magnitude of the input activity from objects at the fovea is greatest due to the higher magnification factor of the fovea incorporated into the model. This results in smaller receptive fields of IT neurons in complex scenes, because the object tends to need to be close to the fovea to trigger the attractor into the state representing that object. (In other words, if the object is far from the fovea, then it will not trigger neurons in IT which represent it, because neurons in IT are preferentially being activated by another object at the fovea.) This may be described as an attractor model in which the competition for which attractor state is retrieved is weighted towards objects at the fovea.

Attentional top-down object-based inputs can bias the competition implemented in this attractor model, but have relatively minor effects (in for example increasing receptive field size) when they are applied in a complex natural scene, as then as usual the stronger forward inputs dominate the states reached. In this network, the recurrent collateral connections may be thought of as implementing constraints between the different inputs present, to help arrive

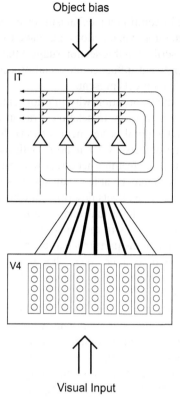

Fig. 2.71 A model of receptive field size of inferior temporal visual cortex (IT) neurons in natural scenes and the effects of top-down attention. The architecture of the inferior temporal cortex (IT) model of Trappenberg, Rolls and Stringer (2002) operating as an attractor network with inputs from the fovea given preferential weighting by the greater cortical magnification factor of the fovea. The model also has a top-down object-selective bias input. The model was used to analyze how object vision and recognition operate in complex natural scenes. (After Trappenberg,T.P., Rolls, E. T. and Stringer,S.M. 2002. Effective size of receptive fields of inferior temporal cortex neurons in natural scenes. Pp. 293–300 in Advances in Neural Information Processing Systems 14, Volume 1, Eds. T.G. Dietterich, S. Becker, Z. Ghahramani. MIT Press: Cambridge, MA.)

at firing in the network which best meets the constraints. In this scenario, the preferential weighting of objects close to the fovea because of the increased magnification factor at the fovea is a useful principle in enabling the system to provide useful output. The attentional object biasing effect is much more marked in a blank scene, or a scene with only two objects present at similar distances from the fovea, which are conditions in which attentional effects have frequently been examined. The results of the investigation (Trappenberg, Rolls and Stringer, 2002) thus suggest that top-down attention may be a much more limited phenomenon in complex, natural, scenes than in reduced displays with one or two objects present. The results also suggest that the alternative principle, of providing strong weight to whatever is close to the fovea, is an important principle governing the operation of the inferior temporal visual cortex, and in general of the output of the visual system in natural environments. This principle of operation is very important in interfacing the visual system to action systems, because the effective stimulus in making inferior temporal cortex neurons fire is in natural scenes usually on or close to the fovea. This means that the spatial coordinates of where the object is in the scene do not have to be represented in the inferior temporal visual cortex, nor passed from it to the action selection system, as the latter can assume that the object making IT neurons fire is close to the fovea in natural scenes.

There may of course be in addition a mechanism for object selection that takes into account the locus of covert attention when actions are made to locations not being looked at. However, the simulations described in this section suggest that in any case covert attention is likely to be a much less significant influence on visual processing in natural scenes than in reduced scenes with one or two objects present.

Given these points, one might question why inferior temporal cortex neurons can have such large receptive fields, which show translation invariance. At least part of the answer to this may be that inferior temporal cortex neurons must have the capability to be large if they are to deal with large objects. A V1 neuron, with its small receptive field, simply could not receive input from all the features necessary to define an object. On the other hand, inferior temporal cortex neurons may be able to adjust their size to approximately the size of objects, using in part the interactive effects described in Chapter 13, and need the capability for translation invariance because the actual relative positions of the features of an object could be at different relative positions in the scene. For example, a car can be recognized whichever way it is viewed, so that the parts (such as the bonnet or hood) must be identifiable as parts wherever they happen to be in the image, though of course the parts themselves also have to be in the correct relative positions, as allowed for by the hierarchical feature analysis architecture described in this chapter.

Some details of the simulations follow. Each independent module within 'V4' in Fig. 2.71 represents a small part of the visual field and receives input from earlier visual areas represented by an input vector for each possible location which is unique for each object. Each module was 6 degrees in width, matching the size of the objects presented to the network. For the simulations Trappenberg, Rolls and Stringer (2002) chose binary random input vectors representing objects with $N^{V4}a^{V4}$ components set to ones and the remaining $N^{V4}(1-a^{V4})$ components set to zeros. N^{V4} is the number of nodes in each module and a^{V4} is the sparseness of the representation which was set to be $a^{V4} = 0.2$ in the simulations.

The structure labelled 'IT' represents areas of visual association cortex such as the inferior temporal visual cortex and cortex in the anterior part of the superior temporal sulcus in which neurons provide distributed representations of faces and objects (Booth and Rolls, 1998; Rolls, 2000a). Nodes in this structure are governed by leaky integrator dynamics (similar to those used in the mean field approach described in Section B.8.1) with time constant τ

$$\tau \frac{dh_i^{IT}(t)}{dt} = -h_i^{IT}(t) + \sum_j (w_{ij}^{IT} - c^{IT}) y_j^{IT}(t) + \sum_k w_{ik}^{IT-V4} y_k^{V4}(t) + k^{IT\_BIAS} I_i^{OBJ}. \quad (2.45)$$

The firing rate y_i^{IT} of the ith node is determined by a sigmoidal function from the activation h_i^{IT} as follows

$$y_i^{IT}(t) = \frac{1}{1 + \exp\left[-2\beta(h_i^{IT}(t) - \alpha)\right]}, \quad (2.46)$$

where the parameters $\beta = 1$ and $\alpha = 1$ represent the gain and the bias, respectively.

The recognition functionality of this structure is modelled as an attractor neural network (ANN) with trained memories indexed by μ representing particular objects. The memories are formed through Hebbian learning on sparse patterns,

$$w_{ij}^{IT} = k^{IT} \sum_\mu (\xi_i^\mu - a^{IT})(\xi_j^\mu - a^{IT}), \quad (2.47)$$

where k^{IT} (set to 1 in the simulations) is a normalization constant that depends on the learning rate, $a^{IT} = 0.2$ is the sparseness of the training pattern in IT, and ξ_i^μ are the components of the pattern used to train the network. The constant c^{IT} in Equation 2.45 represents the strength of the activity-dependent global inhibition simulating the effects of inhibitory interneurons. The external 'top-down' input vector I^{OBJ} produces object-selective inputs, which are used as the attentional drive when a visual search task is simulated. The strength of this object bias is modulated by the value of $k^{IT\text{-}BIAS}$ in equation (2.45).

The weights w_{ij}^{IT-V4} between the V4 nodes and IT nodes were trained by Hebbian learning of the form

$$w_{ij}^{IT-V4} = k^{IT-V4}(k) \sum_{\mu} (\xi_i^{\mu} - a^{V4})(\xi_j^{\mu} - a^{IT}). \tag{2.48}$$

to produce object representations in IT based on inputs in V4. The normalizing modulation factor $k^{IT-V4}(k)$ allows the gain of inputs to be modulated as a function of their distance from the fovea, and depends on the module k to which the presynaptic node belongs. The model supports translation invariant object recognition of a single object in the visual field if the normalization factor is the same for each module and the model is trained with the objects placed at every possible location in the visual field. The translation invariance of the weight vectors between each 'V4' module and the IT nodes is however explicitly modulated in the model by the module-dependent modulation factor $k^{IT-V4}(k)$ as indicated in Fig. 2.71 by the width of the lines connecting V4 with IT. The strength of the foveal V4 module is strongest, and the strength decreases for modules representing increasing eccentricity. The form of this modulation factor was derived from the parameterization of the cortical magnification factors given by Dow et al. (1981)[8].

To study the ability of the model to recognize trained objects at various locations relative to the fovea the system was trained on a set of objects. The network was then tested with distorted versions of the objects, and the 'correlation' between the target object and the final state of the attractor network was taken as a measure of the performance. The correlation was estimated from the normalized dot product between the target object vector that was used during training the IT network, and the state of the IT network after a fixed amount of time sufficient for the network to settle into a stable state. The objects were always presented on backgrounds with some noise (introduced by flipping 2% of the bits in the scene which were not the test stimulus) in order to utilize the properties of the attractor network, and because the input to IT will inevitably be noisy under normal conditions of operation.

In the first simulation only one object was present in the visual scene in a plain (blank) background at different eccentricities from the fovea. As shown in Fig. 2.72a by the line labelled 'blank background', the receptive fields of the neurons were very large. The value of the object bias $k^{IT\text{-}BIAS}$ was set to 0 in these simulations. Good object retrieval (indicated by large correlations) was found even when the object was far from the fovea, indicating large IT receptive fields with a blank background. The reason that any drop is seen in performance as a function of eccentricity is because flipping 2% of the bits outside the object introduces some noise into the recall process. This demonstrates that the attractor dynamics can support translation invariant object recognition even though the translation invariant weight vectors between V4 and IT are explicitly modulated by the modulation factor k^{IT-V4} derived from the cortical magnification factor.

In a second simulation individual objects were placed at all possible locations in a natural and cluttered visual scene. The resulting correlations between the target pattern and the asymptotic IT state are shown in Fig. 2.72a with the line labelled 'natural background'. Many objects in the visual scene are now competing for recognition by the attractor network, and

---

[8]This parameterization is based on V1 data. However, it was shown that similar forms of the magnification factor hold also in V4 (Gattass, Sousa and Covey, 1985). Similar results to the ones presented here can also be achieved with different forms of the modulation factor such as a shifted Gaussian.

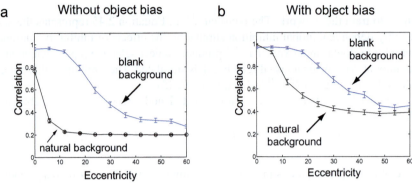

Fig. 2.72 A model of receptive field size of inferior temporal visual cortex neurons in natural scenes and the effects of top-down attention. Correlations as measured by the normalized dot product between the object vector used to train IT and the state of the IT network after settling into a stable state with a single object in the visual scene (blank background) or with other trained objects at all possible locations in the visual scene (natural background). There is no object bias included in the results shown in graph a, whereas an object bias is included in the results shown in b with $k^{\text{IT-BIAS}}$=0.7 in the experiments with a natural background and $k^{\text{IT-BIAS}}$=0.1 in the experiments with a blank background. (After Trappenberg,T.P., Rolls, E. T. and Stringer,S.M. 2002. Effective size of receptive fields of inferior temporal cortex neurons in natural scenes. Pp. 293–300 in Advances in Neural Information Processing Systems 14, Volume 1, Eds. T.G. Dietterich, S. Becker, Z. Ghahramani. MIT Press: Cambridge, MA.)

the objects around the foveal position are enhanced through the modulation factor derived from the cortical magnification factor. This results in a much smaller size of the receptive field of IT neurons when measured with objects in natural backgrounds.

In addition to this major effect of the background on the size of the receptive field, which parallels and may account for the physiological findings outlined above and in Section 2.8.9.1, there is also a dependence of the size of the receptive fields on the level of object bias provided to the IT network. Examples are shown in Fig. 2.72b where an object bias was used. The object bias biases the IT network towards the expected object with a strength determined by the value of $k^{\text{IT-BIAS}}$, and has the effect of increasing the size of the receptive fields in both blank and natural backgrounds (see Fig. 2.72b compared to a). This models the effect found neurophysiologically (Rolls, Aggelopoulos and Zheng, 2003a)[9].

Some of the conclusions are as follows (Trappenberg, Rolls and Stringer, 2002). When single objects are shown in a scene with a blank background, the attractor network helps neurons to respond to an object with large eccentricities of this object relative to the fovea of the agent. When the object is presented in a natural scene, other neurons in the inferior temporal cortex become activated by the other effective stimuli present in the visual field, and these forward inputs decrease the response of the network to the target stimulus by a competitive process. The results found fit well with the neurophysiological data, in that IT operates with almost complete translation invariance when there is only one object in the scene, and reduces the receptive field size of its neurons when the object is presented in a cluttered environment. The model described here provides an explanation of the responses of real IT neurons in natural scenes.

In natural scenes, the model is able to account for the neurophysiological data that the IT neuronal responses are larger when the object is close to the fovea, by virtue of fact that objects close to the fovea are weighted by the cortical magnification factor related modulation $k^{\text{IT-V4}}$.

---

[9] $k^{\text{IT-BIAS}}$ was set to 0.7 in the experiments with a natural background and to 0.1 with a blank background, reflecting the fact that more attention may be needed to find objects in natural cluttered environments because of the noise present than in blank backgrounds. Equivalently, a given level of attention may have a smaller effect in a natural scene than in a blank background, as found neurophysiologically (Rolls, Aggelopoulos and Zheng, 2003a).

The model accounts for the larger receptive field sizes from the fovea of IT neurons in natural backgrounds if the target is the object being selected compared to when it is not selected (Rolls, Aggelopoulos and Zheng, 2003a). The model accounts for this by an effect of top-down bias which simply biases the neurons towards particular objects compensating for their decreasing inputs produced by the decreasing magnification factor modulation with increasing distance from the fovea. Such object-based attention signals could originate in the prefrontal cortex and could provide the object bias for the inferior temporal visual cortex (Renart, Parga and Rolls, 2000) (see Section 2.12).

Important properties of the architecture for obtaining the results just described are the high magnification factor at the fovea and the competition between the effects of different inputs, implemented in the above simulation by the competition inherent in an attractor network.

We have also been able to obtain similar results in a hierarchical feedforward network where each layer operates as a competitive network (Deco and Rolls, 2004). This network thus captures many of the properties of our hierarchical model of invariant object recognition (Rolls, 1992a; Wallis and Rolls, 1997; Rolls and Milward, 2000; Stringer and Rolls, 2000; Rolls and Stringer, 2001a; Elliffe, Rolls and Stringer, 2002; Stringer and Rolls, 2002; Rolls and Deco, 2002; Stringer, Perry, Rolls and Proske, 2006; Rolls and Stringer, 2006a,b; Rolls, 2012d, 2016b, 2021d), but incorporates in addition a foveal magnification factor and top-down projections with a dorsal visual stream so that attentional effects can be studied, as shown in Fig. 2.73.

Deco and Rolls (2004) trained the network shown in Fig. 2.73 with two objects, and used the trace learning rule (Wallis and Rolls, 1997; Rolls and Milward, 2000) in order to achieve translation invariance. In a first experiment we placed only one object on the retina at different distances from the fovea (i.e. different eccentricities relative to the fovea). This corresponds to the blank background condition. In a second experiment, we also placed the object at different eccentricities relative to the fovea, but on a cluttered natural background. Larger receptive fields were found with the blank as compared to the cluttered natural background.

Deco and Rolls (2004) also studied the influence of object-based attentional top-down bias on the effective size of the receptive field of an inferior temporal cortex neuron for the case of an object in a blank or a cluttered background. To do this, they repeated the two simulations but now considered a non-zero top-down bias coming from prefrontal area 46v and impinging on the inferior temporal cortex neuron specific for the object tested. When no attentional object bias was introduced, a shrinkage of the receptive field size was observed in the complex vs the blank background. When attentional object bias was introduced, the shrinkage of the receptive field due to the complex background was somewhat reduced. This is consistent with the neurophysiological results (Rolls, Aggelopoulos and Zheng, 2003a). In the framework of the model (Deco and Rolls, 2004), the reduction of the shrinkage of the receptive field is due to the biasing of the competition in the inferior temporal cortex layer in favour of the specific IT neuron tested, so that it shows more translation invariance (i.e. a slightly larger receptive field). The increase of the receptive field size of an IT neuron, although small, produced by the external top-down attentional bias offers a mechanism for facilitation of the search for specific objects in complex natural scenes (see further Section 2.12).

I note that it is possible that a 'spotlight of attention' (Desimone and Duncan, 1995) can be moved covertly away from the fovea as described in Section 2.12. However, at least during normal visual search tasks in natural scenes, the neurons are sensitive to the object at which the monkey is looking, that is primarily to the object that is on the fovea, as shown by Rolls, Aggelopoulos and Zheng (2003a) and Aggelopoulos and Rolls (2005), and described in Sections 2.8.9.1 and 2.8.10.

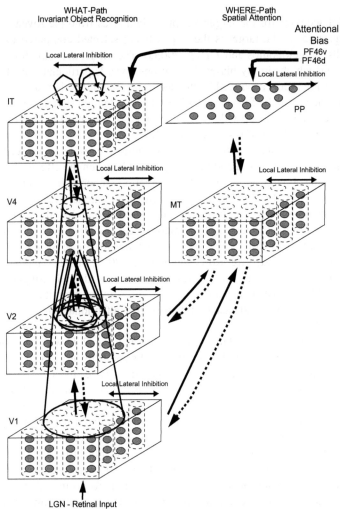

Fig. 2.73 Cortical architecture for hierarchical and attention-based visual perception. The system has five modules structured such that they resemble the two main visual paths of the primate visual cortex. Information from the retino–geniculo-striate pathway enters the visual cortex through area V1 in the occipital lobe and proceeds into two processing streams. The occipital-temporal stream leads ventrally through V2–V4 and IT (inferior temporal visual cortex), and is mainly concerned with object recognition. The occipito-parietal stream leads dorsally into PP (posterior parietal complex), and is responsible for maintaining a spatial map of an object's location. The solid lines with arrows between levels show the forward connections, and the dashed lines the top-down backprojections. Short-term memory systems in the prefrontal cortex (PF46) apply top-down attentional bias to the object or spatial processing streams. (After Deco,G. and Rolls, E. T. (2004) A neurodynamical cortical model of visual attention and invariant object recognition. Vision Research 44: 621–644. © Elsevier Ltd.)

2.8.10 The representation of multiple objects in a scene

When objects have distributed representations, there is a problem of how multiple objects (whether the same or different) can be represented in a scene, because the distributed representations overlap, and it may not be possible to determine whether one has an amalgam of several objects, or a new object (Mozer, 1991), or multiple instances of the same object, let alone the relative spatial positions of the objects in a scene. Yet humans can determine the relative spatial locations of objects in a scene even in short presentation times without eye movements (Biederman, 1972) (and this has been held to involve some spotlight of attention). Aggelopoulos and Rolls (2005) analyzed this issue by recording from single inferior temporal

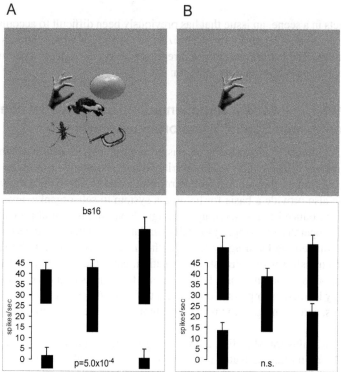

Fig. 2.74 Object-selective receptive fields of inferior temporal cortex neurons that allow the positions of multiple objects close to the fovea to be encoded. (A). The responses (firing rate with the spontaneous rate subtracted, means ± sem) of an inferior temporal cortex neuron when tested with 5 stimuli simultaneously present in the close (10 deg) configuration with the parafoveal stimuli located 10 degrees from the fovea. (B). The responses of the same neuron when only the effective stimulus was presented in each position. The firing rate for each position is that when the effective stimulus (in this case the hand) for the neuron was in that position. The p value is that from the ANOVA calculated over the four parafoveal positions. (After Aggelopoulos,N.C. and Rolls, E. T. (2005) Natural scene perception: inferior temporal cortex neurons encode the positions of different objects in the scene. European Journal of Neuroscience 22: 2903–2916. © Federation of European Neuroscience Societies and John Wiley and Sons Ltd.)

cortex neurons with five objects simultaneously present in the receptive field. They found that although all the neurons responded to their effective stimulus when it was at the fovea, some could also respond to their effective stimulus when it was in some but not other parafoveal positions 10 degrees from the fovea. An example of such a neuron is shown in Fig. 2.74. The asymmetry is much more evident in a scene with 5 images present (Fig. 2.74A) than when only one image is shown on an otherwise blank screen (Fig. 2.74B). Competition between different stimuli in the receptive field thus reveals the asymmetry in the receptive field of inferior temporal visual cortex neurons.

The asymmetry provides a way of encoding the position of multiple objects in a scene. Depending on which asymmetric neurons are firing, the population of neurons provides information to the next processing stage not only about which image is present at or close to the fovea, but where it is with respect to the fovea. This information is provided by neurons that have firing rates that reflect the relevant information, and stimulus-dependent synchrony is not necessary. Top-down attentional biasing input could thus, by biasing the appropriate neurons, facilitate bottom-up information about objects without any need to alter the time relations between the firing of different neurons. The exact position of the object with respect to the fovea, and effectively thus its spatial position relative to other objects in the scene, would then be made evident by the subset of asymmetric neurons firing.

This is thus the solution that these experiments indicate is used for the representation of multiple objects in a scene, an issue that has previously been difficult to account for in neural systems with distributed representations (Mozer, 1991) and for which 'attention' has been a proposed solution. The learning of invariant representations of objects when multiple objects are present in a scene is considered in Section 2.8.6.2.

2.8.11 Learning invariant representations using spatial continuity: Continuous Spatial Transformation learning

The temporal continuity typical of objects has been used in an associative learning rule with a short-term memory trace to help build invariant object representations in the networks described previously in this chapter. Stringer, Perry, Rolls and Proske (2006) showed that spatial continuity can also provide a basis for helping a system to self-organize invariant representations. They introduced a new learning paradigm 'continuous spatial transformation (CT) learning' which operates by mapping spatially similar input patterns to the same postsynaptic neurons in a competitive learning system. As the inputs move through the space of possible continuous transforms (e.g. translation, rotation, etc.), the active synapses are modified onto the set of postsynaptic neurons. Because other transforms of the same stimulus overlap with previously learned exemplars, a common set of postsynaptic neurons is activated by the new transforms, and learning of the new active inputs onto the same postsynaptic neurons is facilitated.

The concept is illustrated in Fig. 2.75. During the presentation of a visual image at one position on the retina that activates neurons in layer 1, a small winning set of neurons in layer 2 will modify (through associative learning) their afferent connections from layer 1 to respond well to that image in that location. When the same image appears later at nearby locations, so that there is spatial continuity, the same neurons in layer 2 will be activated because some of the active afferents are the same as when the image was in the first position. The key point is that if these afferent connections have been strengthened sufficiently while the image is in the first location, then these connections will be able to continue to activate the same neurons in layer 2 when the image appears in overlapping nearby locations. Thus the same neurons in the output layer have learned to respond to inputs that have similar vector elements in common.

As can be seen in Fig. 2.75, the process can be continued for subsequent shifts, provided that a sufficient proportion of input cells stay active between individual shifts. This whole process is repeated throughout the network, both horizontally as the image moves on the retina, and hierarchically up through the network. Over a series of stages, transform invariant (e.g. location invariant) representations of images are successfully learned, allowing the network to perform invariant object recognition. A similar CT learning process may operate for other kinds of transformation, such as change in view or size.

Stringer, Perry, Rolls and Proske (2006) demonstrated that VisNet can be trained with continuous spatial transformation learning to form view invariant representations. They showed that CT learning requires the training transforms to be relatively close together spatially so that spatial continuity is present in the training set; and that the order of stimulus presentation is not crucial, with even interleaving with other objects possible during training, because it is spatial continuity rather the temporal continuity that drives the self-organizing learning with the purely associative synaptic modification rule.

Perry, Rolls and Stringer (2006) extended these simulations with VisNet of view invariant learning using CT to more complex 3D objects, and using the same training images in human psychophysical investigations, showed that view invariant object learning can occur when spatial but not temporal continuity applies in a training condition in which the images of different objects were interleaved. However, they also found that the human view invariance

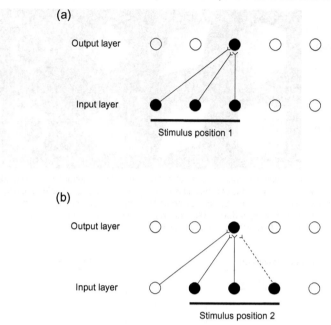

Fig. 2.75 Continuous spatial transformation learning of transform-invariant visual representations of objects. This illustrates how continuous spatial transformation (CT) learning would function in a network with a single layer of forward synaptic connections between an input layer of neurons and an output layer. Initially the forward synaptic weights are set to random values. The top part (a) shows the initial presentation of a stimulus to the network in position 1. Activation from the (shaded) active input cells is transmitted through the initially random forward connections to stimulate the cells in the output layer. The shaded cell in the output layer wins the competition in that layer. The weights from the active input cells to the active output neuron are then strengthened using an associative learning rule. The bottom part (b) shows what happens after the stimulus is shifted by a small amount to a new partially overlapping position 2. As some of the active input cells are the same as those that were active when the stimulus was presented in position 1, the same output cell is driven by these previously strengthened afferents to win the competition again. The rightmost shaded input cell activated by the stimulus in position 2, which was inactive when the stimulus was in position 1, now has its connection to the active output cell strengthened (denoted by the dashed line). Thus the same neuron in the output layer has learned to respond to the two input patterns that have similar vector elements in common. As can be seen, the process can be continued for subsequent shifts, provided that a sufficient proportion of input cells stay active between individual shifts. (After Stringer,S.M., Perry,G., Rolls, E. T. and Proske,H. (2006) Learning invariant object recognition in the visual system with continuous transformations. Biological Cybernetics 94: 128–142. © Springer Nature.)

learning was better if sequential presentation of the images of an object was used, indicating that temporal continuity is an important factor in human invariance learning.

Perry, Rolls and Stringer (2010) extended the use of continuous spatial transformation learning to translation invariance. They showed that translation invariant representations can be learned by continuous spatial transformation learning; that the transforms must be close for this to occur; that the temporal order of presentation of each transformed image during training is not crucial for learning to occur; that relatively large numbers of transforms can be learned; and that such continuous spatial transformation learning can be usefully combined with temporal trace training as explored further (Spoerer, Eguchi and Stringer, 2016).

2.8.12 Lighting invariance

Object recognition should occur correctly even despite variations of lighting. In an investigation of this, Rolls and Stringer (2006b) trained VisNet on a set of 3D objects generated with OpenGL in which the viewing angle and lighting source could be independently varied (see Fig. 2.76). After training with the trace rule on all the 180 views (separated by 1 deg, and rotated about the vertical axis in Fig. 2.76) of each of the four objects under the left lighting

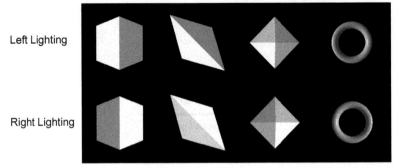

Fig. 2.76 Lighting invariance. VisNet was trained on a set of 3D objects (cube, tetrahedron, octahedron and torus) generated with OpenGL in which for training the objects had left lighting, and for testing the objects had right lighting. Just one view of each object is shown in the Figure, but for training and testing 180 views of each object separated by 1 deg were used. (After Rolls, E. T. and Stringer,S.M. (2007) Invariant visual object recognition: a model, with lighting invariance. Journal of Physiology - Paris 100: 43–62. © Elsevier Ltd.)

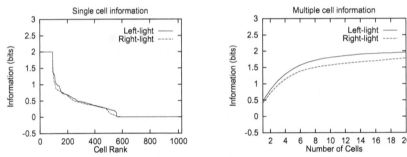

Fig. 2.77 Lighting invariance. The performance of the network after training with 180 views of each object lit from the left, when tested with the lighting again from the left (Left-light), and when tested with the lighting from the right (Right-light). The single cell information measure shows that many single neurons in layer 4 had the maximum amount of information about the objects, 2 bits, which indicates that they responded to all 180 views of one of the objects, and none of the 180 views of the other objects. The multiple cell information shows that the cells were sufficiently different in the objects to which they responded invariantly that all of the objects were perfectly represented when tested with the training images, and very well represented (with nearly 2 bits of information) when tested in the untrained lighting condition. (After Rolls, E. T. and Stringer,S.M. (2007) Invariant visual object recognition: a model, with lighting invariance. Journal of Physiology - Paris 100: 43–62. © Elsevier Ltd.)

condition, we tested whether the network would recognize the objects correctly when they were shown again, but with the source of the lighting moved to the right so that the objects appeared different (see Fig. 2.76). Figure 2.77 shows that the single and multiple cell information measures for the set of objects tested with the light source in the same position as during training (Left-light), and that the measures were almost as good with testing with the light source moved to the right position (Right-light). Thus lighting invariant object recognition was demonstrated (Rolls and Stringer, 2006b).

Some insight into the good performance with a change of lighting is that some neurons in the inferior temporal visual cortex respond to the outlines of 3D objects (Vogels and Biederman, 2002), and these outlines will be relatively consistent across lighting variations. Although the features about the object represented in VisNet will include more than the representations of the outlines, the network may because it uses distributed representations of each object generalize correctly provided that some of the features are similar to those present during training. Under very difficult lighting conditions, it is likely that the performance of the network could be improved by including variations in the lighting during training, so that the trace rule could help to build representations that are explicitly invariant with respect to lighting.

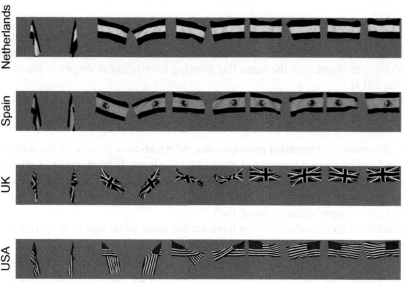

Fig. 2.78 Deformation-invariant object recognition. The flag stimuli used to train VisNet. Each flag is shown with different wind forces and rotations. Starting on the left the first pair, both the 0° and 180° views are shown for windspeed 0, and each successive pair is shown for wind force increased by 50 Blender units. (After Webb,T.J. and Rolls, E. T. (2014) Deformation-specific and deformation-invariant visual object recognition: pose vs identity recognition of people and deforming objects. Frontiers in Computational Neuroscience 8: 37.)

2.8.13 Deformation-invariant object recognition

When we see a human sitting down, standing up, or walking, we can recognise one of these poses independently of the individual, or we can recognise the individual person, independently of the pose. The same issues arise for deforming objects. For example, if we see a flag deformed by the wind, either blowing out or hanging languidly, we can usually recognise the flag, independently of its deformation; or we can recognise the deformation independently of the identity of the flag.

We hypothesized that these types of recognition can be implemented by the primate visual system using temporo-spatial continuity as objects transform as a learning principle. In particular, we hypothesized that pose or deformation can be learned under conditions in which large numbers of different people are successively seen in the same pose, or objects in the same deformation. We also hypothesized that person-specific representations that are independent of pose, and object-specific representations that are independent of deformation and view, could be built, when individual people or objects are observed successively transforming from one pose or deformation and view to another (Webb and Rolls, 2014).

These hypotheses were tested in VisNet. The images to be learned consisted of for example a set of flags with different deformations. The deformation invariant recognition of flags was investigated with a set of 4 flags (each with 5 deformations each with two views, as illustrated in Fig. 2.78). Another set of stimuli consisted of three different people shown with three different poses (sitting, standing, or walking), all presented with 12 different views. It was found that depending on the statistics of the visual input, two types of representation could be built by VisNet.

Pose-specific or deformation-specific representations could be built that were invariant with respect to individual and view, if the statistics of the inputs included in temporal proximity the same pose or deformation. This might occur for example if one saw a scene with several people sitting down, and the people were successively fixated.

Identity-specific representations could be built that were invariant with respect to pose or deformation and view, if the statistics of the inputs included in temporal proximity the same person in different poses, or the same flag in different deformations. This might occur for example if one saw an individual person moving through different poses (sitting, standing up, and walking); or if one saw the same flag blowing into different shapes in the wind (Webb and Rolls, 2014).

We proposed that this is how pose-specific and pose-invariant, and deformation-specific and deformation-invariant, perceptual representations are built in the brain (Webb and Rolls, 2014).

This illustrates an important principle, that information is present in the statistics of the inputs, and can be taken advantage of by the brain to learn different types of representation. This was powerfully illustrated in this investigation in that the functional architecture and stimuli were identical, and it was just the temporal statistics of the inputs that resulted in different types of representation being built.

The utility of these statistics of the input are not taken advantage of in current deep learning models of object recognition (Section B.14).

2.8.14 Learning invariant representations of scenes and places

The primate hippocampal system has neurons that respond to a view of a spatial scene, or when that location in a scene is being looked at in the dark or when it is obscured (Georges-François et al., 1999; Robertson et al., 1998; Rolls et al., 1997a, 1998b; Rolls and Xiang, 2006; Rolls, 2023c). The representation is relatively invariant with respect to the position of the macaque in the environment, and of head direction, and eye position. The requirement for these spatial view neurons is that a position in the spatial scene is being looked at (see Chapter 9). (There is an analogous set of place neurons in the rat hippocampus that respond in this case when the rat is in a given place in space, relatively invariantly with respect to head direction (McNaughton et al., 1983; Muller et al., 1991; O'Keefe, 1984).) How might these spatial view neurons be set up in primates?

Before addressing this, it is useful to consider the difference between a spatial view or scene representation, and an object representation. An object can be moved to different places in space or in a spatial scene. An example is a motor car that can be moved to different places in space. The object is defined by a combination of features or parts in the correct relative spatial position, but its representation is independent of where it is in space. In contrast, a representation of space has landmarks or objects in defined relative spatial positions, which cannot be moved relative to one another in space. An example might be Trafalgar Square, in which Nelson's column is in the middle, and the National Gallery and St Martin's in the Fields church are at set relative locations in space, and cannot be moved relative to one another. This draws out the point that there may be some computational similarities between the construction of an object and of a scene or a representation of space, but there are also important differences in how they are used. The evidence that the hippocampus represents spatial views and not objects is described in Section 9.2.4.1. In the present context we are interested in how the brain may set up a spatial view representation in which the relative position of the objects in the scene defines the spatial view. That spatial view representation may be relatively invariant with respect to the exact position from which the scene is viewed (though extensions are needed if there are central objects in a space through which one moves). The spatial scene representations described here built in the ventral visual system may provide part of the input to the hippocampus that contributes to the presence there of allocentric spatial view cells (Section 9.2.4.1).

It is now possible to propose a unifying hypothesis of the relation between the ventral visual system, and primate hippocampal spatial view representations (Rolls, 2016b; Rolls,

Tromans and Stringer, 2008f), which is introduced in Section 9.3.12. Let us consider a computational architecture in which a fifth layer is added to the VisNet architecture, as illustrated in Fig. 9.35. In the anterior inferior temporal visual cortex, which corresponds to the fourth layer of VisNet, neurons respond to objects, but several objects close to the fovea (within approximately $10°$) can be represented because many object-tuned neurons have asymmetric receptive fields with respect to the fovea (Aggelopoulos and Rolls, 2005) (see Section 2.8.10). If the fifth layer of VisNet performs the same operation as previous layers, it will form neurons that respond to combinations of objects in the scene with the positions of the objects relative spatially to each other incorporated into the representation (as described in Section 2.8.5). The result will be spatial view neurons in the case of primates when the visual field of the primate has a narrow focus (due to the high resolution fovea), and place cells when as in the rat the visual field is very wide (Critchley and Rolls, 1996a; Rolls, 2016b) (Fig. 9.34). The trace learning rule in layer 5 should help the spatial view or place fields that develop to be large and single, because of the temporal continuity that is inherent when the agent moves from one part of the view or place space to another (Rolls, 2021d), in the same way as has been shown for the entorhinal grid cell to hippocampal place cell mapping (Rolls, Stringer and Elliot, 2006c; Rolls, 2016b) (Section 9.3.3).

The hippocampal dentate granule cells form a network expected to be important in this competitive learning of spatial view or place representations based on visual inputs. As the animal navigates through the environment, different spatial view cells would be formed. Because of the overlapping fields of adjacent spatial view neurons, and hence their coactivity as the animal navigates, recurrent collateral associative connections at the next stage of the system, CA3, could form a continuous attractor representation of the environment (Rolls, 2016b). We thus have a hypothesis for how the spatial representations are formed as a natural extension of the hierarchically organised competitive networks in the ventral visual system. The expression of such spatial representations in CA3 may be particularly useful for associating those spatial representations with other inputs, such as objects or rewards (Rolls, 2016b, 2023c) (Chapter 9).

We have performed simulations to test this hypothesis with VisNet simulations with conceptually a fifth layer added (Rolls, Tromans and Stringer, 2008f). Training now with whole scenes that consist of a set of objects in a given fixed spatial relation to each other results in neurons in the added layer that respond to one of the trained whole scenes, but do not respond if the objects in the scene are rearranged to make a new scene from the same objects. The formation of these scene-specific representations in the added layer is related to the fact that in the inferior temporal cortex (Aggelopoulos and Rolls, 2005), and in the VisNet model (Rolls et al., 2008f), the receptive fields of inferior temporal cortex neurons shrink and become asymmetric when multiple objects are present simultaneously in a natural scene. This also provides a solution to the issue of the representation of multiple objects, and their relative spatial positions, in complex natural scenes (Rolls, 2016b, 2012d).

A key concept here is that spatial scenes are built by associating together ventral visual stream features in scenes in a continuous attractor network (Stringer, Rolls and Trappenberg, 2005; Rolls, Tromans and Stringer, 2008f). It is proposed that these spatial scene representations are built in regions such as the retrosplenial scene area and parahippocampal scene area in the Ventromedial Visual Cortical stream (Rolls et al., 2023e; Rolls, 2023c), as described for humans in Section 9.2.8.1 and illustrated in Fig. 9.18. The parahippocampal scene area is proposed to implement its spatial representations using spatial view cells, and in this way to provide the spatial input to the hippocampus for episodic memory (Rolls et al., 2023e; Rolls, 2023c). This is a key proposal for how the 'where' spatial representations for episodic memory are built in primates including humans (Rolls et al., 2023e; Rolls, 2023c), and is in contrast to what is envisaged in the rat where spatial 'where' representations of place not spatial view are assumed to involve the parietal cortex as well as the hippocampus (Hartley, Lever, Burgess and O'Keefe, 2014; Bicanski and Burgess, 2018).

Consistently, in a more artificial network trained by gradient ascent with a goal function that included forming relatively time invariant representations and decorrelating the responses of neurons within each layer of the 5-layer network, place-like cells were formed at the end of the network when the system was trained with a real or simulated robot moving through spatial environments (Wyss, Konig and Verschure, 2006), and slowness as an asset in learning spatial representations has also been investigated by others (Wiskott and Sejnowski, 2002; Wiskott, 2003; Franzius, Sprekeler and Wiskott, 2007; Schonfeld and Wiskott, 2015; Weghenkel and Wiskott, 2018). It will be interesting to test whether spatial view cells develop in a VisNet fifth layer if trained with foveate views of the environment, or place cells if trained with wide angle views of the environment (cf. Critchley and Rolls (1996a), and the utility of testing this with a VisNet-like architecture is that it is embodies a biologically plausible implementation based on neuronally plausible competitive learning and a short-term memory trace learning rule.

2.8.15 Finding and recognising objects in natural scenes: complementary computations in the dorsal and ventral visual systems

Here I consider how the brain solves the major computational task of recognising objects in complex natural scenes, still a major challenge for computer vision approaches.

One mechanism that the brain uses to simplify the task of recognising objects in complex natural scenes is that the receptive fields of inferior temporal cortex neurons change from approximately 70° in diameter when tested under classical neurophysiology conditions with a single stimulus on a blank screen to as little as a radius of 8° (for a 5° stimulus) when tested in a complex natural scene (Rolls, Aggelopoulos and Zheng, 2003a; Aggelopoulos and Rolls, 2005) (with consistent findings described by Sheinberg and Logothetis (2001)) (see Section 2.8.9 and Fig. 2.70). This greatly simplifies the task for the object recognition system, for instead of dealing with the whole scene as in traditional computer vision approaches, the brain processes just a small fixated region of a complex natural scene at any one time, and then the eyes are moved to another part of the screen. During visual search for an object in a complex natural scene, the primate visual system, with its high resolution fovea, therefore keeps moving the eyes until they fall within approximately 8° of the target, and then inferior temporal cortex neurons respond to the target object, and an action can be initiated towards the target, for example to obtain a reward (Rolls et al., 2003a). The inferior temporal cortex neurons then respond to the object being fixated with view, size, and rotation invariance (Rolls, 2012d, 2021d), and also need some translation invariance, for the eyes may not be fixating the centre of the object when the inferior temporal cortex neurons respond (Rolls et al., 2003a).

The questions then arise of how the eyes are guided in a complex natural scene to fixate close to what may be an object; and how close the fixation is to the centre of typical objects for this determines how much translation invariance needs to be built into the ventral visual system. It turns out that the dorsal visual system (Ungerleider and Mishkin, 1982; Ungerleider and Haxby, 1994) (Chapter 3) implements bottom-up saliency mechanisms by guiding saccades to salient stimuli, using properties of the stimulus such as high contrast, color, and visual motion (Miller and Buschman, 2013). (Bottom-up refers to inputs reaching the visual system from the retina.) One particular region, the lateral intraparietal cortex (LIP), which is an area in the dorsal visual system, seems to contain saliency maps sensitive to strong sensory inputs (Arcizet, Mirpour and Bisley, 2011). Highly salient, briefly flashed, stimuli

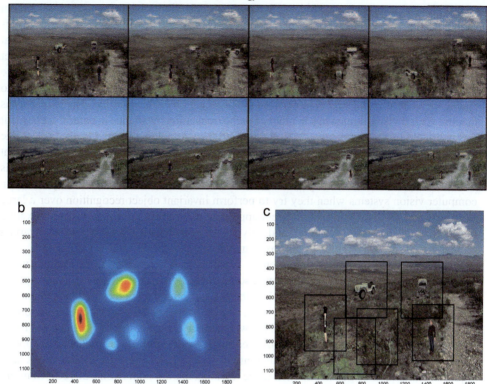

Fig. 2.79 Finding and recognising objects in natural scenes. a. Eight of the 12 test scenes. Each scene has 4 objects, each in one of its four views.
b. The bottom up saliency map generated by the GBVS code for one of the scenes. The highest levels in the saliency map are red, and the lowest blue.
c. Rectangles (384x384 pixels) placed around each peak in the scene for which the bottom-up saliency map is illustrated in (b). (Reproduced from Rolls, E.T. and Webb,T.J. (2014) Finding and recognizing objects in natural scenes: complementary computations in the dorsal and ventral visual systems. Frontiers in Computational Neuroscience 8: 85.)

capture both behavior and the response of LIP neurons (Goldberg et al., 2006; Bisley and Goldberg, 2003, 2006). Inputs reach LIP via dorsal visual stream areas including area MT, and via V4 in the ventral stream (Miller and Buschman, 2013; Soltani and Koch, 2010). Although top-down attention using biased competition can facilitate the operation of attentional mechanisms, and is a subject of great interest (Desimone and Duncan, 1995; Rolls and Deco, 2002; Deco and Rolls, 2004; Miller and Buschman, 2013), top-down object-based attention makes only a small contribution to visual search in a natural scene for an object, increasing the receptive field size from a radius of approximately 7.8° to approximately 9.6° (Rolls, Aggelopoulos and Zheng, 2003a), and is not considered further here.

In research described by Rolls and Webb (2014) we investigated computationally how a bottom-up saliency mechanism in the dorsal visual stream reaching for example area LIP could operate in conjunction with invariant object recognition performed by the ventral visual stream reaching the inferior temporal visual cortex to provide for invariant object recognition in natural scenes. The hypothesis is that the dorsal visual stream, in conjunction with structures such as the superior colliculus (Knudsen, 2011), uses saliency to guide saccadic eye movements to salient stimuli in large parts of the visual field, and that once a stimulus has been fixated, the ventral visual stream performs invariant object recognition on the region being fixated. The dorsal visual stream in this process knows little about invariant object recognition, so cannot identify objects in natural scenes. Similarly, the ventral visual stream cannot perform the whole process, for it cannot efficiently find possible objects in a large natural scene, because its receptive fields are only approximately 9° in radius in complex natural scenes. It is how the dorsal and ventral streams work together to implement invariant object recognition in natural scenes that we investigated. By investigating this computationally, we were able to test whether the dorsal visual stream can find objects with sufficient accuracy to enable the ventral visual stream to perform the invariant object recognition. The issue here is that the ventral visual stream has in practice some translation invariance in natural scenes, but this is limited to approximately 9° (Rolls et al., 2003a; Aggelopoulos and Rolls, 2005). The computational reason why the ventral visual stream does not compute translation invariant representations over the whole visual field as well as view, size and rotation invariance, is that the computation is too complex. Indeed, it is a problem that has not been fully solved in computer vision systems when they try to perform invariant object recognition over a large natural scene. The brain takes a different approach, of simplifying the problem by fixating on one part of the scene at a time, and solving the somewhat easier problem of invariant representations within a region of approximately 9°.

For this scenario to operate, the ventral visual stream needs then to implement view-invariant recognition, but to combine it with some translation invariance, as the fixation position produced by bottom up saliency will not be at the centre of an object, and indeed may be considerably displaced from the centre of an object. In the model of invariant visual object recognition that we have developed, VisNet, which models the hierarchy of visual areas in the ventral visual stream by using competitive learning to develop feature conjunctions supplemented by a temporal trace or by spatial continuity or both, all previous investigations have explored either view or translation invariance learning, but not both (Rolls, 2012d). Combining translation and view invariance learning is a considerable challenge, for the number of transforms becomes the product of the numbers of each transform type, and it is not known how VisNet (or any other biologically plausible approach to invariant object recognition) will perform with the large number, and with the two types of transform combined. Indeed, an important part of the research was to investigate how well architectures of the VisNet type generalize between both trained locations and trained views. This is important for setting the numbers of different views and translations of each object that must be trained. Rolls and Webb (2014) described an investigation that takes these points into account, and measured the performance of a model of the dorsal visual system with VisNet to test how the system would perform to implement view-invariant object recognition in natural scenes.

The operation of the dorsal visual system in providing a saliency map that would guide the locations to which visual fixations would occur was simulated with a bottom up saliency algorithm that is one of the standard ones that has been developed, which adopts the Itti and Koch (2000) approach to visual saliency, and implements it by graph-based visual saliency (GBVS) algorithms (Harel, Koch and Perona, 2006a,b). The basis for the saliency map consists of features such as high contrast edges, and the system knows nothing about objects, people, vehicles etc. This system performs well, that is similarly to humans, in many bottom-up saliency tasks. With the scene illustrated in Fig. 2.79a, the saliency map that was produced is illustrated in Fig. 2.79b. The peaks in this saliency map were used as the site of successive 'fixations', at each of which a rectangles (of 384x384 pixels) was placed, and was used as the input image to VisNet as illustrated in Fig. 2.79c. VisNet had been trained on four views spaced 45° apart of each of the 4 objects as illustrated in Fig. 2.80.

VisNet was trained on a 25-location grid with size 64×64 with spacing of 16 pixels, and with 4 different views of each object, as it was not expected that the peak of a saliency map would be the centre of an object. Part of the aim was to investigate how much translation invariance needs to be present in the ventral visual system, in the context of where the dorsal

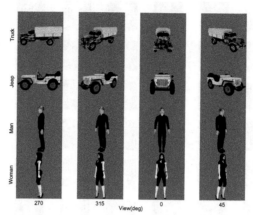

Fig. 2.80 Finding and recognising objects in natural scenes. Training images for the identification of objects in a natural scene: 4 views of each of 4 objects were used. Each image was 256x256 pixels. (Reproduced from Rolls, E.T. and Webb,T.J. (2014) Finding and recognizing objects in natural scenes: complementary computations in the dorsal and ventral visual systems. Frontiers in Computational Neuroscience 8: 85.)

visual system found salient regions in a scene. We found that performance was reasonably good, 90% correct where chance was 25% correct, for which object had been shown. That is, even when the fixation was not on the centre of the object, performance was good. Moreover, the performance was good independently of the view of the person or object, showing that in VisNet both view and position invariance can be trained into the system (Rolls and Webb, 2014). Further, the system also generalized reasonably to views between the training views which were 45° apart. Further, this good performance was obtained when inevitably what was extracted as what was close to the fovea included parts of the background scene within the rectangles shown in Fig. 2.79c.

This investigation elucidated how the brain may solve this major computational problem of recognition of multiple objects seen in different views in complex natural scenes, by moving the eyes to fixate close to objects in a natural scene using bottom-up saliency implemented in the dorsal visual system, and then performing object recognition successively for each of the fixated regions using the ventral visual system modelled to have both translation and view invariance in VisNet. The research described by Rolls and Webb (2014) emphasises that because the eyes do not locate the centre of objects based on saliency, then translation invariance as well as view, size etc invariance needs to be implemented in the ventral visual system. The research showed how a model of invariant object recognition in the ventral visual system, VisNet, can perform the required combination of translation and view invariant recognition, and moreover can generalize between views of objects that are 45° apart during training, and can also generalize to intermediate locations when trained in a coarse training grid with the spacing between trained locations equivalent to 1–3°. Part of the utility of this research is that it helps to identify how much translation invariance needs to be incorporated into the ventral visual system to enable object recognition with successive fixations guided by saliency to different positions in a complex natural scene (Rolls and Webb, 2014).

2.8.16 Non-accidental properties, and transform invariant object recognition

Non-accidental properties (NAPs) of images of objects are those that are relatively invariant over rotations in depth, and can be distinguished from metric properties (MPs), such as the

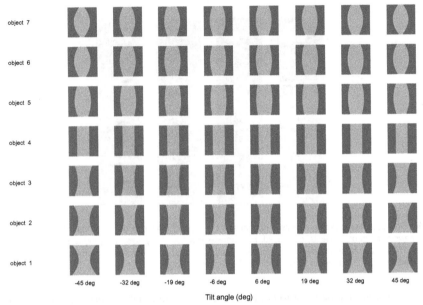

Fig. 2.81 Encoding of non-accidental properties. Stimuli used to investigate non-accidental properties (NAP) vs metric properties (MP). Each object is shown as white on a grey background. Objects 1–3 have the non-accidental property of concave edges. Object 4 has the non-accidental property of parallel edges. Objects 5–7 have the non-accidental property of convex edges. The vertical view of each object was at 0 deg, with the images at -6 and 6 deg of tilt illustrated. Different amounts of tilt of the top towards or away from the viewer are shown at the tilt angles indicated. Each object was thin, and was cut off at the top and bottom to ensure that any view of the top or bottom of the object did not appear, so that the type of curvature of the edges (concave, straight, or convex) was the main cue available. (After Rolls, E. T. and Mills, W.P.C. (2018) Non-accidental properties, metric invariance, and encoding by neurons in a model of ventral stream visual object recognition, VisNet. Neurobiology of Learning and Memory 152: 20–31. © Elsevier Ltd.)

aspect ratio of a part or the degree of curvature of a contour, which do vary continuously with rotation in depth (Biederman, 1987), as described next.

It has been proposed that non-accidental properties of objects as they transform into different views are useful for view-invariant object recognition processes, and that metric properties are much less useful (Biederman, 1987; Biederman and Gerhardstein, 1993; Kayaert, Biederman and Vogels, 2005a; Amir, Biederman and Hayworth, 2011; Kayaert, Biederman, Op de Beeck and Vogels, 2005b). Non-accidental properties (NAPs) are relatively invariant over rotations in depth (Biederman, 1987). A NAP is an image property, such as the linearity of a contour or the cotermination of a pair of contours, that is unaffected by rotation in depth, as long the surfaces manifesting that property are still present in the image (Lowe, 1985). NAPs can be distinguished from metric properties (MPs), such as the aspect ratio of a part or the degree of curvature of a contour, which do vary continuously with rotation in depth. There is psychophysical and functional neuroimaging evidence that supports this distinction (Kayaert et al., 2005a; Amir et al., 2011; Kayaert et al., 2005b). In addition, there is evidence that neurons in the lateral occipital cortex and inferior temporal visual cortex of the macaque are tuned more to non-accidental than to metric properties (Kim and Biederman, 2012; Vogels, Biederman, Bar and Lorincz, 2001).

These concepts are illustrated in Fig. 2.81. If we take object 1 as an example (Fig. 2.81), then we can see that it is approximately cylindrical but with concave sides. Its appearance when vertical is at 0 deg (close to the view illustrated of -6 and 6 deg). As the object is tilted towards or away from the viewer, the degree of curvature appears larger. The degree of curvature is thus a metric property (MP) of the object which is not very useful in transform-invariant object recognition. On the other hand, the fact that object 1 has concave sides is apparent across all these transforms, and therefore is a non-accidental property (NAP) used in identifying an object. This is made evident by a comparison with object 7, which has convex edges, which are always convex through these transforms, while the degree of curvature is a metric property and again varies as a function of the tilt transform. Further, object 4, a cylinder, always has straight sides whatever its tilt, so having straight sides is in this case also a NAP.

We tested VisNet with these sets of stimuli to investigate whether it would learn to represent the three cylinder types based on the non-accidental properties, and would treat the metric properties as transforms, and we found that VisNet did indeed operate in this way (Rolls and Mills, 2018).

Consideration of what is illustrated in Fig. 2.81 leads in fact to a new theory about how Non-Accidental Properties are learned, and how they are relatively invariant with respect to metric changes (Rolls and Mills, 2018; Rolls, 2021d). If we look at object 1, we see that a range of curvatures are shown as the object transforms. These different curvatures are all learned as properties of this class of object by the temporal trace learning rule, because those different views were presented close together in time so that the trace learning rule could learn that these were transforms of the same object. But if we then look at object 2, we see that some of the degrees of curvature in some of its views are similar to what has already been learned for object 1. So without further training of any association between object 1 and object 2, there will be some generalization across these two objects with different degrees of curvature, because some of the degrees of curvature are similar for some of the views of these two objects. *It is in this way, Rolls and Mills (2018) proposed, that non-accidental properties are learned by the brain, and generalize across a range of objects with the same non-accidental property (e.g. concave sides), even though the degree of curvature, the metric property, may be quite different.*

2.9 Further approaches to invariant object recognition

2.9.1 Other types of slow learning

In a more artificial network trained by gradient ascent with a goal function that included forming relatively time invariant representations and decorrelating the responses of neurons within each layer of the 5-layer network, place-like cells were formed at the end of the network when the system was trained with a real or simulated robot moving through spatial environments (Wyss, Konig and Verschure, 2006), and slowness as an asset in learning spatial representations has also been investigated by others (Wiskott and Sejnowski, 2002; Wiskott, 2003; Franzius, Sprekeler and Wiskott, 2007; Schonfeld and Wiskott, 2015; Weghenkel and Wiskott, 2018). It will be interesting to test whether spatial view cells develop in a VisNet fifth layer if trained with foveate views of the environment, or place cells if trained with wide angle views of the environment (cf. Critchley and Rolls (1996a), and the utility of testing this with a VisNet-like architecture is that it is embodies a biologically plausible implementation based on neuronally plausible competitive learning and a short-term memory trace learning rule.

2.9.2 HMAX

A related approach to invariant object recognition is HMAX (Riesenhuber and Poggio, 1999b,a, 2000; Serre, Oliva and Poggio, 2007b; Serre, Wolf, Bileschi, Riesenhuber and Poggio, 2007c),

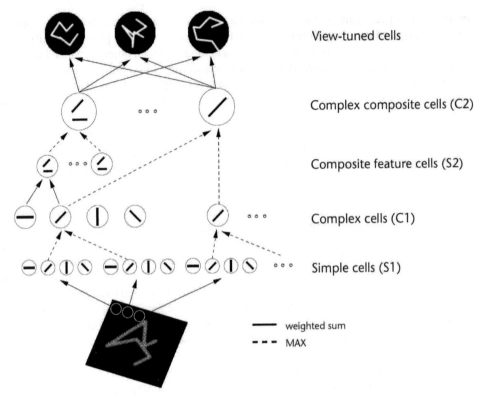

Fig. 2.82 Sketch of Riesenhuber and Poggio's (1999a,b) HMAX model of invariant object recognition. The model includes layers of 'S' cells which perform template matching (solid lines), and 'C' cells (solid lines) which pool information by a non-linear MAX function to achieve invariance (see text). (After Riesenhuber,H. and Poggio,T. (1999) Hierarchical models of object recognition in cortex. Nature Neuroscience 2: 1019–1025. © Springer Nature.)

which builds on the hypothesis that not just shift invariance (as implemented in the Neocognitron of Fukushima (1980)), but also other invariances such as scale, rotation and even view, could be built into a feature hierarchy system such as VisNet (Rolls, 1992a; Wallis, Rolls and Földiák, 1993; Wallis and Rolls, 1997; Rolls and Milward, 2000; Rolls and Stringer, 2006a; Rolls, 2016b, 2012d). HMAX is a feature hierarchy approach that uses alternate 'simple or S cell' and 'complex or C cell' layers in a way analogous to Fukushima (1980) (see Fig. 2.82). The inspiration for this architecture (Riesenhuber and Poggio, 1999b) may have come from the simple and complex cells found in V1 by Hubel and Wiesel (1968).

The function of each S cell layer is to represent more complicated features from the inputs, and works by template matching. In particular, when images are presented to HMAX, a set of firings is produced in a patch of S cells, and this patch is propagated laterally so that the same processing is performed throughout the layer. The use of patches of activity produced by an input image to select synaptic weights for the patch while not typical learning, does mean that the synaptic weights in the network are set up to reflect some effects produced by input images. Learning within the model is performed by sampling patches of the C layer output that are produced by a randomly selected image from the training set, and setting the S neurons that receive from the patch to have the weights that would enable the S neuron to be selective for that patch. Then in forward passes, a C layer set of firings is convolved with the S filters that follow the C layer to produce the next S level activity. The convolution is a non-local operator that acts over the whole C layer and effectively assumes that a given type of S neuron has identical connectivity throughout the spatial extent of the layer.

The function of each 'C' cell layer is to provide some translation invariance over the features discovered in the preceding simple cell layer (as in Fukushima (1980)), and operates by performing a MAX function on the inputs. The non-linear MAX function makes a complex cell respond only to whatever is the highest activity input being received, and is part of the process by which invariance is achieved according to this proposal. This C layer process involves 'implicitly scanning over afferents of the same type differing in the parameter of the transformation to which responses should be invariant (for instance, feature size for scale invariance), and then selecting the best-matching afferent' (Riesenhuber and Poggio, 1999b). Brain mechanisms by which this computation could be set up are not part of the scheme.

The final complex cell layer (of in some instantiations several S-C pairs of layers) is then typically used as an input to a non-biologically plausible support vector machine or least squares computation to perform classification of the representations of the final layer into object classes. This is a supervised type of training, in which a target is provided from the outside world for each neuron in the last C layer. The inputs to both HMAX and VisNet are Gabor-filtered images intended to approximate V1. One difference is that VisNet is normally trained on images generated by objects as they transform in the world, so that view, translation, size, rotation etc invariant representations of objects can be learned by the network. In contrast, HMAX is typically trained with large databases of pictures of different exemplars of for example hats and beer mugs as in the Caltech databases, which do not provide the basis for invariant representations of objects to be learned, but are aimed at object classification.

Robinson and Rolls (2015) compared the performance of HMAX and VisNet in order to help identify which principles of operation of these two models of the ventral visual system best accounted for the responses of inferior temporal cortex neurons. The aim was to identify which of their different principles of operation might best capture the principles of cortical computation. The outputs of both systems were measured in the same way, with a biologically plausible pattern association network receiving input from the final layer of HMAX or VisNet, and with one neuron for each class to be identified. That is, a non-biologically plausible support vector machine or least squares regression were not used to measure the performance. A standard HMAX model (Mutch and Lowe, 2008; Serre, Wolf, Bileschi, Riesenhuber and Poggio, 2007c; Serre, Oliva and Poggio, 2007b) was used in the implementation by Mutch and Lowe (2008) which has two S-C layers. I note that an HMAX family model has in the order of 10 million computational units (Serre, Oliva and Poggio, 2007b), which is at least 100 times the number contained within the current implementation of VisNet (which uses 128x128 neurons in each of 4 layers, i.e. 65,536 neurons).

First, Robinson and Rolls (2015) tested the performance of both nets on an HMAX type of problem, learning to identify classes of object (e.g. hats vs bears) from a set of exemplars, chosen in this case from the CalTech database. The performance of the nets in terms of percentage correct was similar, but a major difference was that it was found that the final layer C neurons of HMAX have a very non-sparse representation (unlike that in the brain or in VisNet) that provides little information in the single neuron responses about the object class. This highlighted an important principle of cortical computation, that the neuronal representation must be in a form in which it can be read, by for example a pattern association network, which is what the cortex and VisNet achieve by producing a sparse distributed representation.

Second, when trained with different views of each object, HMAX performed very poorly because it has no mechanism to learn view invariance, i.e. that somewhat different images produced by a single object seen in different views are in fact of the same object. In contrast, VisNet learned this well, because its short-term memory trace learning rule enabled the different views of the same object appearing in short time periods to be associated together. This highlighted another important principle of cortical computation, that advantage is taken of

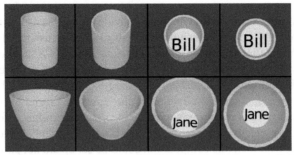

Fig. 2.83 View invariant representations of cups. The two objects, each with four views. HMAX of Riesenhuber and Poggio (1999) fails to categorize these objects correctly, because, unlike VisNet, it has no mechanism to associate together different views of the same object. (After Robinson,L. and Rolls, E. T. (2015) Invariant visual object recognition: biologically plausible approaches. Biological Cybernetics 109: 505–535.)

the statistics of inputs from the world to help learning, with in this case temporal and spatial continuity being relevant.

Third, it was shown that VisNet neurons, like many neurons in the inferior temporal visual cortex (Rolls, Tovee, Purcell, Stewart and Azzopardi, 1994b; Perrett, Rolls and Caan, 1982), do not respond to scrambled images of faces, and thus encode shape information. HMAX neurons responded with similarly high rates to the unscrambled and scrambled faces, indicating that low level features including texture may be relevant to HMAX performance. The VisNet and inferior temporal cortex neurons at the same time encoded the identity of the unscrambled faces. Some other neurons in the inferior temporal visual cortex respond to parts of faces such as eyes or mouth (Perrett, Rolls and Caan, 1982; Issa and DiCarlo, 2012), and this is consistent with the hypothesis that the inferior temporal visual cortex builds configuration-specific whole face or object representations from their parts, helped by feature combination neurons learned at earlier stages of the ventral visual system hierarchy (Rolls, 1992a, 2012d, 2021d). HMAX has no learning to enable it to respond to non-linear combinations of features in the correct relative spatial positions (Robinson and Rolls, 2015). This highlights another important principle of cortical architecture, that neurons learn to respond to non-linear combinations of their inputs using processes such as competitive learning (Section B.4), and that this is essential for correct operation of most sensory systems.

Fourth, it was shown that VisNet can learn to recognise objects even when the view provided by the object changes catastrophically as it transforms, whereas HMAX has no learning mechanism in its S-C hierarchy that provides for view-invariant learning. The objects used in the experiment are shown in Fig. 2.83. There were two objects, two cups, each with four views, constructed with Blender. VisNet was trained with all views of one object shown in random permuted sequence, then all views of the other object shown in random permuted sequence, to enable VisNet to use its temporal trace learning rule to learn about the different images that occurring together in time were likely to be different views of the same object. VisNet performed 100% correct in this task by forming neurons in its layer 4 that responded either to all views of one cup (labelled 'Bill') and to no views of the other cup (labelled 'Jane'), or vice versa. HMAX neurons did not discriminate between the objects, but instead responded more to the images of each object that contained text. This dominance by text is consistent with the fact that HMAX is operating to a considerable extent as a set of image filters, the activity in which included much produced by the text. HMAX has no mechanism within its S-C layers that enables it to learn which input images belong to one object vs another, whereas VisNet can solve this computational problem, by using temporal and spatial continuity present in the way that objects are viewed in a natural environment.

These investigations (Robinson and Rolls, 2015) draw out a fundamental difference between VisNet and HMAX. The output layer neurons of VisNet can represent transform-invariant properties of objects, and can form single neurons that respond to the different views of objects even when the images of the different views may be quite different, as is the case for many real-world objects when they transform in the world. Thus basing object recognition on image statistics, and categorisation based on these, is insufficient for transform-invariant object recognition. VisNet can learn to respond to the different transforms of objects using the trace learning rule to capture the properties of objects as they transform in the world. In contrast, HMAX up to the C2 layer sets some of its neurons to respond to exemplars in the set of images, but has no way of knowing which exemplars may be of the same object, and no way therefore to learn about the properties of objects as they transform in the real world, showing catastrophic changes in the image as they transform (Koenderink, 1990), exemplified in the example in experiment 4 by the new views as the objects transform from not showing to showing writing in the base of the cup (Fig. 2.83). Moreover, because the C2 neurons reflect mainly the way in which all the Gabor filters respond to image exemplars, the firing of C2 neurons is typically very similar and non-sparse to different images, though if the images have very different statistics in terms of for example text or not, it is these properties that dominate the firing of the C2 neurons.

For all these reasons, HMAX is ruled out as a model of invariant visual object recognition for further consideration here (Rolls, 2021d).

Further evidence consistent with the approach developed in the investigations of VisNet described in this chapter comes from psychophysical studies. Wallis and Bülthoff (1999) and Perry, Rolls and Stringer (2006) describe psychophysical evidence for learning of view invariant representations by experience, in that the learning can be shown in special circumstances to be affected by the temporal sequence in which different views of objects are seen.

Some other approaches to biologically plausible invariant object recognition are being developed with hierarchies that may allow unsupervised learning (Pinto, Doukhan, DiCarlo and Cox, 2009; DiCarlo, Zoccolan and Rust, 2012; Yamins, Hong, Cadieu, Solomon, Seibert and DiCarlo, 2014). For example, a hierarchical network has been trained with unsupervised learning, and with many transforms of each object to help the system to learn invariant representations in an analogous way to that in which VisNet is trained, but the details of the network architecture are selected by finding parameter values for the specification of the network structure that produce good results on a benchmark classification task (Pinto et al., 2009). However, formally these are convolutional networks, so that the neuronal filters for one local region are replicated over the whole of visual space, which is computationally efficient but biologically implausible. Further, a general linear model is used to decode the firing in the output level of the model to assess performance, so it is not clear whether the firing rate representations of objects in the output layer of the model are very similar to that of the inferior temporal visual cortex. In contrast, with VisNet (Rolls and Milward, 2000; Rolls, 2012d) the information measurement procedures that we use (Rolls et al., 1997d,b) are the same as those used to measure the representation that is present in the inferior temporal visual cortex (Rolls and Treves, 2011; Tovee et al., 1993; Rolls and Tovee, 1995b; Tovee and Rolls, 1995; Abbott et al., 1996; Rolls et al., 1997b; Baddeley et al., 1997; Rolls et al., 1997d; Treves et al., 1999; Panzeri et al., 1999b; Rolls et al., 2004; Franco et al., 2004; Aggelopoulos et al., 2005; Franco et al., 2007; Rolls et al., 2006b; Rolls, 2012d).

In addition, an important property of inferior temporal cortex neurons is that they convey information about the individual object or face, not just about a class such as face vs non-face, or animal vs non-animal (Rolls and Tovee, 1995b; Rolls, Treves and Tovee, 1997b; Abbott, Rolls and Tovee, 1996; Rolls, Treves, Tovee and Panzeri, 1997d; Baddeley, Abbott, Booth,

Sengpiel, Freeman, Wakeman and Rolls, 1997; Rolls, 2016b; Rolls and Treves, 2011; Rolls, 2011d, 2012d). This key property is essential for recognising a particular person or object, and is frequently not addressed in models of invariant object recognition, which still typically focus on classification into e.g. animal vs non-animal, or classes such as hats and bears from databases such as the CalTech (Serre, Wolf, Bileschi, Riesenhuber and Poggio, 2007c; Serre, Oliva and Poggio, 2007b; Mutch and Lowe, 2008; Serre, Kreiman, Kouh, Cadieu, Knoblich and Poggio, 2007a; Yamins, Hong, Cadieu, Solomon, Seibert and DiCarlo, 2014). It is clear that VisNet has this key property of representing individual objects, faces, etc., as is illustrated in the investigations of Robinson and Rolls (2015), and previously (Rolls and Milward, 2000; Stringer and Rolls, 2000, 2002; Rolls and Webb, 2014; Webb and Rolls, 2014; Stringer, Perry, Rolls and Proske, 2006; Perry, Rolls and Stringer, 2006, 2010; Rolls, 2012d, 2021d). VisNet achieves this by virtue of its competitive learning, in combination with its trace learning rule to learn that different images are of the same object. The investigations of Robinson and Rolls (2015) provide evidence that HMAX categorises together images with similar low level feature properties (such as the presence of text), and does not perform shape recognition relevant to the identification of an individual in which the spatial arrangements of the parts is important.

An important point here is that testing whether networks categorise images into different classes of object is insufficient as a measure of whether a network is operating biologically plausibly (Yamins, Hong, Cadieu, Solomon, Seibert and DiCarlo, 2014), for there are many more criteria that must be satisfied, including many highlighted here, including correct identification of individuals with all the perceptual invariances, operation using combinations of features in the correct spatial configuration, and producing a biologically plausible sparse distributed representation, all without an external teacher for the output neurons (Rolls, 2021d) (cf. Pinto, Cox and DiCarlo (2008), Pinto, Doukhan, DiCarlo and Cox (2009), DiCarlo et al. (2012), Cadieu, Hong, Yamins, Pinto, Ardila, Solomon, Majaj and DiCarlo (2014), and Yamins, Hong, Cadieu, Solomon, Seibert and DiCarlo (2014)). More recently, unsupervised training of deep convolutional neural networks has advanced (Zhuang, Yan, Nayebi, Schrimpf, Frank, DiCarlo and Yamins, 2021), but these still implement convolution and deep learning using non-local learning rules including backpropagation of error to optimize representations, so are still biologically implausible.

These investigations (Robinson and Rolls, 2015) thus highlighted several principles of cortical computation. One is that advantage is taken of the statistics of inputs from the world to help learning, with for example temporal and spatial continuity being relevant. Another is that neurons need to learn to respond to non-linear combinations of their inputs, in the case of vision including their spatial arrangement which is provided by the convergent topology from area to area of the visual cortex. Another principle is that the system must be able to form sparse distributed representations with neurons that encode perceptual and invariance properties, so that the next stage of cortical processing can read the information using dot product decoding as in a pattern associator, autoassociator, or competitive network. None of these properties are provided by HMAX, and all are provided by VisNet, highlighting the importance of these principles of cortical computation (Rolls, 2021d).

2.9.3 Minimal recognizable configurations

Ullman and colleagues have suggested that minimal recognizable configurations (MIRCs) may be building blocks of object and face recognition (Nam et al., 2021; Gruber et al., 2021; Holzinger et al., 2019). This approach is based on empirical investigations which show that some small patches of images can be used to represent how human perception builds up from components. Reducing these components by image cropping or reducing their resolution leads to different responses. The theory of how the whole system would be computed, and how it would learn invariances, does not appear to be well developed, but the approach is consistent which the feature hierarchy approach used in VisNet.

2.9.4 Hierarchical convolutional deep neural networks

A different approach has been to compare neuronal activity in visual cortical areas with the neurons that are learned in artificial models of object recognition such as hierarchical convolutional deep neural networks (HCNN) (Yamins and DiCarlo, 2016; Rajalingham, Issa, Bashivan, Kar, Schmidt and DiCarlo, 2018). Convolutional networks are described in Section B.14 (see also Section 2.6.5). They involve non-biologically plausible operations such as error backpropagation learning, and copying what has been set up in one part of a layer to all other parts of the same layer (see Section 19.4), which is also a non-local operation. They also require a teacher for each output neuron, which again is biologically implausible (see Section 2.6.5). The parameters of the hierarchical convolutional deep neural network are selected or trained until the neurons in the artificial neural network become similar to the responses of neurons found in the brain. The next step of the argument then seems to need some care. The argument that appears to be tempting (Yamins and DiCarlo, 2016; Rajalingham, Issa, Bashivan, Kar, Schmidt and DiCarlo, 2018) is that because the neurons in the HCNN are similar to those in for example the inferior temporal visual cortex, the HCNN provides a model of how the computations are performed in the ventral visual system. But of course the model has been trained so that its neurons do appear similar to those of real neurons in the brain. So the similarity of the artificial and real neurons is not surprising. What would be surprising is if it were proposed that the HCNN is a model of how the ventral visual stream computes (Yamins and DiCarlo, 2016; Rajalingham, Issa, Bashivan, Kar, Schmidt and DiCarlo, 2018), given that a HCNN with its non-local operation does not appear to be biologically plausible (Section 19.4). VisNet, in contrast, utilises only local information such as the presynaptic and postsynaptic firing rates and a slowly decaying traces of previous activity (that could be implemented by a local attractor network using the recurrent collateral connections), so is a biologically plausible approach to invariant visual object recognition.

As noted above, unsupervised training of deep convolutional neural networks has advanced (Zhuang, Yan, Nayebi, Schrimpf, Frank, DiCarlo and Yamins, 2021), but these networks still implement convolution and deep learning using non-local learning rules including backpropagation of error to optimize representations, so are still biologically implausible.

Importantly, as noted earlier, comparing neurons recorded in the brain with the units found in deep learning algorithms tuned to produce neurons that resemble those in the brain (Cadieu, Hong, Yamins, Pinto, Ardila, Solomon, Majaj and DiCarlo, 2014; Yamins, Hong, Cadieu, Solomon, Seibert and DiCarlo, 2014; Yamins and DiCarlo, 2016; Rajalingham, Issa, Bashivan, Kar, Schmidt and DiCarlo, 2018; Jia, Hong and DiCarlo, 2021; Zhuang, Yan, Nayebi, Schrimpf, Frank, DiCarlo and Yamins, 2021) seems like a poorly founded exercise, for two reasons.

First, the solutions found by deep convolution networks and other machine learning algorithms for image to category mapping may be very different to those found in a system such as the brain that uses only local learning rules and is restricted to only 4–5 layers in the hierarchy.

Second, it is difficult to know what can be learned about how primate including human vision works computationally from deep learning and related machine learning algorithms, given that the understanding of exactly how these machine learning algorithms reach their mapping is almost un-understood, apart from the recipe that makes them work (Plebe and Grasso, 2019).

A different approach is to use unsupervised learning with a spike-timing dependent local synaptic learning rule, with a winner-take-all algorithm, and to transmit spikes, and this is reported to enable features to be extracted that are useful for classification (Ferre, Mamalet and Thorpe, 2018). This has been extended to deep convolutional neural networks for object recognition (Kheradpisheh, Ganjtabesh, Thorpe and Masquelier, 2018).

2.9.5 Sigma-Pi synapses

Another approach to the implementation of invariant representations in the brain is the use of neurons with Sigma-Pi synapses. Sigma-Pi synapses, described in Section A.2.3, effectively allow one input to a synapse to be multiplied or gated by a second input to the synapse. The multiplying input might gate the appropriate set of the other inputs to a synapse to produce the shift or scale change required. For example, the x^c input in Equation A.14 could be a signal that varies with the shift required to compute translation invariance, effectively mapping the appropriate set of x_j inputs through to the output neurons depending on the shift required (Mel, Ruderman and Archie, 1998; Mel and Fiser, 2000; Olshausen, Anderson and Van Essen, 1993, 1995). Local operations on a dendrite could be involved in such a process (Mel, Ruderman and Archie, 1998). The explicit neural implementation of the gating mechanism seems implausible, given the need to multiply and thus remap large parts of the retinal input depending on shift and scale modifying connections to a particular set of output neurons. Moreover, the explicit control signal to set the multiplication required in V1 has not been identified. Moreover, if this was the solution used by the brain, the whole problem of shift and scale invariance could in principle be solved in one layer of the system, rather than with the multiple hierarchically organized set of layers actually used in the brain, as shown schematically in Fig. 2.2. The multiple layers actually used in the brain are much more consistent with the type of scheme incorporated in VisNet. Moreover, if a multiplying system of the type hypothesized by Mel, Ruderman and Archie (1998), Olshausen, Anderson and Van Essen (1993) and Olshausen, Anderson and Van Essen (1995) was implemented in a multilayer hierarchy with the shift and scale change emerging gradually, then the multiplying control signal would need to be supplied to every stage of the hierarchy. A further problem with such approaches is how the system is trained in the first place (Mel et al., 2017).

2.9.6 A principal dimensions approach to coding in the inferior temporal visual cortex

Doris Tsao and colleagues have adopted a principal dimensions approach to what is encoded by neurons in the inferior temporal visual cortex to represent faces and objects (Hesse and Tsao, 2020; Chang and Tsao, 2017; Chang, Egger, Vetter and Tsao, 2021). They started with the face patch system, in which there are a number of face patches distributed from posterior to anterior in the inferior temporal visual cortex with the most anterior in the perirhinal cortex (Tsao, 2014). The more anterior patches have greater invariance, e.g. more view invariance. A descriptive set of 50 measures of face parameters such as the distances between different parts of the face and appearance / texture was used to measure many faces, and then principal components analysis was performed to obtain 25 shape and 25 appearance principal components. When testing many face cells, they found that the neurons were tuned to a subset of the principal component features. In particular, it was found that some neurons had linear responses to one of these principal components, with either a linearly graded ramping increase of firing related to the principal component, or a linearly graded decrease of firing related to the component (Hesse and Tsao, 2020; Chang and Tsao, 2017). Different neurons responded to one of the different principal components. Because this was a linear systems analysis, any face could be represented by linearly combining all of the relevant principal components each encoded by different neurons. In that way, it was shown that an image of any person's face, and the identity of the person could be encoded by a sample of 205 neurons in the ML-MF and AM inferior temporal visual cortex face patches (Hesse and Tsao, 2020; Chang and Tsao, 2017; Chang et al., 2021).

The approach was extended to other patches of neurons in the inferior temporal visual cortex (Hesse and Tsao, 2020). By using a large number of test stimuli, and again a dimension reduction approach that included AlexNet and principal components analysis, it was found that neurons in patches X1, X2 and X3 encoded for stubby vs spiky objects, with an example of an object low on this 'stubby' dimension a chair with four protruding legs. This was termed an X dimension. Another dimension coded for body parts, such as hands, legs, etc. (Hesse and Tsao, 2020).

By measuring the responses of several hundred inferior temporal visual cortex neurons in different patch types, it was found that many objects / faces / body parts could be reasonably well represented by such neurons, by reconstructing the image from the linear components encoded by the different neurons, in which each neuron encodes one of these principal dimensions (Hesse and Tsao, 2020; Chang et al., 2021). The approach has been described as 'analysis by synthesis' in that the different components are used together ('synthesised') to describe an object, and in that an image of the object being seen can be generated from the neuronal responses. This approach can account for the responses of inferior temporal cortex neurons better than deep learning models, which fail for example because they do not take into account other relevant variables such as illumination (Chang et al., 2021), and perhaps because they overfit the data provided.

A strength of the approach is that this type of principal dimensions representation with linear combinations used to read out the information can work for objects / faces / body parts where continuously variable properties along these dimensions can be used to describe objects.

A possible limitation of this approach is that other information may be needed to specify objects, such as the relative spatial location of the parts, or the number of protruding parts, and how they protrude from objects, to distinguish for example a chair with four legs, from a chair with three legs, from a table with five legs and one protrusion on top such as an umbrella pole. And of course many other dimensions, such as color, and visual texture, that are encoded by inferior temporal cortex neurons, need to be included in the components that are utilised for the encoding. So it is not clear so far that this approach can deal with all that is required for object representation, identification, and description.

Another potential limitation is about how the code is read out not by a scientist who can estimate the weighting of a large number of linearly varying principal components, but by the receiving neurons in brain regions such as the orbitofrontal cortex and hippocampus for which a sparse distributed code is useful so that they can perform associations in the way implemented in pattern association and autoassociation networks (Sections B.2 and B.3). Neurons that respond to possibly non-linear combinations of the linear components advocated in this approach (Hesse and Tsao, 2020) may be useful, and indeed combinations of features that are orthogonal to other combinations can be useful building blocks in feature hierarchies (Section 2.6.6). We found in our information theoretic analyses that the responses of inferior temporal cortex neurons are well suited for the readout by such associative neuronal networks, in that the information about the identity of which face was presented increased linearly with the number of neurons in the population, at least up to reasonable numbers of neurons (Rolls, Treves and Tovee, 1997b; Abbott, Rolls and Tovee, 1996). This shows that the number of face identities that can be decoded from the firing of inferior temporal cortex neurons increases exponentially with the number of neurons in the population, even with biologically plausible dot-product decoding (Rolls, Treves and Tovee, 1997b; Abbott, Rolls and Tovee, 1996).

Another area needing further exploration is how such a system might be built in the brain. It is possible that competitive networks of the type used in VisNet (Rolls, 2021d), which can help to encode independent components if not principal components, may be part of a solution, it is proposed. Competitive networks do perform a type of dimension reduction (Section B.4). Moreover, competitive networks of the type used in VisNet (Rolls, 2021d) learn to respond to combinations of features such as the relative spatial position of several features that are likely to be key in enabling more details of objects to be represented than in a system using only a restricted set of principal components.

In the inferior temporal cortex patch system, it is also proposed that after an initial forward pass from early visual cortical regions up to the anterior inferior temporal cortex, top-down backprojections to the earlier patches my help to stabilize the system in consistent activity at all levels of the hierarchy or system (Hesse and Tsao, 2020). Exactly this has been proposed as a key function for cortico-cortical top-down backprojections, which can help to bias what is represented at earlier processing stages in a hierarchy to be consistent with a possible high level interpretation (Chapter 11 of Rolls (2016b); see also Sections 4.3.5, 13.6.2, B.3.5 and B.9). This can help with ambiguous figures, such as Necker cubes, and with binocular rivalry, and with degraded scenes such as the Dalmation dog or face example illustrated in Fig. 2.15. In the system proposed for this (Rolls, 2016b), associatively modifiable back-projection top-down synapses may be sufficient to implement this functionality, and are also consistent with using the same synapses for memory recall. In the system considered by Tsao and colleagues (Hesse and Tsao, 2020) it is suggested that there may be repeated forward and backward passes, but in a system of this general type described by Rolls (2016b), the top-down effects can operate continuously in time, and 'flips' or alternations between states should only be necessary when there is an alteration of the interpretation. Such an alteration of the high-level interpretation might be caused for example by adaptation of neuronal firing at a high level in the hierarchy, which would then make an alternative account for the bottom-up input emerge from the neuronal noise (in the decision-making mechanism described in this book), to cause a 'flip' at first at the high, and then the lower levels, in the hierarchy. This could apply for example in ambiguous figure-ground illusions, or in binocular rivalry.

2.10 Visuo-spatial scratchpad memory, and change blindness

Given the fact that the responses of inferior temporal cortex neurons are quite locked to the stimulus being viewed, it is unlikely that IT provides the representation of the visual world that we think we see, with objects at their correct places in a visual scene. In fact, we do not really see the whole visual scene, as most of it is a memory reflecting what was seen when the eyes were last looking at a particular part of the scene. The evidence for this statement comes from change blindness experiments, which show that humans rather remarkably do not notice if, while they are moving their eyes and cannot respond to changes in the visual scene, a part of the scene changes (O'Regan, Rensink and Clark, 1999; Rensink, 2000, 2014, 2018). A famous example is that in which a baby was removed from the mother's arms during the subject's eye movement, and the subject failed to notice that the scene was any different. Similarly, unless we are fixating the location that is different in two alternated versions of a visual scene, we are remarkably insensitive to differences in the scene, such as a glass being present on a dining table in one but not another picture of a dining room. Given then that much of the apparent richness of our visual world is actually based on what was seen at previously fixated

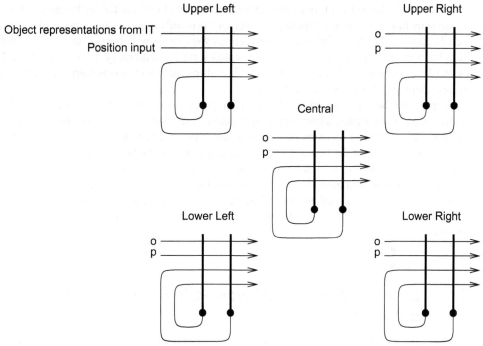

Fig. 2.84 A schematic model of a visuo-spatial scratchpad memory: multiple separate attractor networks could form associations between objects and their place in a scene, and maintain the activity of all the attractors active simultaneously. IT, inferior temporal visual cortex.

positions in the scene (with this being what the inferior temporal visual cortex represents), we may ask where this 'visuo-spatial' scratchpad (short-term, iconic, memory) (Rensink, 2014) is located in the brain. One possibility is in the right parieto-occipital area, for patients with lesions in the parieto-occipital region have (dorsal) simultanagnosia, in which they can recognize objects, but cannot see more than one object at a time (Farah, 2004). Alternatively, the network could be in the left inferior temporo-occipital regions, for patients with (ventral) simultanagnosia cannot recognize but can see multiple objects in a scene (Farah, 2004).

The computational basis for this could be a number of separate, that is local, attractors each representing part of the space, and capable of being loaded by inputs from the inferior temporal visual cortex. According to this computational model, the particular attractor network in the visuo-spatial scratchpad memory would be addressed by information based on the position of the eyes, of covert attention, and probably the position of the head. While being so addressed, inputs to the scratch-pad from the inferior temporal cortex neurons would then provide information about the object at the fovea, together with some information about the location of objects in different parafoveal regions (see Section 2.8.10), and this would then enable object information to be associated by synaptic modification with the active neurons in the attractor network representing that location (see Fig. 2.84). Because there are separate spatially local attractors for each location, each of the attractors with its associated object information could be kept active simultaneously, to maintain for short periods information about the relative spatial position of multiple objects in a scene. The attractor for each spatial location would need to represent some information about the object present at that location (as otherwise a binding problem would arise between the multiple objects and the multiple locations), and this may be a reason why the object information in the visuo-spatial scratchpad is not detailed. The suggestion of different attractors for different regions of the scene is consistent with the architecture of the cerebral neocortex, in which the high density of connections including those of inhibitory interneurons is mainly local, within a range of 1–2 mm (see Section 1.14). (If the inhibitory connections were more widespread, so that the inhibition became more global within the visuo-spatial scratchpad memory, the system would be more like a continuous attractor network with multiple activity packets (Stringer, Rolls and Trappenberg, 2004) (see Section B.5.4).)

It may only be when the inferior temporal visual cortex is representing objects at or close to the fovea in a complex scene that a great deal of information is present about an object, given the competitive processes described in this chapter combined with the large cortical magnification factor of the fovea. The perceptual system may be built in this way for the fundamental reasons described in this chapter (which enable a hierarchical competitive system to learn invariant representations that require feature binding), which account for why it cannot process a whole scene simultaneously. The visual system can, given the way in which it is built, thereby give an output in a form that is very useful for memory systems, but mainly about one or a few objects close to the fovea.

2.11 Different processes involved in different types of object identification

To conclude this chapter, it is proposed that there are (at least) three different types of process that could be involved in object identification. The first is the simple situation where different objects can be distinguished by different non-overlapping sets of features (see Section 2.6.1). An example might be a banana and an orange, where the list of features of the banana might include yellow, elongated, and smooth surface; and of the orange its orange color, round shape, and dimpled surface. Such objects could be distinguished just on the basis of a list of the properties, which could be processed appropriately by a competitive network, pattern associator, etc. No special mechanism is needed for view invariance, because the list of properties is very similar from most viewing angles. Object recognition of this type may be common in animals, especially those with visual systems less developed than those of primates. However, this approach does not describe the shape and form of objects, and is insufficient to account for primate vision. Nevertheless, the features present in objects are valuable cues to object identity, and are naturally incorporated into the feature hierarchy approach.

A second type of process might involve the ability to generalize across a small range of views of an object, that is within a generic view, where cues of the first type cannot be used to solve the problem. An example might be generalization across a range of views of a cup when looking into the cup, from just above the near lip until the bottom inside of the cup comes into view. This type of process includes the learning of the transforms of the surface markings on 3D objects which occur when the object is rotated, as described in Section 2.8.7. Such generalization would work because the neurons are tuned as filters to accept a range of variation of the input within parameters such as relative size and orientation of the components of the features. Generalization of this type would not be expected to work when there is a catastrophic change in the features visible, as for example occurs when the cup is rotated so that one can suddenly no longer see inside it, and the outside bottom of the cup comes into view. VisNet, with its temporal trace learning rule, is able to learn that quite different views may be views of the same object, as illustrated in Section 2.9.2.

The third type of process is one that can deal with the sudden catastrophic change in the features visible when an object is rotated to a completely different view, as in the cup example just given (cf. Koenderink (1990)). Another example, quite extreme to illustrate the point, might be when a card with different images on its two sides is rotated so that one face and then the other is in view. This makes the point that this third type of process may involve arbitrary pairwise association learning, to learn which features and views are different aspects of the same object. Another example occurs when only some parts of an object are visible. For example, a red-handled screwdriver may be recognized either from its round red handle, or from its elongated silver-colored blade. Again, VisNet, with its temporal trace learning rule, is able to learn that quite different views may be views of the same object, as illustrated in Section 2.9.2 (Rolls, 2021d).

The full view-invariant recognition of objects that occurs even when the objects share the same features, such as color, texture, etc. is an especially computationally demanding task which the primate visual system is able to perform with its highly developed temporal lobe cortical visual areas. The neurophysiological evidence and the neuronal networks described in this chapter provide clear hypotheses about how the primate visual system may perform this object recognition task in which shape is important, and which is the major computation performed by the ventral visual stream described in this chapter (Rolls, 2021d).

2.12 Top-down attentional modulation is implemented by biased competition

Top-down modulation of visual and other processing by attention is probably implemented by biased competition. In top-down selective attention, a short-term memory holds online what is to be attended to, for example in vision the location or the object that is the target of attention. This short-term memory is used to bias neurons at earlier stages of processing to help them to respond to competing locations or competing objects on the visual field.

In more detail, the **biased competition hypothesis** of attention proposes that multiple stimuli in the visual field activate populations of neurons that engage in competitive interactions. Attending to a stimulus at a particular location or with a particular feature biases this competition in favour of neurons that respond to the feature or location of the attended stimulus. This attentional effect is produced by generating signals in cortical areas outside the visual cortex that are then fed back (or down) to extrastriate areas, where they bias the competition such that when multiple stimuli appear in the visual field, the neurons representing the attended stimulus 'win', thereby suppressing neurons representing distracting stimuli (Duncan and Humphreys, 1989; Desimone and Duncan, 1995; Duncan, 1996).

A modern neuronal network diagram of how the biased competition theory of attention operates is provided in Fig. 2.85 (Rolls, 2016b). There is usually a single attractor network that can enter different attractor states to provide the source of the top-down bias (as shown). If it is a single network, there can be competition within the short-term memory attractor states, implemented through the local GABA inhibitory neurons. The top-down continuing firing of one of the attractor states then biases in a top-down process some of the neurons in a 'lower' cortical area to respond more to one than the other of the bottom-up inputs, with competition implemented through the GABA inhibitory neurons (symbolized by a filled circle) that make feedback inhibitory connections onto the pyramidal cells (symbolized by a triangle) in the 'lower' cortical area.

We have seen in Fig. 2.85 how given forward (bottom-up) inputs to a network, competition between the principal (excitatory) neurons can be implemented by inhibitory neurons

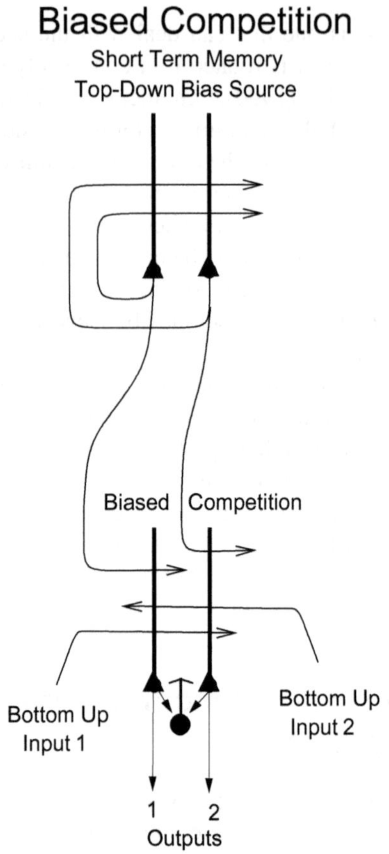

Fig. 2.85 Biased competition mechanism for top-down attention. There is usually a single attractor network that can enter different attractor states to provide the source of the top-down bias (as shown). If it is a single network, there can be competition within the short-term memory attractor states, implemented through the local GABA inhibitory neurons. The top-down continuing firing of one of the attractor states then biases in a top-down process some of the neurons in a cortical area to respond more to one than the other of the bottom-up inputs, with competition implemented through the GABA inhibitory neurons (symbolized by a filled circle) which make feedback inhibitory connections onto the pyramidal cells (symbolized by a triangle) in the cortical area. The thick vertical lines above the pyramidal cells are the dendrites. The axons are shown with thin lines and the excitatory connections by arrow heads. (After Rolls, E. T. (2013) A biased activation theory of the cognitive and attentional modulation of emotion. Frontiers in Human Neuroscience 7: 74.)

which receive from the principal neurons in the network and send back inhibitory connections to the principal neurons in the network. This competition can be biased by a top-down input to favour some of the populations of neurons, and this describes the biased competition hypothesis.

The implementation of biased competition in a computational model can be at the mean-field level, in which the average firing rate of each population of neurons is specified. Equations to implement the dynamics of such a model are given in Section B.8.4. The advantages of this level of formulation are relative simplicity, and speed of computation. The architecture of Fig. B.38 is that of a competitive network (described in Section B.4) but with top-down backprojections as illustrated in Fig. B.19. However, the network could equally well include associatively modifiable synapses in recurrent collateral connections between the excitatory (principal) neurons in the network, making the network into an autoassociation or attractor network capable of short-term memory, as described in Section B.3. The competition between the neurons in the attractor network is again implemented by the inhibitory feedback neurons.

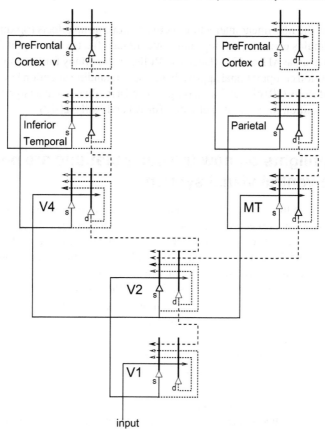

Fig. 2.86 The overall architecture of the model of object and spatial processing and attention, including the prefrontal cortical areas that provide the short-term memory required to hold the object or spatial target of attention active. Forward connections are indicated by solid lines; backprojections, which could implement top-down processing, by dashed lines; and recurrent connections within an area by dotted lines. The triangles represent pyramidal cell bodies, with the thick vertical line above them the dendritic trees. The cortical layers in which the cells are concentrated are indicated by s (superficial, layers 2 and 3) and d (deep, layers 5 and 6). The prefrontal cortical areas most strongly reciprocally connected to the inferior temporal cortex 'what' processing stream are labelled v to indicate that they are in the more ventral part of the lateral prefrontal cortex, area 46, close to the inferior convexity in macaques. The prefrontal cortical areas most strongly reciprocally connected to the parietal visual cortical 'where' processing stream are labelled d to indicate that they are in the more dorsal part of the lateral prefrontal cortex, area 46, in and close to the banks of the principal sulcus in macaques (see text). (After Deco,G. and Rolls, E. T. (2004) A neurodynamical cortical model of visual attention and invariant object recognition. Vision Research 44: 621–644.)

The implementation can also be at the level of the spiking neuron by using an integrate-and-fire simulation (see Section B.6). The integrate-and-fire level allows single neuron findings to be modelled, allows more details of the neuronal implementation to be incorporated, and also allows statistical effects related to the probability that spikes from different neurons will occur at different times to be investigated. Integrate-and-fire simulations are more difficult to set up, and are slow to run. Equations for such simulations are given in Section B.6, and as applied to a biased competition model of attention by Deco and Rolls (2004).

The computational investigations can be extended to systems with many interacting modules, as described in Section B.8.5.

Using these approaches, Deco and Rolls (2004) described a cortical model of visual attention for object recognition and visual search with the architecture illustrated in Fig. 2.86. The model has been extended to the level of spiking neurons which allows biophysical properties of the ion channels affected by synapses, and of the membrane dynamics, to be incorporated, and shows how the non-linear interactions between bottom-up effects (produced for example by altering stimulus contrast) and top-down attentional effects can account for neurophysiological results in areas MT and V4 (Deco and Rolls, 2004). Many further applications of these biased competition computational approaches to understanding attention have been described in Chapter 6 of Rolls (2016b), and we have produced a mathematical analysis of the operation of biased competition for a simple network (Turova and Rolls, 2019).

2.13 Highlights on how the computations are performed in the ventral visual system

1. We have seen in this chapter that the feature hierarchy approach has a number of advantages in performing object recognition over other approaches (see Section 2.6), and that some of the key computational issues that arise in these architectures have solutions (see Sections 2.7 and 2.8). The neurophysiological and computational approach taken here focuses on a feature hierarchy model in which invariant representations can be built by self-organizing learning based on the statistics of the visual input.
2. The model can use temporal continuity in an associative synaptic learning rule with a short-term memory trace, and/or it can use spatial continuity in Continuous Spatial Transformation learning.
3. The model of visual processing in the ventral cortical stream can build representations of objects that are invariant with respect to translation, view, size, spatial frequency, and lighting.
4. The model uses a feature combination neuron approach with the relative spatial positions of the objects specified in the feature combination neurons, and this provides a solution to the binding problem.
5. The model has been extended to provide an account of invariant representations in the dorsal visual system of the global motion produced by objects such as looming, rotation, and object-based movement (Section 3.3).
6. The model has been extended to incorporate top-down feedback connections to model the control of attention by biased competition in for example spatial and object search tasks (see further Section 2.12).
7. The model has also been extended to account for how the visual system can select single objects in complex visual scenes, how multiple objects can be represented in a scene, and how invariant representations of single objects can be learned even when multiple objects are present in the scene.
8. The model has also been extended to account for how the visual system can select multiple objects in complex visual scenes using a simulation of saliency computations in the dorsal visual system, and then with fixations on the salient parts of the scene perform view-invariant visual object recognition using the simulation of the ventral visual stream, VisNet.
9. It has also been suggested in a unifying proposal that adding a fifth layer to the model and training the system in spatial environments will enable hippocampus-like spatial view neurons or place cells to develop, depending on the size of the field of view (Section 9.3.12).
10. We have thus seen how many of the major computational issues that arise when formulating a theory of object recognition in the ventral visual system (such as feature binding, invariance learning, the recognition of objects when they are in cluttered natural scenes, the representation of multiple objects in a scene, and learning invariant representations of

single objects when there are multiple objects in the scene), could be solved in the cortex, with tests of the hypotheses performed by simulations that are consistent with complementary neurophysiological results.

11. The approach described in this chapter is unifying in a number of ways. First, a set of simple organizational principles involving a hierarchy of cortical areas with convergence from stage to stage, and competitive learning using a modified associative learning rule with a short-term memory trace of preceding neuronal activity, provide a basis for understanding much processing in the ventral visual stream, from V1 to the inferior temporal visual cortex. Second, the same principles help to understand some of the processing in the dorsal visual stream by which invariant representations of the global motion of objects may be formed. Third, the same principles continued from the ventral visual stream onwards to the hippocampus help to show how spatial view and place representations may be built from the visual input. Fourth, in all these cases, the learning is possible because the system is able to extract invariant representations because it can utilize the spatio-temporal continuities and statistics in the world that help to define objects, moving objects, and spatial scenes. Fifth, a great simplification and economy in terms of brain design is that the computational principles need not be different in each of the cortical areas in these hierarchical systems, for some of the important properties of the computations in these systems to be performed.

12. The principles of brain computation that are illustrated include the following:

One is that advantage is taken of the statistics of inputs from the world to help learning, with for example temporal and spatial continuity being relevant.

Another is that neurons need to learn to respond to non-linear combinations of their inputs, in the case of vision including their spatial arrangement which is provided by the convergent topology from area to area of the visual cortex, using principles such as competitive learning.

Another principle is that the system must be able to form sparse distributed representations with neurons that encode perceptual and invariance properties, so that the next stage of cortical processing can read the information using dot product decoding as in a pattern associator, autoassociator, or competitive network.

Another principle is the use of hierarchical cortical computation with convergence from stage to stage, which breaks the computation down into neuronally manageable computations.

Another principle is breaking the computation down into manageable parts, by for example not trying to analyze the whole of a scene simultaneously, but instead using successive fixations to objects in different parts of the scene, and maintaining in short-term memory a limited representation of the whole scene.

13. Comparing neurons recorded in the brain with the units found in deep learning algorithms tuned to produce neurons that resemble those in the brain (Cadieu, Hong, Yamins, Pinto, Ardila, Solomon, Majaj and DiCarlo, 2014; Yamins, Hong, Cadieu, Solomon, Seibert and DiCarlo, 2014; Yamins and DiCarlo, 2016; Rajalingham, Issa, Bashivan, Kar, Schmidt and DiCarlo, 2018; Jia, Hong and DiCarlo, 2021; Zhuang, Yan, Nayebi, Schrimpf, Frank, DiCarlo and Yamins, 2021) seems like a poorly founded exercise, for two reasons. First,

the solutions found by deep convolution networks and other machine learning algorithms for image to category mapping may be very different to those found in a system such as the brain that uses only local learning rules and is restricted to only 4–5 layers in the hierarchy. Second, it is difficult to know what can be learned about how primate including human vision works computationally from deep learning and related machine learning algorithms, given that the understanding of exactly how these machine learning algorithms reach their mapping is almost un-understood, apart from the recipe that makes them work (Plebe and Grasso, 2019).

14. The primate including human ventral visual system is very different to that of rats and mice, partly because of the fovea which simplifies the major computational problem of good invariant visual object including shape recognition by limiting the process to what is at the high resolution fovea, which is usually one or a very few objects, and not the whole scene at any one time. Moreover, the primate including human ventral visual system has a hierarchy of processing into the large temporal lobe, with specialized populations of neurons for different categories, including faces. Moreover, the primate visual system requires a whole set of specializations for moving the eyes to foveate an object, and also to track a moving object such as a hand that is about to pick up an object. These factors result in the rodent visual system being a poor model of the primate including human visual system.

15. In conclusion, we have seen in this chapter how a major form of perception, the invariant visual recognition of objects, involves not only the storage and retrieval of information, but also major computations to produce invariant representations. Once these invariant representations have been formed, they are used for many processes including not only recognition memory (see Section 9.2.7), but also associative learning of the rewarding and punishing properties of objects for emotion and motivation (see Chapter 11), the memory for the spatial locations of objects and rewards (see Chapter 9), the building of spatial representations based on visual input (Section 9.3.12), and as an input to short-term memory (Section 13.6.1), attention (Chapter 13), and decision systems (Section 11.5.1).

16. A tutorial version of VisNet written in Matlab is described in Section D.6, and is made available as part of the publication of this book at https://www.oxcns.org.

3 The dorsal visual system

3.1 Introduction, and overview of the dorsal cortical visual stream

The *'dorsal'* or *'where'* or *'action'* visual processing stream shown in Figs. 3.1, 1.8, 2.3 and 3.12 is that from V1 to MT, MST and then to the parietal cortex (Ungerleider, 1995; Ungerleider and Haxby, 1994; Rolls and Deco, 2002; Perry and Fallah, 2014; Rolls et al., 2023e). This 'dorsal' pathway for primate (including human) vision is involved in representing where stimuli are relative to the individual (i.e. in egocentric space), and the motion of these stimuli, and in performing actions on objects at these locations in space (Gallivan and Goodale, 2018; Rolls et al., 2023e,d). Neurons here respond, for example, to stimuli in visual space around

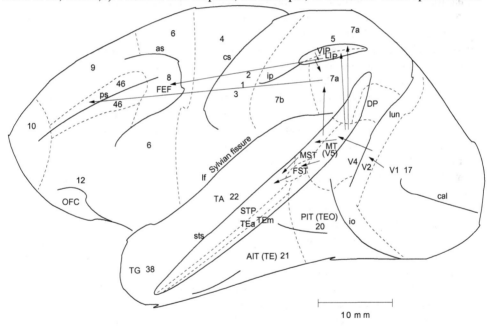

Fig. 3.1 Lateral view of the macaque brain showing the connections in the 'dorsal or where visual pathway' from V1 to V2, MST, LIP, VIP, and parietal cortex area 7a, with some connections then reaching the dorsolateral prefrontal cortex. ip - intraparietal sulcus; LIP - lateral intraparietal area; VIP - ventral intraparietal area; FEF - frontal eye field. Other abbreviations: as, arcuate sulcus; cal, calcarine sulcus; cs, central sulcus; lf, lateral (or Sylvian) fissure; lun, lunate sulcus; ps, principal sulcus; io, inferior occipital sulcus; ip, intraparietal sulcus (which has been opened to reveal some of the areas it contains); sts, superior temporal sulcus (which has been opened to reveal some of the areas it contains). AIT, anterior inferior temporal cortex; FST, visual motion processing area; LIP, lateral intraparietal area; MST, visual motion processing area; MT, visual motion processing area (also called V5); OFC, orbitofrontal cortex; PIT, posterior inferior temporal cortex; STP, superior temporal plane; TA, architectonic area including auditory association cortex; TE, architectonic area including high order visual association cortex, and some of its subareas TEa and TEm; TG, architectonic area in the temporal pole; V1–V4, visual areas 1–4; VIP, ventral intraparietal area; TEO, architectonic area including posterior visual association cortex. The numbers refer to architectonic areas, and have the following approximate functional equivalence: 1, 2, 3, somatosensory cortex (posterior to the central sulcus); 4, motor cortex; 5, superior parietal lobule; 7a, inferior parietal lobule, visual part; 7b, inferior parietal lobule, somatosensory part; 6, lateral premotor cortex; 8, frontal eye field; 12, inferior convexity prefrontal cortex; 46, dorsolateral prefrontal cortex.

Brain Computations and Connectivity. Edmund T. Rolls, Oxford University Press. © Edmund T. Rolls 2023.
DOI: 10.1093/oso/9780198887911.003.0003

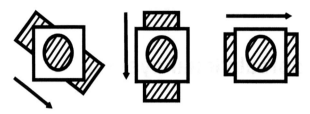

Fig. 3.2 The aperture problem. A large grating moving in three different directions can produce the same physical stimulus when viewed with a small circular aperture, so that the direction of motion within the aperture appears in all three cases to be the same, in this case at right angles to the grating orientation. (After Rolls, E. T. and Deco,G. (2002) Computational Neuroscience of Vision. Oxford University Press: Oxford.)

the individual, including the distance from the observer, and also respond to optic flow or to moving stimuli. Outputs of this system control eye movements to visual stimuli (both slow pursuit and saccadic eye movements). These outputs proceed partly via the frontal eye fields, which then project to the striatum, and then via the substantia nigra reach the superior colliculus (Goldberg and Walker, 2013; Sendhilnathan, Basu, Goldberg, Schall and Murthy, 2021). Other outputs of these dorsal visual system regions are to the dorsolateral prefrontal cortex, area 46, which is important as a short-term memory for where fixation should occur next, as shown by the effects of lesions to the prefrontal cortex on saccades to remembered targets, and by neuronal activity in this region (Goldman-Rakic, 1996; Passingham, 2021). The dorsolateral prefrontal cortex short-term memory systems in area 46 with spatial information received from the parietal cortex plays an important role in attention, by holding on-line the target being attended to, as described in Chapter 13.

Some neurons in the dorsal visual system respond to object-based motion (not to retinal optic flow), and mechanisms for this computation are described in Section 3.3.

A key feature of the dorsal visual system is that the representations start in retinal coordinates, but a coordinate transform takes place to head-based coordinates, which is useful for the interface to sound direction, which is in head-based coordinates.

After this in the hierarchy, a transform to world-based, or allocentric, coordinates, occurs in parietal cortex areas, and this is useful for idiothetic (self-motion) update of spatial view cells in the hippocampal system via the projections from the dorsal visual stream to the parahippocampal gyrus (Rolls, 2020b; Rolls et al., 2023e,d; Rolls, 2023c).

These spatial coordinate transforms up through the parietal cortex are implemented by gain modulation, probably assisted by a trace learning rule as new representations with invariance in a different coordinate system are being computed, as described in Sections 3.4 and 3.5. Other coordinate transforms are also implemented, for example into arm reaching coordinates, useful for actions to locations in space involving dorsal stream connectivity to the parietal cortex (Rolls et al., 2023d), described further in Chapter 10.

3.2 Global motion in the dorsal visual system

The motion or 'where' or 'magnocellular' pathway (see Fig. 2.4) starts in the M-type ganglion cells of the retina which project through the magnocellular (M) layers of the lateral geniculate nucleus to layer 4Cα in V1, from there to layer 4B, then to the thick stripes of V2, then both directly and through V3 on to MT (V5), and finally from there to area MST (V5a) in the parietal cortex. The retinal M-type ganglion cells are not motion sensitive, but they respond more rapidly to change in stimulation than P-type cells, they are strongly sensitive to contrast and contrast variation, have large receptive fields, and have low spatial resolution. These make

M-type retinal ganglion cells specially suitable for pre-processing for motion. In the primary visual cortex (V1), some neurons are selective to a particular direction of motion.

In areas MT and MST, motion processing is further elaborated. Neurons in these areas show high selectivity to direction of motion and speed. In particular, Movshon and his colleagues (Movshon, Adelson, Gizzi and Newsome, 1985) found that there are two different types of motion-sensitive neurons in area MT: component direction-selective neurons, and (global) pattern direction-selective neurons. Component direction-selective neurons are similar to motion-sensitive neurons in V1, in the sense that they respond only to motion perpendicular to their axis of orientation. Thus, their responses provide information about only one-dimensional local components of motion of a global pattern or object, which of course can be ambiguous with respect to the real state of global motion of the whole pattern. This ambiguity can be understood by considering the so-called aperture problem. Figure 3.2 shows this phenomenon.

A large grating moving in three different directions can produce the same physical stimulus when viewed through a small circular aperture (or by the small receptive field of a neuron), so that the direction of motion within the aperture appears in all three cases to be the same. Movshon and his colleagues used a similar set up for distinguishing the detection of global motion versus component motion. They used plaid images, produced by overlapping two moving gratings (see Fig. 3.3), which make the aperture problem explicit. The global motion of the plaid pattern is different from the motion of the two component gratings. The responses of V1 neurons, and of component direction-selective neurons in MT, detect only the motion of each grating component and not the global motion of the plaid.

Movshon, Adelson, Gizzi and Newsome (1985) found that a small population of neurons in MT (about 20%), which they called pattern direction-selective neurons, responds to the perceived global motion of the plaid. These neurons integrate information about two- (or three-) dimensional global object motion by combining the output responses of component direction-selective neurons, for example of V1 neurons that extract just the motion of the components in different one-dimensional directions.

Further, Newsome, Britten and Movshon (1989) demonstrated experimentally that the responses of MT motion-sensitive neurons correlate with the perceptual judgements about motion performed by a monkey that has to report the direction of motion in a random dot display.

The implication of these findings is that the aperture problem is solved in MT primarily by summing motion direction-selective V1 afferents to produce larger receptive fields (Zaharia, Goris, Movshon and Simoncelli, 2019). The presence of a hierarchy in the dorsal visual system with convergence from stage to stage to generate larger receptive fields is a key part of the organisation that enables new representations to be formed, in a way similar to that implemented in the ventral visual stream.

These results are consistent with neuropsychological evidence on human motion perception. Zihl, Von Cramon and Mai (1983) described a patient with damage in an extrastriate brain region homologous to the MT and MST areas of monkeys who was unable to perceive motion. She reported that the world appeared to her as a series of frozen snapshots. Her primary visual cortex was intact, and this was the reason why she was able to detect simple one-dimensional motion in the plane, but unable to integrate this information to infer global motion.

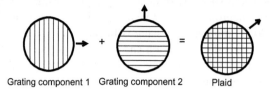

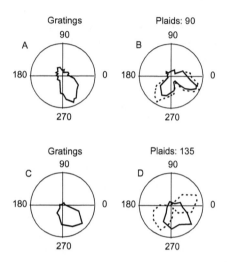

Fig. 3.3 Directional selectivity of component direction-selective neurons and (global) pattern direction-selective neurons in area MT to single versus plaid gratings. The combination of two gratings to produce a single plaid showing global motion is shown in the top part of the diagram. (A) Polar graph of a component direction-selective neuron responding to a single grating moving in different directions. (B) Polar graph of the same component direction-selective neuron responding to a plaid grating (solid line), together with how it should respond if it was responding to each single component (dashed line). (C) and (D) the same as (A) and (B) but for a pattern (or global) direction-selective neuron. (Reproduced from Movshon,J.A., Adelson,E.H., Gizzi,M.S. and Newsome,W.T. (1985) The analysis of moving visual patterns. In Chagas,C., Gattass,R. and Gross,C. (eds.) Pattern Recognition Mechanisms. Experimental Brain Research Series : 117--151. © Springer Nature.)

3.3 Invariant object-based motion in the dorsal visual system

A key issue in understanding the cortical mechanisms that underlie motion perception is how we perceive the motion of objects such as a rotating wheel invariantly with respect to position on the retina, and size. For example, we perceive the wheel shown in Fig. 3.4a rotating clockwise independently of its position on the retina. This occurs even though the local motion for the wheels in the different positions may be opposite. How could this invariance of the visual motion perception of objects arise in the visual system?

Invariant motion representations are known to be developed in the cortical dorsal visual system. Motion-sensitive neurons in V1 have small receptive fields (in the range 1–2 deg at the fovea), and can therefore not detect global motion, and this is part of the aperture problem. Neurons in MT, which receives inputs from V1 and V2 (see Fig. 2.3), have larger receptive fields (e.g. 5 degrees at the fovea), and are able to respond to planar global motion (Movshon et al., 1985; Newsome et al., 1989). One example is a field of small dots in which the majority (in practice as few as 55%) move in one direction. Another example is the overall direction of a moving plaid, the orthogonal grating components of which have motion at 45 degrees to the overall motion. Further on in the dorsal visual system, some neurons in macaque visual area MST (but not MT) respond to rotating flow fields or looming with considerable translation

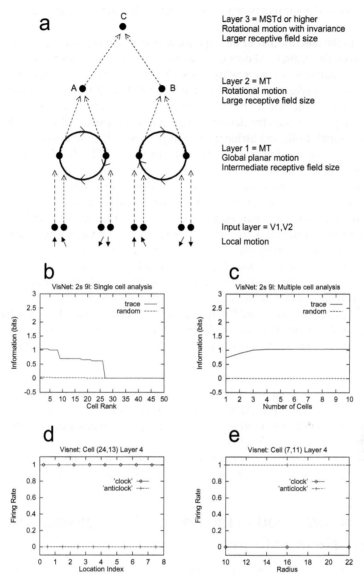

Fig. 3.4 Invariant global motion in the dorsal visual system. (a) Two rotating wheels at different locations rotating in opposite directions. The local flow field is ambiguous. Clockwise or counterclockwise rotation can only be diagnosed by a global flow computation, and it is shown how the network is expected to solve the problem to produce position invariant global motion-sensitive neurons. One rotating wheel is presented at any one time, but the need is to develop a representation of the fact that in the case shown the rotating flow field is always clockwise, independently of the location of the flow field. (b–d) Translation invariance, with training on 9 locations. (b) Single cell information measures showing that some layer 4 neurons have perfect performance of 1 bit (clockwise vs anticlockwise) after training with the trace rule, but not with random initial synaptic weights in the untrained control condition. (c) The multiple cell information measure shows that small groups of neurons have perfect performance. (d) Position invariance illustrated for a single cell from layer 4, which responded only to the clockwise rotation, and for every one of the 9 positions. (e) Size invariance illustrated for a single cell from layer 4, which after training with three different radii of rotating wheel, responded only to anticlockwise rotation, independently of the size of the rotating wheels. (After Rolls, E. T. and Stringer,S.M. (2007) Invariant global motion recognition in the dorsal visual system: a unifying theory. Neural Computation 19: 139–169. © MIT.)

invariance (Graziano et al., 1994; Geesaman and Andersen, 1996; Mineault et al., 2012), with MST especially involved in the representation of object motion in the visual field (Galletti and Fattori, 2018).

In the cortex in the anterior part of the superior temporal sulcus, which is a convergence zone for inputs from the ventral and dorsal visual systems, some neurons respond to object-based motion, for example to a head rotating clockwise but not anticlockwise, independently of whether the head is upright or inverted which reverses the optic flow across the retina (Hasselmo, Rolls, Baylis and Nalwa, 1989b) (see Section 2.4.6 and Fig. 2.12).

In a unifying hypothesis with the design of the ventral cortical visual system about *how* this might be computed, Rolls and Stringer (2006a) proposed that the dorsal visual system uses a hierarchical feedforward network architecture (V1, V2, MT, MSTd, parietal cortex) with training of the connections with a short-term memory trace associative synaptic modification rule to capture what is invariant at each stage. The principle is illustrated in Fig. 3.4a. Simulations showed that the proposal is computationally feasible, in that invariant representations of the motion flow fields produced by objects self-organize in the later layers of the architecture (see examples in Fig. 3.4b–e). The model produces invariant representations of the motion flow fields produced by global in-plane motion of an object, in-plane rotational motion, and looming vs receding of the object. The model also produces invariant representations of object-based rotation about a principal axis, of the type illustrated in Fig. 2.12 on page 71. Thus it is proposed that the dorsal and ventral visual systems may share some unifying computational principles (Rolls and Stringer, 2006a). Indeed, the simulations of Rolls and Stringer (2006a) used a standard version of VisNet, with the exception that instead of using oriented bar receptive fields as the input to the first layer, local motion flow fields provided the inputs.

The interesting and quite original principle proposed is that some of the same mechanisms including trace rule learning and hierarchical organisation that are used in the ventral visual system to compute invariant representations of stationary objects may also be used in the dorsal visual system to compute representations of the global motion of a moving object (Rolls and Stringer, 2006a; Rolls, 2021d).

This may well be an example of a *principle of cortical operation: the re-use of the same principles of cortical operation for different computations in different cortical areas.*

3.4 What is computed in the dorsal visual system: visual coordinate transforms

The dorsal visual system starts with representations that are in retinal coordinates. But to represent a position in space where we might wish to remember an object, it would be better if the representation was in world coordinates, so that we could remember that position in space even if we saw it later with a different eye position, or a different head direction, or indeed from a different place. There might be something valuable at that position in world space, and it would be highly non-adaptive if we could only remember that place in space with the original eye position, head direction, and from the same place. (Eye position refers to the angle of the eye in the head in the horizontal and vertical plane – looking left vs right, or up vs down. World coordinates for places are termed allocentric, meaning 'other-centred', to contrast them with egocentric coordinates, which are coordinates relative to the body or head. Another, perhaps better term for world based coordinates is 'exocentric', where exo is from the Greek word meaning 'outside', which captures the idea that the representation in not in ego or self-centred coordinates, but in outside-centred or world coordinates.) The top of the dorsal visual system, which we can identify as parietal area 7a in Fig. 3.1, has connections

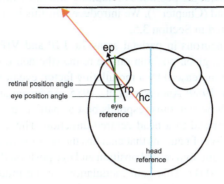

Fig. 3.5 Gain modulation of retinal position by eye position to produce a head-centered representation. The eye position (ep) is the angle between straight ahead with respect to the head (indicated by the green line labelled head reference) and the direction of the eye (indicated by the black arrow labelled ep). A direction in head-centered space (labelled hc) is represented by all combinations of retinal position (rp) and eye position that reach a given head-centered direction indicated by the red arrow tip, with one combination of eye position and retinal position shown. This coordinate transform may be computed by gain modulation of retinal position by eye position. (After Rolls, E. T. (2020) Spatial coordinate transforms linking the allocentric hippocampal and egocentric parietal primate brain systems for memory, action in space, and navigation. Hippocampus 30: 332–353.)

via areas such as the retrosplenial cortex (RSC) and posterior cingulate cortex (PCC) into the hippocampal system (Fig. 9.1), where it has been shown that visual space is represented in primates in allocentric coordinates (Georges-François, Rolls and Robertson, 1999; Rolls and Xiang, 2006; Rolls, 2016b; Rolls and Wirth, 2018; Rolls, 2023c), as described in Chapter 9. There is evidence that the computations in the dorsal visual system involve a series of coordinate transforms from retinal towards allocentric visual coordinates, to provide inputs to the hippocampal system. En route, other coordinate transforms are also computed, into for example a space suitable for directing arm movements to locations in egocentric space, relative to the body. One situation in which coordinate transforms are required is in reaching for targets relative to visual landmarks, in which allocentric information must be transformed into egocentric information to implement the reaching (Chen and Crawford, 2020). Some of the evidence for what is being computed with respect to these coordinate transforms is described later.

3.4.1 The transform from retinal to head-based coordinates

Neurons in area LIP are active in visual, attentional and saccadic processing (Gnadt and Andersen, 1988; Colby et al., 1996; Munuera and Duhamel, 2020). The ventral part of LIP (LIPv) has strong connections with two oculomotor centres, the frontal eye field and the deep layers of the superior colliculus, and may be especially involved in the generation of saccades (Chen et al., 2016b). The dorsal part (LIPd) may be more involved in visual processing, responding for example to visual targets for saccades.

Neurons in area VIP represent the direction and speed of visual motion (Colby et al., 1993), and may be useful in for example tracking moving visual stimuli, and encoding optic flow which can be useful in assessing self-motion and thereby in navigation. These neurons do not respond in relation to saccades. In humans, VIP may have expanded into three sub-regions that code for the head or self in the environment, visual heading direction, and the peripersonal environment around the head (Foster et al., 2022).

A very interesting property of many neurons in both LIP and VIP is that they respond in relation to direction with respect to the head, i.e. use a head-based or head-centred coordinate system, rather than in retinal coordinates, as described next. One advantage of this is that this simplifies associations with the positions of auditory stimuli, with auditory space represented with respect to the head (Chapter 7). We introduce *how* this is computed next, with the concepts developed and tested in Section 3.5.

The response of some neurons in parietal areas 7a, LIP and VIP (areas shown in Fig. 3.1) to a visual stimulus at a given position on the retina (the neuron's receptive field) can be modulated (decreased or increased) by a modulating factor, eye position (the angle of the eye in the head) (Andersen, 1989; Andersen et al., 1985; Andersen and Mountcastle, 1983; Duhamel et al., 1997). Each neuron thus responds best to particular combinations of retinal and eye position that correspond to a head-centred direction. The gain modulation by eye position produces a population of neurons that encodes the position of the stimulus relative to the head, by taking into account both retinal position and eye position (Salinas and Sejnowski, 2001; Salinas and Abbott, 2001). This gain modulation can be thought of as shifting the retinal receptive fields of the population of neurons so that they represent direction relative to the head, which is a spatial coordinate transform (see illustration in Fig. 3.5). The term gain field is used to refer to this process by which a representation (in this case retinal position) can be modulated by another (in this case eye position) to produce a coordinate transform (see further Section 3.5).

3.4.2 The transform from head-based to allocentric bearing coordinates

There is evidence that some neurons in parietal cortex regions respond in allocentric coordinates. Allocentric representations are where the reference frame is the world, for example a particular location in the world, or a bearing direction. A bearing direction is a direction to a stimulus or landmark from the place where one is located. The bearing is with reference to the world, that is, is in allocentric coordinates, and is usually provided as the angle relative to North, which provides an allocentric reference frame. (Bearing direction is well known to navigators, who use the bearings of several landmarks to identify the place in the world where they are located. The bearing direction of a landmark is different from head direction; and from the direction of motion or course travelled of the individual, vessel, etc.) Egocentric representations are where the reference frame is with respect to the head, body, etc, independently of where the organism is, or objects are, in allocentric space.

An allocentric representation has been described in primate parietal area 7a (Snyder et al., 1998) and a region to which it projects the posterior cingulate cortex (Dean and Platt, 2006).

The population of area 7a neurons was described as responding in a world-based coordinate frame, on the basis that they responded in a particular allocentric direction from the macaque when visually evoked or delayed saccades were made after combined head-and-body rotation in the dark (Snyder, Grieve, Brotchie and Andersen, 1998). The important point is that when the head was rotated, the area 7a neurons were gain modulated by the head direction. The parsimonious interpretation is that this 'world-based' or allocentric representation is thus in the coordinate frame of bearing direction to a stimulus or landmark. This could facilitate saccade-making in a given bearing direction, that is, independently of the head direction gain modulating factor. This evidence for area 7a is thus consistent with the hypothesis that some neurons in it code for (allocentric) bearing direction, in that the neuronal responses are gain modulated by head direction (Snyder, Grieve, Brotchie and Andersen, 1998) (see Fig. 3.6). The requisite signal for this gain modulation is head direction, which is represented by neurons in the primate presubiculum (Robertson, Rolls, Georges-François and Panzeri, 1999).

Similar results were found by Dean and Platt (2006) for the posterior cingulate cortex (which receives inputs from the parietal cortex including area 7a), who showed that for most

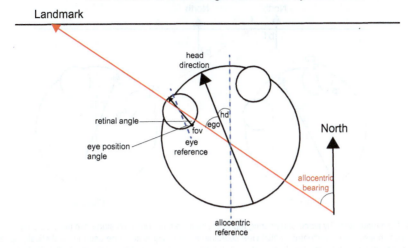

Fig. 3.6 Gain modulation by head direction (hd) to produce a representation in allocentric bearing coordinates (relative to North) to a location in space at which there is a landmark. The head direction is the angle between North (indicated by the long blue line) and the direction of the head (indicated by the long black arrow). A bearing coordinate to a landmark L is represented by all combinations of head direction, eye position (ep) and retinal position that correspond to a given bearing from the individual to a landmark in allocentric space indicated by the line with a red arrow. The large circle is the head, and the two small circles are the eyes. The allocentric bearing to the landmark L is given by the angle between North and the red line from the individual (observer) to the landmark. In this case the allocentric reference frame (indicated by the blue dashed line) is aligned with North, but it could be specified by dominant environmental cues in a particular environment. The large black arrow labelled 'head direction' specifies the direction relative to the allocentric reference framework in which the head is facing, with the head direction angle 'hd' as shown. The head direction (hd) is thus in allocentric coordinates. The egocentric bearing to a landmark ('ego') is the angle between the head direction and the line of sight to the landmark. (As the diagram makes clear, combining the egocentric bearing of the landmark and the head direction yields the allocentric bearing to a landmark.) The diagram also shows how the eye position (the angle between the eye reference frame which is aligned with the head direction as shown), and the retinal angle (the angle between the fovea ('fov') and the place on the retina of the image of the landmark) are relevant. (Modified from Rolls, E. T. (2020) Spatial coordinate transforms linking the allocentric hippocampal and egocentric parietal primate brain systems for memory, action in space, and navigation. Hippocampus 30: 332–353. © Wiley Periodicals Inc.)

neurons, tuning curves aligned more closely when plotted as a function of target position in the room than when plotted as a function of target position with respect to the monkey.

To make an arm reach movement, a transform into body-centred space is needed, as the arms are anchored to the body. Visual neurons that respond in body-centered coordinates have been recorded in area LIP (Snyder, Grieve, Brotchie and Andersen, 1998).

3.4.3 A transform from allocentric bearing coordinates to allocentric spatial view coordinates

A further interesting experiment to those described for area 7a (Snyder, Grieve, Brotchie and Andersen, 1998) and posterior cingulate cortex (Dean and Platt, 2006) would be to move the macaque sideways (or the world at which the monkey was looking), to distinguish bearing direction to a landmark in allocentric space from location of a landmark in allocentric space (see Fig. 3.7). That manipulation was in fact used by Feigenbaum and Rolls (1991), and showed that many hippocampal spatial view neurons code for location in allocentric space, with further experiments involving movement of the macaque to different places relative to the location being viewed providing evidence consistent with this (Rolls and O'Mara, 1995; Georges-François, Rolls and Robertson, 1999). It would be very interesting to try this experiment on neurons in the parietal cortex, and the areas connected to it including the posterior cingulate cortex and retrosplenial cortex. It is shown in Section 3.5 that such a

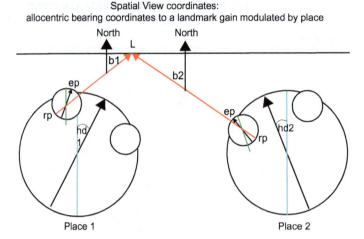

Fig. 3.7 Gain modulation by place of a bearing representation from the previous stage can produce a representation of a landmark L in a scene in allocentric spatial view coordinates. This signal could be used to idiothetically update spatial view cells. b1: bearing of the landmark from place 1; b2: bearing of the landmark from place 2; hd1: head direction 1; hd2: head direction 2; ep: eye position; rp: retinal position. A landmark L at a location being viewed in allocentric space, that is, a spatial view, is represented by transforms over all places, building on transforms over head direction learned in the previous stage, and transforms over eye position learned in the layer before that. Other conventions as in Figs. 3.5 and 3.6. (After Rolls, E. T. (2020). Spatial coordinate transforms linking the allocentric hippocampal and egocentric parietal primate brain systems for memory, action in space, and navigation. Hippocampus 30: 332–353. © Wiley Periodicals Inc.)

transform could be performed by the same type of mechanism that enables other coordinate transforms to take place in the dorsal visual system.

What use might such a transform to allocentric spatial view coordinates at the top of the primate dorsal visual system have? It has been proposed that the dorsal visual system, for whatever combination of retinal and eye positions, head direction, and place is present, generates representations in an allocentric coordinate framework that can be easily interfaced to hippocampal processing which is in the same allocentric spatial view / spatial location coordinate frame (Rolls, 2020b). For example, looking at one location in allocentric space as defined by the current status of the dorsal visual system could provide the allocentric spatial input to the hippocampal memory system via the retrosplenial cortex and/or posterior cingulate cortex (see Fig. 9.1) for location-object memory retrieval by hippocampal mechanisms including recall of the object when an appropriate allocentric spatial location cue is applied. Indeed, something like this is exactly what is proposed to account for the fact that hippocampal spatial view neurons update the allocentric location in space 'out there' to which they respond when eye movements, head direction changes, or even locomotion are performed in the dark (Robertson, Rolls and Georges-François, 1998). The idiothetic update could be performed in the dorsal visual system based on the vestibular, proprioceptive, and corollary discharge related signals that reach the dorsal stream visual areas and update spatial representations in it, with examples including the update of representations made for example by eye movements described here, and by vestibular signals (Chen, DeAngelis and Angelaki, 2018; Avila, Lakshminarasimhan, DeAngelis and Angelaki, 2019). Further, in virtual reality, some macaque hippocampal neurons can respond to a view location towards which eye movements are made even before the view has actually appeared on the screen (Wirth et al., 2017). This idiothetic update of an allocentric view location (Robertson et al., 1998; Wirth et al., 2017) is potentially adaptive, by speeding up the operation of the system, and enabling the system to operate in darkness or when a barrier obscures the spatial view location. This idiothetic update of hippocampal spatial view locations, can, it is proposed (Rolls, 2020b;

Rolls et al., 2023e,d; Rolls, 2023c), be produced by the input from the dorsal visual system (which has information about eye movements etc) but is converted into the correct allocentric view representation by mechanisms of the type illustrated in Fig. 3.7 and described in Section 3.5. Indeed, the empirical evidence for idiothetic update of hippocampal spatial view representations (Robertson et al., 1998; Wirth et al., 2017) is very much in support of the need for a system for coordinate transforms to the allocentric level in the dorsal visual system of the type proposed by Rolls (2020b).

3.5 How visual coordinate transforms are computed in the dorsal visual system

3.5.1 Gain modulation

A new theory of a whole set of hierarchically organised coordinate transforms that are performed in the primate dorsal visual system has been presented in Section 3.4 (Rolls, 2020b).

In this section (3.5), I consider **how** visual coordinate transforms are performed in the dorsal visual system, and describe how they have been tested with a new computational model (Rolls, 2020b).

Gain modulation to produce coordinate transforms is a well-established principle of operation of neuronal systems in the dorsal visual system, and has been applied in particular to the coordinate transform from retinal to head-based coordinates using modulation by eye position (Salinas and Sejnowski, 2001; Salinas and Abbott, 2001, 1996, 1995). The gain modulation by eye position occurs in a spatially systematic and nonlinear way such that the output of the population of neurons encodes the position of the stimulus relative to the head, by taking into account both retinal position and eye position (Salinas and Sejnowski, 2001; Salinas and Abbott, 2001). This gain modulation can be thought of as shifting the retinal receptive fields of the population of neurons so that they represent direction relative to the head, which is a spatial coordinate transform (see illustration in Fig. 3.5).

A problem with the gain modulation mechanism in practice is that it may not be perfect at each stage (Graf and Andersen, 2014), and when successive stages involving other coordinate transforms follow, the imperfections at each stage combine to make a system that operates very imperfectly, as is shown by the simulations described later. It has been proposed that a temporal trace synaptic learning mechanism can help by using the statistics of the natural world across time to help with the learning (Rolls, 2020b, 2021d), as described next.

3.5.2 Mechanisms of gain modulation using a trace learning rule

The new mechanism that has been proposed is to add to gain modulation a trace learning rule, similar to that utilized in the ventral visual system (Rolls, 2020b). The trace rule operates over for example the many combinations of retinal position and eye position that correspond to a given location in head-centred space. That corresponds to a primate (and that includes humans, of course), looking at a location in space relative to the head while the eyes move around the stimulus, so that a number of different retinal and eye positions occur that correspond to the stimulus being in the same position in head-centred space. The trace learning rule helps to ensure that the same neurons learn to encode a single position in head-centred space, in a sense learning invariances over a whole set of retinal and eye position combinations (Rolls, 2020b).

In more detail, a visual stimulus might be steady at a given position relative to the head for several seconds during which many eye movements would occur. The eye movements

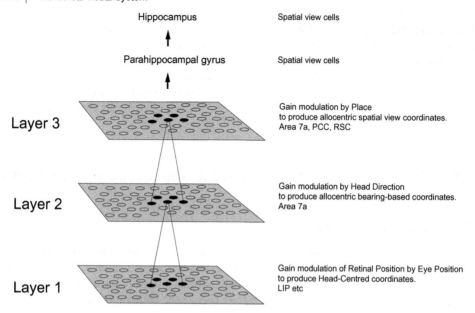

Fig. 3.8 Coordinate transforms in the primate dorsal visual system. Three principal computational stages of coordinate transforms from retinal coordinates via head-centred coordinates and then via allocentric bearing-based coordinates to spatial view coordinates are shown, together with the brain regions in which the different types of neuron are found. The diagram shows the architecture of the VisNetCT model in which gain modulation combined with short-term memory trace associative learning was shown to implement these transforms (see text). Each neuron in a layer (or cortical area in the hierarchy) receives from neurons in a small region of the preceding layer. PCC - posterior cingulate cortex; RSC - retrosplenial cortex. (Modified from Rolls, E. T. (2020) Spatial coordinate transforms linking the allocentric hippocampal and egocentric parietal primate brain systems for memory, action in space, and navigation. Hippocampus 30: 332–353. © Wiley Periodicals Inc.)

would result in different combinations of eye position and retinal position occurring in those few seconds. If the active neurons maintained a short-term memory trace of recent neuronal or synaptic activity for a short period, of even a few hundred ms, the neurons could then learn about what was constant over short periods (such as the position of the visual stimulus relative to the head). The trace learning mechanism itself is very simple and biologically plausible, for it can be included in a competitive network, a standard network in cortical systems, just by utilizing for example the long time constant of NMDA receptors, or the continuing firing of cortical neurons for 100 ms or more that is characteristic of cortical networks with recurrent connections to form attractor networks (Földiák, 1991; Rolls, 1992a; Wallis and Rolls, 1997; Rolls, 2012d, 2016b; Wyss et al., 2006; Wiskott and Sejnowski, 2002; Franzius et al., 2007; Zhao et al., 2019; Eguchi et al., 2016). Exactly these cortical processes provide a theory and model for transform-invariant object representations in the ventral visual system as described in Chapter 2, and have recently been proposed to play an important role in several stages of the dorsal visual system, in relation to learning spatial coordinate transforms (Rolls, 2020b). The uses of these neural mechanisms for each stage of processing in the dorsal visual stream hierarchy are described next.

The following set of spatial coordinate transforms have been investigated in the 3-layer model of successive coordinate transforms, VisNetCT, illustrated in Fig. 3.8 (Rolls, 2020b). Each layer in the model corresponds to a different cortical processing area. The principles may, it is postulated, apply to other spatial coordinate transforms present in these and other cortical areas. The architecture and operation of the model is similar to that of VisNet as described in Chapter 2, except that gain modulation is performed for each presentation of a stimulus with a particular combination of input representation to be gain modulated (e.g. retinal position of the stimulus), and the modulator (e.g. eye position). The gain modulation

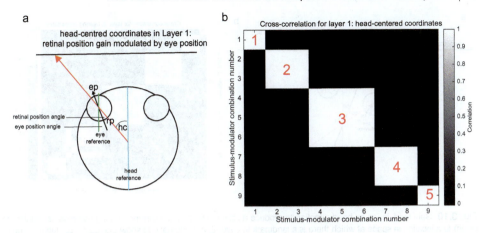

Fig. 3.9 Gain modulation by eye position to produce a head-centered representation in Layer 1. a. Schematic to show that gain modulation by eye position can produce a representation in head-centered coordinates in Layer 1. The abbreviations are as in Fig. 3.5. b. The correlation matrix represents the correlation of the firing between all the neurons in Layer 1 for every one of the five head centred positions (numbered in red) at which a stimulus was presented, after training Layer 1. During training, all combinations of eye position and retinal position that corresponded to one head-centred position were presented together enabling the trace rule to help with the learning, then another head-centred position was selected for training, as described by Rolls (2020). In the correlation matrix, the large white block in the middle thus indicates that the neurons across the whole of Layer 1 that responded to all three combinations of retinal and eye position for head-centred position 3 encoded only head-centred position 3, with no interference from or response to any other retinal and eye position combination that corresponded to other positions in head-centred space. (After Rolls, E. T. (2020) Spatial coordinate transforms linking the allocentric hippocampal and egocentric parietal primate brain systems for memory, action in space, and navigation. Hippocampus 30: 332–353. © Wiley Periodicals Inc.)

was performed in the general way described elsewhere (Salinas and Sejnowski, 2001; Salinas and Abbott, 2001), and was implemented by a convolution of firing in a layer with the gain modulation signal. In addition, the forward connections to a neuron in one layer came from a small region of the preceding layer defined by the radius that will contain approximately 67% of the connections from the preceding layer. This radius was set in VisNetCT to 2 for each layer of 32x32 neurons per layer, and each neuron received 100 synaptic connections from the neurons in the preceding layer. This resulted in the maintenance of some topology through the different layers of VisNetCT, which is different from VisNet, in which the aim is to produce neurons in the final layer with full translation (shift) invariance as well as other invariances.

3.5.3 Gain modulation by eye position to produce a head-centered representation in Layer 1 of VisNetCT

Retinal position is the input to Layer 1, where it is gain modulated by eye position to produce position with respect to the head. The coordinate framework thus becomes head-centred, as illustrated in Fig. 3.9a. Competitive learning with a temporal trace learning rule to select the Layer 1 neurons with good responses for each position with respect to the head occurs, learning over all combinations of retinal position and eye position that correspond to a given position in head-based coordinates. This enables neurons to respond to a given position in head-centred space over many combinations of retinal and eye position that correspond to that position in head-centred space, as found in macaque VIP and LIP.

The results of this training for Layer 1 are illustrated with the correlation matrix shown in Fig. 3.9b. This represents the correlation of the firing between all the neurons in Layer 1 for each of the five head-centred positions at which a stimulus was presented. This shows that the 5 different head-centred positions for a stimulus each produced different firing of Layer 1

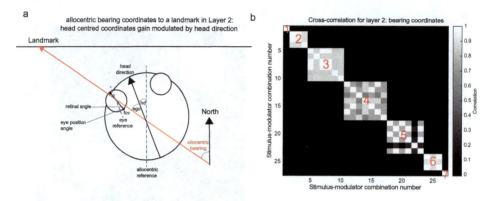

Fig. 3.10 Gain modulation by head direction to produce a representation in allocentric bearing coordinates (relative to North) to a location in space at which there is a landmark in Layer 2. a. Schematic to show that gain modulation by head direction (hd) can produce a representation in allocentric bearing coordinates to a stimulus or landmark (L) in Layer 2. The head direction is the angle between North (indicated by the long blue line) and the direction of the head (indicated by the long black arrow). A bearing coordinate to a landmark L is represented by all combinations of head direction, eye position (ep) and retinal angle that correspond to a given bearing from the individual to a landmark in allocentric space indicated by the line with a red arrow. Other conventions as in Fig. 3.6. b. The correlation matrix represents the correlation of the firing between all the neurons in Layer 2 for every for every one of the seven bearing directions (numbered in red) relative to the agent at which a stimulus was presented, after training Layers 1 and 2. There was one combination of retinal position, eye position, and head direction that corresponded to bearing direction of X=-15 and +15; three for each of X=-10 and +10; six for X=-5 and +5; and seven combinations for bearing direction 4 at X=0. During training, all combinations of head direction, eye position and retinal position that corresponded to one allocentric bearing to a landmark were presented to enable the trace rule to operate usefully; and each of the other allocentric bearings to a landmark were then trained similarly in turn. (After Rolls, E. T. (2020) Spatial coordinate transforms linking the allocentric hippocampal and egocentric parietal primate brain systems for memory, action in space, and navigation. Hippocampus 30: 332–353. © Wiley Periodicals Inc.)

neurons, even though each head-centred position was produced by a number of combinations of retinal stimulus and eye position, as explained in the legend to Fig. 3.9.

The simulation of Layer 1 thus shows that the competitive learning in Layer 1 using a short-term memory trace in combination with gain modulation by eye position can learn to allocate different neurons to respond to each head-centred position in space.

3.5.4 Gain modulation by head direction to produce an allocentric bearing to a landmark in Layer 2 of VisNetCT

For Layer 2, the five head-centred outputs of Layer 1 were gain-modulated by head direction to produce firing that was related to the bearing to a landmark L as illustrated in Fig. 3.10a, using the trace learning rule in the competitive network of Layer 2. There were three head-direction modulators, corresponding to the head directed towards X=-5, X=0, and X=+5. This produced seven possible bearing directions each to a different landmark L, from the single place where the viewer was located. The correlation matrix shown in Fig. 3.10b represents the correlation of the firing between all the neurons in Layer 2 for every one of the seven bearing directions to a landmark relative to the agent at which a stimulus was presented, after training Layers 1–2. This shows that the 7 different bearing directions for a stimulus each produced different firing of Layer 2 neurons, even though each bearing direction was produced by a number of combinations of retinal stimulus, eye position, and head direction.

This then provides a theory and model for how 'allocentric bearing to a landmark cells' can be produced (Rolls, 2020b). Such cells may correspond to those described in area 7a (Snyder, Grieve, Brotchie and Andersen, 1998) and posterior cingulate cortex (Dean and Platt, 2006).

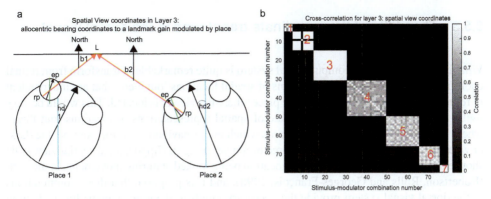

Fig. 3.11 Gain modulation by place to produce an allocentric spatial view representation in Layer 3. a. Schematic to show that gain modulation by place of a bearing representation from Layer 2 can produce a representation of a landmark L in a scene in spatial view coordinates in Layer 3. b1: bearing of the landmark from place 1; b2: bearing of the landmark from place 2; hd1: head direction 1; hd2: head direction 2; ep: eye position; rp: retinal position. A landmark L at a location being viewed in allocentric space, that is, a spatial view, is represented by transforms over all places in Layer 3, building on transforms over head direction learned in Layer 2, and transforms over eye position learned in Layer 1. Other conventions as in previous Figures. b. The correlation matrix represents the correlation of the firing between all the neurons in Layer 3 for 7 spatial views (numbered in red) presented, after training Layers 1–3. During training, all combinations of bearing to a landmark, head direction, eye position and retinal position that corresponded to one spatial view of a landmark from one place were presented to enable the trace rule to operate usefully; and each of the other places were then trained similarly in turn. The results show that the Layer 3 neurons responded selectively and only to all combinations of bearing and place that corresponded to each allocentric spatial view. (After Rolls, E. T. (2020) Spatial coordinate transforms linking the allocentric hippocampal and egocentric parietal primate brain systems for memory, action in space, and navigation. Hippocampus 30: 332–353. © Wiley Periodicals Inc.)

3.5.5 Gain modulation by place to produce an allocentric spatial view representation in Layer 3 of VisNetCT

For Layer 3, the seven bearing direction outputs of Layer 2 to different locations L were gain-modulated by place to produce an allocentric view-based representation using the trace learning rule in the competitive network of Layer 3. This might be produced by walking from one place to another while watching the same location in a scene. Fig. 3.11a shows a schematic for a single location L in the scene. Each location was encoded by spatial view cells that encoded the location in the scene, independently of the place where the viewer was located. There were three place modulators. This produced representations of 7 allocentric, world-based, views each of a different location in the scene. Each of the spatial view representations learned was of a different location L in the scene. Each spatial view representation was independent of the place where the viewer was located.

Fig. 3.11b shows that after training Layers 1–3, the firing of neurons in Layer 3 represented each of the spatial locations in the scene separately and independently. The correlation matrix represents the correlation of the firing between all the neurons in Layer 3 for every spatial location presented. Fig. 3.11 thus shows that the firing of Layer 3 represented each of the 7 spatial locations in the scene almost orthogonally to the other spatial locations, which is good performance.

In an important control condition, it was shown that training using gain modulation but no trace learning rule produced very much poorer performance (Rolls, 2020b). This shows the value of combining trace rule learning with gain modulation.

A neuron that responds allocentrically to a single location in the scene and relatively independently of the place where the viewer is located is termed an allocentric spatial view cell (Rolls, Robertson and Georges-François, 1997a; Georges-François, Rolls and Robertson, 1999; Rolls, 1999c; Rolls and Xiang, 2006; Rolls and Wirth, 2018; Rolls, 2023c), and neurons in these coordinates are what is produced in Layer 3 of VisNetCT (Rolls, 2020b, 2021d).

3.5.6 The utility of the coordinate transforms in the dorsal visual system

What is computed by this computational system is quite remarkable: a transform from retinal coordinates to allocentric representations of spatial locations 'out there' that are independent of retinal position, eye position, and the place where the viewer is located. This would be very useful for idiothetic (self-motion) update of spatial representations of locations 'out there' where there might be a goal object towards which one is navigating, in for example the dark, or when the view of the goal was obscured or not yet in sight. Hippocampal spatial view cells show exactly this type of update of the location being looked at during movements in the dark (Robertson, Rolls and Georges-François, 1998), and it is proposed that these computations in the dorsal visual system provide the necessary inputs to the hippocampus for navigation in the dark (Rolls, 2021f,d), using the pathways from parietal areas via brain regions such as the posterior cingulate cortex and retrosplenial cortex which project via the parahippocampal gyrus (areas TF and TH) into the hippocampal system, as shown in Figs. 9.1 and 3.12 (Rolls, 2021d; Rolls et al., 2023e,d; Rolls, 2023c). The same computation would account for the fact that some macaque hippocampal neurons can respond to a view location towards which eye movements are made even before the view has actually appeared on the projection screen in the virtual reality environment (Wirth et al., 2017).

Brain systems for navigation in primates including humans that make use of computations of the type described here are considered in Chapters 10 and 9 (Rolls, 2021f, 2023c).

The computations described here also account for the representation of allocentric bearing direction, which appears to be implemented by neurons in the primate parietal cortex area 7a (Snyder, Grieve, Brotchie and Andersen, 1998) and a region to which it projects the posterior cingulate cortex (Dean and Platt, 2006). (These allocentric bearing direction neurons are different from head direction cells, in that allocentric bearing cells to a location are independent of head direction.)

To make an arm reach movement, a transform into body-centred space is needed, as the arms are anchored to the body. Visual neurons that respond in body-centered coordinates have been recorded in area LIP (Snyder et al., 1998), and it is proposed that their responses are computed using similar mechanisms (Rolls, 2020b).

The rat has no fovea, and does not have the same mechanisms as those described here in primates for the control of foveation (Bisley and Goldberg, 2010), and probably can not represent transform-invariant locations in viewed scenes which are such important properties of the primate including human visual system. The rat therefore provides a poor model for the computations performed in this part of the primate brain, the dorsal visual system. There is however a model of coordinate transforms based on neurons found in rodents such as boundary-vector cells and object-vector cells (Bicanski and Burgess, 2018), and this is described in Section 9.3.14.3. A description of the model is: "Perceived and imagined egocentric sensory experience is represented in the 'parietal window' (PW), which consists of two neural populations - one coding for extended boundaries ('PWb neurons'), and one for discrete objects ('PWo neurons')". That model holds that "the transformation between egocentric (parietal) and allocentric (medial temporal lobe, MTL) reference frames is performed by a gain-field circuit in retrosplenial cortex" and uses head direction. In comparison, the present model introduces a new approach to coordinate transforms that includes a memory trace learning rule in competitive networks that is combined with gain modulation for multiple stages of the dorsal visual system; and specifically deals with the spatial transforms and representations known to be implemented in the primate dorsal visual system, and in areas such as the posterior cingulate cortex (not known to be present in rodents).

The issues of spatial representations in the parietal cortex, and a region to which it projects the hippocampus, and their involvement in navigation, are considered further in Chapters 10 and 9.

3.6 The human Dorsal Visual Cortical Stream for visual motion leading to the intraparietal visual areas, and then to parietal area 7 regions for actions in space

The human Dorsal Visual Cortical Stream pathways described here lead via dorsal visual system cortical regions to regions in the intraparietal sulcus and parietal cortex area 7. This stream has visual motion outputs to the superior STS semantic system. This stream includes a dorsal 'where' / action system in which idiothetic update of spatial representations is performed.

The effective connectivity of the human Dorsal Visual Stream is shown in Fig. 3.12 (Rolls et al., 2023e). Effective connectivity from regions such as V2, V3, V3A and V3B, V6A and V7 reach the MT+ complex regions (FST, LO1, LO2, LO3, MST, MT, PH, V3CD and V4t) (Fig. 3.12). The MT+ complex regions then have effective connectivity to the intraparietal regions (AIP, LIPd, LIPv, MIP, VIP IP0, IP1 and IP2), which in turn have effective connectivity to the area 7 regions. Interestingly, in humans there are some inputs to this Dorsal Visual Stream from Ventrolateral Visual Stream regions such as FFC and TE2p, and these are shown with dashed lines in Fig. 3.12.

3.6.1 Dorsal stream visual division regions

V3A and V6 are motion-sensitive areas that project to the regions in the MT+ Complex division (Table 1.1) in what is described in macaques as a dorsolateral visual stream which eventually reaches the cortex in the superior temporal sulcus (Galletti and Fattori, 2018). V6 responds to coherent optic flow stimuli and may thus be useful in egomotion (Sulpizio et al., 2020). In macaques, V6 may also project to V6A which is involved in the fast control of prehension and in selecting appropriate postures during reach-to-grasp behaviors (Pitzalis et al., 2015, 2013; Monaco et al., 2011; Tosoni et al., 2015). V6A then projects to what is described as a dorsomedial visual stream directed towards the intraparietal areas such as MIP which are also involved in reach to grasp behavior (Galletti and Fattori, 2018). Neurons in V6A and VIP are invariant with respect to eye position, that is, they can respond in head-based coordinates (Galletti and Fattori, 2018). Coordinate transforms of this type can be implemented by gain modulation (Salinas and Sejnowski, 2001) (in which for example eye direction modulates retinotopic position) which is greatly helped by slow learning to capture the statistical continuities of an object in a fixed position relative to the head when the eyes move (Rolls, 2020b). The same principle can be extended to account for the next transform to allocentric direction in space, and then to a further transform to allocentric location in space independently of the place where the individual is located (Rolls, 2020b), as represented in the parahippocampal gyrus and hippocampus by spatial view cells (Rolls, 2023c). This dorsomedial part of the dorsal visual system provides for idiothetic (self-motion) update of allocentric spatial representations of the type provided by for example primate spatial view cells (Robertson et al., 1998), and is a key computation performed in the dorsal visual 'where' system enabling idiothetic update of the VentroMedial 'Where' Visual Cortical Stream for building scene representations in the VMV and PHA1-PHA3 parahippocampal areas (see Fig. 3.12) (Rolls et al., 2023e,d; Rolls, 2023c). These scene representations are likely to be involved in human navigation from viewed location to viewed location, which is frequently how navigational

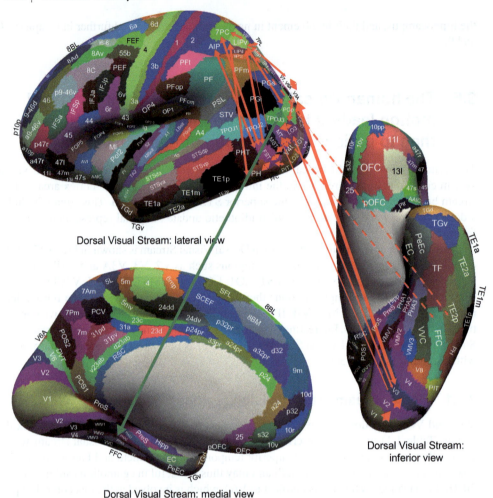

Fig. 3.12 Effective connectivity of the human Dorsal Visual Cortical Stream which reaches (partly via V3, V3A and LO3) the MT+ complex regions (FST, LO1, LO2, LO3, MST, MT, PH, V3CD and V4t), and then the intraparietal regions (AIP, LIPd, LIPv, MIP, VIP IP0, IP1 and IP2) and then the area 7 regions: schematic overview. Connectivity to the inferior parietal cortex region PGp, which in turn has effective connectivity to the parahippocampal scene area in PHA1-3 (Rolls et al., 2023d) is shown. Inputs to this stream from ventral stream regions such as FFC and TE2p are shown with dashed lines. (From Rolls,E.T., Deco,G., Huang,C-C. and Feng,J. (2023) Multiple cortical visual streams in humans. Cerebral Cortex 33: 3319-3349. doi: 10.1093/cercor/bhac276. Copyright © Oxford University Press.)

instructions are provided in humans (Rolls, 2021f). The idiothetic update of scene representations is likely to be important for navigation if the view details are temporarily obscured, or in the dark (Rolls, 2021f, 2023c).

3.6.2 MT+ complex regions (FST, LO1, LO2, LO3, MST, MT, PH, V3CD and V4t)

In macaques, MT neurons compute global motion aided by their receptive fields being about 10 times larger than V1 neurons (Newsome, Britten and Movshon, 1989; Zaharia, Goris, Movshon and Simoncelli, 2019). In MST, the receptive fields are larger (e.g. 40°), and some neurons respond to more complex types of motion such as expanding optic flow consistent with moving forwards in an environment, or rotation of the optic flow in a clockwise vs anticlockwise direction, and therefore useful in analysing self-motion or the motion of an object, disparity may be encoded, and vestibular inputs related to self-motion can influence some neurons (Wild and Treue, 2021).

In a unifying hypothesis with the design of the ventral cortical visual system about how these types of encoded motion might be computed, Rolls and Stringer (2006a) proposed that the dorsal visual system uses a hierarchical feedforward network architecture (V1, V2, MT, MST, parietal cortex) with training of the synaptic connections with a short-term memory trace associative synaptic modification rule to compute what is invariant at each stage by utilizing the temporal continuity inherent in the statistics of the visual inputs (Section 3.3). The same principle (Rolls and Stringer, 2006a) can account for the responses of neurons in the cortex in the superior temporal sulcus (which may receive from these dorsal visual stream regions) which it was discovered can respond to object-based rotation about a principal axis, for example to a head rotating clockwise, invariantly with respect to whether the head was upright or inverted (Hasselmo et al., 1989b).

3.6.3 Intraparietal sulcus posterior parietal cortex, regions (AIP, LIPd, LIPv, MIP, VIP; with IP0, IP1 and IP2)

Neurons in macaques in area VIP represent the direction and speed of visual motion (Colby et al., 1993), and may be useful in for example tracking moving visual stimuli, and encoding optic flow which can be useful in assessing self-motion and thereby in navigation. These neurons do not respond in relation to saccades. Neurons in macaques in LIP are active in visual, attentional and saccadic processing (Gnadt and Andersen, 1988; Colby et al., 1996; Munuera and Duhamel, 2020). The ventral part of LIP (LIPv) has strong connections with two oculomotor centres, the frontal eye field and the deep layers of the superior colliculus, and may be especially involved in the generation of saccades (Chen et al., 2016b). The dorsal part (LIPd) may be more involved in visual processing, responding for example to visual targets for saccades (Chen et al., 2016b). Neurons in MIP (which may be the parietal reach region, PRR (Connolly et al., 2003)) are related to arm movement preparation and execution (Passarelli et al., 2021; Prado et al., 2005; Filimon et al., 2009; Cavina-Pratesi et al., 2010; Gallivan et al., 2011). They are implicated in the sensory-to-motor transformations required for reaching toward visually defined targets (Gamberini et al., 2020). AIP is activated by grasping objects, for which shaping of the hand based on the visual properties of objects is needed (Culham et al., 2006, 2003).

As shown in Fig. 3.12, these regions have strong effective connectivity from early visual cortical areas including from several MT+ complex visual regions in which neurons respond to global optic flow (MST, FST, PH and V3CD), intraparietal sulcus area 1 (IPS1), V3B, V6A (which is a visuo-motor region involved in grasping seen objects (Gamberini et al., 2020)), V7, and superior parietal area 7 regions involved in visuo-motor actions. These intraparietal regions also receive in humans from ventral stream visual cortical areas including the fusiform face cortex (FFC), from inferior temporal cortex regions PIT, PHT, TE1p and TE2p (Fig. 3.12). These ventral stream regions are likely to bring shape / visual form information to the intraparietal cortex regions important in shaping the hand to grasp and manipulate objects and tools. Consistent with this, neurons in regions such as AIP in macaques can respond to 2D and 3D shape information which could be helpful in tool use (Kastner et al., 2017). These intraparietal and also area 7 regions may provide information to the inferior parietal cortex regions such as PFt, PF and PGi that have developed so greatly in humans and that are involved in human tool use (Rolls et al., 2023d). These intraparietal regions also have connectivity with the inferior frontal gyrus and with the dorsolateral prefrontal cortex (especially 46, 8C, a9-46, i6-8 and p9-46v), which are likely to be important when there is a delay between the visual input and when the action can be performed (Funahashi, Bruce and Goldman-Rakic, 1989). These connectivities are stronger to these prefrontal areas, as is appropriate for the operation of short-term memory systems so that the memory does not dominate sensory inputs (Rolls, 2016b, 2021b). There is also connectivity directed towards the parahippocampal TH cortex (PHA3) which may be useful in providing information about visuo-motor actions to the hippocampal memory system. There is also connectivity with the frontal pole p10p, which is likely to be important when sequencing and planning is involved in actions (Shallice and Cipolotti, 2018; Shallice and Burgess, 1996; Gilbert and Burgess, 2008).

The connectivity from the intraparietal areas is strongly towards premotor cortical areas including especially 6a, and to the frontal eye field FEF and prefrontal eye field PEF (from especially AIP, LIPd, LIPv and VIP), which provide action-related outputs from these visuo-motor intraparietal regions. There is also connectivity especially for IP1 and IP2 from the orbitofrontal cortex (medial regions, 11 and OFC) which may provide reward feedback (Rolls, 2019e,f) of potential utility in learning whether actions made are correct, and with the frontal pole. There is also connectivity with inferior parietal regions including PGp and PGs, with PGp having effective connectivity to the parahippocampal scene area PHA1-3 to provide, it is proposed here, for idiothetic update of parahippocampal and hippocampal spatial view representations (Rolls et al., 2023d; Rolls, 2023c). Interestingly, this intraparietal part of the parietal cortex has relatively little effective connectivity with the posterior or anterior (or mid) cingulate cortex. The connectivity from MT+ regions such as MT and MST to intraparietal regions from auditory cortical regions such as A4 and A5, and from somatosensory regions such as 5L and 5m, provides a basis for the auditory and somatosensory responses evident is some macaque intraparietal neurons that also respond to visual stimuli (Kastner et al., 2017).

The functional connectivity is largely consistent with the effective connectivity (Rolls et al., 2023e), but indicates more interactions with early visual cortical areas; with somatosensory/premotor areas; with the hippocampal system; with TE1p and TE2p, with posterior cingulate including DVT; and with supragenual anterior cingulate 33pr and p24pr (Rolls et al., 2023c). The diffusion tractography (Rolls et al., 2023e) is also consistent, but suggests in addition connections with auditory cortex that may be useful in orienting gaze towards sounds.

The intraparietal cortical regions in humans thus are likely in terms of their connectivity (Rolls et al., 2023e) to perform visuomotor functions (without substantial somatosensory processing unlike area 7 regions), and the extensive research on these regions in macaques provides a guide to their functions in humans, including the control of eye movements to acquire and track visual stimuli given the outputs to the FEF and PEF. There are also outputs to regions 6a and 6r that might produce head and body movements to help stabilize images for the visual system. The output to the posterior inferior temporal visual cortex PHT is of interest, and might be involved in the stabilization of images for processing in later parts of the ventral visual system.

3.6.4 Area 7 regions

Area 7 regions in the posterior parietal cortex receive from the intraparietal areas, and are involved in actions in space, and their connectivity in humans is considered in Chapter 10 (Rolls et al., 2023d).

4 The taste and flavor system

4.1 Introduction and overview

4.1.1 Introduction

There are taste receptors in the mouth for at least five tastes, sweet (e.g. sucrose), salt (e.g. sodium chloride), bitter (e.g. quinine), sour (e.g. citric acid and hydrochloric acid), and umami (e.g. monosodium glutamate). The taste receptors project by three gustatory (taste) nerves (facial 7, glossopharyngeal 9, and vagus 10) to the nucleus of the solitary tract (NTS) in the brainstem. From there, the taste pathways project differently in primates and rodents, as shown in Fig. 4.1. As we are concerned in this book with the computations in the primate including human brain, we will focus on the macaque pathways shown in the left of Fig. 4.1, and how they converge with other pathways later on as shown in Fig. 11.1. The points made refer to the primate including human unless otherwise stated, as the connections and functioning of the rodent taste system are so different. Somatosensory information about the texture of food in the mouth, and its temperature, are represented in the primary taste cortex in the anterior insula; and beyond that, convergence with olfactory and visual information in the primate orbitofrontal cortex enables the full flavor of a food to be represented.

4.1.2 Overview of what is computed in the taste and flavor system

What is computed in the taste system is described in Sections 4.2.1 to 4.2.9 with an overview here.

1. The rostral part of the nucleus of the solitary tract contains taste neurons that are not very specifically tuned to individual tastes (Scott et al., 1986b; Rolls, 1989d), and which do not reduce their responses during feeding to satiety (Yaxley et al., 1985).
2. Neurons in the primary taste cortex in the anterodorsal insula and adjoining frontal operculum respond more selectively to tastes, but not to only one taste: it is a sparse distributed code. Neurons in these regions do not reduce their responses during feeding to satiety, so the reward value of taste is not represented in the primary taste cortex. Instead, their firing rates are usually related to the concentration of the tastant, and thus to the intensity of the taste.
3. Some neurons in the primary taste cortex respond to oral texture, including food thickness which is related to viscosity, and the texture of fat which is related to the coefficient of sliding friction. Some neurons combine taste and/or oral texture and/or oral temperature. Neurons in the primary taste cortex do not respond to odor or to visual stimuli (although if a taste is recalled in humans by for example an olfactory stimulus some activation may be found). These features of the insular primary taste cortex allow tastes independently of visual and olfactory associations to be identified, and learned about, and this can occur even if hunger is not present.
4. Neurons in the primary taste cortex project into the orbitofrontal cortex, which thus ranks in the taste hierarchy as secondary taste cortex. Some orbitofrontal cortex neurons are more specifically tuned to taste than in earlier taste processing stages in the hierarchy.

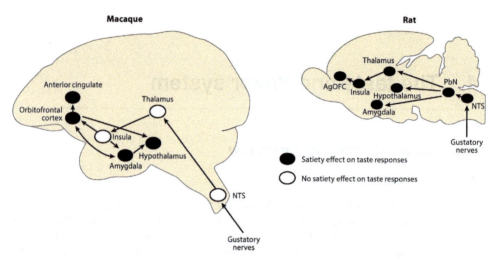

Fig. 4.1 Taste pathways in the macaque and rat. In the macaque, gustatory information reaches the nucleus of the solitary tract (NTS), which projects directly to the taste thalamus (ventral posteromedial nucleus, pars parvocellularis, VPMpc) which then projects to the taste cortex in the anterior insula (Insula). The insular taste cortex then projects to the orbitofrontal cortex and amygdala. The orbitofrontal cortex projects taste information to the anterior cingulate cortex. Both the orbitofrontal cortex and the amygdala project to the hypothalamus (and to the ventral striatum). In macaques, feeding to normal self-induced satiety does not decrease the responses of taste neurons in the NTS or taste insula (and by inference not VPMpc) (see text). In the rat, in contrast, the NTS projects to a pontine taste area, the parabrachial nucleus (PbN). The PbN then has projections directly to a number of subcortical structures, including the hypothalamus, amygdala, and ventral striatum, thus bypassing thalamo-cortical processing. The PbN in the rat also projects to the taste thalamus (VPMpc), which projects to the rat taste insula. The taste insula in the rat then projects to an agranular orbitofrontal cortex (AgOFC), which probably corresponds to the most posterior part of the primate OFC, which is agranular. (In primates, most of the orbitofrontal cortex is granular cortex, and the rat may have no equivalent to this.) In the rat, satiety signals such as gastric distension and satiety-related hormones decrease neuronal responses in the NTS (see text), and by inference therefore in the other brain areas with taste-related responses, as indicated in the Figure. (After Rolls, E. T. (2016) Reward systems in the brain and nutrition. Annual Review of Nutrition 36: 435–470. Reproduced with permission from the Annual Reviews, Volume 36 © 2016 by Annual Reviews, http://www.annualreviews.org.)

5. Some orbitofrontal cortex neurons respond not only to taste but also to olfactory and/or visual stimuli, with these multimodal responses learned by associative learning, and providing a representation of flavor in the brain. Some of these neurons also respond to oral texture and/or temperature. The resulting neurons can respond to specific combinations of their inputs which allow selectivity for particular foods. Convergence of the taste, olfactory, and visual pathways in the orbitofrontal cortex, as shown in Fig. 11.1, provides the anatomical basis for these multimodal responses.

6. Most orbitofrontal cortex neurons decrease their responses to a food that is eaten to satiety, providing evidence that the reward value of taste and more generally food is represented in the orbitofrontal cortex.

7. The effect of feeding to satiety on neurons in the orbitofrontal cortex is relatively specific to the food eaten to satiety, and this is termed sensory-specific satiety. This is one of the most important principles of operation of the flavor system, and indeed more generally of reward systems in the brain. Because of this selectivity of the reward systems in relation to satiety, made possible by the selective tuning of orbitofrontal cortex neurons, presenting a wide variety of foods can lead to overeating, and is likely to be an important contributor to obesity in humans.

8. Human functional neuroimaging investigations provide consistent evidence for humans. They also show that activations in the insular primary taste cortex are related to the subjective intensity but not pleasantness of taste; and that top-down attention to intensity can increase the activations in the primary taste cortex. Activations in the human orbitofrontal

cortex are related to the subjective pleasantness but not intensity of taste; and top-down attention to pleasantness can increase activations in the orbitofrontal cortex. Top-down cognitive modulation of pleasantness, for example describing at the word level a stimulus as rich and delicious, can also enhance activations in the human olfactory cortex to flavor and other reward stimuli.

9. The orbitofrontal cortex projects to the anterior cingulate cortex, in which taste and also multimodal flavor neurons are found (Rolls, 2008c). The pregenual anterior cingulate cortex represents pleasant flavors and other rewarding stimuli, and the supracallosal anterior cingulate cortex represents unpleasant flavors and other aversive stimuli. The anterior cingulate cortex may provide a route for the orbitofrontal cortex reward system to connect to the goal-directed action system that learns actions to obtain the rewards (Rolls, 2019e,c; Rolls et al., 2023c) (Section 12.2).

4.1.3 Overview of how computations are performed in the taste and flavor system

How the computations are performed in the taste system is described in Section 4.3 with an overview here.

1. The taste system is hierarchically organised, and competitive learning in the cortex (complemented by lateral inhibition in the thalamus) is the probable mechanism that sharpens the tuning through the hierarchy.
2. Multimodal associations of visual and olfactory stimuli with taste are learned in the orbitofrontal cortex, with the probable mechanism pattern association. This learning may also involve competitive learning, helping neurons to become selective for different multimodal combinations of their inputs.
3. Visual to taste associations can be reversed in one trial by orbitofrontal cortex neurons, providing evidence for a rule-based mechanism. This is very adaptive in evolutionary terms, and is not known to be possible in rodents, but is an important computation in primates. A model for this is described in Chapter 11.
4. Sensory-specific satiety is probably implemented in the orbitofrontal cortex by adaptation with a time course of several minutes of the active synapses onto orbitofrontal cortex neurons. A simple model is described.
5. Top-down modulation of orbitofrontal cortex activity by attention and cognition is probably implemented by top-down biassed competition (Sections 2.12 and B.8.4) or top-down biased activation (Section 4.3.5).

4.2 Taste and related pathways: what is computed

4.2.1 Hierarchically organised anatomical pathways

The hierarchical organisation of taste processing in primates is shown in Figs. 4.1, 4.3 and 11.1 (Rolls, 2015d, 2016c,g). The taste nerves lead to the first central synapse of the gustatory system, in the rostral part of the nucleus of the solitary tract (Beckstead and Norgren, 1979; Beckstead et al., 1980). Second-order gustatory projections that arise from rostral NTS project directly to the taste thalamus VPMpc (ventral posteromedial nucleus, pars parvocellularis)in primates (Beckstead, Morse and Norgren, 1980; Pritchard, Hamilton and Norgren, 1989). The taste thalamus then projects to the primary taste cortex in the rostrodorsal part of the insula and the adjoining frontal operculum (Pritchard et al., 1986). The primary taste

224 | The taste and flavor system

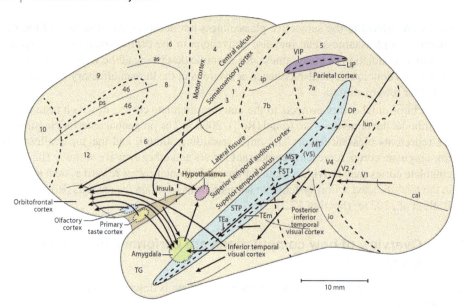

Fig. 4.2 Some of the connections of the primate orbitofrontal cortex and amygdala shown on this lateral view of the brain of the macaque monkey, showing the connections from the primary taste and olfactory cortices. Connections are also shown in the 'ventral visual system' from V1 to V2, V4, the inferior temporal visual cortex, etc., with some connections reaching the amygdala and orbitofrontal cortex. In addition, connections from the somatosensory cortical areas 1, 2, and 3 that reach the orbitofrontal cortex directly and via the insular cortex, and that reach the amygdala via the insular cortex, are shown. as, arcuate sulcus; cal, calcarine sulcus; cs, central sulcus; lf, lateral (or Sylvian) fissure; lun, lunate sulcus; ps, principal sulcus; io, inferior occipital sulcus; ip, intraparietal sulcus (which has been opened to reveal some of the areas it contains); sts, superior temporal sulcus (which has been opened to reveal some of the areas it contains). AIT, anterior inferior temporal cortex; FST, visual motion processing area; LIP, lateral intraparietal area; MST, visual motion processing area; MT, visual motion processing area (also called V5); PIT, posterior inferior temporal cortex; STP, superior temporal plane; TA, architectonic area including auditory association cortex; TE, architectonic area including high order visual association cortex, and some of its subareas TEa and TEm; TG, architectonic area in the temporal pole; V1–V4, visual areas V1–V4; VIP, ventral intraparietal area; TEO, architectonic area including posterior visual association cortex. The numerals refer to architectonic areas, and have the following approximate functional equivalence: 1,2,3, somatosensory cortex (posterior to the central sulcus); 4, motor cortex; 5, superior parietal lobule; 7a, inferior parietal lobule, visual part; 7b, inferior parietal lobule, somatosensory part; 6, lateral premotor cortex; 8, frontal eye field; 12, part of orbitofrontal cortex; 46, dorsolateral prefrontal cortex. (After Rolls, E. T. (2016) Reward systems in the brain and nutrition. Annual Review of Nutrition 36: 435–470. Reproduced with permission from the Annual Review of Nutrition, Volume 36 © 2016 by Annual Reviews, http://www.annualreviews.org.

cortex then projects to the orbitofrontal cortex (Baylis, Rolls and Baylis, 1995), which is secondary taste cortex. The orbitofrontal cortex then has connections with the anterior cingulate cortex (Ongur and Price, 2000; Rolls, 2019c; Du, Rolls, Cheng, Li, Gong, Qiu and Feng, 2020; Hsu, Rolls, Huang, Chong, Lo, Feng and Lin, 2020; Rolls, Deco, Huang and Feng, 2023c) where taste neurons are found (Rolls, 2008c).

This hierarchical architecture provides a foundation for some of the computations revealed in properties of the primate including human taste system that are described in the rest of this chapter. One is the increasing selectivity of neurons as information progresses up through the taste system, which is helped in the orbitofrontal cortex by combining taste with olfactory and visual information. A second is processing of taste, oral texture, and temperature information only in the primary taste cortex, before olfactory and visual information converges with taste information in the orbitofrontal cortex. A consequence is that it is possible for humans to identify a taste separately from the flavor that results after combination of taste and olfactory information. A third type of computation that is afforded by the primary taste cortex is that reward processing is not implemented until satiety and related computations are performed in the orbitofrontal cortex. This enables humans to identify and learn about tastes independently of hunger, which is highly biologically adaptive, if primates encounter a food when they are not hungry.

In humans the primary taste cortex is in the anterior insula (Rolls, 2015d, 2016c, 2019g) in regions that in the HCP-MMP atlas include parts of AVI, FOP5 and FOP4 (Fig. 6.7 see Rolls et al. (2023f) which has coronal slices in the Supplementary Material to show these regions better). The insular and frontal opercular taste regions then have connectivity with the orbitofrontal cortex and anterior cingulate cortex, and also with some prefrontal cortex regions (Rolls et al., 2023f). The lateral orbitofrontal cortex has effective connectivity directed towards language regions in for example Broca's area, and this may provide a route for the representations in orbitofrontal cortex to contribute to the declarative aspects of reward value, subjective emotion, and hedonics (Rolls et al., 2023c,b). Interesting, the amyLgdala has much less connectivity to cortical areas including these language regions, and partly for this reason may play only a small role in experienced, declarative, human emotions and hedonics (Rolls et al., 2023b).

There are major differences in the neural pathways for taste in rodents (Rolls and Scott, 2003; Small and Scott, 2009; Scott and Small, 2009; Rolls, 2015d, 2016c,g) (Fig. 4.1). In rodents the majority of NTS taste neurons responding to stimulation of the taste receptors of the anterior tongue project to the ipsilateral medial aspect of the pontine parabrachial nucleus (PbN), the rodent 'pontine taste area' (Small and Scott, 2009; Cho et al., 2002). From the PbN the rodent gustatory pathway bifurcates into two pathways; 1) a ventral 'affective' projection to the hypothalamus, central gray, ventral striatum, bed nucleus of the stria terminalis and amygdala and 2) a dorsal 'sensory' pathway, which first synapses in the thalamus and then the agranular and dysgranular insular gustatory cortex (Norgren, 1990; Norgren and Leonard, 1971; Norgren, 1974, 1976; Kosar et al., 1986) (Fig. 4.1). These regions, in turn, project back to the PbN to "sculpt the gustatory code" and guide complex feeding behaviors (Norgren, 1990, 1976; Li and Cho, 2006; Li et al., 2002; Lundy and Norgren, 2004; Di Lorenzo, 1990; Scott and Small, 2009; Small and Scott, 2009). It may be noted that there is strong evidence to indicate that the PbN gustatory relay is absent in the human and the nonhuman primate (Small and Scott, 2009; Scott and Small, 2009). First, second-order gustatory projections that arise from rostral NTS appear not to synapse in the PbN and instead join the central tegmental tract and project directly to the taste thalamus in primates (Beckstead, Morse and Norgren, 1980; Pritchard, Hamilton and Norgren, 1989). Second, despite several attempts, no one has successfully isolated taste responses in the monkey PbN (Norgren (1990); and Small and Scott (2009) who cite Ralph Norgren, personal communication and Tom Pritchard, personal communication). Third, in monkeys the projection arising from the PbN does not terminate in the region of ventral basal thalamus that contains gustatory responsive neurons (Pritchard et al., 1989).

It is surprising from an evolutionary perspective that such a fundamental brain system as the taste system should have such different connections (and functioning as shown in Section 4.2.4) in primates and rodents. It is suggested that there are computational reasons for this: the primate visual system has evolved its multiple-layer hierarchy to solve the major computational problem of what object is represented with invariance, and this provides advantage in being able to learn about for example where foods are even when they are not rewarding because no hunger is present. This implies a separation of perceptual from reward value processing in primates. It is suggested that with this evolutionary advance made possible by visual cortical computation, it became advantageous to perform a similar separation of perceptual from reward value processing in other sensory modalities, leading to the advantage in primates of having a primary taste cortex that represents the sensory qualities of taste, so that it can be matched at the object level to perceptual representations in other modalities. Consistent with that, a later stage of processing, the orbitofrontal cortex, then evolved to specialise

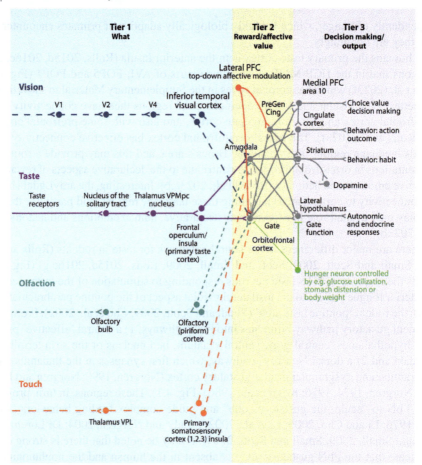

Fig. 4.3 Schematic diagram showing some of the connections of the taste, olfactory, somatosensory, and visual pathways in the primate brain. V1, primary visual (striate) cortex; V2 and V4, further cortical visual areas. PFC, prefrontal cortex. VPL, ventro-postero-lateral nucleus of the thalamus, which conveys somatosensory information to the primary somatosensory cortex (areas 1, 2 and 3). VPMpc, ventro-postero-medial nucleus pars parvocellularis of lthe thalamus, which conveys taste information to the primary taste cortex. Pregen Cing, pregenual cingulate cortex. For purposes of description, the stages can be described as Tier 1, representing what object is present independently of reward value; Tier 2 in which reward value is represented; and Tier 3 in which decisions between stimuli of different value are taken, and in which value is interfaced to behavioral output systems. (After Rolls, E. T. (2016) Reward systems in the brain and nutrition. Annual Review of Nutrition 36: 435–470. Reproduced with permission from the Annual Review of Nutrition, Volume 36 © 2016 by Annual Reviews, http://www.annualreviews.org.)

in reward value processing, for all sensory modalities. In contrast, the rodent taste system sends taste information to many subcortical areas without processing in the taste cortex, and given that even at early stages of taste processing in rodents reward value becomes part of what is encoded, this makes the rodent system not only much more difficult to analyze and understand computationally, but also a poor model of the computations in primates including humans (Rolls, 2015d, 2016c,g, 2019e).

4.2.2 Taste neuronal tuning become more selective through the taste hierarchy

The tuning of taste receptors and the taste nerves has been described as selective for the individual tastes sweet, salt, sour, bitter and umami in mice (Barretto, Gillis-Smith, Chandrashekar, Yarmolinsky, Schnitzer, Ryba and Zuker, 2015). However, there is further evi-

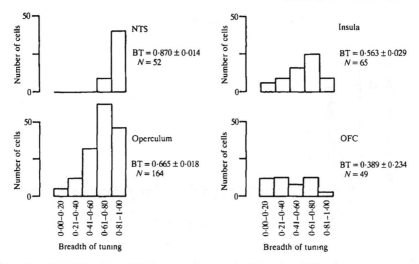

Fig. 4.4 The breadth of tuning index H (see text) for neurons recorded in the nucleus of the solitary tract (NTS), the primary taste cortical areas in the frontal operculum and insula, and the secondary taste cortical area in the caudolateral orbitofrontal cortex (OFC) of macaques is shown. The means ($\pm$ sem) and the number of neurons in the sample for each area are shown. (After Rolls, E. T. (1989) Information processing in the taste system of primates. Journal of Experimental Biology 146: 141–164. © The Company of Biologists Limited.)

dence also in mice that many taste nerves respond to several tastes, especially at midrange concentrations, with a breadth of tuning that was often in the range 0.3 to 0.4, not close to 0 expected of neurons that respond to only one basic taste (Wu et al., 2015; Roper and Chaudhari, 2017)[10]. For comparison, in macaques the tuning in the taste nerves is quite distributed, with values between H= 0.37 and 0.81 (Hellekant et al., 1997). This most of the evidence is that in the periphery, the taste tuning is not of highly selective ('labelled line') encoding, but instead of a more distributed representation.

The first central synapse of the gustatory system is in the rostral part of the nucleus of the solitary tract (Beckstead and Norgren, 1979; Beckstead, Morse and Norgren, 1980; Scott, Yaxley, Sienkiewicz and Rolls, 1986b; Yaxley, Rolls, Sienkiewicz and Scott, 1985), and this projects via the thalamic taste relay to the primary taste cortex in the anterior insula and adjoining frontal operculum (Pritchard et al., 1986). The cortical hierarchy for taste can be thought of as the primary taste cortex in the anterior insula, the secondary taste cortex in the orbitofrontal cortex, and the tertiary taste cortex in the anterior cingulate cortex (Rolls, 2014a, 2015d).

When we consider the different stages of processing in macaques, we find evidence that the breadth of tuning becomes lower, i.e. the neurons become more selective, from the first central relay, the nucleus of the solitary tract, to the primary taste cortex (insula and adjoining frontal operculum), and then to the secondary taste cortex in the orbitofrontal cortex, as shown in Fig. 4.4 (Rolls, 1989d). The tuning of one insula neuron is shown in Fig. 4.5, and its breadth of tuning across the five basic tastes was H=0.4 (with the sparseness a=0.36).

The utility of this computation of a more selective encoding up through the taste hierarchy is that this helps with the computation of sensory-specific satiety, as described in Section 4.2.5; and it facilitates the learning of associations of visual and olfactory with taste stimuli,

[10]The breadth of tuning or entropy measure H used in some taste research is $H = -K\Sigma p_i log_{10} p_i$ where the sum is over the $i = 1$ to n stimuli, p_i is the proportion of the total response over all stimuli to the ith stimulus, and K is set so that if all stimuli produce equal responses, $H = 1$. If the neuron responds to only one stimulus, $H = 0$. The values are numerically similar to the sparseness measure a defined in Equation C.45, except that when a neuron responds to only one stimulus, the lowest value of H is 0, and the lowest value of the sparseness is close to $1/n$.

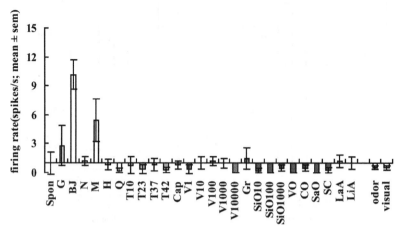

Fig. 4.5 The responses of an insular taste cortex neuron (bo135) with differential responses to taste but no responses to temperature, viscosity, fat, or any of the other stimuli. The neuron did not respond to odor or to the sight of food (visual). The spontaneous (Spon) firing rate is shown by the horizontal line. The taste stimuli were 1 M glucose (G), 0.1 M NaCl (N), 0.1 M MSG (M), 0.01 M HCl (H), and 0.001 M quinine-HCl (Q); the temperature stimuli were T10, T23, T37, and T42 where the number indicates the temperature in degrees celsius; the viscosity stimuli were V1, V10, V100, V1000, and V10000 where the numeral indicates the viscosity in centiPoise at 23°C; fat texture stimuli were SiO10, SiO100, SiO1000 (silicone oil with the viscosity indicated), vegetable oil (VO), coconut oil (CO), and safflower oil (SaO). BJ. fruit juice; Cap, 10 μM capsaicin; LaA, 0.1 mM lauric acid; LiA, 0.1 mM linoleic acid; Gr, the gritty stimulus. (After Verhagen,J.V., Kadohisa,M., and Rolls, E. T. (2004) The primate insular/opercular taste cortex: neuronal representations of the viscosity, fat texture, grittiness, temperature, and taste of foods. Journal of Neurophysiology 92: 1685–1699. © American Physiological Society.)

because the capacity of a pattern associator is higher with sparse representations, as described in Section B.2.

4.2.3 The primary, insular, taste cortex represents what taste is present and its intensity

In the primary gustatory cortex of primates in the frontal operculum and insula, neurons are more sharply tuned to gustatory stimuli than in the nucleus of the solitary tract, with some neurons responding, for example, primarily to sweet, and much less to salt, bitter, or sour stimuli (Scott, Yaxley, Sienkiewicz and Rolls, 1986a; Yaxley, Rolls and Sienkiewicz, 1990) (as illustrated in Figs. 4.5 and 4.4).

Hunger does not influence the magnitude of neuronal responses to gustatory stimuli in the primary taste cortex, so taste reward is not represented in the primary taste cortex (Rolls, Scott, Sienkiewicz and Yaxley, 1988; Yaxley, Rolls and Sienkiewicz, 1988).

The firing rates of the neurons in the primary taste cortex increase with stimulus concentration (Scott et al., 1986a; Yaxley et al., 1990). Consistent with these neuronal findings in macaques, activations in the human insular primary taste cortex are linearly related to the subjective intensity of the taste (which depends on the concentration of the tastant (Rolls, Rolls and Rowe, 1983a)) and not to the pleasantness rating (Fig. 4.13) (Grabenhorst and Rolls, 2008). Further, activations in the human insular primary taste cortex are related to the concentration of the tastant, for example monosodium glutamate (Grabenhorst, Rolls and Bilderbeck, 2008a). Activation of the human insular cortex by taste is illustrated in Fig. 4.6 and is further described in Section 4.2.8.

Some of the computational advantages of what is being computed and represented in the primary taste cortex are described in the second paragraph of Section 4.2.1.

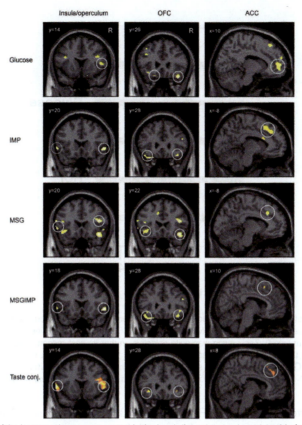

Fig. 4.6 Activation of the human primary taste cortex in the insula/frontal operculum; the orbitofrontal cortex (OFC); and the anterior cingulate cortex (ACC) by taste. The stimuli used included glucose, two umami taste stimuli (monosodium glutamate (MSG) and inosine monophosphate (IMP)), and a mixture of the two umami stimuli. Taste conj. refers to a conjunction analysis over all the taste stimuli. (Reproduced from I. E. T. De Araujo, M. L. Kringelbach, E. T. Rolls, and P. Hobden (2003) Representation of umami taste in the human brain. Journal of Neurophysiology 90: 313–319. © The American Physiological Society.)

4.2.4 The secondary, orbitofrontal, taste cortex, and its representation of the reward value and pleasantness of taste

A secondary cortical taste area has been discovered in the caudolateral orbitofrontal cortex of the primate in which gustatory neurons can be even more finely tuned to particular taste (and oral texture) stimuli (Rolls, Yaxley and Sienkiewicz, 1990; Rolls and Treves, 1990; Rolls, Sienkiewicz and Yaxley, 1989d; Verhagen, Rolls and Kadohisa, 2003; Rolls, Verhagen and Kadohisa, 2003e; Kadohisa, Rolls and Verhagen, 2004, 2005a; Rolls, Critchley, Verhagen and Kadohisa, 2010a) (as illustrated in Figs. 4.7, 4.8, and 4.4). In addition to representations of the 'prototypical' taste stimuli sweet, salt, bitter, and sour, different neurons in this region respond to other taste stimuli including umami or delicious savory taste as exemplified by monosodium glutamate which is present in tomatoes, mushroom, fish and meat, and human mothers' milk (Baylis and Rolls, 1991; Rolls, 1996b; Rolls et al., 1998a), with corresponding activations in humans (De Araujo, Kringelbach, Rolls and Hobden, 2003b). Umami is a component of many foods which helps to make them taste pleasant, especially when the umami taste is paired with a consonant savoury odor (Rolls, Critchley, Browning and Hernadi, 1998a; McCabe and Rolls, 2007; Rolls, 2009b). In addition, water in the mouth activates some orbitofrontal cortex neurons (Rolls et al., 1990).

There is also evidence from functional neuroimaging that taste can activate the human

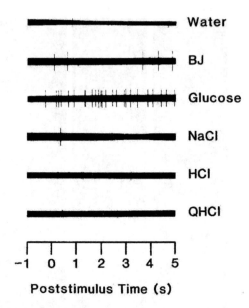

Fig. 4.7 Examples of the responses recorded from one orbitofrontal taste cortex neuron to the six taste stimuli, water, 20% blackcurrant juice (BJ), 1 M glucose, 1 M NaCl, 0.01 M HCl, and 0.001 M quinine HCl (QHCl). The stimuli were placed in the mouth at time 0. The neuron was quite selective, in that its best response was to glucose, even though the complex flavor of the blackcurrant juice included sweet taste. (Reproduced from E. T. Rolls, S. Yaxley and Z. J. Sienkiewicz (1990) Gustatory responses of single neurons in the caudolateral orbitofrontal cortex of the macaque monkey. Journal of Neurophysiology 64: 1055–1066. © The American Physiological Society.)

orbitofrontal cortex. For example, Francis, Rolls, Bowtell, McGlone, O'Doherty, Browning, Clare and Smith (1999) showed that the taste of glucose can activate the human orbitofrontal cortex, and O'Doherty, Rolls, Francis, Bowtell and McGlone (2001b) showed that the taste of glucose and salt activate nearby but separate parts of the human orbitofrontal cortex. De Araujo, Kringelbach, Rolls and Hobden (2003b) showed that umami taste (the taste of protein) as exemplified by monosodium glutamate is represented in the human orbitofrontal cortex as well as in the primary taste cortex as shown by functional magnetic resonance imaging (fMRI) (Fig. 4.6). The taste effect of monosodium glutamate (present in e.g. tomato, green vegetables, fish, and human breast milk) was enhanced in an anterior part of the orbitofrontal cortex in particular by combining it with the nucleotide inosine monophosphate (present in e.g. meat and some fish including tuna), and this provides evidence that the activations found in the orbitofrontal cortex are closely related to subjectively reported taste effects (Rolls, 2009b; Rolls and Grabenhorst, 2008). Small and colleagues have also described activation of the orbitofrontal cortex by taste (Small et al., 1999, 2007).

Another fundamental computation takes place in the primate secondary taste cortex in the orbitofrontal cortex, a transform from the representation about the identity of the taste and texture of stimuli in the primary taste cortex that is independent of reward value and pleasantness, to a representation of the reward value and pleasantness of the taste in the secondary taste cortex. In particular, in the primate orbitofrontal cortex, it is found that the responses of taste neurons to the particular food with which a monkey is fed to satiety decrease to zero (Rolls, Sienkiewicz and Yaxley, 1989d). An example is shown in Fig. 4.8. This neuron reduced its responses to the taste of glucose during the course of feeding as much glucose as the monkey wanted to drink. When the monkey was fully satiated, and did not want to drink any more glucose, the neuron no longer responded to the taste of glucose. Thus the responses of these neurons decrease to zero when the reward value of the food decreases to zero, and

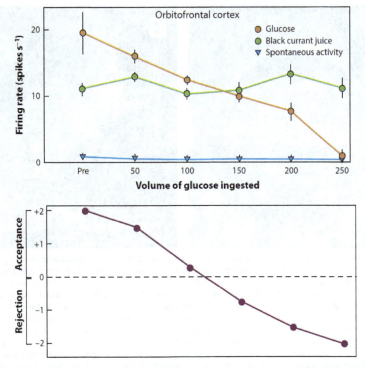

Fig. 4.8 The effect of feeding to satiety with glucose solution on the responses (rate ± s.e.m.) of a neuron in the secondary taste cortex to the taste of glucose (open circles) and of blackcurrant juice (BJ). The spontaneous firing rate is also indicated (SA). Below the neuronal response data, the behavioral measure of the acceptance or rejection of the solution on a scale from +2 (strong acceptance) to −2 (strong rejection) is shown. The solution used to feed to satiety was 20% glucose. The monkey was fed 50 ml of the solution at each stage of the experiment as indicated along the abscissa, until he was satiated as shown by whether he accepted or rejected the solution. Pre is the firing rate of the neuron before the satiety experiment started. (Reproduced with permission from Rolls, E. T., Sienkiewicz, Z. J. and Yaxley, S. (1989) Hunger modulates the responses to gustatory stimuli of single neurons in the caudolateral orbitofrontal cortex of the macaque monkey. European Journal of Neuroscience 1: 53–60. Copyright © Federation of European Neuroscience Societies and John Wiley and Sons.)

they represent reward value. Further evidence that this is a representation of economic value is described in Chapter 11.

4.2.5 Sensory-specific satiety is computed in the orbitofrontal cortex

The neuron illustrated in Fig. 4.8 still responded to another food, blackcurrant juice, after the monkey had been fed to satiety with glucose, and the monkey chose to eat the blackcurrant juice, and other foods. This is typical or orbitofrontal cortex neurons (Rolls et al., 1989d). Thus the modulation of the responses of these orbitofrontal cortex taste neurons occurs in a sensory-specific way, and they represent *reward value in a sensory-specific way*.

In humans, there is evidence that the reward value, and, what can be directly reported in humans, the subjective pleasantness, of food is represented in the orbitofrontal cortex. The evidence comes from an fMRI study in which humans rated the pleasantness of the flavor of chocolate milk and tomato juice, and then ate one of these foods to satiety. It was found that the subjective pleasantness of the flavor of the food eaten to satiety decreased, and that this decrease in pleasantness was reflected in decreased activation in the orbitofrontal cortex (Kringelbach, O'Doherty, Rolls and Andrews, 2003) (see Fig. 4.9). (This was measured in a functional magnetic resonance imaging (fMRI) investigation in which the activation as reflected by the blood oxygenation-level dependent (BOLD) signal was measured, which re-

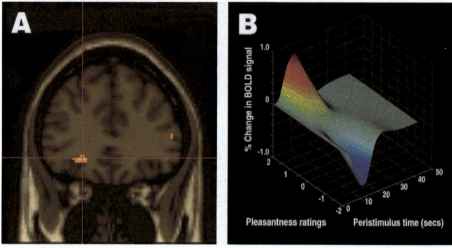

Fig. 4.9 Areas of the human orbitofrontal cortex with activations correlating with pleasantness ratings for food in the mouth. (A) Coronal section through the region of the orbitofrontal cortex from the random effects group analysis showing the peak in the left orbitofrontal cortex (Talairach co-ordinates X,Y,Z=[−22 34 −8], z-score=4.06), in which the BOLD signal in the voxels shown in yellow was significantly correlated with the subjects' subjective pleasantness ratings of the foods throughout an experiment in which the subjects were hungry and found the food pleasant, and were then fed to satiety with the food, after which the pleasantness of the food decreased to neutral or slightly unpleasant. The design was a sensory-specific satiety design, and the pleasantness of the food not eaten in the meal, and the BOLD activation in the orbitofrontal cortex, were not altered by eating the other food to satiety. The two foods were tomato juice and chocolate milk. (B) Plot of the magnitude of the fitted haemodynamic response from a representative single subject against the subjective pleasantness ratings (on a scale from −2 to +2) and peristimulus time in seconds. (Reproduced from M.L. Kringelbach, J.O'Doherty, E.T. Rolls and C. Andrews (2003) Activation of the human orbitofrontal cortex to a liquid food stimulus is correlated with its subjective pleasantness. Cerebral Cortex 13: 1064–1071. Copyright © Oxford University Press.)

flects increased blood flow due to increased neuronal activity (Stephan et al., 2007; Rolls et al., 2009).) Further evidence that the pleasantness of flavor is represented here is that the pleasantness of the food not eaten to satiety showed very little decrease, and correspondingly the activation of the orbitofrontal cortex to this food not eaten in the meal showed little decrease. The phenomenon itself is called sensory-specific satiety, is an important property of reward systems, and is described in more detail below and by Rolls (2014a).

The experiment of Kringelbach, O'Doherty, Rolls and Andrews (2003) was with a whole food, but further evidence that the pleasantness of taste, or at least a stimulus very closely related to a taste, is represented in the human orbitofrontal cortex is that the orbitofrontal cortex is activated by water in the mouth when thirsty but not when satiated (De Araujo, Kringelbach, Rolls and McGlone, 2003c). Thus, the neuroimaging findings with a whole food, and with water when thirsty, provide evidence that the activation to taste *per se* in the human orbitofrontal cortex is related to the subjective pleasantness or affective value of taste and flavor, that is, to *pleasure*. Further evidence on reward value for taste is that in fMRI investigations, activations in the human orbitofrontal cortex are linearly related to the subjective pleasantness of the taste (Grabenhorst and Rolls, 2008) (Fig. 4.12).

Sensory-specific satiety is one of the most important factors that affects reward value, and is therefore described briefly here, in the context that it is computed in the orbitofrontal cortex. Sensory-specific satiety is a decrease in the reward value of a stimulus that is at least partly specific to that reward, and is a result of delivering that reward (Rolls, 2014a). Sensory-specific satiety was discovered during neurophysiological experiments on brain mechanisms of reward and satiety by Edmund Rolls and colleagues in 1974. They observed that if a lateral hypothalamic neuron had ceased to respond to a food on which the monkey had been fed to satiety (a discovery described in *The Brain and Reward* (Rolls, 1975)), then the neuron might still respond to a different food (see Rolls (2014a)). This occurred for neurons with responses associated with the taste (Rolls, 1981a,b; Rolls, Murzi, Yaxley, Thorpe and Simpson, 1986) or sight (Rolls, 1981a; Rolls and Rolls, 1982; Rolls, Murzi, Yaxley, Thorpe and Simpson, 1986) of food. Corresponding to this neuronal specificity of the effects of feeding to satiety, the monkey rejected the food on which he had been fed to satiety, but accepted other foods that he had not been fed. The neurophysiological finding was published for example in Rolls (1981a) and Rolls, Murzi, Yaxley, Thorpe and Simpson (1986). This is now described as a devaluation procedure, and provides evidence that these, and orbitofrontal cortex neurons that provide inputs to the lateral hypothalamus, encode **value**.

Subsequent research showed that sensory-specific satiety is present (and computed (Rolls, 2014a, 2016b)) in the orbitofrontal cortex (Rolls, Sienkiewicz and Yaxley, 1989d; Critchley and Rolls, 1996a; Kringelbach, O'Doherty, Rolls and Andrews, 2003) but not in earlier cortical areas such as the insula (Rolls, Scott, Sienkiewicz and Yaxley, 1988; Yaxley, Rolls and Sienkiewicz, 1988).

Following the neurophysiological discovery of sensory-specific satiety, I initiated a series of studies on sensory-specific satiety in humans, starting with an undergraduate practical class at Oxford, with Barbara Rolls participating, and also my daughter (Rolls and Rolls, 1997). We showed that sensory-specific satiety is one of the most important factors influencing in humans what and how much is ingested in a meal (Rolls and Rolls, 1982; Rolls et al., 1981b,c, 1982c,b; Rolls and Rolls, 1997; Rolls, 1999a, 2014a), showed that olfactory sensory-specific satiety can be produced in part by merely sniffing a food for as long as it would typically be eaten in a meal (Rolls and Rolls, 1997), and showed that there is a long-term form of sensory-specific satiety (Rolls and de Waal, 1985). Sensory-specific satiety is not a sensory adaptation, in that it does not occur in primary taste cortical areas, and the inferior temporal visual cortex (Rolls et al., 1977), and in that there is little decline in the intensity of the stimulus even though the pleasantness declines greatly (Rolls et al., 1983a). The hypothesis is that sensory-specific satiety is produced by adaptation of active afferent synapses onto neurons in the orbitofrontal cortex that represent reward value (Rolls, 2014a). I have argued that it is one of the factors that as a result of variety can overstimulate food intake and be associated with obesity, and is one of many factors that may all need to be taken into account in controlling food intake to prevent or minimize obesity (Rolls, 2016g, 2014a, 2018a, 2012f, 2023f; Rolls et al., 2023g). The evolutionary adaptive value of sensory-specific satiety is that it leads to animals not only eating a variety of food and maintaining good nutrition, but also in performing a whole set of different rewarded behaviors which promote successful reproduction and passing the successful set of genes into the next generation (Rolls, 2014a). Moreover, although sensory-specific satiety is a property of all reward systems, for the reason given, it is not a property of any punishment system, in that aversive stimuli such as a thorn on the foot must be the subject of action, for any single punishing event could threaten reproductive success making any sensory-specific reductions that might occur for punishers highly maladaptive (Rolls, 2014a).

Further evidence on the nature of the taste-related value representations, analyzed in a neuroeconomic framework, is described in Chapter 11.

Some of the computational advantages of what is being computed and represented in the primary taste cortex are described in the second paragraph of Section 4.2.1.

4.2.6 Oral texture is represented in the primary and secondary taste cortex: viscosity and fat texture

Single neurons in the insular primary taste cortex also represent the viscosity (measured with carboxymethylcellulose) and temperature of stimuli in the mouth, and fat texture, but not the sight and smell of food (Verhagen, Kadohisa and Rolls, 2004; Kadohisa, Rolls and Verhagen, 2005a). In humans, the insular primary taste cortex is activated not only by taste (Francis, Rolls, Bowtell, McGlone, O'Doherty, Browning, Clare and Smith, 1999; Small, Zald, Jones-Gotman, Zatorre, Petrides and Evans, 1999; De Araujo, Kringelbach, Rolls and Hobden, 2003b; De Araujo and Rolls, 2004; De Araujo, Kringelbach, Rolls and McGlone, 2003c; Grabenhorst, Rolls and Bilderbeck, 2008a), but also by oral texture including viscosity (with the activation linearly related to the log of the viscosity) and fat texture (De Araujo and Rolls, 2004), and temperature (Guest et al., 2007).

Some orbitofrontal cortex neurons respond to different combinations of taste and related oral texture stimuli. This shows that in the taste system too, in the hierarchy, neurons become tuned to low order combinations of sensory inputs, in order to separate the input space in a way that allows easy decoding by dot product decoding, allows specific tastes to be associated with particular stimuli in other modalities including olfaction and vision, and allows for sensory-specific satiety, as will soon be shown. (The computational mechanisms is probably competitive learning, as described in Section 1.9 and Chapter 2). Examples of the tuning of orbitofrontal cortex neurons to different combinations of taste and oral texture are illustrated in Fig. 4.10. For example, the neuron illustrated in Fig. 4.10 (lower) responded to the taste of sweet (glucose, blackcurrant juice BJ, sour (HCl), and bitter (quinine) but not to the taste of salt (NaCl) or umami (monosodium glutamate, MSG); to viscosity (as altered parametrically using the standard food thickening agent carboxymethylcellulose made up in viscosities of 1–10,000 cPoise (Rolls, Verhagen and Kadohisa, 2003e), where 10,000 cP is approximately the viscosity of toothpaste); did not respond to fat in the mouth (oils); and did respond to capsaicin (chilli pepper). In contrast, the neuron shown in the upper part of Fig. 4.10 had no response to taste; did respond to oral viscosity; did respond to oral fat (see Rolls, Critchley, Browning, Hernadi and Lenard (1999a) and Verhagen, Rolls and Kadohisa (2003)); and did not respond to capsaicin. This combinatorial encoding in the taste and oral texture system is important in the mechanism of the fundamental property of reward systems, sensory-specific satiety, as described in Section 4.2.5.

These findings have been extended to humans, with the finding with fMRI that activation of the orbitofrontal cortex and pregenual cingulate cortex is produced by the texture of fat in the mouth (De Araujo and Rolls, 2004). Moreover, activations in the orbitofrontal cortex and pregenual cingulate cortex are correlated with the pleasantness of fat texture in the mouth (Grabenhorst, Rolls, Parris and D'Souza, 2010b).

Texture in the mouth is an important indicator of whether fat is present in the food, which is important not only as a high value energy source, but also as a potential source of essential fatty acids. In the orbitofrontal cortex, Rolls, Critchley, Browning, Hernadi and Lenard (1999a) discovered a population of neurons that responds when fat is in the mouth. The fat-related responses of these neurons are produced at least in part by the texture of the food rather than by chemical receptors sensitive to certain chemicals, in that such neurons typically respond not only to foods such as cream and milk containing fat, but also to paraffin oil (which is a pure hydrocarbon) and to silicone oil (which contains $Si(CH_3)_2O)_n$) (Rolls et al., 1999a).

To investigate the bases of the responses of fat-sensitive neurons, we measured the correlations between their responses and physical measures of the properties of the set of stimuli, including viscosity and the coefficient of sliding friction (Rolls, Mills, Norton, Lazidis and

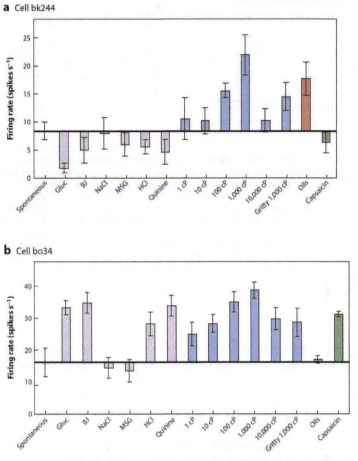

Fig. 4.10 Above. Firing rates (mean ± s.e.m.) of orbitofrontal cortex viscosity-sensitive neuron bk244 which did not have taste responses. The firing rates are shown to the viscosity series (carboxymethylcellulose in the range 1–10,000 centiPoise), to the gritty stimulus (carboxymethylcellulose with Fillite microspheres), to the taste stimuli 1 M glucose (Gluc), 0.1 M NaCl, 0.1 M MSG , 0.01 M HCl and 0.001 M QuinineHCl, and to fruit juice (BJ). Spont = spontaneous firing rate. Below. Firing rates (mean ± s.e.m.) of viscosity-sensitive neuron bo34 which had no response to the oils (mineral oil, vegetable oil, safflower oil and coconut oil, which have viscosities which are all close to 50 cP). The neuron did not respond to the gritty stimulus in a way that was unexpected given the viscosity of the stimulus, was taste tuned, and did respond to capsaicin. (Reproduced from E. T. Rolls, J. V. Verhagen, and M. Kadohisa (2003) Representations of the texture of food in the primate orbitofrontal cortex: neurons responding to viscosity, grittiness, and capsaicin. *Journal of Neurophysiology* 90: 3711–3724, © The American Physiological Society.)

Norton, 2018b). The coefficient of sliding friction is the force required to slide two surfaces divided by the force normal to the surfaces. This is also known as kinetic or dynamic friction. It measures effectively the lubricity or the slipperiness of a substance. We found that some fat-sensitive neurons increased their firing rates linearly as the coefficient of sliding friction of the stimuli became smaller. Another population of neurons had their firing rates non-linearly related to the coefficient of sliding friction, and increased their rates only when the coefficient of sliding friction became less than 0.04, and were thus highly selective to the fats and the non-fat oils (see example in Fig. 4.11) (Rolls et al., 2018b). These neurons were more likely to be found in the orbitofrontal cortex than the primary taste cortex, consistent with the hypothesis of non-linear encoding in hierarchical cortical systems (Rolls, 2016b). Another population of neurons had responses that were inhibited by fat: they had responses that increased linearly with the coefficient of sliding friction. The activity of these fat-sensitive

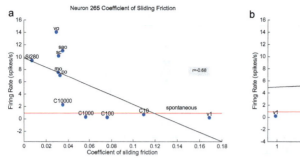
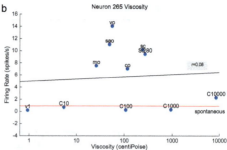

Fig. 4.11 An orbitofrontal cortex neuron with responses non-linearly correlated with decreases in the coefficient of sliding friction (a). The neuron responds almost not at all until the coefficient of sliding friction falls below 0.04. The neuron is thus very selective for fat texture, because of its non-linear response in relation to the coefficient of sliding friction. The linear regression line has a correlation of r = -0.68 (p=0.02). (b): There is a much weaker relation to viscosity (r = 0.08, p=0.82), with the oils producing a larger response than predicted linearly. Further, a regression line through the non-oil stimuli would have a lower slope. C10-C10000: carboxymethyl cellulose with the nominal viscosity of 10, 100, 1000 and 10,000 cP. v1: water (1 cP). co: coconut oil; mo: mineral oil; sao: safflower oil; vo: vegetable oil; sc: single cream. Si280: silicone oil with a nominal viscosity of 280 cP. Li: linoleic acid; La; lauric acid. The horizontal red line indicates the spontaneous firing rate. The Pearson correlation between the firing rate of each neuron and (a) the coefficient of sliding friction, and (b) the viscosity, was calculated to show to what extent the firing of a neuron reflected one or other of these measures. Linear regression lines are shown in the Figure for how the firing rates were related to the coefficient of sliding friction, or to the log of the viscosity. (Reproduced from Edmund T Rolls, Tom Mills, Abigail B Norton, Aris Lazidis, and Ian T Norton (2018) The Neuronal Encoding of Oral Fat by the Coefficient of Sliding Friction in the Cerebral Cortex and Amygdala. Cerebral Cortex 28: 4080-4089.)

neurons was not closely related to viscosity. The responses of these neurons are related to the reward value of fat in the mouth, in that the responses decrease to zero during feeding to satiety (Rolls, Critchley, Browning, Hernadi and Lenard, 1999a). The fat-sensitive neurons did not have responses to lauric or linoleic acid, so their responses were not related to fatty acid sensing. A separate population of neurons did have responses to linoleic or lauric fatty acids, but not to fat in the mouth. Their responses may be related to "off tastes" of food produced for example by butyric acid, which food manufacturers aim to minimize in foods (Rolls, 2020c). Another population of neurons had responses related to the log of viscosity (which correlates with subjective ratings of food thickness (Kadohisa et al., 2005a)), but not with the coefficient of sliding friction (Rolls et al., 2018b).

This new understanding of the representation of oral fat by the coefficient of sliding friction in the cerebral cortex opens the way for the systematic development of foods with the pleasant mouth-feel of fat, together with ideal nutritional content, and has great potential to contribute to healthy eating and a healthy body weight (Rolls et al., 2018b; Rolls, 2020c).

Thus we have seen that what is represented in the primary and secondary taste cortex in terms of texture plays an important role in detecting key nutrients such as fat in a food in the mouth.

4.2.7 Vision and olfaction converge using associative learning with taste to represent flavor in the secondary but not primary taste cortex

As illustrated in Fig. 4.5, the odor and sight of food and other stimuli does not activate neurons in the insular primary taste cortex (Verhagen, Kadohisa and Rolls, 2004). A computational advantage of what is represented is thereby that taste can be represented independently of flavor (where flavor is produced by multimodal inputs that typically involve at least taste and odor), and this is likely to be important in the identification and selection of particular foods.

However, in the secondary taste cortex in the orbitofrontal cortex, many neurons respond to combinations of taste and olfactory stimuli (Rolls and Baylis, 1994), and their tuning to individual food flavors can be selective. These neurons may learn which odor to respond to by olfactory-to-taste association learning. This was confirmed by reversing the taste with which an odor was associated in the reversal of an olfactory discrimination task. It was found that 73% of the sample of neurons analyzed altered the way in which they responded to odor when the taste reinforcer association of the odor was reversed (Rolls, Critchley, Mason and Wakeman, 1996b). Reversal was shown by 25% of the neurons, and 48% altered their activity in that they no longer discriminated after the reversal. These latter neurons thus respond to a particular odor only if it is associated with a taste reward, and not when it is associated with the taste of salt, a punisher. They do not respond to the other odor in the task when it is associated with reward. Thus they respond to a particular combination of an odor, and its being associated with taste reward and not a taste punisher. They may be described as *conditional olfactory-reward neurons*, and may be important in the mechanism by which stimulus–reinforcer (in this case olfactory-to-taste) reversal learning occurs (Deco and Rolls, 2005b), as described in Section 11.5.3.

The human orbitofrontal cortex also reflects the convergence of taste and olfactory inputs, as shown for example by the fact that activations in the human medial orbitofrontal cortex are correlated with both the cross-modal consonance of combined taste and olfactory stimuli (high for example for sweet taste and strawberry odor), as well as for the pleasantness of the combinations (De Araujo, Rolls, Kringelbach, McGlone and Phillips, 2003a). In addition, the combination of monosodium glutamate taste and a consonant savoury odor produced a supralinear effect in the medial orbitofrontal cortex to produce the rich delicious flavor of umami that makes many foods pleasant that are rich in protein (McCabe and Rolls, 2007; Rolls, 2009b).

We have been able to show that there is a major visual input to many neurons in the orbitofrontal cortex, and that what is represented by these neurons is in many cases the reinforcer (reward or punisher) association of visual stimuli. Many of these neurons reflect the relative preference or reward value of different visual stimuli, in that their responses decrease to zero to the sight of one food on which the monkey is being fed to satiety, but remain unchanged to the sight of other food stimuli. In this sense the visual reinforcement-related neurons predict the reward value that is available from the primary reinforcer, the taste. The visual input is from the ventral, temporal lobe, visual stream concerned with 'what' object is being seen, in that orbitofrontal visual neurons frequently respond differentially to objects or images (but depending on their reward association) (Thorpe, Rolls and Maddison, 1983; Rolls, Critchley, Mason and Wakeman, 1996b). The primary reinforcer that has been used is taste.

The fact that these neurons represent the reinforcer associations of visual stimuli and hence the expected value has been shown to be the case in formal investigations of the activity of orbitofrontal cortex visual neurons, which in many cases reverse their responses to visual stimuli when the taste with which the visual stimulus is associated is reversed by the experimenter (Thorpe, Rolls and Maddison, 1983; Rolls, Critchley, Mason and Wakeman, 1996b). An example of the responses of an orbitofrontal cortex neuron that reversed the visual stimulus to which it responded during reward reversal is shown in Fig. 11.5.

This reversal by orbitofrontal visual neurons can be very fast, in as little as one trial, and this is a key computation of the orbitofrontal cortex, for it is rule-based, as described in Chapter 11.

The research described in this section shows that a key computation performed in the orbitofrontal cortex is association of taste with visual and olfactory stimuli, and that this occurs with learning that can allow rapid reversal. These computations are very important for enabling primates with their well developed visual system to find foods based on their sight and odor, which is highly adaptive. It enables the sight of food to be treated as a goal for

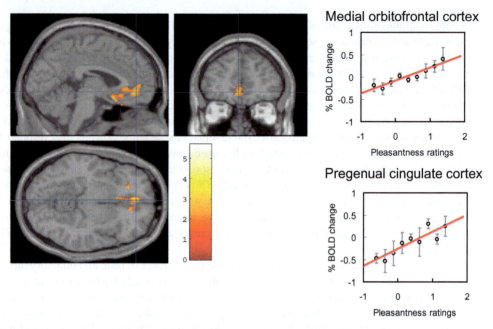

Fig. 4.12 Top-down attention and emotion. Effect of paying attention to the pleasantness of a taste. Left: A significant difference related to the taste period was found in the medial orbitofrontal cortex at [-6 14 -20] z=3.81 p<0.003 (towards the back of the area of activation shown) and in the pregenual cingulate cortex at [-4 46 -8] z=2.90 p<0.04 (at the cursor). Right upper: The correlation between the subjective pleasantness ratings and the activation (% BOLD change) in the orbitofrontal cortex (r=0.94, df=8, p<<0.001). Right lower: The correlation between the pleasantness ratings and the activation (% BOLD change) in the pregenual cingulate cortex r=0.89, df=8, p=0.001). The taste stimulus, monosodium glutamate, was identical on all trials. (Reproduced from Fabian Grabenhorst and Edmund T. Rolls (2008) Selective attention to affective value alters how the brain processes taste stimuli. European Journal of Neuroscience 27: 723–729.)

action, with the action to be performed learned by the cingulate cortex based on the value input from the orbitofrontal cortex, as described in Chapter 12. The same principles of visual to reinforcer learning apply to many stimuli other than taste, making the orbitofrontal cortex a key brain area for the computation of value, as described in Chapter 11.

4.2.8 Top-down attention and cognition can modulate taste and flavor representations in the taste cortical areas

Attentional instructions at a very high, linguistic, level (e.g. 'pay attention to and rate intensity' vs 'pay attention to and rate pleasantness') have a top-down modulatory influence on intensity representations in the primary taste cortex, and on value representations in the orbitofrontal cortex and anterior cingulate cortex. The attentional instructions can bias processing for a stimulus between streams involving sensory processing areas such as the insular taste cortex and pyriform primary olfactory cortex, and a stream through the orbitofrontal and cingulate cortices that processes value and affect.

In an investigation of the effects of selective attention to value and affect vs intensity on taste processing, when subjects were instructed to remember and rate the pleasantness of a savoury taste stimulus, 0.1 M monosodium glutamate, activations were greater in the medial orbitofrontal and pregenual cingulate cortex than when subjects were instructed to remember and rate the intensity of the taste (Grabenhorst and Rolls, 2008) (Fig. 4.12). When the subjects were instructed to remember and rate the intensity, activations were greater in the insular taste cortex and a mid-insular cortex region (Fig. 4.13).

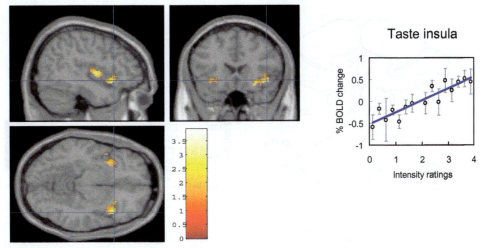

Fig. 4.13 Top-down attention and emotion. Left: Effect of paying attention to the intensity of a taste. Top: A significant difference related to the taste period was found in the taste insula at [42 18 -14] z=2.42 p<0.05 (indicated by the cursor) and in the mid insula at [40 -2 4] z=3.03 p<0.025. Right: The correlation between the intensity ratings and the activation (% BOLD change) in the taste insula (r=0.91, df=14, p<<0.001). The taste stimulus, monosodium glutamate, was identical on all trials. (Reproduced from Fabian Grabenhorst and Edmund T. Rolls (2008) Selective attention to affective value alters how the brain processes taste stimuli. European Journal of Neuroscience 27: 723–729.)

In an investigation of top-down cognitive modulation of affective processing in another modality, taste, it was found that activations related to the affective value of umami (delicious savoury) taste and flavor (as shown by correlations with pleasantness ratings) in the orbitofrontal cortex were modulated by word-level descriptors (Grabenhorst, Rolls and Bilderbeck, 2008a). The cognitive modulation was produced by presenting the taste with a visual word-level descriptor such as 'rich and delicious flavor' or 'boiled vegetable water' to influence the affective value of the taste, with the identical taste or flavor stimulus delivered for the different types of cognitive description. Affect-related activations to taste were modulated in a region that receives from the orbitofrontal cortex, the pregenual cingulate cortex, and to taste and flavor in another region that receives from the orbitofrontal cortex, the ventral striatum. Affect-related cognitive modulations were not found in the insular taste cortex, where the intensity but not the pleasantness of the taste was represented. Thus top-down language-level cognitive effects reach far down into the earliest cortical areas that represent the appetitive value of taste and flavor, and this type of modulation may be important in appetite control (Rolls, 2012f, 2016g).

Thus, depending on the context in which tastes are presented and whether affect is relevant, the brain responds to a taste differently. These findings show that when cognition or attention influences affective value, the brain systems engaged to represent a sensory stimulus are different from those engaged when attention is directed to the physical properties of a stimulus such as its intensity. The computational utility of this is that it provides a mechanism for focussing the activity of the brain on the task at hand to optimize, in the present case, what aspects of stimuli should be enhanced as part of the process of leading to optimized behavioral and subjective responses based on the environmental context. It is also of great interest that these word-level cognitive and attentional modulators have top-down effects on the orbitofrontal cortex, and even the primary taste cortex.

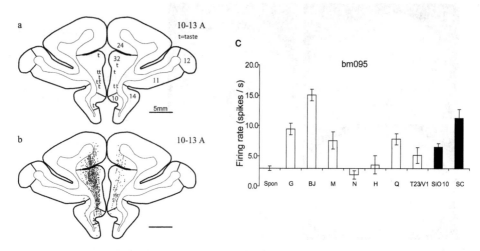

Fig. 4.14 Pregenual cortex taste neurons. The reconstructed positions of the anterior cingulate neurons with taste (t) responses, together with the cytoarchitectonic boundaries determined by Carmichael and Price (1994). Most (11/12) of the taste neurons were in the pregenual cingulate cortex (area 32), as shown. The neurons are shown on a coronal section at 12 mm anterior (A) to the sphenoid reference point. b. The locations of all the 749 neurons recorded in the anterior cingulate region in this study are indicated to show the regions sampled. c. Responses of a pregenual cingulate cortex neuron (bm095) with differential responses to tastes and oral fat texture stimuli. The mean ($\pm$ sem) firing rate responses to each stimulus calculated in a 5 s period over several trials are shown. The spontaneous (Spon) firing rate of 3 spikes/s is shown by the horizontal line, with the responses indicated relative to this line. The taste stimuli were 1 M glucose (G), blackcurrant fruit juice (BJ), 0.1 M NaCl (N), 0.1 M MSG (M), 0.01 M HCl (H) and 0.001 M QuinineHCl (Q); water (T23/V1); single cream (SC); and silicone oil with a viscosity of 10 cP (SiO10). The neuron had significantly different responses to the different stimuli as shown by a one-way ANOVA (F[9,46]=17.7, $p < 10^{-10}$). (Data from E.T.Rolls, P.Gabbott, J.Verhagen, and M.Kadohisa. Reproduced from Rolls, E.T. (2008) Functions of the orbitofrontal and pregenual cingulate cortex in taste, olfaction, appetite and emotion. Acta Physiologica Hungarica 95: 131–164.)

4.2.9 The tertiary taste cortex in the anterior cingulate cortex provides the rewards for action-reward outcome learning

The orbitofrontal cortex projects to the anterior cingulate cortex (Carmichael and Price, 1995a; Morecraft and Tanji, 2009; Vogt, 2009), where taste neurons are also found in what is thereby a tertiary taste cortical area (Rolls, 2008c, 2009a). For example, Gabbott, Verhagen, Kadohisa and Rolls found neurons in the pregenual cingulate cortex that respond to taste (see example in Fig. 4.14), and it was demonstrated that the representation is of reward value, for devaluation by feeding to satiety selectively decreased neuronal responses to the food with which the animal was satiated (Rolls, 2008c, 2014a). Consistently, in humans (pleasant) sweet taste also activates the most anterior part of the anterior cingulate cortex, the pregenual cingulate cortex (De Araujo and Rolls, 2004; De Araujo, Kringelbach, Rolls and Hobden, 2003b). Less pleasant tastes activate an anterior cingulate cortex region just posterior and dorsal to this just above the corpus callosum, the supracallosal anterior cingulate cortex (De Araujo and Rolls, 2004; De Araujo, Kringelbach, Rolls and Hobden, 2003b; Rolls, 2019e; Grabenhorst and Rolls, 2011) (Chapter 12).

So far, this anterior cingulate cortex region appears to be a re-representation of what is already represented in the orbitofrontal cortex. But there is a large difference that occurs in this tertiary level of the taste cortical hierarchy. Whereas the orbitofrontal cortex represents the reward value of the sensory stimulus of taste (and other sensory stimuli) with little activity related to movements, motor events, and actions (Thorpe, Rolls and Maddison, 1983; Rolls, Critchley, Mason and Wakeman, 1996b; Critchley and Rolls, 1996a; Rolls and Baylis, 1994; Rolls, 2005a; Wallis and Miller, 2003; Padoa-Schioppa and Assad, 2006; Rolls, 2014a), in the anterior and midcingulate cortex there are representations also of movements, actions, and errors about actions (Matsumoto et al., 2007; Luk and Wallis, 2009). Moreover, lesions to the cingulate cortex influence action selection when it is guided by the reward value of the goal, and this provides some of the evidence that the anterior cingulate cortex is involved in learning associations between actions and the reward (or punishment) outcome (Rushworth et al., 2004, 2011; Grabenhorst and Rolls, 2011; Rolls, 2014a, 2019e,c).

Thus the anterior cingulate stage of the taste cortical hierarchy can be conceptualized computationally as the level at which the representation of sensory reward value is interfaced to actions (Chapter 12). In primates, stimulus valuation performed in the orbitofrontal cortex is kept separate from motor and action systems. In terms of hierarchical organization, the impact is that the orbitofrontal cortex specialises in reward value representations and learns about the value of sensory stimuli using as we shall see information from all sensory modalities, so it performs one type of computation in which the expected reward value of a visual stimulus can be recomputed in one trial if the taste associated with the visual stimulus changes (Chapter 11). The next stage of the hierarchy, the anterior cingulate cortex, then follows the principle of further convergence as one progresses up the hierarchy, in this case convergence between the value of sensory stimuli and the actions needed to obtain them, which is a separate and typically slower learning process because it involves trial and error learning (Chapter 12), whereas the orbitofrontal cortex can perform its sensory-sensory processes by association in what can be as little as one trial (Rolls, 2019e) (Chapter 11).

4.2.10 Taste, oral texture and flavor provide the rewards for eating, and the gut provides satiety signals

Rewards can be defined as stimuli for which an individual (human or animal) will work instrumentally with an arbitrary action (Rolls, 2014a), and can be shown to be goal-directed in that the actions cease immediately the reward is devalued, for example by feeding to satiety. Reward-guided behavior can thus be distinguished from stimulus-response habits implemented in the basal ganglia (Chapter 16). A reward thus supports goal-directed actions, with brain regions involved in this the anterior cingulate cortex (Section 12.2), which receives information about reward outcome value from the orbitofrontal cortex. The expected value is also signalled by the orbitofrontal cortex, for example by the orbitofrontal cortex neurons that respond to the sight of food (Critchley and Rolls, 1996a; Rolls et al., 1996b).

Oral signals of taste, texture and temperature, and retronasally sensed olfactory effects, implement the reward value of food, with subjective pleasantness or hedonic value correlated with activations in the orbitofrontal cortex and anterior cingulate cortex to taste, olfactory and flavor stimuli, as described above and in Chapters 11 and 5. Part of the evidence comes from sham feeding (Rolls, 2014a). If food that has been eaten just drains out of the stomach or oesophagus and does not reach the intestines, then food remains rewarding, and animals and humans work for long periods for the taste and texture of the food, even though no food reaches the gut (Rolls, 2014a), and the same applies to water reward and drinking when thirsty (Maddison, Wood, Rolls, Rolls and Gibbs, 1980). This provides evidence that gut and postabsorptive signals are necessary for satiety, and indeed if the stomach is drained after eating to satiety, eating resumes again immediately, providing clear evidence that gut signals (gastric distension and intestinal stimulation with food) produce satiety (Gibbs, Maddison and Rolls, 1981).

Complementary evidence is that animals including humans work to obtain small quantities of these oral taste and flavor signals, even a few drops, providing clear evidence that taste and smell provide food reward. The converse type of evidence is that food placed directly into the gut or provided intravenously does not produce immediate unconditioned reward with small quantities: very large quantities of food have to be delivered for food provided into the gut to lead to instrumental actions to obtain such gut infusions (Nicolaidis and Rowland, 1977; Sclafani et al., 2003). That is, a reduction in hunger produced by directly placing food into the gut and bypassing taste and smell is not very rewarding. Consistent with this, turning off hunger-related Agrp neurons in the arcuate nucleus of the hypothalamus is not a good reward for instrumental behavior, though it can produce some conditioned preferences for foods or places with which the hunger reduction is associated (Sternson, 2013). Corresponding evidence in humans is that patients in hospital obtain no food reward value or pleasure from being fed intragastrically.

This type of evidence shows clearly with a double dissociation that oral factors such as the taste, texture and flavor of food produce the reward for which humans and animals work, and that gut and post-absorptive signals produce satiety (Rolls, 2014a). Further evidence for this is that sensory-specific satiety is for the taste, texture and flavor of food, and not for its nutritional content, as shown by experiments in which for example different sensory stimuli with the same nutritional content provide reward value that is related to the sensory properties of the stimuli, and not to the nutritional content (Rolls, Rolls and Rowe, 1980a; Rolls, Rolls, Rowe and Sweeney, 1981b,a; Rolls, Rolls and Rowe, 1982a; Rolls, Rowe and Rolls, 1982b; Rolls, Rolls and Rowe, 1983a), all based on my discovery of sensory-specific satiety when recording from lateral hypothalamic neurons (Rolls, Perrett and Thorpe, 1980c; Rolls, Murzi, Yaxley, Thorpe and Simpson, 1986). One interesting demonstration of this is that just tasting a food for 15 minutes, or even just smelling a food for 15 minutes, can result in some decrease in its reward value, even though no food is swallowed to enter the stomach or gut (Rolls and Rolls, 1997).

This evidence shows that the reward value, and the subjectively reported pleasantness or hedonic value of food, depends on sensory factors such as taste, texture, flavor and smell, and not on signals directly from the gut, which in any case are too slow to implement the reward value and pleasantness of a tiny taste of food in the mouth, before it has even been swallowed. This evidence further shows that the main factor that produces satiety is food in the gut, which produces gastric distension and gut stimulation by food, with of course an additional sensory-specific contribution to satiety (Rolls, 2014a). Thus satiety signals in the gut, and postabsorptively, including the hormones that result from this, produce satiety, and those satiety signals then alter the reward value of food, implemented as shown here by reductions in the responses of neurons in the orbitofrontal cortex and lateral hypothalamus that show smaller responses to the taste, texture, smell, flavor, and sight of food when the food is eaten to satiety (Rolls, Perrett and Thorpe, 1980c; Rolls, Murzi, Yaxley, Thorpe and Simpson, 1986; Rolls, Sienkiewicz and Yaxley, 1989d; Critchley and Rolls, 1996a; Rolls, 2015d, 2016g).

However, food sensed in the gut after ingestion can produce conditioned (learned) appetite or preference for a food, and can also produce conditioned satiety (Booth, 1985). This was demonstrated by David Booth, who fed participants either high energy sandwiches with flavor 1, and low energy sandwiches with flavor 2. After several days with this pairing, when medium energy sandwiches were provided, subjects ate more of those with flavor 2, as it had previously been paired with low energy nutrition sensed after ingestion. This demonstrates how post-ingestive signals in humans can influence flavor preferences by conditioning. It is important to bear in mind these conditioned appetite and satiety effects when designing low-energy foods, for post-ingestive conditioning is likely to produce some compensation by increasing the amount eaten of such foods.

There is considerable interest in how signals sensed in the gut contribute to these post-ingestive effects of nutrients. When ingested food reaches the gastro-intestinal tract, it produces satiety by producing gastric distension and stimulation of intestinal hormone release (as shown by the absence of satiety in sham feeding when food drains from a gastric or duodenal cannula in primates (Gibbs, Maddison and Rolls, 1981), and the gastric distension only occurs if food enters the duodenum where it activates gut receptors so causing closing of the pyloric sphincter. This is probably an unconditioned satiety effect produced by gastric distension and intestinal hormonal release (Seeley, Kaplan and Grill, 1995). If the distension is reduced at the end of a meal, then feeding resumes very quickly, typically within one minute, in primates (Rolls, 2014a; Gibbs et al., 1981). Further evidence is that intraduodenal infusions of food produce satiety (Gibbs et al., 1981). In addition to unconditioned effects of food in the gut, there are also conditioned effects whereby the metabolic and other nutritive consequences of the ingestion of a flavor can influence the reward value of the flavor later, in for example conditioned appetite (Booth, 1985), sometimes referred to as appetition (Sclafani, 2013), with some of the mechanisms described next.

When food enters the gastro-intestinal (GI) tract it activates a wide range of gut receptors including gut taste receptors, which stimulate locally the release of peptides such as CCK, PYY), ghrelin and GLP-1 from endocrine cells (Depoortere, 2014; Kokrashvili et al., 2009b,a; Margolskee et al., 2007), which may be involved in the regulation of food intake (Price and Bloom, 2014; Hussain and Bloom, 2013; Parker et al., 2014), though with the evidence in humans not very clear (Crooks et al., 2021; Lim and Poppitt, 2019). The gut sensing mechanisms, and their role in conditioned appetite, are reviewed elsewhere (Ackroff and Sclafani, 2014; Sclafani, 2013; Kadohisa, 2015; Berthoud, Morrison, Ackroff and Sclafani, 2021). Many of these studies have been on conditioned preferences produced by food in the GI tract. It will be of interest in future research to analyze in addition how visceral signals can produce conditioned satiety for the flavor with which they are paired. It is of interest to develop our understanding of conditioned satiety and conditioned appetite and the role of gut signals in food reward, for this is relevant to food intake control and its disorders (Han, Tellez, Perkins, Perez, Qu, Ferreira, Ferreira, Quinn, Liu, Gao, Kaelberer, Bohorquez, Shammah-Lagnado, de Lartigue and de Araujo, 2018; De Araujo, Schatzker and Small, 2020; Berthoud, Morrison, Ackroff and Sclafani, 2021).

It has been claimed that food reward is produced by gut signals (Han, Tellez, Perkins, Perez, Qu, Ferreira, Ferreira, Quinn, Liu, Gao, Kaelberer, Bohorquez, Shammah-Lagnado, de Lartigue and de Araujo, 2018; De Araujo, Schatzker and Small, 2020). However, that does not fit with the wealth of evidence just described, showing that food reward is produced by the taste, texture, smell and sight of food. Instead, the evidence about the functions of gut signals in the control of food intake is that their main function is to influence satiety, with gut and hormonal signals often operating through conditioned appetite or satiety, rather than by acting directly as rewards (Berthoud, Morrison, Ackroff and Sclafani, 2021). These gut and hormonal signals are likely to act to slowly modulate the reward value of food produced by the taste, texture, flavor and sight of food acting on food reward neurons in the orbitofrontal cortex, with these satiety signals reaching the orbitofrontal cortex (Rolls, 2016g), in part via the visceral representation in the anteroventral insula region AAIC (Rolls et al., 2023c). In this situation, the reward value of food is signalled by the food reward neurons that respond to the taste, texture, smell, flavor and sight of food that relate to the subjective pleasantness / hedonic value of food, described in this book and elsewhere (Rolls, 2016g), and the reward value that they signal is controlled by gut and many other factors as described next.

The factors including gut signals that influence the reward value of food, the amount of food eaten, and thereby influence obesity (Morton et al., 2014; van der Klaauw and Farooqi, 2015; Berthoud et al., 2021) include the following (Rolls, 2016g) (see also Section 19.9.2).

1. Genetic factors. The 'obesity epidemic' that has occurred since 1990 cannot be attributed to genetic changes, for which the time scale is far too short, but instead to factors such as the increased palatability, variety, and availability of food which are some of the crucial

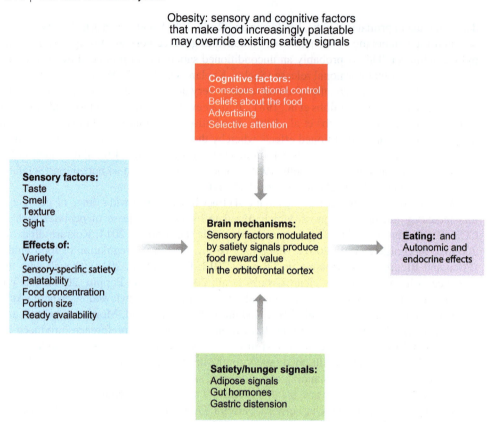

Fig. 4.15 Sensory factors such as the taste, texture, smell, flavor and sight of food are modulated in the orbitofrontal cortex by satiety signals to produce the hedonic, rewarding value of food, which leads to appetite and eating. Cognitive and attentional factors directly modulate the reward system in the orbitofrontal cortex.

drivers of food intake and the amount of food that is eaten in our changed modern environment (Heitmann et al., 2012; Rolls, 2014a, 2016g). Evidence for genetic contributions to body weight comes from family, twin, and adoption studies, which demonstrate that the heritability (fraction of the total phenotypic variance of a quantitative trait attributable to genes in a specified environment) of Body Mass Index is between 0.71 and 0.86 (Silventoinen et al., 2008).

2. Endocrine factors, and their interaction with brain systems. A small proportion of cases of obesity can be related to gene-related dysfunctions of the peptide systems in the hypothalamus, with for example 2-5% of obese people having deficient (MC4) receptors for melanocyte stimulating hormone (van der Klaauw and Farooqi, 2015; Farooqi, 2022). Cases of obesity that can be related to changes in the leptin hormone satiety system are also rare (1-5%) (O'Rahilly, 2009; van der Klaauw and Farooqi, 2015; Farooqi, 2022).

3. Brain processing of the sensory properties and pleasantness / reward value of food. Over the last 30 years, sensory stimulation produced by the taste, smell, texture and appearance of food, as well as its availability, have increased dramatically, yet the satiety signals produced by stomach distension, satiety hormones etc (Cummings and Overduin, 2007; Hussain and Bloom, 2013; Price and Bloom, 2014) have remained essentially unchanged, so that the effect on the brain's control system for appetite (Fig. 4.15) is to lead to a net average increase in the reward value and palatability of food which over-rides the satiety signals, and contributes to the tendency to be overstimulated by food and to overeat.

4. Sensory-specific satiety, and the effects of variety on food intake (Rolls, 2016g).

5. Fixed meal times, and the ready availability of food. The normal control of food intake is by alterations in inter-meal interval but is not readily available in humans because of fixed meal times, and food may be eaten at a meal-time even if hunger is not present (Rolls, 2014a). Even more than this, because of the high and easy availability of food (in the home and workplace) and stimulation by advertising, there is a tendency to start eating again when satiety signals after a previous meal have decreased only a little, and the consequence is that the system again becomes overloaded.
6. Food saliency, and portion size. Making food salient, for example by placing it on display, may increase food selection particularly in the obese (Schachter, 1971), and portion size is a factor, with more being eaten if a large portion of food is presented (Rolls, 2016g).
7. Energy density of food. Gastric emptying rate only partially compensates for the high energy density of food (Rolls, 2016g).
8. Eating rate is typically fast in the obese, and may provide insufficient time for the full effect of satiety signals as food reaches the intestine to operate.
9. Stress (Rolls, 2016g).
10. Food craving and binge eating may be associated with the release of dopamine, which may exacerbate the problem (Rolls, 2016g).
11. Energy output. Although exercise is important for health, it may not have very significant effects on body weight gain and adiposity in the obese or those who become obese (Wilks et al., 2011; Johns et al., 2014; Niemiro et al., 2022).
12. Cognitive factors, and attention. As shown in this book, cognitive descriptions and attention can modulate reward value as represented in the orbitofrontal cortex, and this may influence human liking for a food and how much is eaten (Rolls, 2016g).

4.3 Taste and related pathways: how the computations are performed

4.3.1 Increased selectivity of taste and flavor neurons through the hierarchy by competitive learning and convergence

The taste system is hierarchically organised, and competitive learning in the cortex (complemented by lateral inhibition in the thalamus) is the probable mechanism that sharpens the tuning through the hierarchy. The mechanisms are described in Section B.18 and B.4.

One key feature of taste processing is that because orbitofrontal cortex taste neurons code for some primary reinforcers which must be different for sweet, salt, and bitter, there may need to be genetic specification through the taste pathways from the receptor right through to the orbitofrontal cortex. That is, an orbitofrontal cortex neuron needs to know whether it is connected indirectly to a sweet receptor or a bitter receptor, because in the orbitofrontal cortex the reward / punishment valence is encoded. This is an interesting issue, for although neurons in the insular primary taste cortex have responses that can be moderately tuned to e.g. sweet vs bitter vs salt, their tuning is not fully sparse, but is somewhat distributed.

4.3.2 Pattern association learning of associations of visual and olfactory stimuli with taste

Multimodal associations of visual and olfactory stimuli with taste are learned in the orbitofrontal cortex, with the probable mechanism pattern association as described in Sections B.2. This learning may also involve competitive learning, helping neurons to become selective for different multimodal combinations of their inputs (Section B.4).

4.3.3 Rule-based reversal of visual to taste associations in the orbitofrontal cortex

Visual to taste associations can be reversed in one trial by orbitofrontal cortex neurons, providing evidence for a rule-based mechanism. This is very adaptive in evolutionary terms, and is not known to be possible in rodents, but is an important computation in primates. A model for this is described in Chapter 11.

4.3.4 Sensory-specific satiety is implemented by adaptation of synapses onto orbitofrontal cortex neurons

The findings described in this Chapter lead to the following proposed neuronal mechanism for sensory-specific satiety (see also Rolls and Treves (1990) and Rolls (2014a)). The tuning of neurons becomes more specific for gustatory stimuli through the nucleus of the solitary tract, gustatory thalamus, and frontal opercular taste cortex. Satiety, habituation and adaptation are not features of the responses here. This is what is found in primates (see above). The tuning of neurons becomes even more specific in the orbitofrontal cortex, but here there is some effect of satiety by internal signals such as gastric distension and glucose utilization, and in addition habituation or adaptation with a time course of several minutes which lasts for 1–2 h is a feature of the synapses that are activated. Because of the relative specificity of the tuning of orbitofrontal taste neurons, this results in a decrease in the response to that food, but different foods continue to activate other neurons or even the same neuron. This is an important part of the theory, for it shows the adaptive utility for why different orbitofrontal cortex neurons respond to different combinations of sensory inputs, and in this sense as a population encode a *high-dimensional space of reward value* (Rolls, 2016b). For orbitofrontal cortex neurons that respond to two flavors before satiety, it is suggested that the habituation that results in a loss of the response to the taste eaten to satiety (see e.g. Fig. 4.8, and for sensory-specific satiety for the texture of fat Rolls et al. (1999a)) occurs because of habituation or adaptation of the afferent neurons or synapses onto these orbitofrontal cortex neurons. Because an orbitofrontal cortex neuron can still respond to a food not eaten to satiety, the mechanism can not be neuronal adaptation, and for that reason adaptation of the afferent synapses to a neuron is the mechanism proposed for how the computation is implemented. This would result in the orbitofrontal cortex neurons having the required response properties, and it is then only necessary for other parts of the brain to use the activity of the orbitofrontal cortex neurons to reflect the reward value of that particular taste. One output of these neurons may be to the anterior cingulate cortex; and another to the hypothalamic neurons with food-related responses, for their responses to the sight and/or taste of food show a decrease that is partly specific to a food that has just been eaten to satiety (see above and Rolls (2019e)). Another output may be to the ventral and adjoining striatum, which may provide an important link between reward systems and response habits (see Chapter 16).

It is suggested that the computational significance of this architecture is as follows (see also Rolls (1986b), Rolls (1989d), Rolls and Treves (1990), and Rolls (2016b)). If satiety were to operate at an early level of sensory analysis, then because of the broadness of tuning of neurons, responses to non-foods would become attenuated as well as responses to foods (and this could well be dangerous if poisonous non-foods became undetectable). This argument becomes even more compelling when it is realized that satiety typically shows some specificity for the particular food eaten, with others not eaten in the meal remaining relatively pleasant (see above). Unless tuning were relatively fine, this mechanism could not operate, for reduction in neuronal firing after one food had been eaten would inevitably reduce behavioral responsiveness to other foods. Indeed, it is of interest to note that such a sensory-specific satiety mechanism can be built by arranging for tuning to particular foods to become relatively specific at one level of the nervous system (as a result of categorization processing in earlier stages), and then at this stage (but not at prior stages) to allow habituation to be a property of the synapses, as proposed above.

In summary, the computational hypothesis about how sensory-specific satiety is implemented is in the orbitofrontal cortex by adaptation with a time course of several minutes of the active synapses of specifically tuned neurons onto orbitofrontal cortex neurons. Once adapted, the synapses remain adapted for 1–2 hours (or as long as necessary) to account for the duration of sensory-specific satiety. Sensory-specific satiety applies to all rewards, and to no punishers (Rolls, 2014a).

4.3.5 Top-down cognitive and attentional modulation is implemented by biased activation

We have seen in Section 4.2.8 that whole cortical areas and even processing streams can be biased by top-down selective attention or cognitive modulation. For example, we have seen that paying attention to the pleasantness of a stimulus, or describing a flavor as rich and delicious, can by a top-down language-level bias increase activations in the orbitofrontal cortex. This can occur for example if some processing attributes of stimuli such as reward value are processed in one cortical stream (the orbitofrontal cortex and anterior cingulate cortex), and other attributes such as the intensity and identity of a stimulus in other cortical streams such as the insula (Grabenhorst and Rolls, 2008), and the same occurs for olfactory stimuli, as described in Chapter 5 (Rolls, Grabenhorst, Margot, da Silva and Velazco, 2008b). A biased activation theory of top-down selective attention and cognitive modulation has been described to account for this (Rolls, 2013a).

The way that we think of top-down biased competition as operating normally in for example visual selective attention (Desimone and Duncan, 1995) is that within an area, e.g. a cortical region, some neurons receive a weak top-down input that increases their response to the bottom-up stimuli, potentially supralinearly if the bottom-up stimuli are weak (Rolls and Deco, 2002; Deco and Rolls, 2005b; Rolls, 2016b). The enhanced firing of the biased neurons then, via the local inhibitory neurons, inhibits the other neurons in the local area from responding to the bottom-up stimuli. This is a local mechanism, in that the inhibition in the neocortex is primarily local, being implemented by cortical inhibitory neurons that typically have inputs and outputs over no more than a few mm (Chapter 1, Douglas et al. (2004)). This model of biased competition is described in Sections 2.12 and B.8.4, and is illustrated in Fig. 2.85.

This locally implemented biased competition situation may not apply in the present case, where we have facilitation of processing in a whole cortical area (e.g. orbitofrontal cortex, or pregenual cingulate cortex) or even cortical processing stream (e.g. the linked orbitofrontal and pregenual cingulate cortex) in which any taste neurons may reflect pleasantness and not intensity. So the attentional effect might more accurately be described in this case as biased activation, without local competition being part of the effect. This biased activation theory and model of attention, illustrated in Fig. 4.16 (Rolls, 2013a), is a rather different way to implement attention in the brain than biased competition, and each mechanism may apply in different cases, or both mechanisms in some cases.

The biased activation theory of top-down attentional and cognitive control is as follows (Rolls, 2013a), and is illustrated in Fig. 4.16. There are short-term memory systems implemented as cortical attractor networks with recurrent collateral connections to maintain neuronal activity that provide the source of the top-down activation. The short-term memory systems may be separate (as shown in Fig. 4.16), or could be a single network with diff-

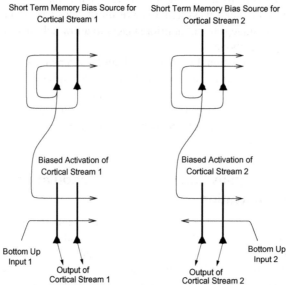

Fig. 4.16 Biased activation mechanism for top-down attention. The short-term memory systems that provide the source of the top-down activations may be separate (as shown), or could be a single network with different attractor states for the different selective attention conditions. The top-down short-term memory systems hold what is being paid attention to active by continuing firing in an attractor state, and bias separately either cortical processing system 1, or cortical processing system 2. This weak top-down bias interacts with the bottom up input to the cortical stream and produces an increase of activity that can be supralinear (Deco and Rolls 2005c). Thus the selective activation of separate cortical processing streams can occur. In the example, stream 1 might process the affective value of a stimulus, and stream 2 might process the intensity and physical properties of the stimulus. The outputs of these separate processing streams then must enter a competition system, which could be for example a cortical attractor decision-making network that makes choices between the two streams, with the choice biased by the activations in the separate streams (see text). The thick vertical lines above the pyramidal cells are the dendrites. The axons are shown with thin lines and the excitatory connections by arrow heads. (Reproduced from Rolls, E. T. (2013) A biased activation theory of the cognitive and attentional modulation of emotion. Frontiers in Human Neuroscience 7: 74.)

erent attractor states for the different selective attention conditions. The top-down short-term memory systems hold what is being paid attention to active by continuing firing in an attractor state, and bias separately either cortical processing system 1, or cortical processing system 2. This weak top-down bias interacts with the bottom-up input to the cortical stream and produces an increase of activity that can be supralinear (Deco and Rolls, 2005b). Thus the selective activation of separate cortical processing streams can occur. In the example, stream 1 might process the affective value of a stimulus, and stream 2 might process the intensity and physical properties of the stimulus.

The top-down bias needs to be weak relative to the bottom-up input, for the top-down bias must not dominate the system, otherwise bottom-up inputs, essential for perception and survival, would be over-ridden. Under such conditions, top-down attentional and cognitive effects will be largest when the bottom-up inputs are not too strong or are ambiguous, and that has been shown to be the case in realistic simulations with integrate-and-fire neurons (Deco and Rolls, 2005b; Rolls, 2016b). The weakness of the top-down biasing input is included as a part of brain design, for the top-down inputs are effectively backprojections from higher cortical areas, and these end on the apical dendrites of cortical pyramidal cells, and so have weaker effects than the bottom up inputs, which make connections lower down the dendrite towards the cell body (Rolls, 2016b). I suggest here that the correct connections could be set up in such a system by the following associative (Hebbian) synaptic learning process. The top-down backprojection synapses would increase in strength when there is activity in a population of short-term memory neurons that by their firing hold attention in one direction (e.g. the short-term memory system for cortical stream 1 shown in Fig. 4.16, and simultaneously there is activity in the neurons that receive the top-down inputs (e.g. in cortical stream 1 shown in Fig. 4.16).

The outputs of the separate processing streams showing biased activation (Fig. 4.16) may need to be compared at a later stage of processing, in order to lead to a single behavior (Rolls, 2013a). One way in which this comparison could take place is by both outputs entering a single network cortical attractor model of decision-making, in which positive feedback implemented by the excitatory recurrent collateral connections leads through non-linear dynamics to a single winner, which is ensured by competition between the different possible attractor states produced through inhibitory neurons (Wang, 2002; Deco and Rolls, 2006; Deco, Rolls, Albantakis and Romo, 2013). A second way in which the competition could be implemented is by that usually conceptualized as important in biased competition (Desimone and Duncan, 1995; Rolls and Deco, 2002; Deco and Rolls, 2005b), in which a feedforward competitive network using inhibition through local inhibitory neurons provides a way for a weak top-down signal to bias the output especially if the bottom-up inputs are weak, and this implementation is what is shown at the bottom of Fig. 2.85. A third way in which the biased activation reflected in the output of the streams shown in Fig. 4.16 could be taken into account is by a mechanism such as that in the basal ganglia, where in the striatum the different excitatory inputs activate GABA (gamma-amino-butyric acid) neurons, which then directly inhibit each other to make the selection (Chapter 16, and Rolls (2014a)).

The difference between biased competition and biased activation may be especially important in the context of functional neuroimaging, for biased activation, in which processing in whole cortical areas is facilitated by selective attention, can be revealed by functional neuroimaging, which operates at relatively low spatial resolution, in the order of mm. In contrast, biased competition may selectively facilitate some pyramidal neurons within a local cortical area which then through the local GABA inhibitory neurons compete with the other pyramidal neurons in the area receiving bottom-up input. In this situation, in which some but not other neurons within a cortical area are showing enhanced firing, functional neuroimaging may not be able to show which local population of pyramidal cells is winning the competition due to the top-down bias. The evidence presented by Grabenhorst and Rolls (2010) is that not only the processing streams, but also even the short-term memory systems in the prefrontal cortex that provide the top-down source of the biased activation, are physically separate (see Fig. 13.8).

A possibility arising from this model is that some competition may occur somewhere in the attentional system before the output stage, and one possible area is within the prefrontal cortex, where it is a possibility that the attractors that implement the short-term memory for attention to pleasantness (at MNI coordinate Y$\approx$50) may inhibit the attractors that implement the short-term memory for attention to intensity (at Y$\approx$37), which could occur if there is some physical overlap between their zones of activation, even if the peaks are well separated. Some evidence for this possibility was found (Grabenhorst and Rolls, 2010), in that the correlation between the % BOLD activations in these two prefrontal cortex regions was r=-0.72 (p=0.0034) on the pleasantness trials; and r=-0.8 (p<0.001) on the intensity trials. In a biased competition model (Fig. 2.85) we would normally think of the short-term memory attractors that provide the source of the bias as being within the same single attractor network, so that there would be competition between the two attractor states through the local inhibitory interneurons. In the biased activation model (Fig. 4.16), it is an open issue about whether the attractors that provide the source of the top-down bias are in the same single network, or are physically separate making interactions between the attractor states difficult through the short-range cortical inhibitory neurons. The findings just described indicate that in the case of top-down control of affective vs intensity processing of taste stimuli, although the two attractors are somewhat apart in the prefrontal cortex, there is some functional inhibitory interaction between them. Further evidence for separate top-down attractor networks for biased activation was found in an investigation in which Granger causality was measured (Ge, Feng, Grabenhorst and Rolls, 2012) (see Section 13.4 and Fig. 13.8).

The principle of biased activation providing a mechanism for selective attention (Rolls, 2013a) probably extends beyond processing in the affective vs sensory coding cortical streams. It may provide the mechanism also for effects in for example the dorsal vs the ventral visual streams, in which attention to the motion of a moving object may enhance processing in the dorsal stream, and attention to the identity of the moving object may enhance processing in the ventral visual stream (Brown, 2009). Similar biased activation may contribute to the different localization in the prefrontal cortex of systems involved in 'what' vs 'where' working memory (Deco, Rolls and Horwitz, 2004; Rottschy, Langner, Dogan, Reetz, Laird, Schulz, Fox and Eickhoff, 2012). Biased activation as a mechanism for top-down selective attention may be widespread in the brain, and may be engaged when there is segregated processing of different attributes of stimuli (Grabenhorst and Rolls, 2010; Rolls, 2013a).

5 The olfactory system

5.1 Introduction

The olfactory pathways are shown in Figs. 4.3, 11.1 on page 476 and 11.4.

In the primate olfactory system, the olfactory bulb projects to the primary olfactory cortex (the pyriform cortex, directly and via the mediodorsal nucleus of the thalamus), which in turn projects to the orbitofrontal cortex, which is thereby defined as a secondary cortical olfactory area, and the orbitofrontal cortex in turn projects to the anterior cingulate cortex (Fig. 11.1) (Price et al., 1991; Morecraft et al., 1992; Barbas, 1993; Carmichael et al., 1994; Price, 2006). The olfactory system is thus organised hierarchically.

Olfactory projections from the olfactory bulb do though reach some other areas, including the olfactory tubercle which is part of the ventral striatum, and the lateral entorhinal cortex, which in turn projects to the hippocampus (Rolls, 2014a; Wilson et al., 2014a; Wilson and Sullivan, 2011). At the hippocampal stage of the hierarchy, the principle of convergence is evident, for in the hippocampus flavor information (which has an olfactory component) can be combined with spatial information to allow learning of where the flavor is in allocentric space (Rolls and Xiang, 2005; Kesner and Rolls, 2015) (see Chapter 9). The principle of convergence in cortical hierarchies is also evident in the fact that olfactory information is combined with taste information to produce flavor in the orbitofrontal cortex, but not at earlier cortical stages (Section 4.2.7).

We should at the outset note that the principles of olfactory as well as taste processing are very different in rodents at least in terms of sensory vs value encoding, in that reward value may influence olfactory processing in the periphery in rodents, so that rodents may not provide a good guide to the principles of olfactory (as well as taste and visual) cortical processing in primates including humans (Rolls, 2015d) (see Section 19.10).

5.1.1 Overview of what is computed in the olfactory system

What is computed in the olfactory system is described in Section 5.2 with an overview here.

1. There are approximately 1000 genes each coding for a different olfactory receptor in the olfactory epithelium in rodents (Buck and Axel, 1991). Each olfactory receptor type projects to a different glomerulus in the olfactory bulb, so that there are 1000 glomeruli in the olfactory bulb (or in fact 2000, as the representation is doubled up in different parts of the olfactory bulb). Although each glomerulus has different encoding of odors, with different glomeruli tuned for example to different carbon chain lengths of aliphatic aldehydes, the tuning of each glomerulus is rather broad, with each glomerulus having a non-sparse representation of odors, and considerable correlations between the response profiles of different glomeruli to a set of odors (Verhagen, Baker, Vasan, Pieribone and Rolls, 2023). In humans, approximately one third of the olfactory receptor genes are disabled. This may be because with other senses such as vision and hearing so much more developed in primates, there is less evolutionary pressure and advantage in maintaining all the 1000 genetically specified olfactory receptor types.

2. In rodents and many other mammals there is an accessory olfactory system that includes the vomeronasal organ and the accessory olfactory bulb, and this system is involved in response to pheromones which are important in sexual and other types of behavior (Wyatt, 2014; Li and Dulac, 2018; Rolls, 2014a). However, this system, and many of its associated genes, are not present or are vestigial at best in humans and Old World monkeys (Meredith, 2001), and whether pheromones operate in humans is questionable (Wyatt, 2020; Cherry and Baum, 2020).

3. Most odors also have trigeminal effects, that is, somatosensory effects that reach the central nervous system via the trigeminal nerve. Although in a much lower dimensional space than in the (up to) 1000 dimensional space encoded by the olfactory receptors, these trigeminal components do differ for different odors, and what is computed to represent an odor may include trigeminal components that are different for different odors. Examples of trigeminal stimuli include air pollutants (e.g. sulphur dioxide), ammonia, ethanol, acetic acid (vinegar), carbon dioxide (in soft drinks), menthol (in some inhalants), and capsaicin (present in chili peppers).

4. The olfactory bulb projects directly to a number of brain regions, including the pyriform cortex. In the pyriform cortex, the tuning may become more selective for odors, partly because neurons learn to respond to combinations of what is encoded in the glomeruli of the olfactory bulb. In humans, activations in the pyriform cortex are related to the subjective intensity of odors, and not to their pleasantness. The coding in the human pyriform cortex is therefore for what the odor is, and its intensity, rather than its reward value.

5. The pyriform, primary olfactory, cortex, projects forward to a part of the orbitofrontal cortex, which is secondary olfactory cortex. In the orbitofrontal cortex, some bimodal neurons are found that respond to olfactory and taste stimuli, so that flavor representations are computed. This association can be reversed, or partially reversed, in some orbitofrontal cortex olfactory neurons. The computation has involved moving the olfactory representation from a space using genetically specified encoding into a space where for some neurons the odor represented depends on the taste with which it is associated.

6. In the secondary olfactory cortex, the reward value of olfactory stimuli is represented, in that some olfactory neurons only respond when hunger is present; and activations in the humans orbitofrontal cortex are correlated with the subjective pleasantness of the odor or flavor. This is a further way in which olfactory representations move beyond a genetically specified code in the periphery, to in this case an olfactory reward value code.

7. The olfactory tubercle is part of the ventral striatum (see Chapter 16) and receives direct olfactory inputs from the olfactory nerve; but is not purely olfactory, for it receives visual inputs in primates.

5.1.2 Overview of how the computations are performed in the olfactory system

How computations are performed in the olfactory system is described in Section 5.3 with an overview here.

1. The olfactory system uses a computationally very simple way of representing different odors: it uses a large number of genes, 1000, approximately 1/30 of the genome, to encode odors. This allows encoding of differences between different odors. There are no invariances to compute, and so it is much simpler computationally than vision and audition.

2. Because the glomeruli are rather poorly tuned to specific odors, the next stage of the olfactory system, the pyriform cortex, primary olfactory cortex, produces more specifically tuned neurons.

3. The pyriform cortex may increase the selectivity of tuning partly by competitive learning, which would encourage pyramidal cells to learn to respond to specific combinations of the odors represented by the glomeruli in the olfactory bulb. This 'feature combination learning' could be achieved in part by competitive learning. But the pyriform cortex is well endowed with recurrent collateral connections, which are likely to operate as attractor networks. The attractor networks in the pyriform cortex may build representations of different categories of odors, and help to ensure that small variations in the odor profile represented by the glomeruli will activate the same subset of pyriform cortex neurons, which thus represent was the odor is, independently of small variations in the profile at the olfactory receptors.

4. Another function of the recurrent collateral connections in the pyriform cortex may be to smooth out the temporal changes in firing with each inhalation that are present in the olfactory bulb (Verhagen, Baker, Vasan, Pieribone and Rolls, 2023), but which are much less evident in the secondary olfactory cortex in the orbitofrontal cortex (Critchley and Rolls, 1996b; Rolls, Critchley, Mason and Wakeman, 1996b; Rolls, Critchley and Treves, 1996a). It is a property of attractor networks that they can act as short-term memories, and this may be the computation. Having a non-phasic odor representation in the olfactory system by the time that it is interfaced to taste and vision in the orbitofrontal cortex may be appropriate, for the information in the visual and taste modalities is represented by neurons with relatively steady firing rate responses over time, and the association with odor would be difficult in terms of synaptic modification if the olfactory representation was phasic with each inhalation, but not the visual, taste, and oral texture representations.

5. The pyriform cortex projects into the orbitofrontal cortex, which is thereby secondary olfactory cortex. But it also receives taste, oral texture, and visual inputs. In the orbitofrontal cortex, at least some neurons remap the olfactory representation from the genetic encoding present in the receptors and olfactory bulb into a space where associations are made to taste, as many orbitofrontal cortex olfactory neurons represent odors by the taste with which they are associated. This is probably learned by pattern association learning (see Section B.2.)

6. Many orbitofrontal cortex olfactory neurons represent odors in terms of their reward value, as shown by the effects of feeding to satiety. Part of this may be implemented by the association with taste, which also represents reward value in the orbitofrontal cortex. Further, olfactory sensory-specific is represented in the orbitofrontal cortex, and this may be computed by synaptic adaptation of the afferent connections to orbitofrontal cortex olfactory neurons, in that it is represented in the orbitofrontal cortex, and because just smelling an odor for several minutes can produce olfactory sensory-specific satiety (Rolls and Rolls, 1997).

5.2 What is computed in the olfactory system

5.2.1 1000 gene-encoded olfactory receptor types, and 1000 corresponding glomerulus types in the olfactory bulb

There are approximately 1000 gene-encoded types of olfactory receptor in the olfactory epithelium in the nose, each specialised to code for different olfactory receptor molecules (Buck and Axel, 1991; Buck and Bargmann, 2013; Mombaerts, 2006; Mori and Sakano, 2011; Zapiec and Mombaerts, 2015; Horowitz et al., 2014). In humans, approximately 300 are disabled. The receptors that are disabled in humans may be somewhat different in different humans, leading to some differences in olfactory perception and hedonics. This reduced number of active olfactory receptor genes in humans may be because with other senses such as vision and hearing so much more developed in primates, there is less evolutionary pressure and advantage in maintaining all the 1000 genetically specified olfactory receptor types.

Each of the 1000 types of olfactory receptor connect to just one type of glomerulus in the olfactory bulb (Mombaerts, 2006; Mori and Sakano, 2011; Zapiec and Mombaerts, 2015). This type of connectivity must rely on a molecular signal that is specific for each genetically encoded receptor type.

In the rodent olfactory bulb, a coding principle is that in many cases each glomerulus (of which there are approximately 1000 types) is tuned to respond to its own characteristic hydrocarbon chain length of odorant (Mori et al., 1992; Imamura et al., 1992; Mori et al., 1999; Mori and Sakano, 2011). Evidence for this was that each mitral/tufted cell in the olfactory bulb has been described as quite sharply tuned, responding for example best to a 5-C length aliphatic odorant (e.g. acid or aldehyde), and being inhibited by nearby hydrocarbon chain-length aliphatic odorants.

The encoding in this early part of the olfactory system may thus be based on the stereochemical structure of the odorant, with receptors that have been produced in a genetically very expensive way, with one gene to build each receptor type. This is a very simple way for a sensory system to operate, with its sensory capability built largely by having one gene that has evolved to produce a single receptor type, with this repeated for 1000 genes, approximately 1/30th of the human genome.

The local inhibition in the olfactory bulb may be seen as a way to spread out (orthogonalize or decorrelate) the olfactory stimulus space by using the contrast enhancement provided by lateral inhibition.

Each olfactory receptor may be tuned to a stereochemical input to some extent, but in practice, even pure chemical stimuli typically activate many glomeruli. This is illustrated in an analysis (Verhagen, Baker, Vasan, Pieribone and Rolls, 2023) of calcium imaging data from the mouse olfactory bulb of the responses of up to 57 glomeruli to 6 olfactory stimuli: amyl acetate, carvone, heptanol, heptanone, hexanal and methyl valerate (Baker et al., 2019). The responses to different odors may be quite correlated over a population of glomeruli, and the coding is non-sparse, with a mean value for the sparseness a for 6 odors of 0.85 (Verhagen, Baker, Vasan, Pieribone and Rolls, 2023). There is a little information in the latencies with which these populations of glomeruli respond to different odors (mean 0.11 bits), but that is small compared to the amount of information conveyed by the firing rate (mean 1.35 bits) (Verhagen et al., 2023). Moreover, the latency information does not add to the rate information (Verhagen et al., 2023) (Fig. C.14), and so the principle that most of the information is conveyed by the firing rate is found in the olfactory system, as it is in most other sensory systems (see Appendix C, Rolls (2016b), and Rolls and Treves (2011)). With 6 stimuli, 2.58 bits of information would be needed to encode correctly the 6 odors, yet these populations of up to 57 glomeruli provided on average only 1.35 bits of information. Putting together the data from all 266 glomeruli in the investigation, the information did rise to the 2.58 bits needed for perfect discrimination between the 6 odors. I hypothesize that the very large number (1000) of gene-encoded olfactory receptors and glomeruli is needed to adequately encode olfactory stimuli, given that even tens of glomeruli provide only a moderate representation of 6 odors. I also suggest that this is the evolutionary background for why approximately 1/30th of the mammalian genome is used to encode olfactory receptors.

5.2.2 The primary olfactory, pyriform, cortex: olfactory feature combinations are what is represented

In the pyriform cortex, neurons may respond to combinations of the inputs received from different glomeruli, and thus to feature combinations of what is encoded by a number of different olfactory receptor genes. This enables neurons to be more selective for odors than in the olfactory bulb. The representations may be built for example by competitive learning (Rolls, 2016b), enabling neurons to learn to represent the co-occurrence of pairs or groups of odorants, so that particular smells in the environment, which typically are produced by combinations of chemical stimuli, are reflected in the responses of pyriform cortex neurons (Wilson and Sullivan, 2011; Barbaro and Shackelford, 2015; Courtiol and Wilson, 2017). Pyriform cortex neurons can for example respond to binary combinations of odors, and much less to the components. Thus what is computed in the olfactory system appears to follow what occurs in other sensory systems, namely that convergence occurs from stage to stage, and new feature combination neurons are formed at each stage of the hierarchy. In the case of the pyriform cortex, the convergence is from the single gene-specified representations in individual glomeruli in the olfactory bulb.

The pyriform cortex has a rich set of recurrent collateral connections between its pyramidal cells, and in line with this the hypothesis is that the pyriform cortex implements an autoassociative memory, which helps to form representations of olfactory mixtures as odor objects, which display a property of completion in which the whole odor may be represented even if some components are missing in the process known as completion (Haberly, 2001; Wilson and Sullivan, 2011) (see Section 5.3.2).

The anterior pyriform cortex is strongly influenced by the olfactory bulb inputs, and in turn influences the posterior pyriform cortex. In both humans (Gottfried et al., 2006; Gottfried, 2010) and rodents (Kadohisa and Wilson, 2006), the anterior piriform cortex may encode information related to structural or perceptual identity of the odor, e.g. 'banana'. More posterior regions, perhaps in accord with the dominance of association fiber input, appear to encode the perceptual category of an odor, e.g. 'fruity' (Wilson and Sullivan, 2011).

In humans, activity in the pyriform cortex appears to be related to 'what' stimulus is present (its identity), and its intensity, and not to its reward value, in that activations in the human pyriform cortex are linearly related to the intensity rating of odorants, and not to their pleasantness (Grabenhorst, Rolls, Margot, da Silva and Velazco, 2007); in that paying attention to the intensity vs the pleasantness of an odor increases activations in the pyriform cortex (Rolls, Grabenhorst, Margot, da Silva and Velazco, 2008b); and in that activations in the pyriform cortex were not decreased by odor devaluation by satiety (Gottfried, 2015).

In contrast, in rodents, reducing reward value by feeding to satiety or by administering leptin reduces the neural activity even in the olfactory bulb (Pager et al., 1972; Sun et al., 2019a). That is further difficult to reconcile with the fact that in humans during olfactory sensory-specific satiety, the pleasantness but much less the intensity of an odor is reduced (Rolls and Rolls, 1997). That finding makes it unlikely that peripheral modulation of olfactory neural responsiveness is a normal mechanism under physiological conditions of olfactory reward value processing in humans. As we will see, there is clear evidence in primates including humans that the reward value of olfactory stimuli is part of what is computed in the orbitofrontal cortex, in what is secondary olfactory cortex.

The effective connectivity of the pyriform cortex in humans can be summarized as follows, based on the research I have been performing on the connectivity of different cortical regions, some of which have connectivity with the pyriform cortex (Rolls et al., 2023c,b,f, 2022a). The human pyriform cortex has strong effective connectivity to the amygdala (0.031, with 0.0 in the reverse direction); strong and bidirectional effective connectivity with AAIC

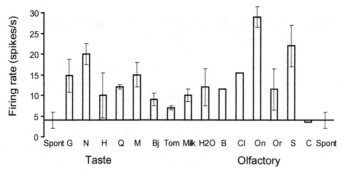

Fig. 5.1 The responses of a bimodal neuron with taste and olfactory responses recorded in the caudolateral orbitofrontal cortex. G, 1 M glucose; N, 0.1 M NaCl; H, 0.01 M HCl; Q, 0.001 M Quinine HCl; M, 0.1 M monosodium glutamate; Bj, 20% blackcurrant juice; Tom, tomato juice; B, banana odor; Cl, clove oil odor; On, onion odor; Or, orange odor; S, salmon odor; C, control no-odor presentation. The mean responses ± s.e.m. are shown. The neuron responded best to the savoury tastes of NaCl and monosodium glutamate and to the consonant odors of onion and salmon. (Reproduced from E. T. Rolls and L. L. Baylis (1994) Gustatory, olfactory and visual convergence within the primate orbitofrontal cortex. Journal of Neuroscience 14: 5437–5452. Copyright © Society for Neuroscience.)

(0.032), the Anterior Agranular Insula Complex which is just posterior to the lateral orbitofrontal cortex and probably the region in which we have shown that convergence between olfactory and taste stimuli occurs to produce flavor (De Araujo, Rolls, Kringelbach, McGlone and Phillips, 2003a); moderate effective connectivity with the medial orbitofrontal cortex (pOFC) and lateral orbitofrontal cortex (47m); some connectivity with posterior insular cortex regions (PoI1, PoI2); stronger effective connectivity towards hippocampal regions (Hipp, PeEc, and TF); and some effective connectivity from the supracallosal anterior cingulate cortex (a24pr and p24pr). The connectivity with the orbitofrontal cortex is consistent with its functions in food flavor, food reward (Chapter 11), and hedonically pleasant and unpleasant odors (Rolls, Kringelbach and De Araujo, 2003c). The connectivity with the hippocampus is useful for remembering odors as components of episodic memories.

5.2.3   Orbitofrontal cortex: olfactory neuronal response selectivity

Some neurons in the macaque orbitofrontal cortex can respond quite selectively to odor, for example with a large response to eugenol but not to the other 7 odors tested (Rolls et al., 1996a). However, for the majority of the neurons, the tuning to a set of odors was quite distributed, with a mean sparseness $a = 0.94$ (Rolls et al., 1996a). However, this value is from neurons measured typically in an olfactory discrimination task in which most odors were associated with reward, and as we will see, the association with taste reward influences how some primate orbitofrontal cortex neurons respond, thus potentially reducing their selectivity for particular odors.

Although the tuning in these experiments was not very sparse, nevertheless each single neuron did convey in its firing rates to the set of stimuli some information about which stimulus had been presented, with the mean mutual information across the set of stimuli 0.06 bits, and the highest information about any one stimulus (the stimulus-specific information, see Appendix 3) in the range 0.02 to 0.08 bits (Rolls, Critchley and Treves, 1996a). Importantly, the response profiles of the neurons to the set of 8 odors were relatively uncorrelated, so that the information increased approximately linearly with the number of neurons (Rolls, Critchley, Verhagen and Kadohisa, 2010a).

5.2.4 Orbitofrontal cortex: olfactory to taste convergence

In the orbitofrontal cortex, some single neurons respond to both gustatory and olfactory stimuli, often with correspondence between the two modalities (Rolls and Baylis, 1994) (see Fig. 5.1; cf. Fig. 11.1). It is probably here in the orbitofrontal cortex of primates that these two modalities converge to produce the representation of flavor (Rolls and Baylis, 1994), and, consistent with this, neurons in the macaque primary taste cortex do not have olfactory responses (Verhagen, Kadohisa and Rolls, 2004). Consistently, in a human fMRI investigation of olfactory and taste convergence in the brain, it was shown that there is a part of the human taste insula that is not activated by odor (De Araujo, Rolls, Kringelbach, McGlone and Phillips, 2003a), though if a taste is recalled by an odor the situation could be different because of the role of cortico-cortical backprojections in recall (Rolls, 2016b, 2015d). The evidence described below indicates that these bimodal representations are built by olfactory–gustatory association learning, an example of stimulus–reinforcer association learning.

The human orbitofrontal cortex also reflects the convergence of taste and olfactory inputs, as shown for example by the fact that activations in the human medial orbitofrontal cortex are correlated with both the cross-modal consonance of combined taste and olfactory stimuli (high for example for sweet taste and strawberry odor), as well as for the pleasantness of the combinations (De Araujo, Rolls, Kringelbach, McGlone and Phillips, 2003a). In addition, the combination of monosodium glutamate taste and a consonant savoury odor produced a supralinear effect in the medial orbitofrontal cortex to produce the rich delicious flavor of umami that makes many foods rich in protein pleasant (McCabe and Rolls, 2007; Rolls, 2009b).

5.2.5 Orbitofrontal cortex: olfactory to taste association learning and reversal

Rolls and colleagues have analyzed the rules by which orbitofrontal olfactory representations are formed and brought together with taste representations in primates as a model of olfactory processing in humans (Rolls, 2001; Rolls and Grabenhorst, 2008; Rolls, 2011a). For 65% of neurons in the orbitofrontal olfactory areas, Critchley and Rolls (1996b) showed that the representation of the olfactory stimulus was independent of its association with taste reward (analyzed in an olfactory discrimination task with taste reward, as some orbitofrontal cortex olfactory neurons are bimodal, with responses also to taste stimuli (Rolls and Baylis, 1994)). For the remaining 35% of the neurons, the odors to which a neuron responded were influenced by the taste (glucose or saline) with which the odor was associated (Critchley and Rolls, 1996b). Thus the odor representation for 35% of orbitofrontal neurons appeared to be built by olfactory-to-taste association learning, and thus by learning the neurons come to encode the **expected value** of olfactory stimuli.

This possibility that the odor representation of some primate orbitofrontal cortex olfactory neurons is built by olfactory-to-taste association learning to encode **expected value** was confirmed by reversing the taste with which an odor was associated in the reversal of an olfactory discrimination task. It was found that 73% of the sample of neurons analyzed altered the way in which they responded to odor when the taste reinforcer association of the odor was reversed (Rolls, Critchley, Mason and Wakeman, 1996b). Reversal was shown by 25% of the neurons (see, for example, Fig. 5.2), and 48% altered their activity in that they no longer discriminated after the reversal. These latter neurons thus respond to a particular odor only if it is associated with a taste reward, and not when it is associated with the taste of salt, a punisher. They do not respond to the other odor in the task when it is associated with reward. Thus they respond to a particular combination of an odor, and its being associated with taste

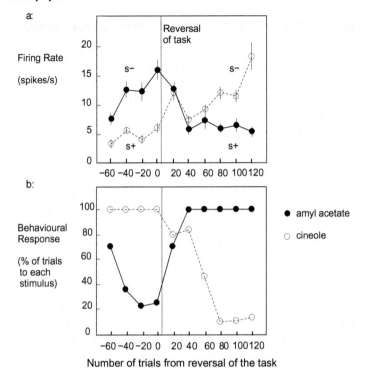

Fig. 5.2 Orbitofrontal cortex: olfactory to taste association reversal. (a) The activity of a single orbitofrontal olfactory neuron during the performance of a two-odor olfactory discrimination task and its reversal is shown. Each point represents the mean poststimulus activity of the neuron in a 500-ms period on approximately 10 trials of the different odorants. The standard errors of these responses are shown. The odorants were amyl acetate (closed circle) (initially S−) and cineole (o) (initially S+). After 80 trials of the task the reward associations of the stimuli were reversed. This neuron reversed its responses to the odorants following the task reversal. (b) The behavioral responses of the monkey during the performance of the olfactory discrimination task. The number of lick responses to each odorant is plotted as a percentage of the number of trials to that odorant in a block of 20 trials of the task. (Reproduced from E. T. Rolls, H. D. Critchley, R. Mason, E. A. Wakeman (1996) Orbitofrontal cortex neurons: role in olfactory and visual association learning. *Journal of Neurophysiology* 75: 1970–1981. Copyright © The American Physiological Society.)

reward and not a taste punisher. They may be described as **conditional olfactory-reward neurons**, and may be important in the mechanism by which stimulus–reinforcer (in this case olfactory-to-taste) reversal learning occurs (Deco and Rolls, 2005d), as described in Chapter 11.

The olfactory to taste reversal was quite slow, both neurophysiologically and behaviorally, often requiring 20–80 trials, consistent with the need for some stability of flavor (i.e. olfactory and taste combination) representations. The relatively high proportion of olfactory neurons with modification of responsiveness by taste association in the set of neurons in this experiment was probably related to the fact that the neurons were preselected to show differential responses to the odors associated with different tastes in the olfactory discrimination task. Thus the rule according to which the orbitofrontal olfactory representation was formed was for some neurons by association learning with taste.

Consistent findings were found in a human fMRI classical conditioning experiment in which odors were paired with a monetary cue, and representations in the orbitofrontal cortex and one of its subregions the ventromedial prefrontal cortex were influenced by this conditioning (Howard et al., 2015, 2016).

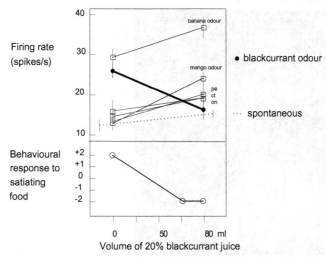

Fig. 5.3 The effect of feeding to satiety on the responses of an olfactory neuron in the orbitofrontal cortex. The monkey was fed to satiety with blackcurrant juice, and the neuronal response to the odor of blackcurrant juice, but not to other odors, decreased as the monkey was being fed to satiety. The neuronal responses reflected the monkey's preference for the blackcurrant juice, as shown in the lower graph. (Reproduced from H. D. Critchley and E. T. Rolls (1996) Hunger and satiety modify the responses of olfactory and visual neurons in the primate orbitofrontal cortex. Journal of Neurophysiology 75: 1673–1686, © The American Physiological Society.)

5.2.6 Orbitofrontal cortex: olfactory reward value is represented

The experiments just described (Rolls, Critchley, Mason and Wakeman, 1996b; Critchley and Rolls, 1996b) show that some olfactory neurons in the primate orbitofrontal cortex represent reward value, in that their responses depend on whether the odor is associated with a rewarding taste or an aversive taste. (Similar findings on associative learning in the mouse orbitofrontal cortex but not pyriform cortex have been reported (Wang, Boboila, Chin, Higashi-Howard, Shamash, Wu, Stein, Abbott and Axel, 2020e)). Further evidence for primates comes from devaluation experiments, in which the odor is devalued by feeding to satiety.

Critchley and Rolls (1996a) measured the responses of olfactory neurons that responded to food while they fed the monkey to satiety in a reward devaluation experiment. They found that the majority of orbitofrontal olfactory neurons reduced their responses to the odor of the food with which the monkey was fed to satiety (see Fig. 5.3). Thus for these neurons, the **expected reward value** of the odor is what is represented in the orbitofrontal cortex. This provides a basis for the olfactory sensory-specific satiety that is found in humans (Rolls and Rolls, 1997).

Consistent with this finding at the neuronal level in non-human primates, activation of a part of the human orbitofrontal cortex is related to the pleasantness and expected value of food odor, in that the activation measured with fMRI produced by one food odor, banana, decreased after banana was eaten for lunch to satiety, but remained strong to another food odor, vanilla, not eaten in the meal (O'Doherty, Rolls, Francis, Bowtell, McGlone, Kobal, Renner and Ahne, 2000). Consistent findings have been reported (Gottfried, O'Doherty and Dolan, 2003; Howard and Gottfried, 2014; Howard, Gottfried, Tobler and Kahnt, 2015).

Further evidence that pleasant odors are represented in the orbitofrontal cortex is that 3 pleasant odors (linalyl acetate [floral, sweet], geranyl acetate [floral], and alpha-ionone [woody, slightly food-related]) had overlapping activations in the medial orbitofrontal cortex in a region not activated by three unpleasant odors (hexanoic acid, octanol, and isovaleric acid) (Rolls, Kringelbach and De Araujo, 2003c) (see Fig. 5.5). Moreover, activation of the medial orbitofrontal cortex was correlated with the subjective pleasantness ratings of the odors, and activation of the lateral orbitofrontal cortex with the subjective unpleasant-

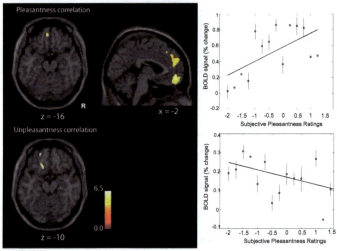

Fig. 5.4 The representation of pleasant and unpleasant odors in the human brain. Random effects group analysis correlation analysis of the BOLD signal with the subjective pleasantness ratings. On the top left is shown the region of the medio-rostral orbitofrontal (peak at [−2 52 −10] z=4.28) correlating positively with pleasantness ratings, as well as the region of the anterior cingulate cortex in the top middle. On the far top-right of the figure is shown the relation between the subjective pleasantness ratings and the BOLD signal from this cluster (in the medial orbitofrontal cortex at Y=52), together with the regression line. The means and s.e.m. across subjects are shown. At the bottom of the figure are shown the regions of left more lateral orbitofrontal cortex (peaks at [−20 54 −14] z=4.26 and [−16 28 −18] z=4.08) correlating negatively with pleasantness ratings. On the far bottom-right of the figure is shown the relation between the subjective pleasantness ratings and the BOLD signal from the first cluster (in the lateral orbitofrontal cortex at Y=54), together with the regression line. The means and s.e.m. across subjects are shown. The activations were thresholded at p<0.0001 for extent. (Reproduced from Edmund T. Rolls, Morten L. Kringelbach, and Ivan E. T. De Araujo (2003) Different representations of pleasant and unpleasant odors in the human brain. European Journal of Neurosciencen 18: 695–703. Copyright © Federation of European Neuroscience Societies and John Wiley and Sons Ltd.)

ness ratings of the odors (see Fig. 5.4). Other studies have also shown activation of the human orbitofrontal cortex by odor (Zatorre, Jones-Gotman, Evans and Meyer, 1992; Zatorre, Jones-Gotman and Rouby, 2000; Royet, Zald, Versace, Costes, Lavenne, Koenig and Gervais, 2000; Anderson, Christoff, Stappen, Panitz, Ghahremani, Glover, Gabrieli and Sobel, 2003; Grabenhorst, Rolls, Margot, da Silva and Velazco, 2007; Rolls, Grabenhorst, Margot, da Silva and Velazco, 2008b).

5.2.7 Cognitive influences on olfactory representations in the orbitofrontal cortex

Cognitive input can bias reward value and emotional states. For example, word level descriptors can influence the subjective pleasantness of olfactory stimuli, and the representation of olfactory stimuli in the human orbitofrontal cortex (De Araujo, Rolls, Velazco, Margot and Cayeux, 2005). The modulation is rather like the top-down effects of attention on perception (Desimone and Duncan, 1995; Rolls and Deco, 2002; Deco and Rolls, 2003, 2005b), not only phenomenologically, as described for taste in Section 4.2.8, but also probably computationally using biased competition or biased activation as described in Section 4.3.5.

In the discovery of top-down effects of cognition on olfactory processing in the brain, a standard test odor, isovaleric acid (with a small amount of cheddar cheese odor added to make it more pleasant), was used as the test olfactory stimulus delivered with an olfactometer during functional neuroimaging with fMRI (De Araujo et al., 2005). This odor is somewhat ambiguous, and might be interpreted as the odor emitted by a cheese-like odor (rather like brie), or might be interpreted as a rather pungent and unpleasant body odor. A word was shown during the 8 s odor delivery. On some trials, the test odor was accompanied by the

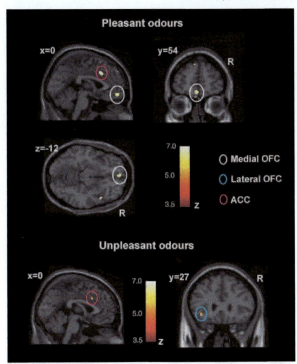

Fig. 5.5 The representation of pleasant and unpleasant odors in the human brain. Above : Group conjunction results for the 3 pleasant odors. Sagittal, horizontal and coronal views are shown at the levels indicated, all including the same activation in the medial orbitofrontal cortex, OFC [0 54 −12] z=5.23). Also shown is activation for the 3 pleasant odors in the anterior cingulate cortex, ACC [2 20 32] z=5.44). These activations were significant at p<0.05 fully corrected for multiple comparisons. Below : Group conjunction results for the 3 unpleasant odors. The sagittal view (left) shows an activated region of the anterior cingulate cortex [0 18 36] z=4.42, p<0.05, svc). The coronal view (right) shows an activated region of the lateral orbitofrontal cortex [−36 27 −8] z=4.23, p<0.05 svc). All the activations were thresholded at p<0.00001 to show the extent of the activations. (Reproduced from Edmund T. Rolls, Morten L. Kringelbach, and Ivan E. T. De Araujo (2003) Different representations of pleasant and unpleasant odors in the human brain. European Journal of Neuroscience 18: 695–703. Copyright © Federation of European Neuroscience Societies and John Wiley and Sons Ltd.)

visually presented word 'Cheddar cheese'. On other trials, the test odor was accompanied by the visually presented word 'Body odor'. A word label was used rather than a picture label to make the modulating input very abstract and cognitive. First, it was found that the word labels influenced the pleasantness ratings of the test odor.

We went on to show that the word label modulated the activation to the odor in brain regions activated by odors such as the orbitofrontal cortex (secondary olfactory cortex), cingulate cortex, and amygdala (De Araujo et al., 2005). For example, in the medial orbitofrontal cortex the word label 'Cheddar cheese' caused a larger activation to be produced to the test odor than when the word label 'Body odor' was being presented. In these medial orbitofrontal cortex regions and the amygdala, and even possibly in some parts of the primary olfactory cortical areas, the activations were correlated with the pleasantness ratings, as shown in Fig. 5.6. This is consistent with the finding that the pleasantness of odors is represented in the medial orbitofrontal cortex (Rolls, Kringelbach and De Araujo, 2003c).

These findings show that cognition can influence and indeed modulate reward-related (affective) processing as far down the human olfactory system as the secondary olfactory cortex in the orbitofrontal cortex, and in the amygdala (De Araujo, Rolls, Velazco, Margot and Cayeux, 2005).

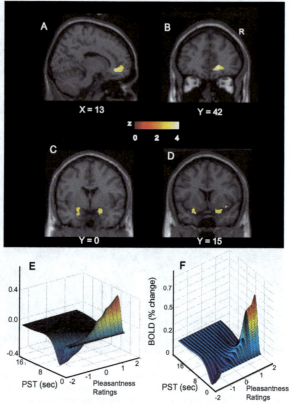

Fig. 5.6 Top-down effects of cognition on olfactory processing. Group (random) effects analysis showing the brain regions where the BOLD signal was correlated with pleasantness ratings given to the test odor. The pleasantness ratings were being modulated by the word labels. (A) Activations in the rostral anterior cingulate cortex, in the region adjoining the medial OFC, shown in a sagittal slice. (B) The same activation shown coronally. (C) Bilateral activations in the amygdala. (D) These activations extended anteriorly to the primary olfactory cortex. The image was thresholded at p<0.0001 uncorrected in order to show the extent of the activation. (E) Parametric plots of the data averaged across all subjects showing that the percentage BOLD change (fitted) correlates with the pleasantness ratings in the region shown in A and B. The parametric plots were very similar for the primary olfactory region shown in D. PST - Post-stimulus time (s). (F) Parametric plots for the amygdala region shown in C. (Reprinted from Neuron, 46 (4), Ivan E. de Araujo, Edmund T. Rolls, Maria Ines Velazco, Christian Margot, and Isabelle Cayeux, Cognitive Modulation of Olfactory Processing, pp. 671–679, Copyright, 2005, with permission from Elsevier.)

5.3 How computations are performed in the olfactory system

5.3.1 Olfactory receptors, and the olfactory bulb

The encoding described in Section 5.2.1 in this early part of the olfactory system is based on the stereochemical structure of the odorant, with receptors that have been produced in a genetically very expensive way, with one gene to build each olfactory receptor type. This is a very simple way for a sensory system to operate, with its sensory capability built largely by having one gene that has evolved to produce a single receptor type, with this repeated for 1000 genes, approximately 1/30th of the human genome.

The convergence from a very large number of olfactory receptors of each type in the olfactory epithelium in the nose, with the different receptor types to some extent intermingled, into a single glomerulus in the bulb for each receptor type shows that the molecular specificity of olfactory encoding is kept largely separate (apart from some lateral inhibition) without feature combinations being formed up to the stage of the glomeruli in the olfactory bulb. The convergence from many receptors onto a single glomerulus must be a way of increasing the signal to noise ratio, by averaging across many receptors of a given type. This, and the molecular specificity of the connectivity is important especially in the context that the olfactory receptor neurons show a constant turnover, being replaced every few days, presumably because in the nose they are in a vulnerable location.

The turnover of olfactory receptors is computationally possible because each glomerulus responds to a single olfactory receptor input, without feature combination neurons being learned at this stage. Once feature combinations have been learned by neurons by associative synaptic modification in for example a competitive network, neuronal turnover is no longer possible, for otherwise the learned combinations will be lost, and later stages of the neural system would not have a reliable input. This is a key reason why the formation of new neurons, neoneurogenesis, and neuronal regeneration, does not happen in the brain. Another is that in a system that operates by learning feature combinations, there is no molecular signal that can inform new neurons about which other neurons to make connections with. The possibility for neuronal turnover in the olfactory epithelium is just because the connections to the olfactory bulb are set by a gene-specified molecular mechanism. There is further discussion of these fundamental computational concepts on how the brain is built, and why neuronal turnover is not possible in the brain except in the dentate gyrus of the hippocampus where information is not stored in these particular synaptic connections, in Rolls (2016b).

The local inhibition in the olfactory bulb may be seen as a way to spread out (orthogonalize or decorrelate) the olfactory stimulus space by using the contrast enhancement provided by lateral inhibition. Feedback from the pyriform cortex may also help to increase the selectivity of neurons in the olfactory bulb (Chae, Banerjee, Dussauze and Albeanu, 2022).

5.3.2 Olfactory (pyriform) cortex

Olfactory (pyriform) cortex is a 3-layer type of cortex termed paleocortex, a type of allocortex (Pandya et al., 2015), with only one layer containing large pyramidal cells. Its structure is shown in Fig. 5.7. This represents my synthesis of what has been described based on these sources (Haberly, 2001; Luskin and Price, 1983) and on discussion with those who work on the pyriform cortex including Joel Price (Washington University School of Medicine), and has some different emphases to those in Figures 9 and 12A2 of Haberly (2001).

The anterior pyriform cortex especially has well-developed recurrent collateral connections, which it is hypothesized enable it to learn as an autoassociation network (Haberly, 2001) which forms combinations of inputs from the glomeruli of the olfactory bulb. Each glomerulus is connected to one of the 1000 types of olfactory receptor each specified by a separate gene, each tuned to a separate range of odors (Buck and Bargmann, 2013; Mombaerts, 2006). The pyriform cortex detects by its autoassociation which combinations of odors tend to occur together as a result of inputs being received from the natural world. This enables discrimination between, and later good recognition of, particular odor combinations.

In more detail, the anatomy suggests that the anterior pyriform cortex acts as an autoassociation or attractor network that can form and remember representations that reflect combinations of simultaneous olfactory inputs. The anterior pyriform cortex has highly developed recurrent collaterals for the autoassociation. (Haberly (2001) distinguished a ventral part which he suggested provided for a first stage of autoassociation, and a dorsal part which provided he postulated a second stage.) The anterior pyriform cortex receives direct inputs from the olfactory bulb and the 'anterior olfactory cortex' (formerly known as the anterior olfactory nucleus). The anterior pyriform cortex necessarily represents the different parts that are being associated together by its recurrent collaterals, and computationally would enable completion of a whole combination from a part, and also short-term memory which might

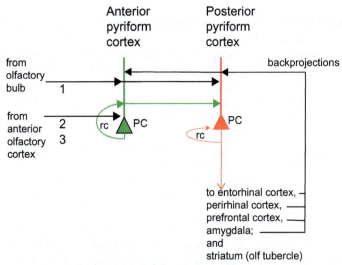

Fig. 5.7 Functional canonical microcircuit of the olfactory (pyriform) cortex. Recurrent collateral connections (rc) are shown as a loop back to a particular population of cells, of which just one neuron is shown. The pyriform cortex has an anterior part, the anterior pyriform cortex (APC), and a posterior part (PPC). Afferents from the olfactory bulb (OB) reach the apical dendrites in layer 1a of APC and PPC. Additional olfactory inputs from an anterior olfactory cortex (AOC) synapse onto the dendrites of the pyramidal cells in layer deep 1b of APC. APC has a highly developed recurrent collateral system, which reaches PPC. There are additional recurrent collaterals on the basal dendrites of the APC (not shown). The APC projects in a feedforward way to PPC, which has a less prominent recurrent collateral system, and which projects on to the recipient olfactory processing regions which include the entorhinal cortex, perirhinal cortex, olfactory tubercle / ventral striatum, prefrontal cortex, and amygdala. (From Rolls, E. T. (2016) Cerebral Cortex: Principles of Operation. Oxford University Press: Oxford.)

be useful in identifying an odor if the concentrations were continually varying, for example with each sniff or because of the wind. I hypothesize that in addition, competitive learning (Section B.4) may also take place in the anterior pyriform cortex, to help the neurons there respond to combinations of glomerular inputs. Consistent with this hypothesis, anterior pyriform cortex neurons do separate overlapping odor combinations better than olfactory bulb neurons (Barnes et al., 2008; Wilson and Sullivan, 2011).

A further useful computation that I propose is performed by the pyriform cortex is the temporal smoothing of the response of the olfactory bulb glomeruli, which is phasically locked to every inhalation, as described above. The proposed mechanism in the pyriform cortex is that an autoassociation network, implemented by the associatively modifiable recurrent collateral connections, provides a short-term memory (Section B.3), which in this case helps to smooth out the activity of pyriform neurons, so that when the outputs are sent to other regions such as the orbitofrontal cortex, they can be easily associated with the non-phasic taste and visual stimuli.

The posterior pyriform cortex receives inputs from the anterior pyriform cortex and also from the olfactory bulb, as shown in Fig. 5.7. Its recurrent collateral system may be less well developed than that of the anterior pyriform cortex (Haberly, 2001) (as indicated by the thinner line in Fig. 5.7), and makes synapses especially with the basal dendrites of the posterior pyriform cortex pyramidal cells (Luskin and Price, 1983). The posterior pyriform cortex then may act (with its feedforward inputs and less highly developed recurrent collateral system), to recode the parts represented in the anterior pyriform cortex into representations that reflect the combinations of the parts, using competitive learning. This corresponds to what I have proposed for the relation between the CA3 recurrent collateral system, and the CA1 competitive network, though the CA1 has essentially no recurrent collaterals (Rolls, 1990b,b; Treves and Rolls, 1994; Rolls, 1996d; Kesner and Rolls, 2015; Rolls, 2018b). The code that is formed in the posterior pyriform cortex thus would be expected on this hypothesis to have different neurons that can respond to different combinations of odors, even when the combinations have overlapping components, and as predicted, this has been found in the Posterior Pyriform Cortex more than in the Anterior Pyriform Cortex, at least in naive animals (Kadohisa and Wilson, 2006). It is also useful to emphasize that the outputs from the pyriform cortex come primarily from the posterior pyriform cortex, which projects to the entorhinal cortex, perirhinal cortex, olfactory tubercle, prefrontal cortex, and amygdala; and not from the anterior pyriform cortex as shown by Haberly (2001).

The implication is that the principle of operation of the pyriform cortex is that it operates primarily as a two-stage system, with the anterior pyriform cortex autoassociation stage followed by a posterior pyriform cortex stage (which may perform competitive learning and some more autoassociation), and that the outputs come primarily from the second stage, the posterior pyriform cortex (see Fig. 5.7). However, the anatomy of the anterior and posterior pyriform cortex shows that any differences in connectivity may be quantitative rather than qualitative, in that some recurrent collaterals from the posterior pyriform cortex reach the anterior pyriform cortex, and the anterior pyriform cortex does have some outputs to other olfactory-related areas (Luskin and Price, 1983). The pyriform cortex does receive backprojections from its target structures, and these end in layer 1, consistent with what is found in neocortex.

The competitive learning proposed for the posterior pyriform cortex is likely to be important in allocating as a category particular combinations of odors that are encountered. This can be described as configural learning, and can result in some neurons responding much more to a combination of inputs than to either of the components (Section B.4). This configural responsiveness is a property of responses to some odor mixtures (Coureaud, Thomas-Danguin, Sandoz and Wilson, 2022). This type of category learning using competition can occur also in systems that in addition implement attractor dynamics related to the recurrent collaterals between the neurons (Rolls, 2021c).

Here is my hypothesis about how the pyriform cortex differs computationally from the neocortex. The pyriform cortex pyramidal cells correspond approximately to the superficial cortical layers of the cerebral neocortex, in which a key computational component is autoassociation or attractor networks, but also competitive learning to form new combination-sensitive representations. Indeed, there is a hint that computationally the anterior pyriform cortex may specialise in autoassociation, and the posterior pyriform cortex, with its less prominent recurrent collateral system, as a competitive learning stage to emphasise encoding of combinations of odor components. The posterior pyriform cortex may thus be analogous to the CA1 neurons of the hippocampus, and to draw out this possibility, both are colored red in Figs. 5.7 and 9.22. Both the posterior pyriform cortex and the CA1 provide the prominent outputs of their cortical region, including projections to the striatum. However, continuing the comparison with the neocortex, the pyriform olfactory cortex evolved before there was any neocortex, or thalamus. So the olfactory cortex in early evolutionary history had no need of a layer 6, because there was no thalamus. Correspondingly, there was no preceding (neo)cortical area for a putative L5 of pyriform cortex to send backprojections to. So effectively, all that the olfactory cortex could do was to perform its autoassociation (and competitive) computation, and send its outputs on to whatever structure was present. There was no neocortex for a forward projection to reach. So the outputs of the pyriform cortex just went to whichever output region for behavior might be present, which was probably the striatum / basal ganglia, which was present at early evolutionary stages. Consistent with this, parts of the output targets of pyriform cortex include regions with a striatal structure, the olfactory tubercle, and parts of the amygdala. At later evolutionary stages, when neocortex was present, outputs from the pyriform cortex then reached neocortical areas such as the entorhinal cortex and prefrontal / orbitofrontal cortex. As in neocortex, the backprojections to the pyriform cortex terminate in layer 1, where they are likely to modulate rather than determine pyramidal cell firing under natural conditions. (This last point is very important. All the analyses that I have performed of cortical processing have been when the system is operating normally in the awake behaving animal, and much of this type of research remains to be performed for the pyriform cortex, instead of under anaesthesia or in slices in which effects may be demonstrated, but with the great need for their significance during normal computation to be evaluated.)

My hypothesis is that the olfactory cortex was then a 'primitive' form of cortex, and was part of the origin of 6-layer neocortex. To lead to neocortex, outputs had to be added in neocortex to drive pyramidal tract neurons with a non-sparse code (L5); and to provide a feedback signal from layer 6 to the thalamus, which of course was not present at early evolutionary stages when most of the cortex was pyriform cortex (Molnar, Kaas, de Carlos, Hevner, Lein and Nemec, 2014). In evolution, the genes that specified the architecture of pyriform cortex might have provided a start to the design of neocortex. Molecular marker / gene comparisons of pyriform cortex with the superficial layers of neocortex might be of interest (Harris and Shepherd, 2015; Bernard et al., 2012; Molnar et al., 2014).

The representation of odors in the anterior pyriform cortex was found to be a little more sparse than in the posterior pyriform cortex in rats familiar with the odors (Kadohisa and Wilson, 2006). This may reflect a principle of cortical design, as follows. In the part of the cortex where the storage of large numbers of memories composed of parts is being performed, in attractor networks, there is an advantage to having a sparse representation, for this will increase the memory capacity. This advantage applies to the anterior pyriform cortex, to the hippocampal CA3 neurons, and to the superficial pyramidal cells (L2/L3) of the neocortex. In contrast, in the part of the cortex following an attractor network where a network operating in part as a competitive network is re-coding the parts of the memory into a single conjunctive representation (in which a neuron might respond to a combination of the parts), the representation may be less sparse, because the advantage here is to convey a large amount of information into a given number of neurons in the whole population, as this information will be used as a recall cue. This could apply to the hippocampal CA1 cells, to the deep layers of the neocortex (L5) which give rise to backprojections used for memory recall, and may apply to the posterior pyriform cortex, where the parts of the memory may no longer be as relevant, just the memory of specific combinations of odors. However, the components were more correlated with each other, and the components were more correlated with the binary mixtures, in the posterior pyriform cortex than in the anterior pyriform cortex (Kadohisa and Wilson, 2006). This does not suggest pattern separation from the anterior to the posterior pyriform cortex, and is consistent with the coding being less sparse in the posterior pyriform cortex. The authors comment that the posterior pyriform cortex encoding may reflect perceptual similarity, in that for example after experiencing a cherry + smoky mixture, the components may become more similar to each other, with for example the cherry being described as having a smoky component. So some recoding may be taking place from anterior to posterior pyriform cortex, but it is not just pattern separation, according to this evidence (Kadohisa and Wilson, 2006). What does appear to be the case is that the posterior pyriform cortex is a later stage in processing, in that it has highly developed axonal connections to entorhinal cortex, perirhinal cortex, prefrontal cortex, amygdala, and striatum (olfactory tubercle) (Haberly, 2001; Luskin and Price, 1983).

In addition, a L4 was not present in olfactory cortex, for there was no thalamus, and the inputs from the glomeruli in the olfactory bulb just appear as forward inputs projecting as they do in most neocortical areas to superficial layers of the cortex. However, an additional key difference (from the hippocampus too) is that there is no granule cell stage in the pyriform cortex to perform pattern separation before the inputs are applied to the pyriform cortex. Taking this concept one step further, the neocortex can be thought of as more advanced computationally (operationally) than the pyriform and hippocampal cortex, in that the neocortex has thalamic inputs, which as suggested above perform a useful and simple stage of pattern separation before inputs reach the primary sensory cortical areas, by virtue of the local lateral inhibition in the topologically mapped thalamic nuclei, which serves to operate as a high pass spatial filter. There is of course no (or very little) spatial topology in the 1000 dimensional odor space spanned by the olfactory receptor genes and glomeruli, and for this reason a thalamus for olfaction acting in the way just described with local lateral inhibition would not be operationally (computationally) very useful.

This provides an answer to why a thalamus evolved in conjunction with the neocortex. My hypothesis is that the thalamus, which performs primarily local lateral inhibition between its neurons, was useful as a cortical preprocessor, for exactly this computation performs hi-pass filtering of the inputs, making them more sparse, which helps the computations performed by the neocortex, including pattern separation and autoassociation (Appendix B).

5.3.3 Orbitofrontal cortex

In the orbitofrontal cortex, at least some neurons remap the olfactory representation from the genetic encoding present in the receptors and olfactory bulb into a space where associations are made to taste, as many orbitofrontal cortex olfactory neurons represent odors by the taste with which they are associated. This is probably learned by pattern association learning (see Section B.2).

The reversal learning implemented for olfactory to taste associations in the orbitofrontal cortex could be implemented by gradual relearning in the pattern association type of network described in Section B.2. The rapid rule-based reversal that can occur in the orbitofrontal cortex for at least visual stimuli (when for example their association with a taste is reversed) is a much more sophisticated system, for it requires a rule-based system, and the rule must be held online. A model for this is described in Chapter 11.

Many orbitofrontal cortex olfactory neurons represent odors in terms of their reward value, as shown by the effects of feeding to satiety. Part of this may be implemented by the association with taste, the reward value of which is represented in the orbitofrontal cortex.

Further, olfactory sensory-specific is represented in the orbitofrontal cortex, and this may be computed by synaptic adaptation of the afferent connections to orbitofrontal cortex olfactory neurons, in that it is represented in the orbitofrontal cortex, and because just smelling an odor for several minutes can produce some olfactory sensory-specific satiety (Rolls and Rolls, 1997).

A summary of what is computed in the olfactory system, and how it is computed, is provided at the start of this Chapter in Sections 5.1.1 and 5.1.2.

6 The somatosensory system

6.1 What is computed in the somatosensory system

The first few subsections (6.1.1–6.1.4) consider somatosensory processing in the parietal somatosensory cortex hierarchy (Delhaye, Long and Bensmaia, 2018), including the interface to visual representations.

Then somatosensory representations in the insular cortex are considered (Section 6.1.5).

The representation of the affective value of touch in the orbitofrontal cortex is described in Section 6.1.6.

Decision-making within the somatosensory system is considered in Section 6.1.7, with the network mechanisms for how the computations are performed to implement decision-making described in Sections 11.5.1 and B.6–B.8.

6.1.1 The receptors and periphery

The main touch receptor types in the skin are shown in Fig. 6.1 (Delhaye et al., 2018). The Meissner corpuscles are superficial, have small receptive fields, are used for fine discrimination, and adapt rapidly. The Pacinian corpuscles are deep, have large receptive fields, and adapt rapidly so respond to mechanical transients. The Merkel corpuscles are superficial and adapt only slowly, so are useful for measuring the force being applied, for example when grasping an object, as well as for fine discrimination. The Ruffini corpuscles are deeper, and adapt only slowly, so are useful for measuring strain forces in the skin and below it. These are relatively similar in glabrous skin (the palms of the hands and the soles of the feet) and non-glabrous skin.

In addition, there are receptors that respond to pain, and others to soft slow stroking movements across the skin (Olausson et al., 2010, 2016), and conduct via the slow C fibres.

Muscles have proprioceptors that signal muscle stretch, and joints have proprioceptors that signal the angle of the joint.

The somatosensory nerves project to the Ventral Posterior (VP) group of thalamic nuclei.

6.1.2 The anterior somatosensory cortex, areas 1, 2, 3a, and 3b, in the anterior parietal cortex

The main somatosensory cortical areas are shown in Fig. 6.2, and the main connections between them are shown in Fig. 6.3 (Delhaye et al., 2018). The ventral posterior (VP) nuclei of the thalamus project most strongly to area 3b, which can be considered as the primary somatosensory cortex, which projects on to areas 1, 2 and 3a. Parts of these anterior parietal cortex areas then project in a dorsal stream to posterior parietal cortex area 5, which in turn projects to area 7b, with this stream related to motor behavior, including reaching and grasping; and in a ventral stream to S2 (sometimes termed secondary somatosensory cortex) and the parietal ventral areas which are in the Sylvian fissure and adjoining insula, and are more involved in higher level feature extraction, attention, and decision-making for tactile stimuli. There is a clear analogy here to the dorsal and ventral visual streams described in Chapters 2 and 3. The system does have hierarchical organisation, even if it is not very strict as shown

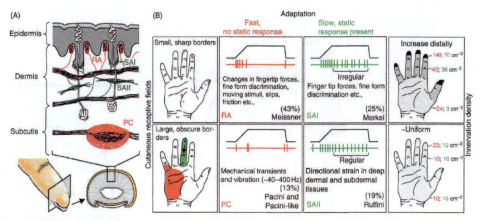

Fig. 6.1 Four classes of receptor in the skin (see text). (Reproduced from Delhaye,B.P., Long,K.H. and Bensmaia,S.J. (2018) Neural basis of touch and proprioception in primate cortex. Comprehensive Physiology 8: 1575–1602. Copyright © American Physiological Society.)

in Fig. 6.3, in that neurons higher is the somatosensory system have more complex and selective properties. There are specializations in each of these parietal areas, as described next (Delhaye et al., 2018).

Neurons in area 3b respond to cutaneous stimulation and have small receptive fields. The receptive fields tend to be elongated (with a mean aspect ratio of 1.7), and thus show orientation tuning analogous to that shown by simple cells in the primary visual cortex.

Neurons in area 1 respond to cutaneous stimulation and have larger receptive fields, which may for example span several digits. These neurons, and also neurons in area 2, have more complex feature selectivity than in 3a, such as a selectivity for curvature, or a shape-invariant selectivity for direction of motion, neither of which are reflected in the spatial structure of their RFs. The receptive fields of neurons in area 1, unlike those in area 3b, solve the aperture problem, in that the receptive fields are sufficiently large for global motion to be encoded, in a similar way to that which occurs in vision in area MT (Section 3.2). They are also sensitive to the speed of motion.

Neurons in area 3a respond to proprioceptive input signalling joint angle and muscle stretch. Some neurons respond to combinations of joint position, and so may respond for a particular reach direction. Some neurons in the head region are tuned to eye position. Some neurons respond to pain (Whitsel et al., 2019).

Neurons in area 2 respond to cutaneous or proprioceptive input or both, and have larger receptive fields than area 3b. Lesions of area 2 impair the coordination of finger movements and the ability to discriminate the shape and size of grasped objects. To determine the shape of a felt object, the tactile input but also the shape of the hand needs to be taken into account, and this process may start in area 2 where both tactile and proprioceptive information are present.

6.1.3 The ventral somatosensory stream: areas S2 and PV, in the lateral parietal cortex

Some neurons in S2 and the parietal ventral area (PV) are orientation tuned and show some position (translation) invariance. Some neurons are tuned to the direction of curved edges (Delhaye et al., 2018). Neurons here may be affected by attention. Some neurons respond to auditory stimuli, such as the sound of hands rubbing together, or to visual stimuli, as considered further below. Some neurons in S2 reflect decision-making about somatosensory stimuli,

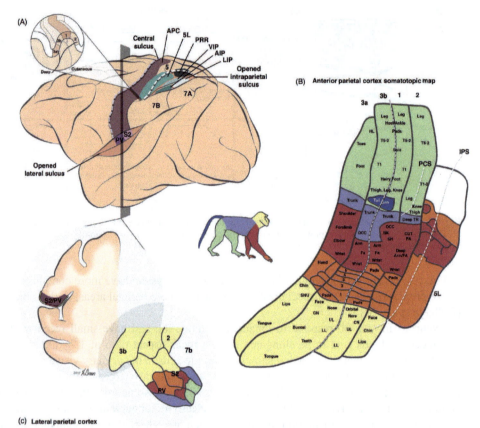

Fig. 6.2 Organization of somatosensory cortical areas. (A) A lateral view of the brain showing the different somatosensory areas in macaque monkey cortex. Inset: Horizontal section of the postcentral gyrus at the level of the hand representation, showing the position of the different APC modules relative to the central and the intraparietal sulci. (B) Detailed view of the somatotopic representation of the body in the four fields of APC (areas 3a, 3b, 1, and 2) and in area 5L. (C) Coronal section showing the location of the lateral parietal cortex (LPC) in the lateral sulcus. Abbreviations: Anterior parietal cortex (APC); second somatosensory area (S2); parietal ventral area (PV); parietal reaching region (PRR); anterior (AIP), ventral (VIP) and lateral (LIP) intraparietal areas; post central sulcus (PCS); intraparietal sulcus (IPS). Somatotopic map: Upper lip (UL); lower lip (LL); chin (CN); snout/jaw (SN/J); digits of the hand (1{5); (cutaneous) forearm ((CUT) FA); occiput (OCC); trunk (TR); toes (T1{5); hindlimb (HL). (Reproduced from Delhaye,B.P., Long,K.H. and Bensmaia,S.J. (2018) Neural basis of touch and proprioception in primate cortex. Comprehensive Physiology 8: 1575–1602. Copyright © American Physiological Society.)

as described in Section 6.1.7. Lesions of the lateral parietal cortex lead to an impairment in shape discrimination, as do lesions in area 2, confirming that these two areas are part of a tactile shape processing pathway.

6.1.4 The dorsal somatosensory stream to area 5 and then 7b, in the posterior parietal cortex

Area 5 receives strongly from area 2, and has a lateral part (5L); and a part with arm reaching neurons, the parietal reaching region (PRR). Neurons in the posterior parietal cortex respond to cutaneous stimulation, and joint movements, and many respond to visual, and some to auditory and vestibular stimuli (Delhaye et al., 2018). These neurons are active during reaching and grasping movements, appear to encode not just limb position but also target locations and motor actions, and have connections with prefrontal, motor, and superior temporal gyrus

What is computed in the somatosensory system | 271

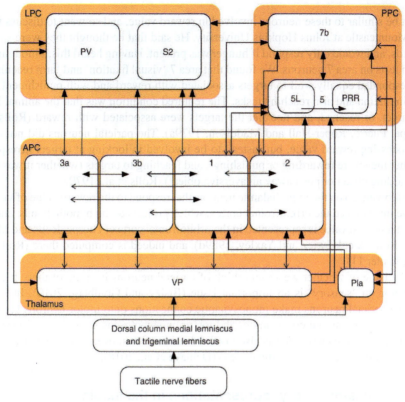

Fig. 6.3 Major connections between somatosensory areas in macaques. Schematic representation of the major connections between somatosensory areas in the central nervous system, split into four major regions: the thalamus, the anterior parietal cortex (APC), the lateral parietal cortex (LPC), and the posterior parietal cortex (PPC). Abbreviations: Ventral posterior nucleus (VP), anterior pulvinar nucleus (PIa), secondary somatosensory cortex (S2), parietal ventral area (PV), parietal reach region (PRR). Area 5 also receives input from the lateral posterior nucleus (LP) in the thalamus. (Reproduced from Delhaye,B.P., Long,K.H. and Bensmaia,S.J. (2018) Neural basis of touch and proprioception in primate cortex. Comprehensive Physiology 8: 1575–1602. Copyright © American Physiological Society.)

areas. Lesions within the posterior parietal cortex impair the ability to reach and grasp objects or to recognize an object's shape through haptic exploration (stereognosis).

Area 7b receives from area 5, and has an anterior part primarily connected to somatosensory areas, and a posterior part that receives visual inputs from MST, temporal visual areas, and the lateral parietal areas. These neurons may respond better during active but also respond during passive movements, and some respond to visual stimuli.

There has been a strong debate about whether neurons in area 7 (7b or 7a) are sensory or motor. Because of their activity during reaching movements to a target in space, the pioneering neuroscientist Vernon Mountcastle and his colleagues described the neurons as 'command neurons', and argued that these neurons represent the value of the goal or target towards which the animal should reach (Mountcastle, Lynch, Georgopoulos, Sakata and Acuna, 1975). They described these neurons as responding 'during eye and hand movements directed towards desired objects, such as food when the animal is hungry'. They described these area 7 neurons as being 'conditional on the nature of the object and the motivational set of the animal' (Mountcastle et al., 1975). At the time, we were discovering neurons in the lateral hypothalamus that responded only to reward-associated objects, and not to aversive objects, and that responded only when hunger was present (Rolls, Burton and Mora, 1976; Burton, Rolls and Mora, 1976; Rolls, Sanghera and Roper-Hall, 1979b). I was sceptical that neurons in the parietal cortex might be similar to these neurons involved in reward value, and so went to discuss with Vernon Mountcastle at Johns Hopkins University. He said that he thought they were specific for rewards, and would only respond if hunger was present. Having heard this, I thought it useful to run tests on area 7 neurons. We found that area 7 'visual fixation' and 'arm reaching' neurons responded equally well to targets associated with reward and with punishment in visual discrimination and arm reaching tasks. The required condition was that the animal looked at the target, or reached, and not that the targets were associated with reward (Rolls, Perrett, Thorpe, Puerto, Roper-Hall and Maddison, 1979a). The parietal neurons did not appear to be processing reward value, but instead to be involved in looking at targets (irrespective of whether they were rewarding or punishing), and reaching to targets (whether it was to obtain a rewarding object or push away an aversive object) (Rolls et al., 1979a).

Following up on the hypothalamic neurons that respond to the reward value of visual stimuli, we investigated the orbitofrontal cortex, which projects to the hypothalamus, and discovered that reward value is represented in the orbitofrontal cortex (Thorpe, Rolls and Maddison, 1983; Rolls, Sienkiewicz and Yaxley, 1989d), and indeed is computed there (Rolls, 2019e) (see Chapter 11).

The issue of whether we should think of parietal neurons in some of these higher areas as 'motor' or 'sensory' is an important issue (Bisley and Goldberg, 2010). In fact, some of these parietal neurons make monosynaptic connections onto motor neurons for the hand, so the posterior parietal cortex although high up in somatosensory and dorsal visual stream sensory processing hierarchies is also involved in initiating movements, both directly, and by its connections to premotor cortical areas (Delhaye et al., 2018).

6.1.5 Somatosensory representations in the insula

The C-tactile afferents that respond to affectively positive soft slow stroking movements across the skin (Olausson et al., 2010, 2016) appear not to project to the anterior parietal cortex, but instead to the insula (Delhaye et al., 2018), which in turn has onward projections to the orbitofrontal cortex (Morecraft et al., 1992; Rolls, 2019e). Pain inputs (also mediated by C-fibres) reach the posterior insula directly from the thalamus (Craig, 2014).

The insula has been described as representing feelings from the body (Craig, 2011). Interestingly, the insula is a brain region that is activated by touch to the arm, but not by the sight of touch to someone else's arm, implicating it in representations of especially one's own body (McCabe, Rolls, Bilderbeck and McGlone, 2008).

The antero-dorsal part of the insula is the primary taste cortex, and has neurons that respond to the texture of food, including its viscosity and fat texture (Verhagen, Kadohisa and Rolls, 2004; Kadohisa, Rolls and Verhagen, 2005a; Rolls, 2016c, 2020c). The antero-ventral insula and nearby parts of the insula are probably visceral / autonomic cortex (Critchley and Harrison, 2013; Strigo and Craig, 2016; Kleckner et al., 2017; Hassanpour et al., 2018), which may account for its activation in some emotion-related processing (Rolls, 2014a, 2016c). The anterior ventral insula has strong interconnections with the orbitofrontal cortex (Baylis, Rolls and Baylis, 1995), which may enable visceral signals involved in for example satiety to reach the orbitofrontal cortex; and the orbitofrontal cortex to produce autonomic responses during emotional processing.

6.1.6 Somatosensory and temperature inputs to the orbitofrontal cortex, affective value, pleasant touch, and pain

In the periphery, C-tactile fibres on non-glabrous skin (most of the skin apart from the hands and feet) respond to soft slowly moving tactile stimuli, and are implicated in affectively positive touch, such as stroking and grooming (Olausson et al., 2016). For glabrous skin, there are no such C-tactile fibres. An interesting distinction may be that touch to non-glabrous skin may be by another individual, whereas for glabrous skin, the touch is more likely to be self-initiated, such as when an object is picked up (Delhaye et al., 2018), leading to different processing in the brain.

Experiments have been performed to investigate where in the human touch-processing system (see Figs. 11.4 and 11.1) tactile stimuli are decoded and represented in terms of their rewarding value or the pleasure they produce. In order to investigate this, Rolls, O'Doherty, Kringelbach, Francis, Bowtell and McGlone (2003d) performed functional magnetic resonance imaging (fMRI) of humans who were receiving pleasant, neutral, and painful tactile stimuli. They found that a weak but very pleasant touch of the hand with velvet produced much stronger activation of the orbitofrontal cortex than a more intense but affectively neutral touch of the hand with wood. In contrast, the pleasant stimuli produced much less activation of the primary somatosensory cortex S1 than the neutral stimuli (see Fig. 6.4). It was concluded that part of the orbitofrontal cortex is concerned with representing the positively affective aspects of somatosensory stimuli. Nearby, but separate, parts of the human orbitofrontal cortex were shown in the same series of experiments to be activated by taste and olfactory stimuli. Thus the pleasantness of tactile stimuli, which can be powerful primary reinforcers (Taira and Rolls, 1996), is correlated with the activity of a part of the orbitofrontal cortex. This part of the orbitofrontal cortex probably receives its somatosensory inputs via the somatosensory cortex both via direct projections and via the insula (Mesulam and Mufson, 1982a,b; Rolls, 2019e, 2006b). In contrast, the pleasantness of a tactile stimulus does not appear to be represented explicitly in the somatosensory cortex. The indication thus is that only certain parts of the somatosensory input, which reflect its pleasantness, are passed on (perhaps after appropriate processing) to the orbitofrontal cortex by the somatosensory cortical areas. It was also notable that the pleasant touch activated the most anterior (pregenual) part of the anterior cingulate cortex (Rolls, O'Doherty, Kringelbach, Francis, Bowtell and McGlone, 2003d) (see Fig. 6.4).

Warm and cold stimuli have affective components such as feeling pleasant or unpleasant, and these components may have survival value, for approach to warmth and avoidance of cold may be reinforcers or goals for action built into us during evolution to direct our behavior to stimuli that are appropriate for survival. Understanding the brain processing that underlies these prototypical reinforcers provides a direct approach to understanding the brain mechanisms of emotion. In an fMRI investigation in humans, it was found that the mid-orbitofrontal and pregenual cingulate cortex and the ventral striatum have activations that are correlated with the subjective pleasantness ratings made to warm (41C) and cold (12C) stimuli, and combinations of warm and cold stimuli, applied to the hand (Rolls, Grabenhorst and Parris, 2008a) (see Fig. 6.5a-c). Activations in the lateral and some more anterior parts of the orbitofrontal cortex were correlated with the unpleasantness of the stimuli. In contrast, activations in the somatosensory cortex and ventral posterior insula were correlated with the intensity but not the pleasantness of the thermal stimuli (see Fig. 6.5d-f).

A principle thus is that processing related to the affective value and associated subjective emotional experience of thermal stimuli that are important for survival is performed in different brain areas to those where activations are related to sensory properties of the stimuli such as their intensity. This conclusion appears to be the case for processing in a number of sensory modalities, including taste and olfaction (see above), and the finding with such prototypical stimuli as warm and cold (Rolls, Grabenhorst and Parris, 2008a) provides strong support for this principle (Rolls, 2014a, 2019f, 2018a).

In another investigation, touch to the forearm (which has unmyelinated C fibre touch (CT) afferents sensitive to light touch) (Olausson et al., 2002) revealed activation in the mid-

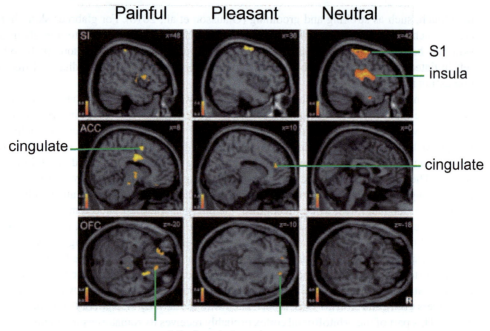

Fig. 6.4 Brain activation to painful, pleasant, and neutral touch of the human brain. The top row shows strongest activation of the somatosensory cortex S1/insula by the neutral touch, on sagittal sections (parallel to the midline). The middle row shows activation of the most anterior part of the anterior cingulate cortex by the pleasant touch, and of a more posterior part by the painful touch, on sagittal sections. The bottom row shows activation of the orbitofrontal cortex by the pleasant and by the painful touch, on axial sections (in the horizontal plane). The activations were thresholded at $p<0.0001$ to show the extent of the activations. (After Rolls, E. T., O'Doherty,J., Kringelbach,M.L., Francis,S., Bowtell,R. and McGlone,F. (2003) Representations of pleasant and painful touch in the human orbitofrontal and cingulate cortices. Cerebral Cortex 13: 308–317. Copyright © Oxford University Press.)

orbitofrontal cortex, providing an indication that the orbitofrontal cortex may be involved in processing the effects of CT afferents, and thus potentially in any positively hedonic effects mediated through CT fibres (McCabe, Rolls, Bilderbeck and McGlone, 2008; Rolls, 2016a).

To investigate how the affective aspects of touch may be modulated by cognitive factors, in an fMRI investigation participants were shown word labels ('rich moisturizing cream' or 'basic cream') while cream was being applied to the forearm, or was seen being applied to a forearm (McCabe, Rolls, Bilderbeck and McGlone, 2008). The subjective pleasantness and richness were modulated by the word labels, and so were the fMRI activations to touch in parietal cortex area 7, the insular somatosensory cortex, and the ventral striatum. The cognitive labels influenced the activations to the sight of touch and also the correlations with pleasantness in the pregenual cingulate / orbitofrontal cortex and ventral striatum.

Comparison of the sight of an arm being rubbed with cream to a visual control with no contact revealed effects in the inferior frontal gyrus (a mirror neuron area, in which neurons respond to motor actions and to the sight of the action being performed (Rizzolatti and Craighero, 2004)), area 7, and even S1, implicating these regions in the imagined or intentional aspects of touch (McCabe et al., 2008). Although neurons in S1 are not activated by most visual or auditory stimuli, effects can be found if these stimuli are relevant to somatosensory processing, such as the sound of a stimulus rubbing the skin (Delhaye et al., 2018). In the experiment of McCabe et al. (2008), when the visual stimulus showed the hand being clearly touched, more brain activation was produced than when a similar visual stimulus was shown not quite touching the hand.

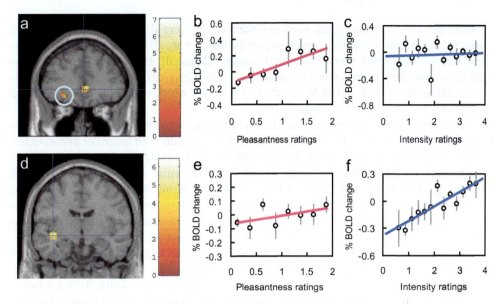

Fig. 6.5 Representation of the pleasantness but not intensity of thermal stimuli in the orbitofrontal cortex (top), and of the intensity but not the pleasantness in the mid ventral (somatosensory) insular cortex (bottom). a. SPM analysis showing a correlation in the mid orbitofrontal cortex (blue circle) at [-26 38 -10] between the BOLD signal and the pleasantness ratings of four thermal stimuli. Correlations are also shown in the pregenual cingulate cortex. For this mid orbitofrontal cortex region, (b) shows the positive correlation between the subjective pleasantness ratings and the BOLD signal ($r=0.84$, $df=7$, $p<0.01$), and (c) shows that there is no correlation between the subjective intensity ratings and the BOLD signal ($r=0.07$, $df=12$, $p=0.8$). d. SPM analysis showing a correlation with intensity in the posterior ventral insula with peak at [-40 -10 -8] between the BOLD signal and the intensity ratings for the four thermal stimuli. For this ventral insula cortex region, (e) shows no correlation between the subjective pleasantness ratings and the BOLD signal ($r=0.56$, $df=7$, $p=0.15$), and (f) shows a positive correlation between the subjective intensity ratings and the BOLD signal ($r=0.89$, $df=12$, $p<0.001$). (Reprinted from Edmund T. Rolls, Fabian Grabenhorst and Benjamin A. Parris (2008) Warm pleasant feelings in the brain. NeuroImage 41: 1504–1513. Copyright © Elsevier Inc.)

It is proposed that the computational principle that operates here is that if an area such as S1 is being activated by touch, and simultaneously there is a top-down backprojected input to S1 from higher cortical areas that is simultaneously being received, such as the sight of the touch, then that backprojected input will be associatively synaptically modified onto S1 (or other active) neurons. Then later, that top-down input alone will be capable of activating these tactile neurons, in for example S1. The same principle could apply to other brain areas receiving visual inputs but also having touch or movement-related firing, in which associative Hebbian synaptic modification could account for touch or movement-related neurons also being activated by the sight of the touch or movement (Keysers and Perrett, 2004). This mechanism might be thought of as a somatosensory mirror neuron system. Similar principles could apply to the findings that neurons with movement-related activity in for example premotor cortex area F5 respond to the sight of grasping an object, as well as to actually grasping an object, in what we might now term the 'motor' mirror neuron system (Rizzolatti and Craighero, 2004; Rizzolatti and Sinigaglia, 2016; Rizzolatti and Rozzi, 2018).

It was notable that this sight of touch did not activate somatosensory regions in the insula, and it was therefore proposed that this area is especially important in representing that one is being actually touched (McCabe, Rolls, Bilderbeck and McGlone, 2008; Rolls, 2016a).

The issue of where the reinforcing and the subjectively unpleasant properties of activation of the pain pathways is represented is complex. There are clearly specialized peripheral nerves (including C fibres, with some activated via VR1 or capsaicin receptors) that convey painful stimulation to the central nervous system (Delhaye et al., 2018). We have seen that area 3a has some neurons that respond to pain (Whitsel et al., 2019) (and loss of pain sensation has been described after a lesion to this region (Marshall, 1951)), and that nociceptive afferents from the thalamus reach the posterior insula (Craig, 2014), which is implicated in pain (Baumgartner et al., 2010; Wiech et al., 2014), and which projects to the orbitofrontal cortex (Morecraft et al., 1992; Rolls, 2019e).

There is evidence that structures as recently developed as the orbitofrontal cortex of primates are important in the subjective aspects of pain, for patients with lesions or disconnection of the orbitofrontal cortex may say that they can identify the input as painful, but that it does not produce the same affective feeling as previously (Freeman and Watts, 1950; Melzack and Wall, 1996). In the fMRI study of Rolls, O'Doherty, Kringelbach, Francis, Bowtell and McGlone (2003d) painful inputs (produced by a stylus) were also applied to the hand, and we found that the orbitofrontal cortex was more strongly activated by the painful touch than by the neutral touch, whereas the somatosensory cortex was relatively more activated by the physically heavier neutral touch (see Fig. 6.4). This provides evidence that negative as well as positive aspects of affective touch are especially represented in the orbitofrontal cortex. In this study, as in many studies (Vogt and Sikes, 2000; Vogt, 2009; Rolls, 2019c), a part of the anterior cingulate cortex in or near to the cingulate motor area which receives from the orbitofrontal cortex was also activated by pain (see example in Fig. 6.4 and Chapter 12).

The activation of parts of the orbitofrontal cortex by painful stimuli (Rolls, O'Doherty, Kringelbach, Francis, Bowtell and McGlone, 2003d; Rolls, Grabenhorst and Parris, 2008a) is likely to have great clinical relevance, for orbitofrontal cortex damage results in individuals knowing that a painful stimulus is being applied, but not feeling the strong negative affective component, of subjective pain (Rolls, 2014a, 2019e). The clinical relevance of these discoveries about the orbitofrontal cortex in relation to pain pathways and pain treatment as well as in subjective aspects of emotion (Rolls, 2019e) is likely to be of great importance, but appears to be under-appreciated at present, with the focus instead on other brain regions such as the posterior insula (Segerdahl, Mezue, Okell, Farrar and Tracey, 2015; Tracey, 2017).

6.1.7 Decision-making in the somatosensory system

The neuronal substrate of the ability to discriminate two sequential vibrotactile stimuli has been investigated by Romo and colleagues (Romo and Salinas, 2001; Hernandez, Zainos and Romo, 2002; Romo, Hernandez, Zainos, Lemus and Brody, 2002; Romo, Hernandez, Zainos and Salinas, 2003; Romo and Salinas, 2003; Romo, Hernandez and Zainos, 2004; de Lafuente and Romo, 2005). They used a task where trained macaques (*Macaca mulatta*) must decide and report which of two mechanical vibrations applied sequentially to their fingertips has the higher frequency of vibration by pressing one of two pushbuttons. This decision-making paradigm requires therefore the following processes: (1) the perception of the first stimulus, a 500 ms long vibration at frequency f1; (2) the storing of a trace of the f1 stimulus in short-term memory during a delay of typically 3 s; (3) the perception of the second stimulus, a 500 ms long vibration at frequency f2; and (4) the comparison of the second stimulus f2 to the trace of f1, and choosing a motor act based on this comparison (f2-f1). The vibrotactile stimuli f1 and f2 utilized were in the range of frequencies called *flutter*, i.e. within approximately 5–50 Hz.

In the primary somatosensory cortex the average firing rates of neurons convey information about the vibrotactile frequency f1 or f2 during the stimulation period. The neuronal responses stop reflecting information about the stimuli immediately after the end of the stimulus. The firing rates increase monotonically with stimulus frequency (Romo and Salinas, 2003). Neurons in the secondary somatosensory area S2 respond to f1 and show significant

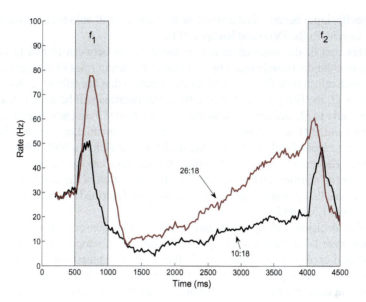

Fig. 6.6 Activity of a single neuron of the 'partially differential' type recorded in the ventral premotor cortex (VPC) during the vibrotactile decision-making task, after Romo et al. (2004), as illustrated in Fig 2JLK of that paper. The f1 period was from 500–1000 ms, there was then a delay period, and the f2 period when f2 was applied and the decision was made was from 4000–4500 ms. f2 was in both cases 18 Hz. When f1 was 26 Hz (red plot), the firing rate during f1, and at the end of the delay period, and during the comparison period when f2 was being applied was higher than when f1 was 10 Hz (black plot). Thus the firing of this type of neuron during f2 helps in the decision that f1>f2 when f1 is 26 Hz, and that f1<f2 when f1 is 10 Hz. Approximately 30 trials were used to generate these peristimulus time histograms for each pair for this single neuron. (Reproduced from Deco,G., Rolls, E. T. and Romo,R. (2010) Synaptic dynamics and decision-making. Proceedings of the National Academy of Sciences of the United States of America 107: 7545–7549.)

delay activity for a few hundred milliseconds after the end of the f1 stimulus (Romo et al., 2002). Some neurons in this region respond if f1>f2; and some to the opposite, and so reflect the decision about which is the higher vibrotactile frequency. Similar neurons are also found in areas to which S2 projects such as the ventral premotor cortex (VPC) (Romo et al., 2004).

In the ventral premotor cortex, some 'partial differential' neurons reflect the memory of f1. The activity of one of these neurons recorded in the ventral prefrontal cortex (Romo et al., 2004) is illustrated in Fig. 6.6. Partial differential neurons respond to f1 during the presentation of f1, do not respond in the first part of the delay period, then gradually ramp up towards the end of the delay period to a firing frequency that reflects f1, and then during the decision period when f2 is presented are influenced by f2 (Romo et al., 2004). The responses of partial differential neurons may be related to the decision-making (Romo et al., 2004), for as shown in Fig. 6.6, if f1>f2 the firing during f2 is higher than when f1<f2, for a given f2.

Part of the mechanism that explains this vibrotactile decision-making reflected in the responses of S2 and VPC 'partial differential' neurons is the 'remembering' during the delay period of the firing that occurred to f1, as the firing rate ramps up again in the delay period, as shown in Fig. 6.6. One mechanism that can account for this is synaptic facilitation produced during f1. This will continue for several seconds into the delay period, and if a non-specific input is applied to the network as the delay period comes to an end, that will lead to reinstatement of the firing just of the neurons with facilitated synapses, thus accounting for the recall (Deco, Rolls and Romo, 2010; Martinez-Garcia, Rolls, Deco and Romo, 2011). This is explained in more detail in Section 11.5.1. Another mechanism is that if some neurons continue to have low firing rates in the delay period which reflect the value of f1 (which is in fact illustrated in Fig. 6.6), then even without synaptic facilitation, the firing rates can be restored by a nonspecific input because just a very few neurons are still active during the delay period (Martinez-Garcia, Rolls, Deco and Romo, 2011).

The other part of the mechanism is how the decision between f1 and f2 is taken. The proposal is that the decision is taken by comparing the firing rates of the partial differential neurons (which reflect both f1 and f2), with other neurons that fire only to f2. As shown in Fig. 6.6, if f1 is $>$ f2, the firing of the partial differential neurons will be higher than of neurons that respond only to f2, and the decision that f1 has a higher frequency than f2 will be taken. On the other hand, if f1 is $<$ f2, the firing of the partial differential neurons will be lower than of neurons that respond only to f2, and the decision that f2 has a higher frequency than f1 will be taken. The attractor decision-making network therefore just has as its two inputs the partial differential neurons, and the f2 neurons. The operation of the whole integrate and fire attractor network that performs the decision-making is described by Deco and Rolls (2006), and in Sections 11.5.1, and B.6–B.8.

In another decision-making investigation using somatosensory stimuli, decisions about pleasantness were taken between a range of pleasant warm temperature stimuli to cold unpleasant stimuli applied with a thermode to the hand. The pleasantness vs the unpleasantness of the stimuli was represented in the orbitofrontal cortex (Rolls, Grabenhorst and Parris, 2008a), but the decision was represented anterior to this, in a part of (ventro) medial prefrontal cortex area 10 (Rolls, Grabenhorst and Deco, 2010b) (see Section 11.5.1). An important conclusion is that decisions can be made in a number of different brain areas depending on exactly what information the decision is about (Rolls and Deco, 2010), with in this case affective touch utilising parts of the human ventromedial prefrontal cortex.

6.1.8 Somatosensory cortical regions and connectivity in humans

It has become possible to understand much better the organisation of the human somatosensory cortical pathways by use of the Human Connectome Project - Multimodal Parcellation (HCP-MMP, Section 1.12), and measuring effective connectivity, complemented by functional connectivity and diffusion tractography (Section 1.13) with data from the Human Connectome Project, as described next (Rolls et al., 2023f). This has implications for understanding what is computed in different somatosensory cortical regions, including their connectivity via the insula to regions in the inferior parietal cortex that develop greatly in humans (Rolls et al., 2023f,d).

Physiological investigations in primates referred to above show that areas 3b and 1 represent cutaneous somatosensory information with area 1 having larger receptive fields, that area 3a represents proprioceptive information, and that neurons in area 2 can respond to cutaneous or proprioceptive information or both (Delhaye et al., 2018). As in humans, the legs are represented at the superior end of the somatosensory cortices 3a-2, and the face at the inferior end close to the operculum (Delhaye et al., 2018). In macaques, ventral to 3a-2 in the operculum are areas S2 and 'parietal ventral' (Fig. 6.2) which are described as a ventral somatosensory stream (Delhaye et al., 2018; Mishkin, 1979). In macaques the pathways to 5 and 7b are described as a dorsal somatosensory stream to the posterior parietal cortex (Delhaye et al., 2018; Gardner, 2008; Mishkin, 1979). It has been suggested that several somatosensory processing streams may be present in humans (de Haan and Dijkerman, 2020).

6.1.8.1 A ventral somatosensory stream via the insula to the inferior parietal cortex

First, the evidence shows that in humans there is a ventral somatosensory stream that connects via Frontal Opercular (FOP) regions to the insula, which in turn has connectivity to the inferior parietal cortex PF regions, as illustrated in Fig. 6.7 (Rolls et al., 2023f). The connectivity from the primary somatosensory cortex 3b to the middle insula is shown with green arrows in Fig. 6.7. The onward connectivity of the middle insula (MI) to for example inferior parietal region PF, the PeriSylvian Language region PSL, and the supracallosal anterior cingulate cortex p32pr, a32pr and a24pr is shown with red arrows. The connectivity of the posterior insular region PoI2 is very similar to that of MI. The pathway in more detail is as follows, where > reflects an effective connectivity but does not exclude effects across levels: (3b + 3a <> 1 + 2) <> OP4 <> 43 <> FOP1 <> FOP3 <> (MI + PoI2 + PoI1) <> PF + PFop.

One of the fascinating features of the connectivity shown in Fig. 6.7 is that it draws out the point that some of the opercular and the frontal opercular (FOP) regions can be considered as a continuation ventrally of somatosensory cortex regions 3a, 3b, 1 and 2; with then a further ventral extension of the cortical sheet into the insula. Another important feature is that this ventral stream is probably a 'what' stream, for it does not have major connectivity with visuo-spatial action regions in area 7, but it does have connectivity with PFop and PF, in which representations appear to be about the properties of objects and one's own body (Rolls et al., 2023d). Indeed part of the function of these PF areas may be related to somatosensory / body image and the sense of body ownership and of self that this provides, consistent with evidence that anosognosia and other disorders of awareness of the body can be produced by PF damage in humans (Ronchi et al., 2018). Another interesting feature is that PF may on its connectivity evidence (Rolls et al., 2023d) not only be the top of a somatosensory hierarchy, but it adds visual and reward inputs to form semantic representations of felt objects, enabling recognition of for example a tool not only by its touch, but also by its sight. Also consistent with the insula to PFop and PF stream being a 'what' stream is that it also has access to language systems, via the PeriSylvian Language Area (Rolls et al., 2022b), thus enabling verbal declarations to be made about what is felt, with declarative systems being 'what' systems in the brain, whereas action systems are typically procedural and not declarative (Squire and Zola, 1996; Squire, 1992; Milner and Goodale, 1995; Goodale and Milner, 1992). Another feature of the connectivity is the very directional input from the reward-related (Rolls, 2019e,f; Grabenhorst and Rolls, 2011) medial orbitofrontal cortex region 111 to the middle insula (Fig. 6.7), leading to the hypothesis that the somatosensory insula may encode some aspects of the reward or aversive value of somatosensory stimuli. Consistent with this, activation of the somatosensory insula was found by painful touch to the hand (Rolls, O'Doherty, Kringelbach, Francis, Bowtell and McGlone, 2003d), with a dorsal posterior insular region implicated in pain (Segerdahl et al., 2015).

An interesting property of insular function is that the insula was activated by touch to the arm, but not to the sight of touch to the arm, whereas the somatosensory cortical areas 1–3 responded to the sight of touch to the arm, as well as to touch to the arm (McCabe, Rolls, Bilderbeck and McGlone, 2008). It was therefore suggested that the insula provides evidence that it is one's own body that is being touched, which might give it special status in body representations (McCabe et al., 2008; Craig, 2011, 2009). Consistent with this, most of the insula (MI, PoI1, PoI2 and also the FOP regions) does not receive connectivity from early cortical visual regions, whereas 3b, 3a, 1, 2, 5L, 5m and 5mv do (Rolls et al., 2023f). Another difference is that the somatomotor and paracentral areas have connectivity with parietal area 7 regions, whereas the insula does not; and the insula has more connectivity with inferior parietal PF regions than do the somatomotor and paracentral regions. Another difference is that as mentioned above the insula has connectivity directed towards language-related areas (the PeriSylvian Language area PSL, STV, TPOJ1, and TPOJ2 (Rolls et al., 2023f, 2022b)), whereas the somatomotor and paracentral regions do not. These findings support the hypothesis that the insula is part of a ventral (or inferior) 'what' stream of somatosensory processing that continues into inferior parietal cortex PF regions (Fig. 6.7); whereas as described next a

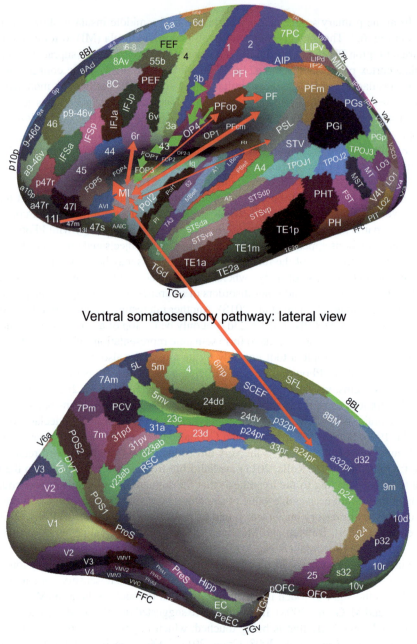

Fig. 6.7 Ventral somatosensory / insula stream effective connectivity. The connectivity from the primary somatosensory cortex 3b to the middle insular area is shown with green arrows. The onward connectivity of the middle insular (MI) to for example inferior parietal region PF, the PeriSylvian Language region PSL, and the supracallosal anterior cingulate cortex p32pr, a32pr and a24pr is shown with red arrows. The connectivity of the posterior insular region PoI2 is very similar to that of MI. The width of the arrows reflects the effective connectivity with the size of the arrowheads reflecting the connectivity in each direction. The pathway in more detail is as follows, where > reflects an effective connectivity but does not exclude effects across levels: (3b + 3a <> 1 + 2) <> OP4 <> 43 <> FOP1 <> FOP3 <> (MI + PoI2 + PoI1) <> PF + PFop. The abbreviations are listed in Section 1.12. (From Rolls,E.T., Deco,G., Huang,C-C. and Feng,J. (2023) Prefrontal and somatosensory-motor cortex effective connectivity in humans. Cerebral Cortex doi: 10.1093/cercor/bhac391. Copyright © Oxford University Press.)

dorsal (or superior) 'action' stream of processing connects from somatomotor (areas 3b, 3a, 1, 2) and paracentral (area 5) cortical regions to posterior parietal cortex area 7 and thereby intraparietal regions (Fig. 6.8).

The supracallosal part of the anterior cingulate cortex is implicated in action-outcome learning, with information about the actions that have been performed available from the somatosensory/motor regions described here, and about the reward outcome received after an action being provided via the pregenual anterior cingulate cortex (Rolls et al., 2023c). This connectivity implicates the insula in this circuitry, and the effective connectivity from the reward-related medial orbitofrontal cortex 11l to the insula could provide reward outcome information to enable the insular cortex to also be involved in action-outcome learning (Rolls et al., 2023f). Consistent with this hypothesis, the insular cortex does have some connectivity to premotor cortex 6 regions, and to the mid-cingulate motor region (Rolls et al., 2023f).

6.1.8.2 A dorsal somatosensory stream

A diagram of a dorsal somatosensory stream connecting via somatosensory area 5 regions to posterior parietal area 7 regions is provided in Fig. 6.8. It should be noted that the area 5 regions in humans appear to be displaced dorsally with respect to their location in macaques such that the area 5 regions roll over to the medial wall of the hemispheres (Fig. 6.8).

In Fig. 6.8 the connectivity from the primary somatosensory cortex area 3b partly via areas 1 and 2 to area 5 somatosensory regions 5m > 5L > 5mv is shown with green arrows. The onward connectivity of 5mv to for example posterior parietal 7AL, 7Am and 7PC which have connectivity with intraparietal regions such as LIP is shown with red arrows. The pathway in more detail is as follows, where > reflects an effective connectivity but does not exclude effects across levels:

(3b + 3a <> 1 + 2) <> 5m <> 5L <> 5mv <> 7AL, 7Am and 7PC.

5mv also has connectivity to 6mp, TPOJ2 and the supracallosal anterior cingulate cortex p32pr, a32pr and a24pr. Given that area 7 is involved in actions in space (Snyder et al., 1998; Rolls, 2020b, 2021f; Dean and Platt, 2006; Vedder et al., 2017; Andersen, 1995b; Avila et al., 2019; Orban et al., 2021b; Passarelli et al., 2021; Gamberini et al., 2020; Rolls et al., 2023d), this dorsal somatosensory stream may be characterized as an 'action' 'where' stream.

Another feature is that the somatosensory cortical areas do have connectivity directed towards motor (area 4), premotor (area 6), or mid-cingulate premotor cortex. This is a principle established in macaques (Rizzolatti and Sinigaglia, 2016), and presumably allows appropriate movements to be made to the somatosensory/ proprioceptive properties analyzed in each somatosensory / proprioceptive region.

6.1.8.3 Taste cortical regions

AVI and FOP3-5 are where in the HCP-MMP atlas (Section 1.12) the human primary taste cortex is located in the anterior dorsal (i.e. superior) insula and adjoining frontal operculum (Rolls, 2016c, 2015d, 2016g).

The taste inputs to these regions are received from the thalamus VPMpc (ventro-postero-medial nucleus pars parvocellularis) (Norgren, 1990; Pritchard et al., 1986). In primates it has been discovered that neurons in the primary taste cortex (in the rostro-dorsal insula and adjoining frontal operculum) have responses to the five primary taste stimuli sweet, salt, bitter, sour and glutamate (umami) (Yaxley et al., 1990; Scott et al., 1986a; Rolls et al., 1996c; Baylis and Rolls, 1991), with each neuron having a different profile of responses to this set of stimuli and thereby encoding information that increases approximately linearly with the number of neurons (Rolls et al., 2010a; Kadohisa et al., 2005a; Rolls and Treves, 2011). The primary taste cortex in macaques has onward connections to the orbitofrontal cortex (Baylis, Rolls and Baylis, 1995), and in this secondary taste cortical area, neurons have also

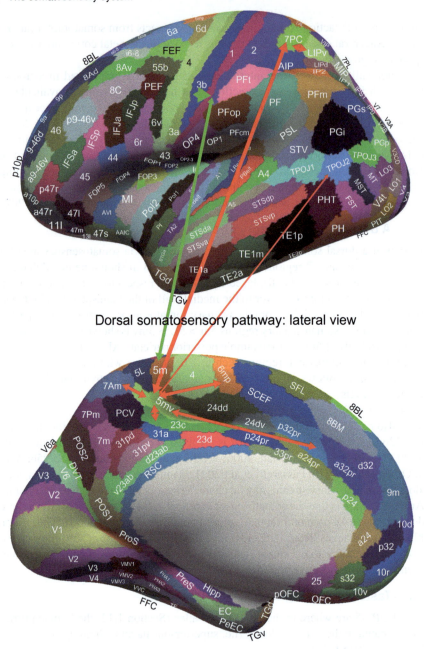

Fig. 6.8 Dorsal somatosensory stream effective connectivity. The connectivity from the primary somatosensory cortex 3b partly via 1 and 2 to area 5 somatosensory regions 5m > 5L > 5mv is shown with green arrows. The onward connectivity of the 5mv to for example posterior parietal 7AL, 7Am and 7PC which have connectivity with intraparietal regions such as LIP is shown with red arrows. The width of the arrows reflects the effective connectivity with the size of the arrowheads reflecting the connectivity in each direction. The pathway in more detail is as follows, where > reflects an effective connectivity but does not exclude effects across levels:

(3b + 3a <> 1 + 2) <> 5m <> 5L <> 5mv <> 7AL, 7Am and 7PC.

5mv also has connectivity to 6mp, TPOJ2 and the supracallosal anterior cingulate cortex p32pr, a32pr and a24pr. The abbreviations are listed in Section 1.12. (From Rolls,E.T., Deco,G., Huang,C-C. and Feng,J. (2023) Prefrontal and somatosensory-motor cortex effective connectivity in humans. Cerebral Cortex doi: 10.1093/cercor/bhac391. Copyright © Oxford University Press.)

been discovered that respond to taste (Rolls, Yaxley and Sienkiewicz, 1990). In the primary taste cortex, feeding to satiety does not reduce the responses of neurons to the taste of the food eaten to satiety, providing evidence that the primary taste cortex represents what the taste is, independently of its reward value (Yaxley, Rolls and Sienkiewicz, 1988; Rolls, Scott, Sienkiewicz and Yaxley, 1988). In contrast, in the orbitofrontal cortex the responses of neurons decrease to zero to the food eaten to satiety, providing evidence that the reward value of the taste is represented in the orbitofrontal cortex (Rolls, Sienkiewicz and Yaxley, 1989d). A similar situation appears to hold in humans, in that feeding to satiety decreases orbitofrontal cortex activations to the food eaten to satiety (Kringelbach, O'Doherty, Rolls and Andrews, 2003), and the orbitofrontal cortex BOLD signal is correlated with the pleasantness of the taste, whereas in the insular taste cortex the BOLD signal is correlated with the intensity of the taste, and not with its pleasantness (Grabenhorst and Rolls, 2008).

However, the taste cortex is even more interesting than this, for it also represents the texture of food, which is a signal of somatosensory origin, in that some macaque neurons in the insula primary taste cortex respond to viscosity, others to rough texture, and others to the texture of fat in the mouth with responses related to the coefficient of sliding friction (Verhagen, Kadohisa and Rolls, 2004), which is how we have discovered that fat in the mouth is sensed (Rolls, Mills, Norton, Lazidis and Norton, 2018b; Rolls, 2016g), with similar encoding of texture as well as taste in the orbitofrontal cortex (Verhagen, Rolls and Kadohisa, 2003). A similar situation appears to hold in humans, in that the BOLD signal in the taste cortical areas can also be related to viscosity; and in some regions there is evidence that fat texture is represented (De Araujo and Rolls, 2004; Kringelbach, O'Doherty, Rolls and Andrews, 2003; Grabenhorst, Rolls, Parris and D'Souza, 2010b).

Part of the interest of these findings (Rolls et al., 2023f) is that they show how the insular and frontal opercular (FOP) regions do receive somatosensory inputs (Rolls et al., 2023f), which are needed if responses are to be found to oral texture stimuli such as the viscosity, roughness, and fat texture of food in the mouth (Rolls, 2020c). These discoveries, including that fat texture is sensed by the coefficient of sliding friction (Rolls et al., 2018b; Rolls, 2020c), help to provide a foundation for understanding the roles of the sensory qualities of food in the control of appetite and food intake (Rolls, 2016g,d, 2018a).

6.1.8.4 Connectivity of somatosensory to motor and premotor frontal cortical regions

Helpful descriptions of the connectivity of motor and premotor cortical regions, and their inputs from intraparietal sulcus and inferior parietal cortex regions for macaques have been provided elsewhere (Gerbella et al., 2017; Rizzolatti and Kalaska, 2013; Rizzolatti and Sinigaglia, 2016) (Fig. 15.1). In this research (Rolls et al., 2023f), the connectivity of these motor and premotor areas with other cortical regions is extended to humans, and in particular to cortical regions as defined in the HCP-MMP atlas (Glasser et al., 2016a; Huang et al., 2022). Highlights of the present results are that the area 6 premotor cortex regions have connectivity not only from postcentral somatosensory cortical regions such as 1,2,3 and 5, but also from parts of parietal area 7 and from the intraparietal regions (Rolls et al., 2023d). The inputs from the latter two parietal systems are likely to be important in functions such as visually guided actions in space (Gerbella et al., 2017; Rizzolatti and Kalaska, 2013; Rizzolatti and Sinigaglia, 2016; Gamberini et al., 2020; Fattori et al., 2017). The area 6 regions also receive from the mid-cingulate premotor regions (24dd, 24dv and 23c), which receive from the supracallosal anterior cingulate cortex and thereby provide a route for action-outcome learning and performance (Rolls et al., 2023c; Rolls, 2022b).

6.2 How computations are performed in the somatosensory system

6.2.1 Hierarchical computation in the somatosensory system

The operations performed in the hierarchically organised somatosensory system are interestingly similar to those in the visual system, and the computations involved may be similar, as follows. The principles of the computations, as for the visual system (Chapter 2), appear to be: convergence from stage to stage; larger receptive fields from stage to stage; responses to feature combinations generated at each stage, including at higher stages combinations of inputs received from different sensory systems, including vision and audition; the computations of shape representations that are invariant with respect to position, which is similar to complex cells in V1, and to what is computed in the inferior temporal visual cortex.

Neurons in area 3a, the primary somatosensory cortex, respond to the orientation of edges, and the receptive field organisation can be predicted from the responses to stimuli applied to different parts of the receptive field. This makes the neurons selective for the position of the edge. This is similar to the responses of simple cells in V1.

Neurons in area 3a have small receptive fields that respond to moving edges, but the direction can only be computed as perpendicular to the edge, because of the aperture problem. This is similar to the responsiveness of V1 neurons that respond to moving visual stimuli.

At the next stage of the hierarchy, in area 1, the receptive fields are larger, and respond to combinations of the inputs from V1, for example to curvature. This can only be achieved by having large receptive fields, and is similar to what can be found in V2.

In area 1 the aperture problem is solved for motion with the larger receptive fields enabling neurons to respond to global motion in a shape-invariant way. This corresponds to the computation performed in MT in the visual system.

Similar feature combination computation through the hierarchy occurs for the proprioceptive system. Neurons in area 3a respond to proprioceptive input signalling joint angle and muscle stretch, and although some combinations may be represented here, there may be more combination-sensitive neurons in area 2, which accordingly can respond to a position of the limb in space relative to the body, and to a particular reach direction. This appears to be further elaborated in area 5 which includes the parietal reach area, where neurons can be well tuned to the direction of reaching in space relative to the body.

Convergence with other sensory modalities also occurs, as in the visual system. In the somatosensory system, convergence with visual, auditory, and vestibular stimuli occurs in area 5, and more in area 7b (Delhaye et al., 2018). These neurons are active during reaching and grasping movements, appear to encode not just limb position but also target locations and motor actions. The coordinate frames in which representations are found is a topic of current interest, with the possible coordinate frames including limb position relative to the body, and visual and reaching coordinate frameworks needed including relative to the body (egocentric), relative to the head (egocentric); and relative to allocentric space (Rolls, 2020b).

6.2.2 Computations for pleasant touch and pain

There is considerable segregation of processing for pain and for positive touch from discriminative and proprioceptive somatosensory processing, even peripherally, with C fibres implicated in negative and positive somatosensory processing.

Partial segregation is maintained into the brain. There are nociceptive inputs to the insula somatosensory areas. However, the full affective value of pain inputs is more evident in the orbitofrontal cortex, damage to which reduces the affective components of pain.

Similarly, positively affective touch are especially represented in the orbitofrontal cortex.

The orbitofrontal cortex is especially involved in representing the reward value of stimuli (Chapter 11), and projects to the cingulate cortex where instrumental actions are chosen to obtain the rewards or avoid painful stimuli (Chapter 12). Subjective feelings of pleasure and pain may be especially related to computations in this system which specializes in reward valuation, and then goal directed instrumental action via its connectivity to the orbitofrontal cortex.

6.2.3 The mechanisms for somatosensory decision-making

The mechanisms for somatosensory and other types of decision-making are considered in Sections 6.1.7, 11.5.1, and B.6–B.8.

7 The auditory system

7.1 Introduction, and overview of computations in the auditory system

The auditory pathways are shown in Fig. 7.1a. The auditory nerves synapse in the cochlear nuclei in the brainstem, which connect to the medial superior olive which detects interaural time difference for auditory localization, and to the lateral superior olivary nucleus which detects interaural intensity differences for auditory localization. The olives project to the inferior colliculi in the midbrain where a map of auditory space is formed. The inferior colliculi project to the medial geniculate nucleus, which is the auditory thalamus, and this in turn projects to the primary auditory cortex in the superior part of the temporal lobe (Oertel and Doupe, 2013; Oertel and Wang, 2021).

Overview

1. Interaural time difference is decoded by delay lines in the medial superior olive. This is useful for left-right sound localisation, and for continuous waveforms is useful up to approximately 1 kHz, which is the maximum frequency with which peaks in the waveform can be detected, given the maximum firing rate of auditory neurons of approximately 1 kHz.
2. Interaural intensity difference is useful for left-right localisation above approximately 1 kHz, the frequency at which the wavelength is sufficiently short that the head starts to act as a baffle.
3. 3D sound localization is possible because we have a pinna that acts as a 3D asymmetric antenna, which performs spectro-temporal filtering that is different for different 3D spatial locations. This is useful for sounds with frequencies above several kHz, due to the size of the pinna; and a broad spectrum helps so that the different filtering performed at different frequencies can be utilised.
4. Because the ears are anchored to the head, the main representation of auditory space is in head-based coordinates. Because we may need to look at locations of sounds that are in head-centred space, there is a mapping of spatial visual inputs to head-centred space, as described in Section 3.4.1.
5. There is a representation of visual space that is for the allocentric position being viewed, and this is implemented by hippocampal spatial view cells as described in Chapter 9 and Section 3.4.3. It is predicted that there will be a representation of auditory space in the same world-based coordinates, but it has not been discovered yet. (This may seem implausible at first, but think of what happens when one rotates one's head while listening to individual singers in an opera or actors in a play: their correct positions in allocentric space remain constant, and this seems to apply to the sounds they make in the 'soundstage', as well as to their allocentric locations in visual space.)
6. There is evidence for dorsal and ventral auditory cortical pathways.

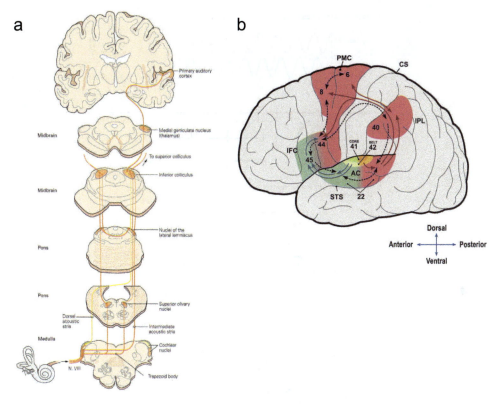

Fig. 7.1 a. The auditory pathways. b. Hierarchical organization of auditory cortical processing. The ventral auditory pathway is shown in green, and the dorsal auditory pathway in red. AC – auditory cortex; CS – central sulcus; IFC – inferior frontal cortex; IPL – inferior parietal lobule; PMC – premotor cortex; STS – superior temporal sulcus. For description, see text. (a. Reproduced from Oertel,D. and Doupe,A.J. (2013) The auditory central nervous system. Chapter 31 pp. 682–711 in Kandel,E.R. et al, 2013, Principles of Neuroscience, 5th Edition. McGraw-Hill: New York. © McGraw-Hill. b. Reprinted from Ina Bornkessel-Schlesewsky, Matthias Schlesewsky, Steven L. Small, and Josef P. Rauschecker (2015) Neurobiological roots of language in primate audition: common computational properties. *Trends in Cognitive Sciences* 19: 142–150. Copyright © Elsevier.)

7. The ventral auditory pathway appears to involve a series of hierarchical stages through the temporal lobe in the superior temporal gyrus. One projection is to the orbitofrontal cortex, where neurons are found that respond for example to the emotional expression in a voice. The ventral auditory pathway in the temporal lobe also projects to the inferior frontal gyrus (area 45), which in humans on the left is Broca's area, a frontal area involved in speech production.

8. The dorsal auditory pathway projects from the auditory cortex to the posterior superior temporal cortex, and then to the inferior parietal lobule (area 40), which in turn projects to the more dorsal part of the inferior frontal cortex (area 44). It is involved in sound localization, and perhaps in processing the dynamic aspects of sounds.

7.2 Auditory Localization

When a sound arises from the right, the right ear detects the sound earlier than the left ear. The difference in the time of arrival at the two ears is the interaural time delay (ITD). Given that the velocity of sound in air is 343 m/s, and the maximum distance between the ears, the time delays can be up to approximately 0.5 ms. For sine waves, nerve fibers can fire in phase

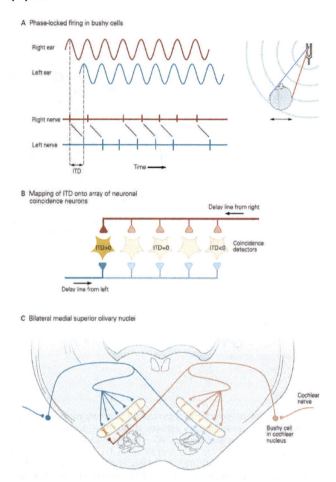

Fig. 7.2 Left-right sound localization. A. Interaural time differences are decoded to provide information about whether a sound source is to the left or right. B. Interaural time differences can be detected with delay lines. C. Mammals use delay lines for signals from the contralateral side to form a map in the superior olive of interaural time differences. (Reproduced from Oertel,D. and Doupe,A.J. (2013) The auditory central nervous system. Chapter 31 pp. 682–711 in Kandel,E.R. et al, 2013, Principles of Neuroscience, 5th Edition. McGraw-Hill: New York. © McGraw-Hill.)

with changes in the sound pressure as shown in Fig. 7.2A. This works up to about 1,000 Hz, which is as fast as the nerves can fire, even if they sometimes miss a beat.

In the medial superior olive, a very nice delay line system is set up to decode the time differences so that different neurons respond to different inter-aural time differences, as illustrated in Fig. 7.2B and C. The bitufted neurons of the medial superior olivary nucleus form a sheet that is contacted on the lateral face by bushy cells from the ipsilateral cochlear nucleus and on the medial face by bushy cells from the contralateral cochlear nucleus. On the ipsilateral side the branches of the bushy cell axons are of equal length and thus deliver synaptic currents to their targets in the medial superior olive simultaneously. On the contralateral side the branches deliver synaptic currents first to the anterior regions, closest to the midline, and then to progressively more posterior regions. When sounds arise from the right side, their early arrival at the right ear is compensated by progressively later arrival at neurons in the posterior region of the left medial superior olive (the mustard-colored cell is activated by a sound from the far right, as in Fig. 7.2B) (Oertel and Doupe, 2013). Thus each medial superior olive forms a map of where sounds arise in the contralateral hemifield.

This system is useful only for frequencies up to approximately 1 kHz, for the reasons described above. However, for frequencies above about 1 kHz, the head acts as a baffle, and sounds that are shadowed by the head reach the far ear with a smaller intensity. These intensity differences are decoded in the lateral superior olivary nucleus, to provide a way to detect left-right differences for high frequency sounds.

However, these two mechanisms implement only left-right localization, and provide no evidence about where the sound source is in front vs behind the listener, or in elevation. It is effectively a one-dimensional system.

Yet humans are quite good at 3D sound localization. 3D sound localization has many evolutionary advantages, but an aesthetic advantage was emphasized in a lecture given on 6 May 1972 that I attended at the Oxford Union by Karlheinz Stockhausen on electronic music. (That lecture is available on YouTube (Stockhausen, 1972).) Stockhausen described experiments he had performed on 3D music. He described that at the World Fair at Osaka in Japan he had made recordings in a spherical hall with 600 people on a metal grid across the middle of the inside of the sphere, with loudspeakers all the way round with 7 circles of speakers arranged in 10 columns vertically to create a sound-field above and below the listeners, with sounds coming potentially from any direction of azimuth or elevation. He described how this enabled him to experiment with 3D sound, which he considered an important aspect of electronic music.

Stockhausen then stated that he greatly regretted not being able to make recordings of the interesting musical effects that he created, because he did not have a 70 channel tape recorder. This started me thinking. How many channels of sound recording were actually needed? Were 70 channels needed? I reasoned that all the information from all the locations in space must be present at the tympanic membrane (the ear drum). I reasoned that therefore with a miniature microphone placed in the external auditory meatus close to the tympanic membrane (ear drum), it should be possible to record all the information that could be used by the brain to localize the source of the sound in space. I tested my hypothesis. I purchased some miniature electret microphones, and made recordings with these placed in my external auditory meatus very close to my tympanic membranes. The recordings were spectacular. When played back through headphones, I could localize the sound source to almost anywhere in 3D space. My hypothesis was that the asymmetric, almost helix-like, shape of the human pinna was acting as an asymmetric antenna that was filtering the sound depending on the direction of the sound source in 3D space. I quantified this by making polar frequency response measurements of the human head including the pinna, and published the results in the Journal of Physiology (Rolls, 1973) (available at https://www.oxcns.org/papers).

I realized the potential for making recordings of music, drama, etc using binaural ear canal recording, for then the exact sound heard by a listener in for example the position of the conductor of a piece of music could be recorded, and played back to the listener, with all the directional and room acoustics faithfully recorded. I therefore registered a UK provisional patent for the method in 1973. I also contacted the BBC Research Department, and demonstrated the system to members of the BBC Research Department at Kingswood Warren at the invitation of D.J.Meares in April 1974. As a result, the BBC broadcast 3D binaural intra-ear sound recordings every week or so for several years. (This recording method, although superb for playback using headphones or earphones, has limitations when listened to through stereo loudspeakers, for then the sound source is less clear, as a second localization occurs for the sound emanating from the loudspeakers.)

Since then, there has been much further research on 3D sound localization (Paul, 2009), with examples of the spectral filtering performed by the ear and head shown in Fig. 7.3. Neurons that encode the location of sounds in 3D space have been found in the ferret auditory cortex (Mrsic-Flogel et al., 2005), but a recent review of sound localization did not

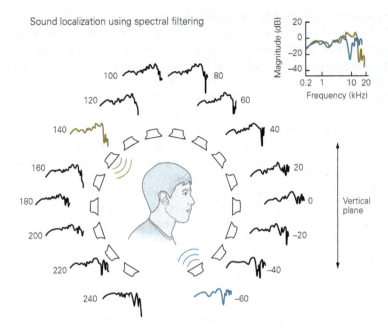

Fig. 7.3 3D sound localization using spectral filtering. When a noise that has equal energy at all frequencies over the human hearing range (white noise) is presented through a speaker, the ear, head, and shoulders cancel energy at some frequencies and enhance others. The amount of sound energy at each frequency at the ear canal is shown by the traces beside each speaker, which plot in decibels the power spectrum of sound that reaches the eardrum relative to the white noise that is produced by the speakers. For a white noise the power spectrum is flat. Note that by the time the noise has reached the bottom of the ear canal its spectrum is no longer flat. The small plot in the upper right compares spectral filtering of sounds coming from low in the front (blue) with sounds coming from behind and above the listener's head (brown). At high frequencies filtering by the ear introduces deep notches into spectra that vary depending on where the sounds arose. Sounds that lack energy at high frequencies and narrowband sounds are difficult to localize in the vertical plane. Spectral filtering also varies in the horizontal plane. (Data from D.Kistler and F.Wightman in Oertel,D. and Doupe,A.J. (2013) The auditory central nervous system. Chapter 31 pp. 682–711 in Kandel,E.R. et al, 2013, Principles of Neuroscience, 5th Edition. McGraw-Hill: New York. © McGraw-Hill.)

identify details of this 3D sound localization in primates including humans, although it did identify areas beyond the primary auditory cortex, in the auditory dorsal cortical stream, in the inferior parietal lobule, and in the dorsolateral prefrontal cortex, that are implicated in sound localization (van der Heijden et al., 2019).

7.3 Ventral and dorsal cortical auditory pathways

Rauschecker and colleagues, building on studies in primates, have described two hierarchical cortical streams of information transfer from auditory cortex (AC) which eventually reach prefrontal cortical regions (Rauschecker, 2012; Bornkessel-Schlesewsky et al., 2015). As illustrated in Fig. 7.1b, there are two streams of auditory processing, a ventral auditory stream (shown in green) that has been compared with the visual ventral stream of object-related processing, and a dorsal auditory stream (shown in red) that has been compared with the dorsal visual cortical stream.

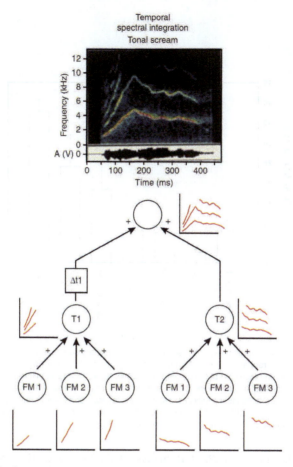

Fig. 7.4 Schematic of a feature hierarchy approach to building communication calls. Communication calls consist of elementary features, such as bandpass noise bursts or frequency-modulated (FM) sweeps. Harmonic calls, such as the vocal scream from the rhesus monkey repertoire depicted here by its spectrogram and time signal amplitude (A, measured as output voltage of a sound meter), consist of fundamental frequencies and higher harmonics. The neural circuitry for processing such calls is thought to consist of small hierarchical networks. At the lowest level, there are neurons serving as FM detectors tuned to the rate and direction of FM sweeps; these detectors extract each FM component (shown in cartoon spectrograms) in the upward and downward sweeps of the scream. The output of these FM detectors is combined nonlinearly at the next level: the target neurons T1 and T2 possess a high threshold and fire only if all inputs are activated. At the final level, a 'tonal-scream detector' is created by again combining output from neurons T1 and T2 nonlinearly. Temporal integration is accomplished by having the output of T1 pass through a delay line sufficient to hold up the input to the top neuron long enough that all inputs arrive at the same time. (Reproduced from J P Rauschecker and S K Scott (2009) Maps and streams in the auditory cortex: nonhuman primates illuminate human speech processing. Nature Neuroscience 12: 718–724. Copyright © Macmillan Publishers Ltd.)

7.4 The ventral cortical auditory stream

The first auditory cortical areas in primates are area 41, a core region, and area 42, a belt region (Pandya et al., 2015).

The ventral auditory stream involves projections to the anterior superior temporal cortex (aST, area 22), which in turn projects to the anterior and ventral parts of the inferior frontal gyrus (IFG, pars triangularis), area 45.

In non-human primates, the ventral stream subserves the recognition of successively more complex auditory objects, ranging from elementary auditory features (e.g., frequency-modulated (FM) sweeps or bandpass noise bursts) in the first auditory cortical areas, to species-specific vocalizations (monkey calls) in higher areas including the ventral prefrontal

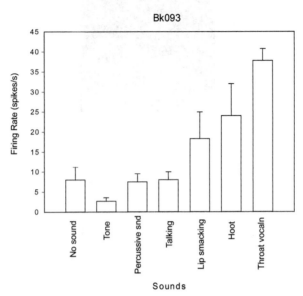

Fig. 7.5 Orbitofrontal cortex neurons respond to socially relevant auditory stimuli. The responses of a mid-orbitofrontal cortex neuron to a set of different auditory stimuli. The mean firing rate ($\pm$SEM) in a 1 s period in which the sounds were made are shown. The neuron responded best to a deep vocalization which may have mimicked a 'grunt' call, second best to a hoot which is a communication call in macaques, and third best to the sound of a monkey lip-smacking, which is a form of social greeting. The 'No sound' condition shows the spontaneous firing rate of the neuron. (From Rolls, E. T., Critchley,H.D., Browning,A.S. and Inoue,K. (2006) Face-selective and auditory neurons in the primate orbitofrontal cortex. Experimental Brain Research 170: 74–87. © Springer-Verlag.)

cortex (Rauschecker and Scott, 2009; Romanski et al., 2005) and orbitofrontal cortex (Rolls, Critchley, Browning and Inoue, 2006a).

A feature hierarchy approach to how neurons with complex auditory properties could be formed is illustrated in Fig. 7.4 (Rauschecker and Scott, 2009).

Evidence for hierarchical processing of speech sounds relevant to language is that in humans, activations associated with the processing of short-timescale patterns (phonemes) are localized to the left mid-superior temporal gyrus, whereas activations associated with the integration of phonemes into temporally complex patterns (words) are localized to the left anterior superior temporal gyrus (DeWitt and Rauschecker, 2012) (see further Chapters 8 and 14).

In an area to which the superior temporal auditory cortex projects, the mid-orbitofrontal cortex areas 13 and 11, we discovered neurons that respond to primate vocalizations (Rolls, Critchley, Browning and Inoue, 2006a). An example is shown in Fig. 7.5, which shows a neuron that responded to the sound of lipsmacking (a social greeting) and a hoot (a contact call), as well as a deep vocalization like a grunt, all of which are important in macaque social communication (Cheney and Seyfarth, 2018). We relate the auditory neurons in this particular part of the auditory cortex hierarchy to decoding the emotional significance of vocalizations, for humans with damage to the orbitofrontal cortex and related areas were found to be impaired at identifying the emotional expression of different human vocalizations (Hornak, Rolls and Wade, 1996).

In the ventrolateral prefrontal cortex of macaques, some neurons respond to the sight of species-specific facial gestures, and to the auditory accompaniment, the vocalization (Romanski et al., 2005). These auditory and visual inputs are being matched, for the neurons respond differently if the visual facial gestures and the auditory vocalization are incongruent (Diehl and Romanski, 2014). Neurons of this type may be important in identity processing and in the integration of multisensory communication information. This ventrolateral prefrontal cortex area includes area 12/47 (Plakke and Romanski, 2014), which is lateral orbitofrontal cortex (Rolls, 2019e).

For auditory short-term memory, the dorso-lateral prefrontal cortex becomes involved in the processing (Plakke and Romanski, 2014), as it does for working memory in other sensory modalities (Chapter 13).

7.5 The dorsal cortical auditory stream

The dorsal auditory stream in primates projects from the first auditory areas 41 and 42 to the posterior superior temporal (pST) cortex, and then to the inferior parietal lobule (IPL, area 40), which in turn projects to the more dorsal part of the inferior frontal gyrus (IFG pars opercularis, area 44), and also to premotor cortical area 6 (PMC) and to area 8 (Fig. 7.1b).

The dorsal auditory stream is implicated for example in the localization of sounds (Rauschecker and Scott, 2009; van der Heijden et al., 2019), and perhaps in processing the dynamic aspects of sounds (Rauschecker, 2012; Bornkessel-Schlesewsky et al., 2015).

So far, the known representations of auditory space are in head-based (egocentric) coordinates (which is natural, as the ears are anchored to the head), and there are mechanisms in the parietal lobe part of the dorsal visual system that match visual coordinates to this space (Oertel and Doupe, 2013), so that the eyes saccade to the source of a sound (see Chapter 3). However, I propose that there is an allocentric representation of auditory space analogous to the allocentric encoding of space 'out there' provided by spatial view cells (Rolls and Wirth, 2018) (see Chapter 9). For example, if the visual scene contains a waterfall in one part of the scene, and a noisy clock tower in another part of the scene, then both the visual and the auditory representations should remain locked in the same allocentric location in the scene when the head is rotated or the individual moves sideways to a different place. Congruency of object representations would thus be expected in visual and auditory space. It would be of interest to investigate this in the primate hippocampus and parahippocampal gyrus. When they are found, neurons coding in this way might be termed 'allocentric sound location cells'.

7.6 Auditory cortical regions and connectivity in humans

It has become possible to understand much better the organisation of the human auditory cortical pathways by use of the Human Connectome Project - Multimodal Parcellation (HCP-MMP, Section 1.12), and measuring effective connectivity, complemented by functional connectivity and diffusion tractography (Section 1.13) with data from the Human Connectome Project, as described next (Rolls et al., 2023h). This has implications for understanding what is computed in different auditory cortical regions, and their connectivity to semantic and language systems involved at least in speech understanding.

Previous evidence for ventral and dorsal auditory streams in macaques, with some consistent evidence in humans, has been described (Rauschecker, 2018b; Rauschecker and Scott, 2009). A summary is that in humans a ventral auditory stream involves anterior auditory temporal cortical regions that connect via the anterior part of the temporal lobe to the inferior frontal gyrus including especially area 45 (Rauschecker, 2012) (Fig. 7.1). A dorsal auditory stream was described as involving the posterior auditory cortical regions connecting via inferior parietal regions to premotor cortex 6, region 44, etc. (Rauschecker, 2012) (Fig. 7.1).

7.6.1 Early Auditory cortical regions

Schematic overviews of the effective connectivity of the human auditory cortical systems are shown in Figs. 7.6 and 7.7 (Rolls et al., 2023h). A simplified schematic organisation is that regions A1 and 52 > LBelt and MBelt > PBelt > A4. (Here > indicates 'has effective connectivity to', though some connectivity may cross levels of the hierarchy.) That part of the connectivity appears to be hierarchical.

In both humans and nonhuman primates, the auditory cortex is described as having core (corresponding to primary and primary-like auditory cortex), then belt (which surrounds the core), and then parabelt fields, all of which contain several subfields (Rauschecker, 2015; Van Essen and Glasser, 2018; Glasser et al., 2016a; van der Heijden et al., 2019; Rauschecker, 2018b,a; Erickson et al., 2017; Leaver and Rauschecker, 2016; DeWitt and Rauschecker, 2016; Bornkessel-Schlesewsky et al., 2015; DeWitt and Rauschecker, 2013; Ahveninen et al., 2013; Rauschecker, 2012; Rauschecker and Scott, 2009; Corcoles-Parada et al., 2019; Scott et al., 2017; Scott and Mishkin, 2016; Petkov et al., 2015; Munoz-Lopez et al., 2015; Karabanov et al., 2015; Scott et al., 2014; Kikuchi et al., 2014; Fukushima et al., 2014; Kravitz et al., 2013; Poremba et al., 2003; Romanski et al., 1999; Moerel et al., 2014; Morel et al., 1993; Rauschecker, 1998b,a; DeWitt and Rauschecker, 2012; Archakov et al., 2020; Rauschecker and Tian, 2000; DeWitt and Rauschecker, 2012; Rauschecker et al., 1995; Kaas and Hackett, 2000). Neurons in the core show responses with narrow tuning to tone frequency; belt neurons respond best to band-passed noise of a specific frequency and bandwidth; and parabelt neurons respond to increasingly complex sounds (Rauschecker, 2015; Leaver and Rauschecker, 2016; Tian et al., 2001).

7.6.2 Ventral auditory cortical streams

After A4 there may be a split in the pathways in humans (Rolls et al., 2023h).

In one ventral stream, A4 has effective connectivity to anterior temporal lobe region TA2, and TA2 given its location is likely to be a ventral stream region (Fig. 7.6). TA2 has interesting connectivity to the parainsular region PI, which also receives visual and somatosensory inputs (Rolls et al., 2023f). TA2 has some effective connectivity to anterior temporal gyrus region STGa. However, STGa cannot be regarded as a region that mainly receives from TA2, for the connectivity to STGa from A5 is ten times stronger than that from TA2. TA2 also has effective connectivity to visual motion regions MT, MST, V6, V3A etc; and with region 1 (somatosensory cortex).

In a second ventral stream, A4 has effective connectivity to A5. A5 is higher in the hierarchy than A4, in that A4 receives from A1 and 52; and A5 receives from PBelt, LBelt, and A4 (Rolls et al., 2023h). A5 then connects to dorsal bank superior temporal sulcus (STS) regions STGa, STSda, and STSdp, which then have onward effective connectivity to TPOJ1, STV, PSL, TGv, TGd and PGi (Fig. 7.6), which are language-related regions (Rolls et al., 2022b).

The dorsal bank superior temporal sulcus regions (STSda and STSdp) also receive visual inputs about, for example, the movements made by the face and mouth during speaking, in that some neurons in these cortical regions of macaques respond perfectly to the small lip and mouth movements made by humans when they speak (Hasselmo, Rolls, Baylis and Nalwa, 1989b; Hasselmo, Rolls and Baylis, 1989a). We also discovered neurons in the same cortical regions that respond to auditory stimuli including vocalisation (Baylis, Rolls and Leonard, 1987), and indeed some neurons in this cortical region respond to both visual and auditory

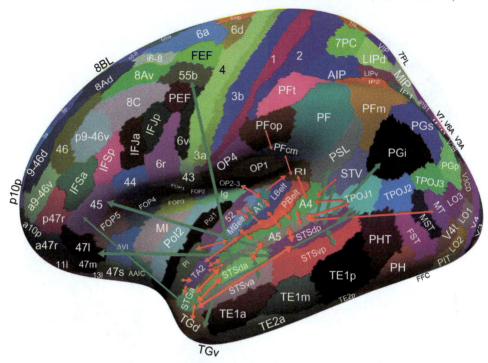

Auditory system: lateral view

Fig. 7.6 Effective connectivity of human auditory cortical regions shown schematically. The widths of the lines and the size of the arrowheads indicate the magnitude and direction of the effective connectivity. Red arrows show the main auditory division connectivity, and green arrows further connectivity. A simplified schematic organisation is that region A1 > LBelt, MBelt and 52 > PBelt > A4 > A5 > STGa, STSda, STSdp > TPOJ1, STV, PGi. (Here > indicates has effective connectivity to, though some connectivity may cross levels of the hierarchy.) Somatosensory cortical regions have connectivity with A1, RI, TA2 etc. MT has connectivity to A5. TPOJ1, STV, PSL, STSdp and STSda are involved in language as analyzed elsewhere (Rolls et al., 2022b). Connections between early cortical auditory regions and area 44 in what may be a dorsal language related auditory stream are found. Lbelt, Pbelt, A4 and A5 have effective connectivity with MT/MST regions as indicated, and this may be part of a dorsal 'where' stream leading to intraparietal and area 7 regions. The abbreviations are listed in Section 1.12. (From Rolls, E. T., Rauschecker,J., Deco,G., Huang,C-C. and Feng,J. (2023) Auditory cortical connectivity in humans. Cerebral Cortex 33: 6207-6227. doi: 10.1093/cercor/bhac496. Copyright © Oxford University Press.)

stimuli (Khandhadia et al., 2021; Belin, 2019). This makes these dorsal bank STS regions important for the decoding of articulator speech movements.

These dorsal bank STS regions are therefore important in linking motion-related changes in the sight of the face to the dynamically changing auditory input, and this is likely to be useful for identifying who in a group is making the vocalisation, in maximising the ability to decode information in noisy environments in order to understand speech, in maximizing the information in social signals by combining the auditory and visual components, etc. In the sense that this processing provides evidence about what the message is, this could be considered as a type of ventral stream 'what' semantic processing. This is developed further in Section 8.4 and in Chapter 14.

7.6.3 Dorsal auditory cortical streams

One stream here is the proposed dorsal 'how' stream for auditory processing related to language (Rauschecker, 2018b; Rauschecker and Scott, 2009) (Fig. 7.1). This auditory dorsal pathway is proposed to be involved in sensorimotor integration and control (Rauschecker, 2011), and in humans plays a role in speech production as well as categorization of phonemes

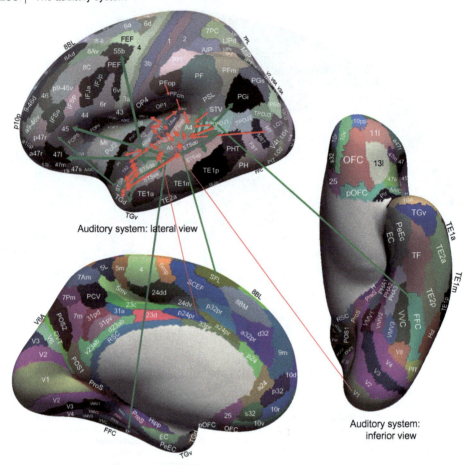

Fig. 7.7 Effective connectivity of human auditory cortical regions shown schematically. The widths of the lines and the size of the arrowheads indicate the magnitude and direction of the effective connectivity. Red arrows show the main auditory division connectivity, and green arrows further connectivity. A simplified schematic organisation is that region A1 > LBelt, MBelt and 52 > PBelt > A4 > A5 > STGa, STSda, STSdp > TPOJ1, STV, PGi. (Here > indicates has effective connectivity to, though some connectivity may cross levels of the hierarchy.) Somatosensory cortical regions have connectivity with A1, RI, TA2 etc. MT has connectivity to A5. TPOJ1, STV, PSL, STSdp and STSda are involved in language as analyzed elsewhere (Rolls et al., 2022b). Connections between early cortical auditory regions and area 44 in what may be a dorsal language related auditory stream are found. Lbelt, Pbelt, A4 and A5 have effective connectivity with MT/MST regions as indicated, and this may be part of a dorsal 'where' stream leading to intraparietal and area 7 regions. The abbreviations are listed in Section 1.12. (From Rolls, E. T., Rauschecker,J., Deco,G., Huang,C-C. and Feng,J. (2023) Auditory cortical connectivity in humans. Cerebral Cortex 33: 6207-6227. doi: 10.1093/cercor/bhac496. Copyright © Oxford University Press.)

during speech processing (Rauschecker, 2012). The pathway is from more posterior auditory cortex regions via the arcuate fasciculus to especially Broca's area 44, with inferior parietal and premotor cortices postulated as part of this dorsal stream network (Rauschecker, 2015). It has been suggested that this dorsal stream evolved as a substrate for sensorimotor processing, connecting sensory and motor cortical systems with each other and the basal ganglia (Rauschecker, 2018b; Archakov et al., 2020), thus permitting the learning of sequences and a foundation for both language and music (Rauschecker, 2018a).

Our diffusion tractography does show connections of PBelt, RI, A4 and A5 with Broca's area 44, and this may be how the dorsal 'how' language-related stream is reflected in our analysis (Rolls et al., 2023h). Corresponding effective or functional connectivity was not identified in our analysis (Rolls et al., 2023h), perhaps because it is functionally relatively weak, or perhaps because the data were acquired in the resting state not during language production.

Considering the connectivity of Broca's area provides some additional relevant evidence to what are ventral vs dorsal language-related auditory streams. The anterior part of Broca's area, 45, in the inferior frontal gyrus pars triangularis, has more effective connectivity than the posterior part of Broca's area, 44, in the inferior frontal gyrus pars opercularis, with STGa, STSda and STSdp and related regions such as TGv (Rolls et al., 2023h, 2022b) which are anterior temporal lobe semantic regions (Rolls et al., 2022b). The diffusion tractography shows more connections of 44 than 45 with PBelt, A4, A5 and STSvp, and with premotor area 6 regions (Rolls et al., 2023h, 2022b). In addition to the hypotheses and this evidence that region 45 which is anterior in the frontal lobes is connected with anterior temporal lobe semantic systems (e.g. in the dorsal bank of the STS), and that region 44 more posteriorly in the frontal lobes is more connected with more posterior temporal lobe auditory regions involved in 'how' processing, it is further proposed that there is information flow from 45 to 44 as part of a route from semantic to language output in terms of speech production and articulation (Rolls et al., 2023h; Rauschecker, 2018b; Rauschecker and Scott, 2009; Rolls et al., 2022b).

A second dorsal auditory stream was found as follows (Rolls et al., 2023h). A4 and A5, and some earlier cortical regions, have effective connectivity to visual motion regions including MT and MST (Rolls et al., 2023h) which in turn have effective connectivity to intraparietal and thereby parietal area 7 regions (Fig. 7.7) (Rolls et al., 2023e). This analysis is supported by the functional connectivity, which is evident between A4, the PBelt etc and parietal 7AL, 7Am and 7PC; and is also supported by the diffusion tractography showing connections between similar regions (Rolls et al., 2023h). These auditory inputs to dorsal-stream parietal areas could be used to shift visual attention and eye position to a source of sound, to help track moving noisy objects such as flying birds and predators (e.g. alarm calls for eagles versus snakes (Seyfarth and Cheney, 2010)), or keeping track of the location of a predator when running away, and performing actions in the dark for objects that can be detected by their sound. This system may be involved not only in detecting the spatial location of sounds, but also to facilitate spatial attention including by moving the eyes and by top-down attentional space-based modulation in what is described for audition as the 'cocktail party' effect.

One point to note is that A4 and A5 are long regions that are likely in future to be subdivided into anterior and posterior parts. Similarly, at earlier stages of auditory processing, single-unit studies in macaques (Rauschecker et al., 1995) have shown that LBelt and PBelt can already be subdivided into subregions with mirror-symmetric target regions.

7.6.4 Other auditory system cortical connectivities

Another feature of the auditory cortical connectivity described here is the connectivity with somatosensory cortical areas, with, for example, connectivity from somatosensory cortical areas 1 and OP2-3 to auditory cortical regions A4 and A5 (Fig. 7.7); and the earlier auditory cortex regions have connectivity with the supracallosal anterior cingulate regions a24pr, a32pr, p24pr and p32pr (Rolls et al., 2023h) (Fig. 7.7) which have somatosensory/motor connectivity (Rolls et al., 2023i). This might relate to directing auditory attention to any touch to the body; to behaviors that might be performed before a highly developed visual system evolved; and to navigation / obstacle avoidance in the dark. Another type of somatosensory feedback may be needed in speech production, especially during early learning of articulation, where it may be crucial for the distinction between different types of consonants (Ohashi and Ostry, 2021).

In addition, there is evidence (Rolls et al., 2023h) for effective connectivity of some auditory cortical regions to the hippocampus, and to the scene-related ventromedial visual region VMV1 (Sulpizio et al., 2020), and the parahippocampal TF, with both types of connectivity involved in episodic memory (Rolls et al., 2023e, 2022a; Rolls, 2023c, 2022b). In addition, auditory cortical region A5 has connectivity with inferior frontal gyrus regions IFJa and IFSp, which are implicated in short-term working memory for the ventral streams (Plakke and Romanski, 2014; Passingham, 2021; Rolls et al., 2023f; Miller et al., 2018) (Chapter 13).

The auditory cortex connectivity with inferior parietal regions is primarily between the STS visual-auditory regions and PGi, with some connectivity also with PGs and PFm (Rolls et al., 2023h) (Fig. 7.7), all of which are visual inferior parietal regions linked considerably to ventral stream processing (Rolls et al., 2022b, 2023d). Inputs related to reward and punishment from, for example, the ventromedial prefrontal cortex (vmPFC) (10r, 10v, 10d) and orbitofrontal cortex (a47r) (Rolls et al., 2023c) reach STS auditory-visual cortical regions where objects, faces, and their semantic meaning are represented (Rolls et al., 2022b), rather than earlier stages of auditory cortical processing (Rolls et al., 2023h). Correspondingly, STS regions have effective connectivity with some orbitofrontal / vmPFC regions in which neurons respond to vocalisation and the face movements that produce them (Rolls, Critchley, Browning and Inoue, 2006a).

7.7 How the computations are performed in the auditory system

The computation of interaural time differences has been described, and the mechanisms for inter-aural intensity differences need not be complicated.

The computation of 3D sound location requires a relatively broad-band signal so that the spectrum can be evaluated. The most important effects are produced by the antenna effects of the pinna, for if the recordings are made from only two artificial pinnae, sound localization in 3D is reasonable. The helical shape of the pinnae is important, as that is asymmetric for sounds at different elevations. Because each individual's pinnae are slightly different shapes, learning in relation to one's own pinnae is needed for accurate sound localization. This is likely to be aided by craniotopic visual representations.

There is evidence for hierarchical processing across cortical areas in primates, and this is likely to proceed by building feature combination neurons from the features represented at the preceding stage. Competitive learning is the mechanism that I propose. This process is likely to be able to lead to neurons tuned to complex sounds including vocalizations that are found in the orbitofrontal and dorsolateral prefrontal cortex. It is likely that the anterior parts of the superior temporal gyrus are involved in this, as described in Chapter 8.

As in vision, there appears to be segregation of two types of computation, one more involved in spatial location and taking place in the dorsal auditory stream, and another computation more involved in analysis of what the sound is, its identity, in the ventral auditory system.

The value of auditory stimuli is represented in the orbitofrontal cortex, as shown by the findings that neurons there represent vocalizations with emotion-related significance, such as lip-smacking; but also by the finding that damage to the human orbitofrontal cortex impairs the ability to identify the emotional expression in the voice, but does not impair identification of sounds in general. Whether the mechanism for value representations for auditory stimuli is by pattern association learning with other reinforcers is not yet known.

8 The temporal cortex

8.1 Introduction and overview

The inferior temporal visual cortex is involved in invariant visual object recognition, as described in Chapter 2 (Rolls, 2021d).

The superior temporal cortex in its mid-part contains the auditory cortex, and the auditory belt cortex, as described in Chapter 7.

Behind the auditory cortex is Wernicke's area in the posterior part of the superior temporal gyrus, part of area 22, which is involved in phonological processing, and its functions are considered in Chapter 14.

The medial temporal lobe includes the parahippocampal gyrus and hippocampus involved in episodic memory, and this system is considered in Chapter 9.

The amygdala, a subcortical part of the anterior temporal lobe involved in emotion, is considered in Chapter 11.

In this Chapter, the focus is on *what* is computed in other parts of the temporal lobe, including the anterior parts of the temporal lobe (Fig. 8.1), which especially in humans are involved in semantic representations. Section 8.5 is about *how* these semantic representations may be set up.

In addition, in humans there is also a middle temporal gyrus, and its functions in face expression and gesture identification, and in theory of mind, are considered first.

8.2 Middle temporal gyrus and face expression and gesture

The cortex in the macaque superior temporal sulcus contains neurons that often combine object selectivity with a preference for moving visual stimuli, as described in Chapter 2. Some of these neurons in the middle to anterior part of the cortex in the superior temporal sulcus respond to moving heads and to face gesture, and some are tuned to face expression (Hasselmo, Rolls, Baylis and Nalwa, 1989b; Hasselmo, Rolls and Baylis, 1989a). With the great expansion of the human temporal lobe, this region may be in the middle temporal gyrus (see Fig. 8.1), which is not present in macaques, for with fMRI, activations are found here to face expression (Critchley et al., 2000).

In this context, it is of interest that a nearby part of the middle temporal gyrus has reduced functional connectivity with the ventromedial prefrontal cortex, precuneus, and posterior cingulate cortex in autism (Cheng, Rolls, Gu, Zhang and Feng, 2015). The reduced functional connectivity of this middle temporal gyrus area in autism spectrum conditions is of great interest, for some of the key typical symptoms of autism spectrum disorder are face processing and especially face expression processing deficits (Lai, Lombardo and Baron-Cohen, 2014), which will impair social and emotional communication (Rolls, 2014a). Further, in a meta-analysis of fMRI studies on the cortex in the superior temporal sulcus / along the middle temporal gyrus, a cluster of activations was identified that reflected motion processing, audiovisual correspondence (e.g. the sound and sight of an utterance), and face processing (Hein

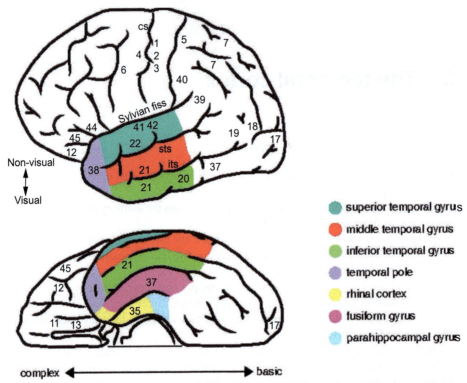

Fig. 8.1 Structures of the anterior temporal lobe of the human brain (in color). Above: lateral view; Below: ventral view. The axes indicate theoretical gradients of differential semantic processes. Along one axis, ventral structures contribute more to the processing of visual information (e.g. object concepts), and dorsolateral structures contribute more to the processing of non-visual information (e.g. abstract concepts, auditory concepts). Along the second axis, posterior structures contribute more to basic object representations, and anterior structures contribute more to the representation of complex conceptual, semantic, associations. Brodmann areas: 1,2,3 somatosensory cortex; 4 motor cortex; 5 superior parietal cortex; 6 premotor cortex; 7 inferior parietal cortex; 11, 13 medial orbitofrontal cortex; 17 primary visual (striate) cortex; 18, 19 prestriate visual cortical areas; 20 posterior inferior temporal cortex; 21 (anterior) inferior temporal cortex; 35 perirhinal cortex; 37 fusiform gyrus; 39 angular gyrus; 40 supramarginal gyrus; 41, 42 auditory cortex; 44 inferior frontal gyrus pars opercularis; 45 inferior frontal gyrus pars triangularis. cs central sulcus; its inferior temporal sulcus; sts superior temporal sulcus; Sylvian fiss Sylvian fissure / lateral sulcus. (Modified from Bonner,M.F. and Price,A.R. (2013) Where is the anterior temporal lobe and what does it do? J. Neurosci 33: 4213–4215.)

and Knight, 2008). The middle temporal gyrus region we identified with reduced functional connectivity in autism also has a more antero-dorsal band. Near this region, activations in the cortex in the superior temporal sulcus are related to speech processing (Hein and Knight, 2008). In addition, activations related to theory of mind were equally distributed over the anterior and posterior clusters (Hein and Knight, 2008). Thus the region that we identified with reduced functional cortical connectivity in autism spectrum disorder in the middle temporal gyrus / cortex in the superior temporal sulcus (Cheng, Rolls, Gu, Zhang and Feng, 2015) has functions related also to theory of mind and even speech processing. This is fascinating, given that there are major impairments of theory of mind and communication in autism spectrum disorder (Lai et al., 2014).

This processing stream in the superior temporal sulcus that performs processing important in social behavior is described further in Sections 2.4.9 and 2.5.3.

8.3 Semantic representations in the temporal lobe neocortex

Humans learn facts about items in the world, and group these items into useful categories and structures as semantic representations. This semantic knowledge is essential for many types of behavior and inferences. An example of a semantic representation might be a map of how cities are situated relative to each other, which could be built using many episodic memories of journeys to different cities. Each node in such a semantic representation might have a set of attributes associated with it, for example one city that was large, with skyscrapers, and beside the sea; whereas another city might have no skyscrapers, be far from the sea, and have a great University. Thus semantic representations, our knowledge about the world, involves a list of attributes or descriptors of each node, where a node might represent an individual person, a particular territory, or a certain type of object, such as a particular yacht or motor car. In the case of a territory, which is a semantic concept, the semantic attributes might include accumulated information, perhaps from many separate episodes, about where it is and its extent, who lives there, who the territory belongs to, whether it is well defended, whether the territory is fertile, prosperous, pleasant to live in, etc. The information used for semantic representations can be accumulated across all times.

Semantic memory is quite distinct from episodic memory, in which we might associate a particular person being in a particular place at a particular time, and that is what the hippocampus is involved in, as described in Chapter 9. Medial temporal lobe damage involving the hippocampus impairs episodic memory, but not previously learned semantic information. The learning of new semantic information is impaired by hippocampal damage, for the recall of episodic information is useful in building new semantic memories in the process of memory consolidation, as described in Chapter 9 (Rolls, 2022b). Semantic memories might be built using information recalled from many different episodic memories about many events each at particular times, as described in Section 9.2.3. Given that the formation of semantic memories is facilitated by the recall of episodic memory from the hippocampus (Section 9.2.8.5), it is proposed that an important contribution of the hippocampus to semantic memories (Section 9.2.8.5) is that pattern separation performed by the hippocampal system including the dentate granule cells (Rolls, 2016f), helps to reduce the correlations between the different semantic memories formed by hippocampus to neocortical recall. Correlations between the components of different semantic memories must be minimized, in order not to degrade the capacity of semantic memories (Ryom, Stendardi, Ciaramelli and Treves, 2023).

8.3.1 Neurophysiology of the medial temporal lobe, including concept cells

In one approach to semantic representations with macaque neurophysiology, two visual stimuli are repeatedly presented together with a short delay of a few seconds between them to set up paired associate learning, with the aim of studying semantic memory, which does involve the organisation of information in which simple associations may play a part. Neurons in the macaque perirhinal cortex were found to respond in relation to this type of visual paired associate learning (Miyashita and Chang, 1988; Fujimichi, Naya, Koyano, Takeda, Takeuchi and Miyashita, 2010; Miyashita, 2019). As described in Chapter 9, the perirhinal cortex is an area that receives multimodal information, and provides a gateway into the hippocampal episodic memory system, in which arbitrary multimodal associations that occur together need to be learned. However, the perirhinal cortex may be more a cortical area that is used in relation to hippocampal episodic memory function, and to recognition and long-term familiarity memory (Section 9.2.7), rather than the semantic system found more laterally and anteriorly in the human anterior temporal lobe.

Neurons that do respond to multimodal associations have been described in the human medial temporal lobe including the parahippocampal gyrus, and some have been described as 'concept cells' (Quian Quiroga, 2012; Quian Quiroga, Reddy, Kreiman, Koch and Fried, 2005; Quian Quiroga, 2023). For example, a neuron that responded to the sight of Jennifer Aniston or the sound of her voice also responded to other actors in the same movie, and the places with which they are associated (Quian Quiroga, 2012; Rey, Ison, Pedreira, Valentin, Alarcon, Selway, Richardson and Quian Quiroga, 2015; Quian Quiroga, Reddy, Kreiman, Koch and Fried, 2005; De Falco, Ison, Fried and Quian Quiroga, 2016). Object-place cells in macaques have some similar multi-attribute properties, in that they can be activated either by the object, or by the location in a viewed spatial scene, in object-location memory tasks (Rolls and Xiang, 2005, 2006; Rolls, 2023d). These neurons in macaques might accordingly also be described as 'concept cells' (Rolls, 2023c,d). Similar properties have been described for human hippocampal neurons, in a task in which a human was associated with the view of a place (Ison, Quian Quiroga and Fried, 2015). Some of these neurons can be described as representing the semantic properties of stimuli and appear to be quite widely distributed in the temporal lobe cortex (Rutishauser, 2019; Fried, Rutishauser, Cerf and Kreiman, 2014). In one study, the similarity of the neuronal responses to different concepts were closely related to the similarity of those concepts for individual participants (De Falco, Ison, Fried and Quian Quiroga, 2016). These findings are consistent with the evidence described in this section (8.3) that semantic representations are found in the temporal lobe cortex. Most of these recordings were made in the medial temporal lobe, and given the other evidence described below, these semantic representations may be especially in the temporal lobe neocortex. It is notable that many of the responses in these regions in humans were relatively small compared to those recorded in the macaque medial temporal lobe, though that could be related to the fact that the majority of these human recordings were made in patients with epilepsy.

Further evidence on what might be described as concept cells in macaques is as follows (Rolls, 2023d). When we discovered neurons in the macaque cortex in the anterior part of the superior temporal sulcus that responded to moving objects such as the sight of a head making or breaking social contact (Rolls, Baylis and Hasselmo, 1987; Hasselmo, Rolls and Baylis, 1989a; Hasselmo, Rolls, Baylis and Nalwa, 1989b), we also discovered nearby neurons that responded to auditory stimuli including vocalization (Rolls, Baylis and Hasselmo, 1987). The concept was that these two representations might be brought together in these cortical regions to form representations that could be activated by the sight of for example the lips moving to vocalize, and by the sound of the vocalization being made (Rolls et al., 1987). That has in fact now been shown to be the case, in that 76% of neurons in face patch AF in the cortex in the superior temporal sulcus were significantly influenced by the auditory component of a movie with faces that elicited neuronal responses, most often through enhancement of visual responses but sometimes in response to the auditory stimulus alone (Khandhadia, Murphy, Romanski, Bizley and Leopold, 2021). This type of neuron in macaques is thus multimodal, and can be activated by corresponding stimuli in the visual and auditory sensory modalities. That would appear to satisfy at least part of what a concept cell is (Rolls, 2023d). The concepts represented by these neurons in the third visual system are often about the social significance of stimuli (Pitcher and Ungerleider, 2021; Pitcher, Ianni and Ungerleider, 2019; Rolls, Deco, Huang and Feng, 2023e; Rolls, 2023a,d).

8.3.2 Neuropsychology

Semantic representations are about general conceptual knowledge about objects and events, including knowledge about their characteristic properties and behaviors, as well as knowledge about the words we use to name and describe objects and events in speech. In contrast, episodic memory encompasses memory for specific episodes or situations in one's life. Semantic representations are of factual knowledge divorced from any specific situational context, for example 'A scallop is an edible sea creature' (semantic) as opposed to 'I ate scallops for dinner yesterday evening' (episodic) (Patterson et al., 2007).

Patients with semantic dementia, a neurodegenerative disease affecting the anterior temporal lobe, and patients with a stroke in this region, have a deficit in semantic knowledge with a relative sparing of most other cognitive domains (Patterson et al., 2007). These patients have little trouble performing episodic recall tasks, visual perceptual tasks, or numerical tasks, and can even retain complex behaviors like performing novel musical pieces – yet they have a striking impairment on nearly all assessments of semantic knowledge. Damage to the left anterior temporal lobe is associated with a decline in object naming ability, providing evidence that it is specialized for the retrieval of unique entity concepts (Swanson et al., 2020).

Neurodegenerative damage to the temporal pole is associated with associative agnosia, semantic forms of primary progressive aphasia and semantic dementia (Mesulam, 2023). Object naming and word comprehension are critically dependent on the language-dominant (usually left) temporopolar region, whereas behavioral control and non-verbal object recognition display a more bilateral representation with a rightward bias (Mesulam, 2023). A first sign of left temporopolar dysfunction takes the form of taxonomic blurring where boundaries between categories are preserved but not boundaries between exemplars of a category (Mesulam, 2023), consistent with what is found in associative neural networks (Virasoro, 1989) which elucidate a mechanism by which these clinical symptoms arise.

8.3.3 Functional neuroimaging

There is evidence that parts of the temporal lobe represent amodal conceptual object knowledge in that they have supramodal representations and play a role in distinguishing between the conceptual representations of different objects (Fairhall and Caramazza, 2013a). In an fMRI study, human participants made category typicality judgments about pictured objects or their names. Activations to supramodal object categories (both the pictures of objects and their names) that reflected the similarity between the categories of objects were found in the posterior middle/inferior temporal gyrus and posterior cingulate/precuneus. Thus the middle/inferior temporal gyri are candidate regions for the amodal representation of the conceptual properties of objects (Fairhall and Caramazza, 2013a).

To investigate further the representations for different types of semantic knowledge, it was shown that access to knowledge of kinds of people (e.g. lawyer, nurse) produced selective activations in the left anterior temporal lobe, posterior middle temporal gyrus and the temporoparietal junction, precuneus, and medial prefrontal cortex (Fairhall and Caramazza, 2013b). For comparison, place-selective activations (e.g. bank, prison) were found in the parahippocampal gyrus and a connected region the retrosplenial cortex. Thus non-perceptual semantic representations about different types of object category appear to involve different parts of the temporal lobe (Fairhall and Caramazza, 2013b).

In an investigation of semantic knowledge about actions, it was found that the left lateral posterior temporal cortex encodes action representations that generalize across observed action scenes and written descriptions (Wurm and Caramazza, 2019). These temporal cortex regions thus are involved in general, conceptual, aspects of actions.

Verbs and nouns are fundamental units of language, and neuropsychological evidence has shown that nouns and verbs can be damaged independently of each other (Hernandez et al., 2014). Also, neuroimaging studies have found regions that are particularly sensitive to a word's grammatical category (Tyler et al., 2008). The grammatical distinction between nouns and verbs is of fundamental importance, because a word's grammatical category determines the types of phrases in which it appears and the morphological transformations it undergoes. For example, 'The boy likes the candies' is correct, but not 'The likes boy the candies'. In another example, 'The boy liked the candies' is correct, but not 'The boyed like the candies'. The semantic-lexical properties of verbs and nouns that underlie their independence may be predication: a core lexical feature involved in binding constituent arguments (boy, candies) into a unified syntactic-semantic structure expressing a proposition (the boy likes the candies). To test whether the intrinsic 'predication-building' function of verbs is what drives the verb-noun distinction in the brain, verb-preferring regions with a localizer experiment including verbs and nouns were first identified. Then, the sensitivity of these regions to transitivity – an index measuring the tendency to select for a direct object – was measured (Hernandez et al., 2014). Transitivity is a verb-specific property lying at the core of its predication function. Neural activity in the left posterior middle temporal and inferior frontal gyri correlated with transitivity, indicating sensitivity to predication. This is evidence that grammatical class preference in the brain is driven by a word's function to build predication structures (Hernandez et al., 2014), and that the temporal lobe plays a key role in this.

Further evidence that temporal lobe semantic systems are involved in language is that left temporal cortex areas and the connected inferior frontal gyrus regions that include Broca's area in the inferior frontal gyrus are specifically involved when listening to syntactically ambiguous sentences such as 'The newspaper reported that bullying teenagers are a problem for the local school' (in which 'bullying teenagers' is syntactically ambiguous) (Campbell and Tyler, 2018). If an additional task was required, then other brain systems related to the task performance were engaged. Thus this temporal lobe - inferior frontal gyrus system may be specifically involved in syntactical processing of semantic information.

8.3.4 Brain stimulation

One type of study in humans possible in the course of surgery for clinical conditions has been electrical stimulation, to provide evidence on the types of function implemented in different parts of the temporal lobe. DeWitt and Rauschecker (2016) review findings from intraoperative stimulation mapping in 90 patients at 2754 cortical sites, extensively sampling the superior temporal gyrus (STG), supramarginal gyrus (SMG), middle temporal gyrus (MTG), and angular gyrus (AG) (Roux et al., 2015). Three findings emerge from the study. First, although the MTG was extensively surveyed, it was found to be uninvolved in auditory single-word comprehension, as indexed by performance on auditory word-to-picture matching (see Fig. 8.2A).

Second, although stimulation of several supramarginal / angular gyrus sites impaired comprehension, the dominant finding was for comprehension to be impaired by superior temporal gyrus stimulation (see Fig. 8.2A, inset).

Third, analysis of error types shows an anterior-oriented processing hierarchy within the superior temporal gyrus. Performance on auditory word-to-picture matching involves (i) auditory word-form recognition, (ii) retrieval of the word-form's semantic referents, and (iii) association of one of the referents to a visual depiction thereof. Roux et al. (2015) classified errors as either 'speech discrimination/word deafness errors', indicating a putative failure to resolve an auditory word-form from sensory input, or 'lexical-semantic errors', indicating putative failure to associate an accurately perceived word-form with a visual depiction of its semantic referent. Word-form analysis (transient word deafness) was associated with the

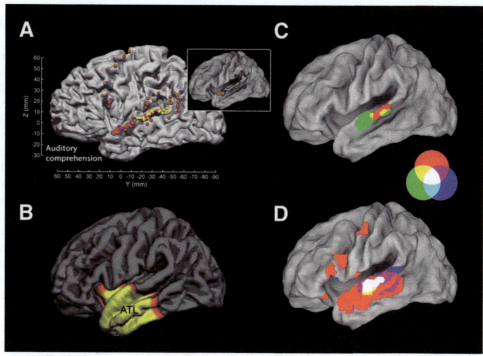

Fig. 8.2 Semantic retrieval in auditory single-word comprehension is associated with the integrity of anterior superior temporal gyrus (STG) function, as found in stimulation mapping (A, orange markers) and lesion-symptom mapping (B). Auditory word-form recognition is associated with mid-to-anterior STG, as found in stimulation mapping (A, yellow markers) and meta-analysis of functional imaging (C, D). The meta-analytic results depicted are RGB overlap maps for effects of repetition suppression for phonemes (C, red shading) and auditory words (C, green shading), as well as for tests of speech-related combination sensitivity (D, red shading), invariant representation (D, green shading) and areal specialization (D, blue shading). Notably, when a probability density function is estimated for the reported stimulation mapping foci (A), peak density is found along STG, excluding the most posterior aspect of STG, with the global peak in anterior STG (A, inset). Together, these results imply a processing hierarchy for phonemes, word-forms and semantic retrieval that extends along STG in an anterior-oriented gradient. (Reprinted from DeWitt,I. and Rauschecker,J.P. (2016) Convergent evidence for the causal involvement of anterior superior temporal gyrus in auditory single-word comprehension. Cortex 77: 164–166. © Elsevier Inc.)

mid-to-anterior superior temporal gyrus (Fig. 8.2A, yellow markers) while semantic retrieval (matching error) was associated with the anterior superior temporal gyrus (Fig. 8.2A, orange markers), indicating that anterior parts of the superior temporal gyrus are especially involved in semantic representations.

The parts of the anterior temporal implicated by all of this evidence in semantic processing are strongly connected with the inferior frontal gyrus ('Broca's area') by the uncinate fasciculus. This connection may enable syntactic operations performed in networks in the inferior frontal gyrus to utilize semantic representations in the anterior temporal lobe (see Section 14.5).

8.4 Connectivity and functions of the human temporal lobe regions related to semantics

In this section evidence is described on semantic systems in and connected to the temporal lobe (Rolls et al., 2022b). The evidence is based on use of the Human Connectome Project - Multimodal cortical Parcellation (HCP-MMP, Section 1.12), and measuring effective connectivity, complemented by functional connectivity and diffusion tractography (Section 1.13) with data from the Human Connectome Project.

Brain areas involved in language and the connectivity between them is a topic of importance for understanding human brain function and in order to minimize language impairments during neurosurgery (Milton et al., 2021; Ding et al., 2016; Hickok and Poeppel, 2015, 2007; Bornkessel-Schlesewsky et al., 2015; DeWitt and Rauschecker, 2013; Rauschecker, 2012; Chang et al., 2015; Bouchard et al., 2013). Earlier views of Wernicke's area and its connections with Broca's area (Geschwind, 1970) have now been re-evaluated (Coslett and Schwartz, 2018) to produce new views on Wernicke's area (DeWitt and Rauschecker, 2013; Binder, 2017), Broca's area (Amunts and Zilles, 2012; Kelly et al., 2010; Gajardo-Vidal et al., 2021), their evolutionary origins (Rauschecker, 2018a), and neuropsychological and neuroimaging investigations of language systems (Kemmerer, 2015; Hagoort, 2017; Hagoort and Indefrey, 2014; Battistella et al., 2020; Friederici et al., 2017). In more recent research utilising the Human Connectome Project Multimodal Parcellation (HCP-MMP) atlas (Glasser et al., 2016a), 157 task-based fMRI studies were analyzed to identify brain regions in the HCP-MMP atlas related to semantics based on categorization of visual words and objects, and auditory words and stories, and the following regions were identified as part of the semantic network: 44, 45, 55b, IFJa, 8C, p32pr, SFL, SCEF, 8BM, STSdp, STSvp, TE1p, PHT and PBelt, and were shown to be interconnected with tractography (Milton et al., 2021).

In the research described next (Rolls et al., 2022b), community analysis was performed on the 360x360 effective connectivity matrix for the HCP-MMP cortical regions, and a community of 26 cortical regions was identified that included most of those or very similar regions to those noted above (Milton et al., 2021) related to language. Analyses were then performed on the connections, functional connectivity, and effective connectivity of these 26 left hemisphere cortical regions with the 360 cortical regions in the HCP-MMP atlas (Glasser et al., 2016a). A community analysis on the effective connectivity of these 26 language-related cortical regions identified the three groups of cortical language-related regions described next.

As background to the connectivity analyses of these three groups of language-related regions, the human temporal lobe semantic regions include cortical regions in the superior temporal sulcus and the adjacent temporal pole regions anteriorly and temporo-parieto occipital regions posteriorly as illustrated in Figs. 8.3 and 8.4. These regions can be placed in their connectional context as follows. The inferior temporal visual cortex, illustrated in Fig. 2.23, has connectivity to the cortical regions in the ventral bank of the Superior Temporal Sulcus (STS) as illustrated in Fig. 2.24. The auditory cortical pathways and other cortical regions have connectivity to the cortical regions in the dorsal bank of the Superior Temporal Sulcus (STS) as illustrated in Figs. 7.7 and 2.25. Some of the functions of these cortical regions in the superior temporal sulcus in responding to socially relevant stimuli such as face expression, head motion, and vocalization have been described in Sections 2.5.3 and 2.5.2. Here these analyses are extended to show how the cortical regions in the superior temporal sulcus are parts of two much more extended systems that are termed here the Group 1 and Group 3 Semantic Regions involved in language (Rolls et al., 2022b). The Group 2 regions of this set include Broca's area regions 44 and 45 that are implicated in syntax, and are described in Chapter 14.

8.4.1 Group 1 semantic regions that include regions in the ventral bank of the Superior Temporal Sulcus

The cortical regions in this group identified by the community analysis are shown in Fig. 8.3 and consist of STSva STSvp TE1a TGd PGi 10v 9m 10pp 47s 8Av 8BL 9a and 9p (Rolls et al., 2022b). The Group 1 network includes inferior (ventral) regions of the cortex

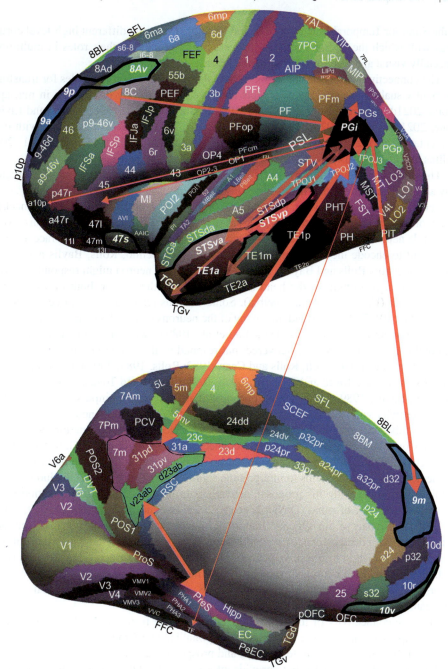

Fig. 8.3 Effective connectivity of region PGi chosen as an example of a Group 1 Semantic region with connectivity with the inferior STS stream, the posterior cingulate cortex, the frontal pole, and the dorsolateral prefrontal cortex. The Group 1 regions are indicated in bold italic font and are outlined in black (including PGi), and are: STSva STSvp TE1a TGd PGi 10v 9m 10pp 47s 8Av 8BL 9a 9p. The widths of the lines and the size of the arrowheads indicate the magnitude and direction of the effective connectivity. 7PM and IP1 connect to PGs which in turn connects to PGi, providing a route for PGi to receive visual motion information, and to connect that to areas such as STSva and STSvp. The thin black outline encloses the postero-ventral memory-related regions of the posterior cingulate cortex, which connect to the hippocampal system (Rolls et al., 2023i). The abbreviations are listed in Section 1.12. (From Rolls,E.T., Deco,G., Huang,C-C. and Feng,J. (2022) The human language effective connectome. Neuroimage 258: 119352.)

in the Superior Temporal Sulcus (STSva and STSvp). The many different high-level cortical areas with which the Group 1 regions have connectivity indicate their roles in multimodal especially visual and value-related semantic representations.

The connectivity with inferior temporal visual cortex TE regions provides for transform-invariant visual representations of objects and faces as shown by discoveries in macaques (Rolls, 2021d,b; Perrett, Rolls and Caan, 1982; Booth and Rolls, 1998; Arcaro and Livingstone, 2021; Freiwald, 2020; Hesse and Tsao, 2020; Lehky and Tanaka, 2016) with complementary evidence from human neuroimaging (Kanwisher et al., 1997; Finzi et al., 2021; Collins and Olson, 2014).

The connectivity with inferior parietal cortex PGi and to a smaller extent PGs regions may allow information about the visual motion of objects, such as a head turning away, or the eyes closing, or the lips moving, to convey a social signal such as a greeting (lip-smack) or threat, or when vocalizing, to reach STS areas (Rolls et al., 2023d). Indeed, it was discovered that single neurons in the macaque STS respond to face expression and also to face and head movement to encode the social relevance of stimuli (Hasselmo, Rolls, Baylis and Nalwa, 1989b; Hasselmo, Rolls and Baylis, 1989a). For example, a neuron might respond to closing of the eyes, or to turning of the head away from facing the viewer, both of which break social contact (Hasselmo et al., 1989b,a). Some neurons respond to the direction of gaze (Perrett et al., 1987). It was found that many of the neurons in the STS respond only or much better to moving faces or objects (Hasselmo et al., 1989a), whereas in the anterior inferior temporal cortex neurons were discovered that respond well to static visual stimuli, and are tuned for face identity (Perrett, Rolls and Caan, 1982; Rolls, 1984, 2000a; Rolls and Treves, 2011; Rolls, Treves, Tovee and Panzeri, 1997d; Rolls, Treves and Tovee, 1997b; Hasselmo, Rolls and Baylis, 1989a). It has been proposed that PGi, with its inputs from PGs which has connectivity with superior parietal and intraparietal regions that encode visual motion, is part of this processing stream for socially relevant face-related information (Rolls et al., 2023d). Consistent with this, the effective connectivity is stronger from PGi to STS regions (Rolls et al., 2022b). In humans, representations of this type could provide part of the basis for the development of systems to interpret the significance of such stimuli, including theory of mind. Consistent with this proposal, activations in the temporo-parietal junction region are related to theory of mind (DiNicola et al., 2020; Buckner and DiNicola, 2019; Schurz et al., 2017). Signals of this type are important in understanding the meaning of seen faces and objects, and indeed evidence about moving objects present in the STS may reach it from PGs and PGi, which in turn receive connectivity from the intraparietal sulcus regions (Rolls et al., 2023d) in which neurons respond to visual motion and to grasping objects which are important in tool use (Maravita and Romano, 2018), which is another fundamental aspect of the meaning or semantics of stimuli.

Effective connectivity of the Group 1 regions with the frontal pole (10pp, 9m, 9a, 9p) regions implicated in planning and sequencing (Shallice and Cipolotti, 2018; Shallice and Burgess, 1996; Gilbert and Burgess, 2008) and prospective as well as retrospective memory (Underwood et al., 2015) is likely to provide information about the temporal order / sequence of events, which is important in interpreting causal interactions in the world (Rolls, 2021e).

Similarly, the connectivity via the parahippocampal TF region (Fig. 8.3) with the hippocampal system implicated in episodic memory (Dere et al., 2008; Ekstrom and Ranganath, 2018; Rolls, 2018b, 2021b; Moscovitch et al., 2016) is likely to be important in building semantic information about the meaning of events by enabling the memory of particular past events to be taken into account. The connectivity of the Group 1 regions with the postero-ventral parts of the posterior cingulate cortex which are implicated in episodic memory (Vann et al., 2009; Leech and Smallwood, 2019; Leech and Sharp, 2014; Rolls et al., 2023i) may, by providing a route to the hippocampal system, in a similar way be important in enabling the

Group 1 regions, especially those in the temporal lobe but also in the inferior parietal cortex (Davis et al., 2018; Papagno, 2018), to build semantic representations by taking particular previous episodes into account. Consistent with this, increasing activation of the angular gyrus in the parietal cortex and decreasing activation of the hippocampus occurs when episodic memories become incorporated into schemas (van der Linden et al., 2017).

The connectivity of the Group 1 regions with the orbitofrontal cortex (regions OFC and pOFC), pregenual anterior cingulate cortex (d32) and some ventromedial prefrontal cortex regions where reward value and emotion are represented (Grabenhorst and Rolls, 2011; Rolls et al., 2023c; Rolls, 2019c,e; Rolls et al., 2020a; Rolls, 2014a; Padoa-Schioppa and Conen, 2017; Cai and Padoa-Schioppa, 2012; Reber et al., 2017; Rolls, 2021h) provides another fundamental type of input for building semantic representations about people and objects.

The extensive connectivity of the Group 1 regions with the prefrontal cortex which is implicated in working memory and planning (Goldman-Rakic, 1996; Baddeley, 2021) (Chapter 13) is likely to enable semantic representations to be held online to facilitate planning, reasoning, and rearrangement of the order of components if a task fails (Rolls, 2020a).

8.4.2 Group 3 semantic regions that include regions in the dorsal bank of the Superior Temporal Sulcus

The cortical regions in Group 3 are shown in Fig. 8.4 and consist of A5 STGa STSda STSdp PSL STV and TPOJ1 (Rolls et al., 2022b).

The Group 3 network includes superior (or dorsal) parts of the cortex in the Superior Temporal Sulcus (STSda and STSdp) in the temporal lobe that have auditory as well as early visual inputs, continues up through the temporo-parietal junction (TPOJ1) into the Superior Temporal Visual region (STV) to the PeriSylvian Language area (PSL), and connects with inferior frontal gyrus areas IFSp and IFJp (rather than dorsolateral prefrontal cortex) and with areas 44 and 45 (Broca's area) (Fig. 8.4). Auditory region A5 (Chapter 7) is adjacent to STSdp.

Region TPOJ1 has robust effective connectivity with auditory association cortex, including A5, A4 and to some extent LBelt, PBelt and TA2 (Fig. 8.4).

The visual input is not from inferior temporal visual cortex (TE regions), but instead with some earlier visual cortical regions involved in motion processing (MST, MT, especially to STV and TPOJ1) and in face processing (the fusiform face cortex FFC and posterior inferior temporal cortex PIT). These inputs are likely to contribute to the neurons discovered in the STS that respond to biological motion such as moving parts of faces such as the lips and eyelids and to the head turning towards vs away from the viewer in object-based coordinates, and also to face expression (Hasselmo, Rolls, Baylis and Nalwa, 1989b; Hasselmo, Rolls and Baylis, 1989a). Activations to corresponding stimuli are found in similar posterior STS regions in humans (Critchley et al., 2000; Bellot et al., 2021). We proposed that this STS region is a third visual system that combines inputs from dorsal and ventral visual streams (Hasselmo, Rolls, Baylis and Nalwa, 1989b; Hasselmo, Rolls and Baylis, 1989a; Baylis, Rolls and Leonard, 1987), and this has recently received support (Pitcher and Ungerleider, 2021). Moreover, the same STS regions also contain neurons that respond to auditory stimuli including in some cases vocalization (Baylis, Rolls and Leonard, 1987). It is likely that neurons in these STS regions respond to combinations of auditory and synchronized visual stimuli such as vocalization and moving lips and are important in speech analysis by the viewer/hearer not only in noisy environments, but also to confirm who is speaking, and to learn associations between the sight of a person's face and the sound of their voice, which is part of what is required for the semantic representation of a person. Neurons of these types, including face expression, underlie the importance of this region in interpreting the social meaning of visual

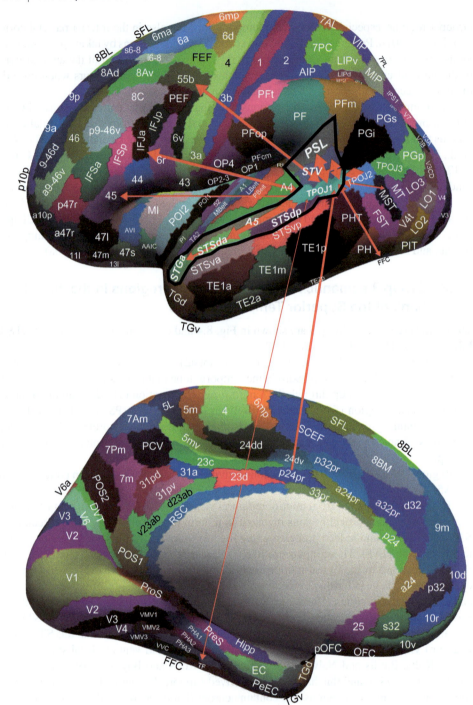

Fig. 8.4 Effective connectivity of region TPOJ1 chosen as an example of the typical effective connectivity of a Group 3 Semantic region with connectivity with a superior STS auditory-visual stream extending from STGA through STSda, A5, STSdp to TPOJ1. The Group 3 regions are indicated in bold italic font and are outlined in black, and are: A5 STGa STSda STSdp PSL STV TPOJ1. TPOJ1 also has effective connectivity with PSL, STV, TPOJ2, the inferior frontal gyrus IFJA and IFSp and 45, and with premotor area 55b and the midcingulate cortex p24pr. There is also effective connectivity with parahippocampal TF. The widths of the lines and the size of the arrowheads indicate the magnitude and direction of the effective connectivity. The abbreviations are listed in Section 1.12. (From Rolls,E.T., Deco,G., Huang,C-C. and Feng,J. (2022) The human language effective connectome. Neuroimage 258: 119352.)

and auditory stimuli, which is a key part of semantic representations implemented in these STS regions, and that contribute to theory of mind, that is, of another individual's intentions and even thoughts.

Another type of influence on these Group 3 regions comes from somatosensory cortical areas, as is especially evident in the functional connectivity (Rolls et al., 2022b). The functional connectivity is not only with 1-3b and 5, but also with frontal opercular and insular cortex, and there is some evidence for this too in the effective connectivity, including with parietal PF which can be considered as the top of the somatosensory hierarchy (Rolls et al., 2023d) (Chapter 6). This may contribute to semantic representations of body image and the sense of self (Rolls et al., 2023d).

The effective connectivity of these Group 3 regions with the inferior frontal gyrus regions and with areas 44 and 45 is proposed to provide inputs to a set of attractor networks in these IFG regions (Rolls and Deco, 2015a), supported by the large number of recurrent collaterals onto each neuron in the inferior frontal gyrus (Elston, 2007; Elston et al., 2006), that are important in some particularly temporal aspects of speech production. Indeed, it is proposed that a set of attractor networks in these inferior frontal gyrus regions are linked by stronger forward than backwards connections, and so naturally implement a temporal trajectory or sequence through the series of attractors that implements by learning the sequential constraints that are a key part of syntax in languages in which word order is important in syntax (Rolls and Deco, 2015a). According to this theory of speech / language production, the biases for the content of what is in each attractor, e.g. the subject attractor=Jane, the verb attractor=jumps over, and the object attractor=John, come from the temporal lobe semantic regions being considered here, and the execution of the learned syntax comes from the temporally linked series of attractors for the parts of a sentence in the inferior frontal gyrus / Broca's area (Rolls and Deco, 2015a) (Section 14.5). The large extent of the inferior frontal gyrus with effective connectivity in humans (IFSp and IFJa, 44 and 45, 47l and 47s) with these temporal lobe semantic regions including TG is consistent with many sequential syntax-related order-dependent attractor networks in these inferior frontal regions, as it is likely that different attractor systems are required for the active vs passive voice and for different languages in which the word order is different (Rolls and Deco, 2015a).

The functions of each of these brain regions is a topic of great interest that is being facilitated by the use of the HCP-MMP atlas (Ekert et al., 2021a). For example, STSdp is implicated in the short-term retention of auditory representations that can be derived from either auditory or visual inputs. The left PeriSylvian Language (PSL) region may hold auditory representations of expected speech on-line until the spoken output is matched to the intended speech. TPOJ1 was not implicated in auditory or phonological short-term memory, but more in motor tasks (Ekert et al., 2021a).

8.5 The mechanisms for semantic learning in the human anterior temporal lobe

One approach to the computations involved in semantics is investigation in connectionist networks, which do not necessarily aim to be biologically plausible, but which can offer insight into what well-defined computations in networks can achieve.

In one such investigation, a deep linear network that displays many of the properties involved in learning semantic representations has been described (Saxe et al., 2019; McClelland et al., 2020). The network has one hidden layer, but is a linear network. It can therefore only compute what a network without a hidden layer can compute (because it is linear, see

Appendix B). However, the network, trained by backpropagation of error, does display interesting non-linear learning dynamics that are beyond what a network without a hidden layer shows. This enables the network to display properties found during semantic development such as the hierarchical differentiation of concepts through rapid developmental transitions, semantic illusions between such transitions, the emergence of item typicality and category coherence as factors controlling the speed of semantic processing, changing patterns of inductive projection over development, and the conservation of semantic similarity in neural representations across species. The network provides analytic insight into how the statistical structure of an environment can interact with nonlinear deep-learning dynamics to give rise to these properties, but the use of error back-propagation (Saxe et al., 2019; McClelland et al., 2020) is a problem in terms of biological plausibility.

Further evidence on semantic representations and how they may be learned is provided in Sections 14.2.4 and 14.4. Hypotheses and a model about how syntactic operations might be performed on semantic representations using a trajectory through a state space of cortical attractor networks are described in Section 14.5.

For semantic memory, different cortical regions may specialize in different attributes of a semantic memory. For example, an individual person might have attributes such as the sight of the face, the sound of the voice, the location where they work, etc. Semantic memories could be formed by coupling many such attractor networks together. An interesting issue arises though that if similar features are present in such compositional memories in the semantic representations of different individuals, this effectively increases the correlations between the items in the whole memory, and this can reduce somewhat the total memory capacity that might be expected (Ryom, Stendardi, Ciaramelli and Treves, 2023). This might occur if for example the sounds of the voices of several of the individuals are similar. How semantic representations are stored using coupled attractor networks each in a different brain region is a topic of current interest.

9 The hippocampus, memory, and spatial function

9.1 Introduction and overview

The hippocampus is involved in episodic memory, which is the memory of particular events in the recent past. An example would be where one was at dinner the preceding evening, who was there, and what one ate for dinner. The hippocampus has to be able to store this information is such a way that it is separate from the memory of what happened the day before. The hippocampus also needs to be able to recall this information, so that it can be used later by the brain to produce appropriate behavior and to help build neocortical semantic memories such as autobiographical memory (Chapter 8). Most episodic memories have a spatial component, and the order in which events happen is also often part of an episodic memory: and spatial and time sequence information is part of what is processed by the hippocampus. Perhaps because the hippocampus processes spatial information, it is also involved in some ways in spatial navigation.

The hippocampal system is extremely interesting to investigate as a brain system, because it has a distinctive set of neural networks, each with it own neural network architecture, which can be related to the computations performed by the hippocampal system.

The focus here is, as throughout this book, on the primate including human hippocampus, as the information processed in the rodent hippocampus is somewhat different. However, investigations of the architecture of the neural networks and how they operate has been performed considerably in rodents, and that information is described for it helps to build an understanding of hippocampal computation. Indeed, many studies in rodents help to test the theory of hippocampal computation that has been developed as described here.

9.1.1 Overview of what is computed by the hippocampal system

1. The hippocampus receives information from the ends of all sensory including spatial processing streams in the brain via the entorhinal cortex, area 28, the gateway to the hippocampus from the neocortex. There are as many backprojections from the hippocampus that return to the top ends of these cortical processing areas.
2. Damage to the human hippocampal system results in anterograde amnesia, in which new episodic memories cannot be formed, but in which previous memory including semantic memory (general knowledge) is relatively intact. The hippocampus may also be involved in prospective memory, of tasks that need to be performed, presumably because these also need the storage of sets of new particular items.
3. The hippocampus is also involved in navigation, but this may be in part when there is a need to store new items for the navigation in for example novel environments, at least in humans. Computations for navigation are described in Chapter 10.
4. The hippocampus contains allocentric (world-based) place cells in rodents and primates. In primates there are also spatial view cells that respond allocentrically to a location in space 'out there' at which the primate is looking. These spatial view cells are likely to be important in remembering what has been seen where in the environment, in that some

spatial view cells respond to a combination of spatial view and object in an 'object-to-place in a scene' memory task. The same is found in a 'reward-to-place in a scene' memory task. The spatial view neurons fire to a viewed location in space relatively independently of eye position, head direction, and the place where the individual is located, which is an important property of a memory system, for this enables correct recall of the object or reward at a viewed location in a scene even if the eye position, head direction, and place are different from when the learning took place. The location in a scene at which spatial view neurons fire can be updated for a few minutes by movements made in the dark, and this may be useful in selecting goals for navigation in the dark. This update by self-motion in for example the dark is referred to as idiothetic update.

5. The primate (including human) hippocampus may utilise information from ventral visual stream areas that respond to scenes to build hippocampal spatial scene representations. 'Where' hippocampal spatial scene representations are thus built by feature combinations in a ventromedial visual cortical stream that reaches the medial parahippocampal cortex (TH or PHA1-3) where spatial view neurons are found. In this situation, the route via the dorsal visual stream and parietal cortex areas to the hippocampal system from human parietal cortex region PGp (and via the retrosplenial scene area and posterior cingulate cortex (Rolls et al., 2023e)) (Section 3.5) is then used for the idiothetic update in the human medial parahippocampal gyrus scene area of where in the allocentric spatial scene we may be looking, for example in the dark or remembering, based on idiothetic information.

6. The primate (including human) hippocampus receives information about 'what' object or person is present via a ventrolateral visual cortical stream that reaches the hippocampus from the inferior temporal visual cortex via lateral parahippocampal gyrus region TF and perirhinal and entorhinal cortex.

7. The primate (including human) hippocampus receives information about the reward value or emotional component of episodic memory from the orbitofrontal cortex / ventromedial prefrontal cortex / pregenual anterior cingulate cortex. Consolidation of information from episodic memory into semantic memory in humans is likely to be influenced by the value component of episodic memory, which leads to enhanced rehearsal of episodic memories that are of potential value to the individual.

8. The primate (including human) hippocampus can then associate together the 'what', 'where' and value / emotional components to form an episodic event memory.

9. The human orbitofrontal cortex (region pOFC) has connectivity to the cholinergic basal forebrain cholinergic neurons that project to the neocortex. The anterior cingulate cortex and vmPFC have connectivity to the septal region which contains cholinergic neurons that project to the hippocampus. These pathways are implicated in memory consolidation in humans, in the context that basal forebrain neurons fire when rewarding, punishing, or novel stimuli are encountered and storage of events may be especially useful.

10. There are also time cells in at least the rodent hippocampus, each of which responds at different times in a delay period, so that they fire in a temporal sequence, which can be up to hundreds or more seconds long. These neurons, when associated with objects or places, are likely to enable the order in which the objects or places occurred to be recalled.

11. The primate hippocampus contains 'whole body motion neurons', which respond to head rotation (angular velocity), and in other cases to linear motion (translation, moving for example forwards). Similar neurons are present in the rodent medial entorhinal cortex, where they have been termed 'speed cells'. They are likely to be involved in the memory of recent movements, and thus in idiothetic navigation.

12. The medial entorhinal cortex contains grid cells in rodents that fire with several peaks of firing as a rodent traverses places. In primates, there are spatial view grid cells, which are

likely to provide inputs to the spatial view cells found in the primate hippocampus. Different entorhinal cortex grid cells operate at different spatial scales. The lateral entorhinal cortex provides a route for object-related information from the ventral cortical systems to reach the hippocampus.

13. The presubiculum contains head direction cells, which use allocentric coordinates. They are found also in many other brain areas, and are likely to be important in navigation and in memory.

14. The perirhinal cortex, a stage before the entorhinal cortex on the route to and from the neocortex, is implicated in recognition memory, the ability to remember having seen an object in the recent past. It is also involved in long-term familiarity memory, with neurons responding with higher firing rates the more familiar a stimulus is.

15. This overview of what is represented in the hippocampal system summarizes evidence that is key to understanding *what* is computed in the hippocampus and connected structures, and *what* this computed information is used for in the hippocampus. *How* the computations are performed to make these representations, and *how* these representations are used in the hippocampus, are summarized in the next section, and are part of what is described in this Chapter.

9.1.2 Overview of how the computations are performed by the hippocampal system

1. A feature of the hippocampal network is that the CA3 system has a highly developed recurrent collateral system that enables it to associate together, operating as an autoassociation or attractor network, places / spatial views with objects. The single attractor network in CA3 enables any object to be associated with any place / spatial view in an episodic or event memory, and for the place to be recalled from the object, and the object from the place. This is completion of a memory in an autoassociation network.

2. The number of memories that can be stored in the hippocampus is determined largely by the number of recurrent collateral connections onto any one CA3 neuron (in the order of 12,000 in the rat) and the sparseness of the representation.

3. The dentate gyrus input to CA3 performs pattern separation of the inputs before CA3 to help achieve the relatively uncorrelated representations that help to achieve high memory capacity in CA3. The dentate granule cells perform this operation by competitive learning; by the low probability of contact of the dentate granule cell to CA3 connections (0.00015 in the rat: a granule cell makes 46 mossy fibre connections and there are 300,000 CA3 cells); and by neurogenesis with the new dentate granule cells helping to ensure that new memories are distinct from old memories by making new random connections to CA3 neurons. The dentate gyrus is the only part of cortex where new neurons can develop in adulthood, for here the premium is on selecting new random sets of neurons in CA3 for new memories distinct from previous memories, whereas elsewhere in cortex the information is stored in the synaptic weights and learned information would be lost if there was any turnover of neurons.

4. The CA1 which follows the CA3 prepares for the recall of memories, completed in CA3 by a partial retrieval cue, back to the neocortex. The CA1 has the architecture of a competitive network, useful for recoding the parts of an episodic memory necessarily represented as separate in CA3 for autoassociation in CA3.

5. Backprojections from the hippocampal system to neocortical areas have a large number of synapses onto each neocortical neuron to achieve high recall capacity of memories from

the hippocampus to the neocortex. This accounts for why there are as many backprojections as forward connections between adjacent cortical areas in a cortical hierarchy. For the recall to work efficiently, the backprojection synapses at one or more stages of the backprojection pathway must be associatively modifiable during the original learning.
6. Once set up in this way, the backprojection connections can also be used for top-down attentional control (see Chapter 13).
7. The medial entorhinal cortex appears to operate as a continuous attractor network that can perform path integration, updating the spatial representation based on motion signals (i.e. idiothetic update). The medial entorhinal cortex neurons reach the dentate and CA3, where competitive network learning can convert the grid cell representation into place cells by leading to different neurons learning combinations of the grid firing present at any one time in the entorhinal cortex. However, in humans the idiothetic update for changes in eye position, head direction, etc take place in the parietal cortex, with mechanisms considered in Section 3.5.
8. The lateral entorhinal cortex includes some neurons with slow ramping changes in firing rates over up to hundreds of seconds. Combinations of the firing of these neurons produced by competitive learning in the hippocampus can produce time cells. The theory for how this computation takes place can account for forward and reverse replay of temporal sequences of firing found in the hippocampus and related brain areas.

9.2 What is computed in the hippocampus

Any theory of the hippocampus must state at the systems level what is computed by the hippocampus. Some of the relevant evidence comes from the systems-level connections of the hippocampus (Section 9.2.1), from the effects of damage to the hippocampus (Section 9.2.2), and from the responses of neurons in the hippocampus during behavior (Section 9.2.4).

9.2.1 Systems-level anatomy

The main cortical connections of the hippocampus are shown in Fig. 9.1 (Rolls and Wirth, 2018), and in schematic form to show the nature of the network connectivity in Fig. 9.2 (Rolls, 2023c). These figures show that the primate hippocampus receives major inputs via the entorhinal cortex (area 28) (Garcia and Buffalo, 2020). These come from the highly developed parahippocampal gyrus (areas TF and TH) and also from the retrosplenial cortex, as well as the perirhinal cortex, and thereby from the ends of many processing streams of the cerebral association cortex, including the visual and auditory temporal lobe association cortical areas, the prefrontal cortex, and the parietal cortex (Van Hoesen, 1982; Amaral, Price, Pitkanen and Carmichael, 1992; Amaral, 1987; Witter, Groenewegen, Lopes da Silva and Lohman, 1989a; Suzuki and Amaral, 1994a; Witter, Wouterlood, Naber and Van Haeften, 2000b; Lavenex, Suzuki and Amaral, 2004; Johnston and Amaral, 2004; Witter, 2007; van Strien, Cappaert and Witter, 2009; Kondo, Lavenex and Amaral, 2009; Somogyi, 2010; Rolls, 2015b, 2018b; Garcia and Buffalo, 2020; Huang, Rolls, Hsu, Feng and Lin, 2021; Ma, Rolls, Huang, Cheng and Feng, 2022a; Rolls, Deco, Huang and Feng, 2022a, 2023e; Rolls, Wirth, Deco, Huang and Feng, 2023i; Rolls, Deco, Huang and Feng, 2023f,d,c; Rolls, 2023c). The hippocampus is thus by its connections potentially able to associate together object representations (from the temporal lobe visual and auditory areas) and spatial representations. In addition, the entorhinal cortex receives inputs from the amygdala, orbitofrontal cortex, and anterior cingulate cortex (Carmichael and Price, 1995b; Suzuki and Amaral, 1994a; Pitkanen et al., 2002; Stefanacci et al., 1996; Rolls, 2015b; Garcia and Buffalo, 2020; Huang et al., 2021; Ma et

What is computed in the hippocampus | 317

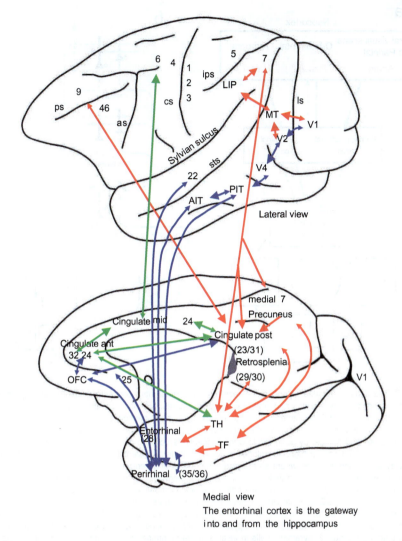

Medial view
The entorhinal cortex is the gateway
into and from the hippocampus

Fig. 9.1 Cortical connections of the primate hippocampus. A medial view of the macaque brain is shown below, and a lateral view is above. The entorhinal cortex area 28 is the main entry for cortical connections to and from the hippocampus. The forward projections to the hippocampus are shown with large arrowheads, and the backprojections with small arrowheads. The main ventral stream connections to the hippocampus that convey information about objects, faces, etc are in blue, and the main dorsal stream connections that convey 'where' information about space and movements are in red. The ventral 'what' visual pathways project from the primary visual cortex V1 to V2, then V4, then posterior inferior temporal visual cortex (PIT), then anterior inferior temporal visual cortex (AIT), then perirhinal cortex (areas 35/36), and thus to entorhinal cortex. The dorsal 'where' visual pathways project from V1 to V2, then MT (middle temporal), then LIP (lateral intraparietal), then parietal area 7 (lateral) and medial (including the precuneus), then to posterior cingulate cortex areas 23/31) including the retrosplenial cortex (areas 29/30) and thus to parahippocampal gyrus (areas TF and TH), and then perirhinal and entorhinal cortex. Area 22 is superior temporal auditory association cortex. The hippocampus enables all the high order cortical regions to converge into a single network in the hippocampal CA3 region. Object information reaches the hippocampus from the temporal cortex parts of the ventral visual system. The parahippocampal place area (Epstein and Baker, 2019), and also the ventral visual stream, may provide visual scene information that drives hippocampal spatial view cells. The retrosplenial cortex (29,30) is the small region in primates including humans behind the splenium of the corpus callosum shaded grey: it is not necessarily homologous with what is termed retrosplenial cortex in rodents (Vann et al., 2009), which may also not have a homologous posterior cingulate cortex (Vogt, 2009). Connections involving the cingulate cortex are in green. Other abbreviations: as–arcuate sulcus; cs–central sulcus; ips–intraparietal sulcus; ios–inferior occipital sulcus; ls–lunate sulcus; sts–superior temporal sulcus. (Modified from Rolls, E. T. and Wirth, S. (2018) Spatial representations in the primate hippocampus, and their functions in memory and navigation. Progress in Neurobiology 171: 90–113.)

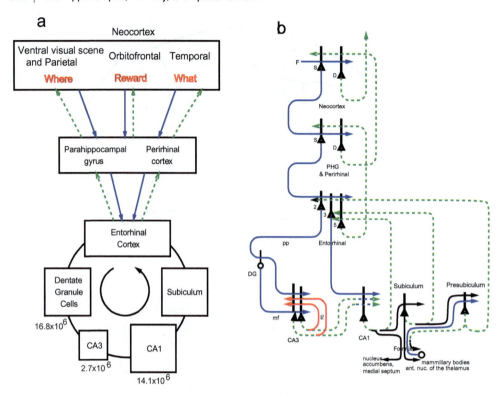

Fig. 9.2 The human / primate hippocampus receives neocortical input connections (blue) not only from the 'what' temporal lobe and 'where' parietal and ventral visual scene areas, but also from the 'reward' prefrontal cortex areas (orbitofrontal cortex, vmPFC, and anterior cingulate cortex) for episodic memory storage; and has return backprojections (green) to the same neocortical areas for memory recall. There is great convergence via the parahippocampal gyrus, perirhinal cortex, and dentate gyrus in the forward connections down to the single network implemented in the CA3 pyramidal cells, which have a highly developed recurrent collateral system (red) to implement an attractor episodic memory by associating the what, where and reward components of an episodic memory. a: Block diagram. b: Some of the principal excitatory neurons and their connections in the pathways. Time and temporal order are also important in episodic memory, and may be computed in the entorhinal-hippocampal circuitry (Rolls and Mills, 2019). Abbreviations - D: Deep pyramidal cells. DG: Dentate Granule cells. F: Forward inputs to areas of the association cortex from preceding cortical areas in the hierarchy. mf: mossy fibres. PHG: parahippocampal gyrus and perirhinal cortex. pp: perforant path. rc: recurrent collateral of the CA3 hippocampal pyramidal cells. S: Superficial pyramidal cells. 2: pyramidal cells in layer 2 of the entorhinal cortex. 3: pyramidal cells in layer 3 of the entorhinal cortex. The thick lines above the cell bodies represent the dendrites. The numbers of neurons in different parts of the hippocampal trisynaptic circuit in humans (Rogers Flattery et al., 2020) are shown in (a), and indicate very many dentate granule cells, consistent with expansion encoding and the production of sparse uncorrelated (pattern separated) representations prior to CA3. (From Rolls, E. T. (2023) Hippocampal spatial view cells for memory and navigation, and their underlying connectivity in humans. Hippocampus doi: 10.1002/hipo.23467.)

al., 2022a; Rolls et al., 2022a, 2023c,b; Rolls, 2023c), which could provide reward-related information to the hippocampus (Rolls, 2018b, 2022b, 2023c). The connections are analogous in the rat, although areas such as the temporal lobe and parietal lobe visual cortical areas are not well developed in rodents, and the parahippocampal gyrus may be represented by the dorsal perirhinal cortex (Burwell, Witter and Amaral, 1995).

Given that some topographic segregation is maintained in the afferents to the hippocampus in the perirhinal, parahippocampal, and entorhinal cortices (Amaral and Witter, 1989; Garcia and Buffalo, 2020; Huang, Rolls, Hsu, Feng and Lin, 2021; Ma, Rolls, Huang, Cheng and Feng, 2022a; Rolls, Deco, Huang and Feng, 2022a), it may be that these areas are able to subserve memory within one of these topographically separated areas, of for example visual object, or spatial, or olfactory information. In contrast, the final convergence afforded by the hippocampus into one network in CA3 (see Fig. 9.2) may be especially appropriate for an episodic memory typically involving arbitrary associations between any of the inputs to the hippocampus, e.g. spatial, vestibular related to self-motion, visual object, olfactory, auditory, and reward (see below). There are also direct subcortical inputs from for example the amygdala and septum (Amaral, 1986; Rolls et al., 2023b).

The primary output from the hippocampus to neocortex originates in CA1 and projects to subiculum, entorhinal cortex, and parahippocampal structures (areas TF-TH) as well as prefrontal cortex (Van Hoesen, 1982; Delatour and Witter, 2002; Witter, 1993; van Haeften et al., 2003; Witter and Amaral, 2021; Huang et al., 2021; Ma et al., 2022a; Rolls et al., 2022a). The subiculum also projects via the fimbria/fornix to subcortical areas such as the mammillary bodies and anterior thalamic nuclei (see Fig. 9.2) (Bubb, Kinnavane and Aggleton, 2017). In addition to the projections originating in CA1, projections out of Ammon's horn also originate in CA3. Many researchers have reported that CA3 projects to the lateral and medial septal nuclei (Amaral and Witter, 1995; Risold and Swanson, 1997; Gaykema et al., 1991). The lateral septum also has projections to the medial septum (Jakab and Leranth, 1995), which in turn projects to subiculum and eventually entorhinal cortex (Amaral and Witter, 1995; Jakab and Leranth, 1995).

Developments in our understanding of the connections and connectivity of the human hippocampal system (Rolls, Deco, Huang and Feng, 2022a; Ma, Rolls, Huang, Cheng and Feng, 2022a; Huang, Rolls, Hsu, Feng and Lin, 2021; Rolls, Deco, Huang and Feng, 2023b; Rolls, 2023c, 2022b) are described in Section 9.2.8.

9.2.2 Evidence from the effects of damage to the hippocampus

Damage to the human hippocampus or some of its major connections such as the fornix can produce anterograde amnesia, which includes an inability to learn new information about events that happen after the damage, while leaving previous memories relatively intact (Corkin, 2002; Burgess et al., 2002; Smith and Milner, 1981; Petrides, 1985; Gaffan and Gaffan, 1991; Bubb et al., 2017). The initial discovery was made in the patient H.M. who was being treated for epilepsy (Scoville and Milner, 1957; Corkin, 2002). Right hippocampal damage is associated with spatial memory impairments (Smith and Milner, 1981; Crane and Milner, 2005). These discoveries have led to analysis of exactly which parts of the human medial temporal lobe are involved in memory, and how memory is implemented in the brain systems here, which include the hippocampus but also other structures.

Damage to the hippocampus or to some of its connections such as the fornix in monkeys produces deficits in learning about the places of objects and about the places where responses should be made (Buckley and Gaffan, 2000). For example, macaques and humans with damage to the hippocampal system or fornix are impaired in object–place memory tasks in which not only the objects seen, but where they were seen, must be remembered (Burgess et al., 2002; Crane and Milner, 2005; Gaffan, 1994; Gaffan and Saunders, 1985; Parkinson et al., 1988; Smith and Milner, 1981). Posterior parahippocampal lesions in macaques impair even a simple type of object–place learning in which the memory load is just one pair of trial-unique stimuli (Malkova and Mishkin, 2003). I further predict that a more difficult object-place learning task with non-trial-unique stimuli and with many object-place pairs would be impaired by neurotoxic hippocampal lesions. Neurotoxic lesions that selectively damage the primate hippocampus impair spatial scene memory (Murray et al., 1998), and spatial location memory (Waters, Basile and Murray, 2023), when for example environmental visual cues are used in foraging and navigation (Hampton, Hampstead and Murray, 2004; Lavenex, Amaral and Lavenex, 2006). Also, fornix lesions impair conditional left–right discrimination learning, in which the visual appearance of an object specifies whether a response is to be made to the left or the right (Rupniak and Gaffan, 1987). A comparable deficit is found in humans

(Petrides, 1985). Fornix sectioned monkeys are also impaired in learning on the basis of a spatial cue which object to choose (e.g. if two objects are on the left, choose object A, but if the two objects are on the right, choose object B) (Gaffan and Harrison, 1989a). Monkeys with fornix damage are also impaired in using information about their place in an environment. For example, Gaffan and Harrison (1989b) found learning impairments when which of two or more objects the monkey had to choose depended on the position of the monkey in the room.

Rats with hippocampal lesions are impaired in using environmental spatial cues to remember particular places (Cassaday and Rawlins, 1997; Martin et al., 2000; O'Keefe and Nadel, 1978; Jarrard, 1993; Kesner et al., 2004; Kesner and Rolls, 2015), to utilize spatial cues or bridge delays (Kesner, 1998; Kesner and Rolls, 2001; Rawlins, 1985; Kesner et al., 2004; Kesner and Rolls, 2015), or it has been argued to perform relational operations on remembered material (Eichenbaum, 1997). The evidence from rats is further considered in Section 9.4, where tests of the theory are described (Kesner and Rolls, 2015).

In humans, functional neuroimaging and neuronal recording show that the hippocampal system is activated by allocentric spatial including scene processing (Burgess, 2008; Chadwick et al., 2013; Hassabis et al., 2009; Maguire, 2014; Zeidman and Maguire, 2016; Mormann et al., 2017; Tsitsiklis et al., 2020) and by object-spatial episodic memory (Ison et al., 2015; Staresina et al., 2019).

One way of relating the impairment of spatial processing to other aspects of hippocampal function is to note that this spatial processing involves a snapshot type of memory, in which one whole scene must be remembered at a particular time. This memory may then be a special case of episodic memory, which involves an arbitrary association of a particular set of events which describe a past episode (Rolls, 2008e, 2010b; Kesner and Rolls, 2015). Further, the non-spatial tasks impaired by damage to the hippocampal system may be impaired because they are tasks in which a memory of a particular episode or context rather than of a general rule is involved (Gaffan et al., 1984). Further, the deficit in paired associate learning in humans may be especially evident when this involves arbitrary associations between words, and when they elicit spatial imagery, for example window – lake (Clark et al., 2018). Consistent with this, single neurons in the human hippocampus may respond not only to the sight or name of a film star, but also to objects associated with them, such as a bicycle (Quian Quiroga, Reddy, Kreiman, Koch and Fried, 2005; Fried, Rutishauser, Cerf and Kreiman, 2014; Rolls, 2015c; Bausch, Niediek, Reber, Mackay, Bostrom, Elger and Mormann, 2021; Rutishauser, Reddy, Mormann and Sarnthein, 2021). The right (spatial) vs left (word) specialization of function in the human hippocampus (Crane and Milner, 2005; Burgess et al., 2002; Amit, 1989; Bonelli et al., 2010; Sidhu et al., 2013), associated in humans with a less well developed hippocampal commissural system, could be related to the fact that arbitrary associations between words and places are not required.

It is suggested that the reason why the hippocampus is used for the spatial and non-spatial types of memory described above, and the reason that makes these two types of memory so analogous, is that the hippocampus contains one stage, the CA3 stage, which acts as an autoassociation memory. It is suggested that an autoassociation memory implemented by the CA3 neurons equally enables whole (spatial) scene or episodic memories to be formed, with a snapshot quality that depends on the arbitrary associations that can be made and the short temporal window which characterises the synaptic modifiability in this system (Rolls, 1990a,b, 1987, 1990b, 1989e, 2016b, 2018b). The hypothesis is that the autoassociation memory enables arbitrary sets of concurrent neuronal firings, representing for example the spatial context where an episode occurred, the people present during the episode, and what was seen during the episode, to be associated together and stored as one event. (The associations are arbitrary in the sense that any representation within CA3 may be associated with any other representation in CA3.) The issue of the types of item, e.g. spatial, for which this type of associativity is hippocampus-dependent is considered below. Later recall of that episode from the hippocampus in response to a partial cue can then lead to reinstatement of the activity in the neocortex that was originally present during the episode. The theory described here shows how the episodic memory could be stored in the hippocampus, and later retrieved from the hippocampus and thereby to the neocortex using backprojections.

It is now evident that recognition memory (tested for example in primates by the ability to recognise a sample visual stimulus in a delayed match to sample task) is not impaired by hippocampal damage, produced for example by neurotoxic lesions (Murray et al., 1998; Baxter and Murray, 2001b,a; Waters et al., 2023). As shown below in Section 9.2.7, perirhinal cortex lesions do impair visual recognition memory in this type of task.

The extensive literature on the effects of hippocampal damage in rats is considered in Section 9.4 and by Kesner and Rolls (2015), in particular the parts of it that involve selective lesions to different subregions of the hippocampus and allow the theory described here to be tested.

The theory described here is intended to be as relevant to rodents as to primates including humans, the main difference being that the spatial representation used in the hippocampus of rats is about the place where the rat is, whereas the spatial representation in primates including humans includes a representation of space "out there", as represented by spatial view cells (see Section 9.2.4).

9.2.3 Episodic memories need to be recalled from the hippocampus, and can be used to help build neocortical semantic memories

The information about episodic events recalled from the hippocampus could be used to help form semantic memories (Rolls, 1990a,b, 1989e,f; Treves and Rolls, 1994). For example, remembering many particular journeys could help to build a geographic cognitive map in the neocortex. The hippocampus and neocortex would thus be complementary memory systems, with the hippocampus being used for rapid, 'on the fly', unstructured storage of information involving activity potentially arriving from many areas of the neocortex; while the neocortex would gradually build and adjust, on the basis of much accumulating information, the semantic representation (Rolls, 1990b; Treves and Rolls, 1994; McClelland et al., 1995). A view close to this in which a hippocampal episodic memory trace helps to build a neocortical semantic memory has also been developed by Moscovitch et al. (2005).

What I mean by an episodic memory of the type in which the hippocampus could be involved is described further next (Rolls and Kesner, 2006b; Kesner and Rolls, 2015; Rolls, 2018b). A hippocampus-dependent episodic memory is unstructured in the sense that the information is stored as an association between representations such as spatial location, objects, and position in a temporal sequence. An episodic memory could be a single event capturing what happens in a time period in the order of 1–10 s (for example a memory of who was present at one's fifth birthday, what they were wearing, where they sat, where the party was, etc), or a sequence of events with some information about the temporal order of the events. A hippocampus-dependent episodic memory includes spatial and/or temporal e.g. sequence information. All this is in contrast to a neocortical semantic memory which might utilize many such episodic memories, for example of separate train journeys, to form a neocortical topological 'cognitive' map. Such a semantic memory might need to benefit from information about exceptions, which contributes to the type of structure needed for a semantic memory. For example we may be told that a bat, although it flies, is not a bird because it is a mammal which nurses its young, and this information allows restructuring of a semantic representation of what constitutes a bird beyond the simple association and generalization from limited experience that birds fly. Because this active restructuring is an important part of semantic memory that may frequently benefit from language, I propose that semantic memories are best formed during waking using thought and reasoning, and not during sleep (Rolls, 2016b). Indeed, I propose that episodic events that are recalled actively in this way from the hippocampus can become incorporated into neocortical representations and thus consolidated into semantic including autobiographical memories (Section 9.2.8.5). If episodic material (such as where and with whom one had dinner three days ago) is not recalled in this way, then it will be gradually overwritten in hippocampal memory in a process of forgetting as new sparse distributed representations are added to the store, in the way that has been analyzed quantitatively (Section B.19).

To make the distinction between an episodic memory in the hippocampus and a semantic memory in the temporal lobe neocortex (Section 8.3) clear, I now provide an example. An association could be built in the hippocampus by synaptic weight modification between coactive neurons some of which represented an individual and others of which represented the place where the individual was located at a particular time. That would form a single memory in an attractor memory network of the type implemented in hippocampal CA3 (Rolls, 1987, 2018b; Kesner and Rolls, 2015). Such a neuron or neurons that have learned this association could be activated later to recall with completion the whole memory by either a location recall cue or a recall cue provided of the individual. This is an object (or person) with place memory for an event at a particular time. These cells, given that the hippocampus is implicated in episodic memory which must be learned as a single event at a particular time, could be set up rapidly, even on a single trial. This memory at a particular time must be kept separate from episodic memories of even quite similar events but at different times. Recall of such recalled episodic representations from the hippocampus to the neocortex could help to build up a semantic memory in the neocortex that would contain knowledge about which spatial locations in the world are associated with which individuals or groups. Such a semantic memory would benefit from recalling a number of episodic memories, for that would establish which individuals were regularly seen in particular locations, which is semantic knowledge, as contrasted with single event episodic memories in the hippocampus. The semantic memory is not about events at a particular time, but in contrast can benefit from many event episodic memories made at particular times. The semantic memory is all the information accumulated across time about the locations, for example. This type of semantic representation would be the representation of a territory in the brain. This semantic representation in the temporal neocortex (Chapter 8) would enable all the properties of each territory to learned, in contrast to hippocampal cells that would represent a single instance of an occasion at a particular time in which the individual or group was in a particular place. Such neurons with these semantic properties in the temporal neocortex might be termed 'territory cells'. Such neocortical semantic representations would be of the attributes or properties that are associated with a particular individual, group, or object etc. Such 'semantic cells' (in this case representing a territory) are likely, in that semantic cells (which were termed 'concept cells') have been recorded in the human temporal cortex, and might respond to many of the attributes of for example Jennifer Aniston (Quian Quiroga, 2012; Rey, Ison, Pedreira, Valentin, Alarcon, Selway, Richardson and Quian Quiroga, 2015; Quian Quiroga, Reddy, Kreiman, Koch and Fried, 2005; De Falco, Ison, Fried and Quian Quiroga, 2016; Bausch, Niediek, Reber, Mackay, Bostrom, Elger and Mormann, 2021; Rutishauser, Reddy, Mormann and Sarnthein, 2021). 'Concept cells' can be activated whenever a concept is brought to mind, including in a memory task (Bausch et al., 2021). As noted in Section 8.3.1, object-location cells in macaques have some similar multi-attribute properties to 'concept cells' in humans, in that they can be activated either by the object, or by the location, in object-location memory tasks

(Rolls and Xiang, 2005, 2006; Rolls, 2023d). These neurons in macaques might accordingly also be described as 'concept cells' (Rolls, 2023c,d).

Moreover, computationally a semantic memory involves associating all the attributes or descriptors of the node (e.g. the territory) obtained across all times in an interactive activation type of network, as shown in Section 14.4. In contrast, an episodic memory is formed in an attractor network in CA3 which associates for example a single location with an object or individual at a particular time, as shown below. It thus follows that the hippocampus could represent a unique location and object at a unique time, but the concept of a territory and all its attributes is a neocortical representation in the anterior temporal lobe (Sections 8.3, 14.4 and 14.2.4).

In summary, this systems-level analysis provides evidence that the hippocampus is involved in associating a viewed location or a place with an object or individual at a particular time. The temporal lobe neocortex is involved in semantic representations with all the attributes accumulated across time to provide a full description. Thus to take an example, a territory is a semantic representation in the temporal neocortex that can represent all of the locations and the individuals who lay claim to the land, which is how a territory is defined. Hippocampal learning instead is about associations between particular locations and particular objects or individuals that occur at a particular time. In line with the hypothesis that the hippocampus is involved in the memory of particular events, hippocampal damage in humans impairs the memory of events that happened for example earlier in the day, but not semantic memory. When these hippocampal episodic event memories are recalled from the hippocampus to the neocortex, the temporal lobe neocortex can accumulate the evidence from many such episodic memories to help form a semantic representation (Rolls, 2022b, 2023d). This is consistent with the evidence from anterograde amnesia produced by hippocampal damage that new semantic memories can only be formed in the neocortex if the hippocampus is present to form its single event memories. The semantic representations, such as a representation of a territory, are neocortical entities, in that they remain after hippocampal damage. Further, as shown in Section 8.3, it is neocortical damage that impairs semantic representations. Thus a territory, in our example, is a neocortical temporal lobe semantic entity and not a hippocampal episodic memory entity. Routes by which semantic information including that represented by concept cells can reach the hippocampus to become incorporated into an episodic memory have been described (Rolls, 2023d).

In contrast to my proposal above that episodic memories would best be recalled from the hippocampus during waking to help build useful structured neocortical semantic memories (Section 9.2.8.5), some have suggested that the transfer of information from the hippocampus to the neocortex occurs especially during sleep (Marr, 1971; Schwindel and McNaughton, 2011; Foster, 2017). (David Marr heard this suggested by Larry Weiskrantz in a Part 2 lecture at Cambridge in 1967.) Indeed, it has been shown that after learning in hippocampal-dependent tasks, neocortical representations may change (Schwindel and McNaughton, 2011). Although this has been interpreted as the transfer of memories from the hippocampus to the neocortex (Schwindel and McNaughton, 2011), it should be noted that if the hippocampal representation changes as a result of learning, then the altered representation in CA1 will, even with fixed synaptic connections back to neocortex, alter neocortical firing, with no learning or actual 'transfer' involved. (This occurs whenever one vector comprised by a population of neurons firing changes and influences another vector of neuronal firing through fixed connections.) Indeed, for the reasons given above, active transfer of episodic memories from the hippocampus to the neocortex to form semantic memories is more likely I propose during the guided construction and correction of semantic memories in the cortex during waking with value taken into account (Section 9.2.8.5).

The actual addition of new information to the neocortical semantic representation could itself be fast, for example when one recalls a particular train journey, and incorporates information from that into a geographical representation. An additional property of hippocampal episodic memories is that when recalled to the neocortex they can be used flexibly for many types of behavioral output (because the information is back in the neocortex). I further note that rapid learning is not a unique feature of episodic memory, with for example the stimulus-reward learning and its reversal implemented in the primate orbitofrontal cortex possible in one trial (Thorpe, Rolls and Maddison, 1983; Rolls, 2014a, 2019e; Rolls, Vatansever, Li, Cheng and Feng, 2020e) (see also Chapter 11).

The quantitative evidence considered below (Section 9.3.5.1) and by Treves and Rolls (1994) on the storage capacity of the CA3 system indicates that episodic memories could be stored in the hippocampus for at least a considerable period. This raises the issue of the possible gradient of retrograde amnesia following hippocampal damage, and of whether information originally hippocampus-dependent for acquisition gradually becomes 'consolidated' in the neocortex and thereby becomes independent of the hippocampus over time (McGaugh, 2000; Debiec, LeDoux and Nader, 2002; Squire, Genzel, Wixted and Morris, 2015). The issue of whether memories stored some time before hippocampal damage are less impaired than more recent memories, and whether the time course is minutes, hours, days, weeks or years is a debated issue (Gaffan, 1993; Squire, 1992; Squire et al., 2015; Barry and Maguire, 2019). (In humans, there is evidence for a gradient of retrograde amnesia; in rats and monkeys, hippocampal damage in many studies appears to impair previously learned hippocampal-type memories, suggesting that in these animals, at least with the rather limited numbers of different memories that need to be stored in the tasks used, the information remains in the hippocampus for long periods.) If there is a gradient of retrograde amnesia related to hippocampal damage, then this suggests that information may be retrieved from the hippocampus if it is needed, allowing the possibility of incorporating the retrieved information into neocortical memory stores. If on the other hand there is no gradient of retrograde amnesia related to hippocampal damage, but old as well as recent memories of the hippocampal type are stored in the hippocampus, and lost if it is damaged, then again this implies the necessity of a mechanism to retrieve information stored in the hippocampus, and to use this retrieved information to affect neural circuits elsewhere (for if this were not the case, information stored in the hippocampus could never be used for anything). The current perspective is thus that whichever view of the gradient of retrograde amnesia is correct, information stored in the hippocampus will need to be retrieved and affect other parts of the brain in order to be used, and the current theory shows how the recall could be implemented.

The other major set of outputs from the hippocampus projects via the subiculum and fimbria/fornix system to the anterior nucleus of the thalamus (both directly and via the mammillary bodies), which in turn projects to the cingulate cortex (Bubb, Kinnavane and Aggleton, 2017). The mammillary bodies do provide a route for vestibular information to enter the hippocampal system. The posterior cingulate cortex and adjoining regions provides a pathway between some neocortical regions and the hippocampus, and, given that connectivity, are implicated in episodic memory (Section 12.3).

9.2.4 Systems-level neurophysiology of the primate including human hippocampus

9.2.4.1 Spatial view neurons

The systems-level neurophysiology of the hippocampus shows what information could be stored or processed by the hippocampus. To understand how the hippocampus works it is not sufficient to state just that it can store information – one needs to know what information.

Discoveries on the systems-level neurophysiology of the primate hippocampus are described next (Rolls and Xiang, 2006; Rolls and Wirth, 2018; Rolls, 2021f, 2023c) that provide a perspective relevant to understanding the function of the human hippocampus that is somewhat different from that provided by the properties of place cells in rodents, which have been reviewed elsewhere (McNaughton, Barnes and O'Keefe, 1983; O'Keefe, 1984; Muller, Kubie, Bostock, Taube and Quirk, 1991; Jeffery and Hayman, 2004; Jeffery, Anderson, Hayman and Chakraborty, 2004; Hartley, Lever, Burgess and O'Keefe, 2014; Howard and Eichenbaum, 2015; Knierim and Neunuebel, 2016) and compared with those in primates (Rolls and Wirth, 2018; Rolls, 2023d).

The primate hippocampus contains spatial cells that respond when the monkey looks at a certain part of space, for example at one quadrant of a video monitor while the monkey is performing an object–place memory task in which he must remember where on the monitor he has seen particular images (Rolls, Miyashita, Cahusac, Kesner, Niki, Feigenbaum and Bach, 1989c). Approximately 9% of the hippocampal neurons have such spatial view fields, and about 2.4% combine information about the position in space with information about the object that is in that position in space (Rolls et al., 1989c). The latter point shows that information from very different parts of the cerebral cortex (medial parahippocampal gyrus and parietal cortex for spatial information, and inferior temporal cortex for visual information about objects) is brought together onto single neurons in the primate hippocampus.

Spatial view cells are allocentric

The reference frames of spatial representations are important to define, in order to understand functions. An egocentric frame of reference (relative to the body or head) is useful for actions made in nearby space. An allocentric frame of reference (i.e. world-based coordinates) is useful for remembering the location of objects and rewards in the world, independently of where one is located or one's body or head orientation. Feigenbaum and Rolls (1991) analyzed whether the spatial view neurons utilize allocentric or egocentric spatial coordinates. They moved the video screen and the macaque relative to each other, and to different places in the room. 46% of the spatial view neurons had firing that occurred in the same position on the display, or in the laboratory, when the macaque was rotated or moved to a different place in the room. Thus these hippocampal cells had spatial representations in allocentric (i.e. world-based) and not in egocentric (relative to the body or head) coordinates (Feigenbaum and Rolls, 1991). 10% of the spatial neurons had firing that stayed in the same place relative to the monkey's body/head axis when the video monitor was displaced, or the macaque was rotated, or was displaced to a different place in the room. Thus 10% of the neurons represented space in egocentric coordinates, that is, relative to the head.

Spatial view cells and place cells in the primate hippocampus

In rats, place cells are found, which respond depending on the place where the rat is in a spatial environment (McNaughton, Barnes and O'Keefe, 1983; O'Keefe, 1984; Muller, Kubie, Bostock, Taube and Quirk, 1991). To analyze whether such cells might be present in the primate hippocampus, Rolls and O'Mara (1993) and Rolls and O'Mara (1995) recorded the responses of hippocampal cells when macaques were moved in a small chair or robot on wheels in a cue-controlled testing environment. The most common type of cell responded to the part of space at which the monkeys were looking, independently of the place where the monkey was. These were termed 'view' neurons, and in some cases it could be shown that the responses moved if the wall cues were moved (Rolls and O'Mara, 1995). As far as I know, nothing like this has been performed in humans. Some testing of this type, with several places from each of which the same parts of a scene are visible, might be practicable in humans, and would be of great interest for understanding human hippocampal function. We

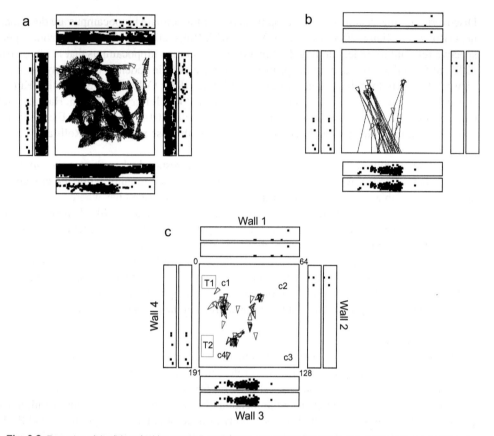

Fig. 9.3 Examples of the firing of a hippocampal spatial view cell when the monkey was walking around the laboratory and looking at the walls of the rich laboratory environment shown in Fig. 9.4. (a) The location in the rich environment at which the cell fired is indicated by the spots in the outer set of 4 rectangles in the Figure, each of which represents one of the walls of the room. There is one spot on the outer rectangle for each action potential. The base of the wall is towards the centre of each rectangle. The positions on the walls fixated during the recording sessions are indicated by points in the inner set of 4 rectangles, each of which also represents a wall of the room. The central square is a plan view of the room, with a triangle printed every 250 ms to indicate the position of the monkey, thus showing that many different places were visited during the recording sessions. (b) A similar representation of the same 3 recording sessions as in (a), but modified to indicate some of the range of monkey positions and horizontal gaze directions when the cell fired at more than 12 spikes/s. (c) A similar representation of the same 3 recording sessions as in (b), but modified to indicate more fully the range of places when the cell fired. The triangle indicates the current position of the monkey, and the line projected from it shows which part of the wall is being viewed at any one time while the monkey is walking. One spot is shown for each action potential. (After Georges-François,P., Rolls, E. T. and Robertson,R.G. (1999) Spatial view cells in the primate hippocampus: allocentric view not head direction or eye position or place. Cerebral Cortex 9: 197–212.)

also discovered that some other hippocampal neurons reflected place encoding, responding for example to the place where the macaque was located, to movement to a place, or to spatial view depending on the place where the monkey was located (Rolls and O'Mara, 1995). Primate hippocampal neurons that respond to place have also been described in virtual navigation tasks (Furuya, Matsumoto, Hori, Boas, Tran, Shimada, Ono and Nishijo, 2014; Wirth, Baraduc, Plante, Pinede and Duhamel, 2017).

Spatial view cells during active locomotion in the primate hippocampus and parahippocampal gyrus

Place cells fire best during active locomotion by the rat (Foster, Castro and McNaughton, 1989; Terrazas, Krause, Lipa, Gothard, Barnes and McNaughton, 2005). To investigate how primate hippocampal formation neurons fire during active locomotion, we recorded from single hippocampal and parahippocampal neurons while monkeys moved themselves round by walking (or running) on all four legs in an open field test environment which was a 2.5m x 2.5m space within a large laboratory that provided a rich spatial environment including doors, windows, equipment, lab benches, etc (Fig. 9.4). The head could rotate in the horizontal plane, and where the monkey was looking in the horizontal and vertical planes as well as where he was facing was measured. We discovered in these investigations **hippocampal spatial view neurons** that responded significantly differently for different allocentric spatial views and had information about spatial view in their firing rate, but conveyed little information about eye position, head direction, or place (Georges-François, Rolls and Robertson, 1999; Robertson, Rolls and Georges-François, 1998; Rolls, Robertson and Georges-François, 1997a; Rolls, Treves, Robertson, Georges-François and Panzeri, 1998b; Rolls, 2023c). An example of such a hippocampal spatial view cell present in the primate hippocampus is shown in Fig. 9.3. The neuron fired primarily while the macaque looked at a part of Wall 3, as emphasized in Fig. 9.3b and c that show a spot on the representation in the Figure of the location on the wall where the monkey was looking when the firing rate was high. (It is emphasized that the monkey was viewing that location in the real rich laboratory environment, and that the spot in the Figure just shows where the monkey was looking in the real rich environment. Part of the rich real environment is illustrated in Fig. 9.6.) Fig. 9.3b illustrates the finding that the neuron responded while the monkey was looking from different places in the room at the spatial view field on Wall 3. The range of different places and head directions over which the neuron fired is illustrated in Fig. 9.3c. Analyses showed that this neuron responded to where the monkey was looking in space relatively independently of the place where the monkey was located, and of head direction and eye position. Moreover, the spatial view fields of the neuron were similar when the monkey was actively walking, and also when he was stationary but actively exploring with eye movements different parts of the spatial environment (Georges-François, Rolls and Robertson, 1999).

Spatial view cells are selective for spatial view much more than for place or head direction or eye position

The firing of a different hippocampal cell is provided in Fig. 9.4, to show with a different type of analysis, how the firing is related primarily to spatial view, rather than to place, or to head direction, or to eye position, or indeed just to the location towards which the monkey was facing (Georges-François, Rolls and Robertson, 1999). The highest firing of the cell, with the macaque at the place and with the head direction shown in Fig. 9.4a, occurred when the macaque looked 10° left. With the monkey in another place and with a different head direction, the highest firing was when the macaque was looking 30° right, but at the same spatial view (Fig. 9.4b). Fig. 9.4c shows the firing with the macaque at a different place (but the same head direction as in Fig. 9.4b), and the firing was now when the monkey looked approximately 30° left. The spatial view field was in the same location on Wall 1 as in Figs. 9.4a and b. Examples of video animations to illustrate the firing of macaque hippocampal spatial view neurons are provided with the Supplementary Material of Rolls and Wirth (2018) and Rolls (2023c) and are available at https://www.oxcns.org/publications.

These experiments show that it is the spatial view towards which the monkey looks that determines the neuronal responses, and not a particular place where the monkey was located, or head direction, or eye position, and this was confirmed with analyses of variance (Georges-François et al., 1999) and information theoretic analyses (Rolls, Treves, Robertson, Georges-François and Panzeri, 1998b). It was found that on average the spatial view cells encoded considerably more information about spatial view (0.47 bits) than about eye position (0.017 bits), head direction (0.005 bits), or place in the room (0.033 bits) (Georges-François

Hippocampal spatial view cells respond to a spatial view independently of place, head direction, and eye position

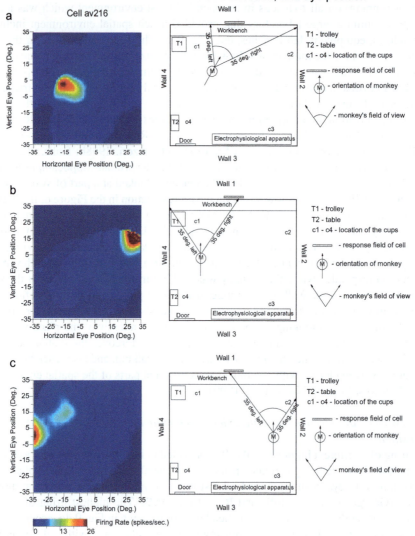

Fig. 9.4 Testing of a hippocampal spatial view neuron (av216) to show that it has allocentric encoding of a spatial view, and that the response does not depend on the place where the monkey is located, or on the allocentric bearing to the effective location in a scene, or on particular eye positions. The firing rate is shown as a function of the horizontal and vertical eye position, where positive values indicate right or up. The neuron responded when the monkey looked towards its view field (indicated with a hatched bar) relatively independently of place, eye position, or head direction. ANOVAs and information theory analyses performed on the same data cast in different ways confirmed this: for spatial view, the ANOVA was $p < 0.001$ with 0.217 bits in a 500 ms period for the average Shannon mutual information; for place $p=0.9$ with 0.001 bits; for head direction $p=0.5$ with 0.0 bits; and for eye position $p=0.8$ with 0.006 bits. (Modified from Georges-François,P., Rolls, E. T. and Robertson,R.G. (1999) Spatial view cells in the primate hippocampus: allocentric view not head direction or eye position or place. Cerebral Cortex 9: 197–212. Note: Colored firing rate plots for the whole series of spatial view cell papers are provided in the .pdfs at https://www.oxcns.org.)

et al., 1999; Rolls et al., 1998b). This shows that the encoding by these primate hippocampal neurons may reflect some information about place etc but is primarily about spatial view.

Another example of a spatial view cell is shown in Fig. 9.5, for cell av083. In this case different vertical angles were investigated. In Fig. 9.5a it is shown that with the head horizontal the neuron responded when the eyes were elevated 15-30°. When the horizontal plane of

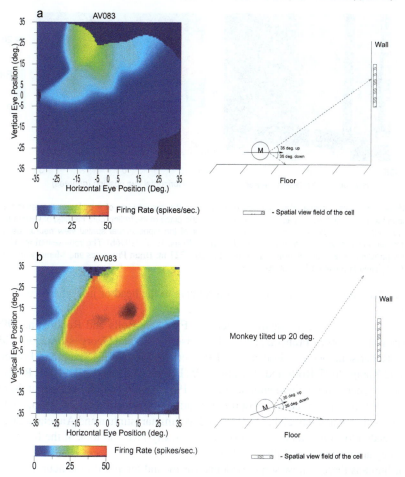

Fig. 9.5 Testing of another hippocampal spatial view neuron (av083) to show that it has allocentric encoding of a spatial view, in this case demonstrated in the vertical plane. The firing rate is shown as a function of the horizontal and vertical eye position, where positive values indicate right or up. The neuron responded when the monkey looked towards its view field (indicated with a hatched bar), independently of the egocentric angle of the spatial view field in the vertical plane. In (a) the head was in the horizontal plane, and some firing occurred when the monkey looked up very high. In (b) the monkey was tilted up $20°$, and the neuron fired when the monkey looked up only a few degrees, and most of the spatial view field can be seen (if the eyes are moved to look at the correct allocentric position on the wall). This was confirmed in one-way ANOVAs, in which the several hundred firing rate and eye position data pairs used to construct (a,b) were sorted according to different hypotheses. When the data were sorted according to where the monkey was looking on the wall, the one-way ANOVA was significant at $P<0.0001$, and the cell provided an average information (about spatial view) of 0.30 bits in a 500 ms epoch. When the same data were sorted according to eye position, the one-way ANOVA was not significant ($P\approx 0.09$), and the cell provided an average information (about eye position) of 0.03 bits in a 500 ms epoch. This analysis leads to the conclusion that the cell responded significantly differently for different allocentric spatial views and had information about spatial view in its firing rate, but did not respond differently just on the basis of eye position. The fact that the cell had different firings even though the monkey was in the same place indicates that the cell was not responding just on the basis of place. (Modified from Georges-François,P., Rolls, E. T. and Robertson,R.G. (1999) Spatial view cells in the primate hippocampus: allocentric view not head direction or eye position or place. Cerebral Cortex 9: 197–212. Note: Colored firing rate plots for the whole series of spatial view cell papers are provided in the .pdfs at https://www.oxcns.org.)

the monkey's head was tilted up, the neuron responded when the eyes were less elevated, corresponding to the same allocentric position on the wall (Fig. 9.5b). Further data for the same cell are provided by Georges-François, Rolls and Robertson (1999). The analysis described for Fig. 9.5 shows that this spatial view cell codes for allocentric spatial view, in the vertical

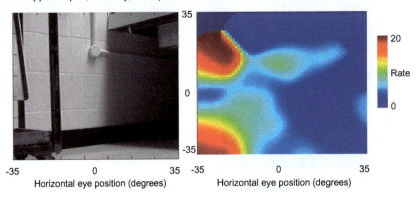

Fig. 9.6 A hippocampal spatial view cell that responded to the spatial view of a trolley in the testing environment, including in this case when the macaque was very close to the place of the trolley. Left: the field of view of the macaque. Right: the firing Rate in spikes per second shown in color of the hippocampal spatial view neuron as a function of the horizontal and vertical eye position. (Modified from Rolls, E. T. (1996b) The representation of space in the primate hippocampus, and its relation to memory. Pp. 203–227 in: Brain Processes and Memory, eds. K.Ishikawa, J.L.McGaugh and H.Sakata. Elsevier: Amsterdam.)

plane, and not for eye position or position relative to the head or just where the monkey was facing.

The same types of investigation (Georges-François, Rolls and Robertson, 1999; Rolls, Robertson and Georges-François, 1997a; Robertson, Rolls and Georges-François, 1998; Rolls, Treves, Robertson, Georges-François and Panzeri, 1998b; Rolls, Xiang and Franco, 2005c; Rolls and Xiang, 2005; Rolls and O'Mara, 1995; Feigenbaum and Rolls, 1991; Rolls, Miyashita, Cahusac, Kesner, Niki, Feigenbaum and Bach, 1989c; Rolls, 2023c) show that these primate hippocampal spatial view cells do not fire in relation to 'facing direction' (Mao, Avila, Caziot, Laurens, Dickman and Angelaki, 2021; Zhu, Lakshminarasimhan and Angelaki, 2023), though care is needed to show this because primates typically face and look at the location towards which they are navigating (Rolls, 2023d).

For humans there is now some evidence for medial temporal lobe neurons with properties like those of spatial view cells (Ekstrom, Kahana, Caplan, Fields, Isham, Newman and Fried, 2003; Miller, Neufang, Solway, Brandt, Trippel, Mader, Hefft, Merkow, Polyn, Jacobs, Kahana and Schulze-Bonhage, 2013; Tsitsiklis, Miller, Qasim, Inman, Gross, Willie, Smith, Sheth, Schevon, Sperling, Sharan, Stein and Jacobs, 2020; Donoghue, Cao, Han, Holman, Brandmeir, Wang and Jacobs, 2023), even though eye position has not usually been measured. For example, in the study by Ekstrom et al. (2003), some cells were found to represent views of landmarks. In a study of human medial temporal lobe neurons (in patients undergoing neurosurgery), it was found that in a virtual reality Treasure Hunt game, some neurons respond to the sight of remote locations rather than the subject's own place (Tsitsiklis et al., 2020; Donoghue et al., 2023) (see Rolls (2023d)). Just like macaque spatial view cells, these neurons in humans respond when the spatial location is seen with different bearings (so they are not allocentric bearing to a landmark neurons, but spatial view neurons, see Section 9.3.15.2) (Donoghue et al., 2023). The locations in the human Treasure Hunt game were in at least some cases within the spatial environment. In the macaque testing, hippocampal spatial view neurons could respond when the macaque was distant from an effective part of the rich 3D environment of a large open laboratory, but also when the macaque was close to the effective part of the environment, as shown for a hippocampal neuron that responded to the part of the environment where there was a trolley, as illustrated in Fig. 9.6 (from Rolls (1996b)). The rich open laboratory testing environment is made evident in Figs. 9.4, 9.6, and 9.7. This is thus somewhat comparable to the way in which the human visual 'spatial target' neurons responded (Tsitsiklis et al., 2020; Donoghue et al., 2023).

The results described by Tsitsiklis, Miller, Qasim, Inman, Gross, Willie, Smith, Sheth, Schevon, Sperling, Sharan, Stein and Jacobs (2020) and Donoghue, Cao, Han, Holman, Brandmeir, Wang and Jacobs (2023) thus appear to confirm the presence of spatial view cells in humans, following their discovery in macaques (Georges-François, Rolls and Robertson, 1999; Rolls, Robertson and Georges-François, 1997a; Robertson, Rolls and Georges-François, 1998; Rolls, Treves, Robertson, Georges-François and Panzeri, 1998b; Rolls, Xiang and Franco, 2005c; Rolls and Xiang, 2005; Rolls and O'Mara, 1995; Feigenbaum and Rolls, 1991; Rolls, Miyashita, Cahusac, Kesner, Niki, Feigenbaum and Bach, 1989c; Rolls, 2023c). However, much work remains to be done on these neurons in humans, including testing whether these neurons signal the location of a reward or goal in space (Rolls and Xiang, 2005), routinely measuring eye position during the recordings, and measuring whether like spatial view cells in macaques they show idiothetic update, which is described below (Robertson et al., 1998).

Further evidence is that in humans some medial temporal lobe neurons reflect the learning of paired associations between views of places, and people or objects (Ison, Quian Quiroga and Fried, 2015; Rutishauser, Reddy, Mormann and Sarnthein, 2021) (just as in macaques (Rolls and Xiang, 2006)), and this shows that views of scenes are important for human hippocampal function. Consistent with these investigations, human functional neuroimaging studies do show hippocampal activation when scenes or parts of scenes are viewed, even when the human is fixed in one place for neuroimaging (Burgess, 2008; Zeidman and Maguire, 2016; Maguire, 2014; Chadwick et al., 2013, 2010; Hassabis et al., 2009; Brown et al., 2016; Epstein and Kanwisher, 1998; O'Keefe et al., 1998; Epstein and Baker, 2019). More evidence is that neurons in the human hippocampus respond differently to different types of scene (landscapes vs buildings), including in a scene-to-object recall association task in which the recall of the object representation in the entorhinal cortex is evident in the neuronal activity (Staresina, Reber, Niediek, Bostrom, Elger and Mormann, 2019). Some human hippocampal neurons also maintain their activity in a working memory task (Rutishauser et al., 2021).

Primate spatial view neurons are found not only in the hippocampus, but also in the parahippocampal gyrus (Georges-François, Rolls and Robertson, 1999; Robertson, Rolls and Georges-François, 1998; Rolls, Robertson and Georges-François, 1997a; Rolls, Treves, Robertson, Georges-François and Panzeri, 1998b). Consistently, in humans, neurons have been recorded in the parahippocampal gyrus that respond preferentially to viewed spatial scenes (Mormann, Kornblith, Cerf, Ison, Kraskov, Tran, Knieling, Quian Quiroga, Koch and Fried, 2017), though it was not possible to analyze whether the neurons respond preferentially to a part of a scene, which is an important property of spatial view neurons. But these observations do confirm that neurons in the parahippocampal gyrus do respond to viewed locations 'out there', rather than the place where the human is located, as shown also by Ekstrom et al. (2003). In human fMRI studies, the parahippocampal place (or scene) area is activated by spatial scenes (Epstein and Baker, 2019).

It is essential to measure the firing rate of a primate hippocampal cell with different head directions so that different spatial views can be compared, as testing with just one head direction (Matsumura et al., 1999) cannot provide evidence that will distinguish a place cell from a spatial view cell. These points will need to be borne in mind in future studies of hippocampal neuronal activity in primates including humans (Ekstrom et al., 2003; Fried et al., 1997; Kreiman et al., 2000; Tsitsiklis et al., 2020), and simultaneous recording of head position, head direction, and eye position, as described by Rolls and colleagues (Georges-François, Rolls and Robertson, 1999; Robertson, Rolls and Georges-François, 1998; Rolls, Robertson and Georges-François, 1997a; Rolls, Treves, Robertson, Georges-François and Panzeri, 1998b) will be needed. To distinguish spatial view from place cells it will be important to test neurons while the primate or human is in one place with all the different rich spatial views visible from that place; and also to test the same neuron when the organism is in a different place, but at least some of the same spatial views are visible, as has been done in our primate single neuron recording (Georges-François, Rolls and Robertson, 1999; Robertson, Rolls and Georges-François, 1998; Rolls, Robertson and Georges-François, 1997a; Rolls, Treves, Robertson, Georges-François and Panzeri, 1998b; Rolls and Xiang, 2006). This type of factorial design is essential if any statement is presented about whether hippocampal neurons respond to spatial view, or place, or a combination of these (Rolls, 2023c,d).

It has been noted (Rolls, 2023d) that neurons that respond to combinations of the location being viewed and the place where the individual is located in what have been described as 'mixed representations' (Wirth et al., 2017; Tan et al., 2021; Wirth, 2023) might arise if training is incomplete, and not all views of a location have been seen from all places. If particular views are seen from only certain places, then hippocampal and related neurons would learn to respond to those views only from those places. Indeed, the evidence that hippocampal neurons learn to respond to particular combinations of the inputs that are present at the same time is likely to be key to understanding hippocampal function for this is ideally suited to episodic memory (Rolls, 2023c,d). Thus we cannot place weight on 'mixed representations' (for example of spatial view from only some places (Wirth et al., 2017; Wirth, 2023)) unless the training has allowed the set of spatial views analysed to be from all the places in the analysis with equal training or experience of all views from all places in the analysis (Rolls, 2023c,d).

Useful confirmation has also recently been obtained that relatively many macaque hippocampal neurons respond to the location "out there" in space (22% of neurons), compared to only 5% of hippocampal neurons that encode the place where the macaque is located (Mao, Avila, Caziot, Laurens, Dickman and Angelaki, 2021; Zhu, Lakshminarasimhan and Angelaki, 2023). Some neurons were classified as spatial view cells and others as 'facing location' cells, but the environment being viewed was simple (a cylindrical arena with a drain on the floor and two touchscreens with food on the walls), and more spatial view cells are likely to be found in a rich spatial environment such as the open lab that we used (Georges-François et al., 1999; Robertson et al., 1998; Rolls et al., 1997a, 1998b; Rolls and Xiang, 2006; Rolls et al., 2005c). Indeed the reason that we moved to a rich open lab visual environment was that we expected to find, and did find, more spatial view cells than in a relatively simple spatial environment with only 4 cues in the testing arena (Rolls and O'Mara, 1995). Some of the cells were described as responding to 'facing direction' (Mao et al., 2021; Zhu et al., 2023), but tests of the type illustrated in Figs. 9.3–9.6 were not reported to clearly dissociate spatial view from facing direction (Rolls, 2023d). In fact, spatial view cells in our testing environments were found to respond to where the macaque was looking in space, and not to the location towards which the individual was facing, by testing these specific hypotheses as illustrated in Figs. 9.4 and 9.5 (Georges-François, Rolls and Robertson, 1999; Rolls, Robertson and Georges-François, 1997a; Rolls and O'Mara, 1995). Further evidence is that in the dark, spatial view cells respond to a remembered spatial view location only when that location is being looked at, with facing location held constant, as illustrated in Fig. 9.7 (Robertson, Rolls and Georges-François, 1998).

In terms of brain computations, it of course makes sense for spatial view cells to respond to viewed locations in a natural scene that has many useful and clear landmarks, even if an individual is not facing those locations but is looking at them, because that information is useful, in the theory of the hippocampus presented here, for remembering where objects or individuals have been seen before in the environment (as described in this Chapter); and for navigation using landmarks as described in Section 9.3.15 (Rolls, 2021f, 2023d). Cells that respond to 'facing direction' (Mao et al., 2021; Zhu et al., 2023) would have little utility for memory and navigation, because primates including humans can search scenes with the eyes and need not face towards a particular location in order to find the location in space (Rolls,

2023d). Spatial view cells are in this sense invariant with respect to facing direction (Rolls, 2023d).

Spatial visual responses during navigation in a virtual environment

To test the nature of hippocampal cell activity in a context requiring that macaques compute a trajectory and move to a goal (at which a hidden reward was given) using visual landmarks, Wirth, Baraduc, Plante, Pinede and Duhamel (2017) measured hippocampal neuronal activity in a virtual environment - a star maze - in which animals navigated using a joystick. The test situation simulated a large environment (radius of 16 meters) and was presented on a large screen that covered 70 percent of the field of view in stereo to provide depth. The virtual environment created a perception of self-motion. The maze had 5 visual landmarks on the walls, and could be used to locate the position of a hidden reward located between two of the landmarks. It was found that 28% (53/189) of hippocampal cells fired when the animals looked at one or sometimes more than one of the visual landmarks, and thus had responses to a viewed location 'out there' in space. Of these view neurons, the responses of 83% were modulated by the position of the animal in the virtual reality environment. This is illustrated by the fact that the majority of cells responded to a landmark when it was viewed from one position only. In addition, 17% of the total population responded when the macaque was in one or more places in the virtual environment without significant modulation by where the animal was looking. Some hippocampal neurons also responded to body turns made during the navigation, and are likely to be whole body motion neurons, some of which respond to optic flow signals of head rotation (O'Mara, Rolls, Berthoz and Kesner (1994) and Section 9.2.4.2) which is the likely input signal given that there is no input from the vestibular system during virtual navigation.

The finding that many of the neurons that responded to the sight of landmarks did so mainly from certain places might have been because the navigational task constrained the individual to stay within the star maze, so that looking at some landmarks from some places, and with a particular view of the star maze in the foreground, might have not provided the opportunity for the landmarks to be seen in the same way from all places (Wirth et al., 2017; Rolls, 2023d), in contrast to the testing in an open field used by Rolls and colleagues (Rolls et al., 1997a; Robertson et al., 1998; Rolls et al., 1998b; Georges-François et al., 1999). Effectively, it could be that in a maze, in which only certain combinations of spatial view, place, body turn etc can occur, neurons can learn to respond only to whatever conjunctions of sensory input actually occur (Rolls, 2023d). Instead, in the real world and in an open field, neurons may be much better able to learn spatial view representations that are invariant with respect to place because each spatial view can be seen from many different places (Rolls, 2023d). In rodents, something like this does happen in a hairpin maze in which the places, head directions and views are constrained by the maze (Derdikman, Whitlock, Tsao, Fyhn, Hafting, Moser and Moser, 2009). This prevents the formation of the usual 2D grid cells in the medial entorhinal cortex found in open field environments, and instead results in grid cells firing at only some parts of the hairpin track being followed, and probably representing the few combinations of place, head direction and view afforded by the hairpin maze (Derdikman et al., 2009). Another and interesting possibility is that some of the macaque neurons (Wirth et al., 2017) only responded to a landmark when it was at a particular bearing, which is how an 'allocentric bearing to a landmark' cell would respond (see Section 9.3.15.2). Another possibility is that testing in the star maze emphasized looking at certain landmarks from certain places, as this is important for the navigation task (Wirth et al., 2017), so the type of combination representation just described of view, place, and head direction may have been formed because that was the sensory input provided in the star maze (Rolls, 2023d) (see Section 9.3.15).

If in the virtual reality navigation task the spatial topology of the star maze was retained, and the goal was retained, but new room cues were introduced, the macaque hippocampal neurons rapidly adapted to the five new room cues which replaced the previously learned room cues (Baraduc, Duhamel and Wirth, 2019). With the new environment, the 'chart' (or 'map') of the environment (Battaglia and Treves, 1998b) may be similar, because of the cues provided by the star maze and by the goal, and the new room cues may be associated onto the same chart (Rolls, 2023d). This parsimonious interpretation is consistent with the concept that remapping of hippocampal neurons in rodents (Schlesiger, Boublil, Hales, Leutgeb and Leutgeb, 2018) occurs mainly when the spatial topology of the test environment is changed, for then the continuous attractor network that forms the 'map' or 'chart' (Samsonovich and McNaughton, 1997; Battaglia and Treves, 1998b) breaks because the links of coactive firing of neurons due to the closeness of the locations to which they respond is no longer present (see Section B.5). It seems likely that the spatial topology of the environment and of possible trajectories through it, the chart or map (Battaglia and Treves, 1998b), defined by the star maze and the goal, remained unchanged when the room cues were substituted (Baraduc, Duhamel and Wirth, 2019), so that no remapping was needed. Remapping occurs when the topology of the space is altered, for example when the shape of the arena is changed (Leutgeb, Leutgeb, Barnes, Moser, McNaughton and Moser, 2005a; Leutgeb, Leutgeb, Moser and Moser, 2006; Leutgeb and Leutgeb, 2007).

Virtual reality testing environments may not allow adequate separation of the different contributions to the firing of primate including human hippocampal spatial representations such as spatial view, place, head direction, and eye position if only a subset of combinations of these are available, and of course do not provide for any normal idiothetic (self-motion) inputs, but have allowed hippocampal neurons with spatial view fields, even if frequently modulated by place in 'mixed representations' (Rolls, 2023d), to be confirmed (Wirth et al., 2017). Further confirmatory investigations relating to spatial view cells are now available (Rolls, 2023d; Yang et al., 2023; Zhu et al., 2023; Corrigan et al., 2023). With these new investigations, the evidence is now very substantial that spatial view cells are a key representation in the primate including human hippocampus, in contrast to the emphasis on place cells that are found in rodents (Rolls, 2023d). This is leading to a re-evaluation of how episodic memory and navigation are performed in primates including humans (Rolls, 2023d).

A very interesting finding in the virtual reality task was that some hippocampal neurons that responded to looking at the room cues could start their firing just before that part of the scene had appeared when the macaque performed a joystick movement to view a new part of the scene (Wirth et al., 2017). This is another example of the evidence for idiothetic update of hippocampal view-responsive neurons that was discovered by Robertson, Rolls and Georges-François (1998), which is described next. Interestingly, this type of memory-related information about scenes may also be reflected in the responses of neurons in parietal cortex region LIP, which can also respond with a memory-related response to what is expected to be present in a location to which a saccade is made, with the coordinates in (at least) craniotopic and not retinal coordinates (Semework, Steenrod and Goldberg, 2018).

Idiothetic (self-motion) update of spatial view cells

If the view details are obscured by curtains and darkness, then some spatial view neurons (especially those in CA1 and less those in CA3) continue to respond when the monkey looks towards the spatial view field (see example in Fig. 9.7). This experiment (Robertson, Rolls and Georges-François, 1998; Rolls, Robertson and Georges-François, 1997a) shows that primate hippocampal spatial view neurons can be updated for at least short periods by idiothetic (self-motion) cues including eye position and head direction signals, and do not necessarily require the view details to be seen (which is different from inferior temporal cor-

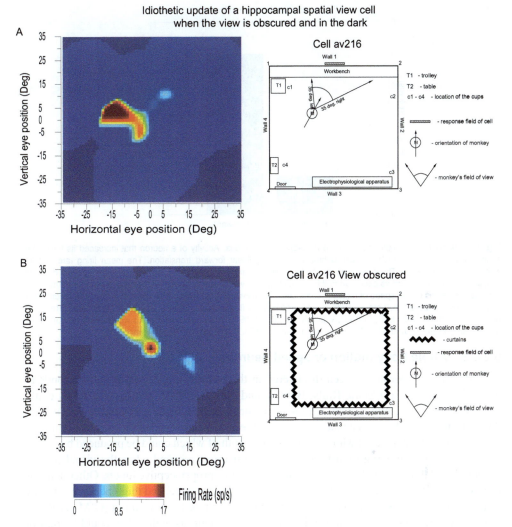

Fig. 9.7 Idiothetic update (by self-motion of the eyes) of the firing of a hippocampal spatial view cell. This cell fired when the macaque looked towards the effective spatial view even when the view was obscured with curtains. The firing is shown with the monkey stationary with his head facing in the direction indicated by the arrow when the curtains were drawn open (A) or were drawn closed (B). Left: firing rate of the cell in spikes/s is indicated by the color (a calibration bar in spikes/s is shown below) projected onto the monkey's field of view. The two-dimensional firing rate profile of the cell was smoothed for clarity using a 2-dimensional Gaussian spatial filter. The space adequately sampled by the eye movements of the monkey is indicated by light blue. The eye position in degrees is shown. Right: a plan view of the room to indicate the monkey's view of the wall is shown. M, position of the monkey. (After Robertson,R.G., Rolls, E. T. and Georges-François,P. (1998) Spatial view cells in the primate hippocampus: Effects of removal of view details. Journal of Neurophysiology 79: 1145-1156. © The American Physiological Society.)

tex object and face neurons). Consistent with this, a small drift is sometimes evident after a delay when the view details are obscured, consistent with inaccuracies in the temporal path integration of these signals, which is then corrected by showing the visual scene again.

This idiothetic update is likely to be important in navigation, especially in the dark, as described in Section 9.3.15, with some of the mechanisms for idiothetic update described in Section 3.4 (Rolls, 2021f).

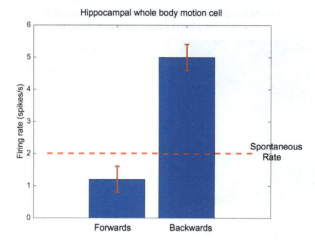

Fig. 9.8 Whole body motion neuron in the macaque hippocampus. Activity of a neuron that increased its firing rate during backward linear translation, and decreased it during linear forward translation. The mean firing rate and its standard error are shown. These neurons responded to velocity, not just speed, in that their responses depended on the direction of motion (forward vs backward in this case; clockwise vs counterclockwise whole body motion for some other neurons, as well as on the speed of motion). Some could be activated if the view of the world was obscured so probably depended on vestibular input; others could be activated by optic flow without the body actually being moved. (Redrawn from O'Mara,S.M., Rolls,E.T., Berthoz,A. and Kesner,R.P. (1994) Neurons responding to whole-body motion in the primate hippocampus. Journal of Neuroscience 14: 6511-6523. © Society for Neuroscience.)

9.2.4.2 Whole body motion or speed neurons

Another type of neuron has been discovered in the primate hippocampus that responds to whole body motion (O'Mara, Rolls, Berthoz and Kesner, 1994), and these neurons could be involved in idiothetic update, and/or in memory, including for example body turns or distances travelled during navigation. Some of these neurons respond to linear motion (e.g. Fig. 9.8), and others to axial whole body rotation (both of which could be produced by sitting the macaque on a moving robot). Some of these neurons respond when the visual field is obscured, and thus respond on the basis of vestibular or proprioceptive inputs. Other neurons respond to rotation of the visual environment round the macaque, and thus encode motion by visual optic flow cues. Some neurons respond to both these types of input (O'Mara, Rolls, Berthoz and Kesner, 1994). The significance of these neurons is that they could be part of the way in which self-motion, i.e. idiothetic, cues are used to update the representation in the hippocampal formation of the current head direction, or the current position, and of the current spatial view, which is likely to be important in navigation, especially in the dark, as described in Section 9.3.15. These whole body motion neurons could also be useful in episodic memory, by encoding the movements that were taking place on a particular occasion.

This discovery of whole body motion cells in the macaque hippocampus (O'Mara, Rolls, Berthoz and Kesner, 1994) has been confirmed for the rat hippocampal system, in which 'speed cells' for linear motion have now been described in the medial entorhinal cortex (Kropff, Carmichael, Moser and Moser, 2015; Hinman, Brandon, Climer, Chapman and Hasselmo, 2016). Experiments have now been performed in rodents to analyze whether 'speed cells' in fact respond to linear velocity as in macaques (in that some macaque whole body motion neurons code for motion direction, with the neuron illustrated in Fig. 9.8 responding to backwards linear motion; and others responding to forwards linear motion); whether there are direction-selective axial rotation cells as in macaques; and about the roles of vestibular, optic flow, or other inputs. Neurons were found that responded to angular or linear velocity in the rat medial entorhinal cortex, presubiculum, and parasubiculum (Spalla, Treves and Boccara, 2022), though the contributions of optic flow vs vestibular inputs were not investigated.

The inputs for whole body motion cells may reach the hippocampus via the mammillary body circuitry which receives inputs from the tegmental nuclei of Gudden (Dillingham et al., 2015; Cullen, 2019). This may provide one route for vestibular inputs, important of course in head direction representation, to reach the presubiculum, where head direction cells are found in primates (Robertson, Rolls, Georges-François and Panzeri, 1999) as well as in rodents (Wiener and Taube, 2005; Cullen and Taube, 2017). The mammillary bodies project to the anterior thalamic nuclei which in turn project to the cingulate and retrosplenial cortex, which in turn project into areas such as the subiculum, and thus can provide inputs to the hippocampal system (see Fig. 9.2 and Aggleton and Nelson (2015)).

The roles of whole body motion cells in navigation in humans and other primates are considered in Section 9.3.15 (Rolls, 2021f).

9.2.4.3 Spatial view grid cells in the primate entorhinal cortex

In the rodent entorhinal cortex, grid cells that represent places by hexagonal place grids and are involved in idiothetic update of place have been described (Moser, Rowland and Moser, 2015; Kropff and Treves, 2008). In macaques, a grid-cell like representation in the entorhinal cortex has been found, but the neurons have grid-like firing as the monkey moves the eyes across a spatial scene (Killian, Jutras and Buffalo, 2012; Rueckemann and Buffalo, 2017; Meister and Buffalo, 2018; Garcia and Buffalo, 2020). Similar competitive learning processes to those suggested for rodents (Rolls, Stringer and Elliot, 2006c) may transform these primate entorhinal cortex 'spatial view grid cells' into primate hippocampal spatial view cells, and may contribute to the idiothetic (eye movement-related) update of spatial view cells (Robertson, Rolls and Georges-François, 1998). The existence of spatial view grid cells in the entorhinal cortex of primates is predicted from the presence of spatial view cells in the primate CA3 and CA1 regions (Kesner and Rolls, 2015; Rueckemann and Buffalo, 2017). Moreover, some of these 'spatial view grid cells' have their responses aligned to the visual image (Meister and Buffalo, 2018), as predicted (Kesner and Rolls, 2015).

In the human entorhinal and cingulate cortex neurons with grid-like response properties are found (Jacobs, Weidemann, Miller, Solway, Burke, Wei, Suthana, Sperling, Sharan, Fried and Kahana, 2013; Nadasdy, Nguyen, Torok, Shen, Briggs, Modur and Buchanan, 2017), and there is neuroimaging evidence that is consistent with this (Nau, Navarro Schroder, Bellmund and Doeller, 2018b; Julian, Keinath, Frazzetta and Epstein, 2018). This is further evidence for the concept that representations of locations being viewed in space 'out there' is a key property of spatial representations in the hippocampal system of primates including humans.

9.2.4.4 Spatial view associated with object neurons in association memory

Primates have a highly developed ventral stream cortical visual system that utilises information from the fovea for object recognition, and a highly developed eye movement control system to bring the fovea to objects, using mechanisms described in Chapters 2 and 3 and elsewhere (Rolls, 2012d; Rolls and Webb, 2014). These developments enable primates to explore and remember information about what is present at locations seen 'out there' in the spatial environment without having to visit those places. Spatial view cells would accordingly be useful as part of a memory system by providing a representation of space that does not depend on where the primate is, and that could be associated with items such as objects or rewards in those viewed spatial locations. This could enable a monkey to remember where it had seen ripe fruit, or a human to remember where in a spatial scene he or she had seen a person. Primate hippocampal system spatial view neurons may therefore be important in forming memories of what has been seen and where it has been seen even on a single occasion, a key component of an episodic memory (Rolls, 2023c). Episodic memories of this type would be useful for spatial navigation or action in space.

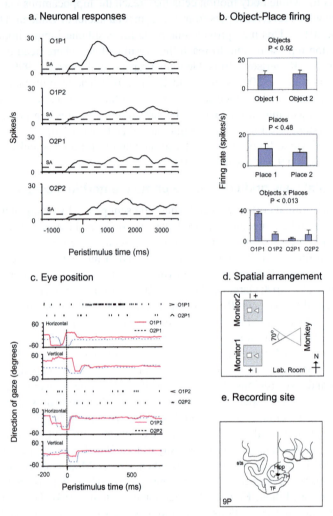

Fig. 9.9 Object–spatial view associations in the primate hippocampus. A hippocampal neuron (BL003c8a) with firing occurring to a particular combination of an object and place being viewed (Object 1–Place 1, O1P1). (a) Peristimulus time histograms showing the response of the neuron to each object–place combination. (b) The firing rate response of the neuron on different trials sorted according to the object that was shown on the trial, the place where the object was shown, and the combination of which object was shown with the place where it was shown. In the object*position bar histograms, O1P1 = Object 1 in Place 1, etc. The mean responses ± sem are shown. (c) Trials to show the eye positions on 4 different trials. (d) Schematic diagram showing the spatial arrangement used in the Go–NoGo object–place combination task in this experiment. + indicates that a Go (lick) response to that object–place combination will be rewarded, and a minus that it will be punished. Only one object was shown on the screen at a time. The room was approximately 4 m x 4 m, and the distance of the monkey from the monitors was typically 1.5–2 m in the different experiments. The triangle labelled monkey shows the position of the monkey, and the angle shows the approximate angle subtended by the video display monitors. (e) The recording site of the neuron. Hipp–hippocampus; Prh–perirhinal cortex; rhs–rhinal sulcus; sts–superior temporal sulcus; TE–inferior temporal visual cortex. 9P = 9 mm Posterior to the sphenoid reference. (After Rolls, E. T., Xiang,J-Z. and Franco,L. (2005) Object, space and object-space representations in the primate hippocampus. Journal of Neurophysiology 94: 833–844. © The American Physiological Society.)

To investigate the fundamental question of whether object information, as well as spatial information, is provided in the primate hippocampus, single hippocampal neurons were recorded during an object-place memory task in which the monkeys had to learn associations between objects and where they were shown in an open laboratory (Rolls, Xiang and Franco, 2005c). Some neurons (10%) responded differently to different objects independently of location; other neurons (13%) responded to the spatial view independently of which object was present at the location; and some neurons (12%) responded to a combination of a particular object and the place where it was shown in the room. An example of a neuron responding to a particular object–place combination is shown in Fig. 9.9. These results show that there are separate as well as combined, conjunctive, representations of objects and their locations in space in the primate hippocampus. This is a property required in an episodic memory system, for which association between objects and the places where they are seen, is prototypical. The results thus show that requirements for a human episodic memory system, separate and combined neuronal representations of objects and where they are seen "out there" in the environment, are present in the primate hippocampus (Rolls, Xiang and Franco, 2005c). These results have been confirmed in humans, in whom association learning between a spatial view and an object or person are reflected in the responses of medial temporal lobe neurons (Ison, Quian Quiroga and Fried, 2015) including hippocampal neurons (Staresina, Reber, Niediek, Bostrom, Elger and Mormann, 2019). When an object is recalled from a spatial scene, firing in the human entorhinal cortex, the route back to ventral stream visual cortical areas in humans (Rolls et al. (2023e), Section 9.2.8), is found to the recalled object (Staresina et al., 2019).

What may be a corresponding finding in rats is that some rat hippocampal neurons respond on the basis of the conjunction of location and odor (Wood et al., 1999). Results consistent with our object-place neurons in primates are that Diamond and colleagues have shown using the vibrissa somatosensory input for the 'object' system, that rat hippocampal neurons respond to object-place combinations, objects, or places, and there is even a reward-place association system in rats (Itskov et al., 2011) similar to that in primates. This brings the evidence from rats closely into line with the evidence from primates of hippocampal neurons useful for object-place episodic associative memory.

It has also been discovered that primate hippocampal neuronal activity is related to the recall of episodic memories. In a one-trial object–place recall task, images of an object in one position on a screen, and of a second object in a different position on the screen, were shown successively. Then one of the objects was shown at the top of the screen, and the monkey had to recall the position in which it had been shown earlier in the trial, and to touch that location (Rolls and Xiang, 2006). In addition to neurons that responded to the objects or places, a new type of neuronal response was found in which 5% of hippocampal neurons had spatial view-related responses when a spatial view was being recalled by an object cue, or vice versa (Rolls and Xiang, 2006; Kesner and Rolls, 2015) (see example in Fig. 9.10). This was like episodic memory, in that it was a one-trial object to spatial view location memory that was being learned and recalled. Consistent with this discovery, in humans, in an object-place recall task in virtual reality, some neurons during recall also reflect the recall of the location when the object recall cue is provided (Miller, Neufang, Solway, Brandt, Trippel, Mader, Hefft, Merkow, Polyn, Jacobs, Kahana and Schulze-Bonhage, 2013). In a complementary way, as noted above, when an object is recalled from a spatial scene, neuronal firing in the human hippocampus and entorhinal cortex is found that reflects the associative recall (Staresina, Reber, Niediek, Bostrom, Elger and Mormann, 2019).

9.2.4.5 Spatial view associated with reward neurons

The primate including human anterior hippocampus (which corresponds to the rodent ventral hippocampus) receives inputs from brain regions involved in reward processing such as the amygdala and orbitofrontal cortex (Carmichael and Price, 1995b; Suzuki and Amaral, 1994a; Pitkanen et al., 2002; Stefanacci et al., 1996; Rolls, 2015b; Rolls et al., 2022a, 2023c,b; Rolls, 2022b). To investigate how this affective input may be incorporated into primate hippocampal function, Rolls and Xiang (2005) recorded neuronal activity while macaques performed a

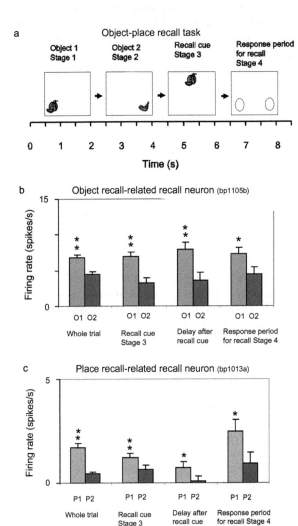

Fig. 9.10 Firing of hippocampal neurons in a one trial object-viewed location recall task. (a) In stage 1, object 1 was shown in a location on the screen being viewed, and in stage 2 object 2 was shown. In stage 3 one of the objects was shown at the top centre of the screen, and the monkey had to touch the location on the screen where that object had been shown in order to obtain a juice reward. (b) A neuron that was selective for object 1 (O1) responded even in stage 4 when the object was not visible but the object and its location had to be recalled. (c) A neuron that was selective for location 1 (P1) responded even in stage 4 when the object was not visible but the object and its location on the screen being viewed had to be recalled. The average firing rate in spikes/s across trials ± sem is shown. ** $p<0.01$; * $p<0.05$. (Modified from Rolls, E. T. and Xiang, J-Z. (2006) Spatial view cells in the primate hippocampus, and memory recall. Reviews in the Neurosciences 17: 175-200.)

reward-place association task in which each spatial scene shown on a video monitor had one location which if touched yielded a preferred fruit juice reward, and a second location which yielded a less preferred juice reward. Each scene had different locations for the different rewards. Of 312 hippocampal neurons analyzed, 18% responded more to the location of the preferred reward in different scenes, and 5% to the location of the less preferred reward (Rolls and Xiang, 2005). An example of one of these neurons, responding to the place in each scene of a preferred reward, is shown in Fig. 9.11.

When the locations of the preferred rewards in the scenes were reversed, 60% of 44

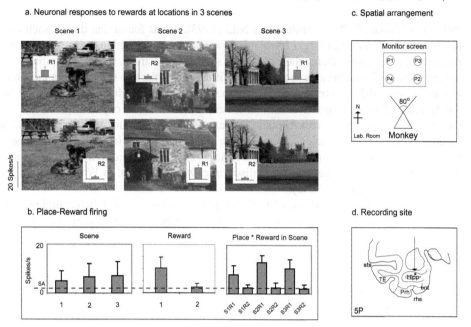

Fig. 9.11 Reward–spatial view associations in the primate hippocampus. A hippocampal neuron that encoded the particular rewards available at different locations in different scenes. On each trial the monkey could touch a circled location in the scene, and, depending on the location, received either a preferred juice reward or a less preferred juice reward. (a) Firing rate inserts to show the firing in 3 different scenes (S1–S3) of the locations associated with reward 1 (R1, preferred) and reward 2 (R2). The mean responses ± sem are shown. SA, spontaneous firing rate. (b) The firing rates sorted by scene, by reward (1 vs 2), and by scene-reward combinations (e.g. scene 1 reward 1 = S1R1). (c) The spatial arrangement on the screen of the 4 spatial locations (P1–P4). (d) The recording site of the neuron. ent–entorhinal cortex; Hipp–hippocampal pyramidal cell field CA3/CA1 and dentate gyrus; Prh–perirhinal cortex; rhs–rhinal sulcus; sts–superior temporal sulcus; TE–inferior temporal visual cortex. (After Rolls, E. T., and Xiang, J-Z. (2005) Reward-spatial view representations and learning in the primate hippocampus. Journal of Neuroscience 25: 6167–6174. © The Society for Neuroscience.)

neurons tested reversed the location to which they responded, showing that the reward-place associations could be altered by new learning in a few trials. The majority (82%) of these 44 hippocampal reward-place neurons tested did not respond to object-reward associations in a visual discrimination object-reward association task. Thus the primate hippocampus contains a representation of the reward associations of places "out there" being viewed, and this is a way in which affective information can be stored as part of an episodic memory, and how the current mood state may influence the retrieval of episodic memories (Rolls and Xiang, 2005). There is consistent evidence that rewards available in a spatial environment can influence the responsiveness of rodent place neurons (Tabuchi et al., 2003; Mizumori and Tryon, 2015).

In another type of task for which the primate hippocampus is needed, conditional spatial response learning, in which the monkeys had to learn which spatial response to make to different stimuli, that is, to acquire associations between visual stimuli and spatial responses, 14% of hippocampal neurons responded to particular combinations of visual stimuli and spatial responses (Miyashita, Rolls, Cahusac, Niki and Feigenbaum, 1989). The firing of these neurons could not be accounted for by the motor requirements of the task, nor wholly by the stimulus aspects of the task, as demonstrated by testing their firing in related visual discrimination tasks. These results showed that single hippocampal neurons respond to combinations of the visual stimuli and the spatial responses with which they must become associated in conditional response tasks, and are consistent with the computational theory described here according to which part of the mechanism of this learning involves associations between visual stimuli and spatial responses learned by single hippocampal neurons. In a following study by Cahusac, Rolls, Miyashita and Niki (1993), it was found that during such conditional spatial response learning, 22% of this type of neuron analyzed in the hippocampus and parahippocampal gyrus altered their responses so that their activity, which was initially equal to the two new stimuli, became progressively differential to the two stimuli when the monkey learned to make different responses to the two stimuli (Cahusac, Rolls, Miyashita and Niki, 1993). These changes occurred for different neurons just before, at, or just after the time when the monkey learned the correct response to make to the stimuli, and are consistent with the hypothesis that when new associations between objects and places (in this case the places for responses) are learned, some hippocampal neurons learn to respond to the new associations that are required to solve the task. These discoveries were confirmed by Wirth, Yanike, Frank, Smith, Brown and Suzuki (2003).

This type of learning may well be relevant to navigation, in which behavioral responses such as a body turn may be needed when a particular visual stimulus identifying a place is seen (see Section 9.3.15).

9.2.5 Spatial view cells in primates including humans, and foveal vision

The discovery that many primate hippocampal neurons respond to the location being viewed 'out there', and not to the place where the individual is located (Rolls et al., 1989c; Feigenbaum and Rolls, 1991; Rolls and O'Mara, 1995; Rolls et al., 1997a; Robertson et al., 1998; Rolls et al., 1998b; Georges-François et al., 1999; Rolls et al., 2005c; Rolls and Xiang, 2005, 2006), is now confirmed by a number of other investigations (Wirth, Baraduc, Plante, Pinede and Duhamel, 2017; Corrigan, Gulli, Doucet, Borna, Abbass, Roussy, Rogelio and Martinez-Trujillo, 2023; Mao, Avila, Caziot, Laurens, Dickman and Angelaki, 2021; Zhu, Lakshminarasimhan and Angelaki, 2023; Yang, Chen and Naya, 2023; Tan, Ng, Owens, Libedinsky and Yen, 2021), with consistent findings in humans (Tsitsiklis, Miller, Qasim, Inman, Gross, Willie, Smith, Sheth, Schevon, Sperling, Sharan, Stein and Jacobs, 2020; Donoghue, Cao, Han, Holman, Brandmeir, Wang and Jacobs, 2023) (see Rolls (2023c), Rolls (2023d) and Rolls and Wirth (2023)). Further properties of primate hippocampal neurons are described by Rolls and Xiang (2006), Rolls and Wirth (2018), Rolls (2021f), Rolls (2023c), and papers in the Special Issue of Hippocampus (2023, issue 5) on View Representations cited by Rolls (2023d), and are fundamental to understanding what is computed in the primate including human hippocampal system.

The difference between a representation of an object and the representation of a spatial scene is considered in Section 2.8.14. That discussion is important for understanding the difference between object representations, and scene representations, and how spatial view cells are important in representing scenes. The idiothetic update of spatial view cells provides further evidence that they are involved in scene representations, for it shows that their representation is in a spatial reference frame.

The very interesting similarities and differences of these primate hippocampal spatial representations, which are influenced by the highly developed primate visual system, from the more place-related representations found in rodents, are considered by Rolls and Wirth (2018) and Rolls (2023d). Ways in which ventral visual stream processing of scenes (Epstein and Baker, 2019) may contribute to the formation of hippocampal spatial view cells are described in Sections 2.8.14 and 9.2.8 (Rolls, Tromans and Stringer, 2008f; Rolls, 2021f, 2023c; Rolls, Deco, Huang and Feng, 2023e; Rolls, 2023d). A key factor is the primate (including human) fovea, which provides for high spatial resolution at the fovea as described next (Rolls, 2023d).

To investigate the difference in what is analysed by the primate and rodent visual systems,

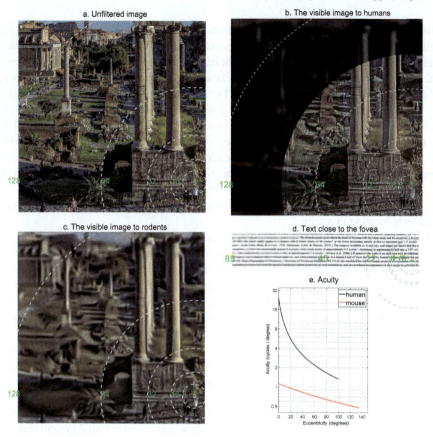

Fig. 9.12 Illustration of how the world is seen differently in terms of their contrast sensitivity functions (Haun, 2021) by rodents and primates including humans. (a) The unfiltered image which has 4096x4096 pixel resolution. The fixation point is just above the head of the man with the white shirt, and the eccentricity in degrees of different parts of the scene is indicated by the scale for the circles. (b) How the scene might appear to a human with a visual acuity of 60 cycles/^{o} at the fovea decreasing rapidly at first to approximately 1.5 cycles/^{o} at 90°. Note that in humans and other primates with forward facing eyes little can be seen beyond 90° of eccentricity from the fovea, which is indicated by the darker region in the figure. (A macaque has a visual acuity of approximately 54 cycles/^{o} at the fovea (Rolls and Cowey, 1970; Srinivasan et al., 2015).) Inspection of the figure shows that the resolution of the filtered image at the fovea is sufficient for face recognition. (c) How the scene might appear to a mouse with visual acuity of approximately 0.5 cycles/^{o}, decreasing to approximately half this at 135° of eccentricity (Prusky et al., 2000; van Beest et al., 2021). (The visual acuity of a rat is close to this, at approximately 1.6 cycles/^{o} (Prusky et al., 2000).) If pasted to the walls of an enclosure with its reflected image too, the visual angle subtended would be approximately 256°, and indicates what a rodent might see, and what a human might see in a human Field of View that would be limited to approximately the central 180° (90° left and right.) (d) To emphasise how the visual acuity keeps increasing in primates close to the fovea, text is shown to be readable in only about the central 3° around the fovea (i.e. to a radius of 1.5^o, with the region shown extending to 8.9^o.) (e) Acuity for humans and mice. Collaboration with Professor Andrew M. Haun (Department of Psychiatry, University of Wisconsin-Madison, WI, USA) who modified his software made available in connection with Haun (2021) at https://osf.io/8xf9w/ is warmly acknowledged. The algorithm takes into account the spatial frequency contrast sensitivity at each eccentricity, and also produces an impression of what might be provided by the rodent colour system. The filtered images in (b-d) show what exceeds the contrast sensitivity threshold at each eccentricity. (After Rolls, E. T. 2023 Hippocampal spatial view cells, place cells, and concept cells: view representations. Hippocampus doi: 10.1002/hipo.23536)

a scene was filtered with the contrast sensitivity function of humans and mice (Haun, 2021), with the results illustrated in Fig. 9.12. The following points can be made. First, the field of view of the rodent is large, approximately 270° (135° each way from the centre), whereas in humans and other primates with forward facing eyes little is visible beyond 90° from the fovea, with calibration circles provided at 64° and 128° in Fig. 9.12, and the invisible region for primates shown as dark in Fig. 9.12. Second, the spatial resolution for the whole of the field of view is poor in rodents, whereas humans have a very high resolution fovea (with approximately 60 cycles/° for the acuity), which, as illustrated in Fig. 9.12b when expanded, is sufficient for face recognition and reading text. The implication for the rodent is that what is analysed by the rodent visual system might be sufficient to process a few, well spread out, visual landmarks to help form rodent place fields (or at least reset them) based on what is visible in the environment, as proposed by De Araujo, Rolls and Stringer (2001) (see Fig. 9.34). The implication for humans and other primates is that very high resolution is available close to the fovea that can enable great detail in a scene available over a relatively small visual angle to be used to associate particular objects or faces or rewards (which as illustrated in Fig. 9.12b might subtend 1° or less) with their location in a scene. This is completely in line with the theory (Rolls, 1989b, 1999c, 2023c,a) and evidence (Rolls and Xiang, 2006, 2005; Rolls et al., 2005c) that an important function of primate including human hippocampal spatial view cells is to participate in forming associations between objects including faces, rewards etc and their location in a scene.

The visual system of primates including humans thus supports this key function in episodic memory, by providing sufficient resolution at the fovea for objects etc together with sufficient resolution more peripherally to represent scenes and landmarks. Further, the high visual spatial resolution of the fovea in primates that provides the ability to use fine detail in a distant scene is also very valuable for navigation that is guided by distant viewed landmarks, for it enables even somewhat similar distant landmarks to be distinguished and used as guides for navigation (Rolls, 2021f, 2023c,d). In contrast, with the relatively poor spatial resolution available in the rodent visual system, rodents could not easily perform object in scene or reward in scene memory for a small object or reward in a large scene, because the rodent visual acuity is too poor to recognise a small object in a very large scene, and learn the location of the small object in the scene.

It is therefore proposed that a key and fundamental difference between the primate including human and rodent hippocampus is that rodents have a poor visual system that cannot implement the memory for where a small object or reward is in a large scene, a key property of primate including human episodic memory (Rolls, 2023d). Instead, rodents are dominated by the place where they are located, given their reliance on somatosensory vibrissa twitching and local olfactory cues, and a visual system that can mainly support place representations of where the individual is located using computations described by De Araujo et al. (2001) and illustrated in Fig. 9.34 in Section 9.3.11. Rodent egocentric visual cells in their hippocampal system may be useful for obstacle avoidance (Rolls, 2023d).

9.2.6 Head direction cells in the presubiculum

Head direction cells found in rats (Ranck, 1985; Taube et al., 1990a, 1996; Muller et al., 1996; Wiener and Taube, 2005) and in primates (Robertson, Rolls, Georges-François and Panzeri, 1999) respond maximally when the animal's head is facing in a particular preferred direction. An example of a primate head direction cell recorded in the presubiculum of the monkey is shown in Fig. 9.13. Similar cells are found in the rat pre-/post-subiculum, but also in a number of connected structures including the anterior thalamic nuclei (Taube et al., 1996; Wiener and Taube, 2005). The firing rate of these cells is a function of the head direction of the monkey, with a response that is typically 10–100 times larger to the optimal as compared to the opposite head direction. The mean half-amplitude width of the tuning of the cells was 76 degrees. The response of head direction cells in the presubiculum was not influenced by the place where the monkey was, there being the same tuning to head direction at different places in a room, and even outside the room. The response of these cells was also independent of the 'spatial view' observed by the monkey, and also of eye position (where the monkey was looking). The cells maintain their tuning for periods of at least several minutes when the

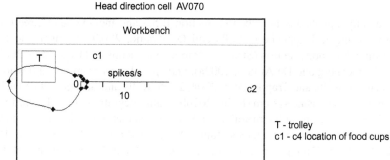
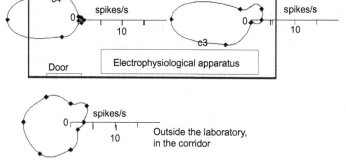

Fig. 9.13 Head direction cell in the primate presubiculum. Polar response plots of the firing rate (in spikes/s) when the monkey was stationary at different positions (shown at the 0 on the firing rate scale) in (and one outside) the room are shown. The monkey was rotated to face in each direction. The mean response of the cell from at least 4 different firing rate measurements in each head direction in pseudorandom sequence are shown. c1–c3: cups to which the monkey could walk on all fours to obtain food. Polar firing rate response plots are superimposed on an overhead view of the square room to show where the firing for each plot was recorded. The plot at the lower left was taken outside the room, in the corridor, where the same head direction firing was maintained. (After Robertson,R.G., Rolls, E. T., Georges-Francois,P. and Panzeri,S. (1999) Head direction cells in the primate pre-subiculum. Hippocampus 9: 206–219. © Wiley-Liss.)

view details are obscured or the room is darkened (Robertson, Rolls, Georges-François and Panzeri, 1999).

This representation of head direction could be useful together with the hippocampal spatial view cells and whole body motion cells found in primates in a number of spatial and memory functions. One is path integration for head direction, the process by which in the absence of visual input one's head direction is updated based on idiothetic, that is self-motion, signals reflecting recent movements or movement 'paths'. The memory mechanism required is an integration over time of self-motion signals produced by for example vestibular inputs or motor commands. Neuronal network computational mechanisms by which this memory function may be performed are described in Section B.5.5. Another memory function for which head direction cells may be important is in episodic memory. An episodic memory might include for example the fact that one had turned right by 90 degrees in the dark, and was therefore facing towards a particular spatial view, which one could later recall. Another spatial / memory function in which head direction cells are implicated is in updating using path integration one's representation of the place where one is located. Indeed, place cells in rats may be updated in the dark through an effect of head direction cells in rotating the place map, and normally the place cell and head direction maps are kept in alignment (Leutgeb, Leutgeb, Treves, Meyer, Barnes, McNaughton, Moser and Moser, 2005b; Wiener and Taube, 2005; Yoganarasimha, Yu and Knierim, 2006).

Self-organizing continuous attractor neural networks that can perform path integration from velocity signals are described in Section B.5.5 and include head direction from head velocity (Stringer, Trappenberg, Rolls and De Araujo, 2002b; Stringer and Rolls, 2006); place from whole body motion (Stringer, Trappenberg, Rolls and De Araujo, 2002b; Stringer, Rolls, Trappenberg and De Araujo, 2002a); and spatial view from eye and whole body motion (Stringer, Rolls and Trappenberg, 2004, 2005; Rolls and Stringer, 2005) using it is now thought the dorsal visual system (Rolls, 2020b). Path integration of head direction is reflected in the firing of neurons in the presubiculum, and mechanisms outside the hippocampus, perhaps in the dorsal tegmental nucleus (Taube, Muller and Ranck, 1990b; Sharp, 1996; Bassett and Taube, 2005; Dillingham, Frizzati, Nelson and Vann, 2015; Cullen and Taube, 2017; Cullen, 2019), probably implement path integration for head direction.

Indeed, one function of the mammillary body circuitry may be to introduce a head direction signal from the tegmental nuclei of Gudden via the anterior thalamic nuclei to the hippocampal circuitry (Dillingham et al., 2015). This may provide one route for vestibular inputs, important of course in head direction representation, to reach the presubiculum, where head direction cells are found in primates (Robertson, Rolls, Georges-François and Panzeri, 1999) as well as in rodents (Wiener and Taube, 2005). Indeed, the anterior thalamic nuclei project to the cingulate and retrosplenial cortex, which in turn project into areas such as the subiculum, and thus can provide inputs to the hippocampal system about for example head direction (see Fig. 9.2 and Aggleton and Nelson (2015)).

Further, there is now evidence that the dorsal visual system leading to the parietal cortex area 7a, and thereby to the retrosplenial and cingulate cortex, which in turn connect via the parahippocampal gyrus to the hippocampus (Fig. 9.1) is one way in which spatial representations are updated idiothetically for use by the hippocampal system (Section 3.4) (Rolls, 2020b, 2021f; Rolls et al., 2023e,d; Rolls, 2023c).

9.2.7 Perirhinal cortex, recognition memory, and long-term familiarity memory

The functions of the perirhinal cortex are different to those of the hippocampus, and are reviewed here partly because the perirhinal cortex (areas 35 and 36) provides ventral stream afferents to the hippocampus via the entorhinal cortex (area 28) (Rolls et al., 2022a, 2023e; Rolls, 2023c), and partly to show that the computations performed in it are different to hippocampal computations. The location of the perirhinal cortex is shown in Fig. 9.16.

The perirhinal cortex is involved in recognition memory in that damage to the perirhinal cortex produces impairments in recognition memory tasks in which several items intervene between the sample presentation of a stimulus and its presentation again as a match stimulus (Malkova, Bachevalier, Mishkin and Saunders, 2001; Zola-Morgan, Squire, Amaral and Suzuki, 1989; Zola-Morgan, Squire and Ramus, 1994). In macaques, damage to the perirhinal cortex rather than to the hippocampus produces deficits in recognition memory measured in a delayed match to sample task with intervening stimuli (Murray, Baxter and Gaffan, 1998; Baxter and Murray, 2001b,a; Buckley and Gaffan, 2006; Waters, Basile and Murray, 2023). Further, damage to the perirhinal cortex rather than to the hippocampus is believed to underlie the impairment in recognition memory found in amnesia in humans associated with medial temporal lobe damage (Buckley and Gaffan, 2000, 2006).

Neurophysiologically, it has been shown that many inferior temporal cortex (area TE) neurons (Rolls, 2016b, 2012d, 2021d), which provide visual inputs to the perirhinal cortex (Suzuki and Amaral, 1994a,b), respond more to the first, than to the second, presentation of a stimulus in a running recognition task with trial-unique stimuli (Baylis and Rolls, 1987). In this running recognition task (originally developed for neurophysiology by Rolls, Perrett, Caan and Wilson (1982d)), there is typically a presentation of a novel stimulus, and after

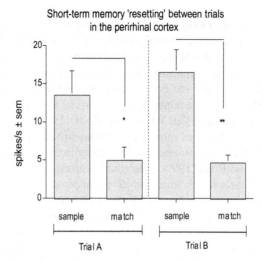

Fig. 9.14 Perirhinal cortex neurons in primates are involved in short-term memory. 'Resetting' of perirhinal cortex neuronal responses between trials in a short-term memory task (delayed match to sample). Neuronal responses are larger to the sample than the match presentation of a particular image within a trial, and are large to the sample on the next trial ('Trial B') even if it is the same image that has just been shown a few seconds earlier as the match image on the preceding trial. * = p<0.01 and ** = p<0.005 in a Wilcoxon post-hoc test. The mean and sem of the responses across neurons are shown. (After Hölscher,C. and Rolls, E. T. (2002) Perirhinal cortex neuronal activity is actively related to working memory in the macaque. Neural Plasticity 9: 41–51.)

a delay which may be in the order of minutes or more and in which other stimuli may be shown, the stimulus is presented again as 'familiar', and the monkey can respond to obtain food reward. Many inferior temporal cortex neurons responded more to the 'novel' than to the 'familiar' presentation of a stimulus, where 'familiar' in this task reflects a change produced by seeing the stimulus typically once (or a few times) before. (A small proportion of neurons respond more to the familiar (second) than to the novel (first) presentation of each visual stimulus.) In the inferior temporal cortex this memory spanned up to 1–2 intervening stimuli between the first (novel) and second (familiar) presentations of a given stimulus (Baylis and Rolls, 1987), and when recordings are made more ventrally, towards and within the perirhinal cortex, the memory span increases to several or more intervening stimuli (Wilson et al., 1990; Brown and Xiang, 1998; Xiang and Brown, 1998). The implication is that the inferior temporal visual cortex can implement a very simple form of recognition memory in which neurons respond more to the first compared to a second presentation of a stimulus with 1–2 intervening stimuli, and that the same rather simple type of recognition process can extend over more intervening stimuli as one moves towards the perirhinal cortex. The underlying mechanism could be a type of habituation or adaptation which is partly stimulus-specific because neurons in these regions can have different responses to different stimuli. For comparison, very few primate hippocampal neurons have activity related to recognition memory (Rolls, Cahusac, Feigenbaum and Miyashita, 1993).

The perirhinal cortex is directly or closely connected with a number of other brain regions involved in the long-term recognition memory for visual stimuli. Relatively far forward in the *orbitofrontal cortex*, in area 11, neurons are activated by novel visual stimuli (Rolls, Browning, Inoue and Hernadi, 2005a), and activations in humans are produced by novel visual stimuli (Frey and Petrides, 2002). The responses of these neurons decrease over on average 5 presentations of a novel stimulus, and may be related to long-term memory in that the responses do not occur to a stimulus that was shown as novel 24 h earlier (Rolls, Browning, Inoue and Hernadi, 2005a). Using the running recognition memory task, Rolls, Perrett, Caan and Wilson (1982d) discovered a population of neurons that responded to familiar visual stimuli and were related to long-term memory at the anterior border of the thalamus, in a region that is at the border of the *ventral anterior thalamic nucleus (VA)* and the reticular nucleus of the thalamus (see also Wilson and Rolls (1990c); cf. Bubb et al. (2017)). Neurons that were also activated in a running recognition memory task by familiar stimuli and that may be related to these thalamic neurons were described by Xiang and Brown (2004) in a *ventromedial prefrontal cortex* region that they termed PFCvm, and a ventrolateral prefrontal region that they termed PFCo. Wilson and Rolls (1993) showed that the activity of some neurons in the amygdala was related to stimulus novelty (with memory spans of 2– 10 intervening other stimuli) and of others to familiarity in monkeys performing recognition memory tasks. Wilson and Rolls (1990c) described neuronal responses related to novel visual stimuli in the *substantia innominata and diagonal band of Broca*. These neurons, also activated in other memory tasks (Wilson and Rolls, 1990b,a), may be the cholinergic neurons that project to the cerebral cortex and that may, by providing acetylcholine to the cerebral cortex, help in the consolidation of memories by the release of acetylcholine at the time that a memory is being formed in the neocortex. Consistent with this, cholinergic basal forebrain lesions produce severe learning impairments in learning visual scenes and in object-reward associations (Easton, Ridley, Baker and Gaffan, 2002), and damage to the cholinergic basal forebrain neurons is implicated in Alzheimer's disease (Whitehouse et al., 1982; Bierer et al., 1995; Fernandez-Cabello et al., 2020). The neurophysiological evidence of Wilson and Rolls (1990c), Wilson and Rolls (1990b) and Wilson and Rolls (1990a) indicates that these *basal forebrain neurons* do change their firing rate during different types of association memory and recognition tasks, and thus the phasic release of acetyl choline to the cortex at the time of memory formation may be important to consolidation, by facilitating LTP (Bear and Singer, 1986; Hasselmo and Sarter, 2011; Zaborszky et al., 2018) (see Section 9.2.8.5).

This interconnected perirhinal cortex / orbitofrontal cortex system may thus be involved in setting up neurons that respond differently to novel and familiar stimuli and thereby implement recognition memory (see also Section 11.3.7 on the ventromedial prefrontal cortex and memory), and may also influence the operation of other memory systems by influences on the basal forebrain cholinergic neurons which have widespread connections to the cerebral cortex (Zaborszky et al., 2018).

A second type of memory in which the perirhinal cortex is involved is the short-term memory for visual stimuli. In a task typically performed with non-trial-unique stimuli, a delayed matching-to-sample task with up to several intervening stimuli, some perirhinal cortex neurons respond more to the match stimulus than to the sample stimulus (Miller et al., 1993). Many other neurons in this task respond more to the sample ('novel') than to the match ('familiar') presentations of the stimuli. There is active engagement of the perirhinal cortex in this delayed matching-to-sample task, in that the response of these neurons is always larger to the sample than to the match stimulus, even if the stimulus shown as the sample has been seen just seconds ago on a previous trial (Hölscher and Rolls, 2002), as shown in Fig. 9.14. Thus this short-term memory in the perirhinal cortex is actively reset at the start of the next trial (Hölscher and Rolls, 2002).

A third type of memory in which the perirhinal cortex is implicated is paired associate learning (a model of semantic long-term memory), which is represented by a population of neurons in a restricted part of area 36 where the neuronal responses may occur to both members of a pair of pictures separated by a delay used in the paired association task (Miyashita et al., 1998, 1996) (see also Section 8.3.1). The learning of this task may be facilitated by the short-term memory-related firing that follows the first member of the pair during the delay period (Hirabayashi et al., 2013). Another very plausible function for these associations across time is not semantic memory but instead view invariant learning, which can be helped

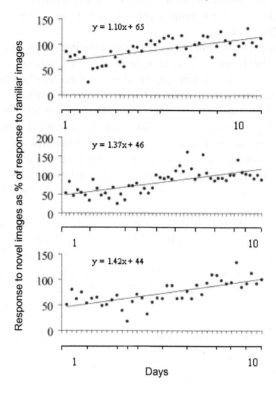

Fig. 9.15 Perirhinal cortex neurons in primates are involved in long-term familiarity memory. The average response of each neuron (shown by a full circle) to a set of 15 novel visual stimuli introduced on day 1 is shown as a proportion of the neuron's response to a very familiar set of stimuli. In each experiment on a neuron, each visual stimulus was shown for approximately 13 1-s periods. Several neurons were analyzed on some days. Thus in the order of 500 exposures to each stimulus in the novel set were required before the response to the initially novel set of stimuli was as large as to the already very familiar set of stimuli. Each stimulus was an image of an object presented on a video monitor. The 3 separate graphs are for 3 separate replications of the whole experiment. (After Hölscher,C., Rolls, E. T. and Xiang,J.-Z. 2003. Perirhinal cortex neuronal activity related to long-term familiarity memory in the macaque. European Journal of Neuroscience 18: 2037–2046. © Federation of European Neuroscience Societies and John Wiley & Sons.)

by associations across time (Rolls, 2021d), as described in Chapter 2, and which may be impaired by perirhinal cortex lesions (Buckley, Booth, Rolls and Gaffan, 2001).

Evidence that the perirhinal cortex is involved in a fourth type of memory, long-term familiarity memory, comes from a neuronal recording study in which it was shown that perirhinal cortex neuronal responses in the rhesus macaque gradually increase in magnitude to a set of stimuli as that set is repeated for 400 presentations each 1.3 s long (Hölscher, Rolls and Xiang, 2003). The single neurons were recorded in the perirhinal cortex in monkeys performing a delayed matching-to-sample task with up to 3 intervening stimuli, using a set of very familiar visual stimuli used for several weeks. When a novel set of stimuli was introduced, the neuronal responses were on average only 47% of the magnitude of the responses to the familiar set of stimuli. It was shown in eight different replications in three monkeys that the responses of the perirhinal cortex neurons gradually increased over hundreds of presentations of the new set of (initially novel) stimuli to become as large as to the already familiar stimuli. Examples of three replications are shown in Fig. 9.15, and the recording sites were in the perirhinal cortex as indicated in Fig. 9.16 (see Hölscher, Rolls and Xiang (2003)). The mean number of 1.3 s presentations to induce this effect was 400 occurring over 7–13 days. These results show that perirhinal cortex neurons represent the very long-term familiarity of visual stimuli (Hölscher, Rolls and Xiang, 2003).

A representation of the long-term familiarity of visual stimuli may be important for many aspects of social and other behavior. For example, long-term familiarity is likely to be a cue about which objects belong to one, who are members of your family, who are members of your social group vs strangers, and which house or village or territory is yours, i.e. about ownership (Hölscher, Rolls and Xiang, 2003; Rolls, Franco and Stringer, 2005b). Indeed, this enhanced processing of highly familiar stimuli by the perirhinal cortex which provides major inputs to the hippocampus is likely to lead to enhanced processing by hippocampal spatial memory systems of information about one's own spatial home environment, which may be adaptive, as individuals spend most of their time there, and may need to defend the environment in which they live which could be enhanced by good spatial knowledge of their home environment.

Indeed, an important aspect of territoriality is a sense of ownership, that the territory belongs to oneself, or to someone else, and it has been proposed that this aspect of territoriality is related to long-term familiarity implemented in the perirhinal cortex (Hölscher, Rolls and Xiang, 2003; Rolls, Franco and Stringer, 2005b). More generally, ownership can be considered to be a semantic attribute of an object, territory, etc. The ownership could signify that we own it, or that someone else owns it. Long-term familiarity is a cue to ownership, but does not in itself encode the attribute about who owns it. A neighbour's garden may be very familiar, but one does not own that territory. So familiarity is a cue, but not all the information needed to specify ownership. The way in which semantic knowledge about for example a territory in the anterior temporal lobe may incorporate attributes such as ownership and familiarity is described in Sections 8.3, 14.2.4, and 14.4.

Another important property of the perirhinal cortex long-term familiarity neurons is that they encode the degree of familiarity of stimuli, as shown by their gradual build-up of responsiveness over 10 days of testing in which the stimuli were seen hundreds of times (Fig. 9.15). This is likely to be important in the build-up of a sense of ownership, for example whether a recently taken territory belongs to you.

Part of the impairment in temporal lobe amnesia may be related to the difficulty of building representations of the degree of familiarity of stimuli in which these perirhinal cortex neurons are implicated. This perirhinal long-term familiarity memory system could also account for the responses of the familiarity neurons discovered in the anterior thalamic region (Rolls et al., 1982d), via the hippocampal–subiculum–fornix–mammillary body–mammillothalamic tract route to the anterior thalamic nuclei, as well as by the direct route from the subiculum via the fornix to the anterior thalamic nuclei (Bubb et al., 2017). This route is involved in memory, in that amnesia can result from damage to the fornix (Gaffan and Gaffan, 1991) and anterior thalamus (Bubb et al., 2017; O'Mara and Aggleton, 2019). The computational roles of these subcortical pathways in memory in primates in not clear. Fornix section will deafferent the hippocampus of cholinergic input, and that will impair memory. It is not surprising if neurons in these diencephalic regions have responses that are similar to those of hippocampal neurons, because of the anatomical connectivity (O'Mara and Aggleton, 2019). The mammillary bodies are likely to be an important relay for vestibular input related to head direction cells (Dillingham et al., 2015). The anterior thalamic nucleus route reaches the cingulate cortex, and that leads me to suggest that this may be part of an evolutionarily early route to enable the hippocampus to influence action (Rolls, 2019c), in which the hippocampal system is implicated as shown by its neuronal activity in conditional spatial responses made to visual stimuli (Cahusac, Miyashita and Rolls, 1989; Miyashita, Rolls, Cahusac, Niki and Feigenbaum, 1989; Cahusac, Rolls, Miyashita and Niki, 1993).

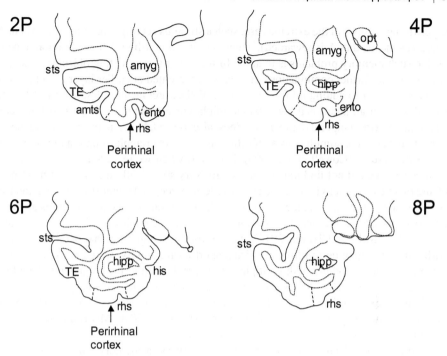

Fig. 9.16 The locations of the perirhinal cortex (areas 35 and 36 in and near the banks of the rhinal sulcus), the entorhinal cortex (area 28), and the hippocampus in macaques. The coronal (transverse) sections are at different distances behind (P, posterior to) an anatomical marker, the sphenoid bone, which is approximately at the anterior–posterior position of the optic chiasm and anterior commissure. amts–anterior middle temporal sulcus; amyg–amygdala; ento–entorhinal cortex; hipp–hippocampus; his–hippocampal sulcus; opt–optic tract; rhs–rhinal sulcus; sts–superior temporal sulcus; TE–inferior temporal visual cortex.

However, in primates the hippocampal backprojection pathways to the neocortex probably provide the main route by which the hippocampus is involved computationally in memory, by implementing memory recall.

It has been shown that long-term familiarity memory for the perirhinal cortex can be modelled by neurons with synapses with a small amount of long-term potentiation which occurs at every presentation of a given stimulus, but which also incorporate hetero-synaptic long-term depression to make the learning self-limiting (Rolls, Franco and Stringer, 2005b).

A fifth type of memory in which the perirhinal cortex is implicated is in tasks in which the stimuli to be discriminated are made up of a small number of features that are combined in different combinations. The features in each stimulus are thus highly overlapping, and the task requires setting up different representations of the different but highly overlapping feature conjunctions in a low-dimensional feature space. This is very different to object representations as they typically occur in the world, in which each object is a particular combination of features from a very high-dimensional feature space, so that the representations of different objects in general have much less overlap in feature space, and the inferior temporal visual cortex can form object representations by forming neurons that respond to different combinations of features from a high-dimensional feature space. In any case, it is argued that perirhinal cortex lesions impair the discrimination between stimuli according to how ambiguous they are in terms of their degree of overlap of a few features (Bussey and Saksida, 2005; Buckley and Gaffan, 2006; Bussey et al., 2002, 2003, 2005). (However, a more mnemonic than perceptual case is made by Hampton (2005) based on the evidence for delay-dependent deficits produced by perirhinal cortex lesions in recognition memory tasks, and reversal-learning impairments which reflect a more associative than perceptual role for the perirhinal cortex.) In the extreme case, such a stimulus set might require A+, B+, but AB– (where A+ means that A is rewarded), which requires a non-linear discrimination. One way to solve such memory problems is to add a further layer to an existing object representation network, where further combinations of what is represented at earlier layers can be formed. This is equivalent to adding a fifth layer to the VisNet architecture described in Chapter 2, and adding such an additional layer, which might correspond to adding a perirhinal cortex layer to an inferior temporal cortex layer, does, as expected, help a network to solve the class of problem where the stimuli consist of different highly overlapping combinations of a small number of features (Cowell et al., 2006). However, when we recorded in the primate perirhinal cortex, we did not find much evidence for very specifically tuned object neurons, but did find that neuronal activity is related to short-term perceptual memory (Hölscher and Rolls, 2002). In the light of this, and the fact that inferior temporal visual cortex neurons do provide very good invariant representations of objects which are complex combinations of features (Rolls, 2012d; Rolls and Treves, 2011), the possibility is suggested that one function of the perirhinal cortex may be to provide a visual short-term memory, which is usually required for the tasks such as oddity with multiple distracters that led to the conjunctive / configural hypothesis (Bussey et al., 2005). Consistently, the visual short-term memory capability of the perirhinal cortex is probably important also for its role in delayed paired-associate learning (Fujimichi, Naya, Koyano, Takeda, Takeuchi and Miyashita, 2010; Miyashita, 2019).

It then becomes a somewhat semantic issue about whether one considers that the perirhinal cortex is involved in object perception as well as in memory (Bussey and Saksida, 2005; Buckley and Gaffan, 2006; Ferko et al., 2022). My own view is that the perirhinal cortex can be thought of as involved in the memory for and discrimination between stimuli when the stimuli are composed of a small number of features with different combinations of features for different stimuli, so that in this way, and perhaps in other ways, the stimuli, which could be objects, are ambiguous. The perirhinal cortex may thus contribute in these special cases, and may be considered to be starting the pattern separation computations that are important in hippocampal computation, as described below. These special cases should be distinguished from object perception that occurs with normal objects in the world, in which each object is composed of a combination of features drawn from a high-dimensional feature space. Object representation in this sense is implemented in the anterior inferior temporal visual cortex, as shown by evidence described in Chapter 2 and Appendix C.

The perirhinal cortex, by receiving from the inferior temporal visual cortex, and perhaps by performing further conjunction learning to that already implemented by the anterior inferior temporal visual cortex (see Chapter 2), thus has visual representations of objects, and some at least of the perirhinal cortex neurons have view-invariant representations.

Another factor that distinguishes the perirhinal cortex is that the perirhinal cortex receives forward inputs from other modalities, including auditory, olfactory and somatosensory (Suzuki and Amaral, 1994a,b; Rolls et al., 2022a, 2023e). This may enable the perirhinal cortex by combining these multimodal inputs to build representations that reflect the convergence of more than visual inputs. The perirhinal cortex, via its projections to the lateral entorhinal cortex and via the lateral perforant path, could thus introduce object information into the hippocampus for object–place associations. The parahippocampal gyrus, in which cells with spatial information are present in macaques (Rolls, Xiang and Franco, 2005c; Rolls and Xiang, 2006), could via connections to the medial entorhinal cortex introduce spatial information into the hippocampus (Section 9.2.8.1), and there is evidence consistent with this in rodents (Hargreaves et al., 2005). In contrast to the perirhinal cortex, the final convergence afforded by the hippocampus into one network in CA3 (see Fig. 9.2) may enable the hippocampus proper to implement an event or episodic memory typically involving arbit-

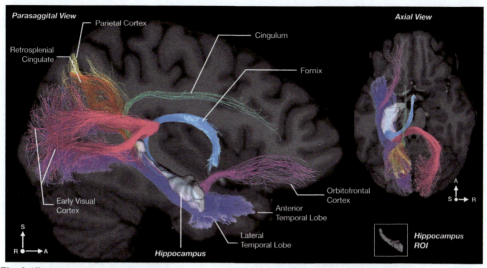

Fig. 9.17 Example of the streamlines showing hippocampal connections using diffusion tractography imaging for a single participant from the Human Connectome Project dataset. The tractography is from a transparent view through the brain, with parasagittal and axial slices of the human brain overlaid to show the trajectory of the pathways in the context of the brain. Voxels in the left hippocampus were seeded for the case illustrated. Streamlines from the hippocampus reach local areas such as the entorhinal and perirhinal cortex, and the parahippocampal gyrus (violet). But in addition streamlines reach more distant areas, including early visual cortical areas bilaterally via the (dorsal) hippocampal commissure (purple, pink); and the parietal cortex (yellow), the orbitofrontal cortex (magenta), the anterior cingulate cortex via the cingulum just above the corpus callosum (light green), and the anterior thalamus and mammillary bodies via the fornix (light blue). The hippocampus is shown in white with slight opacity, and appears small posteriorly just because it rotates laterally. (S - superior/inferior; L - left/right; A - anterior/posterior). (From Huang,C-C., Rolls,E.T., Hsu,C-C.H., Feng,J. and Lin,C-P. (2021) Extensive cortical connectivity of the human hippocampal memory system: beyond the 'what' and 'where' dual stream model. Cerebral Cortex 31: 4652-4669.)

rary associations between any of the inputs to the hippocampus, e.g. spatial, visual object, olfactory, and auditory (see below).

9.2.8 Connectivity of the human hippocampal system

The connections and connectivity of the human hippocampal system have been investigated (Rolls et al., 2022a; Ma et al., 2022a; Huang et al., 2021; Rolls, 2023c, 2022b) using the methods introduced in Section 1.13 and using the HCP-MMP atlas (Section 1.12), and these discoveries, which are leading to new conceptual advances in our understanding of the human hippocampal memory system, are described next. The investigations utilize effective connectivity, functional connectivity, and anatomical connections analyzed with diffusion tractography. The figures in this series of investigations in this book mainly show effective connectivity, but the results that are obtained with diffusion tractography are illustrated for the hippocampus in Fig. 9.17. Connections between the human hippocampus and the lateral and anterior temporal lobe cortex, the orbitofrontal cortex, the anterior cingulate cortex via the cingulum, the retrosplenial cortex, the parietal cortex, and early cortical visual regions are illustrated.

9.2.8.1 A ventromedial visual cortical stream to the hippocampus for visual scene representations

Connectivity is directed to the human hippocampus from a medial posterior part of the parahippocampal gyrus PHA1-3 (which corresponds to TH in macaques) and the adjoining ventromedial visual areas (VMV1-3) (Rolls et al., 2022a, 2023e) (Fig. 9.18). This parahippocampal / VMV region (Sulpizio et al., 2020) is a parahippocampal place area (or Parahippo-

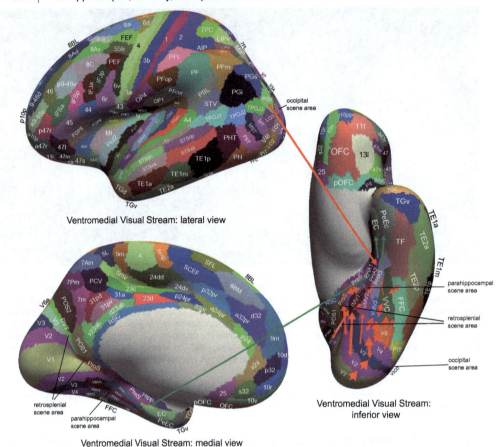

Fig. 9.18 Effective connectivity of the human Ventromedial Visual Cortical Stream which reaches the parahippocampal gyrus PHA1–PHA3 regions via ventromedial (VMV) and Ventral Visual Complex (VVC) and ProStriate regions: schematic overview. Visual scenes are represented in the anterior parts of VMV and the posterior parts of PHA1–PHA3 in what is the Parahippocampal Scene Area PSA (sometimes called the Parahippocampal Place Area, PPA) (Sulpizio et al., 2020). The retrosplenial scene area is in a band of cortex in the Prostriate cortex PRoS and Dorsal Visual Transitional cortex DVT that is posterior to region RSC (Sulpizio et al., 2020). The occipital scene area is in V3CD and borders V4 (Sulpizio et al., 2020). The green arrow shows how the Ventromedial Visual Stream provides 'where' input about locations in scenes to the hippocampal memory system from the medial parahippocampal gyrus PHA1–PHA3 region (which corresponds to TH in macaques). The connectivity from PGp to PHA regions is suggested to be involved in idiothetic update of locations in scenes. The widths of the lines and the size of the arrowheads indicate the magnitude and direction of the effective connectivity. The abbreviations are listed in Section 1.12. (From Rolls, E. T. (2023) Hippocampal spatial view cells for memory and navigation, and their underlying connectivity in humans. Hippocampus doi: 10.1002/hipo.23467.)

campal Scene Area, PSA, as it responds to viewed scenes not the place where the individual is located) (Sulpizio et al., 2020; Natu et al., 2021; Kamps et al., 2016; Epstein and Kanwisher, 1998; Epstein and Baker, 2019; Epstein and Julian, 2013; Epstein, 2008, 2005). My proposal is that the Parahippocampal Scene Area is a route via which hippocampal spatial view cells receive their information about and selectivity for locations in scenes. This direct route (Rolls et al., 2022a, 2023e) is complemented by connectivity via the posterior cingulate cortex (Rolls et al., 2023i) (Section 12.3).

The 'Ventromedial Visual Stream' pathway shown in Fig. 9.18 summarizes how in humans visual information reaches the parahippocampal gyrus PHA1 – PHA3 regions via ventromedial (VMV1-3) and Ventral Visual Complex (VVC) regions (Rolls et al., 2023e). In this stream there is effective connectivity from V1 > V2 > V3 > V4. Then V2, V3 and V4 have effective connectivity to the VMV regions, which in turn have effective connectivity to

PHA1-3, which in turn have effective connectivity directed to the hippocampal system (Fig. 9.18, green arrow) (Rolls et al., 2023e). In addition, V2 has effective connectivity to the transitional visual areas DVT (Dorsal Transitional Visual area) and ProS (the ProStriate region), which in humans are where in the HCP-MMP atlas (Glasser et al., 2016a; Huang et al., 2022) the retrosplenial place area is located (Sulpizio et al., 2020); and these regions in turn have effective connectivity to the PHA1-3 parahippocampal regions (Fig. 9.18) (Rolls et al., 2023e). In humans, the occipital place area OPA is located in V3CD, V3B, and IP0 (Sulpizio et al., 2020) (Fig. 9.18).

It is proposed that scene representations are built using combinations of ventral visual stream features that when overlapping in space are locked together by associative learning and can form a continuous attractor network to encode a visual scene (Rolls et al., 2008f; Stringer et al., 2005; Rolls et al., 2023d; Rolls and Stringer, 2005) using spatial view cells (Rolls and Wirth, 2018; Georges-François et al., 1999; Rolls et al., 1998b; Robertson et al., 1998; Rolls et al., 1997a; Tsitsiklis et al., 2020; Wirth et al., 2017; Rolls, 2022b, 2023c) in the parahippocampal scene (or place) area referred to above, which in turn connects to the hippocampus to provide the 'where' component of episodic memory (Rolls et al., 2022a, 2023d). This connectivity to the hippocampal scene system is considered further elsewhere (Rolls et al., 2023d, 2022a; Rolls, 2022b, 2023c, 2022b). It is proposed below that a contribution of the dorsal visual stream to scene processing is to provide idiothetic update of spatial view representations.

At first sight, this Ventromedial Visual Cortical Stream for 'where', scene, representations, may seem like an unusual proposal. The proposal is that 'where' information, about locations in scenes that are encoded by hippocampal spatial view cells, reaches the hippocampus from the Parahippocampal Scene Area in PHA1-3 and VMV1-3, which has much connectivity with early ventral visual stream cortical areas. Indeed faces are represented near to the Parahippocampal Scene Area in the fusiform gyrus FFC (Pitcher et al., 2019; Natu et al., 2021; Weiner et al., 2017); ideograms (or logograms) of words are represented just lateral to faces in the visual word form area in the fusiform gyrus (Yeatman and White, 2021; Dehaene et al., 2005; Dehaene and Cohen, 2011; Caffarra et al., 2021); and cortical regions that represent objects are nearby and project forward into the inferior temporal visual cortical areas involved in invariant visual object recognition (Grill-Spector et al., 2006; Rolls, 2021b,d). However, scenes are likely to be represented by spatially contiguous scene features that become associated together in the correct topological arrangement because of the statistics of the inputs (Rolls, Tromans and Stringer, 2008f; Stringer, Rolls and Trappenberg, 2005), and thus visual scene representations are likely to be formed from visual features of the type that are represented in ventral stream visual areas.

Highly relevant to these points is that spatial view cells are found in the macaque parahippocampal gyrus as well as the hippocampus (Georges-François et al., 1999; Rolls et al., 1998b; Robertson et al., 1998; Rolls et al., 1997a, 2005c; Rolls and Xiang, 2005; Rolls, 2023c). Indeed, it is proposed and likely that many of the neurons in the Parahippocampal Scene (Place) Area are spatial view cells, and that this is how scenes are represented in the primate including human brain.

These findings are supported by tract-tracing studies in macaques (Kravitz, Saleem, Baker, Ungerleider and Mishkin, 2013; Kravitz, Saleem, Baker and Mishkin, 2011), though more cortical regions are distinguished in the human brain, and the advantage of studying the connectivity in humans with a parcellation such as the HCP-Multimodal Parcellation (Glasser et al., 2016a; Huang et al., 2022) is that we are now dealing with identifiable systems in humans that other studies (fMRI, lesion etc) in humans can directly relate to by reference to the HCP-Multimodal Parcellation, and that the connectivity in humans relates to the strength of connections in both directions between every pair of cortical regions, not only to whether anatomical connections can be traced.

9.2.8.2 The roles of the parietal cortex in the idiothetic update of hippocampal and parahippocampal spatial view cells and scene representations

What has just been proposed in Section 9.2.8.1 raises the question of the role of the parietal cortex, traditionally regarded as the brain region involved in 'where' representations (Ungerleider and Mishkin, 1982; Pitcher and Ungerleider, 2021), in the responses of hippocampal (and parahippocampal gyrus) spatial view cells. As shown in Figs. 3.12 and 9.18, the hippocampal system does receive input from parietal cortex visual regions (Rolls et al., 2023d, 2022a; Ma et al., 2022a; Huang et al., 2021; Rolls et al., 2023e). Inputs are also received via the visuo-motor parts of the posterior cingulate cortex (Rolls et al., 2023i; Baker et al., 2018) (Section 12.3).

In more detail, the effective connectivity of the human Dorsal Visual Cortical Stream is shown in Fig. 3.12 (Rolls et al., 2023e). There is effective connectivity from parietal cortex regions to the parahippocampal scene area, as illustrated in Fig. 3.12. Strong effective connectivity is directed from inferior parietal region PGp to the Parahippocampal Scene Areas (PSA) in PHA1-3 (Figs. 3.12 and 9.18) (Rolls et al., 2023d). PGp receives its inputs from parietal area 7 regions and intraparietal regions (Fig. 3.12) (Rolls et al., 2023e) involved in visual motion analysis and in coordinate transforms from retinal to head-based and then to world-based (allocentric) coordinates (Snyder et al., 1998; Rolls, 2020b; Salinas and Sejnowski, 2001). These coordinate transforms are fundamental for self-motion update of scene representations, so that the spatial view neurons in the parahippocampal scene area can represent where in a scene the individual is looking independently of eye position, head direction, and even the place of the head in the environment, when the view details are obscured or in the dark (Robertson et al., 1998; Rolls, 2020b, 2023c). Given these two lines of evidence, it is proposed that the parietal cortex has the role of idiothetic update of the scene representations in the Parahippocampal Scene Area and thereby in the hippocampus (Rolls et al., 2023e,d; Rolls, 2023c).

Thus the hypothesis is that the 'where' scene representations in the human ventromedial visual stream are built by combinations of ventral stream spatial features, and the viewed position in the scene is idiothetically updated by coordinate transforms to the allocentric level of scenes (Rolls, 2020b, 2023c) by the parietal cortex inputs to the Parahippocampal Scene Area (Rolls et al., 2023e,d; Rolls, 2023c). Optic flow is a signal that can be used in idiothetic update, and in addition it is known that optic flow regions such as V3, V6 and the MT+ complex have functional (Sherrill et al., 2015; Rolls et al., 2023e) and effective (Rolls et al., 2023e) connectivity with regions involved in navigation such as the hippocampus, retrosplenial cortex, and posterior parietal cortex, and that optic flow activates regions that are close to cortical scene regions in the occipital, retrosplenial, and parahippocampal scene regions (Sulpizio et al., 2020).

It is emphasized in this approach that the 'path integration' that is required for idiothetic update in humans and other primates involves eye position as well as head direction and the place where the individual is located, and much takes place in the dorsal visual system regions in the cortex in the intraparietal sulcus and area 7 (Rolls, 2020b; Rolls et al., 2023d). The mechanisms by which these coordinate transforms are implemented in the parietal cortex (Rolls, 2020b) are considered in Section 3.5. A real problem with hypothesizing that path integration of any type occurs within the hippocampus is that the energy landscape of any continuous attractor network representation of place or spatial view in the hippocampus that utilised idiothetic update (Stringer, Rolls and Trappenberg, 2005; Rolls and Stringer, 2005;

Stringer, Rolls, Trappenberg and De Araujo, 2002a) would be so distorted by association with the 'what' and reward information used for episodic memory that it would be very poor at path integration, as the energy landscape would be too bumpy because of the associations (cf. Spalla, Cornacchia and Treves (2021)).

What has been proposed is thus that the primate including human hippocampal 'where' system has two components or parts. One is a ventromedial visual cortical stream scene system with spatial view cells formed by visual feature components locked together in the correct spatial arrangement using overlapping receptive fields and associatively modified synapses of recurrent collaterals of the pyramidal cells that learn from the statistics of the neuronal activity how close the features are in the scene (Rolls et al., 2008f; Stringer et al., 2005). This is located in ventral visual stream areas such as the ventromedial visual areas VMV1-3 and the parahippocampal scene area (Rolls et al., 2022a, 2023e). The second component is the dorsal visual stream areas extending into the intraparietal sulcus areas such as LIP, VIP and MIP, area 7, and PGp (in the HCP-MMP atlas (Glasser et al., 2016a; Huang et al., 2022)), which are involved in idiothetic update of spatial view cells by computing representations of allocentric view that are invariant with respect to retinal position, eye position, head direction, and the place where the individual is located (Rolls et al., 2023d; Rolls, 2020b; Rolls et al., 2023e).

The connectivity from the hippocampus and parahippocampal gyrus to the parietal cortex may further provide a route for allocentric locations in space with associations with rewards, goals, or objects and remembered using hippocampal mechanisms to produce navigation and visuo-motor actions in space that require transforms to egocentric coordinates (Rolls et al., 2023d).

To be clear, this organisation in primates including humans is completely different to anything envisaged for rodents, in which place cells and navigational strategies involving idiothetic update of place representations that can be used in the dark and that might take place at least in part in the hippocampus are invoked (O'Keefe, 1990; Burgess and O'Keefe, 1996; McNaughton, Barnes, Gerrard, Gothard, Jung, Knierim, Kudrimoti, Qin, Skaggs, Suster and Weaver, 1996; Samsonovich and McNaughton, 1997; Royet, Zald, Versace, Costes, Lavenne, Koenig and Gervais, 2000; Bicanski and Burgess, 2018; Edvardsen, Bicanski and Burgess, 2020). In contrast, primates have a highly developed foveate visual system in which eye position, head direction, and even place need to be idiothetically updated for visual scene updates, and this takes place largely in the dorsal visual stream leading to the parietal cortex (Rolls, 2020b) (Chapter 3). This is one example in which the systems-level brain organisation of primates including humans is different from that of rodents (Section 19.10).

9.2.8.3 Ventrolateral visual stream 'What' inputs to the human hippocampal system

To add to the recently developing understanding of human hippocampal system inputs, Fig. 9.19 shows the ventrolateral visual stream in humans progressing via V1 > V2 > V4 > Fusiform Face Cortex FFC (which contains representations of faces, objects and even words in the visual word form area laterally) > the anterior inferior temporal visual cortex TE regions (Rolls et al., 2023e) where invariant representations of objects and faces are built (Rolls, 2000a, 2021b,d). This pathway provides 'what' inputs to the hippocampal memory system via parahippocampal area TF, which is lateral and anterior to the scene area in PHA1-3 (Fig. 9.19) (Rolls et al., 2023e).

Fig. 9.19 also illustrates some of the reward-related inputs to the human hippocampal system with green arrows, and these are considered next.

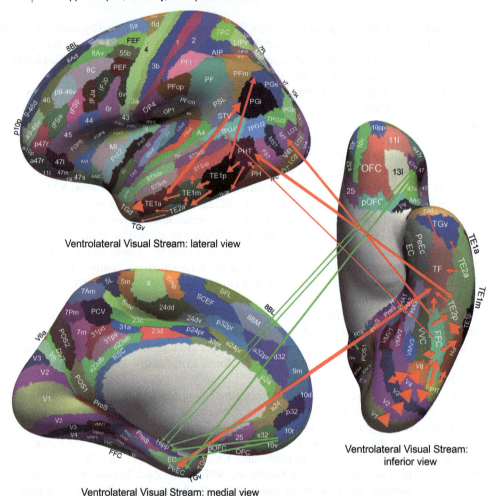

Fig. 9.19 Effective connectivity of the Ventrolateral Visual Stream which reaches inferior temporal cortex TE regions in which objects and faces are represented (red arrows): schematic overview. One of the red arrows shows how the Ventrolateral Visual Stream provides 'what' input to the hippocampal memory system via parahippocampal gyrus TF to perirhinal PeEc connectivity from FFC, PH, TE1p, TE2a and TE2p. The green arrows show how reward regions of the orbitofrontal cortex, vmPFC (pOFC, 10r, 10v) and pregenual anterior cingulate (a24 and p32), and punishment/non-reward regions of the lateral orbitofrontal cortex (47m) have effective connectivity with the hippocampus (Hipp), entorhinal cortex (EC), and perirhinal cortex (PeEC). The Ventrolateral Visual Stream also provides input to the semantic language system via TGd. The Ventrolateral Visual Stream also has connectivity to the inferior parietal visual regions PFm, PGs and PGi as indicated by two red arrows. The widths of the lines and the size of the arrowheads indicate the magnitude and direction of the effective connectivity. The abbreviations are listed in Section 1.12. (From Rolls, E. T. (2023) Hippocampal spatial view cells for memory and navigation, and their underlying connectivity in humans. Hippocampus doi: 10.1002/hipo.23467.)

9.2.8.4 Reward value / emotion-related inputs to the human hippocampus

First, reward value and emotion-related inputs reach the human hippocampal system from the orbitofrontal cortex, ventromedial prefrontal cortex, and anterior cingulate cortex partly via the perirhinal and entorhinal cortex (Figs. 9.19 and 11.28) (Rolls et al., 2022a; Ma et al., 2022a; Rolls et al., 2023c,e), and perhaps even more directly (Huang et al., 2021). This important route for reward to gain access to the human hippocampus in addition to 'what' and 'where' inputs is shown in the hippocampal schematic connection diagram in Fig. 9.2, which shows how reward value information could be associated with 'where' spatial view cell activity in hippocampal CA3, if not before.

The connectivity for these reward value and emotion-related inputs to reach the human hippocampus is shown in more detail in Figs. 9.19 and 11.28 (Rolls et al., 2023c,e). The sensory/perceptual cortical regions on the left of Fig. 11.28 provide visual, taste, olfactory and auditory input not coded in terms of their reward value to the orbitofrontal cortex (Rolls, 2019e,f, 2021b). The representation of these signals in the orbitofrontal cortex is in terms of their reward value, as shown by stimulus-reward learning and reversal; and by satiation which selectively reduces the reward value (Rolls, 2019f; Grabenhorst and Rolls, 2011; Rolls, Cheng and Feng, 2020a; Rolls, 2021h; Rolls, Vatansever, Li, Cheng and Feng, 2020e; Hornak, O'Doherty, Bramham, Rolls, Morris, Bullock and Polkey, 2004; Hornak, Bramham, Rolls, Morris, O'Doherty, Bullock and Polkey, 2003; Hornak, Rolls and Wade, 1996; Rolls, Hornak, Wade and McGrath, 1994a; Berlin, Rolls and Kischka, 2004; Thorpe, Rolls and Maddison, 1983). Reward is represented especially in the human medial orbitofrontal cortex, and punishment and non-reward in the lateral orbitofrontal cortex (Rolls, 2019f,e; Rolls, Cheng and Feng, 2020a; Grabenhorst and Rolls, 2011). The medial and lateral orbitofrontal cortex have effective connectivity to the pregenual anterior cingulate cortex, in part via the ventromedial prefrontal cortex (vmPFC) (Fig. 11.28) (Rolls et al., 2023c). The medial and lateral orbitofrontal cortex, and the vmPFC, then have effective connectivity with the hippocampal system (perirhinal and entorhinal cortex, and perhaps directly with the hippocampus) (Figs. 9.19 and 11.28) (Rolls et al., 2023c). The memory-related part of the posterior cingulate cortex provides additional connectivity between these reward-related regions and the hippocampal system (Rolls et al., 2023i, 2022a).

These neural connectivity investigations provide clear evidence on how reward value and emotion-related information can reach the human hippocampal system. It is proposed that in the hippocampus, including in CA3, reward value information can be associated with spatial view information to enable the reward and emotional aspects of episodic memory to become part of the episodic memory (Rolls et al., 2023c; Rolls, 2022b). The return pathways from the hippocampus to the orbitofrontal cortex, pregenual anterior cingulate cortex, and vmPFC shown in Figs. 9.19, 11.28 and 9.2 provide a route for the reward and emotional value of an episodic memory to be recalled back from the hippocampus to the orbitofrontal and anterior cingulate cortex and vmPFC (Treves and Rolls, 1994; Rolls and Treves, 1994; Rolls, 1995b, 2021b), from which it can influence other brain regions involved in actions (Rolls, 2021b; Rolls et al., 2020a, 2023c).

This connectivity described in humans also shows how a key component of navigation, the goal or reward towards which the navigation is directed, reaches the human hippocampal system, where navigation may be guided by a remembered sequence of spatial view locations encoded by spatial view cells (Rolls et al., 2023c; Rolls, 2021f,b).

9.2.8.5 Human hippocampal system and orbitofrontal / ventromedial prefrontal cortex connectivity involved in memory consolidation

The orbitofrontal cortex and pregenual anterior cingulate cortex have connectivity (yellow in Fig. 11.28) directed to the human cholinergic basal nucleus of Meynert which projects to the neocortex, and septal region which projects to the hippocampus, and these pathways are proposed to influence memory consolidation including consolidation into long-term semantic memory (Rolls et al., 2023c; Rolls, 2022b). It is proposed (Rolls, 2022b) that the orbitofrontal cortex, ventromedial prefrontal cortex (vmPFC), and anterior cingulate regions do not perform spatial computations, but influence them and memory by introducing reward inputs to the hippocampus which are key parts of episodic memory and navigation, and also by influencing the cholinergic system in the septal region that projects to the hippocampus, and in the basal forebrain that projects to the neocortex (Rolls et al., 2023c; Rolls, 2022b), and which are implicated in the synaptic mechanisms involved in memory consolidation (Newman et al.,

2012; Hasselmo and Sarter, 2011; Giocomo and Hasselmo, 2007; Hasselmo and Giocomo, 2006; Hasselmo and McGaughy, 2004; Hasselmo, 1999; Hasselmo and Bower, 1993). This new approach to memory consolidation, which is related to the effective connectivity of the orbitofrontal cortex, vmPFC and anterior cingulate with the hippocampal system directly and via the cholinergic brainstem nuclei (Rolls et al., 2023c) is described next.

Damage to the human vmPFC can impair memory, especially the ability to retrieve vivid autobiographical and episodic memories (McCormick et al., 2018; Bonnici and Maguire, 2018; Barry et al., 2018; Rosenbaum et al., 2014; Moscovitch et al., 2016; Preston and Eichenbaum, 2013; Gilboa and Marlatte, 2017). There is a reduced frequency of mind-wandering; and a reduced focus on future-oriented thoughts and an increased focus on present-related thought (McCormick et al., 2018; Ciaramelli and Treves, 2019). These patients have an inability to initiate internal reflections, including mental visualizations of extended events. In contrast, patients with hippocampal damage seem able to initiate mental events but they are devoid of visual representations of scenes (McCormick et al., 2018; Bonnici and Maguire, 2018). Hippocampal damage seems to particularly impair the spatial coherence of scenes, whereas vmPFC damage leads to a difficulty constructing scenes in a broader sense, with the prediction of what should be in a scene, and the monitoring or integration of the scene elements being particularly compromised (De Luca, McCormick, Mullally, Intraub, Maguire and Ciaramelli, 2018). Schemas can be defined as adaptable associative networks of knowledge extracted over multiple similar experiences (and are an important component of long-term semantic memory (van der Linden, Berkers, Morris and Fernandez, 2017; Farzanfar, Spiers, Moscovitch and Rosenbaum, 2023)), and patients with vmPFC damage appear to have problems in facilitating new encoding by memory schemas, with patients with confabulation (Rosenbaum et al., 2014) having difficulty in reinstating schemas (Ghosh et al., 2014; Ghosh and Gilboa, 2014). The vmPFC is also activated during the learning of new schemas (Gilboa and Marlatte, 2017). (In contrast with the vmPFC, the hippocampus is implicated more in single event memory in which details of the context are encoded (Moscovitch et al., 2016).)

Although the term vmPFC has been used to describe the region implicated in the memory deficits (McCormick et al., 2018; Bonnici and Maguire, 2018), this is not a very precise description, and in fact the overlap of the lesions that produce these problems is in the pregenual anterior cingulate cortex (De Luca, McCormick, Mullally, Intraub, Maguire and Ciaramelli, 2018), and it is activation in the pregenual and supragenual anterior cingulate cortex that precedes activation of the hippocampus during the recall of remote autobiographical memory (McCormick and Maguire, 2021).

The connectivity of the orbitofrontal cortex, vmPFC and pregenual anterior cingulate cortex that connects these reward and punishment emotion-related systems with the hippocampal system is described in Sections 9.2.8.4 and 11.3.10 (Fig. 11.28). A considerable part of the output of the human medial and lateral orbitofrontal cortex value / emotion system is thus directed towards the hippocampal system for memory (Fig. 11.28 (Rolls et al., 2023c)). It is proposed that this connectivity provides a key input about reward / punishment value for the hippocampal episodic memory system, adding to the 'what', 'where', and 'when' information that are also key components of episodic memory. Damage to the vmPFC / anterior cingulate cortex system is likely to contribute to episodic memory impairments produced by damage to these OFC/ vmPFC / ACC regions by impairing a key component of episodic memory, the reward / punishment / emotional value component. Such damage would impair the value information reaching the hippocampal system for storage, and also for later retrieval. Indeed, if one of the possible inputs such as the reward input used for hippocampal memory retrieval by completion in the CA3 attractor network was missing, that would be expected to impair memory retrieval (Treves and Rolls, 1994; Rolls, 2018b; Treves and Rolls, 1991; Rolls, 2021b).

One of the great puzzles of the hippocampal episodic memory system is that hippocampal damage impairs not only episodic memory (the memory for particular events at a particular place and time), but also the learning of new semantic memories, that is knowledge about the world, facts, etc. Already existing semantic memory may show little impairment. A well-known example is that HM, who had bilateral medial temporal lobe damage which included large parts of the hippocampus, could not learn his way to his new house after the bitemporal surgery, but could remember his way to the house he lived in before the surgery. He could never learn who his doctors were (Corkin, 2002). There is much consistent evidence that hippocampal damage can impair new semantic learning (Duff et al., 2019). Why is the hippocampal episodic memory system so importantly involved in learning new semantic information? The new findings on the connectivity of the orbitofrontal cortex / vmPFC / anterior cingulate cortex system with the hippocampus (Rolls et al., 2023c) considered above lead to a new proposal.

During our daily lives, hundreds of events occur to us. We see many people and objects in many places. Some of these events will be associated with some value representation, for example if one of the people is a close friend, who perhaps tells us something useful about a scientific experiment. Most of the daily episodic events will have no value association. In any case, many of these episodic events are stored 'on the fly' in unstructured form in the hippocampus.

Later, when we are not faced with a barrage of incoming information in different episodes, we may have time to reflect on the events of the day. During that recall, the object/people and spatial but also value representations will be recalled by the hippocampus, with activation of neocortical areas that originally provided the object/person, spatial, and value information to the hippocampus for episodic memory storage as described above. If the recalled episodic memory during this time of reflection contains no value component, that is, is not useful to us, or is not very novel as signalled by the orbitofrontal cortex (Rolls et al., 2005a, 2020a; Rolls, 2019e,f), we are likely to think no more about those 'insignificant' events with no value/novelty association. However, if there is a reward/punishment/emotional/novelty component, then we are likely to keep thinking about the whole episode, and what we might learn from that episodic event. It is argued that the prolonged reflection on, and thinking about, episodic events with value associations, is key to learning new semantic memories which are only likely to be formed if they have some utility as reflected in orbitofrontal cortex / vmPFC processing. In reflecting on the episodic events, we try to incorporate them into our knowledge base, including schemas (van der Linden, Berkers, Morris and Fernandez, 2017) and adjust our knowledge base as necessary, that is, to learn new semantic information in neocortical areas such as the anterior temporal lobe, temporo-parietal junction, and angular gyrus (Bonner and Price, 2013; Rolls, 2021b; Rolls et al., 2022b; van der Linden et al., 2017; Farzanfar et al., 2023).

The proposal thus is that if an episodic event has a value component (including a potential value component) as signalled by the vmPFC / anterior cingulate cortex / orbitofrontal cortex, then that value information is likely to make us process the recalled episodic events deeply, and incorporate new information from the hippocampal episodic event into our neocortical knowledge / semantic memory. Evidence supporting this approach is that the depth of processing makes a large difference to how well a memory is encoded and stored (Craik and Tulving, 1975; Xue, 2018). Indeed, I propose that one key factor that influences the depth of processing and the storage of memory, and its conversion into a semantic representation with depth, is the reward value associated with the event, which reflects the utility of that event for long-term memory storage. I propose that the depth of processing tends to remain shallow for daily events with no reward value or emotional component, and that if the event has reward value, we are far more likely to think about the ramifications of the event in depth, and to make use of the event in developing semantic representations and schemas. This provides a clear and testable hypothesis about how episodic memory can be so important in forming new semantic memories; and indeed accords the orbitofrontal cortex / vmPFC / pregenual anterior cingulate cortex a key role in influencing how the operation of episodic memory is related to the formation of new semantic memories, by allowing value to influence the processing and thereby the consolidation. Further support for the approach is that there is increasing acceptance that the vmPFC 'helps refine hippocampal representations to form efficient concept spaces that are tuned based on goal relevance' (Morton and Preston, 2021).

In addition, the medial orbitofrontal cortex (pOFC region) is the only cortical region in humans found to have effective connectivity directed to the basal forebrain magnocellular nucleus of Meynert (yellow in Fig. 11.28 (Rolls et al., 2023c)), which contains cholinergic neurons that project to the neocortex in humans (Mesulam, 1990; Zaborszky et al., 2018, 2008). The human pregenual anterior cingulate cortex (with subgenual 25 and 10r) in humans has effective connectivity directed to the septal nuclei (yellow in Fig. 11.28 (Rolls et al., 2023c)), which contains cholinergic neurons that project to the hippocampus in humans (Mesulam, 1990; Zaborszky et al., 2018, 2008). These pregenual anterior cingulate regions are likely to be important influences on septal neurons, for the only other cortical regions found with substantial effective connectivity to the human septal region (Rolls et al., 2023c) are the hippocampus, subiculum, and v23ab which is part of the posterior cingulate cortex also implicated in episodic memory (Rolls et al., 2023i). In accordance with this, it is proposed that the damage in humans to the orbitofrontal and anterior cingulate cortex regions that impairs episodic memory (Ciaramelli et al., 2019; McCormick et al., 2018) arises in part because of the reduced release of acetylcholine to reward / punishing / salient stimuli, which may impair long-term synaptic potentiation and thus memory storage in both the hippocampus and neocortex (Zaborszky et al., 2018; Newman et al., 2012; Hasselmo and Sarter, 2011; Giocomo and Hasselmo, 2007; Hasselmo and Giocomo, 2006; Rolls, 2021b).

Indeed, it has been discovered that different magnocellular neurons in the basal nucleus which are probably cholinergic respond to reinforcing (rewarding, or punishing), or novel, stimuli (Wilson and Rolls, 1990a,b,c), all represented in the orbitofrontal cortex (Rolls et al., 2005a; Rolls, 2019f,e). Cholinergic activation by these types of 'salient' stimuli can be utilised to enhance memory storage when these rewarding, punishing, or novel stimuli are encountered, which is evolutionarily adaptive by facilitating memory storage when rewarding, punishing, or novel environmental situations are encountered (Rolls and Deco, 2015b; Rolls, 2021b). Consistent with these proposals, depletion of acetylcholine in the forebrain by cholinergic lesions impairs scene memory (Easton, Ridley, Baker and Gaffan, 2002), and in the neocortical / hippocampal system (by depletion in the inferior temporal cortex and fornix transection) also impairs spatial scene memory in macaques (Browning, Gaffan, Croxson and Baxter, 2010).

In terms of the different effects of vmPFC and hippocampal damage on mind-wandering (McCormick et al., 2018; Ciaramelli and Treves, 2019), it is to be expected that damage to the orbitofrontal cortex region will impair neocortically mediated effects because the pOFC region has effective connectivity to the nucleus basalis which in turns connects to neocortical regions where it influences cortical excitability, learning, and thereby semantic memory consolidation (Fig. 11.28) (Rolls et al., 2023c). vmPFC lesions that influence the cholinergic nucleus basalis to neocortex system would thus be expected to impair long-term memory consolidation and remote memory including the use and development of schemata.

The view proposed here is therefore that there is not a major memory system / network in the vmPFC that processes schemata, but that instead the vmPFC can modulate the use and generation of such schemata because of alteration of neocortical function produced by altering the nucleus basalis input to the neocortex. The normal function of this pOFC to nucleus basalis system is proposed, based on the above evidence, to release acetylcholine into the neocortex to facilitate its storage and processing functions when rewarding, punishing, or novel stimuli are encountered, which are important times when consolidation of memory in the neocortex may be useful, to facilitate the memory and semantic processing about those events. In contrast, as expected, damage to the hippocampus impairs mind-wandering about events in 'recent' memory (in the order of the last 6 months) (McCormick et al., 2018; Ciaramelli and Treves, 2019), and if vmPFC damage extends to the pregenual anterior cingulate cortex this hippocampal episodic memory system may also be impaired, because the pregenual anterior cingulate cortex has effective connectivity to the cholinergic septal region, as does the hippocampus, and this system is expected in a comparable way to modulate when the hippocampus stores episodic memory (Fig. 11.28) (Rolls et al., 2023c).

In summary, the following proposals are made in a new approach to memory consolidation in the brain (Rolls, 2022b), and show how better understanding of the connectivity of the human brain is leading to better understanding of what is computed in different brain regions, which in turn has implications for how the computations are performed, including in this case the roles of cholinergic systems.

1. The reward / punishment value system in the human orbitofrontal cortex and regions to which it projects including the vmPFC and pregenual anterior cingulate cortex have effective connectivity with the hippocampus, and provide an important value / emotion-related component of episodic memory used by the hippocampus in addition to 'what', 'where', and 'when' components.

2. Damage to the human vmPFC and anterior cingulate cortex may impair episodic memory implemented by the hippocampal system because it impairs this important component, value information. That may leave the memory system less anchored in goals, and therefore perhaps results in thinking less about the future.

3. Damage to the human orbitofrontal cortex, pregenual anterior cingulate cortex, and vmPFC may also impair activation of brain regions to which they connect, the basal forebrain cholinergic system which connects to the neocortex, and the cholinergic medial septal nuclei which project to the hippocampus, and thereby impair memory consolidation in the neocortex and hippocampus, leading to weaker memories, and thereby to confabulation, a key memory change that follows the medial prefrontal damage.

4. The value / utility component of hippocampal episodic memory representations dependent on the human orbitofrontal cortex / vmPFC / pregenual anterior cingulate cortex may influence the extent to which value-related episodic memories are repeatedly recalled and used in further processing. Greater depth of processing driven by an orbitofrontal cortex / vmPFC / pregenual anterior cingulate cortex value component of a recalled hippocampal episodic event memory is more likely to activate neocortical semantic representations and schemas which then are modified to incorporate new evidence from the episodic event. It is proposed that this is an important way in which the formation or correction of semantic memories depends on the operation of the hippocampal episodic memory system including its value component (Rolls, 2022b).

9.3 How computations are performed in the hippocampal system

Given the systems-level hypothesis that the primate hippocampus is involved in episodic memory, and the neurophysiological evidence about what is represented in the primate hippocampus (described in Section 9.2), we now consider *how* the hippocampus performs its computations. The computations include storing memories that often have a spatial or temporal component, and that can be formed rapidly, and later recalled back to the neocortex. A feature of the theory of hippocampal computation is that it is guided importantly by the neuronal network internal connectivity and synaptic modifiability of the hippocampus that enables it to store and retrieve many memories. Another feature of the theory is that it provides what I think is the only quantitative approach to how memories are retrieved from the hippocampus for later use in the neocortex. The computational theory of the hippocampus is described in this section (9.3), and has been developed in many papers (Rolls, 1989a, 1990b, 1989e,f, 1987; Treves and Rolls, 1994; Rolls, 1990a,b; Treves and Rolls, 1991, 1992; Rolls, 1996d; Rolls and Treves, 1998; Rolls, Stringer and Trappenberg, 2002; Stringer, Rolls and Trappenberg, 2005; Rolls and Stringer, 2005; Rolls and Kesner, 2006b; Rolls, Stringer and Elliot, 2006c; Kesner and Rolls, 2015; Rolls, 2016b, 2018b, 2021f). Ways in which the primate hippocampus could be involved in navigation are described in Section 9.3.15 (Rolls, 2021f).

9.3.1 Historical development of the theory of the hippocampus

Many scientists are interested in how the theory was developed, and a brief account is now provided. Some other approaches to hippocampal computation are considered in Section 9.7.

The theory was preceded by work of Marr (1971) who developed a mathematical model, which although not applied to particular networks within the hippocampus and dealing with binary neurons and binary synapses which utilised heavily the properties of the binomial distribution, was important in utilizing computational concepts. The model was assessed by Willshaw and Buckingham (1990) and Willshaw, Dayan and Morris (2015)[11], who showed that Marr's model did not require any recurrent collateral effect. Early work of Gardner-Medwin (1976) showed how progressive recall could operate in a network of binary neurons with binary synapses.

Rolls (1987) described a theory of the hippocampus that had been presented to the Dahlem conference in 1985 on the Neural and Molecular Bases of Learning in which the CA3 neurons operated as an autoassociation memory to store episodic memories including object and place memories, and could operate using **pattern completion** to recall the whole memory from any part. Rolls (1987) also proposed that the dentate granule cells operated as a preprocessing stage for this by performing **pattern separation** so that the mossy fibres could act to set up different representations for each memory to be stored in the CA3 cells. Rolls (1987) proposed that the CA1 cells operate as a recoder for the information recalled from the CA3

---

[11] Marr (1971) showed how a network with recurrent collaterals could complete a memory using a partial retrieval cue, and how sparse representations could increase the number of memories stored. The analysis of these autoassociation or attractor networks was developed by Kohonen (1977) and Hopfield (1982), and the value of sparse representations was quantified by Treves and Rolls (1991). Marr (1971) did not specify the functions of the dentate granule cells vs the CA3 cells vs the CA1 cells (which were addressed in the Rolls (1989) papers (see e.g. Rolls (1990b) and Rolls 1990b)) and by Treves and Rolls (1992) and Treves and Rolls (1994)), nor how retrieval to the neocortex of hippocampal memories could be produced, for which a theory was developed by Rolls (1990b) and made quantitative by Treves and Rolls (1994). In addition, Treves and Rolls (1994) and Rolls and Treves (1998) have argued that approaches to neurocomputation which base their calculations on what would happen in the tail of an exponential, Poisson, or binomial distribution are very fragile.

cells to a partial memory cue, so that the recalled information would be represented more efficiently to enable recall, via the backprojection synapses, of activity in the neocortical areas similar to that which had been present during the original episode[12]. This theory was developed further (Rolls, 1989a, 1990b, 1989e,f, 1990a,b), including further details about how the backprojections could operate (Rolls, 1990b, 1989e), and how the dentate granule cells could operate as a competitive network and could further produce *pattern separation* by using the very diluted connectivity of the dentate to CA3 neuron mossy fibre synapses (Rolls, 1989a, 1990b, 2013b, 2016f, 2021i). Quantitative aspects of the theory were then developed with Alessandro Treves, who brought the expertise of theoretical physics applied previously mainly to understand the properties of fully connected attractor networks with binary neurons (Amit, 1989; Hopfield, 1982) to bear on the much more diluted connectivity of the recurrent collateral connections found in real biological networks (e.g. 2% between CA3 pyramidal cells in the rat), in networks of neurons with graded (continuously variable) firing rates, graded synaptic strengths, and sparse representations in which only a small proportion of the neurons is active at any one time, as is found in the hippocampus (Treves, 1990; Treves and Rolls, 1991). These developments in understanding quantitatively the operation of more biologically relevant recurrent networks with modifiable synapses were applied quantitatively to the CA3 region (Treves and Rolls, 1991), and to the issue of why there are separate mossy fibre and perforant path inputs to the CA3 cells of the hippocampus (Treves and Rolls, 1992). This whole model of the hippocampus was described in more detail, and a quantitative treatment of the theory of recall by backprojection pathways in the brain was formulated (Treves and Rolls, 1994; Rolls and Treves, 1994).

The speed of operation of the CA3 system, and of the cortico-cortical recall backprojections, was addressed in a number of developments (Battaglia and Treves, 1998b; Panzeri, Rolls, Battaglia and Lavis, 2001; Simmen, Rolls and Treves, 1996a; Treves, 1993). Rolls (1995b) produced a simulation of the operation of the major parts of the hippocampus from the entorhinal cortex through the dentate, CA3, and CA1 cells back to the hippocampus, which established the quantitative feasibility of the whole theory, and raised a number of important issues considered below, including the role of topography within parts of the hippocampal internal connectivity. The simulation also emphasized some of the advantages, for a system that must store many different memories, of a binary representation, in which for any one memory the neurons were either firing or not, as opposed to having continuously graded firing rates. The simulation by Rolls (1995b) also showed how recall, if not perfect at the stage of the CA3 cells, was improved by associative synapses at subsequent stages, including the connections of the CA3 cells to the CA1 cells, and the connections of the CA1 cells to the entorhinal cortex cells.

The theory has been developed further (Stringer, Rolls and Trappenberg, 2005; Rolls, Tromans and Stringer, 2008f; Rolls, 2010b; Webb, Rolls, Deco and Feng, 2011; Rolls and Webb, 2012; Rolls, 2012b, 2013c,b; Kesner and Rolls, 2015; Rolls, 2015a, 2016f,b, 2018b; Rolls and Wirth, 2018; Rolls and Mills, 2019; Rolls, 2020b, 2021d,f, 2022b), as described below.

---

[12]McNaughton and Morris (1987) at about the same time suggested that the CA3 network might be an autoassociation network, and that the mossy fibre to CA3 connections might implement 'detonator' synapses. However, the concepts that the diluted mossy fibre connectivity might implement selection of a new random set of CA3 cells for each new memory, and that a direct perforant path input to CA3 was needed to initiate retrieval, were introduced by Treves and Rolls (1992). The theory of CA1 and of backprojections to the neocortex for memory recall were introduced by Rolls (1990b). Contributions by Levy (1989); McNaughton (1991); Hasselmo et al. (1995); McClelland et al. (1995); and many others, are described below.

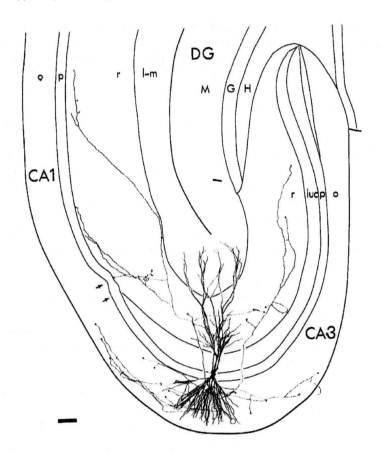

Fig. 9.20 An example of a CA3 neuron from the hippocampus. The thick extensions from the cell body or soma are the dendrites, which form an extensive dendritic tree receiving in this case approximately 12,000 synapses. The axon is the thin connection leaving the cell. It divides into a number of collateral branches. Two axonal branches can be seen in the plane of the section to travel to each end of the population of CA3 cells. One branch (on the left) continues to connect to the next group of cells, the CA1 cells. The junction between the CA3 and CA1 cells is shown by the two arrows. The diagram shows a camera lucida drawing of a single CA3 pyramidal cell intracellularly labelled with horseradish peroxidase. DG, dentate gyrus. The small letters refer to the different strata of the hippocampus. (Reproduced from Norio Ishizuk, Janet Weber and David G. Amaral (1990) Organization of intrahippocampal projections originating from CA3 pyramidal cells in the rat. Journal of Comparative Neurology 295: 580–623. Copyright © Wiley-Liss, Inc.)

Tests of the theory including analysis of the functions of different subregions of the hippocampus are described in Section 9.4 and by Rolls and Kesner (2006b) and Kesner and Rolls (2015).

9.3.2 Hippocampal circuitry

Figs. 9.2 on page 318, 9.20, 9.21 and 9.22 show diagrams of hippocampal circuitry that is described next, based on many sources (Amaral, Ishizuka and Claiborne, 1990; Storm-Mathiesen, Zimmer and Ottersen, 1990; Amaral and Witter, 1989; Amaral, 1993; Naber, Lopes da Silva and Witter, 2001; Lavenex, Suzuki and Amaral, 2004; Witter, Wouterlood, Naber and Van Haeften, 2000b; Johnston and Amaral, 2004; Witter, 2007; van Strien, Cappaert and Witter, 2009; Kondo, Lavenex and Amaral, 2009).

Projections from the entorhinal cortex layer 2 reach the granule cells (of which there are 10^6 in the rat) in the dentate gyrus (DG), via the perforant path (pp) (Witter, 1993).

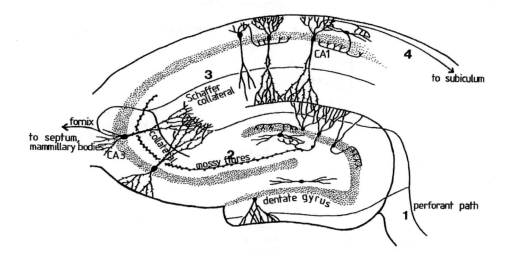

Fig. 9.21 Representation of connections within the hippocampus. Inputs reach the hippocampus through the perforant path (1) which makes synapses with the dendrites of the dentate granule cells and also with the apical dendrites of the CA3 pyramidal cells. The dentate granule cells project via the mossy fibres (2) to the CA3 pyramidal cells. The well-developed recurrent collateral system of the CA3 cells is indicated. The CA3 pyramidal cells project via the Schaffer collaterals (3) to the CA1 pyramidal cells, which in turn have connections (4) to the subiculum.

In the dentate gyrus there is a set of inhibitory interneurons that provide recurrent inhibition between the granule cells. (In addition, there are some excitatory interneurons in the hilus that interconnect granule cells.) The granule cells project to CA3 cells via the mossy fibres (mf), which provide a sparse but possibly powerful connection to the 3×10^5 CA3 pyramidal cells in the rat. Each CA3 cell receives approximately 50 mossy fibre inputs, so that the sparseness of this connectivity is thus 0.005%. By contrast, there are many more – probably weaker – direct perforant path inputs also from layer 2 of the entorhinal cortex onto each CA3 cell, in the rat in the order of 4×10^3. The largest number of synapses (about 1.2×10^4 in the rat) on the dendrites of CA3 pyramidal cells is, however, provided by the (recurrent) axon collaterals of CA3 cells themselves (rc) (see Fig. 9.23). It is remarkable that the recurrent collaterals are distributed to other CA3 cells throughout the hippocampus (Amaral and Witter, 1989, 1995; Amaral, Ishizuka and Claiborne, 1990; Ishizuka, Weber and Amaral, 1990; Witter, 2007), so that effectively the CA3 system provides a single network, with a connectivity of approximately 2% between the different CA3 neurons given that the connections are bilateral.

The CA3–CA3 recurrent collateral system is even more extensive in macaques than in rats (Kondo, Lavenex and Amaral, 2009). This is a clear indication that in primates there is recurrent collateral connectivity within a hemisphere to provide for a single autoassociation / attractor network in the primate CA3. Interestingly, the left and right CA3 neurons in humans are not connected across the midline, so the human has two hippocampi (which doubles the number of memories that can be stored), whereas the rat has a single hippocampus. The neurons that comprise CA3, in turn, project to CA1 neurons via the Schaffer collaterals. In addition, projections that terminate in the CA1 region originate in layer 3 of the entorhinal cortex (see Fig. 9.2).

Some of the neuron numbers in different parts of the circuitry in humans are shown in Fig. 9.2 (Rogers Flattery et al., 2020). Very important for humans would be an estimate of the number of synapses that the CA3 recurrent collaterals make on each CA3 neuron, for that sets the limit on the memory capacity of the hippocampal system, as shown below.

A CA2 group of cells lies between CA3 and CA1. CA2 neurons do not have highly

368 | The hippocampus, memory, and spatial function

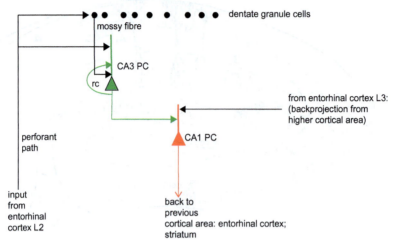

Fig. 9.22 Functional canonical microcircuit of the hippocampal cortex. Recurrent collateral connections (rc) are shown as a loop back to a particular population of cells, of which just one neuron is shown. (From Rolls, E. T. (2016) Cerebral Cortex: Principles of Operation. Oxford University Press: Oxford.)

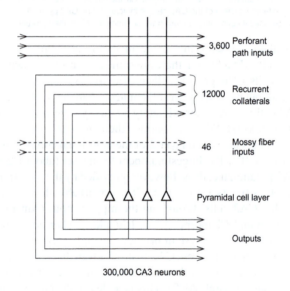

Fig. 9.23 The numbers of connections onto each CA3 cell from three different sources in the rat. (After Treves, A. and Rolls, E. T. (1992) Computational constraints suggest the need for two distinct input systems to the hippocampal CA3 network. Hippocampus 2: 189–199. © Churchill Livingstone Inc; and Rolls, E. T. and Treves, A. (1998) Neural Networks and Brain Function. Oxford University Press: Oxford.)

developed recurrent collaterals that mix with CA3 recurrent collaterals. CA2 does act to disinhibit CA1, where it may act as a general facilitator on CA1 of learning about its CA3 inputs about 'what', 'when' and reward associations, for which CA1 uses competitive learning. The CA2 neurons are influenced by oxytocin (Tirko, Eyring, Carcea, Mitre, Chao, Froemke and Tsien, 2018), and may play a role in the facilitating effects that social interactions have on memory (Oliva, 2022). In this context, CA2 has been proposed to play a role in the facilitation of memories of events that might be relevant to territoriality (Wirth et al., 2021).

9.3.3 Medial entorhinal cortex, spatial processing streams, and grid cells

The entorhinal cortex (area 28) provides inputs to the hippocampus, as well as receiving the outputs of the hippocampus (Garcia and Buffalo, 2020), so its operation is considered briefly first. The medial (/posterior) entorhinal cortex receives spatial inputs from the dorsal 'spatial' processing streams via the parahippocampal gyrus, and provides a route for these to enter the hippocampus; and for the return routes from the hippocampus to send backprojections back via the parahippocampal gyri to the dorsal 'spatial' processing streams (the red pathways in Fig. 9.2). The lateral (/anterior) entorhinal cortex receives inputs from the ventral 'object' processing streams via the perirhinal cortex, and provides a route for these to enter the hippocampus; and for the return routes from the hippocampus to send backprojections back via the perirhinal cortex to the ventral 'object' processing streams (the blue pathways in Fig. 9.2).

The entorhinal cortex performs interesting computations in its own right. In the rodent medial entorhinal cortex, there are grid cells, which have regularly spaced peaks of firing in an environment, so that as a rat runs through an environment, a single neuron increases then decreases its firing a number of times as the rat traverses the environment (Hafting et al., 2005; Moser et al., 2015). Each grid cell responds to a set of places in a spatial environment, with the places to which a cell responds set out in a regular grid. Different grid cells have different phases (positional offsets) and grid spacings or frequencies (Hafting, Fyhn, Molden, Moser and Moser, 2005; Giocomo, Moser and Moser, 2011; Moser, Rowland and Moser, 2015; Kropff and Treves, 2008). The grid cell system appears to provide ring continuous attractors that would be useful for spatial path integration (computing position based on self-motion) (Giocomo et al., 2011; Moser et al., 2014a; Zilli, 2012).

One attractive theory is that different temporal delays in the neural circuitry of the medial entorhinal cortex are related to different temporal adaptation time courses and result in the different sizes of spatial grids that are found in the rodent medial entorhinal cortex (Kropff and Treves, 2008; Soldatkina, Schonsberg and Treves, 2022).

An interesting computational issue is how the grid cells present in the medial entorhinal cortex (Hafting, Fyhn, Molden, Moser and Moser, 2005; Moser, Rowland and Moser, 2015) might help to generate hippocampal place cells in rodents. We have proposed that this could be performed by competitive learning, implemented in the dentate granule cells (or beyond) in the hippocampal system (Rolls, Stringer and Elliot, 2006c). Each grid cell responds to a set of places in a spatial environment, with the places to which a cell responds set out in a regular grid. Different grid cells have different phases (positional offsets) and grid spacings or frequencies (Hafting, Fyhn, Molden, Moser and Moser, 2005; Giocomo, Moser and Moser, 2011; Moser, Rowland and Moser, 2015; Kropff and Treves, 2008). We have simulated the dentate granule cells as a system that receives as inputs the activity of a population of grid cells as the animal traverses a spatial environment, and have shown that the competitive net builds dentate-like place cells from such entorhinal grid cell inputs (Rolls, Stringer and Elliot, 2006c). This occurs because the combination of entorhinal cortex grid cells that are co-active when the animal is in one place become associated together by the action of the competitive net. Each dentate cell represents primarily one place because the dentate representation is kept sparse, thus helping to implement symmetry-breaking. Simulations to demonstrate this are shown next. The operation of competitive nets is described in Section B.4, and the anatomical connectivity is that of a competitive net, with the entorhinal inputs making synaptic connections onto the dendrites of the dentate granule cells, as shown in Figs. 9.2 and 9.21.

Fig. 9.24a and b show examples of two 2D entorhinal cortex (EC) grid cells (with frequencies of 4 and 7 cycles along the X axis) (Rolls, Stringer and Elliot, 2006c). As in the

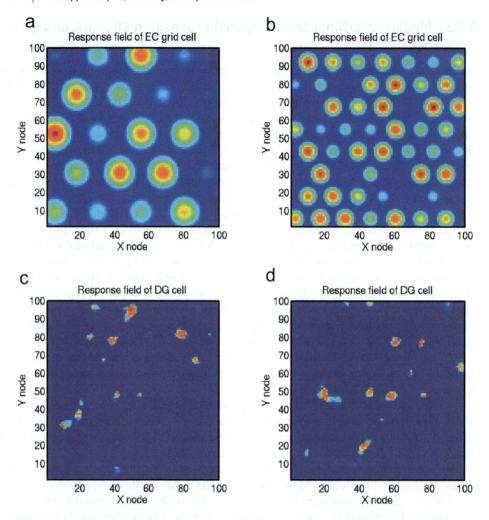

Fig. 9.24 Simulation of competitive learning in the dentate gyrus to produce place cells from the entorhinal cortex grid cell inputs. (a and b) Firing rate profiles of two entorhinal cortex (EC) grid cells with frequencies of 4 and 7 cycles. (c and d) Firing rate profiles of two dentate gyrus (DG) cells with no training. (After Rolls, E. T., Stringer, S.M. and Elliot, T. (2006) Entorhinal cortex grid cells can map to hippocampal place cells by competitive learning. Network: Computation in Neural Systems 17: 447–465. © Informa UK Limited.)

neurophysiological recordings (Hafting et al., 2005), the firing peaks occur at the vertices of a grid of equilateral triangles. Fig. 9.24c and d show the firing rate profiles of two dentate gyrus (DG) cells without training. Multiple peaks in the response profiles are evident, and this shows that the contrast enhancement and the competitive interactions in the DG layer were not sufficient without training and thereby synaptic modification to produce place-like fields in DG.

Fig. 9.25a and b show the firing rate profiles of two Dentate Granule cells after training with the Hebb rule. This type of relatively small 2D place field was frequently found in the simulations. This result shows that competitive learning was sufficient to produce place-like fields in the dentate granule cells. Fig. 9.25c and d show the firing rate profiles of two DG cells after training with the trace rule, which is a modified form of Equation B.32 on page 873 that has a short-term memory trace of previous neuronal activity as specified in Equation 2.3 on page 110. The use of the trace rule is intended to test the concept that by keeping neurons

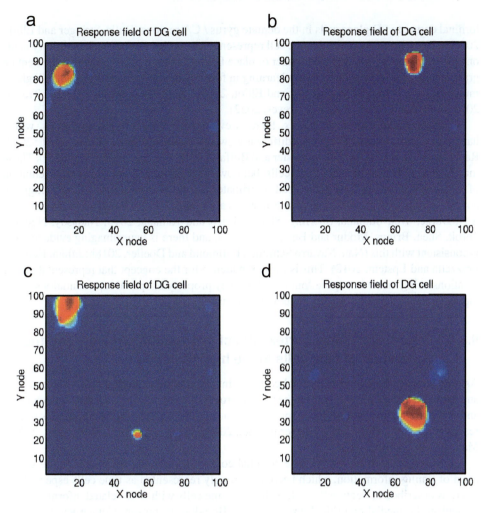

Fig. 9.25 Simulation of competitive learning in the dentate gyrus (DG) to produce place cells from the entorhinal cortex grid cell inputs. (a and b) Firing rate profiles of two DG cells after training with the Hebb associative synaptic modification rule. (c and d) Firing rate profiles of two DG cells after training with the trace rule with $\eta = 0.8$. (After Rolls, E. T., Stringer,S.M. and Elliot,T. (2006) Entorhinal cortex grid cells can map to hippocampal place cells by competitive learning. Network: Computation in Neural Systems 17: 447–465. © Informa UK Limited.)

in a modifiable state for a short time after strong activation (using for example the long time constant of NMDA receptors) the inputs from places near to a recently visited place where the activity of the neuron was high will tend to become associated onto the same postsynaptic neuron, thereby enlarging the place field. In the simulations, the place fields tended to be larger with the trace than with the purely associative Hebb rule shown in Equation 9.8 (Rolls, Stringer and Elliot, 2006c).

Although the Dentate Granule cells illustrated had one main place field, some remaining grid-like firing was sometimes evident in the place fields with both Hebb and trace rule training, and indeed is evident in Fig. 9.25c and d. These are also characteristics of dentate granule cells recorded under the same conditions as the EC grid cell experiments (E. Moser, personal communication). These results were found only with training, with untrained networks showing repeating peaks of firing in large parts of the space as illustrated in Fig. 9.24c and d. These results show that competitive learning can account for the mapping of 2D grid cells in the entorhinal cortex to 2D place cells in the dentate gyrus / CA regions (Rolls, Stringer and Elliot, 2006c). The sparseness of the dentate cell representation, set by the feedback inhibitory neurons in the dentate gyrus, sets the number of place fields that are typically found in the dentate granule cells. The role of competitive learning in forming dentate granule cells with single or multiple place fields (Rolls, Stringer and Elliot, 2006c) has been confirmed (Si and Treves, 2009; Soldatkina, Schonsberg and Treves, 2022).

In the macaque entorhinal cortex, there is evidence for spatial view grid cells, which have peaks and troughs of firing for different viewed locations in space (Killian et al., 2012; Rueckemann and Buffalo, 2017; Meister and Buffalo, 2018; Garcia and Buffalo, 2020). These may be the equivalent of rodent grid cells, but now involved in the continuous representation of visual space, which is so developed in primates. In the human entorhinal and cingulate cortex neurons with grid-like response properties are found (Jacobs, Weidemann, Miller, Solway, Burke, Wei, Suthana, Sperling, Sharan, Fried and Kahana, 2013; Nadasdy, Nguyen, Torok, Shen, Briggs, Modur and Buchanan, 2017), and there is neuroimaging evidence that is consistent with this (Nau, Navarro Schroder, Bellmund and Doeller, 2018b; Julian, Keinath, Frazzetta and Epstein, 2018). This is further evidence for the concept that representations of locations being viewed in space 'out there' is a key property of spatial representations in the hippocampal system of primates including humans.

9.3.4 Lateral entorhinal cortex, object processing streams, and the generation of time cells in the hippocampus

As noted above, the lateral entorhinal cortex is involved in representing object information, and provides a route for inputs from the ventral processing streams to reach the hippocampus, and for return pathways from the hippocampus back to the ventral processing streams (Hargreaves et al., 2005; Witter, 1993; Knierim et al., 2014; Huang et al., 2021; Rolls et al., 2022a; Ma et al., 2022a; Rolls et al., 2023e).

However, in addition the lateral entorhinal cortex may play a special role in the generation of timing information, which becomes strongly represented as time cells especially in CA1, as described in Section 9.3.7.4. Although some cells with time-related information are present in the medial entorhinal cortex (Kraus, Brandon, Robinson, Connerney, Hasselmo and Eichenbaum, 2015), in the lateral entorhinal cortex, temporal information is robustly encoded across time scales from seconds to many minutes within neuronal populations in freely foraging rats (Tsao, Sugar, Lu, Wang, Knierim, Moser and Moser, 2018). In the lateral entorhinal cortex, the neurons that encode time have rather long firing rate timescales in which the firing of individual neurons may ramp down towards zero over many minutes, and in some cases may ramp or jump up from low rates to these high rates before starting another decrease in firing over a long period (Tsao et al., 2018), as illustrated in Fig. 9.26b.

9.3.4.1 The theory of the generation of time in the brain, and of hippocampal time cells

The encoding of the time-related information in the hippocampus appears to use a firing rate code, in that different CA1 hippocampal neurons have short periods of firing at different times in a delay period, and thus reflect which temporal part of the task is current (Macdonald, Lepage, Eden and Eichenbaum, 2011). An example is shown in Fig. 9.26c (Kraus et al., 2013). Some hippocampal neurons in both CA3 and CA1 fire to combinations of time and object or place (Eichenbaum, 2017; Salz et al., 2016; Howard and Eichenbaum, 2015; Eichenbaum, 2014), thus reflecting associations of objects and places with time which enable the sequence of places and/or objects to be remembered (Rolls and Mills, 2019).

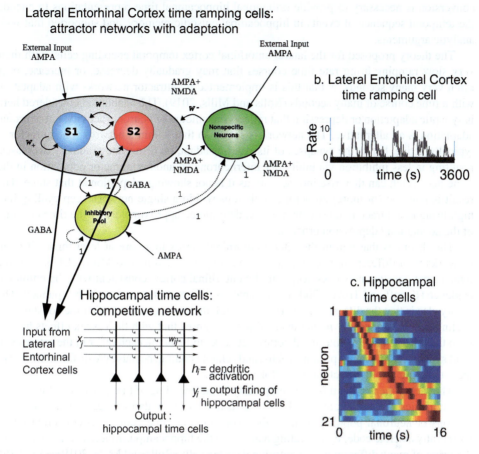

Fig. 9.26 The generation of time in the hippocampal memory system. Model of the lateral entorhinal cortex temporal cells and hippocampal time cells. a. The lateral entorhinal cortex is modelled as an integrate-and-fire attractor neuronal network. The excitatory neurons are divided into two selective populations or pools S1 and S2 either of which can sustain a high firing rate attractor state because of strong synaptic connections w+ within each population. The inhibitory neurons ensure that only one population, S1, or S2, can be active at any one time. In the model, there are three such attractor networks for the lateral entorhinal cortex, each with different time constants for the synaptic depression that occurs in the recurrent collaterals of the attractors networks (indicated by recurrent arrows), so that nets 1–3 tend to cycle with different periods (long, medium, and short). The S1 and S2 pools of all three lateral entorhinal cortex attractor networks send their outputs to a competitive network in the hippocampus (e.g. in CA1 or in the dentate gyrus). The competitive network learns to respond to combinations of the outputs of the lateral entorhinal cortex, and forms thereby hippocampal time cells, as shown in the simulations. b. Example of a lateral entorhinal cortex time ramping cell recorded in the rat by Tsao et al. (2018). The firing rate is in spikes/s. These neurons are characterized by slow ramping changes in their firing rates with a long time period. c. Hippocampal time cells recorded in the rat by Kraus et al (2013). Each neuron of the 21 shown has a high firing rate for a short period of time during a 16 s interval during which the rat was running on a treadmill. The firing rate is indicated by the color with low rates blue, and high rates red/brown. (From Rolls, E. T. and Mills,P. (2019) The generation of time in the hippocampal memory system. Cell Reports 28: 1649–1658. [b from Albert Tsao, Jorgen Sugar, Li Lu, Cheng Wang, James J. Knierim, May-Britt Moser, and Edvard I. Moser (2018) Integrating time from experience in the lateral entorhinal cortex. Nature 561: 57--62. © Springer Nature. c from Benjamin J. Kraus, Robert J. Robinson, John A. White, Howard Eichenbaum, and Michael E. Hasselmo (2013) Hippocampal 'Time Cells': Time versus Path Integration. Neuron 78: 1092. © Elsevier Inc.])

Rolls and Mills (2019) proposed that ramping time cells in the lateral entorhinal cortex can be produced by synaptic adaptation, and demonstrated this in an integrate-and-fire attractor network model. They proposed that competitive networks in the hippocampal system can convert these entorhinal cortex time ramping cells into hippocampal time cells, and demonstrated this in a competitive network (Fig. 9.26). Rolls and Mills (2019) proposed that this conversion is necessary to provide orthogonal hippocampal time representations to encode the temporal sequence of events in hippocampal episodic memory, and supported that with analytic arguments.

The theory proposed for the lateral entorhinal cortex temporal encoding cells, with their very slow ramping firing rate time courses that may gradually decrease, or increase, over often very many seconds, is that this is implemented by attractor networks with adaptation with a time course of many seconds (Rolls and Mills, 2019). The adaptation considered here is synaptic adaptation or depression that reflects the amount of neuronal activity, but neuronal adaptation is an alternative. The network is set up so that within a network, one attractor is typically active, but as the synapses of its neurons adapt, its firing rate gradually decreases, resulting in less inhibition via inhibitory interneurons on another attractor population in the same net, which can then rise into activity as it is not showing adaptation at that stage. The result is that two (or more) attractor populations within a single network keep cycling into high firing rate attractor states with a period determined approximately by the time constant of the adaptation / depression process.

The theory is that within the lateral entorhinal cortex there are at least three different networks with different time constants for the adaptation (Rolls and Mills, 2019), with the longer time constant networks deeper in the entorhinal cortex, consistent with the empirical evidence (Kropff and Treves, 2008). This enables different time periods to be spanned. The theory also is that the different networks, each with their own characteristic time constant and cycling period, are weakly interconnected with synapses that with their weak effects help to keep the different lateral entorhinal cortex networks influencing each other in the interests of mild synchrony helping to produce robust and reliable coding, because the different networks are interacting weakly (Section B.9) (Rolls, 2016b).

The theory then is that this very temporally broad encoding of time, in terms of the temporal dynamics of each cell, and by the very distributed representation because many different neurons or neuronal populations have their own gradual time courses, is converted into a temporally discrete code, by allocating neurons in the hippocampus to learn combinations of the firing of many different lateral entorhinal cortex cells (Rolls and Mills, 2019) (Fig. 9.26). The hippocampal time code is much more time discrete, and is therefore much better suited to making associations between this discrete and sparse time cell code with object representations in the hippocampus. The hippocampal / dentate gyrus network that is proposed to learn these different combinations is a competitive network. By forming neurons that respond differently to different combinations of the different time courses of different populations of entorhinal cortex neurons, a time-unique code suitable for sequential memory can be formed in the hippocampus. This is completely analogous to our theory that a competitive network is used to convert medial entorhinal cortex grid cell firing into hippocampal place cell firing (Rolls et al., 2006c), suitable in a parallel way for object-place associations, and reflecting it is suggested the conservatism in brain design (Rolls, 2016b). The overall architecture is illustrated in Fig. 9.26.

9.3.4.2 The model of lateral entorhinal cortex temporal cells and hippocampal time cells

The theory was tested, illustrated, and analyzed in a simulation that provided a model shown in Fig. 9.26 with biologically plausible characteristics (Rolls and Mills, 2019). The lateral entorhinal cortex was modelled as three networks, each with an integrate-and-fire attractor neuronal network with synaptic adaptation in the recurrent collateral synapses (Rolls and Deco, 2016). In the model as simulated, there are three such attractor networks for the lateral entorhinal cortex, each with different time constants for the synaptic depression that occurs in the recurrent collaterals of the attractor networks, so that Nets 1–3 tend to cycle with different periods (long, medium, and short).

The synaptic depression mechanism used for the recurrent collateral connections between the neurons in each specific pool, i.e. within S1 or within S2, following Dayan and Abbott (2001) and Deco and Rolls (2005c), was as follows. The probability of transmitter release P_{rel} was decreased after each presynaptic spike by a factor $P_{\mathrm{rel}} = P_{\mathrm{rel}} \cdot f_{\mathrm{D}}$ with $f_{\mathrm{D}} = 0.999$. Between presynaptic action potentials the release probability P_{rel} was updated by

$$\tau_P \frac{dP_{\mathrm{rel}}}{dt} = P_0 - P_{\mathrm{rel}} \qquad (9.1)$$

with $P_0 = 1$ and $\tau_P = 25$ s.

Each lateral entorhinal cortex network was a biophysically realistic attractor network, so that the properties of receptors, synaptic currents and the statistical effects related to the probabilistic spiking of the neurons could be part of the model (Brunel and Wang, 2001; Rolls and Deco, 2010) with synaptic adaptation (Rolls and Mills, 2019; Deco and Rolls, 2005c). The S1 and S2 pools of all three lateral entorhinal cortex attractor networks send their outputs to a competitive network in the hippocampus (e.g. in CA1 or in the dentate gyrus) (Fig. 9.26). The competitive network learns to respond to combinations of the outputs of the lateral entorhinal cortex, and forms thereby hippocampal time cells, as shown in the simulations. A description of the operation and properties of competitive networks, together with demonstration simulation software, is provided with this book (see Appendices B and D). The fully connected 2-layer lateral entorhinal cortex (LEC) / hippocampal model has the architecture of a competitive network. There is an input layer of 6 LEC temporal cell populations (S1 and S2 from Nets 1–3) with feedforward associatively modifiable synaptic connections onto an output layer of 20 hippocampal cells (Fig. 9.26).

9.3.4.3 Operation of the entorhinal-hippocampal time generation network

Fig. 9.27a shows a simulation of the lateral entorhinal cortex model with an intermediate value for the time constant of the synaptic adaptation set by fD=0.99960 for Net 2. The firing rates in Nets 1–3 are shown, and within each network, the firing rates of the population of neurons in S1 and S2 are shown. For Net 1, the value of fD=0.99972, producing a longer time constant for the synaptic depression and longer cycle times for the firing of Net 1. For Net 3, the value of fD=0.99800, producing a shorter time constant for the synaptic depression and shorter cycle times for the firing of Net 3.

Fig. 9.27b shows the firing of the hippocampal (e.g. CA1) neurons in the same simulation. The hippocampal neurons have been sorted so that the neuron that fires first in the sequence is in the top row. Each vertical yellow line represents firing by a hippocampal neuron. The first 100 s of the simulation is shown.

Fig. 9.27c shows the simulation of the firing of the hippocampal (e.g. CA1) neurons as illustrated in Fig. 9.27b, but now for the full 1000 s of the simulation. An interesting point emerges, that the hippocampal neurons come back into activity again later on. This is also found by neurons recorded in the lateral entorhinal cortex (Tsao, Sugar, Lu, Wang, Knierim, Moser and Moser, 2018). However, Fig. 9.27c also shows that a reasonable approximation of the 120 s sequence repeats later on in the time period of 1000 s. This is evidence that the whole system is generating a time signature that is reasonably stable over the whole 1000 s time period, in that components of the sequence are replayed later on in time. This 'replay' is more evident in the simulations for shorter time periods described by Rolls and Mills (2019).

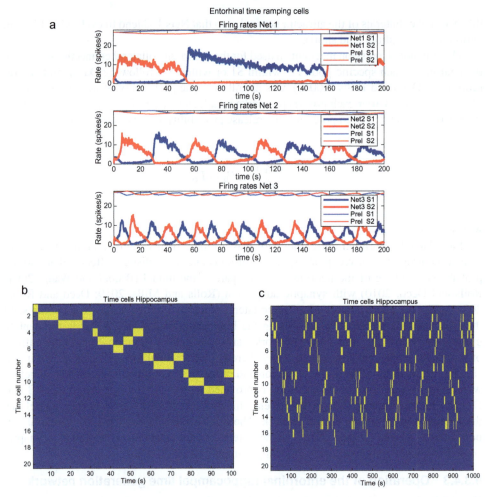

Fig. 9.27 The generation of time in the hippocampal memory system. Simulation of the model with a long value for the time constant set by fD=0.99960 for Net 2. a. The firing rates in Nets 1–3 are shown, and within each network, the firing rates of the population of neurons in S1 and S2 are shown. In addition the value of the variable P_{rel} for pools S1 and S2 is shown, scaled so that a value of $P_{rel}=1$ is shown as 30 on the y axis. For Net 1, the value of fD=0.99972, producing a longer time constant for the synaptic depression and longer cycle times for the firing of Net 1. For Net 3, the value of fD=0.99800, producing a shorter time constant for the synaptic depression and shorter cycle times for the firing of Net 3. The first 200 s period of a 600 s simulation in which similar firing continued is shown. b,c. The firing of the hippocampal neurons in the same simulation. The hippocampal neurons have been sorted so that the neuron that fires first in the sequence is in the top row. Each vertical yellow line represents firing by a hippocampal neuron. The first 100 s of the simulation is shown in (b), and the full 1000 s of the simulation is in (c). The whole 1000 s of the simulation shows that although the neurons may be synchronised to be in a particular order at the start of the simulation (or potentially by an external event), the neurons have further time-ordered bursts of firing later in time. (From Rolls, E. T. and Mills,P. (2019) The generation of time in the hippocampal memory system. Cell Reports 28: 1649–1658.)

9.3.4.4 Forward and reverse replay of temporal sequences by the time generation system

To investigate whether the forward and reverse replay illustrated in Fig. 9.27 is a robust emergent property of this neuronal architecture, we ran the same competitive network simulations, but for the lateral entorhinal cortex replaced the firing of the integrate-and-fire neurons with precisely generated waveforms, for example square waves as shown in Fig. 9.28a (Rolls and Mills, 2019). An example of the perfect play and reverse replay that resulted is shown in Fig. 9.28b.

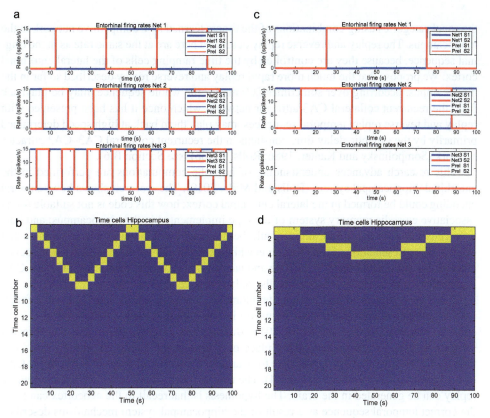

Fig. 9.28 The generation of time in the hippocampal memory system. Simulations to show how replay and reverse replay can be generated. a. Simulated square waves for the lateral entorhinal cortex for Nets 1–3, with a frequency of 2 for Net 1, 4 for Net 2, and 8 for Net 3. b. The hippocampal neurons produced by the lateral entorhinal cortex firing in (a) have been sorted so that the neuron that fires first in the sequence is in the top row. Each vertical yellow line represents firing by a hippocampal neuron. After the initial sequence in which 8 neurons come into successive firing, from 0–25 s, there is a period of reverse replay from 25–50 s. This is followed by a repetition of the initial forward sequence from 50–75 s; and this is followed by reverse replay of the sequence from 75–100 s. c. Simulated square waves for the lateral entorhinal cortex for Nets 1–2, with a frequency of 1 for Net 1, 2 for Net 2, and no firing for Net 3. d. The hippocampal neurons produced by the lateral entorhinal cortex firing in (c) have been sorted so that the neuron that fires first in the sequence is in the top row. After the initial sequence in which 4 neurons come into successive firing, from 0–50 s, there is a period of reverse replay from 50–100 s. (From Rolls, E. T. and Mills,P. (2019) The generation of time in the hippocampal memory system. Cell Reports 28: 1649–1658.)

We explained the mechanism using Fig. 9.28c, d with a simplified system in which only Nets 1 and 2 of the entorhinal cortex are active (Fig. 9.28c). Fig. 9.28d shows that Neuron 1 had learned to respond to the combination of Net 1 population S1 firing, and Net 2 population S1 firing. Neuron 2 had learned to respond to Net 1 S1 and Net 2 S2. Neuron 3 had learned to respond to Net 1 S2 and Net 2 S2. Neuron 4 had learned to respond to Net 1 S2 and Net 2 S1. It is now possible to see that these combinations of firing in Nets 1 and 2 then occur in reverse sequence, generating the reverse replay in the hippocampal neurons. Only four neurons are needed to encode the combinations of firing in Nets 1 and 2, and no other hippocampal neurons have learned to respond, because this is a competitive network (see Section B.4).

This provides a computational account for the frequently studied and observed 'reverse replay' recorded from hippocampal neurons in rodents (Foster and Wilson, 2006; Foster, 2017; Berners-Lee, Feng, Silva, Wu, Ambrose, Pfeiffer and Foster, 2022). The account provided here is that 'reverse replay' may be a simple or mechanistic but emergent property of a set of coupled timers of the type found in the lateral entorhinal cortex which is then recoded into orthogonal categories using combinations of the timers learned by a competitive network in the hippocampus. The replay and reverse replay described here are at the same rate as in the original sequence, because they are controlled by the time ramping cells of the lateral entorhinal cortex. We propose that the much more rapid replay and reverse replay described so far in the hippocampus, occurring over sometimes 200 ms for the whole sequence, may be playback from the recurrent collateral CA3 attractor network, which once it has been presented with replay and reverse replay temporal sequences, may play them back at high speed determined primarily by the synaptic delay time constants in the recurrent collateral CA3–CA3 attractor network (Sompolinsky and Kanter, 1986; Rolls, 2016b) (see Section B.6).

This research advances understanding of how the computations are performed in the entorhinal–hippocampal system (Rolls and Mills, 2019). The research shows how temporal encoding could be formed in the lateral entorhinal cortex; how this code is not suitable for an associative episodic memory system of the type implemented in the hippocampus; and how time cells found in the hippocampus could be produced, with an appropriately sparse and orthogonal representation of time for use in a hippocampal memory system that can associate place and/or time with objects to encode and later retrieve episodic memories, in which CA1 is especially implicated (Kesner and Rolls, 2015) (see Section 9.3.7.4).

It has been suggested that learning temporal sequences of events is an important function of the hippocampus which may be useful in remembering the sequence of events in an episodic memory (Kesner and Rolls, 2015; Buzsaki and Tingley, 2018), and this research shows how synaptic adaptation taking place over time in the lateral entorhinal cortex can then lead to neurons that are appropriate for learning temporal sequences in for example CA1 of the hippocampus (see Section 9.3.7.4). The research also shows how forward and reverse replay can be generated in the brain. The hypothesis is that recall to the neocortex can be in the correct temporal sequence as a result of the hippocampal system mechanisms described here, using the hippocampal to neocortical backprojection system described in Section 9.3.8. The reverse replay described may be a mechanistic consequence of the way in which the memory of temporal sequences is implemented in the brain. Whether the fast reverse replay observed neurophysiologically performs a useful function such as the transfer of information to the neocortex for consolidation (Foster and Wilson, 2006; Foster, 2017; Berners-Lee et al., 2022) is an open issue in the light of the mechanisms described here that generate it as a side effect. Alternative mechanisms that are likely to be involved in memory consolidation are described in Section 9.2.8.5 (Rolls, 2022b).

Part of the interest of this computational approach to how time cells are formed in the hippocampus by competitive learning of inputs from the lateral entorhinal cortex, is that the mechanism is very similar to that involved in transforming medial entorhinal cortex grid cells into dentate and hippocampal place cells. This probably reflects reuse of the same computational mechanism to perform computations using different types of input, and is an example of how evolution often works by reusing similar neural operations to perform different functions and computations (Rolls, 2016b).

9.3.5 CA3 as an autoassociation memory

9.3.5.1 Arbitrary associations, and pattern completion in recall

CA3 recurrent collaterals form a single attractor network

The architecture of the CA3 neurons is shown in Figs. 9.2 and 9.21. There is a highly developed CA3 to CA3 recurrent collateral system forming a single network (see Section 9.3.2).

Moreover, many of the synapses in the hippocampus show associative modification as shown by long-term potentiation, and this synaptic modification appears to be involved in

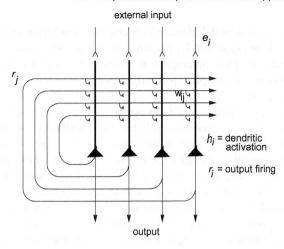

Fig. 9.29 The architecture of an attractor or autoassociation neural network. The architecture of a discrete attractor neural network used for storing discrete patterns is the same as that of a continuous attractor neural network (CANN) used for storing continuous, e.g. spatial, patterns (see further Sections B.3 and B.5).

learning (Morris, 2003, 1989; Morris et al., 2003; Lynch, 2004; Nakazawa et al., 2003, 2004; Andersen et al., 2007; Wang and Morris, 2010; Jackson, 2013; Siegelbaum and Kandel, 2013; Takeuchi et al., 2014) (Section 1.6). On the basis of the evidence summarized above, Rolls has proposed that the CA3 stage acts as an autoassociation memory that enables episodic memories to be formed and stored in the CA3 network, and that subsequently the extensive recurrent collateral connectivity allows for the retrieval of a whole representation to be initiated by the activation of some small part of the same representation (the cue) (Rolls, 1987, 1989a, 1990b, 1989f, 1990a,b). The crucial synaptic modification for this is in the recurrent collateral synapses. (A description of the operation of autoassociative networks is provided in Section B.3 and by Hertz et al. (1991) and Rolls and Treves (1998). The architecture of an autoassociation network is shown in Fig. 9.29.)

Rolls' theory presented at the Dahlem conference in 1985 (Rolls, 1987) is that because the CA3 operates effectively as a single network because of its long-range recurrent collaterals that extend throughout the CA3 region, it can allow arbitrary associations between inputs originating from very different parts of the cerebral neocortex to be formed (Rolls, 1987, 1989a, 1990b, 1989f, 1990a,b). These might involve associations between information originating in the temporal visual cortex about the presence of an object, and information originating in the parietal cortex about where it is. I note that although there is some spatial gradient in the CA3 recurrent connections, so that the connectivity is not fully uniform (Ishizuka et al., 1990; Witter, 2007), nevertheless the network will still have the properties of a single interconnected autoassociation network allowing associations between arbitrary neurons to be formed, given the presence of many long-range connections which overlap from different CA3 cells. It is very interesting indeed that in primates (macaques), the associational projections from CA3 to CA3 travel extensively along the longitudinal axis, and overall the radial, transverse, and longitudinal gradients of CA3 fiber distribution, clear in the rat, are much more subtle in the nonhuman primate brain (Kondo, Lavenex and Amaral, 2009). The implication is that in primates, the CA3 network operates even more as a single network than in rodents.

The autoassociation or attractor memory is different from pattern association memory, in which a visual stimulus might become associated with a taste by associative synaptic modification. Later presentation of the visual stimulus would retrieve the taste representation. However, presentation of the taste would not retrieve the visual representation, and this is an important and fundamental difference between autoassociation and pattern association, as described in detail in Appendix B. Pattern association memories generalize, and autoassociation memories complete incomplete representations. Further, competitive networks can generalize, but may not complete perfectly depending on what input is being clamped into the network (Appendix B).

Tests of the attractor hypothesis of CA3 operation based on the effects of CA3 lesions or CA3 NMDA knockouts on pattern completion are described in Section 9.4 (Kesner and Rolls, 2015). Another type of test of the autoassociation (or attractor) hypothesis for CA3 has been to train rats in different environments, e.g. a square and a circular environment, and then test the prediction of the hypothesis that when presented with an environment ambiguous between these, hippocampal neurons will fall into an attractor state that represents one of the two previously learned environments, but not a mixture of the two environments. Evidence consistent with the hypothesis has been found (Wills, Lever, Cacucci, Burgess and O'Keefe, 2005). In a particularly dramatic example, it has been found that within each theta cycle, hippocampal pyramidal neurons may represent one or other of the learned environments (Jezek, Henriksen, Treves, Moser and Moser, 2011). This was measured by recording in an ambiguous environment, in which it was found that the CA3 representation 'flickered' between two possible environments. This is an indication, predicted by Rolls and Treves (1998) (page 118), that autoassociative memory recall can take place sufficiently rapidly to be complete within one theta cycle (120 ms), and that theta cycles could provide a mechanism for a fresh retrieval process to occur after a reset caused by the inhibitory part of each theta cycle, so that the memory can be updated rapidly to reflect a continuously changing environment, and not remain too long in an attractor state.

Storage capacity

We have performed quantitative analyses of the storage and retrieval processes in the CA3 network (Treves and Rolls, 1991, 1992). We have extended previous formal models of autoassociative memory (Amit, 1989) by analyzing a network with graded response neurons, so as to represent more realistically the continuously variable rates at which neurons fire, and with incomplete connectivity (Treves, 1990; Treves and Rolls, 1991). We have found that in general the maximum number $p_{\max}$ of firing patterns that can be (individually) retrieved is proportional to the number C^{RC} of (associatively) modifiable recurrent collateral synapses per neuron, by a factor that increases roughly with the inverse of the population sparseness a^p of the neuronal representation. The sparseness a^p of the representation can be measured, by extending the binary notion of the proportion of neurons that are firing, as

$$a^p = \frac{(\sum_{i=1}^{N} y_i/N)^2}{\sum_{i=1}^{N} y_i^2/N} \qquad (9.2)$$

where y_i is the firing rate of the ith neuron in the set of N neurons (Treves and Rolls, 1991; Rolls and Treves, 1998; Rolls and Deco, 2002; Franco, Rolls, Aggelopoulos and Jerez, 2007). More precisely, Treves and Rolls (1991) and Rolls, Treves, Foster and Perez-Vicente (1997c) have shown that such a network with graded patterns does operate efficiently as an autoassociative network, and can store (and recall correctly) a number of different patterns p as follows

$$p \approx \frac{C^{RC}}{a^p \ln(\frac{1}{a^p})} k \qquad (9.3)$$

where C^{RC} is the number of synapses on the dendrites of each neuron devoted to the recurrent collaterals from other neurons in the network, and k is a factor that depends weakly on the detailed structure of the rate distribution, on the connectivity pattern, etc., but is roughly in the order of 0.2–0.3. For example, for $C^{RC} = 12{,}000$ and $a^p = 0.02$ (realistic estimates for the rat), p_{max} is calculated to be approximately 36,000. This analysis emphasizes the utility of having a sparse representation in the hippocampus, for this enables many different memories to be stored. Third, in order for most associative networks to store information efficiently, heterosynaptic long term depression (Fazeli and Collingridge, 1996) (as well as LTP) is required (Rolls and Treves, 1990; Treves and Rolls, 1991) (see Section B.3). Simulations that are fully consistent with the analytic theory are provided by Simmen, Treves and Rolls (1996b) and Rolls, Treves, Foster and Perez-Vicente (1997c).

We have also indicated how to estimate I, the total amount of information (in bits per synapse) that can be retrieved from the network. (Information theory applied to what is represented in the brain is described in Appendix C.) I is defined with respect to the information i_p (in bits per cell) contained in each stored firing pattern, by subtracting the amount i_1 lost in retrieval and multiplying by p/C^{RC}:

$$I \approx \frac{p}{C^{RC}}(i_p - i_1) \tag{9.4}$$

The maximal value I_{max} of this quantity was found (Treves and Rolls, 1991) to be in several interesting cases around 0.2–0.3 bits per synapse, with only a mild dependency on parameters such as the sparseness of coding a^p.

We may then estimate (Treves and Rolls, 1992) how much information has to be stored in each pattern for the network to efficiently exploit its information retrieval capacity I_{max}. The estimate is expressed as a requirement on i_p:

$$i_p > a^p \ln(\frac{1}{a^p}) \tag{9.5}$$

As the information content i_p of each stored pattern depends on the storage process, we see how the retrieval capacity analysis, coupled with the notion that the system is organized so as to be an efficient memory device in a quantitative sense, leads to a constraint on the storage process.

A number of points deserve comment. First, if it is stated that a certain number of memories is the upper limit of what could be stored in a given network, then the question is sometimes asked, what constitutes a memory? The answer is precise (Section B.3). Any one memory is represented by the firing rates of the population of neurons that are stored by the associative synaptic modification, and can be correctly recalled later. The firing rates in the primate hippocampus might be constant for a period of for example 1 s in which the monkey was looking at an object in one position in space; synaptic modification would occur in this time period (cf. the time course of LTP, which is sufficiently rapid for this); and the memory of the event would have been stored. The quantitative analysis shows how many such random patterns of rates of the neuronal population can be stored and later recalled correctly. If the rates were constant for 5 s while the rat was at one place or the monkey was looking at an object at one position in space, then the memory would be for the pattern of firing of the neurons in this 5-s period. (The pattern of firing of the population refers to the rate at which each neuron in the population of CA3 neurons is firing.)

Second, the question sometimes arises of whether the CA3 neurons operate as an attractor network. An attractor network is one in which a stable pattern of firing is maintained once it has been started. Autoassociation networks trained with modified Hebb rules can store the number of different memories, each one expressed as a stable attractor, indicated in Equation

B.15. However, the hippocampal CA3 cells do not necessarily have to operate as a stable attractor: instead, it would be sufficient for the present theory if they can retrieve stored information in response to a partial cue initiating retrieval. The partial cue would remain on during recall, so that the attractor network would be operating in the clamped condition (Rolls and Treves, 1998) (see Section B.3). The completion of the partial pattern would then provide more information than entered the hippocampus, and the extra information retrieved would help the next stage to operate. Demonstrations of this by simulations that are fully consistent with the analytic theory are provided by Rolls (1995b), Simmen, Treves and Rolls (1996b), and Rolls, Treves, Foster and Perez-Vicente (1997c).

Third, in order for most associative networks to store information efficiently, heterosynaptic long term depression (as well as LTP) is required (Rolls and Treves, 1990; Treves and Rolls, 1991; Rolls, 1996c). Without heterosynaptic LTD, there would otherwise always be a correlation between any set of positively firing inputs acting as the input pattern vector to a neuron. LTD effectively enables the average firing of each input axon to be subtracted from its input at any one time, reducing the average correlation between different pattern vectors to be stored to a low value (Rolls, 1996c) (see Section B.3).

Fourth, the firing of CA3 cells is relatively sparse, and this helps to decorrelate different population vectors of CA3 cell firing for different memories (Rolls, 2013c,b). (Sparse representations are more likely to be decorrelated with each other (Appendices B and C).) Evidence on the sparseness of the CA3 cell representation in rats includes evidence that CA3 cell ensembles may support the fast acquisition of detailed memories by providing a locally continuous, but globally orthogonal spatial representation, onto which new sensory inputs can rapidly be associated (Leutgeb and Leutgeb, 2007). In the macaque hippocampus, in which spatial view cells are found, for the representation of 64 locations around the walls of the room, the mean single cell sparseness a^s was 0.34, and the mean population sparseness a^p was 0.33 (Rolls, Treves, Robertson, Georges-François and Panzeri, 1998b; Rolls and Treves, 2011). For comparison, the corresponding values for macaque inferior temporal cortex neurons tuned to objects and faces were 0.77 (Franco, Rolls, Aggelopoulos and Jerez, 2007; Rolls and Treves, 2011); for taste and oral texture neurons in the insular cortex the population sparseness was 0.71; for taste and oral texture neurons in the orbitofrontal cortex was 0.61; and for taste and oral texture neurons in the amygdala was 0.81 (Rolls and Treves, 2011). Thus the evidence is that the hippocampal CA3 / pyramidal cell representation is more sparse in macaques than in neocortical areas and the amygdala, and this is consistent with the importance in hippocampal CA3 of using a sparse representation to produce a large memory capacity. Although the value of a for the sparseness of the representation does not seem especially low, it must be remembered that these are graded firing rate representations, and the graded nature appears to increase the value of a (Rolls and Treves, 2011). Moreover, these values were obtained in just one spatial environment, and if measured over many spatial environments, might be more sparse. A further analysis of how to interpret these sparseness measures is provided in Section C.3.1.1, and their potential utility in better understanding hippocampal representations in humans is described by Rolls (2023d).

Fifth, given that the memory capacity of the hippocampal CA3 system is limited, it is necessary to have some form of forgetting in this store, or another mechanism, to ensure that its capacity is not exceeded. (Exceeding the capacity can lead to a loss of much of the information retrievable from the network.) Heterosynaptic LTD could help this forgetting, by enabling new memories to overwrite old memories (Rolls, 1996c) (see Section B.19). The limited capacity of the CA3 system does also provide one of the arguments that some transfer of information from the hippocampus to neocortical memory stores may be useful (see Treves and Rolls (1994)). Given its limited capacity, the hippocampus might be a useful store for only a limited period, which might be in the order of days, weeks, or months. This period may well depend on the acquisition rate of new episodic memories. If the animal were in a constant and limited environment, then as new information is not being added to the hippocampus, the representations in the hippocampus would remain stable and persistent. These hypotheses have clear experimental implications, both for recordings from single neurons and for the gradient of retrograde amnesia, both of which might be expected to depend on whether the environment is stable or frequently changing. They show that the conditions under which a gradient of retrograde amnesia might be demonstrable would be when large numbers of new memories are being acquired, not when only a few memories (few in the case of the hippocampus being less than a few hundred) are being learned.

The potential link to the gradient of retrograde amnesia is that the retrograde memories lost in amnesia are those not yet consolidated in longer term storage (in the neocortex). As they are still held in the hippocampus, their number has to be less than the storage capacity of the (presumed) CA3 autoassociative memory. Therefore the time gradient of the amnesia provides not only a measure of a characteristic time for consolidation, but also an upper bound on the rate of storage of new memories in CA3. For example, if one were to take as a measure of the time gradient in the monkey, say, 5 weeks (about 50,000 min) (Squire, 1992) and as a reasonable estimate of the capacity of CA3 in the monkey e.g $p = 50,000$, then one would conclude that there is an upper bound on the rate of storage in CA3 of not more than one new memory per minute, on average. (This might be an average over many weeks; the fastest rate might be closer to 1 per s, see Treves and Rolls (1994).) These quantitative considerations are consistent with the concept described in Section 9.2.3 that retrieval of episodic memories from the hippocampus for a considerable time after they have been stored would be useful in helping the neocortex to build a semantic memory (Rolls, 1990a, 1989f, 1990b,a; Treves and Rolls, 1994; Moscovitch et al., 2005; McClelland et al., 1995; Rolls, 2022b).

Recall and Completion

A fundamental property of the autoassociation model of the CA3 recurrent collateral network is that the recall can be symmetric, that is, the whole of the memory can be retrieved from any part. For example, in an object–place autoassociation memory, an object could be recalled from a place retrieval cue, and vice versa. This is not the case with a pattern association network. If for example the CA3 activity represented a place / spatial view, and perforant path inputs with associative synapses to CA3 neurons carried object information (consistent with evidence that the lateral perforant path (LPP) may reflect inputs from the perirhinal cortex connecting via the lateral entorhinal cortex (Hargreaves et al., 2005)), then an object could recall a place, but a place could not recall an object.

Another fundamental property is that the recall can be complete even from a small fragment. Thus, it is a prediction that when an incomplete retrieval cue is given, CA3 may be especially important in the retrieval process. Tests of this prediction are described in Section 9.4. Further evidence for pattern completion has been observed using imaging with voltage-sensitive dye in the CA3 region of a rat hippocampal slice. Following the induction of long-term potentiation from two stimulation sites activated simultaneously, stimulation at either of the two sites produced the whole pattern of activation that could be produced from both stimulation sites before LTP, thus demonstrating pattern completion in CA3 (Jackson, 2013).

CA3 as a short term attractor memory

Another fundamental property of the autoassociation model of the CA3 recurrent collateral network is that it can implement a short-term memory by maintaining the firing of neurons using the excitatory recurrent collateral connections. A stable attractor can maintain one memory active in this way for a considerable period, until a new input pushes the attractor to represent a new location or memory (see Section B.3). For example, if one place were being held in a CA3 place short-term memory, then if the rat moved to a new place, the CA3 representation would move to represent the new place, and the short-term memory held in the CA3 network would be lost. It is thus predicted that when the hippocampus is used as a short-term memory with ongoing neuronal activity used to represent the short-term memory, then maintenance of the memory will be very dependent on what happens in the delay period. If the animal is relatively isolated from its environment and does not move around in a well-defined spatial environment (as can be achieved by placing a vertical cylinder / bucket around a rat in the delay period), then the memory may be maintained for a considerable period in the CA3 (and even updated by idiothetic, self-motion, inputs as described below). However, the CA3 short-term memory will be very sensitive to disruption / interference, so that if the rat is allowed to move in the spatial environment during the delay period, then it is predicted that CA3 will not be able to maintain correctly the spatial short-term memory. In the circumstances where a representation must be kept active while the hippocampus (or inferior temporal visual cortex or parietal cortex) must be updating its representation to reflect the new changing perceptual inputs, which must be represented in these brain areas for the ongoing events to have high-level representations, the prefrontal cortex is thought computationally to provide an off-line buffer store, see Section 13.6.1.

The predictions are thus that if there is no task in a delay period (and no need for an off-line buffer store), the hippocampus may be sufficient to perform the short-term memory function (such as remembering a previous location), provided that there is little distraction in the delay period. On the other hand, short-term memory deficits are predicted to be produced by prefrontal cortex lesions if there are intervening stimuli in a delay period in a task. However, the order of items in a hippocampal episodic memory is important, and the mechanism for this is proposed to be the lateral entorhinal cortex / CA1 system that generates time cells, which can then be associated with objects or places to remember the order of the items (see Sections 9.3.4 and 9.3.7.4).

9.3.5.2 Continuous, spatial, patterns and CA3 representations: hippocampal charts

The fact that spatial patterns, which imply continuous representations of space, are represented in the hippocampus has led to the application of continuous attractor models to help understand hippocampal function. This has been necessary, because space is inherently continuous, because the firing of place and spatial view cells is approximately Gaussian as a function of the distance away from the preferred spatial location, because these cells have spatially overlapping fields, and because the theory is that these cells in CA3 are connected by Hebb-modifiable synapses. This specification would inherently lead the system to operate as a continuous attractor network. Such models have been developed with the hippocampus in mind (Samsonovich and McNaughton, 1997; Battaglia and Treves, 1998b; Rolls, Stringer and Trappenberg, 2002; Stringer, Trappenberg, Rolls and De Araujo, 2002b; Stringer, Rolls, Trappenberg and De Araujo, 2002a; Stringer and Rolls, 2002; Stringer, Rolls and Trappenberg, 2004, 2005; Stringer and Rolls, 2006) and are described next (see for detailed description Section B.5).

A class of network that can maintain the firing of its neurons to represent any location along a continuous physical dimension such as spatial position, head direction, etc. is a 'continuous attractor' neural network (CANN). It uses excitatory recurrent collateral connections between the neurons (as are present in CA3) to reflect the distance between the neurons in the state space of the animal (e.g. place or head direction). These networks can maintain the bubble of neural activity constant for long periods wherever it is started to represent the current state (head direction, position, etc) of the animal, and are likely to be involved in many aspects

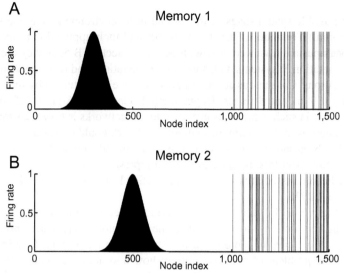

Fig. 9.30 An attractor network can associate continuous spatial patterns with discrete sets of neurons firing to represent for example objects. This provides a basis for the hippocampal CA3 network to associate spatial locations with objects or people. The types of firing patterns stored in continuous attractor networks are illustrated for the patterns present on neurons 1–1,000 for Memory 1 (when the firing is that produced when the spatial state represented is that for location 300), and for Memory 2 (when the firing is that produced when the spatial state represented is that for location 500). The continuous nature of the spatial representation results from the fact that each neuron has a Gaussian firing rate that peaks at its optimal location. This particular mixed network also contains discrete representations that consist of discrete subsets of active binary firing rate neurons in the range 1,001–1,500. The firing of these latter neurons can be thought of as representing the discrete events that occur at the location. Continuous attractor networks by definition contain only continuous representations, but this particular network can store mixed continuous and discrete representations, and is illustrated to show the difference of the firing patterns normally stored in separate continuous attractor and discrete attractor networks. For this particular mixed network, during learning, Memory 1 is stored in the synaptic weights, then Memory 2, etc, and each memory contains a part that is continuously distributed to represent physical space, and a part that represents a discrete event or object. (After Rolls, E. T., Stringer,S.M. and Trappenberg,T.P. (2002) A unified model of spatial and episodic memory. Proceedings of the Royal Society B 269: 1087–1093. © The Royal Society.)

of spatial processing and memory, including spatial vision. Global inhibition is used to keep the number of neurons in a bubble or packet of actively firing neurons relatively constant, and to help to ensure that there is only one activity packet. Continuous attractor networks can be thought of as very similar to autoassociation or discrete attractor networks (see Appendix B), and have the same architecture, as illustrated in Fig. 9.29. The main difference is that the patterns stored in a CANN are continuous patterns, with each neuron having broadly tuned firing which decreases with for example a Gaussian function as the distance from the optimal firing location of the cell is varied, and with different neurons having tuning that overlaps throughout the space. Such tuning is illustrated in Fig. 9.30. For comparison, autoassociation networks normally have discrete (separate) patterns (each pattern implemented by the firing of a particular subset of the neurons), with no continuous distribution of the patterns throughout the space (see Fig. 9.30). A consequent difference is that the CANN can maintain its firing at any location in the trained continuous space, whereas a discrete attractor or autoassociation network moves its population of active neurons towards one of the previously learned attractor states, and thus implements the recall of a particular previously learned pattern from an incomplete or noisy (distorted) version of one of the previously learned patterns. The energy landscape of a discrete attractor network (see Section B.3, Hopfield (1982)) has separate energy minima, each one of which corresponds to a learned pattern, whereas the energy landscape of a continuous attractor network is flat, so that the activity packet remains stable with continuous firing wherever it is started in the state space. (The state space refers to the set of possible spatial states of the animal in its environment, e.g. the set of possible places in a room.) Continuous attractor networks and their application to memory systems in the hippocampus are reviewed next with details in Section B.5, as they are very likely to apply to the operation of systems with spatial representations and recurrent connections, such as the CA3 neurons. Continuous attractor networks have been studied by for example Amari (1977), Zhang (1996), and Stringer, Trappenberg, Rolls and De Araujo (2002b).

One key issue in such continuous attractor neural networks is how the synaptic strengths between the neurons in the continuous attractor network could be learned in biological systems, and it has been shown that associative synaptic modification while navigating the environment can implement this, because the spatial representations of nearby locations overlap and therefore become associatively linked (see Section B.5.3 and Stringer, Trappenberg, Rolls and De Araujo (2002b)).

A second key issue in such continuous attractor neural networks is how the bubble of neuronal firing representing one location in the continuous state space should be updated based on non-visual cues to represent a new location in state space (Section B.5.5). This is essentially the problem of path integration: how a system that represents a memory of where the agent is in physical space could be updated based on idiothetic (self-motion) cues such as vestibular cues (which might represent a head velocity signal), or proprioceptive cues (which might update a representation of place based on movements being made in the space, during for example walking in the dark). Examples of classes of neurons that can be updated idiothetically include head direction cells in rats (Muller et al., 1996; Ranck, 1985; Taube et al., 1996, 1990a; Bassett and Taube, 2005) and primates (Robertson, Rolls, Georges-François and Panzeri, 1999), which respond maximally when the animal's head is facing in a preferred direction and can be updated by head rotation in the dark; place cells in rats (O'Keefe, 1984; Markus et al., 1995; O'Keefe and Dostrovsky, 1971; McNaughton et al., 1983; Muller et al., 1991; Jeffery and Hayman, 2004; Jeffery et al., 2004) that fire maximally when the animal is in a particular location and can be updated by running in a particular direction in the dark; and spatial view cells in primates that respond when the monkey is looking towards a particular location in space (Georges-François, Rolls and Robertson, 1999; Robertson, Rolls and Georges-François, 1998; Rolls, Robertson and Georges-François, 1997a; Rolls, Treves, Robertson, Georges-François and Panzeri, 1998b; Rolls, 2023c) and can be updated by eye movements in the dark (Robertson, Rolls and Georges-François, 1998).

Path integration is described in Section B.5.5, using as an example the update of a head direction representation by a head velocity signal. For example, a proposal about how the synaptic connections from idiothetic inputs to a continuous attractor network can be learned with some biological plausibility, in that the network can be trained by a self-organizing process, was introduced by Stringer, Trappenberg, Rolls and De Araujo (2002b). The mechanism associates a short-term memory trace of the firing of the neurons in the attractor network reflecting recent movements in the state space (e.g. of places), with an idiothetic velocity of movement input (see Fig. B.28). This has been applied to head direction cells (Stringer, Trappenberg, Rolls and De Araujo, 2002b; Stringer and Rolls, 2006), rat place cells (Stringer, Trappenberg, Rolls and De Araujo, 2002b; Stringer, Rolls, Trappenberg and De Araujo, 2002a), and primate spatial view cells (Stringer, Rolls and Trappenberg, 2004, 2005; Rolls and Stringer, 2005). These attractor networks provide a basis for understanding cognitive maps, and how they are updated by learning and by self-motion. The implication is that to the extent that path integration of place or spatial view representations is performed within the hippocampus itself, then the CA3 system is the most likely part of the hippocampus to be involved in this, because it has the appropriate recurrent collateral connections. Consistent with this, Whishaw and colleagues (Wallace and Whishaw, 2003; Maaswinkel et al., 1999; Whishaw et al., 2001) have shown that path integration is impaired by hippocampal lesions.

Part of the neural mechanism for the updating of place by path integration may be in the entorhinal cortex (McNaughton, Battaglia, Jensen, Moser and Moser, 2006; Soldatkina, Schonsberg and Treves, 2022) (see Section 9.3.3). Head direction cells are present in the entorhinal cortex, where grid cells (see Section 9.3.6) are also present (Giocomo et al., 2011; Moser et al., 2014b, 2015), and indeed where some cells respond to combinations of grid and head direction (Leutgeb, Leutgeb, Treves, Meyer, Barnes, McNaughton, Moser and Moser, 2005b; Sargolini, Fyhn, Hafting, McNaughton, Witter, Moser and Moser, 2006). Such combination cells in the entorhinal cortex may be part of the mechanism by which the place map is kept in register with the head direction map. The rodent medial entorhinal cortex grid cells are a strong candidate for path integration over distance and direction travelled, for the repeating nature of the grid (see Section 9.3.6 for details and Fig. 9.24) is likely to be a reflection of a continuous attractor cycling once round its ring for every peak observed. The simplification this offers is that the path integration need be learned only once, as it is just an integration over self-movement, and can be used then in any environment (Soldatkina, Schonsberg and Treves, 2022). Consistent with this, grid cells are relatively little influenced by the details of the visual cues in the environment in which the rat is tested, apart from the rotation of the whole grid by the head direction cells, which can be set by the environment (Hafting, Fyhn, Molden, Moser and Moser, 2005; Fyhn, Molden, Witter, Moser and Moser, 2004; Sargolini, Fyhn, Hafting, McNaughton, Witter, Moser and Moser, 2006).Thus path integration for place may be performed by grid cells in the rodent entorhinal cortex (Giocomo et al., 2011; Moser et al., 2015; Kropff and Treves, 2008; Zilli, 2012; Moser et al., 2014b,a; Soldatkina et al., 2022).

The summary of path integration in the context of grid cells provided by McNaughton et al. (2006) was not self-organizing, that is, the appropriate synaptic strengths for the model to perform the path integration did not become specified as a result of movements in the environment. Self-organizing continuous attractor neural networks that can perform path integration from velocity signals are described in Section B.5.5 and include head direction from head velocity (Stringer, Trappenberg, Rolls and De Araujo, 2002b; Stringer and Rolls, 2006); place from whole body motion (Stringer, Trappenberg, Rolls and De Araujo, 2002b; Stringer, Rolls, Trappenberg and De Araujo, 2002a); and spatial view from eye and whole body motion (Stringer, Rolls and Trappenberg, 2004, 2005; Rolls and Stringer, 2005). Models such as these provide a basis for understanding the principles of operation of medial entorhinal cortex grid cells (Giocomo, Moser and Moser, 2011; Moser, Rowland and Moser, 2015; Kropff and Treves, 2008; Moser, Roudi, Witter, Kentros, Bonhoeffer and Moser, 2014b; Moser, Moser and Roudi, 2014a; Soldatkina, Schonsberg and Treves, 2022).

This leaves open the question of where idiothetic update is performed for where one is looking in space. Is this in the primate medial entorhinal cortex, where spatial view grid cells are found (Killian, Jutras and Buffalo, 2012; Meister and Buffalo, 2018; Garcia and Buffalo, 2020)? The evidence described in Section 3.4 indicates that the dorsal visual stream leading into the parietal cortex area 7a performs much of the self-motion update for visual spatial representations, by using the different mechanism of gain modulation (Rolls, 2020b).

A third key issue is how stability in the bubble of activity representing the current location can be maintained without much drift in darkness, when it is operating as a memory system. A solution is described in Section B.5.6 (Stringer, Trappenberg, Rolls and De Araujo, 2002b).

A fourth key issue is considered in Section B.5.8 in which networks are described that store both continuous patterns and discrete patterns (see Fig. 9.30). These networks can be used to store for example the location in (continuous, physical) space where an object (an item with a discrete representation) is present (Rolls, Stringer and Trappenberg, 2002). *This type of mixed attractor in which discrete representations of objects and continuous representations of space can be combined is important for understanding the operation of the CA3 region of the hippocampus in episodic memory, in which discrete object and continuous spatial representations must be combined.*

A fifth key issue is the capacity of a continuous attractor network for storing many different environments each with many places. It turns out that the capacity is high, for each environment has its own chart of connected set of places, and the charts for different environments are quite uncorrelated with each other (Battaglia and Treves, 1998b) (Section B.5.4). Although the capacity of a continuous attractor network for charts is high, because each chart is relatively uncorrelated with other charts, the capacity is nevertheless more than 100 times lower than for the number of discrete items that can be stored in an attractor network such as CA3 in the hippocampus (Battaglia and Treves, 1998b; Treves, 2016). The smaller number of charts or maps than discrete items is related to a reduction of approximately 0.3 caused by changing from discrete to continuous, spatial, representations; and to the fact that each chart includes many places (Treves, 2016; Papp and Treves, 2008; Cerasti and Treves, 2013; Soldatkina, Schonsberg and Treves, 2022). But that might still mean in the order of 100 charts in the rat hippocampus (Soldatkina et al., 2022).

Continuous attractor networks provide a way to understand spatial maps and charts. The topology of a 2D space through which trajectories have been followed is represented by the connection strengths between neurons, which are high if the neurons are often coactive because they are close together in a space (Stringer, Rolls, Trappenberg and De Araujo, 2002a; Stringer, Rolls and Trappenberg, 2004, 2005; Rolls and Stringer, 2005). In this situation, *remapping* of hippocampal neurons (Schlesiger, Boublil, Hales, Leutgeb and Leutgeb, 2018) occurs mainly when the spatial topology of the test environment is changed, for then the continuous attractor network that forms the map or chart (Battaglia and Treves, 1998b) breaks because the synaptic links formed by coactive firing of neurons due to the closeness of the places to which they respond are no longer applicable (see Section B.5). Then remapping results in a new chart or map being formed for the new space, and after remapping a new arbitrary set of neurons learns to represent the topology of the space in a new chart. The well established concept of a 'map' or 'chart' (Samsonovich and McNaughton, 1997; Battaglia and Treves, 1998b) (also used in *The Hippocampus as a Cognitive Map* (O'Keefe and Nadel, 1978; O'Keefe, 1990)) has also had the term 'schema' applied to it (Baraduc, Duhamel and Wirth, 2019). If the map or chart remains with the same spatial topology, but changes are made that do not affect the topology such as introducing different room cues with the shape of the arena (a star maze) and the goal remaining unchanged, then no remapping need occur in the continuous attractor network map or chart, as has been found (Baraduc, Duhamel and Wirth, 2019). A continuous attractor network or chart is of course just a series of locations that overlap with each other, and thus the parsimonious interpretation of the result (Baraduc, Duhamel and Wirth, 2019) is that the topology of the spatial map or chart of the star maze and goal was not altered by substituting new room cues onto the same chart or topological space. Remapping occurs when the topology of the space is altered, for example when the shape of the arena is changed (Leutgeb, Leutgeb, Barnes, Moser, McNaughton and Moser, 2005a; Leutgeb, Leutgeb, Moser and Moser, 2006; Leutgeb and Leutgeb, 2007). The hippocampus may store in a continuous attractor network a representation of views or places as they are encountered and perhaps associated with objects and rewards and body turns in what is usually termed a chart (Samsonovich and McNaughton, 1997; Battaglia and Treves, 1998b). A schema more usually refers to a full semantic representation in neocortical semantic regions that contains all the information about the cognitive representation (for example about a territory) that may have been obtained over many particular episodes, with the hippocampus contributing because it can store information about particular episodes (Rolls, 2022b; Farzanfar, Spiers, Moscovitch and Rosenbaum, 2023).

Overall, it is argued that the CA3 region is likely to be involved in associating a relatively continuous spatial representation with an object representation as an episodic memory computation, and not with performing a continuous attractor-based idiothetic update of the spatial representation, which latter may be performed by the entorhinal cortex (Rolls, 2013c) and by the dorsal visual system (Rolls, 2020b) (Section 3.5). Consistent with this view, it has been argued that the bumpiness of the CA3 representation of space is more consistent with episodic memory storage, than with spatial path integration using the CA3 system as a continuous attractor network implementing path integration (Cerasti and Treves, 2013; Stella, Cerasti and Treves, 2013).

9.3.5.3 The dynamics of the recurrent network

The analysis described above of the capacity of a recurrent network such as the CA3 considered steady-state conditions of the firing rates of the neurons. The question arises of how quickly the recurrent network would settle into its final state. With reference to the CA3 network, how long does it take before a pattern of activity, originally evoked in CA3 by afferent inputs, becomes influenced by the activation of recurrent collaterals? In a more general context, recurrent collaterals between the pyramidal cells are an important feature of the connectivity of the cerebral neocortex. How long would it take these collaterals to contribute fully to the activity of cortical cells? If these settling processes took in the order of hundreds of ms, they would be much too slow to contribute usefully to cortical activity, whether in the hippocampus or in the neocortex (Rolls and Deco, 2002; Panzeri, Rolls, Battaglia and Lavis, 2001; Rolls, 1992a, 2003, 2016b).

It has been shown that if the neurons are treated not as McCulloch-Pitts neurons that are simply 'updated' at each iteration, or cycle of time steps (and assume the active state if the threshold is exceeded), but instead are analyzed and modelled as 'integrate-and-fire' neurons in real continuous time, then the network can effectively 'relax' into its recall state very rapidly, in one or two time constants of the synapses (Treves, 1993; Rolls and Treves, 1998; Battaglia and Treves, 1998b; Panzeri, Rolls, Battaglia and Lavis, 2001). This corresponds to perhaps 20 ms in the brain. One factor in this rapid dynamics of autoassociative networks with brain-like 'integrate-and-fire' membrane and synaptic properties is that with some spontaneous activity, some of the neurons in the network are close to threshold already before the recall cue is applied, and hence some of the neurons are very quickly pushed by the recall cue into firing, so that information starts to be exchanged very rapidly (within 1–2 ms of brain time) through the modified synapses by the neurons in the network. The progressive exchange of information starting early on within what would otherwise be thought of as an iteration period (of perhaps 20 ms, corresponding to a neuronal firing rate of 50 spikes/s), is the mechanism accounting for rapid recall in an autoassociative neuronal network made biologically realistic in this way. Further analysis of the fast dynamics of these networks if they are implemented in a biologically plausible way with 'integrate-and-fire' neurons is provided in Section B.6.4, in Appendix A5 of Rolls and Treves (1998), by Treves (1993), by Battaglia and Treves (1998b), and by Panzeri, Rolls, Battaglia and Lavis (2001).

9.3.5.4 Memory for sequences

One possibility that has been considered previously is that sequences might be stored in an attractor network such as CA3 by assuming that each 'cycle' round the recurrent collaterals might be a step in a sequential memory (Hopfield, 1982; Kleinfeld, 1986; Sompolinsky and Kanter, 1986). In practice, that does not work well, for the continuous dynamics of integrate-and-fire attractor networks results in them performing the recall in approximately 1.5 time constants of the recurrent collateral synapses, about 15 ms (Battaglia and Treves, 1998a). Moreover, such a system would be very expensive in terms of memory capacity, in that each cycle round the recurrent collateral loop on a discrete update scenario would use up one of the available memories in the network. Consideration of such systems is therefore left to Section B.3.3.10.

Probably the most likely way for the hippocampus to encode sequences to encode the order of items in a memory is to use the time cells generated in the entorhinal cortex to hippocampal system, described in Sections 9.3.4 and 9.3.7.4, and associate a particular time in the sequence with for example a place or object (Rolls and Mills, 2019). This would enable the temporal order to be recalled correctly. This system is known to act over time periods of the order of up to many hundreds of seconds. The evidence described in Section 9.3.7.4 suggests that this is implemented by the time cells in CA1.

9.3.5.5 The dilution of the CA3 recurrent collateral connectivity enhances memory storage capacity and pattern completion

Fig. 9.23 shows that in the rat, there are approximately 300,000 CA3 neurons, but only 12,000 recurrent collateral synapses per neuron. The dilution of the connectivity is thus 12,000 / 300,000 = 0.04. The connectivity is thus not complete, and complete connectivity in an autoassociation network would make it simple, for the connectivity between the neurons would then be symmetric (i.e. the connection strength from any one neuron to another is matched by a connection of the same strength in the opposite direction), and this guarantees energy minima for the basins of attraction that will be stable, and a memory capacity that can be calculated (Hopfield, 1982). We have shown how this attractor type of network can be extended to have similar properties with diluted connectivity, and also with sparse representations with graded firing rates (Treves and Rolls, 1991; Treves, 1990, 1991b; Rolls and Webb, 2012; Webb, Rolls, Deco and Feng, 2011).

However, the question has been asked about whether there are any advantages to diluted autoassociation or attractor networks compared to fully connected attractor networks (Rolls, 2012b). One biological property that may be a limiting factor is the number of synaptic connections per neuron, which is 12,000 in the CA3-CA3 network just for the recurrent collaterals (see Fig. 9.23). The number may be higher in humans, allowing more memories to be stored in the hippocampus than order 12,000. I note that the storage of a large number of memories may be facilitated in humans because the left and right hippocampus appear to be much less connected between the two hemispheres than in the rat, which effectively has a single hippocampus in that the CA3 neurons are connected by commissural connections. In humans, with effectively two separate CA3 networks, one on each side of the brain, the memory storage capacity may be doubled, as the capacity is set by the number of recurrent collaterals per neuron in each attractor network. In humans, the right hippocampus may be devoted to episodic memories with spatial and visual components, whereas the left hippocampus may be devoted to memories with verbal / linguistic components, i.e. in which words may be part of the episode (e.g. who said what to whom and when) (Amit, 1989; Bonelli et al., 2010; Sidhu et al., 2013).

The answer that has been suggested to why the connectivity of the CA3 autoassociation network is diluted (and why neocortical recurrent networks are also diluted), is that this may help to reduce the probability of having two or more synapses between any pair of randomly connected neurons within the network, which it has been shown greatly impairs the number of memories that can be stored in an attractor network, because of the distortion that this produces in the energy landscape (Rolls, 2012b) (Section B.3.4). In more detail, the hypothesis proposed is that the diluted connectivity allows biological processes that set up synaptic connections between neurons to arrange for there to be only very rarely more than one synaptic connection between any pair of neurons. If probabilistically there were more than one connection between any two neurons, it was shown by simulation of an autoassociation attractor network that such connections would dominate the attractor states into which the network could enter and be stable, thus strongly reducing the memory capacity of the network (the number of memories that can be stored and correctly retrieved), below the normal large capacity for diluted connectivity. Diluted connectivity between neurons in the cortex thus has an important role in allowing high capacity of memory networks in the cortex, and helping to ensure that the critical capacity is not reached at which overloading occurs leading to an impairment in the ability to retrieve any memories from the network (Rolls, 2012b). The diluted connectivity is thus seen as an adaptation that simplifies the genetic specification of the wiring of the brain, by enabling just two attributes of the connectivity to be specified (e.g. from a CA3 to another CA3 neuron chosen at random to specify the CA3 to CA3 recurrent collateral connectivity), rather than which particular neuron should connect to which other particular neuron (Rolls, 2012b; Rolls and Stringer, 2000). Consistent with this hypothesis, there are NMDA receptors with the genetic specification that they are NMDA receptors on neurons of a particular type, CA3 neurons (as shown by the evidence from CA3-specific vs CA1-specific NMDA receptor knockouts) (Nakazawa et al., 2002, 2003, 2004; Rondi-Reig et al., 2001). A consequence is that the vector of output neuronal firing in the CA3 region, i.e. the number of CA3 neurons, is quite large (300,000 neurons in the rat). The large number of elements in this vector may have consequences for the noise in the system, as we will see below.

The role of dilution in the connectivity of the CA3 recurrent collateral connectivity includes enabling this large number of separate memories to be recalled from any part of each memory, that is, in pattern completion (Rolls, 2012b) (Section B.3.4).

The dilution of the CA3-CA3 recurrent collateral connectivity at 0.04 may be greater dilution than that in a local neocortical area, which is in the order of 0.1 (Rolls, 2012b). This is consistent with the hypothesis that the storage capacity of the CA3 system is at a premium, and so the dilution is kept to a low value (i.e. great dilution), as then there is lower distortion of the basins of attraction and hence the memory capacity is maximized (Rolls, 2012b) (Section B.3.4).

9.3.5.6 Noise and stability produced by the diluted connectivity and the graded firing rates in the CA3-CA3 attractor network

Many processes in the brain are influenced by the noise or variability of neuronal spike firing (Rolls and Deco, 2010; Faisal, Selen and Wolpert, 2008; Deco, Rolls, Albantakis and Romo, 2013). The action potentials are generated in a way that frequently approximates a Poisson process, in which the spikes for a given mean firing rate occur at times that are essentially random (apart from a small effect of the refractory period), with a coefficient of variation of the interspike interval distribution (CV) near 1.0 (Rolls and Deco, 2010). The sources of the noise include quantal transmitter release, and noise in ion channel openings (Faisal, Selen and Wolpert, 2008). The membrane potential is often held close to the firing threshold, and then small changes in the inputs and the noise in the neuronal operations cause spikes to be emitted at almost random times for a given mean firing rate. Spiking neuronal networks with balanced inhibition and excitation currents and associatively modified recurrent synaptic connections can be shown to possess a stable attractor state where neuron spiking is approximately Poisson too (Amit and Brunel, 1997; Miller and Wang, 2006). The noise caused by the variability of individual neuron spiking which then affects other neurons in the network can play an important role in the function of such recurrent attractor networks, by causing for example an otherwise stable network to jump into a decision state (Wang, 2002; Deco and Rolls, 2006; Rolls and Deco, 2010). Attractor networks with this type of spiking-related noise are used in the brain for memory recall, and for decision-making, which in terms of the neural mechanism are effectively the same process. Noise in attractor networks is useful for memory and decision-making, for it makes them non-deterministic, and this contributes to new solutions to problems, and indeed to creativity (Rolls and Deco, 2010) (Section 18.2).

To investigate the extent to which the diluted connectivity affects the dynamics of attractor networks in the cerebral cortex (which includes the hippocampus), we simulated an integrate-and-fire attractor network taking decisions between competing inputs with diluted connectivity of 0.25 or 0.1 but the same number of synaptic connections per neuron for the recurrent collateral synapses within an attractor population as for full connectivity (Rolls and Webb, 2012). The results indicated that there was less spiking-related noise with the diluted connectivity in that the stability of the network when in the spontaneous state of firing increased, and the accuracy of the correct decisions increased. The decision times were a little slower with diluted than with complete connectivity. Given that the capacity of the network is set by the number of recurrent collateral synaptic connections per neuron, on which there is a biological limit, the findings indicate that the stability of cortical networks, and the accuracy of their correct decisions or memory recall operations, can be increased by utilizing diluted connectivity and correspondingly increasing the number of neurons in the network (which may help to smooth the noise), with little impact on the speed of processing of the cortex. Thus diluted connectivity can decrease cortical spiking-related noise, and thus enhance the reliability of memory recall, which includes completion from a partial recall cue (Rolls and Webb, 2012).

Representations in the neocortex and in the hippocampus are often distributed with graded firing rates in the neuronal populations (Rolls and Treves, 2011) (Appendix C). The firing rate probability distribution of each neuron to a set of stimuli is often exponential or gamma (Rolls and Treves, 2011) (Section C.3.1). These graded firing rate distributed representations are present in the hippocampus, both for place cells in rodents and for spatial view cells in the primate (O'Keefe and Speakman, 1987; O'Keefe, 1979; McNaughton, Barnes and O'Keefe, 1983; Rolls, Robertson and Georges-François, 1997a; Rolls, Treves, Robertson, Georges-François and Panzeri, 1998b; Georges-François, Rolls and Robertson, 1999; Rolls and Treves, 2011). In processes in the brain such as memory recall in the hippocampus or decision-making in the neocortex that are influenced by the noise produced by the close to random spike timings of each neuron for a given mean rate, the noise with this graded type of representation may be larger than with the binary firing rate distribution that is usually investigated.

In integrate-and-fire simulations of an attractor decision-making network, we showed that the noise is indeed greater for a given sparseness of the representation for graded, exponential, than for binary firing rate distributions (Webb, Rolls, Deco and Feng, 2011). The greater noise was measured by faster escaping times from the spontaneous firing rate state when the decision cues are applied, and this corresponds to faster decision or reaction times. The greater noise was also evident as less stability of the spontaneous firing state before the decision cues are applied. The implication is that spiking-related noise will continue to be a factor that influences processes such as decision-making, signal detection, short-term memory, and memory recall and completion (including in the CA3 network) even with the quite large networks found in the cerebral cortex. In these networks there are several thousand recurrent collateral synapses onto each neuron. The greater noise with graded firing rate distributions has the advantage that it can increase the speed of operation of cortical circuitry (Webb, Rolls, Deco and Feng, 2011). The graded firing rates also by operating in a non-linear network effectively increase the sparseness of the representation, and this itself provides a pattern separation effect (Webb, Rolls, Deco and Feng, 2011). The non-linearity is present in the NMDA threshold for synaptic modification, as well as in the threshold for firing of a neuron.

9.3.5.7 Pattern separation of CA3 cell populations encoding different memories

For the CA3 to operate with high capacity as an autoassociation or attractor memory, the sets of CA3 neurons that represent each event to be stored and later recalled need to be as uncorrelated from each other as possible. Correlations between patterns reduce the memory capacity of an autoassociation network (Marr, 1971; Kohonen, 1977, 1989; Kohonen, Oja and Lehtio, 1981; Sompolinsky, 1987; Rolls and Treves, 1998; Boboeva, Brasselet and Treves, 2018; Rolls, 2023d; Ryom, Stendardi, Ciaramelli and Treves, 2023), and because storage capacity is at a premium in an episodic memory system, there are several mechanisms that reduce the correlations between the firing of the population vectors of CA3 neuron firing each one of which represents a different event to be stored in memory. In the theoretical physics approach to the capacity of attractor networks, it is indeed assumed that the different vectors of firing rates to be stored are well separated from each other, by drawing each vector of firing at random, and by assuming very large (infinite) numbers of neurons in each pattern (Hopfield, 1982; Rolls and Treves, 1998) (Section B.3).

We have proposed that there are several mechanisms that help to achieve this pattern separation, namely the mossy fibre pattern separation effect produced by the small number of connections received by a CA3 neuron from mossy fibers which dominate the CA3 cell firing; the expansion recoding, and the sparse representation provided by the dentate granule cells that form the mossy fiber synapses; and the sparseness of the CA3 cell representation. Neurogenesis of dentate granule cells is a fifth potential contributor to achieving pattern separation of CA3 cell firing. These five mechanisms are described here, and elsewhere (Rolls, 2013c,b, 2016f, 2021i). It is remarked that some of this architecture may be special to the hippocampus, and not found in the neocortex, because of the importance of storing and retrieving large numbers of (episodic) memories in the hippocampus. The neocortex in contrast is more concerned with building new representations for which competitive learning is more important, and thus neocortical circuitry does not use a mossy fibre system to produce new random sets of neurons activated.

9.3.5.8 Mossy fibre inputs to the CA3 cells

We hypothesize that the mossy fibre inputs force efficient information storage by virtue of their strong and sparse influence on the CA3 cell firing rates (Rolls, 1987, 1990b, 1989f; Treves and Rolls, 1992). (The strong effects likely to be mediated by the mossy fibres were also emphasized by McNaughton and Morris (1987) and McNaughton and Nadel (1990).) We hypothesize that the mossy fibre input appears to be particularly appropriate in several ways. First of all, the fact that mossy fibre synapses are large and located very close to the soma makes them relatively powerful in activating the postsynaptic cell. (This should not be taken to imply that a CA3 cell can be fired by a single mossy fibre EPSP.)

Second, the firing activity of dentate granule cells appears to be very sparse (Jung and McNaughton, 1993; Leutgeb and Leutgeb, 2007) and this, together with the small number of connections on each CA3 cell, produces a sparse signal, which can then be transformed into an even sparser firing activity in CA3 by a threshold effect[13]. The hypothesis is that the

---

[13] For example, if only 1 granule cell in 100 were active in the dentate gyrus, and each CA3 cell received a connection from 50 randomly placed granule cells, then the number of active mossy fibre inputs received by CA3 cells would follow a Poisson distribution of average $50/100 = 1/2$, i.e. 60% of the cells would not receive any active input, 30% would receive only one, 7.5% two, little more than 1% would receive three, and so on. (It is easy to show from the properties of the Poisson distribution and our definition of sparseness, that the sparseness of the mossy fibre signal as seen by a CA3 cell would be $x/(1 + x)$, with $x = C^{MF} a_{DG}$, assuming equal strengths for all mossy fibre synapses. C^{MF} is the number of mossy fibre connections to a CA3 neuron, and a_{DG} is the sparseness of the representation in the dentate granule cells.) If three mossy fibre inputs were required to fire a CA3 cell and these

mossy fibre sparse connectivity solution performs the appropriate function to enable learning to operate correctly in CA3 (Treves and Rolls, 1992; Cerasti and Treves, 2010, 2013; Soldatkina, Schonsberg and Treves, 2022). The perforant path input would, the quantitative analysis shows, not produce a pattern of firing in CA3 that contains sufficient information for learning (Treves and Rolls, 1992).

Third, non-associative plasticity of mossy fibres (Brown et al., 1989, 1990b) might have a useful effect in enhancing the signal-to-noise ratio, in that a consistently firing mossy fibre would produce non-linearly amplified currents in the postsynaptic cell, which would not happen with an occasionally firing fibre (Treves and Rolls, 1992). This plasticity, and also learning in the dentate, would also have the effect that similar fragments of each episode (e.g. the same environmental location) recurring on subsequent occasions would be more likely to activate the same population of CA3 cells, which would have potential advantages in terms of economy of use of the CA3 cells in different memories, and in making some link between different episodic memories with a common feature, such as the same location in space.

Fourth, with only a few, and powerful, active mossy fibre inputs to each CA3 cell, setting a given sparseness of the representation provided by CA3 cells would be simplified, for the EPSPs produced by the mossy fibres would be Poisson distributed with large membrane potential differences for each active mossy fibre. Setting the average firing rate of the dentate granule cells would effectively set the sparseness of the CA3 representation, without great precision being required in the threshold setting of the CA3 cells (Rolls, Treves, Foster and Perez-Vicente, 1997c). Part of what is achieved by the mossy fibre input may be setting the sparseness of the CA3 cells correctly, which, as shown above and in Section B.3, is very important in an autoassociative memory store.

Fifth, the non-associative and sparse connectivity properties of the mossy fibre connections to CA3 cells may be appropriate for an episodic memory system that can learn very fast, in one trial. The hypothesis is that the sparse connectivity would help arbitrary relatively uncorrelated sets of CA3 neurons to be activated for even somewhat similar input patterns without the need for any learning of how best to separate the patterns, which in a self-organizing competitive network would take several repetitions (at least) of the set of patterns. The mossy fibre solution may thus be adaptive in a system that must learn in one trial, and for which the CA3 recurrent collateral learning requires uncorrelated sets of CA3 cells to be allocated for each (one-trial) episodic memory. The hypothesis is that the mossy fibre sparse connectivity solution performs the appropriate function without the mossy fibre system having to learn by repeated presentations how best to separate a set of training patterns (see further Section 9.4).

The argument based on information suggests, then, that an input system with the characteristics of the mossy fibres is essential during learning, in that it may act as a sort of (unsupervised) teacher that effectively strongly influences which CA3 neurons fire based on the pattern of granule cell activity. This establishes an information-rich neuronal representation of the episode in the CA3 network (Treves and Rolls, 1992; Rolls, 2013b; Kesner and Rolls, 2015; Rolls, 2016f). The perforant path input would, the quantitative analysis shows, not produce a pattern of firing in CA3 that contains sufficient information for learning (Treves and Rolls, 1992; Soldatkina, Schonsberg and Treves, 2022).

The particular property of the small number of mossy fibre connections onto a CA3 cell, approximately 46 (see Fig. 9.23), is that this has a randomizing effect on the representations set up in CA3, so that they are as different as possible from each other (Rolls, 1990b, 1989e; Treves and Rolls, 1992). (This means for example that place cells in a given environment are well separated to cover the whole space.) The result is that any one event or episode will set

were the only inputs available, we see that the activity in CA3 would be roughly as sparse, in the example, as in the dentate gyrus.

up a representation that is very different from other events or episodes, because the set of CA3 neurons activated for each event is random. This is then the optimal situation for the CA3 recurrent collateral effect to operate, for it can then associate together the random set of neurons that are active for a particular event (for example an object in a particular place), and later recall the whole set from any part. It is because the representations in CA3 are unstructured, or random, in this way that large numbers of memories can be stored in the CA3 autoassociation system, and that interference between the different memories is kept as low as possible, in that they are maximally different from each other (Hopfield, 1982; Treves and Rolls, 1991).

This is a key difference from the neocortex, in which new representations should be learned at each stage of the hierarchy that usefully combine information received from earlier cortical stages in the hierarchy. The difference then for the neocortex is that it uses competitive learning for the forward inputs to produce information-enhanced firing of the cortical pyramidal cells (Rolls, 2021c). In contrast, the hippocampus randomly allocates CA3 cells to new memories, to make each memory as different as possible from earlier memories.

The requirement for a small number of mossy fibre connections onto each CA3 neuron applies not only to discrete (Treves and Rolls, 1992) but also to spatial representations, and some learning in these connections, whether associative or not, can help to select out the small number of mossy fibres that may be active at any one time to select a set of random neurons in the CA3 (Cerasti and Treves, 2010). Any learning may help by reducing the accuracy required for a particular number of mossy fibre connections to be specified genetically onto each CA3 neuron. The optimal number of mossy fibres for the best information transfer from dentate granule cells to CA3 cells is in the order of 35–50 (Treves and Rolls, 1992; Cerasti and Treves, 2010). The mossy fibres also make connections useful for feedforward inhibition in CA3 (Acsady et al., 1998), which is likely to be useful to help in the sparse representations being formed in CA3.

On the basis of these points, it has been predicted that the mossy fibres may be necessary for new learning in the hippocampus, but may not be necessary for recall of existing memories from the hippocampus. Experimental evidence consistent with this prediction about the role of the mossy fibres in learning has been found in rats with disruption of the dentate granule cells (Lassalle et al., 2000) (see Section 9.4).

I have hypothesized that non-associative plasticity of mossy fibres (Brown et al., 1989, 1990b) might have a useful effect in enhancing the signal-to-noise ratio, in that a consistently firing mossy fibre would produce nonlinearly amplified currents in the postsynaptic cell, which would not happen with an occasionally firing fibre (Treves and Rolls, 1992). This plasticity, and also learning in the dentate, would also have the effect that similar fragments of each episode (e.g. the same environmental location) recurring on subsequent occasions would be more likely to activate the same population of CA3 cells, which would have potential advantages in terms of economy of use of the CA3 cells in different memories, and in making some link between different episodic memories with a common feature, such as the same location in space. Consistent with this, dentate neurons that fire repeatedly are more effective in activating CA3 neurons (Henze et al., 2002).

As acetylcholine does turn down the efficacy of the recurrent collateral synapses between CA3 neurons (Hasselmo et al., 1995; Giocomo and Hasselmo, 2007), then cholinergic activation also might help to allow external inputs rather than the internal recurrent collateral inputs to dominate the firing of the CA3 neurons during learning, as the current theory proposes. If cholinergic activation at the same time facilitated LTP in the recurrent collaterals (as it appears to in the neocortex), then cholinergic activation could have a useful double role in facilitating new learning at times of behavioral activation, when presumably it may be

9.3.5.9 Perforant path inputs to CA3 cells initiate recall in CA3 and contribute to generalization

By calculating the amount of information that would end up being carried by a CA3 firing pattern produced solely by the perforant path input and by the effect of the recurrent connections, we have been able to show (Treves and Rolls, 1992) that an input of the perforant path type, alone, is unable to direct efficient information storage. Such an input is too weak, it turns out, to drive the firing of the cells, as the 'dynamics' of the network is dominated by the randomizing effect of the recurrent collaterals. This is the manifestation, in the CA3 network, of a general problem affecting storage (i.e. learning) in all autoassociative memories. The problem arises when the system is considered to be activated by a set of input axons making synaptic connections that have to compete with the recurrent connections, rather than having the firing rates of the neurons artificially clamped into a prescribed pattern (Rolls, 2021c).

An autoassociative memory network needs afferent inputs also in the other mode of operation, i.e. when it retrieves a previously stored pattern of activity. We have shown (Treves and Rolls, 1992) that the requirements on the organization of the afferents are in this case very different, implying the necessity of a second, separate, input system, which we have identified with the perforant path input to CA3. In brief, the argument is based on the notion that the cue available to initiate retrieval might be rather small, i.e. the distribution of activity on the afferent axons might carry a small correlation, $q \ll 1$, with the activity distribution present during learning. In order not to lose this small correlation altogether, but rather transform it into an input current in the CA3 cells that carries a sizable signal – which can then initiate the retrieval of the full pattern by the recurrent collaterals – one needs a large number of associatively modifiable synapses. This is expressed by the following formulas that give the specific signal S produced by sets of associatively modifiable synapses, or by non-associatively modifiable synapses: if C^{AFF} is the number of afferents per cell,

$$S_{\text{ASS}} \approx \frac{\sqrt{C^{\text{AFF}}}}{\sqrt{p}} q \tag{9.6}$$

$$S_{\text{NONASS}} \approx \frac{1}{\sqrt{C^{\text{AFF}}}} q \tag{9.7}$$

Associatively modifiable synapses are therefore needed, and are needed in a number C^{AFF} of the same order as the number of concurrently stored patterns p, so that small cues can be effective; whereas non-associatively modifiable synapses – or even more so, non-modifiable ones – produce very small signals, which decrease in size the larger the number of synapses. In contrast with the storage process, the average strength of these synapses does not now play a crucial role. This suggests that the perforant path system is the one involved in relaying the cues that initiate retrieval.

The concept is that to initiate retrieval, a numerically large input (the perforant path system, see Fig. 9.23) is useful so that even a partial cue is sufficient (see Equation 17 of Treves and Rolls (1992)); and that the retrieval cue need not be very strong, as the recurrent collaterals (in CA3) then take over in the retrieval process to produce good recall (Treves and Rolls, 1992). In this scenario, the perforant path to CA3 synapses operate as a pattern associator, the quantitative properties of which are described in Section B.2. If an incomplete recall cue is provided to a pattern association network using distributed input representations, then most of the output pattern will be retrieved, and in this sense pattern association networks generalize between similar retrieval patterns to produce the correct output firing, and this generalization performed at the perforant path synapses to CA3 cells helps in the further completion produced by the recurrent collateral CA3-CA3 autoassociation process.

In contrast, during storage, strong signals, in the order of mV for each synaptic connection, are provided by the mossy fibre inputs to dominate the recurrent collateral activations, so that the new pattern of CA3 cell firing can be stored in the CA3 recurrent collateral connections (Treves and Rolls, 1992).

Before leaving the CA3 cells, it is suggested that the three major classes of excitatory input to the CA3 cells (recurrent collateral, mossy fibre, and perforant path, see Fig. 9.2) could be independently scaled, by virtue of the different classes of inhibitory interneuron which receive their own set of inputs, and end on different parts of the dendrite of the CA3 cells (cf. for CA1 Buhl et al. (1994) and Gulyas et al. (1993)). This possibility is made simpler by having these major classes of input terminate on different segments of the dendrites. Each of these inputs, and the negative feedback produced through inhibitory interneurons when the CA3 cells fire, should for optimal functioning be separately regulated (Rolls, 1995b), and the anatomical arrangement of the different types of inhibitory interneuron might be appropriate for achieving this.

9.3.6 Dentate granule cells

The theory is that the dentate granule cell stage of hippocampal processing which precedes the CA3 stage acts in a number of ways to produce during learning the sparse yet efficient (i.e. non-redundant) representation in CA3 neurons that is required for the autoassociation to perform well (Rolls, 1989a, 1990b, 1989f; Treves and Rolls, 1992; Rolls and Kesner, 2006b; Rolls, 2013b; Kesner and Rolls, 2015; Rolls, 2016f). An important property for episodic memory is that the dentate by acting in this way would perform pattern separation (or orthogonalization), enabling the hippocampus to store different memories of even similar events, and this prediction has been confirmed as described in Section 9.4. By *pattern separation* I mean that the correlations between different memory patterns represented by a population of neurons become reduced (Rolls, 2013b, 2016f).

9.3.6.1 The dentate cells as a competitive network

The first way in which the dentate granule cell stage helps to produce during learning the sparse yet efficient (i.e. non-redundant) representation in CA3 neurons is that the perforant path – dentate granule cell system with its Hebb-like modifiability is suggested to act as a competitive learning network to remove redundancy from the inputs producing a more orthogonal, sparse, and categorised set of outputs (Rolls, 1987, 1989a, 1990b, 1989f, 1990a,b). Competitive networks are described in Section B.4. The non-linearity in the NMDA receptors may help the operation of such a competitive net, for it ensures that only the most active neurons left after the competitive feedback inhibition have synapses that become modified and thus learn to respond to that input (Rolls, 1989a) (see Section B.4.9.3). If the synaptic modification produced in the dentate granule cells lasts for a period of more than the duration of learning the episodic memory, then it could reflect the formation of codes for regularly occurring combinations of active inputs that might need to participate in different episodic memories. Because of the non-linearity in the NMDA receptors, the non-linearity of the competitive interactions between the neurons (produced by feedback inhibition and non-linearity in the activation function of the neurons) need not be so great (Rolls, 1989a) (see Section B.4). Because of the feedback inhibition, the competitive process may result in a relatively constant number of strongly active dentate neurons relatively independently of the number of active perforant path inputs to the dentate cells. The operation of the dentate granule cell system as a competitive network may also be facilitated by a Hebb rule of the form:

$$\delta w_{ij} = \alpha y_i (x_j - w_{ij}) \tag{9.8}$$

where δw_{ij} is the change of the synaptic weight w_{ij} that results from the simultaneous (or conjunctive) presence of presynaptic firing x_j and postsynaptic firing or activation y_i, and α is a learning rate constant that specifies how much the synapses alter on any one pairing (see Rolls (1989a) and Appendix B). Incorporation of a rule such as this which implies heterosynaptic long-term depression as well as long-term potentiation (Levy and Desmond, 1985; Levy et al., 1990) makes the sum of the synaptic weights on each neuron remain roughly constant during learning (Oja, 1982; Rolls and Deco, 2002; Rolls and Treves, 1998; Rolls, 1989a) (see Section B.4).

This functionality could be used to help build dentate gyrus and hippocampal place cells in rats from the grid cells present in the medial entorhinal cortex (Hafting et al., 2005; Moser et al., 2015), as described in Section 9.3.3 (Rolls, Stringer and Elliot, 2006c).

As described above, in primates, there is evidence that there is a grid-cell like representation in the entorhinal cortex, with neurons having grid-like firing as the monkey moves the eyes across a spatial scene (Killian, Jutras and Buffalo, 2012; Meister and Buffalo, 2018). Similar competitive learning processes may transform these entorhinal cortex 'spatial view grid cells' into hippocampal spatial view cells, and may help with the idiothetic (produced in this case by movements of the eyes) update of spatial view cells (Robertson, Rolls and Georges-François, 1998). The presence of spatial view grid cells in the entorhinal cortex of primates (Killian et al., 2012) is of course predicted from the presence of spatial view cells in the primate CA3 and CA1 regions (Rolls and Xiang, 2006). Further support for this type of representation of space being viewed 'out there' rather than where one is located as for rat place cells is that neurons in the human entorhinal cortex with spatial view grid-like properties have now been described (Jacobs, Weidemann, Miller, Solway, Burke, Wei, Suthana, Sperling, Sharan, Fried and Kahana, 2013).

The importance of transforming from a grid cell representation in the entorhinal cortex to a place cell representation (or in primates a spatial view cell representation) in the hippocampus is considered quantitatively next. At least one important function this allows is the formation of memories, formed for example between an object and a place or a viewed spatial location, which is proposed to be a prototypical function of the hippocampus that is fundamental to episodic memory (Rolls, 1996d; Rolls and Treves, 1998; Rolls and Kesner, 2006b; Rolls and Xiang, 2006). For the formation of such object–place memories in an associative network (in particular, an autoassociative network in the CA3 region of the hippocampus), the place must be made explicit in the representation, and moreover, for high capacity, that is the ability to store and retrieve many memories, the representation must be sparse. By made explicit, I mean that information can be read off easily from the firing rates of the neurons, with different places producing very different sets of neurons firing, so that different representations are relatively orthogonal. The entorhinal cortex representations are not only not sparse (in the simulations of Rolls, Stringer and Elliot (2006c), the sparseness a^p was 0.54), but in addition the typical overlap between the sets of firing of the neuronal populations representing two different places was high (with a mean cosine of the angle or normalized dot product of 0.540). In contrast, the sparseness of the representations formed in the dentate granule cells with Hebb rule training was 0.024, and a typical cosine of the angle was 0.000. (Low values of this measure of sparseness, a^p, defined in Equation 9.2, indicate sparse representations. The cosine of the angle between two vectors takes the value 1 if they point in the same direction, and the value 0 if they are orthogonal, as described in Appendix A.) These sparse and orthogonal representations are what is required for high capacity storage of object and place, object and reward, and of in general episodic, memories, and this is the function, I propose, of the mapping from entorhinal cortex to hippocampal cells for which Rolls, Stringer and Elliot (2006c) produced a computational model. This concept maps well onto utility in an environment, for it is the place where we are located or at which we are looking in the world with which we wish to associate objects or rewards, and this is made explicit in the dentate granule cell / hippocampal representation (Rolls, 1999c; Rolls et al., 2005c; Rolls and Xiang, 2005; Rolls and Kesner, 2006b; Rolls and Xiang, 2006; Kesner and Rolls, 2015). In contrast, the medial entorhinal cortex may represent self-motion space in a way that is suitable for idiothetic path integration in *any* environment. Any association of an object with a grid cell representation would not be useful, because no unique place or spatial location would be involved.

9.3.6.2 Separation of overlapping inputs

The second way in which the dentate granule cell stage acts to produce during learning the sparse yet efficient (i.e. non-redundant) representation in CA3 neurons is also a result of the competitive learning hypothesized to be implemented by the dentate granule cells (Rolls, 1987, 1989a, 1990b, 1989f, 1990a,b, 1994b). It is proposed that this allows overlapping (or very similar) inputs to the hippocampus to be separated, in the following way (see also Rolls (1996d)). Consider three patterns B, W, and BW, where BW is a linear combination of B and W. (To make the example very concrete, we could consider binary patterns where B=10, W=01 and BW=11.) Then the memory system is required to associate B with reward, W with reward, but BW with punishment. Without the hippocampus, rats might have more difficulty in solving such problems, particularly when they are spatial, for the dentate / CA3 system in rodents is characterized by being implicated in spatial memory. However, it is a property of competitive neuronal networks that they can separate such overlapping patterns, as has been shown elsewhere (Rolls and Treves, 1998; Rolls, 1989a) (see Section B.4); normalization of synaptic weight vectors is required for this property. It is thus an important part of hippocampal neuronal network architecture that there is a competitive network that precedes the CA3 autoassociation system. Without the dentate gyrus, if a conventional autoassociation network were presented with the mixture BW having learned B and W separately, then the autoassociation network would produce a mixed output state, and would therefore be incapable of storing separate memories for B, W and BW. It is suggested therefore that competition in the dentate gyrus is one of the powerful computational features of the hippocampus, and that could enable it to help solve spatial pattern separation tasks. Consistent with this, rats with dentate gyrus lesions are impaired at a metric spatial pattern separation task (Gilbert, Kesner and Lee, 2001; Goodrich-Hunsaker, Hunsaker and Kesner, 2005) (see Section 9.4). The recoding of grid cells in the entorhinal cortex (Hafting et al., 2005; Moser et al., 2015) into small place field cells in the dentate granule cells that was modelled by Rolls, Stringer and Elliot (2006c) can also be considered to be a case where overlapping inputs must be recoded so that different spatial components can be treated differently.

It is noted that Sutherland and Rudy's configural learning hypothesis was similar, but was not tested with spatial pattern separation. Instead, when tested with for example tone and light combinations, it was not consistently found that the hippocampus was important (O'Reilly and Rudy, 2001; Sutherland and Rudy, 1991). I suggest that application of the configural concept, but applied to spatial pattern separation, may capture part of what the dentate gyrus acting as a competitive network could perform, particularly when a large number of such overlapping spatial memories must be stored and retrieved.

9.3.6.3 Low contact probability of dentate with CA3 neurons

The third way in which the dentate gyrus is hypothesized to contribute to the sparse and relatively orthogonal representations in CA3 arises because of the very low contact probability in the mossy fibre–CA3 connections, and has been explained above in Section 9.3.5.8 and by Treves and Rolls (1992).

9.3.6.4 Dentate mossy fibre synapses to CA3 cells are strong

A fourth way is that as suggested and explained above in Section 9.3.5.8, the dentate granule cell–mossy fibre input to the CA3 cells may be powerful and its use particularly during learning would be efficient in forcing a new pattern of firing onto the CA3 cells during learning.

9.3.6.5 Expansion recoding

Fifth, expansion recoding can decorrelate input patterns, and this can be performed by a stage of competitive learning with a large number of neurons (Appendix B). A mechanism like this appears to be implemented by the dentate granule cells, which are numerous (10^6) in the rat, compared to 300,000 CA3 cells, have associatively modifiable synapses (required for a competitive network), and strong inhibition provided by the inhibitory interneurons. This may not represent expansion of numbers relative to the number of entorhinal cortex cells, but the principle of a large number of dentate granule cells, with competitive learning and strong inhibition through inhibitory interneurons, would produce a decorrelation of signals like that achieved by expansion recoding (Rolls, 2013b).

9.3.6.6 Neurogenesis of dentate granule cells

Sixth, adult neurogenesis in the dentate gyrus may perform the computational role of facilitating pattern separation for new patterns, by providing new dentate granule cells with new sets of random connections to CA3 neurons (Rolls, 2010b; Aimone, Deng and Gage, 2010; Aimone and Gage, 2011; Johnston, Shtrahman, Parylak, Goncalves and Gage, 2016; Toda, Parylak, Linker and Gage, 2019). Consistent with the dentate spatial pattern separation hypothesis reviewed here, in mice with impaired dentate neurogenesis, spatial learning in a delayed non-matching-to-place task in the radial arm maze was impaired for arms that were presented with little separation, but no deficit was observed when the arms were presented farther apart (Clelland et al., 2009). Consistently, impaired neurogenesis in the dentate also produced a deficit for small spatial separations in an associative object-in-place task (Clelland et al., 2009).

The dentate granule cell / mossy fiber system may be one of the few places in the mammalian brain where neurogenesis may occur, because here the proposed computational role of the dentate granule cells is just to select new subsets of CA3 neurons for new learning. That is, the dentate granule cells, according to the theory, do not store the information, which instead is stored by the modification that then occurs in the CA3–CA3 recurrent collateral synapses between the selected CA3 neurons. In contrast, in most other brain areas where memories are stored and learning occurs, the learning is implemented by synaptic modification of the neurons in the circuit, and any loss of existing neurons and replacement by new neurons would result in loss of the learning or memory (Rolls, 2016b, 2021c).

9.3.7 CA1 cells

9.3.7.1 Associative retrieval at the CA3 to CA1 (Schaffer collateral) synapses

The CA3 cells connect to the CA1 cells by the Schaeffer collateral synapses. The following arguments outline the advantage of this connection being associatively modifiable, and apply independently of the relative extent to which the CA3 or the direct entorhinal cortex inputs to CA1 drive the CA1 cells during the learning phase.

The amount of information about each episode retrievable from CA3 has to be balanced off against the number of episodes that can be held concurrently in storage. The balance is regulated by the sparseness of the coding. Whatever the amount of information per episode in CA3, one may hypothesize that the organization of the structures that follow CA3 (i.e. CA1, the various subicular fields, and the return projections to neocortex shown in Fig. 9.2) should be optimized so as to preserve and use this information content in its entirety. This would prevent further loss of information, after the massive but necessary reduction in information content that has taken place along the sensory pathways and before the autoassociation stage in CA3. We have proposed (Treves and Rolls, 1994; Treves, 1995; Schultz and Rolls, 1999) that the need to preserve the full information content present in the output of an autoassociative memory requires an intermediate recoding stage (CA1) with special characteristics. In fact, a calculation of the information present in the CA1 firing pattern, elicited by a pattern of activity retrieved from CA3, shows that a considerable fraction of the information is lost if the synapses are non-modifiable, and that this loss can be prevented only if the CA3 to CA1 synapses are associatively modifiable. Their modifiability should match the plasticity of the CA3 recurrent collaterals. The additional information that can be retrieved beyond that retrieved by CA3 because the CA3 to CA1 synapses are associatively modifiable is strongly demonstrated by the hippocampal simulation described by Rolls (1995b), and quantitatively analyzed by Schultz and Rolls (1999).

9.3.7.2 Recoding in CA1 to facilitate retrieval to the neocortex

An additional factor is that if the total amount of information carried by CA3 cells is redistributed over a larger number of CA1 cells, less information needs to be loaded onto each CA1 cell, rendering the code more robust to information loss in the next stages. For example, if each CA3 cell had to code for 2 bits of information, e.g. by firing at one of four equiprobable activity levels, then each CA1 cell (if there were twice as many as there are CA3 cells) could code for just 1 bit, e.g. by firing at one of only two equiprobable levels. Thus the same information content could be maintained in the overall representation while reducing the sensitivity to noise in the firing level of each cell. In fact, there are more CA1 cells (4×10^5) than CA3 cells in (SD) rats. There are even more CA1 cells (4.6×10^6) in humans (and the ratio of CA1 to CA3 cells is greater). The CA1 cells may thus provide the first part of the expansion for the return projections to the enormous numbers of neocortical cells in primates, after the bottleneck of the single network in CA3, the number of neurons in which may be limited because it has to operate as a single network.

Another argument on the operation of the CA1 cells is also considered to be related to the CA3 autoassociation effect. In this, several arbitrary patterns of firing occur together on the CA3 neurons, and become associated together to form an episodic or 'whole scene' memory. It is essential for this operation that several different sparse representations are present conjunctively in order to form the association. Moreover, when completion operates in the CA3 autoassociation system, all the neurons firing in the original conjunction can be brought into activity by only a part of the original set of conjunctive events. For these reasons, a memory in the CA3 cells consists of several different simultaneously active ensembles of activity. To be explicit, the parts A, B, C, D and E of a particular episode would each be represented, roughly speaking, by its own population of CA3 cells, and these five populations would be linked together by autoassociation. It is suggested that the CA1 cells, which receive these groups of simultaneously active ensembles, can detect the conjunctions of firing of the different ensembles that represent the episodic memory, and allocate by competitive learning neurons to represent at least larger parts of each episodic memory (Rolls, 1987, 1989a, 1990b, 1989f,

1990a,a,b). In relation to the simple example above, some CA1 neurons might code for ABC, and others for BDE, rather than having to maintain independent representations in CA1 of A, B, C, D, and E. This implies a more efficient representation, in the sense that when eventually after many further stages, neocortical neuronal activity is recalled (as discussed below), each neocortical cell need not be accessed by all the axons carrying each component A, B, C, D and E, but instead by fewer axons carrying larger fragments, such as ABC, and BDE; or even ABCDE. This process is performed by competitive networks, which self-organize to find categories in the input space, where each category is represented by a set or combination of simultaneously active inputs (Rolls and Deco, 2002; Rolls and Treves, 1998; Rolls, 2000b) (see Section B.4).

Concerning the details of operation of the CA1 system, I note that although competitive learning may capture part of how it is able to recode, the competition is probably not global, but instead would operate relatively locally within the domain of the connections of inhibitory neurons. This simple example is intended to show how the coding may become less componential and more conjunctive in CA1 than in CA3, but should not be taken to imply that the representation produced becomes more sparse. An example of what might be predicted follows. Given that objects and the places in which they are seen may be associated by learning in the hippocampus, we might predict that relatively more CA3 neurons might be encoding either objects or places (the components to be associated), and relatively more CA1 neurons might be encoding conjunctive combinations of objects and places. Although object, spatial view, and object-spatial view combination neurons have been shown to be present in the primate hippocampus during a room-based object-spatial view task (Rolls, Xiang and Franco, 2005c), the relative proportions of the types of neuronal response in CA3 vs CA1 have not yet been analyzed.

The conjunctive recoding just described applies to any one single item in memory. Successive memory items would be encoded by a temporal sequence of such conjunctively encoded representations. To the extent that CA1 helps to build conjunctively encoded separate memory items, this could help a sequence of such memories (i.e. memory items) to be distinct (i.e. orthogonal to each other). This may be contrasted with successive memory items as encoded in CA3, in which there might be more overlap because each memory would be represented by its components, and some of the components might be common to some of the successive memory items. Episodic memory has been used here to refer to the memory of a single event or item. It can also be used to describe a succession of items that occurred close together in time, usually at one place. CA1 could help the encoding of these successive items that are parts of a multi-item episodic memory by making each item distinct from the next, due to the conjunctive encoding of each item. These arguments suggest that the CA1 could be useful in what is described as temporal pattern separation in Section 9.4.

9.3.7.3 CA1 inputs from CA3 vs direct entorhinal inputs

Another feature of the CA1 network is its double set of afferents, with each of its cells receiving most synapses from the Schaeffer collaterals coming from CA3, but also a proportion (about 1/6 – Amaral et al. (1990)) from direct perforant path projections from the entorhinal cortex. Such projections appear to originate mainly in layer 3 of entorhinal cortex (Witter et al., 1989b), from a population of cells only partially overlapping with that (mainly in layer 2) giving rise to the perforant path projections to DG and CA3. This suggests that it is useful to include in CA1 not only what it is possible to recall from CA3, but also the detailed information present in the retrieval cue itself (Treves and Rolls, 1994).

Another possibility is that the perforant path input provides the strong forcing input to the CA1 neurons during learning, and that the output of the CA3 system is associated with this forced CA1 firing during learning (McClelland, McNaughton and O'Reilly, 1995). During recall, an incomplete cue could then be completed in CA3, and the CA3 output would then produce firing in CA1 that would correspond to that present during the learning. This suggestion is essentially identical to that of Treves and Rolls (1994) about the backprojection system and recall, except that McClelland et al. (1995) suggest that the output of CA3 is associated at the CA3 to CA1 (Schaeffer collateral) synapses with the signal present during training in CA1, whereas in the theory of Treves and Rolls (1994) the output of the hippocampus consists of CA1 firing which is associated in the entorhinal cortex and earlier cortical stages with the firing present during learning, providing a theory of how the correct recall is implemented at every backprojection stage though the neocortex (see Section 9.3.8). There is evidence that the CA3 inputs to CA1 are much stronger than the entorhinal cortex inputs to CA1 (Zhao, Hsu and Spruston, 2022; Zhao, Wang, Spruston and Magee, 2020) (and N. Spruston, personal communication, 2022), so the theory of McClelland, McNaughton and O'Reilly (1995) about CA1 does not receive support.

9.3.7.4 CA1 time cells and sequence memory for objects and odors

Time cells each of which fires at a different time in a temporal sequence are found in CA3 and especially in CA1 (Macdonald et al., 2011; Eichenbaum, 2017; Salz et al., 2016; Howard and Eichenbaum, 2015; Eichenbaum, 2014). An example is shown in Fig. 9.26c (Kraus et al., 2013). These neurons are likely to be involved in remembering the order of events and temporal sequences, in that some hippocampal neurons in both CA3 and CA1 fire to combinations of time and object or place (Eichenbaum, 2017; Salz et al., 2016; Howard and Eichenbaum, 2015; Eichenbaum, 2014).

A theory about how time cells are generated by a competitive network in the hippocampus based on inputs from lateral entorhinal cortex time ramping cells has been described in Section 9.3.4 (Rolls and Mills, 2019). The relevant competitive network could be in any of the dentate gyrus, the CA3 (which although it is an attractor network could still operate to help categorise inputs using competitive mechanisms), and CA1.

Evidence described in Section 9.4.3 and by Kesner and Rolls (2015) indicates that the CA1, but not CA3, subregion is involved in the memory for sequences of objects and odors and spatial locations. For example Hunsaker et al. (2008) trained rats to remember unique sequences of spatial locations along a runway box. Rats with lesions to CA1 had especial difficulty with this spatial sequence memory task. Further, the memory for the temporal order of odors (Kesner et al., 2002, 2011) and visual objects is impaired especially by CA1 lesions (Hoge and Kesner, 2007). In humans, the hippocampus becomes activated when the temporal order of events is being processed (Lehn et al., 2009).

The association of time cell firing with object, or spatial, information could most naturally take place in the CA3 autoassociation network, with different neurons responding to time or object or place becoming associated together, so that when the timing input is represented later, the correct objects or places are recalled in the correct temporal sequence. However, time cell firing with object or place information might also become associated together in CA1.

9.3.7.5 Subcortical, vs neocortical backprojection, outputs from CA1

The CA1 network is on anatomical grounds thought to be important for the hippocampus to access the neocortex, and the route by which retrieval to the neocortex would occur (see Fig. 9.2). However, as also shown in Fig. 9.2, there are direct subcortical outputs of the hippocampus. One route is that outputs that originate from CA3 project via the fimbria directly to the medial septum (Gaykema et al., 1991) or indirectly via the lateral septum to the medial septum (Swanson and Cowan, 1977; Saper et al., 1979). The medial septum in turn provides cholinergic and GABAergic inputs back to the hippocampus, especially the CA3 subregion.

In addition to projecting back to the hippocampus, the medial septum also projects to subiculum, entorhinal cortex and mammillary bodies. In turn, the mammillary bodies project to the anterior thalamus which projects to the cingulate cortex, and also to the entorhinal cortex via the pre- and parasubiculum. The outputs from CA3 in the fimbria can thus potentially send information to the entorhinal cortex via direct projections from the medial septum, and via the anterior thalamus. A second subcortical output route is provided by the subiculum and CA1 projections via the fimbria/fornix to the lateral septum, and from the subiculum to the mammillary bodies and anterior thalamic nuclei, which in turn project to the cingulate cortex as well as to the prelimbic cortex (rat), which could provide a potential output to behavior (Vann and Aggleton, 2004; Bubb, Kinnavane and Aggleton, 2017), and to the entorhinal cortex. A third subcortical output route is that the subiculum and CA1 also project to the nucleus accumbens (Swanson and Cowan, 1977). How might the CA1 to entorhinal cortico-cortical backprojection system, and the different subcortical output routes from the hippocampus, implement different functions?

First, we should note that the CA1 to entorhinal cortico-cortical backprojection system is numerically, in terms of the number of connections involved, large, and this as developed below is likely to be crucial in allowing large numbers of memories to be retrieved from the hippocampus back to the neocortex. This recall operation to the neocortex is described below, but I note here that once a memory has been retrieved to the neocortex, the neocortex then provides a way for hippocampal function to influence behavior. For example, in a place–object recall task, a place cue used to initiate recall of the whole place-object memory in the CA3 would then lead via the backprojections to the object being retrieved (via entorhinal cortex layer 5 and perirhinal cortex) back to the inferior temporal visual cortex (see Fig. 9.2 left), and this object representation could then guide behavior via the other outputs of the inferior temporal visual cortex (Rolls and Deco, 2002; Rolls, 2016b). As objects are represented in the neocortex, it is a strong prediction of the theory that place–object recall will involve this CA1 backprojection pathway back to the neocortex. Backprojections from CA1 via entorhinal cortex to parahippocampal gyrus and thus to parietal cortex or other parts of the neocortex with spatial representations could allow spatial representations to be retrieved in for example an object–place recall task, and this provides a possible route to spatial action (though an alternative subcortical route for spatial action is described below). In addition, there are more direct CA1, subicular, and entorhinal connections to the prefrontal cortex (Jay and Witter, 1991), which could allow the hippocampus to provide inputs to prefrontal cortex networks involved in short-term memory and in planning actions (Deco and Rolls, 2003, 2005a).

Second, I note that the part of the second subcortical pathway that projects from CA1 via the subiculum to the mammillary bodies and anterior thalamus is also numerically large, with in the order of 10^6 axons in the fornix and mammillo-thalamic tract. Although subcortical connections of the hippocampus are well known, their computational functions are not clear (O'Mara and Aggleton, 2019). One hypothesis is that this could provide an information-rich output pathway to regions such as the cingulate cortex (Rolls, 2019c) via which some types of (e.g. spatial) behavioral response could be specified by the hippocampus. This cingulate cortex route may provide an output for more action-directed use of information stored in the hippocampus (Rolls, 2019c). In addition, head direction signals based on vestibular system processing may be introduced into hippocampal circuitry via the mammillary bodies (Dillingham et al., 2015). In contrast, the CA3 projections via the fimbria to the medial septum described as part of the first subcortical route are much less numerous, with indeed for example only approximately 2000 cholinergic neurons in the rat medial septum (Moore et al., 1998). Given further that this first subcortical route returns mainly to the hippocampus and connected structures, this route may be more involved in regulating hippocampal function (via cholinergic and GABAergic influences damage to which impairs hippocampal function), than in directly specifying behavior (cf. Hasselmo et al. (1995)).

9.3.8 Backprojections to the neocortex, episodic memory recall, and consolidation

The need for information to be retrieved from the hippocampus to influence neocortical areas and recall memories from the hippocampus was noted in Section 9.1. David Marr (1971) realised the importance of a theory for this, promised one in his 1971 paper, but never produced a theory. Rolls did produce a theory of how the recall of information to the neocortex could be implemented via cortico-cortical backprojections from the hippocampus to the neocortex (Rolls, 1990b, 1989f, 1990b), and the theory became quantitative (Treves and Rolls, 1994; Rolls and Treves, 1994), and has been tested by simulation (Rolls, 1995b, 2023c,e). The theory and developments of it are described next.

It is suggested that the modifiable connections from the CA3 neurons to the CA1 neurons allow the whole episode in CA3 to be produced in CA1. This may be assisted as described above by the direct perforant path input to CA1. This might allow details of the input key for the recall process, as well as the possibly less information-rich memory of the whole episode recalled from the CA3 network, to contribute to the firing of CA1 neurons. The CA1 neurons would then activate, via their termination in the deep layers of the entorhinal cortex, at least the pyramidal cells in the deep layers of the entorhinal cortex (see Fig. 9.2). These entorhinal cortex layer 5 neurons would then, by virtue of their backprojections (Lavenex and Amaral, 2000; Witter et al., 2000a) to the parts of cerebral cortex that originally provided the inputs to the hippocampus, terminate in the superficial layers of those neocortical areas, where synapses would be made onto the distal parts of the dendrites of the cortical pyramidal cells (Rolls, 1989a, 1990b, 1989f; Markov et al., 2014b; Pandya et al., 2015). The areas of cerebral neocortex in which this recall would be produced could include multimodal cortical areas (e.g. the cortex in the superior temporal sulcus which receives inputs from temporal, parietal and occipital cortical areas, and from which it is thought that cortical areas such as 39 and 40 related to language developed); and the orbitofrontal and anterior cingulate cortex to retrieve the reward / affective aspects of an episodic memory (Rolls, 2014a, 2019e,c); and also areas of unimodal association cortex (e.g. inferior temporal visual cortex).

Thus when an episodic memory is recalled, it is predicted that activity will be reinstated using backprojections in cortical areas that represent the different semantic features of the episodic memory. For example, if a friend on a ski slope was recalled, activity would be recalled in medial temporal scene and related areas that represent spatial scenes (in primates including humans (Rolls, 2023c), in temporal lobe areas that represent faces, and in the orbitofrontal cortex where reward value and emotion are represented. The episodic memory would be represented in CA3. Each of these other cortical areas would have neurons that represent the semantic features of each attribute or component of the episodic memory. The same prediction is made about the effects of words, which similarly from cortical areas where words are represented (Chapters 8 and 14) would by backprojections activate many different cortical areas in which the different semantic features are represented. This prediction has been confirmed using fMRI (Huth, de Heer, Griffiths, Theunissen and Gallant, 2016). The concept is that the episodic memory would be represented in the hippocampus, the word in language areas (in both using sparse distributed representations), and that each of the components that are active when the episodic memory was formed, or word is normally accessed, using forward inputs from the world, would become activated to represent the relevant semantic parts during the memory recall, or during the presentation of the word.

The backprojections, by recalling previous episodic events, could provide information useful to the neocortex in the building of new representations in the multimodal and unimodal association cortical areas, which by building new long-term representations can be considered as a form of memory consolidation (Rolls, 1989a, 1990b, 1989f, 1990a,b, 2022b) (Section 9.2.8.5).

The hypothesis of the architecture with which this would be achieved is shown in Fig. 9.2. The feedforward connections from association areas of the cerebral neocortex (solid lines in Fig. 9.2) show major convergence as information is passed to CA3, with the CA3 autoassociation network having the smallest number of neurons at any stage of the processing. The backprojections allow for divergence back to neocortical areas. The way in which I suggest that the backprojection synapses are set up to have the appropriate strengths for recall is as follows (Rolls, 1989a, 1990b, 1989f, 2016b; Kesner and Rolls, 2015; Rolls, 2015a, 2018b). During the setting up of a new episodic memory, there would be strong feedforward activity progressing towards the hippocampus. During the episode, the CA3 synapses would be modified, and via the CA1 neurons and the subiculum, a pattern of activity would be produced on the backprojecting synapses to the entorhinal cortex. Here the backprojecting synapses from active backprojection axons onto pyramidal cells being activated by the forward inputs to entorhinal cortex would be associatively modified. A similar process would be implemented at (at least some) preceding stages of neocortex, that is in the parahippocampal gyrus/perirhinal cortex stage, and in association cortical areas, as shown in Fig. 9.2.

The concept is that during the learning of an episodic memory, cortical pyramidal cells in at least one of the stages would be driven by forward inputs, but would simultaneously be receiving backprojected activity (indirectly) from the hippocampus which would by pattern association from the backprojecting synapses to the cortical pyramidal cells become associated with whichever cortical cells were being made to fire by the forward inputs. Then later on, during recall, a recall cue from perhaps another part of cortex might reach CA3, where the firing during the original episode would be completed. The resulting backprojecting activity would then, as a result of the pattern association learned previously, bring back the firing in any cortical area that was present during the original episode. Thus retrieval involves reinstating the activity that was present in different cortical areas that was present during the learning of an episode. (The pattern association is also called heteroassociation, to contrast it with autoassociation. The pattern association operates at multiple stages in the backprojection pathway, as made evident in Fig. 9.2.) If the recall cue was an object, this might result in recall of the neocortical firing that represented the place in which that object had been seen previously. As noted elsewhere in this Chapter and by McClelland et al. (1995), that recall might be useful to the neocortex to help it build new semantic memories, which might inherently be a slow process and is not part of the theory of recall. It is an interesting possibility that recall might involve several cycles through the recall process. After the information fed back from the first pass with a recall cue from perhaps only one cortical area, information might gradually be retrieved to other cortical areas involved in the original memory, and this would then act as a better retrieval cue for the next pass.

The timing of the backprojecting activity would be sufficiently rapid for this, in that for example inferior temporal cortex (IT) neurons become activated by visual stimuli with latencies of 90–110 ms and may continue firing for several hundred milliseconds (Rolls, 1992a; Rolls and Deco, 2002; Rolls, 2003); and hippocampal pyramidal cells are activated in visual object-and-place and conditional spatial response tasks with latencies of 120–180 ms (Miyashita, Rolls, Cahusac, Niki and Feigenbaum, 1989; Rolls, Miyashita, Cahusac, Kesner, Niki, Feigenbaum and Bach, 1989c). Thus, backprojected activity from the hippocampus might be expected to reach association cortical areas such as the inferior temporal visual cortex within 60 – 100 ms of the onset of their firing, and there would be a several hundred millisecond period in which there would be conjunctive feedforward activation present with simultaneous backprojected signals in the association cortex.

During recall, the backprojection connections onto the distal synapses of cortical pyramidal cells would be helped in their efficiency in activating the pyramidal cells by virtue of two factors. The first is that with no forward input to the neocortical pyramidal cells, there would be little shunting of the effects received at the distal dendrites by the more proximal effects on the dendrite normally produced by the forward synapses. Further, without strong forward activation of the pyramidal cells, there would not be very strong feedback and feedforward inhibition via GABA cells, so that there would not be a further major loss of signal due to (shunting) inhibition on the cell body and (subtractive) inhibition on the dendrite. (The converse of this is that when forward inputs are present, as during normal processing of the environment rather than during recall, the forward inputs would, appropriately, dominate the activity of the pyramidal cells, which would be only influenced, not determined, by the backprojecting inputs (Rolls, 1990b, 1989e; Deco and Rolls, 2005b).)

The synapses receiving the backprojections would have to be Hebb-modifiable, as suggested by Rolls (1990b) and Rolls (1989e). This would solve the de-addressing problem, which is the problem of how the hippocampus is able to bring into activity during recall just those cortical pyramidal cells that were active when the memory was originally being stored. The solution hypothesized (Rolls, 1990b, 1989e) arises because modification occurs during learning of the synapses from active backprojecting neurons from the hippocampal system onto the dendrites of only those neocortical pyramidal cells active at the time of learning. Without this modifiability of cortical backprojections during learning at some cortical stages at least, it is difficult to see how exactly the correct cortical pyramidal cells active during the original learning experience would be activated during recall. Consistent with this hypothesis (Rolls, 1990b, 1989e), there are NMDA receptors present especially in superficial layers of the cerebral cortex (Monaghan and Cotman, 1985), implying Hebb-like learning just where the backprojecting axons make synapses with the apical dendrites of cortical pyramidal cells.

The quantitative argument that the backprojecting synapses in at least one stage have to be associatively modifiable is that the information retrieved would otherwise be very low, and parallels that applied to the pattern retrieval performed at the entorhinal to CA3 synapses (Treves and Rolls, 1992) and at the CA3 to CA1 synapses (Schultz and Rolls, 1999). The performance of pattern association networks is considered in detail by Rolls and Treves (1990), Rolls and Treves (1998), other authors (Hertz et al., 1991), and in Appendix B. An interesting development is that dilution in the connectivity of pattern association networks by reducing the probability of two synapses onto a neuron from the same backprojecting input helps to maintain high capacity in the backprojecting system (Rolls, 2015a). If there are some instances of two or more synapses onto a neuron from the same input axon in a pattern association network, the capacity of the system degrades because of distortion and interferences between the stored patterns (Rolls, 2015a). It is also noted that the somewhat greater anatomical spread of the backprojections than the forward connections between two different stages in the hierarchy shown in Fig. 9.2 would not be a problem, for it would provide every chance for the backprojecting axons to find co-active neurons in an earlier cortical stage that are part of the representation that is relevant to the current memory being formed.

Rolls' theory of recall of information back to the neocortex from the hippocampus (Rolls, 1990b; Rolls and Treves, 1994; Treves and Rolls, 1994; Rolls, 2016b, 2018b) has been shown to be compatible with new learning in the cortex when forward inputs are present, and with the operation of the neocortex as a system with local attractors implemented by the local recurrent collaterals (Rolls, 2021c). The new model to show this is based on the neocortical canonical circuit shown in Fig. 1.17, is described in Section 19.7, and utilises the architecture shown in Fig. 9.31. It is shown that a population of pyramidal cells can implement new

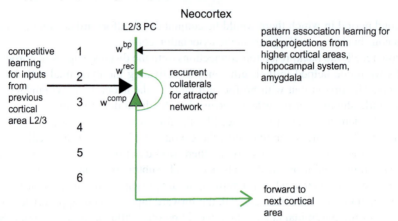

Fig. 9.31 The neocortical model that combines competitive learning using the forward inputs from the preceding cortical region, with associatively modifiable recurrent collateral synapses to form an autoassociation attractor network to maintain neuronal firing for short periods, and with pattern association learning to implement recall or top-down attention using cortico-cortical backprojections. L2/3 PC is a layer 2/3 pyramidal cell. The thick line above the pyramidal cell body is the dendrite, receiving inputs from the previous cortical area that operates by competitive learning using the synapses w^{comp}; from the recurrent collaterals that operate as an attractor network using synapses w^{rec}; and back-projections from higher cortical areas for memory recall and top-down attention that operate by pattern association learning using the synapses w^{bp}. 1-6 : the layers of the neocortex. (Reprinted from Rolls (2021) The connections of neocortical pyramidal cells can implement the learning of new categories, attractor memory, and top-down recall and attention. Brain Structure and Function 226: 2523-2536. © Springer.)

learning based on forward inputs when they are present using competitive learning, and at the same time can train the recurrent collaterals to implement an attractor network for later short-term memory, and can simultaneously train the backprojections as a pattern associator to implement later top-down recall (from e.g. the hippocampus) and top-down attention. Later, when a forward input is not present, recall can be initiated by the backprojections, and the activity can be maintained in short-term memory by the autoassociation recurrent collaterals. The architecture is quite simple, as is shown here in Fig. 9.31 to illustrate that point, with details in Section 19.7 and in Rolls (2021c).

If the backprojection synapses are associatively modifiable, we may consider the duration of the period for which their synaptic modification should persist. What follows from the operation of the system described above is that there would be no point, indeed it would be disadvantageous, if the synaptic modifications lasted for longer than the memory remained in the hippocampal buffer store. What would be optimal would be to arrange for the associative modification of the backprojecting synapses to remain for as long as the memory persists in the hippocampus. This suggests that a similar mechanism for the associative modification within the hippocampus and for that of at least one stage of the backprojecting synapses would be appropriate. It is suggested that the presence of high concentrations of NMDA synapses in the distal parts of the dendrites of neocortical pyramidal cells and within the hippocampus may reflect the similarity of the synaptic modification processes in these two regions (Kirkwood et al., 1993). It is noted that it would be appropriate to have this similarity of time course (i.e. rapid learning within 1–2 s, and slow decay over perhaps weeks) for at least one stage in the series of backprojecting stages from the CA3 region to the neocortex. Such stages might include the CA1 region, subiculum, entorhinal cortex, and perhaps the parahippocampal gyrus / perirhinal cortex. However from multimodal cortex (e.g. the parahippocampal gyrus) back to earlier cortical stages, it might be desirable for the backprojecting synapses to persist for a long period, so that some types of recall and top-down processing (Rolls, 1990b, 1989e, 2016b) mediated by the operation of neocortico-neocortical backprojecting synapses could be stable, and might not require modification during the learning of a new episodic memory.

An alternative hypothesis to that above is that rapid modifiability of backprojection synapses would be required only at the beginning of the backprojecting stream. Relatively fixed associations from higher to earlier neocortical stages would serve to activate the correct neurons at earlier cortical stages during recall. For example, there might be rapid modifiability from CA3 to CA1 neurons, but relatively fixed connections from there back (McClelland, McNaughton and O'Reilly, 1995). For such a scheme to work, one would need to produce a theory not only of the formation of semantic memories in the neocortex, but also of how the operations performed according to that theory would lead to recall by setting up appropriately the backprojecting synapses. It is suggested that they could be learned by the same associative processes between the backprojections and the neuronal firing in the preceding cortical area as just described. Also, as noted above, there is evidence that the CA3 inputs to CA1 are much stronger than the entorhinal cortex inputs to CA1 (Zhao, Hsu and Spruston, 2022; Zhao, Wang, Spruston and Magee, 2020) (and N. Spruston, personal communication, 2022), so the theory of McClelland, McNaughton and O'Reilly (1995) about CA1 does not receive support.

We have noted elsewhere that backprojections, which included cortico-cortical backprojections, and backprojections originating from structures such as the hippocampus and amygdala, may have a number of different but compatible functions (Rolls and Deco, 2002; Rolls, 2005a, 1990a,b, 1989e, 1990b, 1989a, 1992a, 2016b) including implementing top-down attention by biased competition (see Chapter 13). The particular function with which we have been concerned here is how memories stored in the hippocampus might be recalled in regions of the cerebral neocortex.

Rolls' theory of how the recall of information to the neocortex could be implemented via cortico-cortical backprojections from the hippocampus to the neocortex (Rolls, 1990b, 1989f, 1990b) was a key conceptual discovery and theory, because it showed how the deaddressing problem could be solved of how the hippocampus could retrieve information to the correct neurons in the neocortex. In a sense, the theory shows how the hippocampus 'points to' the correct neurons in the neocortex for the hippocampal recall. The concept of how the hippocampus could point to the correct neurons in the neocortex had been raised by Teyler and DiScenna (1986), and they used the word 'pointer', but had no theory of how a hippocampal pointer might be implemented or how information might be recalled from the hippocampus back to the correct neurons in the neocortex. That was the theory that Rolls developed (Rolls, 1990b, 1989f, 1990b), and the theory became quantitative (Rolls and Treves, 1994; Treves and Rolls, 1994), and has been tested by simulation (Rolls, 1995b, 2023c,e). The high capacity of memory recall with sparse representations in associative networks (Rolls and Treves, 1990; Treves and Rolls, 1991; Rolls and Treves, 1994; Treves and Rolls, 1994) has been confirmed (Schonsberg, Roudi and Treves, 2021).

9.3.9 Backprojections to the neocortex – quantitative aspects

How many backprojecting fibres does one need to synapse on any given neocortical pyramidal cell, in order to implement the mechanism outlined above? Clearly, if neural network theory were to produce a definite constraint of that sort, quantitative anatomical data could be used for verification or falsification.

Attempts to come up with an estimate of the number of synapses required have sometimes followed the simple line of reasoning presented next, which is shown to be unsatisfactory. [The type of argument to be described has been applied to analyze the capacity of pattern association and autoassociation memories (see for example Marr (1971) and Willshaw and

Buckingham (1990)), and to show that there are limitations in that type of approach, that approach is considered in this paragraph.] Consider first the assumption that hippocampo-cortical connections are monosynaptic and not modifiable, and that all existing synapses have the same efficacy. Consider further the assumption that a hippocampal representation across N cells of an event consists of $a_h N$ cells firing at the same elevated rate (where a_h is the sparseness of the hippocampal representation), while the remaining $(1-a_h)N$ cells are silent. If each pyramidal cell in the association areas of neocortex receives synapses from an average C^{HBP} hippocampal axons, there will be an average probability $y = C^{\mathrm{HBP}}/N$ of finding a synapse from any given hippocampal cell to any given neocortical one. Across neocortical cells, the number A of synapses of hippocampal origin activated by the retrieval of a particular episodic memory will follow a Poisson distribution of average $ya_h N = a_h C^{\mathrm{HBP}}$

$$P(A) = (a_h C^{\mathrm{HBP}})^A \exp(-a_h C^{\mathrm{HBP}})/A! \tag{9.9}$$

The neocortical cells activated as a result will be those, in the tail of the distribution, receiving at least T active input lines, where T is a given threshold for activation. Requiring that $P(A > T)$ be at least equal to a_{nc}, the fraction of neocortical cells involved in the neocortical representation of the episode, results in a constraint on C^{HBP}. This simple type of calculation can be extended to the case in which hippocampo-cortical projections are taken to be polysynaptic, and mediated by modifiable synapses. In any case, the procedure does not appear to produce a very meaningful constraint for at least three reasons. First, the resulting minimum value of C^{HBP}, being extracted by looking at the tail of an exponential distribution, varies dramatically with any variation in the assumed values of the parameters a_h, a_{nc}, and T. Second, those parameters are ill-defined in principle: a_h and a_{nc} are used having in mind the unrealistic assumption of binary distributions of activity in both the hippocampus and neocortex (although the sparseness of a representation can be defined in general, as shown above, it is the particular definition pertaining to the binary case that is invoked here); while the definition of T is based on unrealistic assumptions about neuronal dynamics (how coincident does one require the various inputs to be in time, in order to generate a single spike, or a train of spikes of given frequency, in the postsynaptic cell?). Third, the calculation assumes that neocortical cells receive no other inputs, excitatory or inhibitory. Relaxing this assumption, to include for example non-specific activation by subcortical afferents, makes the calculation extremely fragile. This argument applies in general to approaches to neurocomputation which base their calculations on what would happen in the tail of an exponential, Poisson, or binomial distribution. Such calculations must be interpreted with great care for the above reasons (Rolls and Treves, 1998).

An alternative way to estimate a constraint on C^{HBP}, still based on very simple assumptions, but which is more robust with respect to relaxing those assumptions, is the following.

Consider a polysynaptic sequence of backprojecting stages, from hippocampus to neocortex, as a string of simple (hetero-)associative memories in which, at each stage, the input lines are those coming from the previous stage (closer to the hippocampus) (Treves and Rolls, 1994) (Fig. 9.2). Implicit in this framework is the assumption that the synapses at each stage are modifiable and have been indeed modified at the time of first experiencing each episode, according to some Hebbian associative plasticity rule. A plausible requirement for a successful hippocampo-directed recall operation is that the signal generated from the hippocampally retrieved pattern of activity, and carried backwards towards neocortex, remains undegraded when compared to the noise due, at each stage, to the interference effects caused by the concurrent storage of other patterns of activity on the same backprojecting synaptic systems. That requirement is equivalent to that used in deriving the storage capacity of such a series of heteroassociative memories, and it was shown in Treves and Rolls (1991) that the maximum number of independently generated activity patterns that can be retrieved is given, essentially, by the same formula as Equation 9.3 above

$$p \approx \frac{C}{a \ln(\frac{1}{a})} k' \qquad (9.10)$$

where, however, a is now the sparseness of the representation at any given backprojection stage, and C is the average number of (back-)projections each cell of that stage receives from cells of the previous one[14]. (k' is a similar slowly varying factor to that introduced above.) If p is equal to the number of memories held in the hippocampal memory, it is limited by the retrieval capacity of the CA3 network, $p_{\max}$. Putting together the formula for the latter with that shown here, one concludes that, roughly, the requirement implies that the number of afferents of (indirect) hippocampal origin to a given neocortical stage (C^{HBP}) must be $C^{\text{HBP}} = C^{\text{RC}} a_{\text{nc}} / a_{\text{CA3}}$, where C^{RC} is the number of recurrent collaterals to any given cell in CA3, the average sparseness of a neocortical representation is a_{nc}, and a_{CA3} is the sparseness of memory representations in CA3.

The above requirement is very strong: even if representations were to remain as sparse as they are in CA3, which is unlikely, to avoid degrading the signal, C^{HBP} should be as large as C^{RC}, i.e. 12,000 in the rat. Moreover, other sources of noise not considered in the present calculation would add to the severity of the constraint, and partially compensate for the relaxation in the constraint that would result from requiring that only a fraction of the p episodes would involve any given cortical area. If then C^{HBP} has to be of the same order as C^{RC}, one is led to a very definite conclusion: a mechanism of the type envisaged here could not possibly rely on a set of monosynaptic CA3-to-neocortex backprojections. This would imply that, to make a sufficient number of synapses on each of the vast number of neocortical cells, each cell in CA3 has to generate a disproportionate number of synapses (i.e. C^{HBP} times the ratio between the number of neocortical and that of CA3 cells). The required divergence can be kept within reasonable limits only by assuming that the backprojecting system is polysynaptic, provided that the number of cells involved grows gradually at each stage, from CA3 back to neocortical association areas (Treves and Rolls, 1994) (cf. Fig. 9.2).

Although backprojections between any two adjacent areas in the cerebral cortex are approximately as numerous as forward projections, and much of the distal parts of the dendrites of cortical pyramidal cells are devoted to backprojections, the actual number of such connections onto each pyramidal cell may be on average only in the order of thousands. Further, not all might reflect backprojection signals originating from the hippocampus, for there are backprojections which might be considered to originate in the amygdala (Amaral et al., 1992) or in multimodal cortical areas (allowing for example for recall of a visual image by an auditory stimulus with which it has been regularly associated). In this situation, one may consider whether the backprojections from any one of these systems would be sufficiently numerous to produce recall. One factor which may help here is that when recall is being produced by the backprojections, it may be assisted by the local recurrent collaterals between nearby ($\approx$1 mm) pyramidal cells which are a feature of neocortical connectivity. These would tend to complete a partial neocortical representation being recalled by the backprojections into a complete recalled pattern. (Note that this completion would be only over the local information present within a cortical area about e.g. visual input or spatial input; it provides a local 'clean-up'

---

[14] The interesting and important insight here is that multiple iterations through a recurrent autoassociative network can be treated as being formally similar to a whole series of feedforward associative networks, with each new feedforward network equivalent to another iteration in the recurrent network (Treves and Rolls, 1991). This formal similarity enables the quantitative analysis developed in general for autoassociation nets (see Treves and Rolls (1991)) to be applied directly to the series of backprojection networks (Treves and Rolls, 1994).

mechanism, and could not replace the global autoassociation performed effectively over the activity of very many cortical areas which the CA3 could perform by virtue of its widespread recurrent collateral connectivity.) There are two alternative possibilities about how this would operate. First, if the recurrent collaterals showed slow and long-lasting synaptic modification, then they would be useful in completing the whole of long-term (e.g. semantic) memories. Second, if the neocortical recurrent collaterals showed rapid changes in synaptic modifiability with the same time course as that of hippocampal synaptic modification, then they would be useful in filling in parts of the information forming episodic memories which could be made available locally within an area of the cerebral neocortex.

This theory of recall by the backprojections thus provides a quantitative account of why the cerebral cortex has as many backprojection as forward projection connections (Treves and Rolls, 1994; Rolls and Treves, 1994; Rolls, 2016b). I know of no alternative quantitative account for this key feature of neocortical design (Rolls, 2016b).

A development of the theory has been in understanding the diluted connectivity in the back-projection pathways. The backprojection pathways have diluted connectivity in that each neocortical neuron may receive up to in the order of 10,000 backprojection synapses, yet the total number of neurons at each neocortical stage in the backprojection hierarchy shown in Fig. 9.2 has very many more neurons than this, at least 10 times as many neurons as there are synapses per neuron. This diluted connectivity in the backprojection pathways is likely to reduce the probability of more than one connection onto a receiving neuron in the backprojecting pathways. It has now been shown that if there were more than one connection onto each neuron in a pattern associator, this would reduce the capacity of the system, which in this case is the number of memories that can be recalled from the hippocampus to the neocortex (Rolls, 2015a). However, given that there is dilution in the connectivity of the backprojection pathways in the neocortex, it may be useful to have the representations not very sparse in the backprojection pathways, for otherwise the pattern association computation that implements the recall may be downgraded (Rolls, 2023e).

These concepts show how the backprojection system to neocortex can be conceptualized in terms of pattern completion, as follows. The information that is present when a memory is formed may be present in different areas of the cerebral cortex, for example of a face in a temporal cortex face area (Rolls, 2012d), of a spatial location in a neocortical scene location area, and of a reward received in the orbitofrontal cortex (Rolls, 2014a, 2023c; Rolls et al., 2023e,c). To achieve detailed retrieval of the memory, reinstatement of the activity during recall of the neuronal activity during the original memory formation may be needed. This is what the backprojection system described could achieve, and is a form of completion of the information that was represented in the different cortical areas when the memory was formed. In particular, the concept of completion here is that if a recall cue from a visual object area is provided and the hippocampus recalls the other components of the episodic memory, then the emotional parts of the episodic memory can be recalled in the orbitofrontal cortex, and the spatial parts in medial temporal lobe cortical areas, with the result that a complete memory is retrieved, with activity recalled into several higher-order cortical areas. Because such a wide set of different neocortical areas must be content-addressed, a multistage feedback system from the hippocampus is required, to keep the number of synapses per neuron in the back-projection pathways down to reasonable numbers (Treves and Rolls, 1994; Rolls and Treves, 1994). (Having CA1 directly address neocortical areas would require each CA1 neuron to have tens of millions of synapses with cortical neurons. That is part of the computational problem solved by the multistage backprojection system shown in Fig. 9.2.) Thus, the back-projection system with its series of pattern associators can each be thought of as retrieving the complete pattern of cortical activity in many different higher-order cortical areas that was present during the original formation of the episodic memory.

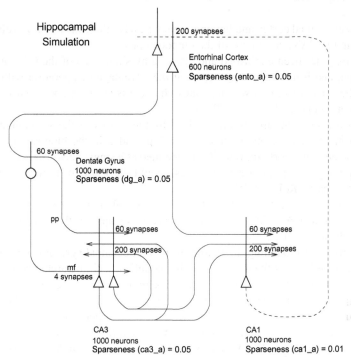

Fig. 9.32 Simulation of a scaled down model of the hippocampus and recall to the neocortex. The numbers of synapses and the sparseness values used are shown. (After Rolls, E. T. (1995) A model of the operation of the hippocampus and entorhinal cortex in memory. International Journal of Neural Systems 6, Supplement: 51–70. © World Scientific Publishing Company.)

9.3.10 Simulations of hippocampal operation

In order to test the operation of the whole system for individual parts of which an analytic theory is available (Rolls and Treves, 1998; Treves and Rolls, 1994, 1992; Schultz and Rolls, 1999), Rolls (1995b) simulated a scaled down version of the part of the architecture shown in Fig. 9.2 from the entorhinal cortex to the hippocampus and back to the entorhinal cortex. The network included competitive learning in the dentate gyrus to form a sparse representation, using this to drive the CA3 cells by diluted non-associative mossy fibre connectivity during learning, competitive learning in CA1, and pattern association in the retrieval back to entorhinal cortex (Fig. 9.32). The analytic approaches to the storage capacity of the CA3 network, the role of the mossy fibres and of the perforant path, the functions of CA1, and the operation of the backprojections in recall, were all shown to be computationally plausible in the computer simulations. In the simulation, during recall, partial keys are presented to the entorhinal cortex, completion is produced by the CA3 autoassociation network, and recall is produced in the entorhinal cortex of the original learned vector. The network, which has 1,000 neurons at each stage, can recall large numbers of different sparse random vectors, which approach the calculated storage capacity.

One of the points highlighted by the simulation is that the network operated much better if the CA3 cells operated in binary mode (either firing or not), rather than having continuously graded firing rates (Rolls, 1995b). The reason for this is that given that the total amount of information that can be stored in a recurrent network such as the CA3 network is approximately constant independently of how graded the firing rates are in each pattern (Treves, 1990), then if much information is used to store the graded firing rates in the firing of CA3 cells, fewer patterns can be stored. The implication of this is that in order to store many memories in the hippocampus, and to be able to recall them at later stages of the system in for example the entorhinal cortex and beyond, it may be advantageous to utilize relatively binary firing rates in the CA3 part at least of the hippocampus.

This finding has been confirmed and clarified by simulation of the CA3 autoassociative system alone, and it has been suggested that the advantage of operation with binary firing rates may be related to the low firing rates characteristic of hippocampal neurons (Rolls, Treves, Foster and Perez-Vicente, 1997c).

Another aspect of the theory emphasized by the results of the simulation was the importance of having effectively a single network provided in the hippocampus by the CA3 recurrent collateral network, for only if this operated as a single network (given the constraint of some topography present at earlier stages), could the whole of a memory be completed from any of its parts (Rolls, 1995b).

Another aspect of the theory illustrated by these simulations was the information retrieval that can occur at the CA3–CA1 (Schaeffer collateral) synapses if they are associatively modifiable (Schultz and Rolls, 1999).

The approach to modelling the whole of the hippocampal system has been extended to allow recall as far back as the neocortex to be modelled, with the architecture shown in Fig. 9.33 (Rolls, 2023c,e). The model has separate regions in the neocortex and entorhinal cortex for the prototypical 'where' and 'what' inputs to the hippocampus. When trained with 'where' and 'what' pairs of inputs to the neocortex, the hippocampal system modelled can recall the correct 'where' pattern back to the neocortex if the recall cue is a 'what' neocortical input, and vice versa. This type of symmetric recall of a whole memory from any part is made possible because of the autoassociation network in CA3. This type of symmetric recall could of course not be achieved by a pattern association network (Appendix B). An interesting aspect emphasised by the operation of the model is that the backprojection patterns to the neocortex that implement recall by pattern association should not be very sparse, for otherwise given the diluted connectivity in the neocortical backprojection pathways the recall to the neocortex can be degraded (Rolls, 2023e). In the hierarchical organisation of the neocortex the sparseness of the activity patterns can be more sparse in the forward direction, because the forward connectivity up through the network operates by competitive learning, which in fact benefits from diluted connectivity and sparse patterns (Rolls, 2016f,b) (Section B.4.3.3).

9.3.11 The learning of spatial view and place cell representations from visual inputs

In the ways just described, the dentate granule cells could be particularly important in helping to build and prepare spatial representations for the CA3 network. The actual representation of space in the primate hippocampus includes a representation of spatial view, whereas in the rat hippocampus it is of the place where the rat is. The representation in the rat may be related to the fact that with a much less developed visual system than the primate, the rat's representation of space may be defined more by the olfactory and tactile as well as distant visual cues present, and may thus tend to reflect the place where the rat is. However, the spatial representations in the rat and primate could arise from essentially the same computational process as follows (Rolls, 1999c; Critchley and Rolls, 1996a).

The starting assumption is that in both the rat and the primate, the dentate granule cells (and the CA3 and CA1 pyramidal cells) respond to combinations of the inputs received. In the case of the primate, a combination of visual features in the environment will, because of the fovea providing high spatial resolution over a typical viewing angle of perhaps 10–20 degrees, result in the formation of a spatial view cell, the effective trigger for which will thus be a combination of visual features within a relatively small part of space. In contrast,

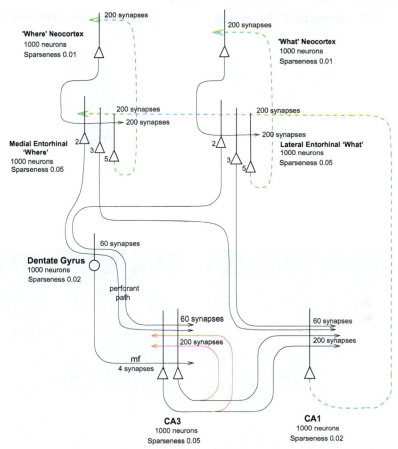

Fig. 9.33 Simulation of neocortical 'what' and 'where' inputs to the hippocampus for the storage of episodic memory, and for the recall of 'what' (object) and 'where' (spatial view) information back to the 'what' and 'where' neocortex. The pyramidal cells bodies are shown as triangles, the dendrites as the thick lines above the cell bodies, and the axons as thin lines terminated with an arrow. The backprojection pathways for memory recall are shown in dashed green lines, and in red the CA3 recurrent collaterals via which 'what' and 'where' representations present at the same time can be associated during episodic memory storage, and via which completion of a whole memory from a part can occur during recall. All synapses are associatively modifiable except for the dentate Gyrus (DG) mossy fibre (mf) synapses on the CA3 pyramidal cells. The dentate granule cells, the CA1 cells, and the entorhinal cortex inputs from the neocortex operate as competitive networks. The CA3 cells operate as an autoassociation attractor network to implement completion. The backprojection connections shown in green operate as pattern association networks. (After Rolls, E. T. (2023) Hippocampal spatial view cells for memory and navigation, and their underlying connectivity in humans. Hippocampus doi: 10.1002/hipo.23467.)

in the rat, given the very extensive visual field subtended by the rodent retina, which may extend over 180–270 degrees, a combination of visual features formed over such a wide visual angle would effectively define a position in space that is a place (see Fig. 9.34). The actual processes by which the hippocampal formation cells would come to respond to feature combinations could be similar in rats and monkeys, involving for example competitive learning in the dentate granule cells, as utilized in the simulations of Critchley and Rolls (1996a) which produced neurons with place-like and spatial view-like tuning. This competitive learning has the required properties, of associating together co-occurrent features, and of ensuring by the competition that each feature combination (representing a place or spatial view) is very different from that of other places or spatial views (pattern separation, and orthogonalizing effect), and is also a sparse representation. Consistent with this, dentate place fields in rats are small (Jung and McNaughton, 1993). Although this computation could be performed to some extent also by autoassociation learning in CA3 pyramidal cells, and competitive learning in

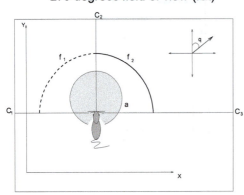
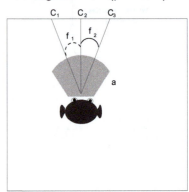
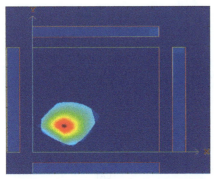
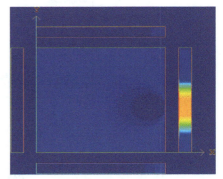

Fig. 9.34 Place cells can be formed in animals such as rodents with a wide field of view, and spatial view neurons can be formed with a small high resolution field of view as provided in primates including humans by the fovea. Simulation of rodent place cells (left) vs primate spatial view cells (right). The agent moved through a grid of all 200x200 places x, y. At each place the head direction θ was rotated in 5 degree increments. Hippocampal cells are activated by a set of 3 or more landmark visual cues within the field of view of the agent α. The firing rates of the hippocampal neurons depended on the angles ϕ subtended by the landmarks. The top left shows that for a rodent with a 270° field of view a combination of such cues defines a place. The top right shows that for a primate with a 30° view the combination of cues in the scene defines a spatial view. The sizes of the fields of view are shown by shading. The bottom left shows that in the simulations place fields arise with a 270° field of view, and the bottom right that spatial view fields arise on one of the walls indicated by the rectangles when the view is 30°. High firing rates are indicated by yellow-red. (Modified from Araujo,I.E.T., Rolls, E. T. and Stringer,S.M. (2001) A view model which accounts for the spatial fields of hippocampal primate spatial view cells and rat place cells. Hippocampus 11: 699–706. © Wiley-Liss Inc.)

CA1 pyramidal cells (Rolls and Treves, 1998; Treves and Rolls, 1994), the combined effect of the dentate competitive learning and the mossy fibre low probability but strong synapses to CA3 cells would enable this part of the hippocampal circuitry to be especially important in separating spatial representations, which as noted above are inherently continuous. The prediction thus is that during the learning of spatial tasks in which the spatial discrimination is difficult (for example because the places are close together), then the dentate system should be especially important. Tests of this prediction are described in Section 9.4.

9.3.12 Linking the inferior temporal visual cortex to spatial view and place cell representations

It is now possible to propose a unifying computational hypothesis of the relation between the ventral visual system, and hippocampal spatial representations (Rolls, Tromans and Stringer, 2008f). Let us consider a computational architecture in which a fifth layer is added to the

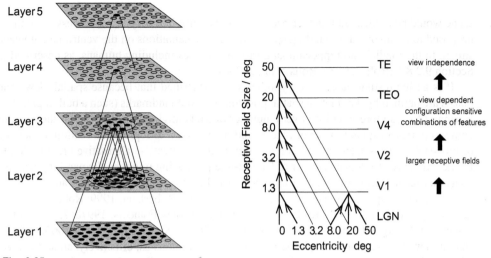

Fig. 9.35 Adding a fifth layer, corresponding to the parahippocampal gyrus / hippocampal system, after the inferior temporal visual cortex (corresponding to layer 4) may lead to the self-organization of spatial view / place cells in layer 5 when whole scenes are presented (see text). Convergence in the visual system is shown in the earlier layers (see Chapter 2). Right – as it occurs in the brain. V1, visual cortex area V1; TEO, posterior inferior temporal cortex; TE, inferior temporal cortex (IT). Left – as implemented in VisNet (layers 1–4). Convergence through the network is designed to provide fourth layer neurons with information from across the entire input retina. (From Rolls, E. T., Tromans, J. and Stringer, S.M. (2008) Spatial scene representations formed by self-organizing learning in a hippocampal extension of the ventral visual system. European Journal of Neuroscience 28: 2116–2127. © Federation of European Neuroscience Societies and Blackwell Publishing Ltd.)

VisNet architecture described in Chapter 2, as illustrated in Fig. 9.35. In the anterior inferior temporal visual cortex, which corresponds to the fourth layer of VisNet, neurons respond to objects, but several objects close to the fovea (within approximately 10°) can be represented because many object-tuned neurons have asymmetric receptive fields with respect to the fovea (Aggelopoulos and Rolls, 2005) (see Section 2.8.10). If the fifth layer of VisNet performs the same operation as previous layers, it will form neurons that respond to combinations of objects in the scene with the positions of the objects relative spatially to each other incorporated into the representation (as described in Section 2.8.5). It was found that training now with whole scenes that consist of a set of objects in a given fixed spatial relation to each other results in neurons in the added, fifth, layer that respond to one of the trained whole scenes, but do not respond if the objects in the scene are rearranged to make a new scene from the same objects (Rolls, Tromans and Stringer, 2008f). The formation of these scene-specific representations in the added layer is related to the fact that in the inferior temporal cortex, and, we showed, in the VisNet model, the receptive fields of inferior temporal cortex neurons shrink and become asymmetric when multiple objects are present simultaneously in a natural scene. This also provides a solution to the issue of the representation of multiple objects, and their relative spatial positions, in complex natural scenes (Rolls, Tromans and Stringer, 2008f). The implication of the findings is that in a unifying computational approach, competitive network processes operating in areas such as the parahippocampal cortex, the entorhinal cortex, and/or the dentate granule cells could form unique views of scenes by forming a sparse representation of these object or feature tuned inferior temporal cortex ventral visual stream representations which have some spatial asymmetry into spatial view cells in the hippocampus (Rolls, Tromans and Stringer, 2008f) (see further Section 2.8.14).

It is proposed that this type of learning could be complemented by recurrent collateral connections between the Layer 5 neurons, which would form a continuous attractor network which would encode the relations between parts of the scene, in that nearby parts of the scene would be associated together because of coactivity. These types of processes are those proposed to be involved in building spatial scene representations on the ventromedial visual stream to the medial parahippocampal gyrus in primates including humans, as described in Section 9.2.8.1 (Rolls, 2023c; Rolls et al., 2023e).

It is an interesting part of the hypothesis just described that because spatial views and places are defined by the relative spatial positions of fixed landmarks (such a buildings), slow learning of such representations over a number of trials might be useful, so that the neurons come to represent spatial views or places, and do not learn to represent a random collection of moveable objects seen once in conjunction. In this context, an alternative brain region to the dentate gyrus for this next layer of VisNet-like processing might be the parahippocampal areas that receive from the inferior temporal visual cortex. Spatial view cells are present in the parahippocampal areas (Georges-François, Rolls and Robertson, 1999; Robertson, Rolls and Georges-François, 1998; Rolls, Robertson and Georges-François, 1997a; Rolls, Treves, Robertson, Georges-François and Panzeri, 1998b; Rolls, Xiang and Franco, 2005c). These spatial view representations could be formed in these regions as, effectively, an added layer to VisNet. Moreover, these cortical regions have recurrent collateral connections that could implement a continuous attractor representation. Alternatively, it is possible that these parahippocampal spatial representations reflect the effects of backprojections from the hippocampus to the entorhinal cortex and thus to parahippocampal areas. In either case, it is an interesting and unifying hypothesis that an effect of adding an additional layer to VisNet-like ventral stream visual processing might with training in a natural environment lead to the self-organization, using the same principles as in the ventral visual stream, of spatial view or place representations in parahippocampal or hippocampal areas (Rolls, Tromans and Stringer, 2008f).

The ventral visual stream inputs that could be used to help build hippocampal spatial view representations of scenes include ventral stream temporal cortex representations of scenes (Kornblith et al., 2013; Nasr et al., 2011; Kamps et al., 2016; Epstein and Julian, 2013; Troiani et al., 2014; Epstein and Baker, 2019). My current hypothesis is that these ventral visual stream inputs are what is used to build hippocampal spatial scene representations. Consistent with this, microstimulation of the occipito-temporal scene area of macaques activated the macaque parahippocampal gyrus (Kornblith et al., 2013) in a parahippocampal region in which we recorded spatial view cells (Georges-François et al., 1999; Robertson et al., 1998; Rolls et al., 1997a, 1998b, 2005c; Rolls, 2023c).

In this situation, the route via the dorsal visual stream and parietal cortex areas to the hippocampal system via the retrosplenial cortex and posterior cingulate cortex (Rolls, 2019c) (Section 3.5) is then used for the idiothetic update of where in the allocentric spatial scene we may be looking, for example in the dark or remembering based on idiothetic information (Rolls, 2021f, 2023c; Rolls et al., 2023e).

9.3.13 A scientific theory of the art of memory: scientia artis memoriae

Simonides of Ceos lived to tell the story of how when a banquet hall collapsed in an earthquake, he could identify all the victims by recalling from each place at the table who had been sitting there (Cicero, 55 BC). This way of remembering items was developed into what has become known as *ars memoriae* by Roman senators, who presented the steps of a complex legal argument in a speech that might last a whole day by associating each step in the argument with a location in a spatial scene through which their memory could progress from one end to the other during the speech to recall each item in the correct order (Yates, 1992).

Why is *ars memoriae* so successful in helping to remember complex series of points or arguments or people or objects?

The theory is proposed that *ars memoriae* in implemented in the CA3 region of the hippocampus where there are spatial view cells in primates that allow a particular view to be associated with a particular object in an event or episodic memory. Given that the CA3 cells with their extensive recurrent collateral system connecting different CA3 cells, and associative synaptic modifiability, form an autoassociation or attractor network, the spatial view cells with their approximately Gaussian view fields become linked in a continuous attractor. In this continuous attractor network, the strength of the connections thus reflects the proximity of two spatial views. As the view space is traversed (for example by self-motion), the views are therefore successively recalled in the correct order, with no view missing. Given that each view has been associated with a different discrete item, the items are recalled in the correct order, with none missing (Rolls, Stringer and Trappenberg, 2002). There is some forgetting in the system, so the same view can be used on a later occasion to associate each view in the scene with a new set of items. This is the theory proposed for *ars memoriae* (Rolls, 2017d).

9.3.14 How navigation is performed

9.3.14.1 Navigation using a hippocampal allocentric Euclidean cognitive map

One approach is to use place cells to provide an allocentric representation of space, and to postulate that the space is Euclidean (O'Keefe and Nadel, 1978; O'Keefe, 1990). Head direction cells, which are allocentric, and anchored to the landmarks, for example the room cues, can then potentially help the animal to move in the correct direction to reach a place in allocentric space. If turns need to be made en route, the situation may become more complicated if sufficient allocentric room / landmark cues are not visible for example in a cluttered environment, for then the distance travelled needs to be estimated, and that typically involves self-motion, that is idiothetic, update, based for example on how many steps have been taken, or on integrating over velocity cues computed in the vestibular system.

An approach to how this might work in rodents has been described (Edvardsen, Bicanski and Burgess, 2020). In this model, the CA3 cells respond to places, and the recurrent collaterals in CA3 enable neighbourhood relationships between locations in the explored environment to be retrieved using the recurrent collaterals. Such a system could implement a topological navigation strategy whereby the agent navigates to its goal location by calculating the shortest path in this internal representation of the environment and then following the resultant sequence of place cells' firing fields as its itinerary. The operation of this type of system, which is a continuous attractor network (described in Section B.5), and how it can be moved from place to place has been described previously (Stringer, Rolls, Trappenberg and De Araujo, 2002a). However, such a system must have explored the environment well, so that the shortest path to the goal can be found, for this system relies on the overlapping of the place fields for previously traversed routes. Also, this system is susceptible to difficulties if an unexpected obstacle is found, for that breaks the route in the continuous attractor network. A further problem is that any CA3 spatial continuous attractor could be too bumpy (with valleys in the energy landscape) because of associations with objects etc to implement a continuous spatial chart, and may accordingly be more suitable for episodic memory (Cerasti and Treves, 2013) (see above).

9.3.14.2 Navigation using an entorhinal cortex goal vector system

Partly because of these difficulties, Edvardsen, Bicanski and Burgess (2020) complemented the hippocampal CA3 place cell system with an entorhinal cortex grid cell system to support goal vector representations (Poulter et al., 2018). Given grid cell activity for the present location and a trace of the grid cell activity for the goal location, the appropriate straight-line vector across two-dimensional space can be determined with the grid cell system. The agent can then find the correct bearing toward the goal location even across large stretches of unexplored space due to the metric properties of grid cells. This could support navigation in the correct direction across unexplored territory, but would fail if there was an obstacle in the direct path that required a detour. In a combined model, 'replay' from a hippocampal CA3 model (described in Section 9.3.4.4) using place cells is used to dynamically adjust the target for the vector navigation process. The whole system uses rodent border cells which respond when a border is encountered (Solstad, Boccara, Kropff, Moser and Moser, 2008), and rodent boundary vector cells (which signal the bearing and distance to a border (Lever et al., 2009)) to help with obstacle avoidance. The system is then programmed with a graph data structure that uses a graph search algorithm for the place cell system, and the agent's high-level control logic is represented by explicit rules, so it is not clear how the system would operate biologically. Further, in the model, each visited place field is associated with and can recall when useful the unique entorhinal grid cell activity pattern associated with that place cell firing, in order in the model for any location to become the start or end point for vector navigation. Also, the applicability of the system to primates including humans is not clear, as some of the cell types utilized in the model are not known to be present in primates, and some of the types of spatial representation found in the primate hippocampal system (Rolls and Wirth, 2018; Rolls, 2023c) are not part of the approach.

9.3.14.3 Transforms between allocentric and egocentric representations

Because the parietal cortex utilizes in part egocentric coordinates (e.g. direction relative to the head), and the hippocampal system uses allocentric coordinates (e.g. allocentric place cells and allocentric head direction cells), it is important to be able to transform between these representations. For example, if we are in one place in allocentric space, what will the egocentric view look like? Conversely, if we see a set of landmarks in head-based (i.e. egocentric) coordinates, can we work out where we are in allocentric space? Transforms of this type are likely to be important in navigation as well as in spatial memory and in imagery which is typically egocentric. Three approaches to this are described.

One approach utilizes types of neuron found in the rat, and argues that the transform takes place in the retrosplenial cortex (Bicanski and Burgess, 2018) (Fig. 9.36). The model uses boundary vector cells, known in the rat and which respond to the allocentric bearing and distance to a boundary such as a wall, to specify the allocentric place. The egocentric parietal representation used is in head-based coordinates, and the model specifies neurons that respond to extended boundaries ('PWb neurons'), and neurons that respond to discrete objects ('PWo neurons'). The receptive fields of both these populations lie in peri-personal space, that is are tuned to distances and egocentric directions ahead, left or right of the agent. Then gain modulation by head direction can be used to convert the egocentric view representation into an allocentric representation, using principles described in Section 3.4.2. It is suggested that the reverse transform could also be performed in the retrosplenial cortex, but the mechanism would be very different. This model does not deal with how eye movements affect spatial vision which is a major part of what is implemented in the primate dorsal visual system in areas such as LIP, VIP, and area 7a together with mechanisms for reaching into space. (Eye movements and reaching into space are poorly developed and understood in rodents, and no set of highly developed dorsal visual stream cortical areas is found in rodents). The proposal (Bicanski and Burgess, 2018) also relies on boundary-vector cells found in rodents. The model does not account for the types of neuron found in the primate dorsal visual system through the parietal hierarchy which even before the retrosplenial cortex show evidence of encoding in allocentric coordinates, as described in Chapter 3.

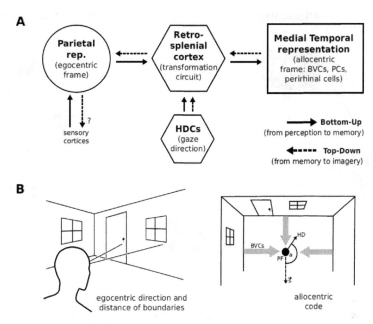

Fig. 9.36 Schematic of the Bicanski and Burgess approach to egocentric to allocentric coordinate transforms. (A) Processed sensory inputs reach parietal areas and support an egocentric representation of the local environment (in a head-centered frame of reference). Retrosplenial cortex uses current head or gaze direction to perform the transformation from egocentric to allocentric coding. At a given location, environmental layout is represented as an allocentric code by activity in a set of Boundary Vector Cells (BVCs), the place cells (PCs) corresponding to the location, and perirhinal neurons representing boundary identities. (In a familiar environment, all these representations are associated via Hebbian learning to form an attractor network.) Black arrows indicate the flow of information during perception and memory encoding (bottom-up). Dotted arrows indicate the reverse flow of information, reconstructing the parietal representation from view-point invariant memory (imagery, top-down). (B) Illustration of the egocentric (left panel) and allocentric frame of reference (right panel), where the vector s indicates South (an arbitrary reference direction) and the angle a is coded for by head direction cells (HDCs), which modulate the transformation circuit. This allows Boundary Vector Cells and Place Cells to code for location within a given environmental layout irrespective of the agent's head direction (HD). The place field (PF, black circle) of an example Place Cell is shown together with possible Boundary Vector Cell inputs driving the Place Cell (broad grey arrows). (Reproduced from Bicanski,A. and Burgess,N. (2018) A neural-level model of spatial memory and imagery. Elife 7: e33752.))

A second approach makes an interesting point about the mathematics of the relation between egocentric and allocentric space, as shown in Fig. 9.37 (Ekstrom et al., 2017; Ekstrom and Ranganath, 2018). This approach is much more closely related to the ability of humans to visualize what they see when in different allocentric locations. It discusses evidence that allocentric and egocentric representations are found in quite a large set of brain areas, and argues that navigation is performed by this very distributed system. However, this approach is not developed into a formal computational model that specifies how the computations are performed, that is, what the types of neuron are that are involved, and what computation enables the transforms between different neuron types. Also, as shown below, it is helpful to consider separate navigational strategies that are implemented when the navigation is idiothetic, that is, based on self-motion in the dark or when landmarks cannot be seen, compared to navigation when landmarks can be seen.

The third approach to coordinate transforms builds on the types of neuron actually found at different stages of the hierarchically organised primate dorsal visual system (Rolls, 2020b), is described in Chapter 3, and summarized next in the context of navigation. The parietal cortex hierarchy transforms from egocentric retinal representations to allocentric bearing to a landmark and spatial view representations. The system starts with representations in retinal coordinates, and transforms these into head-based egocentric representations in LIP and VIP

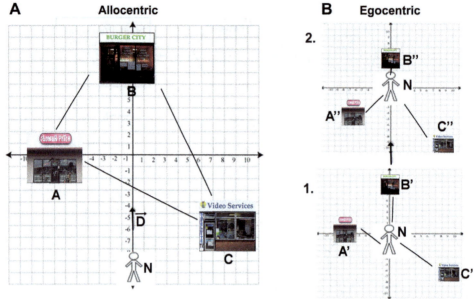

Fig. 9.37 Similarities between allocentric and egocentric coordinate systems. A: within an allocentric coordinate system, A, B, and C are landmark coordinates, N is the position of the navigator, and D is the displacement vector (movement of the navigator). AB, AC, and BC are therefore vectors that indicate both the direction and distance of landmarks to each other. The positions of landmarks stay stable with displacements of the navigator. B: in an egocentric coordinate system, in contrast, the positions of landmarks change continuously with movements of the navigator (i.e., movement from frame 1 to frame 2). The position of the navigator, however, is always centered at the origin. A', B', and C' are positions of landmarks in egocentric frame 1, A", B", and C" are positions of landmarks in egocentric frame 2. These correspond to vectors A'N, B'N, C'N, etc. Within this framework, egocentric to allocentric conversion can be accomplished many different ways. For example, AB, BC, AC in allocentric coordinates can be approximated with vector subtraction (A'N - B'N or A'N - B'N); see McNaughton et al. (1991) for more details. This conversion can also be solved using estimation of the Pythagorean theorem [e.g., $AB = \sqrt{(A'N^2 + B'N^2)}$ or $AB = \sqrt{(A''N^2 + B''N^2)}$]. This is because vectors AB = A'B' = A"B" and the displacement vector (D) are the same in allocentric (A) and egocentric (B) space. This also means the two subspaces have the same basis set. (Reproduced from Ekstrom,A.D., Huffman,D.J. and Starrett,M. (2017) Interacting networks of brain regions underlie human spatial navigation: a review and novel synthesis of the literature. Journal of Neurophysiology 118: 3328–3344. © American Physiological Society.)

using gain modulation by eye position. Then the head-centred representation is transformed into an 'allocentric bearing to a landmark' from the primate using gain modulation by head direction (Rolls, 2020b). This type of representation is potentially of great use in navigation, as described below.

Then the 'allocentric bearing to a landmark' representation is transformed into an allocentric *spatial view* representation by gain modulation using translation of the animal to different places (Rolls, 2020b) (see Chapter 3). This builds a representation in the same spatial coordinates used in the primate hippocampus, namely allocentric spatial view that represents a location in allocentric space 'out there', independently of the bearing of the landmark and of the exact place where the individual is located, as well as its head direction and eye position. This type of representation is ideal for the episodic memory functions of the primate hippocampus, for it enables memories to be formed of where in allocentric space an object or person was seen. Because the memory is independent of the exact place where the animal is located, if the same location is seen from a different place, the hippocampal memory system will correctly recall the object or person that was at that location. Similarly, if the object or person is the recall cue, the location in allocentric space where they were seen can be recalled from the CA3 network in the hippocampus, and that memory is suitable for navigation to that location, because it does not depend on the place where the animal is, which would be very restrictive indeed in a memory system (Rolls, 2020b) (see Chapter 3).

This system is likely to apply just as much to humans as to macaques, given the considerable similarity of their visual systems, and the use of a retina with a high resolution fovea that enables particular locations in viewed scenes 'out there' and possibly at a considerable distance to be encoded.

How would such a system operate if an egocentric view was being recalled from an allocentric representation? One possibility would be to use the hippocampal spatial view cells, which as a continuous attractor network are effectively a set of viewed items linked in the correct order (Rolls, Stringer and Trappenberg, 2002; Rolls, 2017d). The information is already there in the way that spatial view cells are implemented in the primate hippocampus. This is part of the utility of the primate allocentric spatial view cell system: that it provides a natural route to imagery. This great utility would not apply if only allocentric bearing to a landmark cells were computed in primates. This also may be a useful concept to bear in mind by those who believe that episodic memory is viewpoint dependent. Spatial view cells would make a scene maintain its parts in the correct spatial relationship when viewed from many places, all on the same side of the scene.

It might be more difficult to utilise this type of hippocampal representation to imagine the scene seen from the other side if we have never seen it from the other side before. But for that case, the order would still be present in the hippocampal spatial view continuous attractor, and that could be used to reconstruct in a type of 'perspective-taking' what the scene would look like from the other side. This is an interesting way to link human spatial imagery to the representations of scenes 'out there' provided in the primate hippocampus by spatial view cells (Rolls, 2018b; Rolls and Wirth, 2018; Rolls, 2023d).

9.3.15 Navigational computations using neuron types found in primates including humans

The analysis of coordinate transforms in the primate dorsal visual system described here (see Chapter 3 and Rolls (2020b)) and referred to above deals with particular types of neuron known to be present in primates, and these neuron types provide very interesting possibilities for different navigational strategies in primates, some of which are described next, based on the types of neuron found in primates, which are relevant to better understanding navigation in humans (Rolls, 2021f). Indeed, exactly the computations described here could be involved in different types of human navigation (Rolls, 2021f). As a reminder, neurotoxic lesions that selectively damage the primate hippocampus impair spatial scene memory (Murray et al., 1998), and spatial location memory (Waters, Basile and Murray, 2023), when for example environmental visual cues are used in foraging and navigation (Hampton, Hampstead and Murray, 2004; Lavenex, Amaral and Lavenex, 2006). Some of the mechanisms involved that are likely to use hippocampal spatial view cells are considered next.

9.3.15.1 Navigation using spatial view cells

In this strategy, navigation is implemented by proceeding via a series of landmarks, to which spatial view cells respond. This is allocentric navigation, as spatial view cells are allocentric. It is illustrated in Fig. 9.38. The individual learns the sequence of landmarks, either by previous trial and error learning, or by following another individual, or in humans by being told the list of landmarks and holding them in working memory. The individual looks for the next landmark in the list (e.g. L2 if at L1), and locomotes to approach it, and then looks for the next landmark, and locomotes towards it (Rolls, 2021f).

If this is the first time the route has been followed in humans, the list of sequential landmarks could be implemented in the hippocampal episodic memory system. The sequence could be stored by using the time-cells described in Chapter 9, and associating each land-

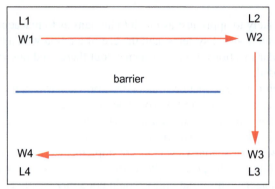

Fig. 9.38 An example of navigation using spatial view cells. The task is to start at Landmark 1 (L1), and to reach Landmark 4 (L4). There is a barrier so that Landmark 4, and for that matter Landmark 3, cannot be seen from Landmark 1. The course followed is shown by red arrows. Each landmark can be thought of as having a waypoint (e.g. W2), or intermediate step in the whole route, associated with it. (After Rolls, E. T. (2020) Neurons and navigation in primates including humans.)

mark with a different time in the time-cell system. Another possibility is that the sequence of landmarks is stored in short-term / working memory in the prefrontal cortex (Chapter 13).

Each step in the sequence could have additional information associated with it. One example at W2 could be 'turn right', which is egocentric information, and is available in whole body motion cells in the primate hippocampus (O'Mara, Rolls, Berthoz and Kesner, 1994) (known as speed cells in rodents (Kropff et al., 2015)); or 'turn South', which is allocentric information, and is available in head direction cells in the primate presubiculum (Robertson, Rolls, Georges-François and Panzeri, 1999). This is exactly the type of information that could be associated together in the primate hippocampus, utilizing especially CA3 cells (see Chapter 9). Another type of information that could also be associated with each step of the sequence is the distance to be travelled between the landmarks, which could be implemented by idiothetic update. The idiothetic update mechanisms are described in Section 9.3.15.4, and could utilize the whole body motion cells (O'Mara et al., 1994).

If the route becomes well learned, it could be implemented by a continuous attractor network in the hippocampus, which would implement the spatial views as being adjacent in the sequence because of overlap of the spatial view fields (Chapter 9). Each step of the continuous attractor could have additional information associated with it, in the way just described. Continuous attractor networks are described in Section B.5, and their use for hippocampal spatial view cell navigation networks has been described (Stringer, Rolls and Trappenberg, 2005; Rolls and Stringer, 2005; Rolls, Tromans and Stringer, 2008f).

Part of the utility of spatial view cells for this computational role in navigation is that they are largely place invariant, as well as invariant with respect to head direction and eye position, and of the bearing of the landmark (Georges-François, Rolls and Robertson, 1999), so are able to guide the animal irrespective of the exact place, head direction, etc from which the next landmark is viewed. Moreover, if the landmark is temporarily obscured, by a barrier, darkness etc, then spatial view cells can still be used to guide the agent to the next landmark, because they can be updated for a few minutes by self-motion (Robertson, Rolls and Georges-François, 1998). A major advantage of navigation using spatial view cells is that this does not require path integration of for example head direction to maintain a sense of direction, and so very long routes with many legs can be followed (Rolls, 2021f).

This type of navigation is illustrated in program NavSVC.m described in Appendix D, and by Rolls (2021f). It is proposed that this is the most common type of navigational strategy used in humans and other primates (Rolls, 2021f).

Humans normally navigate to a viewed object or reward in a scene such as a building, and non-human primates might locomote to particular locations in the viewed environment with local cues where there are sources of food, water, shelter and a place to sleep etc. In these cases, identifiable environmental features identify each location, and spatial view cells encode the features in these locations, and their spatial overlap with features of nearby locations (Rolls, 2023d). Hippocampal spatial view cells are ideal for this type of navigation. In this context the type of navigation to an unmarked place without local visual cues and relying on relatively distant environmental cues (as in the Morris rodent water maze (Morris, Garrud, Rawlins and O'Keefe, 1982)) is unusual in humans and other primates (Rolls, 2023d). It is like looking for a needle in a haystack using distant hills as navigational cues. What is often studied in rodents as a model of navigation without any local cues as in the Morris water maze may not be at all commonly how humans and other primates navigate. Spatial view cells provide the mechanism often used for navigation in humans and other primates which is typically towards visible landmarks such as a building, the top of a hill, etc (Rolls, 2021f, 2023d). Navigation may thus be performed in primates including humans (Rolls, 2021f, 2023a,d) in very different ways to those utilised in rodents, in which local place-associated cues sensed with the vibrissae or olfactory system define places, and idiothetic navigation between such places often in the dark may be important (McNaughton, Barnes, Gerrard, Gothard, Jung, Knierim, Kudrimoti, Qin, Skaggs, Suster and Weaver, 1996; Moser, Rowland and Moser, 2015; Moser, Moser and McNaughton, 2017). Moreover, because of the limited visual acuity of rodents illustrated in Fig. 9.12 in Section 9.2.5, navigation in rodents is unlikely to be towards small objects or rewards located at distant locations in visual scenes, whereas this is typical of navigation in primates including humans implemented using spatial view cells (Rolls, 2023d).

The type of navigation based on spatial view cells can be considered as a true navigational strategy, because the strategy would include a sequential list of landmarks, with each landmark in the list potentially being associated with for example a body turn or a change of allocentric heading (using head direction cells) to head for example South, to help find the next landmark. Moreover, the navigation can be to a hidden landmark goal, as illustrated in Fig. 9.38 (Rolls, 2021f).

9.3.15.2 Navigation using allocentric bearing to a landmark cells

Neurons that appear to respond to an allocentric bearing to a stimulus in space (an example of which might be a landmark) have been described in the macaque parietal cortex area 7a (Snyder, Grieve, Brotchie and Andersen, 1998) and in the posterior cingulate cortex (Dean and Platt, 2006) (which receives inputs from the parietal cortex including area 7a) (see Section 3.4.2). Neurons that may respond in the same way are found in the primate hippocampus, in that some neurons respond when the macaque looks at a spatial view, but from only some places in a virtual environment (Wirth et al., 2017). Moreover, allocentric bearing to a landmark neurons are generated naturally in a theory and model of spatial coordinate transforms in the dorsal visual system (Rolls, 2020b) (see Chapter 3 and Fig. 3.6).

Navigation that could be implemented by allocentric bearing to a landmark (ABL) neurons is illustrated in Fig. 9.39. The route to be followed is from Waypoint 1 (W1) to Waypoint 4, as shown by the red arrows, and as before a barrier prevents the goal from being seen at the start of the navigation. The individual starts at W1, with the information that it must start with a head direction of East, and locomote until the bearing to landmark L2 becomes 45 degrees. For this, information from only head direction cells and allocentric bearing to a landmark cells is needed. At Waypoint 2 in the sequence, information is associated that a right turn should be made (using whole body motion cells), or that a turn should be made to head in direction South (using head direction cells). The individual then locomotes South until the bearing to landmark L3 becomes 135 degrees. (Of course, the bearings to the other

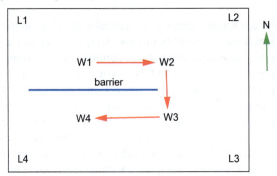

Fig. 9.39 An example of navigation using allocentric bearing to a landmark cells. The task is to start at Waypoint 1 (W1), and to reach Waypoint 4 (W4). There is a barrier so that Waypoint 4, and for that matter Waypoint 3, cannot be seen from Waypoint 1. The course followed is shown by red arrows. The landmarks used are L1–L4. North is indicated by N. (After Rolls, E. T. (2020) Neurons and navigation in primates including humans.)

visible landmarks, L2 and L4, could also be used.) At Waypoint 3 in the sequence, information is associated that a right turn should be made (using whole body motion cells), or that a turn should be made to head direction West (using head direction cells), and that locomotion should continue in that direction. The final instruction is that the goal has been reached at W4 when the bearing to landmark L4 is 225 degrees.

The sequence of steps, and the information associated with all steps, could be implemented in the same ways as described for spatial view cells in Section 9.3.15.1.

The interest of this illustration is that it involves navigation to places that are not at landmarks, and uses just two types of neuron found in primates, allocentric bearing to a landmark cells, and head direction or whole body motion cells.

This type of navigation (Rolls, 2021f) is illustrated in program NavABL.m described in Appendix D.

It is noted that if the distance to a landmark is part of what is encoded by allocentric bearing to a landmark cells, then this is helpful, though not essential. In rodents, cells that reflect the bearing and distance to an object have been described (Hoydal et al., 2019), and the primate equivalent that would be useful in navigation is allocentric bearing to a landmark vector cells that encode distance to a landmark as well as allocentric bearing to a landmark.

If more than one 'allocentric bearing to a landmark' cell is used at any one time in this type of navigation, then the navigation can be thought of as navigation from place to place, where each place is defined by a combination of active 'allocentric bearing to a landmark' cells. Navigation with such a system is considered next.

9.3.15.3 Navigation using combinations of allocentric bearing to a landmark cells, and triangulation

As just noted, if combinations of active allocentric bearing to a landmark cells are formed, these would represent places. Navigation using this type of triangulation is harder to implement in the brain, but is practiced by mariners, and is described for comparison with the methods previously described (Rolls, 2021f).

One way to implement this can be described using the route illustrated in Fig. 9.39. The environment could be defined as a Euclidean allocentric topological space as envisaged for rodent place cells (O'Keefe and Nadel, 1978), with X and Y coordinates to define each place. To locomote from W1 to W2, the agent would calculate its place at every small step of the locomotion, using triangulation based on combinations of the active 'allocentric bearing to a landmark' cells. It would then calculate with trigonometry the (allocentric) compass bearing to W2 using its current X,Y position, and its knowledge of the X,Y position of W2, and set off in that direction using head direction cells. This type of navigation works if a topological map is stored in the head, and if trigonometric calculations can be performed, but may not be biologically plausible without the ability to calculate directions in topological maps. (This type of navigation is illustrated in program NavTRI.m described in Appendix D (Rolls, 2021f).) This type of navigation by triangulation is thus very different from that performed using spatial view cells, which does not require trigonometry in a Euclidean topological space.

Instead of using geometrical computation in a Euclidean space of the type implemented using triangulation as implemented in NavTRI.m, it is suggested that in primates including humans, simultaneously active spatial view cells for different landmarks in a scene can be associated together to form a spatial representation of a scene, seen from a particular place. As a primate traverses through different places and the scene defined by the landmarks gradually changes, storage of a few such scenes (using for example the hippocampus to store such episodic memories) could enable later recall of the place, given the set of spatial view cells that are active by comparison with the stored representations. It is proposed that such a neural mechanism might enable spatial view cells to contribute to the lookup in an association memory of a place where the individual is located. This is proposed as another biologically plausible way for spatial view cells to be involved in navigation, by using the viewed scene to recall a place. Such a mechanism might operate to provide useful accuracy even without the need to store too many scenes. Although allocentric bearing to a landmark cells (which might also encode distance) might be used in addition to or as an alternative to spatial view cells, there is the considerable disadvantage that very many allocentric bearing to a landmark cells could be required, as a number of bearings need to be specifiable for each landmark.

For these reasons, navigation in primates using spatial view cells or 'allocentric bearing to a landmark' cells as described in Sections 9.3.15.1 and 9.3.15.2, *or combinations of these approaches*, is more likely to be the type of computation that is typically used in humans, and other primates. Navigation using approach to landmarks has been described as navigation using beacons (Ekstrom and Isham, 2017), though no neural mechanism was proposed. I propose (Rolls, 2021f) that spatial view cells provide an important and natural component of the neural mechanism, and this has been illustrated in Fig. 9.38, with a computational model of this (illustrated in program NavSVC.m). The approach using 'bearing to a landmark' cells just described goes beyond navigation to beacons, because it involves the computationally more specific navigation involving taking bearings to beacons, and using that information to make a turn in an allocentric or egocentric direction that is held in memory (Rolls, 2021f).

As soon as one has combinations of primate cells encoding allocentric bearings to landmarks in an environment, as proposed here, then this can provide a key part, it is proposed, of a topological allocentric navigational system. Another important aspect of the approach to navigation in humans and primates described here is that it does not have to be 'egocentric' *or* 'allocentric' (Ekstrom and Isham, 2017), but can use egocentric whole body motion and/or allocentric head direction cells, in combination with (allocentric) spatial view cells and/or 'allocentric bearing to a landmark' cells (Rolls, 2021f).

9.3.15.4 Idiothetic navigation in primates

A very different strategy for navigation to the use of visual cues about locations in scenes is idiothetic navigation, that is, navigation based on self-motion. This is an important strategy in the dark or when visual landmarks cannot be seen. Idiothetic information may also be combined with information based on visual (or for that matter auditory) inputs as part of a navigational strategy.

Three principal types of neuron in primates provide idiothetic information useful for navigation. The first type is head direction cells found in the primate presubiculum (Robertson, Rolls, Georges-François and Panzeri, 1999) (and probably elsewhere) (Section 9.2.6). These neurons continue to encode head direction even when the monkey is moved from a familiar room to a relatively unfamiliar corridor (Fig. 9.13), and maintain their directionality for a few minutes in the dark, after which they drift. This is important, for these cells can only maintain head directionality for a relatively short period without visual cues to lock them back into the correct directionality. Their inputs are derived from velocity signals produced in the vestibular nuclei in the brainstem, and reach the parietal vestibular cortical areas (Grusser et al., 1990; Ventre-Dominey, 2014). The direction signal thus reflects a great deal of integration over time, and this is imprecise and noisy resulting in drift. This means that only short-term idiothetic navigation is possible. Similar head direction cells are well known in rodents (Taube et al., 1990a; Cullen and Taube, 2017). Vestibular signals influence neurons in a number of parietal cortex areas including VIP, with neurons that respond to head position (i.e. head direction) or head acceleration, in addition to the many neurons with head velocity tuning (Klam and Graf, 2003). Neurons that respond to vestibular inputs produced by head rotation or translation are also found in area 7a (Avila, Lakshminarasimhan, DeAngelis and Angelaki, 2019).

The second type of neuron that provides idiothetic information useful for navigation in primates are hippocampal whole body motion cells (O'Mara, Rolls, Berthoz and Kesner, 1994) (Section 9.2.4.2). Some of these neurons respond to angular head rotation, and others to linear translation. Some of these neurons respond to vestibular cues, some to the corresponding visual optic flow cues, and some to both. The vestibular inputs are evident when the movements are in the dark. In the light, rotation of the environment to produce optic flow was able to activate some of these neurons. Some of this testing was performed while the monkey was moved on a robot (O'Mara et al., 1994). There may be similar neurons in rodents in the medial entorhinal cortex termed 'speed cells' which respond to translation (i.e. linear motion) (Kropff, Carmichael, Moser and Moser, 2015), and neurons that respond to angular velocity (i.e. head rotation) have also been described in the rat parietal cortex (Wilber et al., 2017, 2014), but the roles of visual vs vestibular inputs for these rodent neurons are not yet clear. It is neurons that respond to vestibular inputs that are important for idiothetic update in the dark. Of course the visual cues produced by the corresponding motion may be used for idiothetic navigation in the light.

Neurons of these two types could be used as follows for navigation in the dark, or without visible landmarks (Rolls, 2021f). We can consider the route illustrated in Fig. 9.39. If the individual starts off with an Easterly head direction at Waypoint 1, then navigation would use head direction cells to keep the direction constant, and integration over linear whole body motion cells (which encode velocity) to locomote for the distance to Waypoint 2. At Waypoint 2, the sequence generator would have associated with it an egocentric 'turn right' signal calibrated by head rotation whole body motion cells; or an allocentric head direction signal to turn to face South. The distance to W3 would then be traversed using integration over the linear whole body motion cells. After the correct distance, the sequence generator would specify an egocentric 'turn right' signal calibrated by head rotation whole body motion cells; or an allocentric head direction signal to turn to face East; etc.

This navigation could thus be performed using only primate head direction and whole body motion cells. The sequence of steps, and the information associated with each step, could be implemented in the same ways as described for spatial view cells in Section 9.3.15.1.

This idiothetic navigation would be suitable for only a few minutes, for after that time the integration required to compute head direction, and distance travelled based on whole body motion / vestibular inputs, becomes inaccurate.

Importantly, this idiothetic type of navigation could be used as a supplement with the strategies described previously using spatial view cells (Section 9.3.15.1) or allocentric bearing to a landmark cells (Section 9.3.15.2) (Rolls, 2021f). For example, when navigation using bearing to a landmark cells described in Section 9.3.15.2 is being used, it could be helpful to use the known distance between W1 and W2 to help provide information about when W2 had been reached (see Fig. 9.39). The implementation could use the self-motion cues to update the position in a spatial continuous attractor in the ways described by Stringer, Rolls, Trappenberg and De Araujo (2002a) and Stringer, Rolls and Trappenberg (2005).

A third type of neuron, spatial view cells, could also be useful in idiothetic navigation in primates including humans. As described in Section 9.2.4.1, spatial view cells can be updated in the dark and without visual landmarks by the idiothetic signals head direction and eye position, and probably by whole body motion (Robertson, Rolls and Georges-François, 1998). Mechanisms for this idiothetic update are described in Chapter 3 (Rolls, 2020b). Accordingly, navigation could be towards a remembered spatial view location even when the view is not visible. As with other types of idiothetic navigation, it would probably be useful for only a few minutes, due to the inaccuracy of the path integration over the idiothetic signals.

In more detail, the dorsal visual system plays an important role in the idiothetic update of spatial representations, as described in Section 3.4, and indeed this route is likely to be involved in the idiothetic update of hippocampal and parahippocampal spatial view cells (Rolls, 2020b). The idiothetic updates are for eye position, head direction, and place, and allow representations to be formed that are in allocentric spatial view coordinates. This is useful for navigation when visual inputs are not available, for it provides a recall cue to the hippocampal system via the parahippocampal cortex (see Fig. 9.1) that enables the object at a spatial view location to be recalled even when the spatial view is not visible (Rolls, 2021f). That is an important way for identifying the goals for navigation even when vision is not possible. The implication of this is that much of the idiothetic update for spatial representations and navigation is performed in the primate dorsal visual system. This idiothetic update can then communicate with the hippocampal memory system via brain areas such as the retrosplenial cortex and posterior cingulate cortex, as illustrated in Fig. 9.1 (Rolls, 2021f).

9.3.15.5 Conclusions on navigation in primates including humans

The new proposal has been made that key principles of navigation in primates use spatial view cells (Rolls, 2021f). The great development of the primate visual system with its foveate representations that are capitalised on to enable neurons on the hippocampus, parahippocampal gyrus and probably connected brain regions to respond to viewed locations 'out there' in space enables navigational strategies to be used very frequently based on spatial view cells. The fact that spatial view cells are allocentric (see Section 9.2.4.1) has important implications for navigation, for it means that independently of the place where the human is located, or of the egocentric coordinates relative to the human observer of a landmark being viewed, or the allocentric bearing of a landmark, navigation can be based on movement towards (or away from) a landmark or sequence of landmarks (Rolls, 2021f).

This type of navigation based on spatial view cells can be considered as a true navigational strategy, because the strategy would include a sequential list of landmarks, with each landmark in the list potentially being associated with for example a body turn or a change of allocentric heading (using head direction cells) to head for example South, to help find the next landmark (Rolls, 2021f). Such a computation could be implemented in a continuous attractor network forming a chart (Battaglia and Treves, 1998b) of linked spatial view cells with associated primate egocentric body turn ('whole body motion' cells (O'Mara et al., 1994) or allocentric head direction cells (Robertson et al., 1999) in ways that have been investigated computationally (Rolls and Stringer, 2005; Stringer, Rolls and Trappenberg, 2005; Rolls, Tromans and Stringer, 2008f). Moreover, if the landmarks were temporarily obscured, idiothetic update of them based on self motion could occur (Robertson et al., 1998) using the gain modulation mechanisms in the dorsal visual system described in Section 3.4 (Rolls, 2020b). An alternative to a continuous attractor network for spatial view cell based navigation could be a short-term or working memory system implemented in the prefrontal cortex (see Chapter 13) to remember the sequence of landmarks, and this could be particularly advantageous for new routes for which a continuous attractor representation has not already been set up by learning.

Geometrical computation using triangulation for navigation in primates including humans could it is proposed be based on the allocentric bearing to a landmark cells as exemplified in Sections 9.3.15.2 and 9.3.15.3 and as described further by Rolls (2021f).

It is proposed that this type of visually guided navigation based on spatial view cells and perhaps allocentric bearing to a landmark cells is the prototypical method used for navigation in humans and other primates (Rolls, 2021f). Humans given instruction about how to find a location are typically given a series of instructions about what to look for as they navigate, often supplemented with body turn information such as 'turn left when you see Notre Dame' or heading information such as 'turn South when you see Notre Dame'. This is not the method of navigation that is typically described based on the place and other neuron types found in rodents (O'Keefe and Nadel, 1978; McNaughton et al., 1996; Bicanski and Burgess, 2018). Those systems in rodents can work almost as well in the dark, yet humans find navigation in the dark without views of spatial scenes very difficult for more than a very few minutes.

The spatial view cell approach to navigation proposed here has considerable advantages over navigation using 'allocentric bearing to a landmark' cells, which require a sense of allocentric direction to be maintained while the bearings are being made, which becomes difficult because of inaccuracies in the idiothetic update of the sense of direction for more than a few minutes, with reset being required based for example on a dominant landmark, or on the set of currently viewable landmarks. As a list of waypoints defined by spatial view cells does not suffer from this problem of maintaining a sense of direction, and because of its simplicity as described here, it is proposed that this is the most common type of navigational strategy used in humans and other primates (Rolls, 2021f).

The force of this proposal (Rolls, 2021f) about the use of spatial view cells for navigation in humans and other primates is made evident when we consider navigation by humans without vision, for example in complete darkness, when humans have to fall back on the path integration mechanisms for place using direction and distance traversed of the type that are typically described as being important in rodents (Stringer et al., 2002a; Bicanski and Burgess, 2018). This approach is used for example by mariners as 'dead-reckoning navigation' when out of the sight of land. Mariners rely for this type of navigation on a compass, for humans without landmarks can perform idiothetic navigation for only short periods, because head direction cells then quickly lose their sense of direction.

The new proposal for navigation using spatial view cells in primates including humans (Rolls, 2021f) is very different from the much more complex systems for navigation using place cells in rodents that requires a idiothetic update using a topological map of space (O'Keefe and Nadel, 1978; O'Keefe, 1990; Poulter, Hartley and Lever, 2018; Bicanski and Burgess, 2018; Edvardsen, Bicanski and Burgess, 2020). Rodents have poor vision, and rely on local sensing of the place where they are located using touch sensing by vibrissae, olfactory cues, etc, and often navigation underground or in the dark. The rodent place cell system (O'Keefe and Nadel, 1978; Morris et al., 1982; O'Keefe et al., 1998; Hartley et al., 2014) may be specialized for that. But primates including humans have highly developed visual systems that enable completely different types of navigation, using spatial view neurons and mechanisms of the type described here, and only fall back on the very different idiothetic mechanisms when they have to navigate for example in the dark, which most humans know is a very different type of navigation, which often does rely on somatosensory input to guide the navigation.

These points underline the importance of the spatial view cell navigational strategies described here for humans, rather than the navigational strategies based on place cell idiothetic update proposed for rodents.

The exact brain regions in which navigation using spatial view cells is implemented is a topic for future research. As noted above, the hippocampal system may be involved in relatively new environments when new memories must be formed. Spatial view cells in the medial parahippocampal gyrus (Rolls, 2023c; Rolls et al., 2023e) are likely to be important. For well established navigational routes, brain areas such as the parietal cortex are likely to be involved in processing motion and avoiding obstacles, and semantic parts of the anterior temporal lobe and inferior parietal cortex, may be involved (Chapters 8 and 10). For very well learned routes, for which the strategy may be somewhat different, the habit system (Chapter 16) may be involved.

9.3.15.6 Synthesis: different functions of the parahippocampal scene area and hippocampus in navigation in primates including humans

The Parahippocampal Scene Area (PSA, also known as the Parahippocampal Place Area (PPA)) may in primates including humans build scene representations in the ventromedial visual stream (Fig. 9.18, Rolls et al. (2023e) and Rolls (2023c)). These scene representations could be in the form of continuous attractor networks, in which the features in a scene are associated together based on overlap between the features (or of features held in a local short term memory if the landmark features are too distant). The operation of continuous attractor networks is described in Section B.5, and their implementation of spatial scenes using spatial view cells is described by Rolls and Stringer (2005) and Stringer, Rolls and Trappenberg (2005). Very different scenes, for example scenes in different countries, need not be stored in the same attractor network in the parahippocampal scene area, which is sufficiently large to include many cortical local attractor networks each 1–2 mm in diameter.

These Parahippocampal Scene Area networks would be appropriate for scene representations, but need not implement navigation from one place to another, which in any case might best be kept separate, for many different navigational routes might need to be computed, and it would be advantageous to keep the actual representations of scenes considerably independent of and not distorted by all the particular navigational routes an individual might learn.

The actual navigation from place to place using scene landmark cues encoded by spatial view cells (Rolls, 2023c) could then be implemented in a different network, for example the single attractor network in hippocampal CA3. The advantage of using CA3 for the navigation is that having a single continuous attractor network for a whole route would ensure continuity of the route from location to location. Interestingly, the navigational route might not be in metric Euclidean space, as what is stored for the landmarks in the parahippocampal scene area and connected to the hippocampus might well not be equally spaced landmark cues, but instead just prominent landmark cues, which might not be equally spaced. Accordingly I do not accept the claim made by O'Keefe and Nadel (1978) and O'Keefe (1990) that the navigational space as implemented in the brain is Euclidean and would permit mathematical geometric calculations. Instead, I have suggested above that the navigation is implemented by a trajectory through a continuous attractor network that contains scene information but also other information such as body turn and head direction information (Rolls, 2021f).

It would be appropriate to have the navigational system in the hippocampus separate from the spatial scene system in the parahippocampal scene area, for the navigational system would benefit greatly from information about body turns made at particular points in the route (Rolls, 2021f), which is exactly what is represented in the hippocampus as shown by whole body motion cells (O'Mara et al., 1994). Similarly head direction information present in the primate presubiculum (Robertson et al., 1999; Rolls, 2023c) would be important for the hippocampal navigational system implemented in the hippocampus.

In humans, long-term semantic representations, perhaps language based, in the neocortex could also be useful in navigation for well known environments and routes, and need to be taken into account when considering effects of hippocampal damage on navigation.

9.4 Tests of the theory of hippocampal cortex operation

Empirical evidence that tests the theory comes from a wide range of investigation methods, including the effects of selective lesions to different subregions of the hippocampal system mainly in rodents, the activity of single neurons in different subregions of the hippocampal system, pharmacological and genetic manipulations of different parts of the system, the detailed neuroanatomy of the system, and functional neuroimaging studies and clinical neuropsychological studies in humans (Kesner and Rolls, 2015).

Because the theory makes predictions about the functions of different parts of the hippocampal system (e.g. dentate, CA3, and CA1), evidence from subregion analysis is very relevant to testing the theory, and such evidence is included in the following assessment, which starts from the dentate gyrus, and works through to CA1. The evidence comes from the effects of selective lesions to different subregions of the hippocampal system, the activity of single neurons in different subregions, together with pharmacological and genetic manipulations of different parts of the system (Kesner and Rolls, 2015).

9.4.1 Dentate gyrus (DG) subregion of the hippocampus

Based on the anatomy of the DG, its input and output pathways, and the development of a computational model, it has been suggested (see Section 9.3, Rolls (1990b), and Rolls (1996d)) that the DG can act as a competitive learning network with Hebb-like modifiability to remove redundancy from the inputs producing a more orthogonal, sparse, and categorized set of outputs. One example of this in the theory is that to the extent that some entorhinal cortex neurons represent space as a grid (Moser et al., 2015), the correlations in this type of encoding are removed by competitive learning to produce a representation of place, with each place encoded differently from other places (Rolls, Stringer and Elliot, 2006c)[15]. To the extent then that DG acts to produce separate representations of different places, it is predicted that the DG will be especially important when memories must be formed about similar places. To form spatial representations, learned conjunctions of sensory inputs including vestibular, olfactory, visual, auditory, and somatosensory may be involved. DG may help to form orthogonal representations based on all these inputs, and could thus help to form orthogonal non-spatial as well as orthogonal spatial representations for use in CA3. In any case, the model predicts that for spatial information, the DG should play an important role in hippocampal memory functions when the spatial information is very similar, for example, when the places are close together. As we will see, there is evidence that the DG is involved in several types of pattern separation, including social pattern separation (Kesner and Rolls, 2015; Kesner, 2018).

---

[15] Indeed, it was a prediction of the theory that the mapping from entorhinal cortex grid cells to dentate / CA place cells could be achieved by competitive learning, and this prediction was verified by simulation (Rolls, Stringer and Elliot, 2006c).

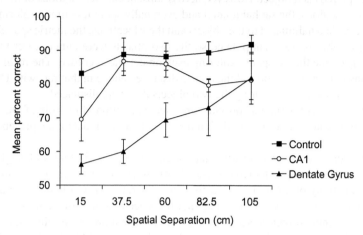

Fig. 9.40 Spatial pattern separation impairment produced by dentate gyrus lesions. Mean percent correct performance as a function of spatial separation of control group, CA1 lesion group, and dentate gyrus lesion group on postoperative trials. A graded impairment was found as a function of the distance between the places only following dentate gyrus lesions. (After Gilbert,P.E., Kesner,R.P. and Lee,I. (2001) Dissociating hippocampal subregions: double dissociation between dentate gyrus and CA1. Hippocampus 11: 626–636. © Wiley-Liss Inc.)

9.4.1.1 Spatial pattern separation

To examine the contribution of the DG to spatial pattern separation, Gilbert, Kesner and Lee (2001) tested rats with DG lesions using a paradigm that measured one-trial short term memory for spatial location information as a function of spatial similarity between two spatial locations (Gilbert, Kesner and DeCoteau, 1998). Rats were trained to displace an object that was randomly positioned to cover a baited food well in 1 of 15 locations along a row of food wells. Following a short delay, the rats were required to choose between two objects identical to the sample phase object. One object was in the same location as the sample phase object and the second object was in a different location along the row of food wells. A rat was rewarded for displacing the object in the same position as the sample phase object (correct choice) but received no reward for displacing the foil object (incorrect choice). Five spatial separations, from 15 cm to 105 cm, were used to separate the correct object from the foil object on the choice phase. The results showed that rats with DG lesions were significantly impaired at short spatial separations; however, the performance of the DG lesioned rats increased as a function of increased spatial separation between the correct object and the foil on the choice phases. The performance of rats with DG lesions matched controls at the largest spatial separation. The graded nature of the impairment and the significant linear increase in performance as a function of increased separation illustrate the deficit in pattern separation produced by DG lesions (see Fig. 9.40). Based on these results, it can be concluded that lesions of the DG decrease efficiency in spatial pattern separation, which resulted in impairments on trials with increased spatial proximity and hence increased spatial similarity among working memory representations (Gilbert, Kesner and Lee, 2001). In the same study it was found that CA1 lesions do not produce a deficit in this task.

Additional evidence comes from a study (Goodrich-Hunsaker, Hunsaker and Kesner, 2008) using a modified version of an exploratory paradigm developed by Poucet (1989), in which rats with DG lesions and controls were tested on tasks involving a metric spatial manipulation. In this task, a rat was allowed to explore two different visual objects that were separated by a specific distance on a cheese-board maze. On the initial presentation of the objects, the rat explored each object. However, across subsequent presentations of the objects in their respective locations, the rat habituated and eventually spent less time exploring the objects. Once the rat had habituated to the objects and their locations, the metric spatial distance between the two objects was manipulated so the two objects were either closer together or further apart. The time the rat spent exploring each object was recorded. The results showed that DG lesions impaired detection of the metric distance change in that rats with DG lesions spent significantly less time exploring the two objects that were displaced.

The results of both experiments provide empirical validation of the role of DG in spatial pattern separation, and support the prediction from the computational model presented in this chapter.

There are neurophysiological results that are also consistent, in that McNaughton et al. (1989) found that following colchicine-induced lesions of the DG, there is a significant decrease in the reliability of CA3 place-related firing. Therefore, if CA3 cells display less reliability following DG lesions, the cells may not form accurate representations of space due to decreased efficiency in pattern separation. Also consistent are the findings that the place fields of DG cells and specifically dentate granular cells (Jung and McNaughton, 1993; Leutgeb et al., 2007) are small and highly reliable, and this may reflect the role of DG in pattern separation.

These studies thus indicate that the DG plays an important role in spatial pattern separation in spatial memory tasks. Building and utilizing separate representations for other classes of stimuli engage other brain areas, including for objects the inferior temporal visual cortex (Rolls, 2000a, 2012d), for reward value the orbitofrontal cortex (Rolls, 2014a) and amygdala (Gilbert and Kesner, 2002), and for motor responses the caudate nucleus (Kesner and Gilbert, 2006).

9.4.1.2 Pattern separation and neurogenesis

Based on the observation that neurogenesis occurs in the DG and that new DG granule cells can be formed across time, it has been proposed that the dDG mediates a spatial pattern separation mechanism as well as generates patterns of episodic memories within remote memory (Aimone and Gage, 2011). Thus far, it has been shown in mice that disruption of neurogenesis using low-dose x-irradiation was sufficient to produce a loss of newly born dDG cells. Further testing indicated impairments in spatial learning in a delayed non-matching-to-place task in the radial-arm maze. Specifically, impairment occurred for arms that were presented with little separation, but no deficit was observed when the arms were presented farther apart (Clelland et al., 2009), suggesting a spatial pattern separation deficit. These results are similar to those described for rats in the study by Morris et al. (2012). Another study in mice provided evidence that the disruption of neurogenesis using lentivirus expression of a dominant Wnt protein produced a loss of newly born dDG cells; and these mice were tested in an associative object-in-place task with different spatial separations and observed to be impaired as a function of the degree of separation, again suggesting a spatial pattern separation deficit (Clelland et al., 2009). In another study (Kesner et al., 2014) it was shown that DNA methyltransferase 1-c knockout mice are impaired relative to controls in the spatial pattern separation task (Goodrich-Hunsaker, Hunsaker and Kesner, 2008). These data suggest that neurogenesis in the dDG may contribute to the operation of spatial pattern separation. Thus, spatial pattern separation may play an important role in the acquisition of new spatial information, and there is a good possibility that the dDG may have been the subregion responsible for the impairments in the various tasks described above.

Impaired DG neurogenesis may be involved in some neurological diseases such as Alzheimer's disease and in the relation between aging and memory in humans (Toda, Parylak, Linker and Gage, 2019).

9.4.1.3 Encoding versus retrieval

The theory postulates that the dentate / mossy fibre system is necessary for setting up the appropriate conditions for optimal storage of new information in the CA3 system (which could be called encoding); and that (especially when an incomplete cue is provided) the retrieval of information from CA3 is optimally cued by the direct entorhinal to CA3 connections.

In strong support of the role of the DG in encoding, a study conducted in mice showed that the mossy fibre projections to CA3 are essential for the encoding of spatial information in a water maze reference memory task, but are not necessary for retrieval (Lassalle, Bataille and Halley, 2000).

Another type of evidence comes from a study in which rats had 10 learning trials per day in a Hebb–Williams maze. Lee and Kesner (2004b) found that based on a within-day analysis DG lesions (but not lesions of the perforant path input to CA3) impaired the acquisition of this task, consistent with an encoding or learning impairment. However, when tested using a between-days analysis, retrieval of what had been learned previously was not impaired by DG lesions, but was impaired by lesions of the perforant path input to CA3. This double dissociation is consistent with the hypothesis that the DG is important for optimal encoding, and the entorhinal to CA3 connections for optimal retrieval.

Further evidence for a DG mediation of spatial encoding comes from the observation that rats with DG lesions are impaired in learning the Morris water maze task when the start location varied on each trial (Nanry et al., 1989; Sutherland et al., 1983; Xavier et al., 1999). Under these conditions, spatial pattern separation may be at a premium, for different, partially overlapping, subsets of spatial cues are likely to be visible from the different starting locations.

Further evidence consistent with the hypothesis that the DG is important in spatial learning (acquisition) is that rats with DG lesions are impaired on acquisition of spatial contextual fear conditioning (Lee and Kesner, 2004a).

However, I note that in the studies described in this section (encoding vs retrieval), during acquisition of these tasks over a number of trials both the storage and the retrieval processes are likely to influence the rate of behavioral learning. Thus, even though in behavioral tasks the deficit can be described as an encoding deficit because it is apparent during initial learning, it is not easy to separate the actual underlying processes by which the DG may be important for setting up the representations for new learning in the CA3 system, and the perforant path to CA3 connections for initiating retrieval especially with a partial cue from CA3.

9.4.2 CA3 subregion of the hippocampus

In Rolls' theory of the hippocampus the CA3 system acts as an autoassociation system. This enables arbitrary (especially spatial in animals and probably language for humans as well) associations to be formed between whatever is represented in the hippocampus, in that for example any place could be associated with any object, and in that the object could be recalled with a spatial recall cue, or the place with an object recall cue. The same system must be capable of fast (one-trial) learning if it is to contribute to forming new episodic memories, though it could also play an important role in the encoding of new information requiring multiple trials. The same system is also predicted to be important in retrieval of hippocampus-dependent information when there is an incomplete retrieval cue. The same system has the property that it can maintain firing activity because of the associative recurrent collateral connections, and for this reason is likely to be important in hippocampus-dependent delay / short-term memory tasks. The CA3 recurrent collateral system could also make a contribution to the learning of sequences if it has some temporal asymmetry in its associative synapses, as described in Section 9.3.5.4. The CA3 system might also contribute to spatial path integration, though this could be performed outside the hippocampus. Tests of these proposed functions are described next.

9.4.2.1 Rapid encoding of new information

The theory proposes that associative learning in the CA3 recurrent collateral connections can occur rapidly, in as little as one trial, so that it can contribute to episodic memory. Evidence for one-trial learning between places and objects or odors, in the hippocampal CA3 is provided in Section 9.4.2.5.

The situation is a little different in a task in which there is one-trial learning of just a spatial location. In one such task, delayed non-matching-to-place (DNMP) for a single spatial location in an 8-arm maze, Lee and Kesner (2002) and Lee and Kesner (2003a) showed that blockade of CA3 NMDA receptors with AP5 or CA3 (neurotoxic) lesions did not impair one-trial learning in a familiar environment, but did impair it in an initial period in a novel environment. The implication is that a place can be remembered over a 10 s delay even without the CA3, but that learning of new spatial environments does require the CA3 subregion. Consistent with this observation is the finding that hippocampal CA3 (dorsal plus ventral) lesions disrupt learning of the standard 8-arm maze where the rats have to learn not to go back to arms previously visited (Handelmann and Olton, 1981). Rats tend to use different sequences on every trial, thus requiring new learning on every trial. When learning a new spatial environment, associations may be made between the different visual cues and their spatial locations, and this type of learning is computationally similar to that involved in object–place or odor–place association learning, providing a consistent interpretation of CA3 function.

Nakazawa, Sun, Quirk, Rondi-Reig, Wilson and Tonegawa (2003) also reported similar findings with mice in which the function of CA3 NMDA receptors was disrupted. These mice were impaired in learning a novel platform location in a working memory water maze task, whereas they were normal in finding familiar platform locations.

Evidence that rapid learning is reflected in the responses of CA3 neurons comes from a study in which it was found that CA3 neurons alter their responses rapidly when rats encounter novel configurations of familiar cues for the first time (Lee et al., 2004). Specifically, rats were trained to run clockwise on a ring track whose surface was composed of four different texture cues (local cues). The ring track was positioned in the centre of a curtained area in which various visual landmarks were also available along the curtained walls. To produce a novel cue configuration in the environment, distal landmarks and local cues on the track were rotated in opposite directions (distal landmarks were rotated clockwise and local cues were rotated counterclockwise by equal amounts).

In sum, these results and those in Section 9.4.2.5 strongly suggest that rapid plastic changes in the CA3 network are essential in encoding novel information involving associations between objects and places, odors and places, or between landmark visual cues and spatial locations, and NMDA receptor-mediated plasticity mechanisms appear to play a significant role in the process.

9.4.2.2 The types of information associated in CA3

A prediction is that the CA3 recurrent collateral associative connections enable arbitrary associations to be formed between whatever is represented in the hippocampus, in that, for example, any place could be associated with any object. Arbitrary in this context refers to the possibility of what is provided for by non-localized connectivity within the CA3–CA3 system, in that any one representation in CA3 can potentially become associated with any other representation in CA3. The prediction is neutral with respect to what is actually represented in the CA3 system, which I note from the effects of lesions almost always includes space, at least in animals, but could include language in humans. The object representations might originate in the temporal cortical visual areas, and the spatial representations might utilize some information from the parietal cortex such as vestibular inputs related to self-motion (see Section 9.3). Two important issues need to be clarified. First, is the hippocampus the only neural system that supports all types of stimulus-stimulus associations (Eichenbaum and Cohen, 2001)? Based on the observations that the primate orbitofrontal cortex is involved in some types of stimulus–stimulus association, including visual-to-taste and olfactory-to-taste association learning and more generally in rapid and reversible stimulus–reinforcer association learning (Rolls, 2014a; Grabenhorst and Rolls, 2011; Rolls, 2019e,f), there appear to be other neural systems that can learn stimulus-stimulus associations. Second, what is the nature of the information that can be associated in this arbitrary way in the CA3 recurrent collateral system? The studies described next indicate that at least the non-human hippocampus is involved in associations when one of the components is spatial.

In order to directly test the involvement of the CA3 subregion of the hippocampus in spatial paired-associate learning, rats were trained on a successive discrimination Go/No-Go task to examine object–place and odor–place paired associate learning. Normal rats learn these tasks in approximately 240 trials. CA3 lesions impaired the learning of these object–place and odor–place paired associations (Gilbert and Kesner, 2003). Furthermore, lesions of DG or CA1 did not produce a deficit, and the reasons for this are considered later.

In contrast, object–odor paired associate learning was not impaired by CA3 lesions (even with a delay between the object and the odor) (Kesner et al., 2005). Thus, not all types of paired associate learning require the rat hippocampus. This conclusion is supported by the fact that (large or total) hippocampal lesions do not impair the following types of association including odor–odor (Bunsey and Eichenbaum, 1996; Li et al., 1999), odor–reward (Wood et al., 2004), auditory–visual (Jarrard and Davidson, 1990), and object–object associations (Cho and Kesner, 1995; Murray et al., 1993). Thus, in rats paired associate learning appears to be impaired by CA3 lesions only when one of the associates is place. This is consistent with the theory of episodic memory in which the hippocampus is important because the associates of a particular episodic memory and that have therefore to be represented in the hippocampus include place and/or the time at which the event occurred (Rolls, 2018b).

9.4.2.3 Acquisition/encoding associated with multiple trials

The CA3 subregion also appears to be necessary in some tasks that require multiple trials to acquire the task, and a common feature of these tasks is that a new environment must be learned. For example, lesions of the CA3 (but not the CA1) subregion impair the acquisition of object–place and odor–place paired associate learning, a task that requires multiple trials to learn (Gilbert and Kesner, 2003). Another multiple trial task in which a learning set is needed that is affected by CA3, but not by CA1, lesions is acquisition of a non-match to sample one-trial spatial location task on an 8-arm maze with 10 s delays (delayed non-match to place, DNMP). In this case the output from CA3 is via the fimbria, in that fimbria lesions that interrupt the CA3 hippocampal output without affecting the input also impair acquisition of this task. Finally, CA3 lesioned rats are impaired in the standard water maze task which requires multiple trials (Brun et al., 2002; Florian and Roullet, 2004) (although mice that lacked NMDA receptors in CA3 do not appear to be impaired in learning the water maze (Nakazawa et al., 2002)). These findings are consistent with the hypothesis that when a new environment is learned this may involve multiple associations between different environmental cues, both with each other and with idiothetic (self-motion cues), and that this type of learning depends on new associations formed in the CA3–CA3 connections (see Section 9.3.5.2).

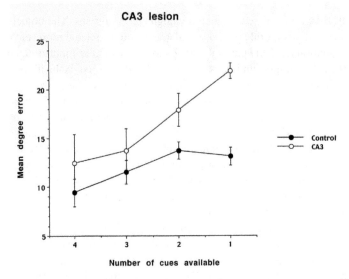

Fig. 9.41 Pattern completion impairment produced by CA3 lesions. The mean (and sem) degree of error in finding the correct place in the cheese-board task when rats were tested with 1, 2, 3 or 4 of the cues available. A graded impairment in the CA3 lesion group as a function of the number of cues available was found. The performance of the control group is also shown. (After Gold,A.E. and Kesner,R.P. 2005. The role of the CA3 subregion of the dorsal hippocampus in spatial pattern completion in the rat. Hippocampus 15: 808–814. See further Kesner,R.P. and Rolls, E. T. 2015. A computational theory of hippocampal function, and tests of the theory: new developments. Neuroscience and Biobehavioral Reviews 48: 92–147.)

9.4.2.4 Pattern completion in CA3

The CA3 system is predicted to be important in the retrieval of hippocampus-dependent information when there is an incomplete retrieval cue. Support for the pattern completion process in CA3 can be found in lesion studies. In one study (Gold and Kesner, 2005), rats were tested on a cheese board with a black curtain with four extramaze cues surrounding the apparatus. (The cheese board is like a dry land water maze with 177 holes on a 119 cm diameter board.) Rats were trained to move a sample phase object covering a food well that could appear in one of five possible spatial locations. During the test phase of the task, following a 30 s delay, the animal needs to find the same food well in order to receive reinforcement with the object now removed. After reaching stable performance in terms of accuracy to find the correct location, rats received lesions in CA3. During post-surgery testing, four extramaze cues were always available during the sample phase. However, during the test phase zero, one, two, or three cues were removed in different combinations. The results indicate that controls performed well on the task regardless of the availability of one, two, three, or all cues, suggesting intact spatial pattern completion. Following the CA3 lesion, however, there was an impairment in accuracy compared to the controls especially when only one or two cues were available, suggesting impairment in spatial pattern completion in CA3 lesioned rats (Gold and Kesner, 2005) (see Fig. 9.41). A useful aspect of this task is that the ability to remember a spatial location learned in one presentation can be tested with varying number of available cues, and many times in which the locations vary, to allow for accurate measurement of pattern completion ability when the information stored on the single presentation must be recalled. Based on the observation that the lateral perforant path input into the dentate gyrus mediates visual object information via activation of opioid receptors, it was shown that naloxone (a μ opioid receptor antagonist) injected into the CA3 produced the same pattern completion problem (Kesner and Warthen, 2010).

In another study Nakazawa, Quirk, Chitwood, Watanabe, Yeckel, Sun, Kato, Carr, Johnston, Wilson and Tonegawa (2002) trained CA3 NMDA receptor-knockout mice in an analogous task, using the water maze. When the animals were required to perform the task in an environment where some of the familiar cues were removed, they were impaired in performing the task. The result suggests that the NMDA receptor-dependent synaptic plasticity mechanisms in CA3 are critical to perform the pattern completion process in the hippocampus.

9.4.2.5 Recall and arbitrary associations in CA3

A prediction of the theory is that the CA3 recurrent collateral associative connections enable arbitrary associations to be formed between whatever is represented in the hippocampus, in that for example any place could be associated with any object, and in that the object could be recalled with a spatial recall cue, or the place with an object recall cue.

In one test of this, Day, Langston and Morris (2003) trained rats in a study phase to learn in one trial an association between two flavors of food and two spatial locations. During a recall test phase they were presented with a flavor which served as a cue for the selection of the correct location. They found that injections of an NMDA blocker (AP5) or AMPA blocker (CNQX) to the dorsal hippocampus prior to the study phase impaired encoding, but injections of AP5 prior to the test phase did not impair the place recall, whereas injections of CNQX did impair the place recall. The interpretation is that somewhere in the hippocampus NMDA receptors are necessary for forming one-trial odor–place associations, and that recall can be performed without further involvement of NMDA receptors.

In a development related to the Day, Langston and Morris (2003) experiment, Kesner et al. (2008) designed a task in which a visual object could be recalled from a spatial location, and in an important extension, a spatial location could be recalled from an object. In this task, after training to displace objects, rats in the study phase are placed in the start box and when the door in front of the start box is opened the rats are allowed to displace one object in one location, and then after returning to the start box, the door is opened again and the rats are allowed to displace a second object in another location. There are 50 possible objects and 48 locations. In the test phase, the rat is shown one object (first or second randomized) in the start box as a cue, and then, after a 10-s delay, the door is opened and the rats must go to the correct location (choosing and displacing one of two identical neutral objects). The rats receive a reward for selecting the correct location that was associated with the object cue. A spatial location-recall for a visual object task was also used. For the spatial recall for a visual object task, the study phase is the same, but in this case in the test phase when the door is opened the rat is allowed to displace a neutral object in one location (first or second randomized) on the maze as a location cue, return to the start box, and then, after a 10 s delay, the door is opened and the rats must select the correct object (choosing and displacing one of two visual objects). The rats received a reward for selecting the correct visual object that was associated with the location cue. It was found that CA3a,b lesions produce chance performance on both the one-trial object-place recall task, and on the one-trial place-object recall task (Kesner et al., 2008). The potential implications of such results are that indeed the CA3a,b supports arbitrary associations as well as episodic memory based on one-trial learning. A control fixed visual conditional to place task with the same delay was not impaired, showing that it is recall after one-trial (or rapid) learning that is impaired.

Additional support comes from the finding that in a similar one-trial object–place learning followed by recall of the spatial position in which to respond when shown the object, Rolls and Xiang (2005) showed that some primate hippocampal (including CA3) neurons respond to an object cue with the spatial position in which the object had been shown earlier in the trial. Thus, some hippocampal neurons appear to reflect spatial recall given an object recall cue.

Evidence that the CA3 is not necessarily required during recall in a reference memory spatial task, such as the water maze spatial navigation for a single spatial location task, is that CA3 lesioned rats are not impaired during recall of a previously learned water maze task (Brun et al., 2002; Florian and Roullet, 2004). However, if completion from an incomplete cue is needed, then CA3 NMDA receptors are necessary (presumably to ensure satisfactory CA3–CA3 learning) even in a reference memory task (Nakazawa, Quirk, Chitwood, Watanabe, Yeckel, Sun, Kato, Carr, Johnston, Wilson and Tonegawa, 2002). Thus, the CA3 system appears to be especially needed in rapid, one-trial object–place recall, and when completion from an incomplete cue is needed.

9.4.2.6 Functional analysis of mossy fibre vs direct perforant path input into CA3

The computational model suggests that the dentate granule cell / mossy fibre pathway to CA3 may be important during the learning of new associations in the CA3 network, and that part of the way in which it is important is that it helps by pattern separation to produce relatively sparse and orthogonal representations in CA3 (see Section 9.3.5.8). In contrast, the theory predicts that the direct perforant path input to CA3 is important in initiating retrieval from the CA3 autoassociation network, especially with an incomplete retrieval cue (see Section 9.3.5.9).

Support for this hypothesis comes from the findings of Lee and Kesner (2004b) and Jerman et al. (2006) that lesions of the DG or CA3 (or a crossed lesion) disrupt within-day learning on the Hebb–Williams maze, but that retrieval of information at the start of the following day is not impaired. In contrast, lesions of the perforant path input to CA3 from entorhinal cortex disrupt retrieval (i.e. initial performance on the following day), but not learning within a day (Lee and Kesner, 2004b). These findings support the hypothesis that the CA3 processes both inputs from the DG to support pattern separation; and inputs from the entorhinal cortex via the perforant path to support pattern completion.

The perforant path can be divided into a medial and lateral component. It has been suggested that the medial component processes spatial information and that the lateral component processes non-spatial (e.g objects, odors) information (Hargreaves et al., 2005; Witter et al., 1989a). In one study, Ferbinteanu et al. (1999) showed that lesions of the medial perforant path (MPP) disrupted water maze learning, whereas lateral perforant path (LPP) lesions had no effect. As predicted by the theory, there is associative LTP between the medial or lateral perforant path and the intrinsic commissural/associational-CA3 synapses) (Martinez et al., 2002). Either place or object recall cues could thus be introduced by the associative MPP and LPP connections to CA3 cells.

In addition, Martinez et al. (2002) demonstrated associative (cooperative) LTP between the medial and lateral perforant path inputs to the CA3 neurons. This could provide a mechanism for object (LPP) – place (MPP) associative learning, with either the object or the place during recall activating a CA3 neuron. However, this LPP to MPP cooperative LTP onto a CA3 neuron would be a low capacity memory system, in that there are only 3,300 PP inputs to a CA3 cell, compared to 12,000 recurrent collaterals in the CA3–CA3 connections, and these numbers are the leading term in the memory capacity of pattern association and autoassociation memory systems (see Appendix B).

I note that disruption of DG and mossy fibre input into CA3 does not produce a disruption in the acquisition of the object–place paired associate task unless the stimuli are close together, implying that the DG contribution is important particularly when pattern separation is needed (Gilbert and Kesner, 2003). The implication is that sufficient input for object–place learning can be introduced into the CA3 system (which is required for this object–place learning) by the perforant path inputs provided that spatial pattern separation is not at a premium (or perhaps the storage of large numbers of different object–place associations is not at a premium, as this is the other condition for which the computational theory indicates that the DG is needed to help produce sparse and orthogonal representations in the CA3 system).

9.4.2.7 Orthogonal representations in CA3

The CA3 subregion may have more distinct representations of different environments than CA1. This may be consistent with the computational point that if CA3 is an autoassociator, the pattern representations in it should be as orthogonal as possible to maximize memory capacity and minimize interference. The actual pattern separation may be performed, the theory holds, as a result of the operation of the dentate granule cells as a competitive net, and the nature of the mossy fibre connections to CA3 cells. Some of the empirical evidence is as follows.

Tanila (1999) showed that CA3 place cells were able to maintain distinct representations of two visually identical environments, and selectively reactivate either one of the representation patterns depending on the experience of the rat. Also, Leutgeb et al. (2004) showed that when rats experienced a completely different environment, CA3 place cells developed orthogonal representations of those different environments by changing their firing rates between the two environments, whereas CA1 place cells maintained similar responses. Evidence on the sparseness of the CA3 cell representation in rats includes evidence that CA3 cell ensembles may support the fast acquisition of detailed memories by providing a locally continuous, but globally orthogonal spatial representation, onto which new sensory inputs can rapidly be associated (Leutgeb and Leutgeb, 2007). Further, CA3 cells are very sensitive to the place where the rat is, and so potentially help to provide a basis for object-place memory in which the place is precisely specified (Leutgeb and Leutgeb, 2007).

In the computational account, each environment would be a separate chart, and the number of charts that could be stored in CA3 would be high if the representations in each chart are relatively orthogonal to those in other charts (see Section B.5.4 and Battaglia and Treves (1998b)), and further, the charts could operate independently (Stringer, Rolls and Trappenberg, 2004). Any one chart of one spatial environment can be understood as a continuous attractor network, with place cells with Gaussian shaped place fields, which overlap continuously with each other. In different charts (different spatial environments) the neurons may represent very different parts of space, and neurons representing close places in one environment may represent distant places in another environment (chart).

9.4.2.8 Short-term memory, path integration, and CA3

The CA3 recurrent collateral associative connections suggest that the CA3 system can operate as an attractor network which can be useful in some types of working memory. Support for this idea comes from a variety of studies analyzed by Kesner and Rolls (2001), including a study where in the short-term (30 s delay) memory for spatial location task to measure spatial pattern separation, it was shown that CA3 lesioned rats were impaired for all pattern separations, consistent with the hypothesis that the rats could not remember the correct spatial location (Gilbert and Kesner, 2006). Furthermore, in the short-term memory-based delayed non-matching to sample place task mentioned above (Lee and Kesner, 2003b), lesions of CA3 impaired the acquisition of this task with 10 s delays. Also single neuron activity has been recorded in CA3 during the delay period in rats in a spatial position short-term memory task (Hampson et al., 2000) and in monkeys in an object–place and a location-scene association short-term memory task (Cahusac et al., 1989). The finding that neuronal representations in the hippocampus switch abruptly from representing a square vs a circular environment on which rats have been trained when the environment changes incrementally between the two ('remapping') has also been suggested as evidence that the hippocampus implements attractor dynamics (Wills et al., 2005). The flickering (alternation) between place-cell maps in the hippocampus in an ambiguous environment also provides evidence for an attractor system in the hippocampus, which can be reset by theta (Jezek et al., 2011).

In a task in which rats were required to remember multiple places, CA3 and CA1 lesions produced a deficit. In the task, during the study phase rats were presented with four different places within sections that were sequentially visited on a newly devised maze (i.e. Tulum maze). Each place was cued by a unique object that was specifically associated with each location within the section during the study phase. Following a 15-s delay and during the test phase in the absence of the cued object, rats were required to recall and revisit the place within one section of the maze that had been previously visited. Both CA1 and CA3 lesions disrupted accurate relocation of a previously visited place (Lee et al., 2005). Thus, short-term memory for multiple places in a one-trial multiple place task depends on both CA3 and CA1. As an attractor network can in general hold only one item active in a delay period by maintained firing, this type of multiple item short-term memory is computationally predicted to require synaptic modification to store each item, and both CA3 and CA1 appear to contribute to this.

The other mechanism in the hippocampus that is likely to be involved in short-term memory is the time cell system described in Sections 9.3.4 and 9.3.7.4.

9.4.2.9 Cholinergic modulation of CA3 towards storage vs recall including pattern completion

Acetylcholine may act to facilitate memory storage by increasing LTP in the CA3–CA3 recurrent collaterals, and reducing the recurrent collateral synaptic recall of previous interfering memories (Hasselmo et al., 1995; Giocomo and Hasselmo, 2007). Consistent with this, scopolamine (which blocks muscarinic cholinergic receptors), but not physostigmine, infusions, into CA3 disrupt encoding. In contrast, physostigmine (which inhibits acetylcholinesterase and thereby increases acetylcholine), but not scopolamine infusions, into CA3 disrupt recall. This was observed during a spatial exploration paradigm (Hunsaker et al., 2007), during Hebb-Williams maze learning (Rogers and Kesner, 2003), and during delay fear-conditioning (Rogers and Kesner, 2004).

These findings are consistent with the hypothesis that acetylcholine in CA3 when low supports recall which involves pattern completion implemented by the recurrent collaterals; and that acetylcholine when high facilitates new learning. Acetylcholine influences the hippocampus via the septum, and the neocortex (including the parietal cortex) via the basal forebrain cholinergic neurons. There are influences of both these cholinergic systems on memory, spatial function, and navigation (Solari and Hangya, 2018). Neurons in the basal forebrain may play a role in increasing memory consolidation, for they are activated in primates by novel and rewarding and punishing stimuli (Wilson and Rolls, 1990c,b,a), which facilitate consolidation. Consistent with this, cholinergic basal forebrain lesions produce severe learning impairments in learning visual scenes and in object-reward associations (Easton, Ridley, Baker and Gaffan, 2002), and damage to the cholinergic basal forebrain neurons is implicated in Alzheimer's disease (Zaborszky et al., 2018).

9.4.3 CA1 subregion of the hippocampus

The CA1 subregion of the hippocampus receives inputs from two major sources: the Schaffer collateral inputs from CA3, and the perforant path inputs from the entorhinal cortex (see Fig. 9.2). CA1 outputs are directed towards the subiculum, entorhinal cortex, prefrontal cortex and many other neural regions including the lateral septum, anterior thalamus, and the mammillary bodies (Amaral and Witter, 1995). The anatomical and physiological characteristics suggest that the CA1 can operate as a competitive network and have triggered the development of computational models of CA1 in which for example the CA1 system is involved in the recall process by which backprojections to the cerebral neocortex allow neuronal activity during recall to reflect that present during the original learning (see Section 9.3.8). In this terminology, cortico-cortical backprojections originate from deep (layer 5) pyramidal cells, and terminate on the apical dendrites of pyramidal cells in layer 1 of the preceding cortical area (see Fig. 9.2). In contrast, cortico-cortical forward projections originate from superficial (layers 2 and 3) pyramidal cells, and terminate in the deep layers of the hierarchically next cortical area (see Fig. 9.2). Within this context, the projections from the entorhinal cortex to DG, CA3 and CA1 can be thought of as forward projections; and from CA1 to entorhinal cortex, subiculum etc. as the start of the backprojection system (see Fig. 9.2).

The evidence reviewed next of the effects of selective damage to CA1 indicates that it makes a special contribution to temporal aspects of memory including associations over a delay period, and sequence memory. There is also evidence relating it to intermediate memory as well as consolidation (see for more detail Rolls and Kesner (2006b)). The effects of damage to the CA1 may not be identical to the effects of damage to CA3, because CA1 has some inputs that bypass CA3 (e.g. the direct entorhinal / perforant path input); and CA3 has some outputs that bypass CA1. In particular, the CA3 output through the fimbria projects directly to the lateral septum and then to the medial septum or directly to the medial septum (Amaral and Witter, 1995; Risold and Swanson, 1997). The medial septum, in turn, provides cholinergic and GABAergic inputs to the hippocampus (Amaral and Witter, 1995).

9.4.3.1 Sequence memory and CA1

In Sections 9.3.5.4 and 9.3.7.4 I describe how a sequence memory could be implemented by pairing places with time cells to implement spatial sequence learning.

To test this, Hunsaker et al. (2008) trained rats to remember unique sequences of spatial locations along a runway box. Rats with lesions to either CA3 or CA1 had difficulty with this spatial sequence memory task, although CA1 lesioned animals had a much greater deficit. However, when animals were trained on a non-episodic version of the same task, hippocampal lesions had no effect. The results suggest that the CA3 and CA1 contribute to episodic based spatial sequence memory and pattern completion (Hunsaker et al., 2008). Further results are described by Kesner and Rolls (2015).

9.4.3.2 Associations across time, and CA1

There is evidence implicating the hippocampus in mediating associations across time (Rawlins, 1985; Kesner, 1998), and hypotheses on the mechanisms including time cells are described in Sections 9.3.5.4 and 9.3.7.4.

The CA1 subregion of the hippocampus may play a role in influencing the formation of associations whenever a time component (requiring a memory trace) is introduced between any two stimuli that need to be associated. Support for this idea comes from studies based on a classical conditioning paradigm. Lesions of the hippocampus in rabbits or rats disrupt the acquisition of eye-blink trace conditioning. In trace conditioning a short delay intervenes between the conditioned stimulus (CS) and the unconditioned stimulus (UCS). When, however, a UCS and CS overlap in time (delay conditioning), rabbits with hippocampal damage typically perform as well as normals (Moyer et al., 1990; Weiss et al., 1999). Based on a subregional analysis, it has been shown that ventral, but not dorsal, CA1 lesions impair at least the retention (tested after 48 h) of trace fear conditioning (Rogers et al., 2006). Similar learning deficits in trace fear conditioning (but not in conditioning without a delay between the CS and UCS), were observed for mice that lacked NMDA receptors in both dorsal and ventral CA1 subregions of the hippocampus (Huerta et al., 2000).

Based on a previous finding that the acquisition of an object-odor association is not dependent on the hippocampus, would adding a temporal component to an object-odor association task recruit the hippocampus and more specifically the CA1 region? To test this idea rats were given dorsal CA1, CA3, or control lesions prior to learning an object-delay-odor task. Rats that had dorsal CA1 lesions were unable to make the association and never performed above chance, however CA3 lesioned rats displayed no deficit (Kesner, Hunsaker and Gilbert, 2005). The observation of time cells during the trace in the object-trace-odor task supports the idea that the CA1 supports temporal processing of object and odor information. These results support the idea that the CA1 region is at least on the route for forming arbitrary associations across time even when there is no spatial component.

9.4.3.3 Temporal order memory, and CA1

There are also data on temporal order memory, which does not necessarily imply that a particular sequence has been learned, and could be recalled. Estes (1986) summarized data demonstrating that in human memory there are fewer errors for distinguishing items (by specifying the order in which they occurred) that are far apart in a sequence than those that are temporally adjacent. Other studies have also shown that order judgements improve as the number of items in a sequence between the test items increases (Banks, 1978; Chiba et al., 1994; Madsen and Kesner, 1995). This phenomenon is referred to as a temporal distance effect (sometimes referred to as a temporal pattern separation effect). It is assumed to occur because there is more interference for temporally proximal events than temporally distant events. Hypotheses on the mechanisms involved including time cells are described in Sections 9.3.5.4 and 9.3.7.4.

Based on these findings, Gilbert, Kesner and Lee (2001) tested memory for the temporal order of items in a one-trial sequence learning paradigm. In the task, each rat was given one daily trial consisting of a sample phase followed by a choice phase. During the sample phase, the animal visited each arm of an 8-arm radial maze once in a randomly predetermined order and was given a reward at the end of each arm. The choice phase began immediately following the presentation of the final arm in the sequence. In the choice phase, two arms were opened simultaneously and the animal was allowed to choose between the two arms. To obtain a food reward, the animal had to enter the arm that occurred earliest in the sequence that it had just followed. Temporal separations of 0, 2, 4, and 6 were randomly selected for each choice phase. These values represented the number of arms in the sample phase that intervened between the two arms that were to be used in the test phase. After reaching criterion rats received CA1 lesions. Following surgery, control rats matched their preoperative performance across all temporal separations. In contrast, rats with CA1 lesions performed at chance across 0, 2, or 4 temporal separations and a little better than chance in the case of a 6 separation. The results suggest that the CA1 subregion is involved in memory for spatial location as a function of temporal separation of spatial locations and that lesions of the CA1 decrease efficiency in temporal pattern separation. CA1 lesioned rats cannot separate events across time, perhaps due to an inability to inhibit interference that may be associated with sequentially occurring events. The increase in temporal interference impairs the rat's ability to remember the order of specific events.

The hippocampus is known to process spatial and temporal information independently (O'Keefe and Nadel, 1978; Kesner, 1998). In the previous experiments sequence learning and temporal pattern separation were assessed using spatial cues. Therefore, one possibility is that the CA1 and CA3 deficits were due to the processing of spatial rather than non-spatial temporal information. To determine if the hippocampus is critical for processing all domains of temporal information, it is necessary to use a task that does not depend on spatial information. Since the hippocampus does not mediate short-term (delayed match to sample) memory for odors (Dudchenko et al., 2000; Otto and Eichenbaum, 1992), it is possible to test whether the hippocampus plays a role in memory for the temporal sequence of odors (i.e. temporal separation effect). Memory for the temporal order for a sequence of odors was assessed in rats based on a varied sequence of five odors, using a similar paradigm described for sequences of spatial locations. Rats with hippocampal lesions were impaired relative to control animals for memory for all temporal distances for the odors, yet the rats were able to discriminate between the odors (Kesner et al., 2002). In a further subregional analysis, rats with dorsal CA1 lesions show a mild impairment, but rats with ventral CA1 lesions show a severe impairment in memory for the temporal distance for odors (Kesner et al., 2011). Thus, the CA1 appears to be involved in separating events in time for spatial and non-spatial information, so that one event can be remembered distinct from another event, but the dorsal CA1 might play a more important role than the ventral CA1 for spatial information, and conversely ventral CA1 might play a more important role than the dorsal CA1 for odor information (Kesner and Rolls, 2015).

In a more recent experiment using a paradigm described by Hannesson et al. (2004), it was shown that temporal order information for visual objects is impaired only by CA1, but not CA3 lesions (Hoge and Kesner, 2007). Thus, with respect to sequence learning or memory for order information one hypothesis that would be consistent with the data is that the CA1 is the critical substrate for sequence learning and temporal order or temporal pattern separation. This would be consistent with CA1 deficits in sequence completion of a spatial task and CA1 deficits in temporal order for spatial locations, odor, and visual objects. Dorsal CA3 contributes to this temporal order or sequence process whenever spatial location is also important. When visual objects are used the CA3 region does not play a role.

These findings support the hypothesis that time cells in these regions are involved in order memory (see Sections 9.3.5.4 and 9.3.7.4).

Many more tests of the theory of hippocampal operation, and a summary of the interactions and dissociations between CA3 and CA1, are provided by Kesner and Rolls (2015), with an update on the dentate gyrus by Kesner (2018). In addition, there is a Special Issue of *Neurobiology of Learning and Memory* devoted to pattern separation and pattern completion in the hippocampal system (Rolls and Kesner, 2016).

9.5 Comparison of spatial processing and computations in primates including humans vs rodents

9.5.1 Similarities and differences between the spatial representations in primates and rodents

Despite the major differences in the spatial representations in the primate and rodent hippocampus, there are important similarities between the operation of the rodent and primate hippocampus, which indicate that the computational operation of these neural systems is comparable in rodents and primates, even though what is represented is different. Some of the similarities of the hippocampal system in primates and rodents were set out as follows (Rolls and Wirth, 2018; Rolls, 2023c,d).

First, the spatial representations are in both cases by most spatial view and place cells primarily allocentric. In monkeys, hippocampal spatial view cells during active locomotion in an open environment respond allocentrically to the view of a position in a spatial scene, relatively independently of the place where the monkey is in the open environment, of head direction, of eye position, and of where the spatial view field is relative to the monkey (Georges-François et al., 1999; Rolls and O'Mara, 1995).

Second, the spatial representations can be updated idiothetically, by one's body or eye motion in primates, as in the rat.

Third, in both cases the firing rates are low: in primates with a typical mean rate of 0.5 spikes/s, and a typical peak response rate of 17-20 spikes/s (Rolls et al., 1997a; Wirth et al., 2017). This matches numerous accounts of firing properties in the rat hippocampus.

Fourth, spatial view cells may fire just before the eyes reach the centre of the spatial view field, and may have their maximal response soon after the eyes reach the spatial view field, and decrease somewhat after that, i.e. show some adaptation (Wirth et al., 2017). Analogous findings have been described for rodent hippocampal cells which generate spike sequences lasting about 2 seconds as rats traverse a place field. The firing rate in the place field shows an asymmetry which changes with experience: as rats become familiar with an environment; cells show an increase in rate before animals reach the place field, followed by a gradual decrease as rats leave the field (Mehta et al., 2000).

Fifth, in macaques, there is evidence for independent representation about spatial view by hippocampal neurons, in that the information rises linearly with the number of neurons (Rolls et al., 1998b). This independence arises when the response profiles of the neurons are uncorrelated (Rolls and Treves, 2011; Rolls, 2021b). This is a powerful encoding, because the number of stimuli (e.g. spatial views) rises exponentially with the number of neurons. (Of course this independence applies only in a high-dimensional environment, and saturates to the limit in lower dimensional environments (Rolls and Treves, 2011; Rolls, 2016b, 2021b).) Ensemble encoding by populations of neurons is found in rodents (Wilson and McNaughton, 1993), and it would be interesting to know whether the coding by different neurons is also independent in rodents.

Sixth, rodent place cells may respond differently on the trajectory to approach a goal depending on the state of the animal (Fyhn et al., 2002; Wood et al., 2000; Ferbinteanu et al., 2011), as in primates (Wirth et al., 2017). This implies that place cells support cognition in both species.

Seventh, in macaques, object-spatial view neurons are found (Rolls et al., 2005c), and one-trial object-place learning and recall can occur (Rolls and Xiang, 2006). In rodents object-place or odor-place neurons have been described (Kim et al., 2011; Komorowski et al., 2009). The presence of a barrier or boundary, which might be thought of as an object, in a place, may also be encoded by rodent hippocampal (Rivard et al., 2004; Wang et al., 2020b,a) and retrosplenial (Alexander et al., 2020) neurons.

Eighth, in macaques, reward-spatial view neurons are found (Rolls and Xiang, 2005), and cells are found to encode reward outcomes (Wirth et al., 2009; Brincat and Miller, 2015). In rodents reward-place neurons have been described (Tabuchi, Mulder and Wiener, 2003), and it was found that place cells are more active after the receipt of a reward (Singer and Frank, 2009).

Ninth, in rodents, distal room cues can influence place cells (Shapiro et al., 1997; Acharya et al., 2016; Aronov and Tank, 2014; Knierim and Rao, 2003). However, this is different to the encoding of a location in a scene that is provided by primate spatial view cells, in that in rodents the distal room cues are used to encode the place where the rodent is located.

Tenth, in both primates and rodents, restricting the view of the environment may have analogous effects. In primates navigating through spatial trajectories in a star maze, many neurons had their responses influenced by place, the direction in which the macaque was facing, and by the part of the trajectory being performed (Wirth et al., 2017). In rats tested in an open foraging environment in which all places and head directions occur, rat place cells tend to have only small directional selectivity. However, in rats tested in linear runways in which a task may be performed and in which only some combinations of head direction and place are common, place cells may be quite directional (Acharya et al., 2016). A possibility is that in the foraging situation used by Rolls and colleagues (Georges-François et al., 1999; Rolls et al., 1998b; Robertson et al., 1998; Rolls et al., 1997a), all places, views, and head directions occurred, and the cells were dominated by where the animal looked, and not by place or head direction. In contrast, if the macaque in a VR environment was constrained by the star maze to visit only certain places with particular spatial views and head directions that were frequently viewed from each of those places, and was performing a task that required a trajectory to a goal, then the neurons might reflect not only where the macaque was looking in the environment, but also the place from which the looking occurred etc. (Wirth et al., 2017). That is, if certain combinations of spatial view and place are common in an environment, then hippocampal neurons would be likely to encode primarily the combinations of spatial views and the places from which they are primarily seen.

Eleventh, whole body motion cells which respond to either linear velocity or angular velocity are present in the macaque hippocampus (O'Mara, Rolls, Berthoz and Kesner, 1994), and have more recently been described as speed cells in the rodent entorhinal cortex (Kropff et al., 2015; Spalla et al., 2022).

Twelfth, macaques (Rolls, 2005b; Robertson et al., 1999), as well as rodents (Taube et al., 1996, 1990a), have head direction cells in the presubiculum / subiculum.

These considerable similarities between the responses of neurons found in the rodent and primate hippocampal system provide evidence that the systems operate in similar ways in primates and rodents, but with different spatial representations (Rolls and Wirth, 2018). The different representations can be related to the evolution of the primate fovea, and its effects on object representations in the ventral cortical visual stream, and on systems in the primate dorsal visual stream for eye movements to produce foveation and for an interface to produce visually guided actions in the connected parietal cortical areas (Rolls et al., 2023e,d). Moreover, foveation of an object in primates is an efficient way to transmit the coordinates from a visually fixated object to the dorsal visuomotor system (Rolls et al., 2003a; Rolls and Deco, 2002) in the parietal cortex (Rolls et al., 2023d; Gamberini et al., 2020; Galletti and Fattori, 2018; Andersen and Cui, 2009). Further, the saccadic system of primates (including humans) enables a primate in one place to look towards one part of a scene and recall the object there, and then to saccade to another point in the scene and recall the object there. There is no evidence for anything similar in rodents, and this highlights an important difference between primate and rodent hippocampal spatial representation and memory systems that arises because of the primate fovea (Rolls, 2023d).

9.5.2 Hippocampal computational similarities and differences between primates and rodents

Although the spatial representations in the primate and rodent hippocampus are different, it is proposed that the underlying computations performed are similar (Rolls and Wirth, 2018; Rolls, 2023c).

A quantitative and detailed theory and model of how the hippocampus operates as a memory system, and of the way in which information stored in the hippocampus could be recalled back to the neocortex, has been developed (Rolls, 1989b; Treves and Rolls, 1994; Kesner and Rolls, 2015; Rolls, 2016b; Treves and Rolls, 1992; Rolls, 2018b, 2021b), with the architecture illustrated in Fig. 9.2. In the theory, the CA3 network forms an autoassociative or attractor memory, given the associatively modifiable recurrent connectivity between CA3 neurons. According to this theory, this system operates similarly in rodents and primates, to allow arbitrary associations between places in rodents, or spatial views in primates, and objects or rewards, to be rapidly formed, and later the whole memory to be recalled from a part. For example, the location of an object might be recalled in CA3 when an object recall cue was presented.

Temporal sequences for episodic memory may be remembered by replacing the location cells with the timing cells described by Eichenbaum and colleagues (Howard and Eichenbaum, 2015; Howard et al., 2014; Eichenbaum, 2014; Macdonald et al., 2011; Kraus et al., 2015, 2013), and this applies to primates (Naya et al., 2017) including humans (Umbach et al., 2020) too. A theory of the generation of hippocampal time cells (Rolls and Mills, 2019) from entorhinal cortex cells with time courses of their firing changing over tens or hundreds of seconds (Tsao et al., 2018) could apply equally to primates as rodents. Indeed, consistent with this, neurons in the monkey entorhinal cortex have a spectrum of time constants of their firing (Bright et al., 2020). The theory of the operation of time cells shows a mechanism by which forward and reverse replay of memories could be produced (Rolls and Mills, 2019), and rather than these phenomena being involved in memory consolidation, it is proposed that at least in humans the reward value of episodic memories helps to influence their recall and whether therefore they are retrieved in the neocortex and reorganized for semantic storage and consolidation in the neocortex (Rolls, 2022b). The temporal order of events in an episodic memory might also be implemented using a temporal asymmetry of the synaptic modification in for example the CA3 recurrent collaterals, but such models are expensive in terms of memory capacity and can probably only be used for short sequences in the order of 2 s (Sompolinsky and Kanter, 1986; Hasselmo, Giocomo, Brandon and Yoshida, 2010; Akrami, Russo and Treves, 2012; Spalla, Cornacchia and Treves, 2021).

The leading factor in the number of memories that can be stored and successfully recalled in this system is the number of synapses onto any one CA3 neuron by the associatively modifiable synapses from the recurrent collaterals of other CA3 neurons. With sparse representations, the number of memories that can be stored is in the order of the number of synapses onto each CA3 neuron (Treves and Rolls, 1991). It is interesting that an important difference in evolution arises in humans, in which the CA3 neurons are not well connected across the midline by the hippocampal commissure, given what is found in macaques (Amaral et al., 1984). In rodents, the CA3-CA3 in the two hippocampi are as much connected as within the hippocampus on one side in the brain, and this enables the rodent CA3 hippocampal network to operate as a single hippocampus (Rolls, 2016b, 2021b). In humans, there appear to be effectively separate left and right CA3 hippocampal networks given the poor commissural connectivity. Consistent with this point, there is evidence that the right human hippocampus specialises in spatial including object-place and reward-place memories, and the left hippocampus specialises in more language/word-related memory processes (Crane and Milner, 2005; Burgess et al., 2002; Barkas et al., 2010; Sidhu et al., 2013; Bonelli et al., 2010). The adaptation here is that humans have twice the memory capacity of a hippocampal system connected across the midline as in rodents; and that associations are not typically made between words and their position in space, for the latter are not part of what is implemented for human language. The implication for spatial view neurons in humans is that they may be found more in the right hippocampus and possibly more in the right parahippocampal scene area.

Key points made here are that the primate parietal cortex may implement idiothetic update of hippocampal and parahippocampal spatial view neurons; and that recall of spatial view information from the hippocampus to neocortical areas such as the parietal cortex may be involved in navigation and in visuo-motor processing to reach for and grasp objects or rewards at recalled locations in the world. A possible implication is that the primate including human hippocampus may be especially involved in episodic memory, but that the actual computations for navigation and movements in the environment for navigation and visuo-motor function may be implemented outside the hippocampus, in neocortical areas such as the parietal cortex. Consistent with this hypothesis, lesions of the human neocortex can produce topographical agnosia and inability to navigate (Kolb and Whishaw, 2021; Barton, 2011), and the retrosplenial cortex is implicated in navigation (Vedder et al., 2017; Alexander and Nitz, 2015; Byrne et al., 2007; Epstein, 2008; Vann et al., 2009). In more detail, lesions restricted to the hippocampus in humans result only in slight navigation impairments in familiar environments, but rather strongly impair learning or imagining new trajectories (Bohbot and Corkin, 2007; Teng and Squire, 1999; Spiers and Maguire, 2006; Maguire et al., 2016; Clark and Maguire, 2016). In contrast, lesions in regions such as the parietal cortex or the retrosplenial cortex produce strong topographical disorientation in both familiar and new environments (Aguirre and D'Esposito, 1999; Habib and Sirigu, 1987; Takahashi et al., 1997; Maguire, 2001; Kim et al., 2015b). This suggests that the core navigation processes (which may include transformations from allocentric representations to egocentric motor commands) is performed independently by neocortical areas outside the hippocampus, which may utilize hippocampal information related to recent memories (Ekstrom et al., 2014; Miller et al., 2013).

Further, and consistent with the spatial view cells found in non-human primates, regions of the human hippocampal formation can become activated when people look at spatial views (Epstein and Kanwisher, 1998; O'Keefe et al., 1998; Epstein and Baker, 2019). Moreover, the right human hippocampus is activated during mental navigation in recently learned but not in highly familiar environments (Hirshhorn et al., 2012). Mental navigation in familiar environments produces activation of cortical areas such as the lateral temporal cortex, posterior parahippocampal cortex, lingual gyrus, and precuneus (Hirshhorn et al., 2012). Further, as noted above, patients with anterograde amnesia may not be impaired in navigation in familiar environments, as contrasted with new environments (Clark and Maguire, 2016; Maguire et al., 2016). The implication is that, at least in primates, the hippocampus may be involved in episodic memory, and that neocortical regions implement navigation (helped when it is useful by recent memories recalled from the hippocampus).

In contrast, the view has often been held that the rodent hippocampus implements navigation. Indeed, in rodents, the existence of place cells has led to hypotheses that the rodent hippocampus provides a spatial cognitive map, and can implement spatial computations to perform navigation (O'Keefe and Nadel, 1978). These navigational hypotheses could not account for what is found in the primate hippocampus. An alternative that is suggested is that, in both rodents and primates, hippocampal neurons provide a representation of space (which for rodents is the place where the rat is located, and for primates includes positions "out there" in space), which are used as part of an episodic memory system. In primates this would enable formation of a memory of where an object was seen (Rolls, 1987, 1989b; Rolls and Kesner, 2006a; Rolls, 2016b, 2018b, 2021b). In rodents, this would enable the formation of memories of where particular objects (defined by olfactory, tactile, and taste inputs for instance) were found (Kesner and Rolls, 2015). Consistent with this theory of hippocampal function, one-trial object-place memory in rodents requires the hippocampus (Takeuchi et al., 2014; Day et al., 2003; Kesner and Rolls, 2015); texture sensed by whiskers and the places of rewards are reflected in neuronal firing (Itskov et al., 2011); some hippocampal neurons respond to behavioral, perceptual, or cognitive events, independently of the place where these events occurred, and may thus be useful for memory functions (Wood et al., 1999; Komorowski et al., 2009; Wood et al., 2000); hippocampal neurons may be activated following relocation of a target object to a new place (Fyhn et al., 2002); some hippocampal neurons alter their response when a different recording chamber is placed in the same location in the room (Leutgeb et al., 2005a); and another continuous dimension than place, namely auditory frequency, can be mapped by rodent hippocampal neurons (Aronov et al., 2017). Thus in primates, and probably also in rodents, the hippocampal representation of space may be appropriate for the formation of memories of episodic events (for which there is typically a spatial component). These memories would be of use in spatial navigation.

9.6 Synthesis: the hippocampus: memory, navigation, or both?

Much of the evidence described above indicates that the hippocampus is involved in memory, and especially in episodic memory. But some, starting with rodent place cells, propose that the hippocampus is a cognitive map for navigation (O'Keefe and Nadel, 1978; Hartley et al., 2014; Bicanski and Burgess, 2018). I now provide a synthesis, with much of the evidence described above in this Chapter.

1. The evidence is that the hippocampus provides a memory network, with the CA3 recurrent collateral network operating as an autoassociation network with attractor dynamics providing for recall of a whole memory from any part (Rolls, 1989b; Kesner and Rolls, 2015; Rolls, 2018b). Because CA3 is a single network, any input to the hippocampus can be associated with any other input. That is a special property of CA3 not found elsewhere in the brain.
2. Because the CA3 operates with Hebbian associative learning, it associates events that occur within a short time window of 1 to a few seconds. That makes it specialize in single event memory, typical of episodic memory, where the components of the episodic memory are simultaneously present. The hippocampal system uses pattern separation to help somewhat similar episodes to be stored as separate episodic memories (Rolls, 2016f).
3. Because of time cells in the hippocampus, the hippocampus can also be involved in the temporal order of events in an episodic memory, by associating objects, people, or spatial information with the firing of particular time cells (Eichenbaum, 2017; Rolls and Mills, 2019).
4. One of the key inputs to the hippocampus is from spatial view cells in the primate including human medial parahippocampal gyrus PHA1-3 (Rolls et al., 2023e; Rolls, 2023c). Thus spatial information about locations in for example scenes is a prototypical part of human episodic memory.
5. Other key inputs are about objects and people, from the inferior temporal visual cortex via the lateral parahippocampal cortex TF and the perirhinal cortex; and are about reward, value, and emotion from the orbitofrontal cortex (Rolls et al., 2023e; Rolls, 2023c; Rolls et al., 2023c). This enables the human hippocampus to include in a prototypical episodic memory where the events happened, who or what was present and where they were located, and value.
6. The spatial scene input in primates including humans in the hippocampus is built from ventral visual stream features and combinations of features in a scene (Rolls et al., 2023e; Rolls, 2023c). The mechanism for this is associations of features in each foveated part of a scene which form spatial view cells that respond to only a small part of a scene. That was clearly set out and modelled by De Araujo, Rolls and Stringer (2001). As clearly explained in that paper, the spatial view cells formed are relatively independent of the place where the individual is located, because the scene looks similar from different places on the same side of the scene. For example a hill will always be on the left side of a lake as long as the individual is on one side of the scene. That is the sense in which spatial view cells are allocentric with respect to place, as well as of head direction and eye position (Rolls, 2023c). This is because it is the features in the spatial scene that have been associated together in a particular spatial order (e.g. hill then lake then house), and

when those features are seen in that spatial arrangement, the spatial view cell will fire (De Araujo, Rolls and Stringer, 2001). Of course if the individual crosses over and goes behind the viewed scene, then the egocentric view will change (the hill may change from being on the left of the scene to being on the right of the scene. Does that mean that the locations in the scene do not form a cognitive allocentric map of the type envisaged in many models of navigation (O'Keefe and Nadel, 1978; Hartley et al., 2014; Bicanski and Burgess, 2018)? To think about this, let us consider the situation in rodents.

7. The situation is different in rodents, in that they have place cells (O'Keefe, 1979). The computational argument, clearly specified and modelled by De Araujo, Rolls and Stringer (2001), is that place cells are formed because the rodent has such a wide field of view, perhaps 270 degrees, that a combination of features 'out there' (for example the room cues) will define a place where the individual is located. The place field should then be mainly but not completely invariant with respect to head direction, because a rat cannot see the whole 360 degrees of the environment at one time, and as the head rotates, somewhat different features in the environment may become more prominent. In the sense that environmental (e.g. room) cues determine where a place cell fires, rodent place cells are responsive to spatial cues 'out there', which is a feature of what spatial view cells in primates respond to (Rolls and Wirth, 2018; Rolls, 2023c,d).

8. Let us consider further how the parts of a scene are stitched together in primates. When a primate including human with spatial view cells is on one side of a scene, then the nearby parts of the scene become associated together by co-firing of neurons that produce synaptic modification based on how much co-firing there is, and therefore the distance between the spatial view fields. (I assume some sort of Gaussian shaped receptive field spatial sensitivity, as shown for primate hippocampal spatial view cells (Rolls, 2023c).) That forms a continuous attractor network for spatial view in primates (Stringer, Rolls and Trappenberg, 2005; Rolls and Stringer, 2005; Rolls, Tromans and Stringer, 2008f). Exactly the same computational mechanism in rodents potentially builds a continuous attractor network for place fields (Samsonovich and McNaughton, 1997; Stringer, Rolls, Trappenberg and De Araujo, 2002a). Now a continuous attractor network (described in Section B.5) can be regarded as a type of map, for nearby locations in the map are represented by co-firing neurons, and one can imagine moving through a series of nearby items in a trajectory, which may be thought of as a type of navigation (Stringer, Rolls and Trappenberg, 2005; Rolls and Stringer, 2005; Stringer, Rolls, Trappenberg and De Araujo, 2002a). Indeed, if one continued the navigation to get behind the scene, the order in which the landmarks in the scene are linked would be the same (e.g. house then lake then hill), so the representation of the scene would be allocentric, world-based, in that the parts of the map would be linked together in the correct order independently of which side of the scene it was viewed from. The viewpoint-dependent relations, e.g. which landmark was on the left, would change, but not the allocentric world-based representation in which the landmarks are linked in the same order regardless of the exact viewpoint. Thus spatial view cells could be linked in a continuous attractor network to provide an allocentric representation of the structure of the scene (Rolls, 2023d). That allocentric representation could be useful for navigation from landmark to landmark (Rolls, 2021f).

For this analysis, it is important to be clear about different coordinate frameworks (Rolls, 2023d). If the locations of the stimuli are in coordinates relative to the head (craniotopic) or body, these representations are in an **egocentric spatial coordinate framework**. If the representations of the locations of things such as parts of a scene are fixed relative to other parts of a scene, and are encoded provided that location in the world is viewed, independently of the location relative to the head, body, or retinal position, then this is in an **allocentric spatial coordinate framework**. These are coordinate frameworks for spatial relationships. Completely different are **viewpoint-dependent spatial frameworks** for relationships, for which left-right is reversed when a scene is viewed from different sides, but that is independent of whether what is viewed is represented in an egocentric spatial framework relative to the head in craniotopic coordinates, or in an allocentric framework that is independent of position relative to the craniotopic egocentric head-based framework (Rolls, 2023c,d).

The following are some implications for understanding the representation of space 'out there' in the hippocampus and parahippocampal scene area by spatial view neurons (Rolls, 2023c,d). First, spatial view neurons are allocentric in that they do not depend on the exact place from where a scene is viewed (Georges-François, Rolls and Robertson, 1999; Rolls, 2023c). Second, spatial view cells do not depend on head direction (provided of course that the scene can be viewed), so spatial view cells are not egocentric (Georges-François et al., 1999; Rolls, 2023c). Third, spatial view neurons are spatial in the sense that they can be idiothetically updated in the dark to fire when the individual looks towards the spatial view field (Robertson, Rolls and Georges-François, 1998; Rolls, 2023c). That is not a property of inferior temporal cortex neurons that respond to objects and faces. Fourth, spatial view neurons are allocentric in that they represent features in a scene stitched together in the correct spatial organisation with respect to each other: this more formally is implemented by the continuous attractor network formed because of the cofiring of nearby spatial view neurons with spatially overlapping receptive fields (Rolls and Stringer, 2005; Stringer, Rolls and Trappenberg, 2005). Some of the clear evidence for this is that spatial view neurons start to respond in virtual reality to a part of the scene towards which a movement is being performed even before the view of the scene has even appeared on the VR screen (Wirth et al., 2017). That is evidence that there is a hippocampal representation that has information about the spatial relations of parts of a scene. The same point is made by the idiothetic update of hippocampal spatial view neurons in the dark, in that they fire even in the dark and when the scene is hidden by curtains but the eyes look towards the spatial view field of the spatial view neuron (Robertson, Rolls and Georges-François, 1998). All of this is consistent with the theory that spatial view neurons are in a sense viewing-point dependent, in that they are formed by looking at scenes that are being viewed when the individual is on one side of the scene (Rolls, 2023d). In such a representation part 1 of the scene may be to the left of part 2 of a scene, part 2 may be to the left of part 3, etc, and that relationship will remain as long as the individual is on that side of a scene. In that sense, hippocampal spatial view neurons may have an allocentric world based representation, based in the evidence above, which may nevertheless be stored with the scene viewed from one side, in a viewer-based framework. However, if one moves to the other side of the scene, a continuous attractor network representation already built could still reflect the closeness of the landmarks in a scene, in that part 1 would be close to part 2 but not part 3, etc, and that could still potentially be used in terms of the closeness of parts of a scene, even though when viewed from the other side the left/right relations will be reversed consistent with a viewer-based framework. The closeness of the parts of a scene will still be useful for truly allocentric navigation independently of which side the scene is viewed from (Rolls, 2023d).

Thus it is proposed that spatial view cells form allocentric representations of scenes, even though the left-right viewpoint-dependent relationships are different on different sides of the scene when the viewpoint changes. The spatial representation provided by spatial view cells is allocentric in that it is not craniotopic, even when it may look "egocentrically" different from a "first person perspective" to a viewer who is on different sides of a scene (Wirth, 2023), in what should most clearly be described as a view-dependent allocentric representation (Rolls, 2023d). Moreover that allocentric representation even though it may have viewpoint dependence may however also have important viewpoint-independent topological properties, for example about the closeness of the different parts of the scene, which is important for navigation (Rolls, 2023d). Thus viewpoint dependence of scenes is important (Rolls, 2023d), but is completely different from egocentric vs allocentric encoding (Rolls, 2023d), and it is important to be clear about this (Wirth, 2023).

9. However, as noted above, a continuous attractor network of this type might not operate very well for navigation, because the association of items and rewards with spatial locations might make the energy landscape too bumpy and the attractor might be likely to become stuck (Soldatkina, Schonsberg and Treves, 2022; Ryom, Stendardi, Ciaramelli and Treves, 2023).

10. Given the evidence described above that navigation may not be impaired in familiar environments in humans with hippocampal damage, and is only impaired in new environments since the hippocampal damage, there may be brain regions outside the hippocampus (for example the retrosplenial cortex) that play key roles in navigation, with the hippocampus specialising primarily in event memory, in line with the evidence just summarized.

11. In summary, the evidence is that the hippocampal system in primates including humans is primarily for episodic memory, with the ability to retrieve a whole memory in CA3 from any part, and then to retrieve the components back to the relevant regions of neocortex, where they can be used to help form semantic memories in memory consolidation, where an important modulating factor is likely to be the value of the episodic memory (Rolls, 2022b). The hippocampal system contributes to navigation in novel environments because it can learn about the organisation of the features/landmarks in a novel environment. The hippocampus is likely to be involved in human navigation that proceeds from landmark to landmark, because landmarks are encoded by parahippocampal and hippocampal spatial view cells (Rolls, 2021f). Whether the hippocampus implements geometrical computations on place cell maps to organize novel trajectories involving novel short cuts through a place cell topology remains to be shown.

What is shown in this section is that spatial view cells are allocentric in the sense that they respond to features in scenes relatively independently of the place where the individual is located, because what is viewed in a distant scene is not very dependent on exactly where the individual is located, or on head direction.

Further, it is shown that a continuous attractor network of spatial view cells could be allocentric, world-based, in that the neighbourhood relations between parts of a scene would be useful on either side of the scene to implement a trajectory from landmark to landmark. The viewpoint-dependent representation would be reversed on different sides of a scene, with what is to the left of what reversed, but the allocentric map useful for trajectories would still be useful as an allocentric map useful for navigation from landmark to landmark (Rolls, 2023d, 2021f).

9.7 Comparison with other theories of hippocampal function

The theory described here is quantitative, and supported by both formal analyses and quantitative simulations. Many of the points made, such as on the number of memories that can be stored in autoassociative networks, the utility of sparse representations, and the dynamics of the operation of networks with recurrent connections, are quite general, and will apply to networks in a number of different brain areas. With respect to the hippocampus, the theory specifies the maximum number of memories that could be stored in it, and this has implications for how it could be used biologically. It indicates that if this number is approached, it will be useful to have a mechanism for recalling information from the hippocampus for incorporation into memories elsewhere. With respect to recall, the theory provides a quantitative account for why there are as many backprojections as forward projections in the cerebral cortex. Overall, the theory provides an explanation for how this part of the brain could work, and even if this theory needs to be revised, it is suggested that a fully quantitative computational theory along the lines proposed which is based on the evidence available from a wide range of techniques will be essential before we can say that we understand how a part of the cortex operates. This theory is almost unique in being a *quantitative* theory of hippocampal function.

Hypotheses have been described in this chapter about how a number of different parts of hippocampal and related circuitry might operate. Although these hypotheses are consistent with a theory of how the hippocampus operates, some of these hypotheses could be incorporated into other views or theories. In order to highlight the differences between alternative theories, and in order to lead to constructive analyses that can test them, the theory described above is compared with other theories of hippocampal function in this section. Although the differences between the theories are highlighted in this section, the overall view described here is close in different respects to the views of a number of other investigators (Marr, 1971; Brown and Zador, 1990; Eichenbaum, Otto and Cohen, 1992; McNaughton and Nadel, 1990; Squire, 1992; McClelland, McNaughton and O'Reilly, 1995; Moscovitch, Rosenbaum, Gilboa, Addis, Westmacott, Grady, McAndrews, Levine, Black, Winocur and Nadel, 2005; Wang and Morris, 2010; Preston and Eichenbaum, 2013; Winocur and Moscovitch, 2011) and of course priority is not claimed on all the propositions put forward here.

Some theories postulate that the hippocampus performs spatial computation. The theory of O'Keefe and Nadel (1978) that the hippocampus implements a cognitive map, placed great emphasis on spatial function. It supposed that the hippocampus at least holds information about allocentric space in a form which enables rats to find their way in an environment even when novel trajectories are necessary, that is it permits an animal to "go from one place to another independent of particular inputs (cues) or outputs (responses), and to link together conceptually parts of the environment which have never been experienced at the same time". O'Keefe (1990) extended this analysis and produced a computational theory of the hippocampus as a cognitive map, in which the hippocampus performs geometric spatial computations. Key aspects of the theory are that the hippocampus stores the centroid and slope of the distribution of landmarks in an environment, and stores the relationships between the centroid and the individual landmarks. The hippocampus then receives as inputs information about where the rat currently is, and where the rat's target location is, and computes geometrically the body turns and movements necessary to reach the target location. In this sense, the hippocampus is taken to be a spatial computer, which produces an output which is very different from its inputs. This is in contrast to the present theory, in which the hippocampus is a memory device, which is able to recall what was stored in it, using as input a partial cue. The theory of O'Keefe postulates that the hippocampus actually performs a spatial computation. The well-deserved award of a Nobel prize to John O'Keefe and colleagues explicitly recognized the spatial aspects of his approach, referring to an "inner GPS" in the brain. Updates to the theory (Burgess, Recce and O'Keefe, 1994; Burgess, Jackson, Hartley and O'Keefe, 2000; Edvardsen, Bicanski and Burgess, 2020) also make the same postulate, but now the firing of place cells is determined by the distance and approximate bearing to landmarks, and the navigation is performed by increasing the strength of connections from place cells to "goal cells", and then performing gradient-ascent style search for the goal using the network. Rolls' discoveries and theory are thus somewhat different from those of O'Keefe and colleagues, in that Rolls has shown that spatial view cells may be especially relevant to the operation of the hippocampus in primates including humans; and in that the roles of the hippocampal system in memory are emphasized. Further, Rolls has developed theories about how the spatial view and other cells found in the primate hippocampal and related parietal cortex systems could be involved in navigation (Section 9.3.15).

McNaughton et al. (1991) have also proposed that the hippocampus is involved in spatial computation. They propose a "compass" solution to the problem of spatial navigation along novel trajectories in known environments, postulating that distances and bearings (i.e. vector quantities) from landmarks are stored, and that computation of a new trajectory involves vector subtraction by the hippocampus. They postulate that a linear associative mapping is performed, using as inputs a "cross-feature" (combination) representation of (head) angular velocity and (its time integral) head direction, to produce as output the future value of the integral (head direction) after some specified time interval. The system can be reset by learned associations between local views of the environment and head direction, so that when later a local view is seen, it can lead to an output from the network which is a (corrected) head direction. They suggest that some of the key signals in the computational system can be identified with the firing of hippocampal cells (e.g. local view cells) and subicular cells (head direction cells). It should be noted that this theory requires a (linear) associative mapping with an output (head direction) different in form from the inputs (head angular velocity over a time period, or local view). This is pattern association (with the conditioned stimulus local view, and the unconditioned stimulus head direction), not autoassociation, and it has been postulated that this pattern association can be performed by the hippocampus (cf. McNaughton and Morris (1987)). This theory is again in contrast to the present theory, in which the hippocampus operates as a memory to store events that occur at the same time, and can recall the whole memory from any part of what was stored. (A pattern associator uses a conditioned stimulus to map an input to a pattern of firing in an output set of neurons which is like that produced in the output neurons by the unconditioned stimulus. A description of pattern associators and autoassociators in a neurobiological context is provided in Appendix B. The present theory is fully consistent with the presence of 'spatial view' cells and whole body motion cells in the primate hippocampus (Rolls and Xiang, 2006; Rolls, 1999c; Rolls and O'Mara, 1993) (or place or local view cells in the rat hippocampus, and head direction cells in the presubiculum), for it is often important to store and later recall where one has been (views of the environment, body turns made, etc), and indeed such (episodic) memories are required for navigation by "dead reckoning" in small environments.

The present theory thus holds that the hippocampus is used for the formation of episodic memories using autoassociation. This function is often necessary for successful spatial computation, but is not itself spatial computation. Instead, we believe that spatial computation is more likely to be performed in the neocortex (utilising information if necessary recalled from the hippocampus). Consistent with this view, hippocampal damage impairs the ability to learn new environments but not to perform spatial computations such as finding one's way to a place in a familiar environment, whereas damage to the parietal cortex and parahippocampal cortex can lead to problems such as topographical and other spatial agnosias, in humans (Grusser and Landis, 1991; Kolb and Whishaw, 2021; Maguire et al., 2016; Rolls and Wirth, 2018) (see Section 10.6). This is consistent with spatial computations normally being performed in the neocortex. (In monkeys, there is evidence for a role of the parietal cortex in allocentric spatial computation. For example, monkeys with parietal cortex lesions are impaired at performing a landmark task, in which the object to be chosen is signified by the proximity to it of a "landmark" (another object) (Ungerleider and Mishkin, 1982).)

A theory closely related to the present theory of how the hippocampus operates has been developed by McClelland, McNaughton and O'Reilly (1995). It is very similar to the theory we have developed (Rolls, 1987, 1989a, 1990b, 1989f; Treves and Rolls, 1992, 1994; Rolls, 1996d; Rolls and Treves, 1998; Rolls and Kesner, 2006b; Rolls, 2008e, 2010b; Kesner and Rolls, 2015) at the systems level, except that it takes a stronger position on the gradient of retrograde amnesia, emphasises that recall from the hippocampus of episodic information is used to help build semantic representations in the neocortex, and holds that the last set of synapses that are modified rapidly during the learning of each episode are those between the CA3 and the CA1 pyramidal cells (see Fig. 9.2). It also emphasizes the important point that the hippocampal and neocortical memory systems may be quite different, with the hippocampus specialized for the rapid learning of single events or episodes, and the neocortex for the slower learning of semantic representations which may necessarily benefit from the many exemplars needed to shape the semantic representation. In the formulation by McClelland, McNaughton and O'Reilly (1995), the entorhinal cortex connections via the perforant path onto the CA1 cells are non-modifiable (in the short term), and allow a representation of neocortical long-term memories to activate the CA1 cells. The new information learned in an episode by the CA3 system is then linked to existing long-term memories by the CA3 to CA1 rapidly modifiable synapses. All the connections from the CA1 back via the subiculum, entorhinal cortex, parahippocampal cortex etc. to the association neocortex are held to be unmodifiable in the short term, during the formation of an episodic memory. The formal argument that leads us to suggest that the backprojecting synapses are associatively modifiable during the learning of an episodic memory is similar to that which we have used to show that for efficient recall, the synapses which initiate recall in the CA3 system (identified above with the perforant path projection to CA3) must be associatively modifiable if recall is to operate efficiently (Treves and Rolls, 1992). The present theory holds that it is possible that for several stages back into neocortical processing, the backprojecting synapses should be associatively modifiable, with a similar time course to the time it takes to learn a new episodic memory. It may well be that at earlier stages of cortical processing, for example from inferior temporal visual cortex to V4, and from V4 to V2, the backprojections are relatively more fixed, being formed (still associatively) during early developmental plasticity or during the formation of new long-term semantic memory structures. Having such relatively fixed synaptic strengths in these earlier cortical backprojection systems could ensure that whatever is recalled in higher cortical areas, such as objects, will in turn recall relatively fixed and stable representations of parts of objects or features. Given that the functions of backprojections may include many top-down processing operations, including attention (Deco and Rolls, 2005a) and priming, it may be useful to ensure that there is consistency in how higher cortical areas affect activity in earlier "front-end" or preprocessing cortical areas. Indeed, the current theory shows that at least one backprojection stage, the hippocampo-cortical connections must be associatively modifiable during the learning of an episodic memory, but does not require the associative backprojection learning to occur at all backprojection stages during the learning of the episodic memory. Crucial stages might include CA1 to subiculum or to entorhinal cortex (see Fig. 9.2), or entorhinal cortex to parahippocampal gyrus and perirhinal cortex. It would be interesting to test this using local inactivation of NMDA receptors at different stages of the backprojection system to determine where this impairs the learning of for example place–object recall, i.e. a task that is likely to utilize the hippocampo-cortical backprojection pathways.

If a model of the hippocampal / neocortical memory system could store only a small number of patterns, it would not be a good model of the real hippocampal / neocortical memory system in the brain. Indeed, this appears to be a major limitation of another model presented by Alvarez and Squire (1994). The model specifies that the hippocampus helps the operation of a neocortical multimodal memory system in which all memories are stored by associative recurrent collaterals between the neocortical neurons. Although the idea worked in the model with twenty neurons and two patterns to be learned (Alvarez and Squire, 1994), the whole idea is computationally not feasible, because the number of memories that can be stored in a single autoassociative network of the type described is limited by the number of inputs per neuron from other neurons, not by the number of neurons in the network (Treves and Rolls, 1991, 1994). This would render the capacity of the whole neocortical multimodal (or amodal) memory store very low (in the order of the number of inputs per neuron from the other neurons, that is in the order of 5,000–10,000) (O'Kane and Treves, 1992). This example makes it clear that it is important to take into account analytic and quantitative approaches when investigating memory systems. The current work is an attempt to do this.

The discovery of hippocampal time cells (Macdonald et al., 2011; Eichenbaum, 2017; Salz et al., 2016; Howard and Eichenbaum, 2015; Eichenbaum, 2014) has transformed our understanding of how the order of items in a memory could be implemented. A mechanism for the generation of time cells has been described (Rolls and Mills, 2019) (Section 9.3.4). A side effect of the way in which time cells are generated in the model is the generation of reverse replay, as well as forward replay. There have been many discoveries about these forward and reverse replay phenomena, in the context that they may be involved in the transfer of memories from the hippocampal system to the neocortex (Wilson and McNaughton, 1994; Foster and Wilson, 2006; Foster, 2017). The concept advocated there is for a type of undirected burst of replay in the hippocampus, which would transfer the information, presumably in its raw episodic form, to the neocortex. Sharp wave ripples are associated with these 'replay' events and are generated for example in CA1 during slow wave sleep and quiescent wakefulness (Buzsaki, 2015), and occur in humans when memories are being stored or recalled (Norman, Yeagle, Khuvis, Harel, Mehta and Malach, 2019). However, my view is that recall of episodic information to the neocortex could best be initiated by a recall cue from the neocortex, which would lead to completion of the whole episodic memory from the hippocampus, which would then recall the whole memory to the neocortex in the quantitative way described in Section 9.3.8. This recall would reinstate activity in the cortical neurons that had been present during learning of the original episodic memory. It would then be up to the cortex to use that information, in conjunction with much semantic information it already has, to add to that semantic (including autobiographical) memory in a way that could usefully extend the semantic memory. The example I provided was of recalling a train journey, and using the particular information from that, to help build a semantic geographical map. In humans, this would best be performed when thinking about the sematic information, recalling the episode from the hippocampus, and then actively adjusting the semantic map in the light of the episodic information. Memory consolidation guided by value is described in Section 9.2.8.5 (Rolls, 2022b).

A different type of sequence memory uses synaptic adaptation to effectively encode the order of the items in a sequence (Deco and Rolls, 2005c). This could be implemented in recurrent networks such as the prefrontal cortex.

The proposal that acetylcholine could be important during encoding by facilitating CA3–CA3 LTP, and should be lower during retrieval (Hasselmo, Schnell and Barkai, 1995; Hasselmo and Sarter, 2011; Zaborszky, Gombkoto, Varsanyi, Gielow, Poe, Role, Ananth, Rajebhosale, Talmage, Hasselmo, Dannenberg, Minces and Chiba, 2018), is a useful concept. This has been extended by the concept that memory consolidation in humans is influenced by the posterior orbitofrontal cortex that influences the basal forebrain cholinergic system that projects to the neocortex; and by the vmPFC and anterior cingulate cortex that influences the cholinergic septal system that projects to the hippocampus (Rolls, 2022b; Rolls et al., 2023c)(Section 9.2.8.5).

An approach linked to neuropsychology and neuroimaging is that the hippocampus is involved in the construction of spatial scenes, and that patients with hippocampal damage are devoid of visual representations of scenes (Maguire et al., 2016; McCormick et al., 2018; Zeidman et al., 2015; Clark et al., 2019). That is of course very close to the view developed in this chapter, that the primate including human hippocampal system is especially involved in the construction of visual scenes using spatial view cells, with the 'construction' being implemented by continuous attractor networks, which provide a way in which the brain builds cognitive maps where there is continuity of the representations, as is the case for spatial representations. Moreover, the present approach links to the evidence that other types of continuous space are natural candidates for implementation as continuous attractors in the entorhinal cortex / hippocampal attractor networks (Constantinescu et al., 2016; Bellmund et al., 2018; Nau et al., 2018b).

Teyler and DiScenna (1986) proposed that the hippocampus stores pointers to neocortical areas, and uses those pointers to recall memories in the cortex. The present theory is different, for it emphasizes that spatial and temporal order representations are present in the hippocampus, and can be combined with object information to store episodic memories in the hippocampus by forming associations between these components. However, the theory also shows how recall of these episodic memories within the hippocampus can then using backprojections to neocortical areas allow neocortical representations present at the time of the encoding to be retrieved, and then potentially stored in the neocortex in a schema or semantic memory. The actual retrieval process to neocortex is implemented by using associatively modified synapses in at least one stage of the backprojection system, and this provides a deaddressing method for the hippocampus to retrieve a content-addressable neocortical memory. This deaddressing process for recall to the neocortex that is part of the current theory can be likened to the use of a pointer, but rather than being a metaphor as in Teyler and DiScenna (1986), the current theory specifies a mechanism by which the correct set of neurons in the neocortex can be brought into activity during recall, and provides the only solution I know to how information is correctly retrieved from the hippocampus to the correct set of neurons in the neocortex. The present theory (Rolls, 1990b, 1996d, 2010b; Rolls and Kesner, 2006b; Kesner and Rolls, 2015; Rolls, 2016b, 2018b, 2023c, 2022b) is I believe unique in that it enables both the hippocampal storage process, and the recall to the neocortex, to be understood quantitatively.

The aim of this comparison of the present theory with other theories has been to highlight differences between the theories, to assist in the future assessment of the utility and the further development of each of the theories.

Overall, the approach taken in this chapter shows how it is now possible to understand quantitatively how the circuitry in a major brain system could actually operate to store and later recall memories.

10 The parietal cortex, spatial functions, and navigation

10.1 Introduction and overview

10.1.1 Overview of what is computed in the parietal cortex

1. The dorsal visual stream projects up into the parietal cortex to intraparietal sulcus regions such as LIP, VIP, and MIP, and then to area 7 regions, as shown in Fig. 3.1 and Fig. 10.2 (see Chapter 3 and Sections 10.3 and 10.4). This system includes neurons that link visual responsiveness with action such as grasping an object (Galletti and Fattori, 2018; Bisley and Goldberg, 2010) (see also Chapter 15).

2. One of the visual coordinate frames that is represented in some parietal cortex areas is head-based. That facilitates coordination between spatial representations in the visual and auditory systems using bimodal visual-auditory neurons that respond to the same position in head-centred space, because auditory space is necessarily in head-based coordinates in primates including humans. This facilitates for example saccades towards positions in space where a sound was heard.

3. Visual regions in the greatly developed inferior parietal cortex PG regions (PGi, PGs, PGp and also PFm) receive visual motion-related inputs from some of the more superior intraparietal sulcus and area 7 regions, and have connectivity also with inferior temporal visual 'what' cortex to produce motion-related representations of objects, faces and the body, which communicate with superior temporal sulcus regions with similar activity.

4. The primary somatosensory cortex areas 1, 2 and 3 are in the parietal cortex, and project via a 'ventral somatosensory stream' (Section 6.1.8.1) through frontal opercular (FOP) regions and the insula to parietal PF regions that reach finally region PF itself where somatosensory representations about felt objects and the body image can be combined with visual inputs to provide multimodal representations.

5. The primary somatosensory cortex areas 1, 2 and 3, also project into parietal areas 5 and 7, in a 'dorsal somatosensory stream' (Section 6.1.8.2) in which somatosensory information is brought together with visual information for functions such as reaching for and grasping objects. Neurons with movement-related activity in the parietal cortex as well as in premotor cortex area F5 respond to the sight of grasping an object, as well as to actually grasping an object, in the mirror neuron system (Rizzolatti and Craighero, 2004; Rizzolatti and Sinigaglia, 2016; Rizzolatti and Rozzi, 2018) (Section 15.3).

6. Somatosensory including proprioceptive inputs are represented in parietal cortex areas BA 1, 2 and 3a, which then project to area 5, and thus to 7 in the 'dorsal somatosensory stream'. The representations in early stages may be of single joint positions, but become more complex up through the hierarchy because neurons come to represent combinations of joint positions, which can then represent for example the position of the arm in egocentric space, for example relative to the trunk.

7. The human inferior parietal cortex multimodal regions including PGi and PF provide inputs to and are part of the semantic language-related regions that extend through the

temporo-parieto-occipital junction (TPOJ) regions and the superior temporal sulcus (STS) regions that extend to the temporal pole that are further described in Chapter 14.

10.1.2 Overview of how the computations are performed in the parietal cortex

1. A feature hierarchy for proprioceptive information through the parietal cortex from the primary somatosensory cortex through area 5 to macaque area 7b is proposed to lead to representations of the egocentric position in space relative to the body of for example an arm. This would be appropriate for movements made to positions in egocentric space. The feature hierarchy it is proposed performs this computation by forming combinations of the positions of single joints that are represented at early stages of the hierarchy.
2. Similarly a feature hierarchy for touch information is proposed to lead to combinations of local touch information in for example several parts of the hand to enable tactile object recognition. Whether a trace synaptic learning rule is used in making such object representations show position invariance (even across the right and left hands) is an interesting but untested possibility. A different mechanism might be use of invariant visual object recognition to help set up by association the correct invariant touch object representations in a multimodal region, which might be more in a ventral stream area such as the anterior temporal lobe.
3. Visual and proprioceptive information, both in egocentric coordinates, could combine by pattern association learning, or by competitive learning with a mixture of visual and somatosensory inputs, to form neurons that could respond in egocentric coordinates, to help guide arm movements to a viewed target. In this way, the parietal cortex is involved in actions in space (Goodale, 2014).
4. Visual information and auditory information about spatial location in head-based coordinates could be combined by pattern association learning, or by competitive learning with a mixture of visual and auditory inputs.
5. The coordinate transforms present in the parietal lobe could be performed by gain field modulation, made more efficient it is suggested by the memory trace synaptic modification rule described in Chapter 3.
6. These coordinate transforms are used to help control eye movements, and it is proposed to provide update of parahippocampal gyrus spatial view representations as described in Section 9.2.8.2.

10.2 Inferior parietal cortex somatosensory stream, PF regions

The somatosensory cortex in the superior anterior parts of the parietal cortex (regions 3b, 3a, 1, and 2) connect via frontal opercular (FOP) and opercular (OP) regions to the insula, which then has connectivity to anterior inferior parietal cortex regions such as PFop and PF, as described in Section 6.1.8 and illustrated in Fig. 6.7. The stream that involves anterior inferior parietal cortex regions PFcm, PFop, PFt, and PF is described in this section (Rolls et al., 2023d). The connectivity of the last stage of this somatosensory hierarchy, region PF, where information from other modalities is also received, is shown in Fig. 10.1. A key concept is that the top of this parietal somatosensory stream, PF, integrates somatosensory and proprioceptive information with visual object information from inferior temporal visual cortex region PHT. This is highly appropriate for tool use. As shown in Yokoyama, Autio, Ikeda,

Inferior parietal cortex somatosensory stream, PF regions | 461

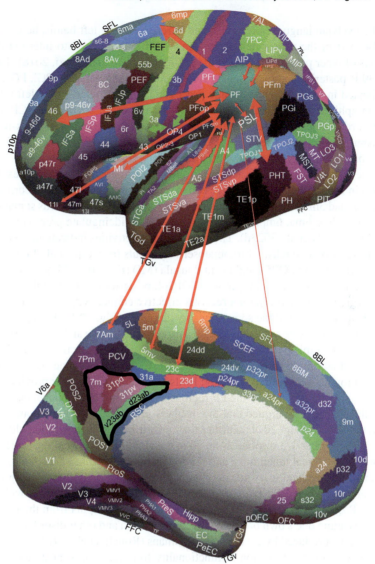

Fig. 10.1 Effective connectivity of region PF in the human brain. The widths of the red lines and the size of the arrowheads indicate the magnitude and direction of the effective connectivity with PF. The black outline encloses the postero-ventral memory-related regions of the posterior cingulate cortex. PF receives somatosensory inputs from many cortical regions including PFop which in turn receives from somatosensory 5 and fronto-opercular regions such as OP4 which in turn receive from somatosensory cortex such as 3a. (The green arrows help to illustrate the somatosensory hierarchy from for example 3a etc via OP4 to PFop to PF.) PF also receives some visual inputs from AIP, LIPd, IP2 and 7Pm. PF has outputs to premotor cortical areas (6) including the mid-cingulate cortex. The abbreviations are listed in Section 1.12. (From Rolls,E.T., Deco,G., Huang,C-C. and Feng,J. (2023) The human posterior parietal cortex: effective connectome, and its relation to functions. Cerebral Cortex 33: 3142-3170. doi: 10.1093/cercor/bhac266. Copyright © Oxford University Press.)

Sallet, Mars, Van Essen, Glasser, Sadato and Hayashi (2021), these PF regions in humans correspond approximately to area 7b in macaques.

Topologically (Caspers et al., 2008; Caspers and Zilles, 2018), PF areas are more anterior in the inferior parietal cortex, and the PG areas are more posterior (Fig. 10.1). In terms of alternative terminology in common use for the inferior parietal cortex, the supramarginal gyrus BA40 is mainly represented in the HCP-MMP (Glasser et al., 2016a) by PF, PFt, and the PeriSylvian language area PSL, and is related in the left hemisphere to phonology, and is also part of the mirror neuron system which may be used to interpret the gestures and actions of other people (Caspers et al., 2008; Rizzolatti and Rozzi, 2018). The angular gyrus BA 39 is posterior and may include HCP-MMP regions IP1, IP0, PGi, PGs, and PFm and is implicated in memory and semantic processing, with damage on the left related to dyslexia and agraphia and on the right to body image (Davis et al., 2018). The HCP-MMP, based as it is on cortical thickness and myelination, functional connectivity, and task-related activations (Glasser et al., 2016a) (Section 1.12), thus provides a more detailed parcellation than BA 40 the supramarginal gyrus, and BA 39 the angular gyrus.

The PF areas (which are anterior in the inferior parietal cortex, and excluding PFm), as shown in Fig. 10.1 receive effective connectivity from somatosensory cortical areas (including 2, 5L and 5mv), and have effective connectivities directed towards somatomotor premotor areas including 6ma, 6mp, 6a, 6d, 6r and 6v and midcingulate premotor regions 23c, 24dd and 24dv (Rolls et al., 2023d). The effective connectivities indicate that PF is at the top of a somatosensory hierarchy, with somatosensory inputs from especially PFop, frontal opercular 4 and 5 (FOP4 and FOP5), and the mid insula (MI) (Fig. 10.1). PFop receives input from PFt and somatosensory Frontal Opercular FOP2-4, posterior Opercular OP4, 5l and 5mv and the insula (green in Fig. 10.1). OP4 receives effective connectivity from somatosensory 1, 2, 3a and 3b at the bottom of the somatosensory hierarchy (Fig. 10.1). Thus part of the function of these PF areas may be related to somatosensory / body image and the sense of body ownership and of self that this bestows (Ronchi et al., 2018). The connectivity with the somatosensory insula and adjoining frontal operculum (FOP regions) (in which somatosensory responses are also found (Verhagen et al., 2004; Rolls et al., 2015b)), further provides a foundation for understanding a function of the PF regions as involving body image, and indeed consistent with this, it has been argued that the insula is involved in the human awareness of feelings from the body (Craig, 2011). Further than this, it has been shown that although somatosensory cortical areas 1-3 respond as much to the sight of touch as to the touch itself, the insula responds to the real touch only, and not to the sight of touch, which led to the proposal that the insula is involved in awareness that it is one's own body that is being touched, and not someone else's body (Rolls, 2010a; McCabe et al., 2008). This then fits with the concept that the PF Posterior Parietal Cortex regions (which receive inputs from the insula) are involved in representing one's own body, and that anosognosia and other disorders of awareness of the body can be produced by PF damage in humans (Ronchi et al., 2018).

There is a clear transition of functionality from anterior to posterior within the PF regions. PFcm and PFop have mainly somatosensory inputs, and premotor outputs. PFcm has inputs from OP1-4, and is further implicated in responsiveness to vestibular inputs (Huber et al., 2022). Indeed, OP1-4 correspond approximately to the parieto-insular vestibular cortex (Huber et al., 2022; Grusser et al., 1990), and may make a contribution to heading direction useful for navigation (Chen et al., 2016a). PFt (which is more dorsal, and closer to parietal visual areas) also receives effective connectivity from superior parietal (7Al, 7Am, 7PC and 7PL) and intraparietal (AIP, LIPv, MIP and VIP) regions, and so is implicated in visuo-motor as well as somatosensory functions. Indeed, the combination of visual and somatosensory inputs is likely to be important for reaching with the correct shape of the hand to grasp an object, and when the object is felt that provides further information relevant to the action being performed. These regions (PFcm, and PFop) also receive inputs from the supracallosal anterior cingulate cortex, which is a region with somatosensory inputs that responds to many aversive stimuli (Rolls et al., 2023c; Grabenhorst and Rolls, 2011).

More posteriorly, and in a sense higher up the inferior parietal somatosensory hierarchy, PF (Fig. 10.1) (which receives from PFop) also has somatosensory and premotor and visuospatial inputs relating to 7Am and intraparietal AIP, but adds to these, beyond what is found for earlier stages, strong effective connectivity from the posterior inferior temporal visual cortex (PHT, which is likely to introduce visual information about the shape of objects useful for performing actions on objects), from the reward-related medial orbitofrontal cortex 11l (which will provide reward-related information useful in building a semantic representation of felt objects and in influencing whether actions should be performed to obtain them), and, consistent with this concept, PF has effective connectivity directed towards language-related regions - the PeriSylvian language area (PSL), TPOJ2, STSvp (Rolls et al., 2022b), and to prefrontal cortex areas involved in short-term memory related functions IFsa and 46 (Rolls et al., 2023d). The diffusion tractography (Rolls et al., 2023d) further emphasizes connections with language-related areas 44, 45 and PSL. PF also adds extensive connectivity to dorsolateral prefrontal 46 regions, implicated in short-term memory (Goldman-Rakic, 1996; Passingham, 2021; Miller et al., 2018) (Chapter 13), and appropriate for maintaining a memory of a tactile object active during delays.

PF may on this connectivity evidence (Fig. 10.1) be the top of a somatosensory hierarchy which adds visual and reward inputs to form semantic representations of felt objects, which can then gain access to language systems, as well as having outputs to superior parietal and intraparietal areas involved in performing actions such as reaching and grasping for felt or seen objects. PF may thus build a multimodal, semantic, representation of felt objects. The PeriSylvian Language region (PSL) is very interesting, because it receives somatosensory inputs from PF, and has connections to STS semantic areas, so PSL may be a route for tactile inputs to become part of object representations (Rolls et al., 2022b). All of the somatosensory-related inferior parietal areas are conspicuous in not having effective connectivity with the posterior cingulate cortex and in having little connectivity with the hippocampal memory system.

Consistent with this connectivity, damage to the human inferior parietal cortex can result in tactile agnosia (also termed stereognosis), which is the inability to recognize objects through palpation in the absence of elementary sensory deficits (Klingner and Witte, 2018). Recognition through the visual modality is preserved, and this aspect of semantics is suggested to rely on object/semantic representations in the temporal lobe (Rolls et al., 2022b). The inferior parietal deficit can be interpreted as a failure of the associative-semantic system to match the tactile features identifying an object with its meaning (Berti et al., 2015; Berti and Neppi-Modona, 2012).

The input to PF regions (mainly to PF itself) from anterior cingulate regions including a24pr, d32, p24pr; and orbitofrontal OFC, 11l which are involved in punishment and reward (Grabenhorst and Rolls, 2011; Rolls et al., 2023c; Rolls, 2019c,e,f) deserves further consideration. It is found that the pleasantness and painfulness of touch is related to activations of the orbitofrontal cortex, whereas activations of somatosensory cortex are related to physical aspects of the stimuli such as their intensity (Rolls, O'Doherty, Kringelbach, Francis, Bowtell and McGlone, 2003d). Further evidence that the reward value of touch and related visual stimuli are not represented in parietal cortex is that 'visual fixation neurons' (Mountcastle, Lynch, Georgopoulos, Sakata and Acuna, 1975) do not reflect the reward value of visual stimuli measured by a devaluation experiment in which macaques were fed to satiety, and the neurons did not reverse the visual stimulus to which they responded when the reward value of the two stimuli was reversed in a visual discrimination task (Rolls, Perrett, Thorpe, Puerto, Roper-Hall and Maddison, 1979a). (This was tested following a visit to Vernon Mountcastle's lab in which he confirmed his view that reward value was represented by the parietal "command" neurons (Mountcastle et al., 1975).) Evidence that parietal neurons are related to decision-making (Platt and Glimcher, 1999) does not contradict the hypothesis presented above, for the decision-making need not be about reward value but could be about the physical properties of the stimuli. Evidence about the fact that a stimulus is harmful could of course be

464 | The parietal cortex, spatial functions, and navigation

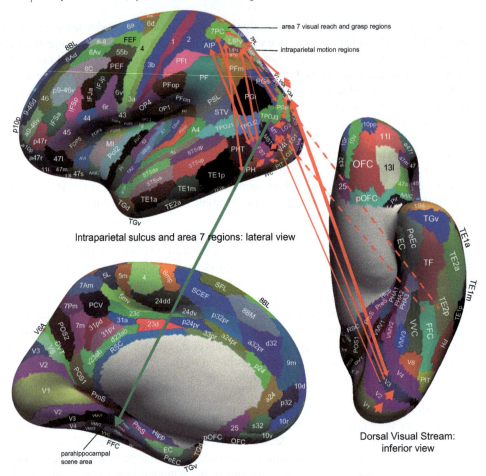

Fig. 10.2 Effective connectivity of the human Dorsal Visual Cortical Stream which reaches (partly via V3, V3A and LO3) the MT+ complex regions (FST, LO1, LO2, LO3, MST, MT, PH, V3CD and V4t), and then the intraparietal regions (AIP, LIPd, LIPv, MIP, VIP IP0, IP1 and IP2) and then the area 7 regions: schematic overview. Connectivity to the inferior parietal cortex region PGp, which in turn has effective connectivity to the parahippocampal scene area in PHA1-3 (Rolls et al., 2023d) is shown. Inputs to this stream from ventral stream regions such as FFC and TE2p are shown with dashed lines. (From Rolls,E.T., Deco,G., Huang,C-C. and Feng,J. (2023) Multiple cortical visual streams in humans. Cerebral Cortex 33: 3319-3349. doi: 10.1093/cercor/bhac276. Copyright © Oxford University Press.)

useful in the parietal cortex to facilitate withdrawal, and about reward and punishment could be useful to provide evidence that an action has been successfully completed (or not), which could occur in the absence of a primary representation of the reward and painful affective value of touch, which appears to be in the human orbitofrontal and anterior cingulate cortex (Rolls, O'Doherty, Kringelbach, Francis, Bowtell and McGlone, 2003d; McCabe, Rolls, Bilderbeck and McGlone, 2008).

10.3 Intraparietal sulcus posterior parietal cortex, regions AIP, LIPd, LIPv, MIP, VIP, IP0, IP1, and IP2

Fig. 10.2 shows the effective connectivity of some of the human parietal cortex regions in the cortex in the intraparietal sulcus, and in area 7 (Rolls et al., 2023d,e). This figure shows the same effective connectivity as in Fig. 3.12, but here it is emphasised that this is relevant to understanding the connectivity and functions of these posterior parietal cortex visual motion and visuo-motor regions.

As shown in Fig. 10.2, these regions in the intraparietal sulcus that respond to visual motion have strong effective connectivity from dorsal visual stream cortical regions (Chapter 3) including from several MT+ complex visual regions in which neurons respond to global optic flow (Kolster et al., 2010; Galletti and Fattori, 2018) (MST, FST, PH and V3CD), intraparietal sulcus area 1 (IPS1), V3B, V6A (which is a visuo-motor region involved in grasping seen objects (Gamberini et al., 2020)), V7, and superior parietal area 7 regions involved in visuo-motor actions. These intraparietal regions also receive in humans from ventral stream visual cortical regions including the fusiform face cortex (FFC), and inferior temporal cortex regions PIT, PHT, TE1p and TE2p (Fig. 10.2). These ventral stream regions are likely to bring shape / visual form information (Rolls, 2021d; Rolls et al., 2023e; Rolls, 2021b) to the intraparietal cortex regions important in shaping the hand to grasp and manipulate objects and tools. These intraparietal sulcus regions also have connectivity with the inferior frontal gyrus and with the dorsolateral prefrontal cortex (especially 46, 8C, a9-46, i6-8 and p9-46v), which are likely to be important when there is a delay between the visual input and when the action can be performed (Funahashi, Bruce and Goldman-Rakic, 1989). These connectivities are stronger to these prefrontal areas (Rolls et al., 2023d), as is appropriate for the operation of short-term memory systems so that the memory does not dominate sensory inputs (Rolls, 2016b, 2021b). There is also connectivity directed towards the parahippocampal TH cortex (PHA3) which may be useful in providing information about visuo-motor actions to the hippocampal memory system (Rolls et al., 2022a; Rolls, 2018b). There is also connectivity with the frontal pole p10p, which is likely to be important when sequencing and planning is involved in actions (Shallice and Cipolotti, 2018; Shallice and Burgess, 1996; Gilbert and Burgess, 2008). The connectivity from the intraparietal areas is strongly towards premotor cortical areas including especially 6a, and to the frontal eye field FEF and prefrontal eye field PEF (from especially AIP, LIPd, LIPv and VIP) (Rolls et al., 2023d) (Fig. 10.2), which provides action-related outputs from these visuo-motor intraparietal regions. There is also connectivity especially for IP1 and IP2 from the orbitofrontal cortex (medial regions, 11l and OFC) which may provide reward/no-reward feedback (Rolls, 2019e,f) of potential utility in learning whether actions made are correct, and with the frontal pole. There is also some connectivity with inferior parietal regions including PGp and PGs. Interestingly, this intraparietal part of the parietal cortex has relatively little effective connectivity with the posterior or anterior (or mid) cingulate cortex (Rolls et al., 2023d), though in the right hemisphere IP1 has effective connectivity with 31a, d23ab and POS2.

The functional connectivity is largely consistent (Rolls et al., 2023d), but indicates more interactions with early visual cortical areas; with somatosensory/premotor areas; with the hippocampal system; with TE1p and TE2p, with posterior cingulate including DVT; and with supracallosal anterior cingulate 33pr and p24pr (Rolls et al., 2023c). The diffusion tractography is also consistent, but suggests in addition connections with auditory cortex that may be useful in orienting gaze towards sounds (Rolls et al., 2023d,h).

Neurons in macaques in area VIP represent the direction and speed of visual motion (Colby, Duhamel and Goldberg, 1993), and may be useful in for example tracking moving visual stimuli, and encoding optic flow which can be useful in assessing self-motion and thereby in navigation. These neurons do not respond in relation to saccades. Neurons in macaques in LIP are active in visual, attentional and saccadic processing (Gnadt and Andersen, 1988; Colby et al., 1996; Munuera and Duhamel, 2020). The ventral part of LIP (LIPv) has strong connections with two oculomotor centres, the frontal eye field and the deep layers of the superior colliculus, and may be especially involved in the generation of saccades (Chen et al., 2016b). The dorsal part (LIPd) may be more involved in visual processing, responding for example to visual targets for saccades (Chen et al., 2016b). Neurons in MIP (which may be the parietal reach region, PRR) are related to arm movement preparation and execution (Passarelli et al., 2021). They are implicated in the sensory-to-motor transformation required for reaching toward visually defined targets (Gamberini et al., 2020; Andersen, 1995b; Huang and Sereno, 2018; Urgen and Orban, 2021; Orban et al., 2021b).

The intraparietal cortical regions in humans thus are likely in terms of their connectivity (Rolls et al., 2023d,e) to perform visuomotor functions (without somatosensory processing unlike area 7 regions), and the extensive research on these regions in macaques provides a guide to their functions in humans, including the control of eye movements to acquire and track visual stimuli given the outputs to the Frontal Eye Fields (FEF) and Premotor Eye Fields (PEF). There are also outputs to regions 6a and 6r that might produce head and body movements to help stabilize images for the visual system. The output to the posterior inferior temporal visual cortex PHT is of interest, and might be involved in the stabilization of images for processing in later parts of the ventral visual system.

10.4 Posterior superior parietal cortex, regions 7AL, 7Am, 7PC, 7PL, and 7Pm

The connectivity of some of the area 7 regions, involved in visuo-motor functions, are shown in Fig. 10.2, and are considered here. Region 7Pm is in the medial parietal cortex and is part of the precuneus (together with the Precuneus Visual region PCV), and as it is included in the Posterior Cingulate Division of the HCP-MMP atlas (Section 1.12), it is considered in Chapter 12.

The more posterior parts of this group (7PC, 7PL) receive inputs strongly from VIP, and from LIP and MIP (Rolls et al., 2023d). 7PC and 7PL also have some inputs from early visual cortical areas including intraparietal sulcus area 1 (IPS1), V6A, MT, MST and LO3 and FST; somatosensory/premotor areas (regions 1, 2, 5 and 6); some inputs from inferior parietal PF and PG; some inputs from the posterior cingulate cortex (including DVT, the Dorsal Visual Transitional region) (Rolls et al., 2023i); from the supracallosal anterior cingulate cortex (p24pr) which has much somatosensory/motor connectivity and is involved in aversive events (Rolls et al., 2023c; Grabenhorst and Rolls, 2011); and the dorsolateral prefrontal cortex (46 and 9-46d). Interestingly, there are also inputs from ventral visual stream regions including the posterior inferior temporal cortex PHT. Thus some information about the shape of objects reaches these regions, and that may be important for the control of grasping. In turn, there is effective connectivity from the posterior regions of the superior parietal cortex to premotor cortical and somatosensory cortical areas (6, 5) and the midcingulate cortex, which in most cases is stronger from the posterior parietal cortex than to it (see Fig. 10.2) (Rolls et al., 2023d).

These area 7 regions therefore have connectivity that seems appropriate for making visually guided arm reach and grasp responses that are shaped properly because of shape inputs from the ventral visual system to seen objects. The more anterior parts of area 7 (7AL and 7Am) have more connectivity with somatosensory cortical areas (which are immediately anterior to them), and less with early visual cortical areas (Fig. 2), so may be involved more in proprioceptive and somatosensory integration than visuo-motor functions. 7Pm (which is medial) has connectivity with the nearby posterior cingulate regions DVT, POS1 and RSC, which are implicated in spatial including scene processing (Rolls et al., 2023i). This may be an interesting and telling difference in the connectivity of lateral vs medial posterior parietal area 7 regions, with the lateral regions more involved in somatomotor functions, and the medial area 7 regions more involved in visuo-spatial functions, which would be in line with minimising connection length as a principle that influences the topology of the cerebral cortex (Rolls, 2016b). These area 7 regions also have effective connectivity directed to the hippocampal system, especially to parahippocampal gyrus TH (PHA2-3), and to the temporo-parietal-occipital junction area (TPOJ2-3) (Rolls et al., 2023d).

The functional connectivity and diffusion tractography also provide evidence for some connectivity with auditory cortical areas, and this may be related to auditory cues being signals for orientation in space. They also provide further evidence (Rolls et al., 2023d) for connectivity with the posterior cingulate cortex especially the antero-dorsal part involved in visuo-spatial functions (Rolls et al., 2023i) (Chapter 12).

The area 7 parietal regions thus combine visuomotor with somatosensory functions, and the extensive research on these regions in macaques (Snyder et al., 1998; Orban et al., 2021b; Passarelli et al., 2021; Gamberini et al., 2020) provides a guide to their functions in humans, including reaching for, grasping, and manipulating objects in space and tool use. These area 7 regions are also implicated in coordinate transforms from egocentric eye-based frames to allocentric world-based frames suitable for idiothetic update of hippocampal spatial representations (Snyder et al., 1998; Rolls, 2020b, 2021f; Dean and Platt, 2006; Vedder et al., 2017; Andersen, 1995b) (see further Section 3.4). Consistent with this, vestibular as well as optic flow signals influence neurons in macaque 7a (Avila, Lakshminarasimhan, DeAngelis and Angelaki, 2019). How these coordinate transforms are performed is considered in Section 3.5.

10.5 Inferior parietal cortex, visual regions PFm, PGi, PGs and PGp

These regions are implicated in humans in a number of functions, including visual object and face motion analysis for social functions, theory of mind, and memory, and their connectivity and functions (Rolls et al., 2023d) are described in this section. The effective connectivities of two key regions, PGi and PGp, are illustrated in Figs. 10.3 and 10.4.

The PG areas and PFm, located posteriorly (Figs. 10.3 and 10.4), and compared to PF areas, have more effective connectivity with visual cortical areas and have less connectivity than the PF regions with somatosensory and premotor cortical areas. This fits with the location in the brain of the PG areas, and the importance of minimizing connection length in the brain, so that brain regions with many interconnections are found close together in the brain, where possible (Rolls, 2016b). However, the connectivity of PGi, PGs, PFm, and PGp are all quite different, suggesting different functions for each of these regions, so they are considered separately.

In this context, a key concept is that visual motion information in the intraparietal and area 7 regions can connect in part via IP1 and IP2 to regions such as PFm and PGs (green arrows in Fig. 10.3) which in turn have connectivity to PGi and thus to the visual motion regions in the cortex in the superior temporal sulcus (STS) (Rolls et al., 2023d). Support for this concept comes also from the functional connectivity and from the connections shown with diffusion tractography (Rolls et al., 2023d). The IP1 and IP2 regions may be new in humans, and in providing this connectivity may be connecting the well-developed intraparietal and area 7 systems also present in other primates to the PGs, PFm and then PGi regions of the inferior parietal cortex that are so highly developed in humans.

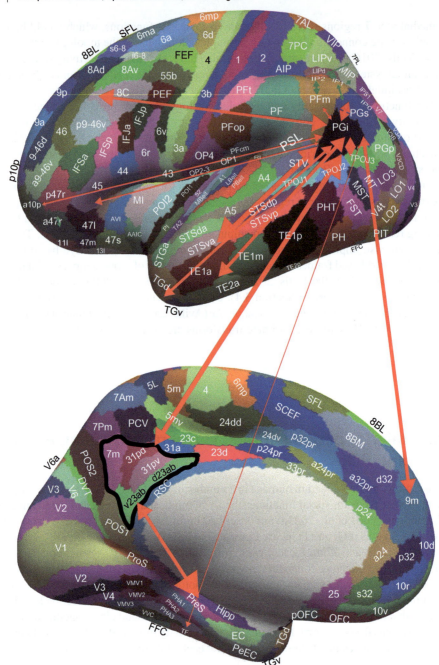

Fig. 10.3 Effective connectivity of region PGi (red arrows). The widths of the lines and the size of the arrowheads indicate the magnitude and direction of the effective connectivity. 7Pm and IP1 connect to PGs which in turn connects to PGi, providing a route for PGi to receive visual motion information, and to connect that to areas such as STSda, STSva, STSdp and STSvp. The green arrows show some of the ways in which visual motion information in the intraparietal and area 7 regions can connect in part by IP1 and IP2 to regions such as PFm and PGs which in turn have connectivity to PGi and thus to the STS visual motion regions. The black outline encloses the postero-ventral memory-related regions of the posterior cingulate cortex, which connect to the hippocampal system (Rolls et al., 2023i). (Modified from Rolls,E.T., Deco,G., Huang,C-C. and Feng,J. (2023) The human posterior parietal cortex: effective connectome, and its relation to functions. Cerebral Cortex 33: 3142-3170. doi: 10.1093/cercor/bhac266. Copyright © Oxford University Press.)

10.5.1 Region PGi

This most inferior part of the inferior parietal lobule is closest to ventral stream areas, and has connectivity (Rolls et al., 2023d) very interestingly with object / 'what' brain regions including for vision the anterior inferior temporal TE1a, TE1m, TE1p, and TE2a regions; from all the superior temporal sulcus (STS) auditory - visual association / semantic areas (Section 8.4); and from the anterior temporal lobe TG semantic regions (Price et al., 2015; Bonner and Price, 2013) (Fig. 10.3). It also has connectivity with the temporo-parieto-occipital junction region TPOJ3 implicated in semantic processing, theory of mind, and social behavior (DiNicola et al., 2020; Buckner and DiNicola, 2019; Schurz et al., 2017; Quesque and Brass, 2019). TPOJ regions and PGi are activated by faces (including face expression and other socially relevant visual representations (Patel et al., 2019)) vs other visual stimuli, as are the TE1a and superior temporal sulcus (STS) regions that have effective connectivity with PGi (Yokoyama, Autio, Ikeda, Sallet, Mars, Van Essen, Glasser, Sadato and Hayashi, 2021). It is important to recognise that regions in the STS include not only auditory responsiveness dorsally, but in much of the STS visual responsiveness, so STS regions should not be considered as only 'auditory association cortex'. Indeed, it was discovered that single neurons in the macaque STS respond to face expression and also to face and head movement to encode the social relevance of stimuli (Hasselmo, Rolls, Baylis and Nalwa, 1989b; Hasselmo, Rolls and Baylis, 1989a; Robin, Hirshhorn, Rosenbaum, Winocur, Moscovitch and Grady, 2015). For example, a neuron might respond to closing of the eyes, or to turning of the head away from facing the viewer, both of which break social contact (Hasselmo et al., 1989b,a). Some neurons respond to the direction of gaze (Perrett et al., 1987). It was assumed that some of the movement-related information required to account for the neuronal responses in the cortex in the STS came from the dorsal visual stream and could be combined in the STS with ventral stream information about the identity of the faces. It was found that many of the neurons in the STS respond only or much better to moving faces or objects (Hasselmo, Rolls and Baylis, 1989a), whereas in the anterior inferior temporal cortex neurons were discovered that responded well to static visual stimuli, and were tuned for face identity (Perrett, Rolls and Caan, 1982; Rolls, 1984, 2000a; Rolls and Treves, 2011; Rolls, Treves, Tovee and Panzeri, 1997d; Rolls, Treves and Tovee, 1997b; Hasselmo, Rolls and Baylis, 1989a).

It is now proposed that PGi, with its inputs from PGs which has connectivity with superior parietal and intraparietal regions that encode visual motion, is part of this processing stream for socially relevant face-related information. Consistent with this, PGi, and some temporo-parieto-occipital regions, are activated by faces (Yokoyama et al., 2021). Also consistent with this proposal, the effective connectivity is strong from PGi to STS regions, though there is some effective connectivity also from PGs and PFm to STS regions (Fig. 10.3). In humans, representations of this type could provide part of the basis for the development of systems to interpret the social and emotional significance of such stimuli, including theory of mind. Consistent with this, PGi and PGs receive inputs from PCV (the precuneus visual area) and 7m which are regions of medial parietal cortex related to the precuneus (Rolls et al., 2023i), which is implicated in visual and self-referential processing (Cavanna and Trimble, 2006; Freton, Lemogne, Bergouignan, Delaveau, Lehericy and Fossati, 2014). Connectivity with the pregenual reward-related anterior cingulate cortex introduces reward value into this region, potentially useful in forming semantic including social representations of objects and faces. Very interestingly, there is also connectivity with the postero-ventral parts of the posterior cingulate cortex (31pd, 31pv, 7m, d23ab, v23ab) that are implicated in episodic memory (Rolls et al., 2023i), and with the hippocampal system (parahippocampal TF) and PGi is thus likely to be involved in the memory-related functions of the inferior parietal cortex (Davis et al., 2018). Consistent with this, the functional connectivity reveals some interactions with the hippocampal system (hippocampus, entorhinal cortex, parahippocampal TF and TH (PHA1-3)) (Rolls et al., 2023d). The tractography provides some evidence for connections with the Peri-Sylvian Language area (PSL), and with Broca's area region 44 (Rolls et al., 2023d). PGi also has very extensive connectivity with dorsolateral prefrontal cortex regions (8BL, 8Ad, 8Av, 9a, 9b, s6-8) implicated in short-term memory (Fig. 10.3).

10.5.2 Region PGs

PGs is posterior to PGi (and therefore closer to visual cortical areas), and is superior to PGp (Fig. 10.3). In contrast to PGi, PGs has connectivity with visuo-motor areas that are intraparietal (IP1) and in area 7 (e.g. 7Pm), but it does also (as PGi) have connectivity with object areas such as the visual inferior temporal cortex (TE1a, TE1m, TE1p) (Fig. 10.3). PGs also has connectivity with the Frontal pole (10d, p10p), regions implicated in planning and sequencing (Shallice and Cipolotti, 2018; Shallice and Burgess, 1996; Gilbert and Burgess, 2008) and prospective as well as retrospective memory especially about the self (Underwood et al., 2015). It also has connectivity with the postero-ventral (7m, 31pd, 31pv, d23ab, d23ab) part of the posterior cingulate cortex, which has effective connectivity to the hippocampal episodic memory system (Rolls et al., 2023i), and connectivity directly to the hippocampal memory system (hippocampus, entorhinal cortex, presubiculum, and parahippocampal PHA2), to PF and PGi, and with the dorsolateral prefrontal cortex. The functional connectivity provides an indication in addition of some interactions with STS regions, and the tractography is consistent with this and with some connections with TPOJ regions (Rolls et al., 2023d). The effective connectivity from PGs to PGi may provide PGi with visual motion information, where it can be combined with object and face information. PGi in turn has connectivity to STS regions (Fig. 10.3), and may provide a route for dorsal visual stream information to reach the STS areas where neurons often respond primarily to moving faces, heads, or objects (Hasselmo, Rolls, Baylis and Nalwa, 1989b; Hasselmo, Rolls and Baylis, 1989a). Consistent with this, PGi does have strong effective connectivity to STSda, STSdp, STSva and STSvp (Rolls et al., 2023d).

10.5.3 Region PFm

PFm is not a somatosensory area (unlike other PF areas). PFm receives from high order visual (TE1m, TE1p, TE2a) and visual / auditory (STSvp) areas that represent objects and faces and (for the STS) their motion and face expression (Hasselmo, Rolls and Baylis, 1989a). It has some intraparietal visuo-motor inputs (IP1 and IP2), and has connectivity with the visuo-motor (dorsal / anterior) parts of the posterior cingulate cortex (23d, 31a) and not the memory related parts; it also receives from the frontal pole (a10p, p10p and 10pp); and it has effective connectivity with the reward related regions (orbitofrontal cortex region OFC and pregenual anterior cingulate d32) and punishment-related orbitofrontal cortex a47r (Grabenhorst and Rolls, 2011; Rolls et al., 2023c). PFm thus appears to be a part of the parietal cortex that communicates with the visuo-spatial part of the posterior cingulate cortex (Rolls et al., 2023i), and could thereby reach the hippocampus for visuo-spatial functions. In particular, the retrosplenial complex in the posterior cingulate cortex visuo-spatial part is especially important with respect to the location of landmarks (Persichetti and Dilks, 2019) (Chapter 12); and posterior cingulate area 31 is implicated by neuroimaging in representing heading direction (Baumann and Mattingley, 2021). A small region in the parieto-occipital sulcus (POS) that has been considered in connection with the posterior cingulate cortex (Rolls et al., 2023i) has also been described as in the medial parietal cortex directly anterior to the visually scene-selective medial place area (Silson et al., 2016), and has strong functional connectivity with anterior portions of the scene-selective parahippocampal place area (Epstein, 2008) (aPPA), located in the medial temporal cortex. This connectivity-defined region overlaps with regions of the medial parietal cortex engaged during memory recall, and there may be distinct regions for people and places (Silson et al., 2019). PFm has extensive connectivity with the dorsolateral and inferolateral prefrontal cortex regions, and is likely to be involved in short-term memory, which plays a key role in top-down attention by providing the continuing top-down bias for biased competition in the cortical regions linked to these prefrontal cortical areas enabling attentional interactions between the spatial and object streams (Rolls, 2016b, 2021b; Deco and Rolls, 2005b,a).

PFm thus appears to combine visual motion with temporal lobe object / face information, and has connectivity with posterior cingulate areas involved in scene (/place) processing. It also has connectivity with language-related areas (Broca's area 44).

10.5.4 Region PGp

PGp is a far posterior part of PG (Fig. 10.4), and it has effective connectivity (Rolls et al., 2023d) with some early visual cortical areas related to scene processing (e.g. VMV2 and LO3) (Sulpizio et al., 2020; Rolls et al., 2022a; Kamps et al., 2016); and with intraparietal (e.g. MIP, VIP, IP0) and superior parietal 7 (e.g. 7Pm, 7PL) visuo-motor regions, both of which distinguish PGp from PGi and PGs and PFm (Fig. 10.4). However, PGp also has connectivity to parahippocampal TH areas PHA1-3 and with posterior cingulate DVT and ProS, all of which with VMV areas are implicated in visual scene processing (Rolls et al., 2023i, 2022a; Sulpizio et al., 2020) (Fig. 9.18). Functional connectivity between PGp in the human angular gyrus and the parahippocampal scene area, hippocampus, and retrosplenial complex (Boccia et al., 2017) is consistent with and supports what is described here and elsewhere (Rolls et al., 2023i). PGp also has connectivity with TPOJ3 and TE2p, and has no connectivity with the orbitofrontal cortex, or with prefrontal areas involved in short-term memory. The functional connectivity provides evidence for, in addition, interactions with early visual cortical regions including other VMV regions, and with more intraparietal and area 7 regions, and the diffusion tractography provides additional indications of this (Rolls et al., 2023d).

The connectivity of PGp, because it has connectivities with scene and egomotion regions, and with the parahippocampal cortex in which spatial view cells are found (Rolls and Wirth, 2018; Georges-François et al., 1999; Rolls et al., 1998b; Robertson et al., 1998; Rolls et al., 1997a; Tsitsiklis et al., 2020; Wirth et al., 2017; Rolls, 2023c), implicates PGp in navigation (Rolls, 2020b, 2021f, 2023c). PGp may be involved together with its connected intraparietal regions in the coordinate transforms necessary to map from retinal inputs to scenes which require representations of these types (Rolls, 2020b, 2021f) (see further Sections 3.4 and 3.5).

It is thus proposed that PGp provides a route for visuo-spatial parietal cortex regions involved in spatial coordinate transforms (Snyder et al., 1998; Rolls, 2020b) (see further Sections 3.4 and 3.5) to provide the hippocampal system with information useful in the idiothetic (self-motion) update of hippocampal spatial view representations of allocentric space (Robertson et al., 1998; Rolls, 2021f; Rolls and Wirth, 2018; Wirth et al., 2017; Rolls, 2023c, 2022b). Consistent with this, PGp also receives from visual scene-related areas (Sulpizio et al., 2020) DVT and ventromedial visual cortex (VMV2) (Fig. 10.4).

Supporting evidence is that the caudal inferior parietal lobule (cIPL, which includes PGp) has functional connectivity with the anterior part of the parahippocampal place (or scene) area (Baldassano et al., 2016), and although not strongly responsive to standard scene localizers showing sequences of unfamiliar and unrelated scene images (Baldassano et al., 2016; Sulpizio et al., 2020), cIPL is activated by familiar places. For example, cIPL is involved in

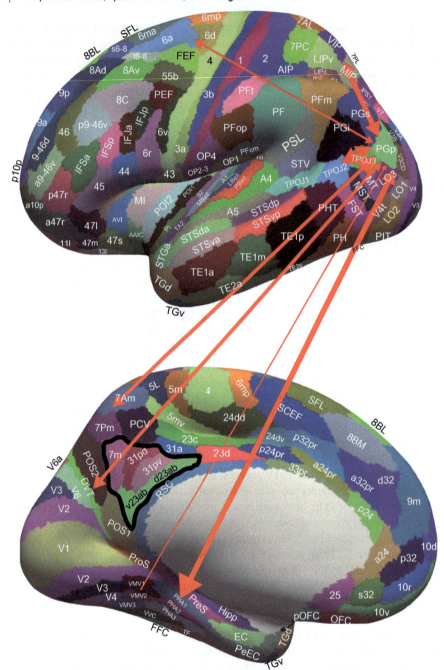

Fig. 10.4 Effective connectivity of region PGp. The widths of the lines and the size of the arrowheads indicate the magnitude and direction of the effective connectivity. PGp has effective connectivity from area 7 and intraparietal regions, and has effective connectivity directed to parahippocampal TH (PHA1-3). It is proposed that this provides a route for visuo-spatial parietal cortex regions involved in spatial coordinate transforms to provide the hippocampal system with information useful in the idiothetic (self-motion) update of hippocampal spatial representations of allocentric space. Consistent with this, PGp also receives from visual scene-related areas DVT (part of the retrosplenial scene area (Sulpizio et al., 2020)) and ventromedial visual cortex (VMV2). (From Rolls,E.T., Deco,G., Huang,C-C. and Feng,J. (2023) The human posterior parietal cortex: effective connectome, and its relation to functions. Cerebral Cortex 33: 3142-3170. doi: 10.1093/cercor/bhac266. Copyright © Oxford University Press.)

memory for visual scenes (Montaldi et al., 2006; Takashima et al., 2006; Elman et al., 2013; van Assche et al., 2016), object-place associations in a virtual reality environment (Burgess et al., 2001), and imagining past events or future events in familiar places (Hassabis et al., 2007; Szpunar et al., 2009).

10.6 Navigation: What computations are performed in the parietal and related cortex

The hippocampus plays an important role in episodic memory, as described in Chapter 9. Key components of the episodic memories implemented by the hippocampus include spatial locations, and/or time. Given that spatial processing is an important component of what computations are performed by the hippocampus, it has been implicated in the important spatial function of navigation, especially by research in rodents (O'Keefe, 1991; Burgess and O'Keefe, 1996; Buzsaki and Moser, 2013; Aronov and Tank, 2014) (see Chapter 9).

The situation is not as clear in humans, in which some of the evidence indicates that the hippocampus is involved in navigation when recent memories are required for the navigation, but is less involved when navigation is being performed when the spatial information is well known, and does not need to be memorized (Maguire et al., 2016; Rolls and Wirth, 2018). An implication is that some of the key computations involved in navigation may take place in the neocortex, in areas that include and are connected to parietal cortex areas, and not in the hippocampus. The role of the hippocampus in navigation in humans may be to store new information, which of course may be needed if the navigation is in a novel environment. Evidence on this is considered next.

Lesions to the human neocortex can produce topographical agnosia and inability to navigate (Kolb and Whishaw, 2021; Barton, 2011), and the retrosplenial cortex is implicated in navigation (Vedder et al., 2017; Alexander and Nitz, 2015; Byrne et al., 2007; Epstein, 2008; Vann et al., 2009). In more detail, lesions restricted to the hippocampus in humans result only in slight navigation impairments in familiar environments, but rather strongly impair learning or imagining new trajectories (Bohbot and Corkin, 2007; Teng and Squire, 1999; Spiers and Maguire, 2006; Maguire et al., 2016; Clark and Maguire, 2016). In contrast, lesions in regions such as the parietal cortex or the retrosplenial cortex produce strong topographical disorientation in both familiar and new environments (Aguirre and D'Esposito, 1999; Habib and Sirigu, 1987; Takahashi, Kawamura, Shiota, Kasahata and Hirayama, 1997; Maguire, 2001; Kim, Aminoff, Kastner and Behrmann, 2015b). This suggests that some of the core navigation processes (which may include transformations from allocentric representations to egocentric motor commands) are performed independently by neocortical areas outside the hippocampus, which may utilize hippocampal information related to recent memories (Ekstrom et al., 2014; Miller et al., 2013).

It was suggested in Chapter 3 that the dorsal visual system with its coordinate transforms to what may be allocentric bearing and spatial view coordinates provides a useful input to the hippocampal system via the parahippocampal gyrus (see Fig. 9.1) for idiothetic (self-motion) update of hippocampal spatial representations related to where one is currently looking in allocentric space, in for example the dark. Given the role of the entorhinal cortex grid cell system in idiothetic update of place, at least in rodents (see Chapter 9), it may be that the hippocampus receives its idiothetic update for place from the entorhinal cortex system. However, in primates including humans the idiothetic updates required to perform the coordinate transforms from retinal to head-centred coordinates, from head-centred to allocentric bearings to landmarks, and to allocentric representations of spatial view, are performed in the dorsal visual system and its extensions into the parietal cortex, as described in Sections 3.4

and 3.5, in Chapter 3, and using in part pathways in the posterior cingulate cortex, retrosplenial regions, and medial parietal cortex (Chapter 12) (Fig. 9.1).

10.7 How the computations are performed in the parietal cortex

Key computations performed in the parietal cortex include coordinate transforms. Some of these involve the coordinate transforms just described from retinal representations to allocentric spatial view representations (Section 3.4). Other coordinate transforms are needed for controlling arm movements to reach for and grasp objects in peripersonal space. The principles of how transforms of these types may be performed are described in Section 3.5.

Hierarchical organisation is another key computational process evident in the parietal lobe as well as elsewhere. One example of the somatosensory hierarchy to reach region PF, which appears to be at the top of the somatosensory 'what' hierarchy for representing what object is being touched, and to represent the body image.

Another example is the hierarchy from MT+ regions to intraparietal regions involved in visual motion analysis, and in the control of eye movements such as saccades and visual tracking. That hierarchy continues to the area 7 regions where somatosensory information is combined with visual information to perform the computations required to reach for and grasp objects and to manipulate them.

Another parietal hierarchy is that involving visual regions such as PFm, PGs and PGi, in which visual representation of motion are combined with ventral visual stream information about what object is present to produce representations that appear to involve combinations of object 'what' and motion information. Indeed, it is quite remarkable how these inferior parietal cortex regions, which develop so greatly in humans, are connected to inferior temporal cortex including TE regions involved in representing objects, and to regions in the cortex in the superior temporal sulcus (STS) that represent movements of objects, faces, and bodies that are likely to be produced in these parietal cortex visual regions.

Another aspect of the parietal hierarchy is that regions such as PGi provide information about moving objects, faces and bodies, and PF provides information from the somatosensory system about felt objects and about body image, to the semantic systems involved in language which include the whole suite of regions from PGi and probably PF through the temporo-parieto-occipital junction TPOJ regions to the superior temporal sulcus STS regions and the temporal pole, as described in Chapter 14.

Another principle of cortical computation evident in the parietal cortex as well as elsewhere is that after a hierarchy of mainly unimodal processing, information is then combined from different modalities to form multimodal representations.

One example is that in the parietal somatosensory 'what' hierarchy, it is especially in PF at the top of the hierarchy that 'what' visual information from the inferior temporal cortical regions is introduced to form multimodal representations.

Another example is that in the inferior parietal visual areas PFm, PGs and PGi, it is especially in PGi at the top of this hierarchy which receives visual motion information from intraparietal and area 7 regions that this information is combined with visual object 'what' information from the visual inferior temporal cortex.

Another example is that it is especially the information in these multimodal areas that has connectivity into the semantic systems for language that have just been referred to and are described in Chapters 8 and 14.

11 The orbitofrontal cortex, amygdala, reward value, emotion, and decision-making

11.1 Introduction and overview

11.1.1 Introduction

The orbitofrontal cortex receives from the ends of all sensory processing systems, and converts these representations of what the stimuli are into representations of their reward value (Fig. 11.1 and 4.2). The orbitofrontal cortex is therefore a key brain region in emotions, which can be defined as states elicited by rewards and punishers (Rolls, 2000e, 2014a, 2023b). Indeed, orbitofrontal cortex activations are linearly related to the subjectively reported pleasantness (or unpleasantness) of stimuli.

The orbitofrontal cortex then projects this reward value information to other structures, which implement behavioral output. One output region is the anterior cingulate cortex, which learns actions to obtain the reward outcomes signalled by the orbitofrontal cortex (see Chapter 12).

Another output region is the basal ganglia, which learn stimulus-response associations where a stimulus is linked directly to a response to produce a habit. This type of reinforcement learning may benefit from projections of reward and non-reward information from the orbitofrontal cortex to the dopamine neurons in the midbrain, which help with such stimulus-response habit learning by relaying a reward prediction error signal to the basal ganglia and some other brain regions.

The Orbitofrontal Cortex (Rolls, 2019e) provides a description of the functions of the orbitofrontal cortex, and as that is available, this Chapter focuses particularly on computational aspects, especially what is computed in the orbitofrontal cortex, and how it is computed.

11.1.2 Overview of what is computed in the orbitofrontal cortex

1. The orbitofrontal cortex is the first stage of processing to represent reward value. A representation of value is shown by rapid (one-trial) reversal of visual responses to stimuli when the reward value is reversed, and by a decrease to zero of the responses of orbitofrontal cortex neurons when the stimulus is devalued. The reward value is that of each particular stimulus, as shown by the discovery that sensory-specific satiety is computed in the orbitofrontal cortex. This systems-level organisation of reward value is not the case in rodents, which have a much less developed orbitofrontal cortex than in primates including humans, and in which value appears to be represented much earlier in processing hierarchies. Indeed, most of the evidence described in this Chapter, and in this book, is about the operation of brain systems in primates including humans, because the systems-level functional organisation of most brain systems is so different in rodents, as set out in Section 19.10.

476 | The orbitofrontal cortex, amygdala, reward value, emotion, and decision-making

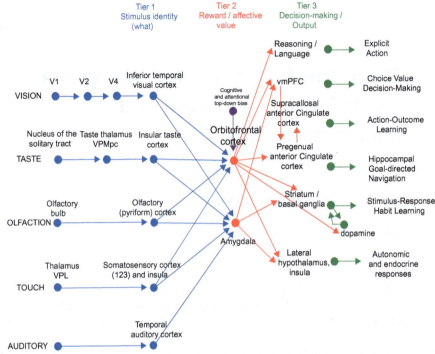

Fig. 11.1 The systems level organization of the brain for emotion in primates including humans. In Tier 1, representations are built of visual, taste, olfactory and tactile stimuli that are independent of reward value and therefore of emotion. In Tier 2, reward value and emotion are represented. A pathway for top-down attentional and cognitive modulation of emotion is shown in purple. In Tier 3 actions are learned in the supracallosal (or dorsal) anterior cingulate cortex to obtain the reward values signaled by the orbitofrontal cortex and amygdala that are relayed in part via the pregenual anterior cingulate cortex and vmPFC. Decisions between stimuli of different reward value can be taken in the ventromedial prefrontal cortex, vmPFC. In Tier 3, orbitofrontal cortex inputs to the reasoning / language systems enable affective value to be incorporated and reported. In Tier 3, stimulus-response habits can also be produced using reinforcement learning. In Tier 3 autonomic responses can also be produced to emotion-provoking stimuli. Auditory inputs also reach the amygdala. V1: primary visual (striate) cortex; V2 and V4: further cortical visual areas. PFC: prefrontal cortex. The Medial PFC area 10 is part of the ventromedial prefrontal cortex (vmPFC). VPL: ventro-postero-lateral nucleus of the thalamus, which conveys somatosensory information to the primary somatosensory cortex (areas 1, 2 and 3). VPMpc: ventro-postero-medial nucleus pars parvocellularis of the thalamus, which conveys taste information to the primary taste cortex.

2. The orbitofrontal cortex represents the expected value, outcome value, and negative reward prediction error for particular stimuli.

3. The orbitofrontal cortex represents neuroeconomic value: the representations reflect for example the quantity available, the probability, and the reward value of each good.

4. The orbitofrontal cortex is involved in reward value and emotional experience, in that activations in the orbitofrontal cortex are often linearly related to the conscious subjective pleasantness (or unpleasantness) of stimuli. Connectivity from the orbitofrontal cortex to language regions is likely to be involved in declarative reports about subjective emotional state (Rolls et al., 2023b).

5. The orbitofrontal cortex is involved in social and emotional behavior, in that face expression and face identity are both represented in the orbitofrontal cortex, and in that social and emotional behavior are severely impaired by damage to the human orbitofrontal cortex.

6. A key computational capacity of the orbitofrontal cortex is one-trial object-reward associations, which are rule-based. This enables very rapid changes in behavior when the current reinforcement contingencies change, and this is very likely to be important in primate

social behavior, in which rapid sensitivity to social / rewarding feedback can be very important. This type of one-trial rule-based reversal learning appears not to occur in rodents.
7. Negative reward prediction error (nRPE) is represented by primate orbitofrontal cortex neurons that increase their firing rates when an expected reward is not obtained. The nRPE neurons may be important in changing reward behavior when expected rewards are no longer obtained, in for example one-trial reward reversal.
8. The orbitofrontal cortex provides a common scale for the reward value for different rewards, but does not convert to a common currency. A common scale is important for the inputs to decision-making networks. Conversion to a common currency would not be adaptive, because the decision-making system needs to keep the particular reward that has won in the competition active, while goal-directed action is performed to obtain the reward. A common currency would not specify the winning reward and goal for action. The dopamine system in contrast may use a common currency for its reinforcement learning of stimulus-response habits.
9. Relative and absolute value are both represented in the orbitofrontal cortex. Absolute value is important for consistent long-term choice and transitive preferences. Relative value is useful for short-term choice, for example on a particular trial or a block of trials.
10. Top-down cognition and attention, even from the level of language, exert effects on the orbitofrontal cortex, and bias its representations of value.
11. Decision-making about value is represented in the ventromedial prefrontal cortex, VMPFC. Whereas much of the orbitofrontal cortex represents value on a continuous scale, in a more anterior part which may be part of medial prefrontal cortex area 10 and which may be described as the ventromedial prefrontal cortex, decisions are made between stimuli of different reward value.
12. The orbitofrontal cortex plays a key role in emotion, which can be defined as states elicited by rewards and punishers, which are what is represented in the orbitofrontal cortex.
13. The orbitofrontal cortex does not represent actions or behavioral responses: the orbitofrontal cortex contains representations of sensory stimuli in terms of their reward value. It sends this information to the anterior cingulate cortex which learns actions to obtain rewarding outcomes signalled by the orbitofrontal cortex; and to the striatum which interfaces stimuli to responses, using reinforcement information provided in part by the dopamine neurons which receive inputs from the orbitofrontal cortex.
14. Reward value information is also sent from the orbitofrontal cortex to the hippocampus, where reward and emotional value can become part of an episodic memory. In addition, the reward value component of an episodic memory may influence how often it is retrieved and processes that are then involved in memory consolidation.
15. The pOFC region of the human medial orbitofrontal cortex has effective connectivity to the basal forebrain cholinergic nucleus of Meynert, which in turn provides the cholinergic input to the neocortex. This is likely to provide a key route that enables value representations decoded in the orbitofrontal cortex to influence memory consolidation.
16. Region OFC of the human medial orbitofrontal cortex has effective connectivity directed towards the substantia nigra pars compacta (SNpc) and ventral tegmental area (VTA), which contain dopaminergic neurons, and this is a key way in which, in part via the ventral striatum and habenula, reward information can reach dopamine neurons to enable their representation of reward prediction error.
17. The amygdala in humans has effective connectivity from anterior temporal lobe regions, has little backprojection to the cortex, and overall has much less cortical connectivity than the orbitofrontal cortex. Damage to the amygdala in humans has much smaller effects than damage to the orbitofrontal cortex on reported emotion, and may be involved in

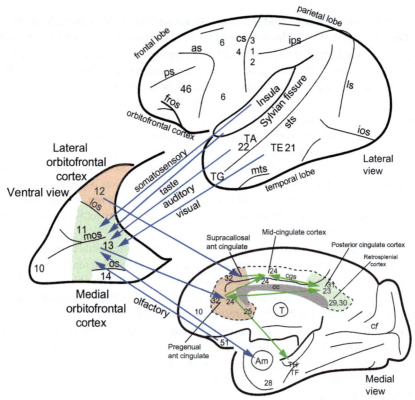

Fig. 11.2 The orbitofrontal cortex forms the ventral (lower) part of the frontal lobes of the primate (illustrated) including human brain. This diagram shows some of the gustatory, olfactory, visual, and auditory pathways to the orbitofrontal cortex, and some of the outputs of the orbitofrontal cortex. The secondary taste cortex and the secondary olfactory cortex are within the orbitofrontal cortex. The medial orbitofrontal cortex (areas 13 and 11) is shaded green, and the lateral orbitofrontal cortex (area 12) is shaded red. V1, primary visual cortex. V4, visual cortical area V4. Abbreviations: as, arcuate sulcus; cc, corpus callosum; cf, calcarine fissure; cgs, cingulate sulcus; cs, central sulcus; ls, lunate sulcus; ios, inferior occipital sulcus; mos, medial orbital sulcus; os, orbital sulcus; ots, occipito-temporal sulcus; ps, principal sulcus; rhs, rhinal sulcus; sts, superior temporal sulcus; the Sylvian (or lateral) fissure has been opened to reveal the insula; Am, amygdala; ant cingulate, anterior cingulate cortex (shaded red); T, thalamus; TE (21), inferior temporal visual cortex; TA (22), superior temporal auditory association cortex; TF and TH, parahippocampal cortex; TG, temporal pole cortex; 3,1,2, somatosensory cortex; 4, motor cortex; 6, premotor cortex; 14, gyrus rectus; 28, entorhinal cortex; 51, olfactory (prepyriform and periamygdaloid) cortex. (From Rolls, E. T. (2019) The Orbitofrontal Cortex. Oxford University Press: Oxford.)

humans as in rodents more in autonomic and related behavioral responses such as freezing implemented via brainstem outputs.

11.1.3 Overview of how the computations are performed by the orbitofrontal cortex

1. Some stimuli, such as food and water, have their reward value modulated in the orbitofrontal cortex by internal homeostatic signals, such as gastric distension, and the effects of absorbed nutrients and water. One route for these satiety signals to reach the orbitofrontal cortex is via the visceral insula. This is part of the mechanism that influences the reward value of a number of stimuli in the orbitofrontal cortex.
2. Sensory-specific satiety, a key process by which the reward value of a particular reward that is being received diminishes over time, is implemented in the orbitofrontal cortex using it is suggested temporal adaptation of the synapses transmitting information to

orbitofrontal cortex neurons. This is a key process with a time course of minutes or more that ensures that animals switch occasionally to different rewards, which is evolutionarily adaptive. Sensory-specific decreases in activity are not a property of orbitofrontal cortex neurons that respond to aversive stimuli, which again is evolutionarily adaptive.

3. The learning of associations between visual and other stimuli and primary reinforcers (such as taste or pleasant touch or pain) can be implemented by pattern association learning.

4. An attractor network mechanism for the computation involved in generating non-reward (negative reward prediction error, nRPE) neurons in the orbitofrontal cortex is described.

5. The one-trial rule-based reversal of orbitofrontal cortex neurons is non-associative, and requires a short-term memory network to hold online which stimuli are currently associated with rewards. Neural network models of this computation are described, and utilise a non-reward (negative reward prediction error) signal to initiate the reversal of the rule attractor network.

6. Part of how the computations work in this system must be that the systems such as the anterior cingulate cortex that receive inputs from the orbitofrontal cortex must be organized to learn actions that will promote behavior to work for the stimuli when the reward neurons are firing, and to work to escape from or avoid the stimuli if neurons that respond to aversive stimuli are active.

7. Evidence that decisions between different rewards are taken in the anterior orbitofrontal cortex / VMPFC by attractor networks in which the decision variables compete to win is described. Decision-making attractor networks, which are probably implemented in a number of different cortical areas for different types of decision, are described, with an integrate-and-fire model analyzed. These attractor decision-making networks are probabilistic, because they are influenced by the almost Poisson (random) spiking times for a given mean firing rate of the neurons in the network. The confidence in the decision can be read out from these networks by the final firing rate, which reflects the difference between the decision variables. The attractor network can maintain its decision to act as a goal for behavior because of the positive feedback within the network.

11.2 The topology and connections of the orbitofrontal cortex

The orbitofrontal cortex is on the lower (ventral) surface of the frontal lobes. The topology and many connections of the orbitofrontal cortex are shown in Fig. 11.2. The term **medial orbitofrontal cortex** refers to areas 13 and 11 shown in Figs. 11.2 and 11.3, and **lateral orbitofrontal cortex** refers to area 12 (12/47 in humans) (Rolls, 2019e; Rolls, Cheng and Feng, 2020a). The medial orbitofrontal cortex in humans tends to represent rewards, and the lateral orbitofrontal cortex punishers (Rolls, 2019e; Rolls et al., 2020a). Also shown in Fig. 11.3 on the medial view (above) is the anterior cingulate cortex areas 24 and 32. On the medial view of the human brain (left), areas 14r (the gyrus rectus) and 10m and 10r can be described as the ventromedial prefrontal cortex. Fig. 11.3 also shows that the macaque orbitofrontal cortex has relatively similar areas to humans, but the rodent appears to have no granular orbitofrontal cortex (Wise, 2008; Passingham and Wise, 2012; Rolls, 2019e; Passingham, 2021) (see Section 19.10). (Granular cortex, light gray or colored in Fig. 11.3, has small cells in layer 4 that give it a granular appearance, and cytoarchitectural differences such as this, as well as differences of the connections, are what make the primate including human orbitofrontal cortex appear different to what is present in rodents.)

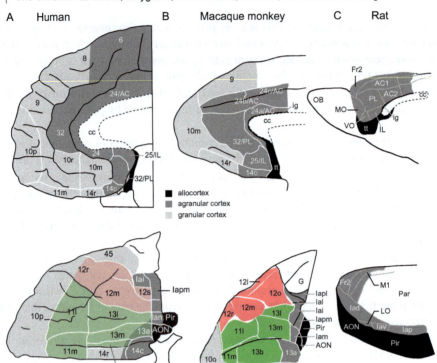

Fig. 11.3 Comparison of the orbitofrontal (below) and medial prefrontal (above) cortical areas in humans, macaque monkeys, and rats. (A) Medial (top) and orbital (bottom) areas of the human frontal cortex (Ongur et al. 2003). The medial orbitofrontal cortex is shown in green (areas 13 and 11), and the lateral orbitofrontal cortex in red (area 12). Almost all of the human orbitofrontal cortex except area 13a is granular. Agranular cortex is shown in dark grey. The part of area 45 shown is the orbital part of the inferior frontal gyrus pars triangularis. (B) Medial (top) and orbital (bottom) areas of the macaque frontal cortex (Carmichael and Price 1994). (C) Medial (top) and lateral (bottom) areas of rat frontal cortex (Palomero-Gallagher and Zilles 2004). Rostral is to the left in all drawings. Top row: dorsal is up in all drawings. Bottom row: in (A) and (B), lateral is up; in (C), dorsal is up. Not to scale. Abbreviations: AC, anterior cingulate cortex; AON, anterior olfactory 'nucleus'; cc, corpus callosum; Fr2 second frontal area; Ia, agranular insular cortex; ig, induseum griseum; IL, infralimbic cortex; LO, lateral orbital cortex; MO, medial orbital cortex: OB, olfactory bulb; Pir, piriform (olfactory) cortex; PL, prelimbic cortex; tt, tenia tecta; VO, ventral orbital cortex; Subdivisions of areas are labelled caudal (c); inferior (i), lateral (l), medial (m); orbital (o), posterior or polar (p), rostral(r), or by arbitrary designation (a, b). (Modified from Passingham and Wise (2012). (a) Modified from Dost Ongur, Amon T. Ferry, and Joseph L. Price (2003) Architectonic subdivision of the human orbital and medial prefrontal cortex. Journal of Comparative Neurology 460: 425–449. Copyright © Wiley-Liss. (b) Adapted from S. T. Carmichael and J. L. Price (1994) Architectonic subdivision of the orbital and medial prefrontal cortex in the macaque monkey. Journal of Comparative Neurology 346: 366–402. Copyright © Wiley-Liss Inc. (c) Adapted from Nicola Palomero-Gallagher and Karl Zilles (2004) Isocortex. In Paxinos, George ed., The Rat Nervous System, 3e, pp. 729–757, doi.org/10.1016/B978-012547638-6/50024-9. Copyright © Elsevier Inc.)

11.2.1 Inputs to the orbitofrontal cortex

Some of the connections of the orbitofrontal cortex (Price, 2006; Ongur and Price, 2000) are shown in Figs. 11.1, 11.2, and 11.4. A brief summary will be provided here, with citations of many of the original papers available (Rolls, 2019f,e). Although much of the literature is based on tract tracing in macaques, consistent data are now becoming available from humans in studies using functional connectivity (in which correlations between the signal in different brain regions are used to infer connectivity, even if some of it may be trans-synaptic (Du, Rolls, Cheng, Li, Gong, Qiu and Feng, 2020; Rolls, Deco, Huang and Feng, 2023c), from diffusion tensor neuroimaging which can show direct connections (Hsu, Rolls, Huang, Chong, Lo, Feng and Lin, 2020; Rolls, Deco, Huang and Feng, 2023c), and from effective connectivity which can show the strength in both directions of the connectivity, and which can

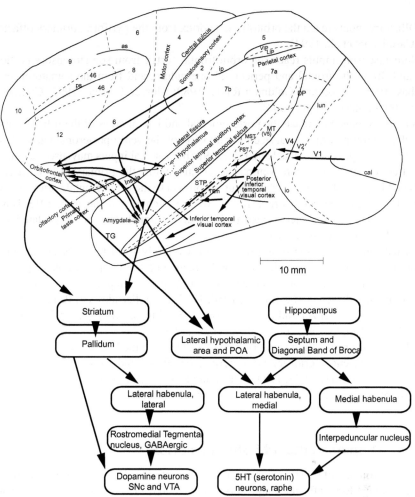

Fig. 11.4 Possible routes for reward and non-reward related information from the primate orbitofrontal cortex and amygdala to reach the brainstem dopamine and serotonin (5-HT) neurons (see text). One route is via the ventral striatum and ventral pallidum. A second route is via the ventral striatum, ventral pallidum, lateral habenula, and rostromedial tegmental nucleus. as, arcuate sulcus; cal, calcarine sulcus; cs, central sulcus; lf, lateral (or Sylvian) fissure; lun, lunate sulcus; ps, principal sulcus; io, inferior occipital sulcus; ip, intraparietal sulcus (which has been opened to reveal some of the areas it contains); sts, superior temporal sulcus (which has been opened to reveal some of the areas it contains). AIT, anterior inferior temporal cortex; FST, visual motion processing area; LIP, lateral intraparietal area; MST, visual motion processing area; MT, visual motion processing area (also called V5); PIT, posterior inferior temporal cortex; POA, preoptic area; SNc, substantia nigra pars compacta; STP, superior temporal plane; TA, architectonic area including auditory association cortex; TE, architectonic area including high order visual association cortex, and some of its subareas TEa and TEm; TG, architectonic area in the temporal pole; V1–V4, visual areas V1–V4; VIP, ventral intraparietal area; TEO, architectonic area including posterior visual association cortex; VTA, ventral tegmental area. The numerals refer to architectonic areas, and have the following approximate functional equivalence: 1,2,3, somatosensory cortex (posterior to the central sulcus); 4, motor cortex; 5, superior parietal lobule; 7a, inferior parietal lobule, visual part; 7b, inferior parietal lobule, somatosensory part; 6, lateral premotor cortex; 8, frontal eye field; 12, part of orbitofrontal cortex; 46, dorsolateral prefrontal cortex. (Modified from Rolls, E. T. (2017) The roles of the orbitofrontal cortex via the habenula in non-reward and depression, and in the responses of serotonin and dopamine neurons. Neuroscience and Biobehavioral Reviews 75: 331–334. © Elsevier Ltd.)

be described as causal, partly in the sense that it provides a generative model for functional connectivity (Rolls et al., 2023c). Evidence on the connectivity of the orbitofrontal cortex in humans (Rolls et al., 2023c) is described in Section 11.3.10.

Taste inputs reach the orbitofrontal cortex from the insular primary taste cortex (Baylis, Rolls and Baylis, 1995).

Olfactory inputs reach the orbitofrontal cortex from the pyriform, primary olfactory, cortex (Carmichael et al., 1994).

Somatosensory inputs reach the orbitofrontal cortex from somatosensory cortical areas 1, 2 and SII in the frontal and pericentral operculum, and from the somatosensory insula (Barbas, 1988; Preuss and Goldman-Rakic, 1989; Morecraft et al., 1992; Carmichael and Price, 1995b; Saleem et al., 2008).

Visceral inputs may reach the posteromedial and lateral areas of the orbitofrontal cortex from the ventral part of the parvicellular division of the ventroposteromedial nucleus of the thalamus (VPMpc) (Carmichael and Price, 1995b). Visceral inputs may also reach the orbitofrontal cortex from the antero-ventral insula (just below the primary taste cortex) (Baylis, Rolls and Baylis, 1995), from which neurons project to the orbitofrontal cortex, and which is probably an area of visceral cortex (Rolls, 2016c; Critchley and Harrison, 2013; Hassanpour et al., 2018). (In humans, there is also a mid-insular region that has activity related to visceral effects (Hassanpour et al., 2018).)

Visual inputs reach the orbitofrontal cortex directly from the inferior temporal visual cortex, the cortex in the superior temporal sulcus, and the temporal pole, especially from areas TEav and the fundus and ventral bank of the superior temporal sulcus, and the temporal pole (Jones and Powell, 1970; Barbas, 1988, 1993, 1995; Petrides and Pandya, 1988; Barbas and Pandya, 1989; Seltzer and Pandya, 1978, 1989; Morecraft et al., 1992; Carmichael and Price, 1995b; Kondo et al., 2003; Saleem et al., 2008, 2014).

There are corresponding auditory inputs, which reach the lateral orbitofrontal cortex area 12 and the adjacent inferior temporal gyrus areas BA45 and BA44 from temporal cortical auditory areas (Barbas, 1988, 1993; Plakke and Romanski, 2014).

The inputs to the human orbitofrontal cortex (Rolls et al., 2023c) are described in Section 11.3.10.

11.2.2 Outputs of the orbitofrontal cortex

The orbitofrontal cortex has major outputs to the anterior cingulate cortex (Carmichael and Price, 1995a; Morecraft and Tanji, 2009; Vogt, 2009; Garcia-Cabezas and Barbas, 2017; Rolls, 2019c; Du, Rolls, Cheng, Li, Gong, Qiu and Feng, 2020; Hsu, Rolls, Huang, Chong, Lo, Feng and Lin, 2020) and to the ventral striatum (Choi et al., 2017), as well as projections back to many of the areas that send afferents to it.

The caudal orbitofrontal cortex (area 13) has strong reciprocal connections with the amygdala (Price et al., 1991; Carmichael and Price, 1995a; Barbas, 2007; Garcia-Cabezas and Barbas, 2017).

Some of the output pathways of the orbitofrontal cortex (and amygdala) reward processing systems to the subcortical systems that utilize dopamine and serotonin (5-hydroxytryptamine) as neurotransmitters are considered next. The operation of the dopamine systems is considered further in Section 16.4.3.

A somewhat unaddressed issue is how the dopamine neurons in the midbrain, implicated in positive reward prediction error signalling to brain regions such as the striatum (Schultz, 2013, 2016b) (Section 16.4.3), and in addiction (Koob and Volkow, 2016), receive their information about rewards. In this context, it has now been suggested that reward and non-reward areas of the brain such as the orbitofrontal cortex and amygdala do provide a source of relevant inputs to the dopamine neurons (Rolls, 2017c). Pathways that provide a route for reward and emotion-related information to reach the dopamine neurons in the midbrain are shown in Fig. 11.4. One pathway is via a basal ganglia route (striatum, ventral pallidum, and globus pallidus / bed nucleus of the stria terminalis) to influence the Lateral Habenula, lateral part, which in turn via the GABAergic Rostromedial Tegmental nucleus can influence dopamine neurons in the Substantia Nigra pars compacta and ventral Tegmental Area (SNc and VTA). This provides a route for reward, non-reward, and reward prediction error signals of largely cortical origin to influence the dopamine neurons. Details of some of these anatomical connections are provided elsewhere (Haber, 2014; Proulx et al., 2014; Loonen and Ivanova, 2016), and the operation of this dopamine system and the source of its inputs is considered in Chapter 16.

Serotonin neurons, whose cell bodies are in the raphe nucleus in the brainstem, also have widespread projections throughout the brain, and serotonin is implicated in the effects of some antidepressants (Rolls, 2018a). The origin of the relevant inputs to the serotonin neurons is also a somewhat unaddressed question: how do the serotonin neurons in the raphe nucleus in the midbrain receive inputs that might influence depression in the first place? In this context, it has now been suggested that reward and non-reward areas of the brain such as the orbitofrontal cortex and amygdala do provide a source of relevant inputs to the 5-HT neurons, via brain regions such as the habenula and ventral striatum (Proulx et al., 2014; Loonen and Ivanova, 2016; Rolls, 2017c) (Fig. 11.4). Many antidepressant drugs may influence this cortical to brainstem pathway by influencing the effects of the 5-HT neurons, which terminate in many brain areas.

The outputs of the human orbitofrontal cortex (Rolls et al., 2023c) are described in Section 11.3.10.

11.3 What is computed in the orbitofrontal cortex

11.3.1 The orbitofrontal cortex represents reward value

An overall framework for helping to understand the functions of the orbitofrontal cortex is shown in Fig. 11.1 on page 476, which shows three tiers of processing, with the orbitofrontal cortex in Tier 2.

In Tier 1 (Fig. 11.1) in primates, information is processed to a level at which the neurons represent 'what' the stimulus is, independently of the reward or punishment and hence emotional value of the stimulus. In Tier 2 in the orbitofrontal cortex in particular, reward value is represented, as shown for example by the effects of devaluation by feeding a food to satiety, reversal of neuronal responses when the reward value of stimuli is reversed, and correlations of activations with subjectively reported pleasantness. Some of the evidence (Rolls, 2019e) is summarized next.

11.3.1.1 Orbitofrontal cortex representations of the reward value for taste, olfaction, oral texture, and touch

Neurons in the insular primary taste cortex represent what the taste is, but not its reward value, as shown by the findings that neurons in the primary taste cortex do not decrease their responses to zero when the macaque is fed to satiety, with consistent fMRI evidence in humans. Correspondingly, activations in the insular primary taste cortex are correlated with the subjective intensity but not the subjective pleasantness of the taste (Section 4.2.3). In contrast, the reward value of taste is represented in the orbitofrontal cortex, as shown by devaluation (Section 4.2.4) and sensory-specific satiety effects (Section 4.2.5) (Rolls, 2016g, 2019f).

Similarly, the reward value and pleasantness of oral texture, is represented in the orbitofrontal cortex (Rolls et al., 1999a; Grabenhorst et al., 2010b), and so is temperature (Kadohisa et al., 2004; Rolls et al., 2008a; Grabenhorst et al., 2010a).

In the human primary olfactory (pyriform) cortex, activations are correlated with the subjective intensity but not pleasantness of odors (Rolls, Grabenhorst, Margot, da Silva and

Velazco, 2008b). In the orbitofrontal cortex, activations are correlated with the subjective pleasantness of odors (Rolls, Kringelbach and De Araujo, 2003c; Rolls, Grabenhorst, Margot, da Silva and Velazco, 2008b) (Fig. 5.4 and Section 5.2.6). Further, neurons in the orbitofrontal cortex stop responding to a food odor after devaluation and implement olfactory sensory-specific satiety (Section 5.2.6), and show olfactory-to-taste reversal (Section 5.2.5).

The pleasantness of touch is also represented in the orbitofrontal cortex (Section 6.1.6).

11.3.1.2 The expected value of visual stimuli is represented in the orbitofrontal cortex, and can be reversed in one trial

For visual stimuli, the identity but not the reward value is represented at the end of the ventral visual stream in the inferior temporal cortex, in that neurons here do not reverse during visual-to-taste visual discrimination reversal, and do not reduce their response during devaluation by feeding to satiety (Rolls, Judge and Sanghera, 1977) (Section 2.4.1, Fig. 2.6).

We have been able to show that there is a major visual input to many neurons in the orbitofrontal cortex, and that what is represented by these neurons is in many cases the reinforcer (reward or punisher) association of visual stimuli (Thorpe, Rolls and Maddison, 1983; Rolls, Critchley, Mason and Wakeman, 1996b). Many of these neurons reflect the relative preference or reward value of different visual stimuli, in that their responses decrease to zero to the sight of one food on which the monkey is being fed to satiety, but remain unchanged to the sight of other food stimuli (Critchley and Rolls, 1996a). In this sense the visual reinforcement-related neurons predict the reward value that is available from the primary reinforcer, the taste.

The fact that these neurons represent the reinforcer associations of visual stimuli and hence the expected value has been shown to be the case in formal investigations of the activity of orbitofrontal cortex visual neurons, which in many cases reverse their responses to visual stimuli when the taste with which the visual stimulus is associated is reversed by the experimenter (Thorpe, Rolls and Maddison, 1983; Rolls, Critchley, Mason and Wakeman, 1996b). An example of the responses of an orbitofrontal cortex neuron that reversed the visual stimulus to which it responded during reward reversal is shown in Fig. 11.5.

Visual reversal to compute expected value can be rapid and rule-based in primates including humans

This reversal by orbitofrontal visual neurons can be very fast, in as little as one trial, that is a few seconds (see for example Fig. 11.6). The significance of the visual stimulus, a syringe from which the monkey was fed, was altered during the trials. On trials 1–5, no response of the neuron occurred to the sight of the syringe from which the monkey had been given glucose solution to drink from the syringe on the preceding trials. On trials 6–9, the neuron responded to the sight of the same syringe from which he had been given aversive hypertonic saline drink on the preceding trial. Two more reversals (trials 10–15, and 16–17) were performed. The reversal of the neuron's response when the significance of the visual stimulus was reversed shows that the responses of the neuron only occurred to the stimulus when it was associated with aversive saline and not when it was associated with glucose reward.

It is of great importance for understanding the functions of the primate including human orbitofrontal cortex that this reward reversal learning can be very fast, in one trial. This is shown by the fact that after an expected reward was not obtained due to a reversal contingency being applied, on the very next trial the macaque selected the previously non-rewarded stimulus. This occurred despite the fact that the stimulus now chosen had been previously associated with punishment. This shows that rapid reversal can be performed by a non-associative process, and must be rule-based. The primate must learn the rule that if one stimulus is no longer rewarded, then the other stimulus will be rewarded on the next trial. More generally,

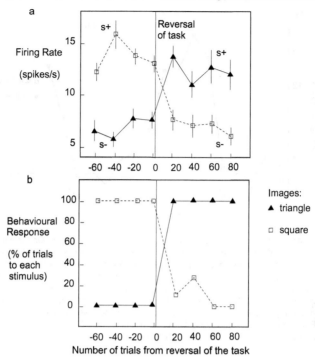

Fig. 11.5 Orbitofrontal cortex: visual discrimination reversal. The activity of an orbitofrontal visual neuron during performance of a visual discrimination task and its reversal. The stimuli were a triangle and a square presented on a video monitor. (a) Each point represents the mean poststimulus activity in a 500 ms period of the neuron based on approximately 10 trials of the different visual stimuli. The standard errors of these responses are shown. After 60 trials of the task the reward associations of the visual stimuli were reversed. s+ indicates that a lick response to that visual stimulus produces fruit juice reward; s– indicates that a lick response to that visual stimulus results in a small drop of aversive tasting saline. This neuron reversed its responses to the visual stimuli following the task reversal. (b) The behavioral response of the monkey to the task. It is shown that the monkey performs well, in that he rapidly learns to lick only to the visual stimulus associated with fruit juice reward. (Reproduced from E. T. Rolls, H.D.Critchley, R.Mason, and E.A.Wakeman (1996) Orbitofrontal cortex neurons: role in olfactory and visual association learning. Journal of Neurophysiology 75: 1970–1981. © The American Physiological Society.)

if a stimulus is no longer rewarded, then behavior should change to another stimulus. This is of great adaptive value for many aspects of primate (including human) behavior, including social behavior, in which it may be appropriate to adjust behavior after even a subtle change in reinforcing feedback (outcome) is received. An example of this demonstrated in an fMRI study is shown in Fig. 11.15. This one-trial, rule-based, reversal activates especially the human right lateral orbitofrontal cortex (Rolls, Vatansever, Li, Cheng and Feng, 2020e), which supports the hypotheses that a lateral orbitofrontal cortex non-reward mechanism is involved in depression (Section 18.5). A model for this rule-based reversal is the subject of Section 11.5.3.

This rapid stimulus-reward learning and reversal, so important in primate behavior, has not been demonstrated in rodents as far as I know (and see Hervig et al. (2020)), and may be one of the fundamental advances provided for by the great evolution of the primate including human orbitofrontal cortex, especially in the context of the representations of social reinforcers that are described in Section 11.3.3. For the slower type of reversal found in rodents, the rodent lateral orbitofrontal cortex is involved, as shown by pharmacological inactivation (Hervig et al., 2020).

Consistent with this evidence that the responses of some orbitofrontal cortex neurons reflect the learned predictive reward value of visual stimuli, Thorpe, Rolls and Maddison

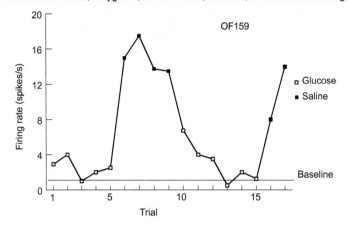

Fig. 11.6 Orbitofrontal cortex: one-trial visual discrimination reversal by a neuron. On trials 1–5, no response of the neuron occurred to the sight of a 2 ml syringe from which the monkey had been given orally glucose solution to drink on the previous trial. On trials 6–9, the neuron responded to the sight of the same syringe from which he had been given aversive hypertonic saline to drink on the previous trial. Two more reversals (trials 10–15, and 16–17) were performed. The reversal of the neuron's response when the significance of the same visual stimulus was reversed shows that the responses of the neuron only occurred to the sight of the visual stimulus when it was associated with a positively reinforcing and not with a negatively reinforcing taste. Moreover, it is shown that the neuronal reversal took only one trial. (Reproduced from S.J.Thorpe, E.T. Rolls, and S.Maddison (1983) The orbitofrontal cortex: Neuronal activity in the behaving monkey. Experimental Brain Research 49: 93–115. © Springer Nature.)

(1983) and Tremblay and Schultz (2000) found that orbitofrontal cortex neurons learned to respond differently to new stimuli that did or did not predict reward. Different neurons in the orbitofrontal cortex are tuned to different learned or conditioned reinforcers, with for example approximately 5% responding to visual stimuli associated with taste reward, and 3% to visual stimuli associated with taste punishment (Thorpe, Rolls and Maddison, 1983; Rolls, Critchley, Mason and Wakeman, 1996b).

Although using a somewhat different test situation, classical conditioning, Saez, Saez, Paton, Lau and Salzman (2017) found consistent evidence: they found that neuronal responses to reward-predictive cues update more rapidly in the macaque orbitofrontal cortex than amygdala, and activity in the orbitofrontal cortex but not the amygdala was modulated by recent reward history.

Visual stimulus-selective expected value neurons

In the visual discrimination reversal task, a second class of neuron was found that codes for particular stimuli only if they are associated with reward, and not if they are associated with punishment. Such a neuron might respond to a green stimulus associated with reward; after reversal not respond to the green stimulus when it was associated with punishment; and not respond to a blue stimulus irrespective of whether it was associated with reward or punishment (Thorpe, Rolls and Maddison, 1983) (see example in Fig. 11.7). They may be described as *conditional visual stimulus-to-taste reward neurons* or *conditional expected value neurons* (Rolls et al., 1996b), and are analogous to their olfactory counterparts (Rolls et al., 1996b). These neurons are probably important in the mechanisms that implement rapid reversal, as described in Section 11.5.3. More generally, they are part of a mechanism that enables the orbitofrontal cortex to specify individual objects or individuals who may be currently associated with reward, or not.

In addition to selectivity for which stimulus or class of stimulus is currently associated with reward, the fact that many different types of primary reinforcer are present in the orbito-

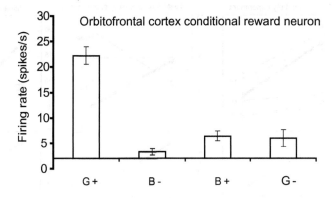

Fig. 11.7 A conditional reward neuron recorded in the orbitofrontal cortex. The neuron responded only to the Green stimulus when it was associated with reward (G+), and not to the Blue stimulus when it was associated with Reward (B+), or to either stimuli when they were associated with a punisher, the taste of salt (G− and B−). The mean firing rate ± the s.e.m. is shown. (Reproduced from S.J.Thorpe, E.T. Rolls, and S.Maddison (1983) The orbitofrontal cortex: Neuronal activity in the behaving monkey. Experimental Brain Research 49: 93–115. © Springer Nature.)

frontal cortex enables it to represent the expected value of many different types of primary reinforcer.

This reversal learning found in orbitofrontal cortex neurons probably is implemented in the orbitofrontal cortex, for it does not occur one synapse earlier in the visual inferior temporal cortex (Rolls, Judge and Sanghera, 1977), and it is in the orbitofrontal cortex that there is convergence of visual and taste pathways on to the same neurons (Thorpe, Rolls and Maddison, 1983; Rolls, Critchley, Mason and Wakeman, 1996b).

Devaluation shows that orbitofrontal cortex visual neurons represent expected value

Another way in which it has been shown that the visual neurons in the orbitofrontal cortex reflect the expected value predicted by visual stimuli is by reducing the reward value by feeding to satiety in devaluation experiments. With this sensory-specific satiety (or reward devaluation) paradigm, it has been shown that the visual (as well as the olfactory and taste) responses of orbitofrontal cortex neurons in the macaque decrease to zero as the monkey is fed to satiety with one food, but remain unchanged to another food not eaten in the meal (Critchley and Rolls, 1996a) (see example in Fig. 11.8). In that these neurons parallel the changing preference of the monkey for the food being eaten to satiety vs the food not being eaten to satiety, they reflect the relative preference for different visual stimuli, that is the expected value (Thorpe, Rolls and Maddison, 1983; Rolls, Critchley, Mason and Wakeman, 1996b) (as found also by Tremblay and Schultz (1999) and Wallis and Miller (2003)).

All this evidence shows that the great majority of neurons in the orbitofrontal cortex encode stimuli, frequently in terms of the (outcome) value or expected value, and do not reflect the actions or responses or spatial responses being performed by the macaques (Thorpe, Rolls and Maddison, 1983; Rolls, Critchley, Mason and Wakeman, 1996b; Critchley and Rolls, 1996a; Rolls and Baylis, 1994; Rolls, 2014a; Wallis and Miller, 2003; Padoa-Schioppa and Assad, 2006; Grattan and Glimcher, 2014). Indeed, most orbitofrontal cortex neurons that we have recorded do not respond in relation to movements or actions (such as the lick instrumental responses made in a visual discrimination task), and in this sense reflect the value of sensory stimuli, though some do respond to oral or perioral somatosensory stimuli (Thorpe et al., 1983; Rolls et al., 1996b; Critchley and Rolls, 1996a; Rolls and Baylis, 1994; Rolls, 2014a). Consistent with this, orbitofrontal cortex neurons were found to respond to rewards but not to the eye movements being made to obtain the rewards (Grattan and Glimcher, 2014).

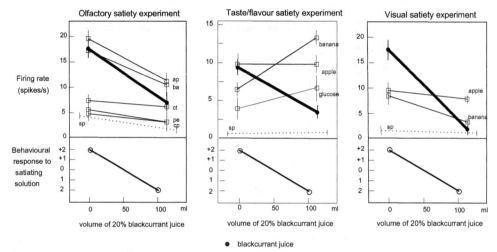

Fig. 11.8 Orbitofrontal cortex neuron with visual, olfactory and taste responses, showing the responses before and after feeding to satiety with blackcurrant juice. The solid circles show the responses to blackcurrant juice. The olfactory stimuli included apple (ap), banana (ba), citral (ct), phenylethanol (pe), and caprylic acid (cp). The spontaneous firing rate of the neuron is shown (sp). (Reproduced from H.D.Critchley and E. T. Rolls (1996) Hunger and satiety modify the responses of olfactory and visual neurons in the primate orbitofrontal cortex. Journal of Neurophysiology 75: 1673–1886. © The American Physiological Society.)

These findings are consistent with the hypothesis that expected reward value is represented in the orbitofrontal cortex, reflects stimulus–reinforcer (sensory–sensory) association learning, and that this information is projected to other structures such as the cingulate cortex for action–outcome learning (Chapter 12), or to the basal ganglia for stimulus-response habit learning (Chapter 16). Outputs of the orbitofrontal cortex to the dorsolateral prefrontal cortex may be used in tasks requiring planning, for example where rewarding stimuli must be flexibly linked to particular actions, and where delays may be involved, in ways that have been modelled by Deco and Rolls (2003) and Deco and Rolls (2005d).

Given that reward value and not action is implemented in the orbitofrontal cortex, it is an interesting further question about whether the reward value represented in the orbitofrontal cortex is influenced by the costs of actions. Some evidence for this was that in the macaque orbitofrontal cortex, some (but not other) neurons responded less to an expected reward if the cost involved in obtaining it was high (Cai and Padoa-Schioppa, 2019). The neurons that represent value independently of cost are important, for in a sense they represent the absolute value of the good, which is necessary for long-term economic choice. The neurons that have their value representation affected by the cost of the action to obtain the reward correspond more to relative value representations, which may be useful to guide choice in the current session especially when the costs for different rewards are altered. In a lesion study, monkeys with medial orbitofrontal cortex lesions were impaired in estimating the 'desirability' of food (in updating their choices based on changes in reward value manipulated by sensory-specific satiety), while monkeys with lateral orbitofrontal cortex lesions (termed ventrolateral prefrontal cortex lesions) were impaired in updating choices in response to changes in reward availability (as manipulated by the probability of obtaining food) (Rudebeck, Saunders, Lundgren and Murray, 2017).

The types of visual–taste reward associations that have been studied in primates have been confirmed as applying in humans in an fMRI study (O'Doherty et al., 2002). However in humans it was very interesting to investigate whether the orbitofrontal cortex is involved in more abstract rewards, such as monetary rewards, or points. In an fMRI study, O'Doherty, Kringelbach, Rolls, Hornak and Andrews (2001a) used a visual discrimination task in which one

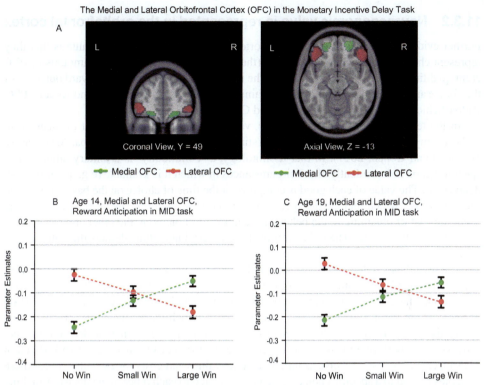

Fig. 11.9 The lateral orbitofrontal cortex is activated by not winning, and the medial orbitofrontal cortex by winning, in the monetary incentive delay task. The lateral orbitofrontal cortex region in which activations increased towards no reward (No Win) in the monetary incentive delay task are shown in red in 1140 participants at age 19 and in 1877 overlapping participants at age 14. The conditions were Large win (10 points) to Small Win (2 points) to No Win (0 points) (at 19; sweets were used at 14). The medial orbitofrontal cortex region in which activations increased with increasing reward from No Win to Small Win to High Win) is shown in green. The parameter estimates are shown from the activations for the participants (mean ± sem) with the lateral orbitofrontal in red and medial orbitofrontal cortex in green. The interaction term showing the sensitivity of the medial orbitofrontal cortex to reward and the lateral orbitofrontal cortex to non-reward was significant at $p = 10^{-50}$ at age 19 and $p < 10^{-72}$ at age 14. In a subgroup with depressive symptoms as shown by the Adolescent Depression Rating Scale, it was further found that there was a greater activation to the No Win condition in the lateral orbitofrontal cortex; and the medial orbitofrontal cortex was less sensitive to the differences in reward value. (Modified from Xie,C., Jia,T., Rolls, E. T. et al, (2021) Reward vs non-reward sensitivity of the medial vs lateral orbitofrontal cortex relates to the severity of depressive symptoms. Biological Psychiatry: Cognitive Neuroscience and Neuroimaging 6: 259-269. doi: 10.1016/j.bpsc.2020.08.017.)

stimulus was associated with monetary reward, and a different visual stimulus with monetary loss (punishment). The actual amounts of money won on reward trials and lost on punishment trials were probabilistic. This part of the design, and the fact that unexpected visual discrimination reversals occurred so that there were trials on which money was lost, enabled us to show that the magnitude of the activation of the medial orbitofrontal cortex was correlated with the amount of money won on each trial, and the magnitude of the activation of the lateral orbitofrontal cortex was correlated with the amount of money lost on each trial (O'Doherty, Kringelbach, Rolls, Hornak and Andrews, 2001a).

These findings have been extended by showing that the medial orbitofrontal cortex has greater activation as reward increases, and that the lateral orbotofrontal cortex has increasing activations as reward decreases to zero, in an investigation in 1,877 participants, as shown in Fig. 11.9 (Xie, Jia, Rolls et al (2021)).

11.3.2 Neuroeconomic value is represented in the orbitofrontal cortex

Further evidence that these orbitofrontal cortex neurons encode expected value is that they represent choices made when the 'offers' (the visual stimuli) are different amounts or different qualities of the 'goods' (for example the type of fruit juice that is the reward outcome of the choice and different probabilities of obtaining reward) (Padoa-Schioppa and Assad, 2006; Padoa-Schioppa, 2011; Padoa-Schioppa and Conen, 2017).

In the terminology of neuroeconomics, value represents a common unit of measure to make a comparison between the reinforcing stimuli or 'goods' (Padoa-Schioppa, 2011; Padoa-Schioppa and Conen, 2017). In that terminology, a 'commodity' is a unitary amount of a specified good independently of the circumstances in which it is available (e.g. quantity, cost, delay, etc.). The value of each good is computed at the time of choice on the basis of multiple 'determinants', which include the specific commodity, its quantity, the current motivational state, the cost of obtaining it, the behavioral context of choice (i.e. the other choices that are currently available), etc. The collection of these determinants thus defines the value of the 'good'.

The hypothesis is that while choosing, individuals compute the values of different options independently of one another. It is argued that the 'net reward value', i.e. the value of each good minus the cost of obtaining it, must be computed and represented on a common scale of value as the input to the decision-making process, which makes the choice (Grabenhorst and Rolls, 2011). The reason that the net value must be computed is that the decision-making process itself, performed it is suggested by an attractor decision-making network (Section 11.5.1), cannot by itself receive as inputs separate values and costs for each choice, for these variables related to a specific choice could not be related to each other in the decision-making attractor network.

A brain region that does appear to compute the actions needed to obtain a stimulus with the particular value, and which takes into account the costs of actions (which we have termed the extrinsic costs (Grabenhorst and Rolls, 2011)), is the cingulate cortex (Rushworth et al., 2011; Grabenhorst and Rolls, 2011; Rolls, 2019c), which receives value information about the goods in its anterior cingulate part from the orbitofrontal cortex (Rolls, 2005a, 2009a; Grabenhorst and Rolls, 2011). It is argued that the computation of net value in the orbitofrontal cortex does not depend on the sensori-motor contingencies of choice (the spatial configuration of the offers or the specific action that will implement the choice outcome), for the behavioral responses and actions are not represented in the orbitofrontal cortex, which represents the value of stimuli, and does not represent actions and responses (Thorpe, Rolls and Maddison, 1983; Rolls, 2005a; Padoa-Schioppa, 2011; Padoa-Schioppa and Conen, 2017). These action contingencies may, however, affect values in the form of action costs. In particular, the actions necessary to obtain different goods often bear different costs. There is evidence that these 'extrinsic costs' (the costs of the actions necessary to obtain a reward (Grabenhorst and Rolls, 2011)) are represented in the orbitofrontal cortex (Cai and Padoa-Schioppa, 2019).

The *extrinsic factors* that influence the value of a good and the value of a choice include:
1. The action costs, including the difficulty of the actions needed to obtain the good;
2. the time delay (with future rewards being discounted as a function of the length of the delay, and differently discounted by different individuals);
3. the 'risk', i.e. the probability that the reward will be obtained;
4. the amount of the good obtained if it is chosen;
5. the quality of the good, e.g. one juice may be preferred over another;
6. ambiguity (i.e. poor knowledge about the probability that a reward will be obtained).

The *intrinsic or internal factors* that influence the value of stimuli include (Grabenhorst and Rolls, 2011; Padoa-Schioppa, 2011; Padoa-Schioppa and Conen, 2017):
1. motivational state;
2. patience vs impatience or impulsiveness;
3. risk attitude, that is choice when the outcome is probabilistic, for example whether one is likely to gamble;
4. ambiguity attitude;
5. whether the stimulus which may have pleasant components has in addition unpleasant components.

Further factors important in understanding choices in the field of neuroeconomics, many described in more detail below, are:
1. The value of each good must be computed 'online' at the time of choice, for value is influenced by for example motivational state.
2. While choosing, individuals normally compute the values of different goods independently of one another. Such 'menu invariance' implies transitive preferences (Padoa-Schioppa, 2011; Padoa-Schioppa and Conen, 2017).
3. Absolute value is important for long-term choice and transitive preferences. This may be represented in the orbitofrontal cortex.
4. Relative value is useful for short-term choice, for example on a particular trial or a block of trials, and may be separately represented in the orbitofrontal cortex.

In one neuroeconomics study that illustrates how the responses of orbitofrontal cortex neurons encode the value of a stimulus or choice, the value of the choice was manipulated by providing different numbers of drops of juice (quantity) of different quality (e.g. grape juice (A) and peppermint tea (B), which were termed commodities) to monkeys (Padoa-Schioppa and Assad, 2006). The monkey preferred juice A. When offered one drop of juice A versus one drop of juice B (offer 1A:1B), the animals chose juice A. However, the animals were thirsty: they generally preferred larger amounts of juice to smaller amounts of juice. The amounts of the two juices offered against each other varied from trial to trial, which induced a commodity quantity trade-off in the choice pattern. For example in one session (Fig. 11.10), offer types (indicated by the number of small squares on a screen that were available for A and for B) included 0B:1A, 1B:2A, 1B:1A, 2B:1A, 3B:1A, 4B:1A, 6B:1A, 10B:1A and 3B:0A. The monkey generally chose 1A when 1B or 2B were available as the alternative, it was roughly indifferent between the two juices when offered 3B:1A, and it chose B when 4B, 6B or 10B were available (Fig. 11.10). In other words, the monkey assigned to 1A a value roughly equal to the value it assigned to 3B. A neuron recorded in the orbitofrontal cortex responded with a low rate (several spikes/s) when the offer was 2B or less, at an intermediate rate (approximately 10 spikes/s) when the offer was 3B or 4B, and at a high rate (approximately 17 spikes/s) when the offer was 6B or higher relative to 1A (Fig. 11.10). The neuron thus encoded the value of the offer, where the value assigned by the monkey reflected a commodity × quantity tradeoff.

The offer value neurons respond when the visual stimulus indicating the taste/flavor reward that will be obtained is shown (Padoa-Schioppa and Assad, 2006; Padoa-Schioppa, 2011; Padoa-Schioppa and Conen, 2017). They thus correspond to the orbitofrontal cortex neurons described by Rolls and colleagues that respond to a visual stimulus, for example in a visual discrimination task, that indicates the value of the reward or punisher that will be obtained (Thorpe, Rolls and Maddison, 1983; Rolls, Critchley, Mason and Wakeman, 1996b; Critchley and Rolls, 1996a). These visual neurons reflect expected reward value in that they respond to a particular visual stimulus when the value is high, and gradually respond less

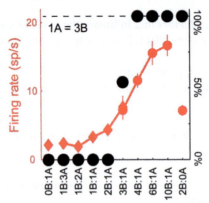

Fig. 11.10 Orbitofrontal cortex neuron encoding the offer value. On individual trials, the monkey was offered different numbers of drops of peppermint tea (juice B) versus 1 drop of grape juice (juice A). Black circles indicate the behavioral choice pattern (relative value in the upper left) and red symbols indicate the neuronal firing rate when the offer of different amounts of juice B was made vs 1 drop of juice A (1A). Red diamonds and circles refer, respectively, to trials in which the animal chose juice A and juice B. There is a sigmoid relationship between the firing rate of the neuron and the quantity of juice B offered to the monkey. (Reproduced from Camillo Padoa-Schioppa (2009) Range-adapting representation of economic value in the orbitofrontal cortex. Journal of Neuroscience 29: 14005. © Society for Neuroscience.)

to the visual stimulus as gradually it becomes devalued by feeding to satiety (Critchley and Rolls, 1996a) (Fig. 11.8). These visual neurons also respond to a visual stimulus when it signifies a high value, and do not respond when it is devalued by visual discrimination reversal learning so that it signifies after learning a low reward value (Rolls, Critchley, Mason and Wakeman, 1996b) (Fig. 11.5). In addition, these studies show that other neurons reflect the punisher value of a visual stimulus, responding for example to a visual stimulus when it signifies the punisher of a taste of saline if the visual stimulus is selected (Fig. 11.6) (Thorpe, Rolls and Maddison, 1983; Rolls, Critchley, Mason and Wakeman, 1996b).

Padoa-Schioppa and Assad (2006) also described neurons that in the same task responded when the juice taste reward was delivered. Their taste neurons reflected value, in that they had for example a large response when 4B or greater was delivered, an intermediate response when 3B was delivered, and no response when 2B or less was delivered (Fig. 11.10) (Padoa-Schioppa, 2011). These neurons again correspond to the taste reward neurons of Rolls and colleagues analyzed in the orbitofrontal cortex (Rolls, Yaxley and Sienkiewicz, 1990; Rolls, Critchley, Verhagen and Kadohisa, 2010a), which respond to a taste when it has a high value, and gradually respond less to that taste when it is gradually devalued by feeding to satiety (Rolls, Sienkiewicz and Yaxley (1989d), e.g. Fig. 4.8).

11.3.3 A representation of face and voice expression and other socially relevant stimuli in the orbitofrontal cortex

Socially relevant stimuli, such as the emotional expression on a face, and in the voice, are represented in the orbitofrontal cortex. There is a population of orbitofrontal cortex face-selective neurons (Rolls, Critchley, Browning and Inoue, 2006a) that respond in many ways similarly to those in the temporal cortical visual areas (Rolls, 1984, 1992a, 2000a, 2007e, 2008b, 2011d, 2012d, 2016b). The orbitofrontal face-responsive neurons, first observed by Thorpe, Rolls and Maddison (1983), then by Rolls, Critchley, Browning and Inoue (2006a), tend to respond with longer latencies than temporal lobe neurons (140–200 ms typically, compared with 80–100 ms); they also convey information about which face is being seen, by having different responses to different faces; and are typically rather harder to activate strongly than temporal cortical face-selective neurons, in that many of them respond much

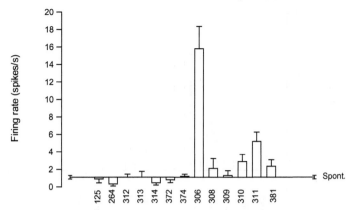

Fig. 11.11 Orbitofrontal cortex face-selective neuron tuned to face identity in the macaque. Firing rate histogram of cell be009 to different face stimuli (306-311 and 381) and different non-face stimuli (125, 264, 312, 313, 314, 372 and 374). Stimuli 305–308 and 381 were macaque faces with different identities, 309-311 were human face stimuli with different identities, and the other stimuli were different non-face stimuli (25=hand, 372=triangle, 374=saline-associated square, 312 - Fourier boundary curvature descriptor, 313 grating, 314 shirt). The means and standard error of the mean (sem) of the responses in spikes/s are shown as changes from the spontaneous rate (Spont.) (Reproduced from Rolls, E. T., Critchley,H.D., Browning,A.S. and Inoue,K. (2006) Face-selective and auditory neurons in the primate orbitofrontal cortex. Experimental Brain Research 170: 743–787. © Springer Nature.)

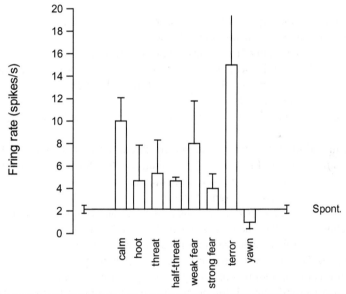

Fig. 11.12 Orbitofrontal cortex face-selective neuron tuned to face expression in the macaque. A firing rate histogram of cell aq045 to different face expressions is shown. The means and standard error of the mean (sem) of the responses in spikes/s are shown as changes from the spontaneous rate (Spont.) (Reproduced from Rolls, E. T., Critchley,H.D., Browning,A.S. and Inoue,K. (2006) Face-selective and auditory neurons in the primate orbitofrontal cortex. Experimental Brain Research 170: 743–787. © Springer Nature.)

better to real faces than to two-dimensional images of faces on a video monitor (cf. Rolls and Baylis (1986)). As shown in Fig. 11.11, some orbitofrontal cortex neurons respond to face identity.

Other orbitofrontal cortex face-selective neurons are tuned to the emotional expression of a face, as illustrated in Fig. 11.12.

We hypothesized that both face identity and face expression information is represented in the macaque orbitofrontal cortex because it is important to take into account both the identity

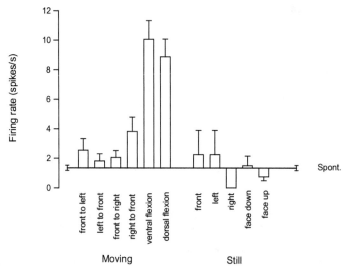

Fig. 11.13 Orbitofrontal cortex face-selective neuron tuned to some movements of a head, but with no response when the head was still. (Reproduced from Rolls, E. T., Critchley,H.D., Browning,A.S. and Inoue,K. (2006) Face-selective and auditory neurons in the primate orbitofrontal cortex. Experimental Brain Research 170: 743–787. © Springer Nature.)

of the individual and the expression on a face in order to produce an appropriate emotional and social response to a face (Rolls et al., 2006a).

In addition to categorising face expression, some orbitofrontal cortex neurons categorise faces by their social significance, such as young faces (Barat, Wirth and Duhamel, 2018). In another study, it was reported that some orbitofrontal cortex face-selective neurons are sensitive to the rank of the individual being viewed in the social hierarchy, with neurons also reflecting social hierarchy in the amygdala and anterior cingulate cortex (Munuera et al., 2018).

Some of the orbitofrontal cortex face-selective neurons are responsive to face gesture or movement, as illustrated in Fig. 11.13 (Rolls et al., 2006a). Such neurons are very likely to be involved in social situations, when for example the turn of a head towards or away from the viewer may have great social significance.

The discovery of face-selective neurons in the primate orbitofrontal cortex is consistent with the likelihood that these neurons are activated via the inputs from the temporal cortical visual areas in which face-selective neurons are found (see Fig. 11.1). The significance of the neurons is likely to be related to the fact that faces convey information that is important in social reinforcement, both by conveying face expression (cf. Hasselmo, Rolls and Baylis (1989a)), which can indicate reinforcement, and by encoding information about which individual is present, also important in evaluating and utilizing reinforcing inputs in social situations (Rolls, Critchley, Browning and Inoue, 2006a; Rolls, 2011d).

Consistent with these findings in macaques, and as described above, in humans, activation of the lateral orbitofrontal cortex occurs when a rewarding smile expression is expected, but an angry face expression is obtained, in a visual discrimination reversal task (Kringelbach and Rolls, 2003). This is an example of the operation of a social reinforcer, and, consistent with these results, Farrow et al. (2001) have found that activation of the orbitofrontal cortex is found when humans are making social judgements. In addition, activation of the medial orbitofrontal cortex is correlated with face attractiveness (O'Doherty et al., 2003b).

These orbitofrontal cortex face-selective neurons are frequently found close to the lateral orbitofrontal sulcus (Rolls, Critchley, Browning and Inoue, 2006a), and with fMRI in humans, activation of this region by faces is found (area PO) (D'Urso et al., 2017). Face selective neurons have also been found in the inferior prefrontal cortex below the principal sulcus (O'Scalaidhe et al., 1997; Romanski and Diehl, 2011; Diehl and Romanski, 2014) (area PL), and in the anterior bank of the arcuate sulcus (O'Scalaidhe et al., 1997) (area PA).

We also discovered that some orbitofrontal cortex neurons are activated by auditory stimuli, such as socially relevant vocalization (Fig. 7.5) (Rolls, Critchley, Browning and Inoue, 2006a). This has been confirmed (Plakke and Romanski, 2014), and indeed in the ventrolateral prefrontal cortex (which includes areas 12, 45, and 44) neurons may be tuned to the type of call or to the identity of the caller (Plakke et al., 2013; Plakke and Romanski, 2014). Neurons in this ventrolateral prefrontal cortex region can also be influenced by the sight or the sound of a vocalization, and by mismatches between these (Diehl and Romanski, 2014). Auditory stimuli may have similar representations in the orbitofrontal cortex related to their affective value. For example, Blood et al. (1999) found a correlation between subjective ratings of dissonance and consonance of musical chords and the activations produced in the orbitofrontal cortex (see also Blood and Zatorre (2001) and Frey et al. (2000)). The transition of harmony towards a pleasant resolution also activates the orbitofrontal cortex (Fujisawa and Cook, 2011).

In one study in a social situation it was found that neurons in the macaque orbitofrontal cortex predominantly encoded rewards that were delivered to the self (Chang et al., 2013). But in a social situation in which rewards were given to the self and to another monkey, some orbitofrontal cortex neurons reflected not only the value of the reward, but also the identity and social status of the other monkey (Azzi et al., 2012).

We were able to confirm the importance of this system for face expression analysis and social behavior in a group of patients with ventral frontal lobe damage who had impairments in the identification of facial and vocal emotional expression, and who had socially inappropriate behavior (Hornak, Rolls and Wade, 1996; Rolls, 1999b).

11.3.4 Negative reward prediction error neurons in the orbitofrontal cortex, and visual stimulus–reinforcer association learning and reversal during decision-making

In addition to the neurons that encode the reward value of visual stimuli, other neurons (3.5%) in the orbitofrontal cortex detect different types of non-reward, i.e. negative reward prediction error, the difference between the expected value and the reward outcome value (Thorpe, Rolls and Maddison, 1983). For example, some neurons responded in extinction, immediately after a lick had been made to a visual stimulus that had previously been associated with fruit juice reward, but no reward was obtained. Other neurons responded in a reversal task, immediately after the monkey had responded to the previously rewarded visual stimulus, but had obtained the punisher of salt taste rather than reward (see example in Fig. 11.14). Other orbitofrontal cortex neurons respond to other types of non-reward, including the removal of a formerly approaching taste reward, and the termination of a taste reward (Thorpe, Rolls and Maddison, 1983). Thus the error neurons can be specific to different tasks, and this could provide a mechanism for reversal in one task to be implemented, while at the same time not reversing behavior in another task. Neurons selective for different types of error have been found in a region to which the orbitofrontal cortex projects, the anterior cingulate cortex (Oemisch et al., 2019).

The existence of neurons in the middle part of the macaque orbitofrontal cortex that respond to non-reward (Thorpe, Rolls and Maddison, 1983) (originally described by Thorpe, Maddison and Rolls (1979) and Rolls (1981b)) is confirmed by recordings that revealed 10 such non-reward neurons (of 140 recorded, or approximately 7%) found in delayed match to

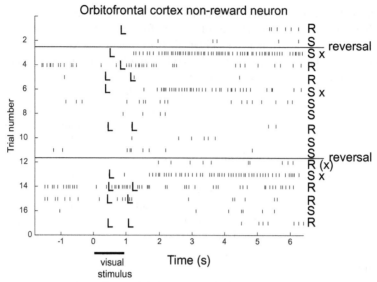

Fig. 11.14 Error neuron: Responses of an orbitofrontal cortex neuron that responded only when the monkey licked to a visual stimulus during reversal, expecting to obtain fruit juice reward, but actually obtaining the taste of aversive saline because it was the first trial of reversal. Each single dot represents an action potential; each vertically arranged double dot represents a lick response. The visual stimulus was shown at time 0 for 1 s. The neuron did not respond on most reward (R) or saline (S) trials, but did respond on the trials marked x, which were the first trials after a reversal of the visual discrimination on which the monkey licked to obtain reward, but actually obtained saline because the task had been reversed. It is notable that after an expected reward was not obtained due to a reversal contingency being applied, on the very next trial the macaque selected the previously non-rewarded stimulus. This shows that rapid reversal can be performed by a non-associative process, and must be rule-based. A model for this is the subject of Section 11.5.3. (Redrawn from S.J.Thorpe, E.T.Rolls, and S.Maddison (1983) The orbitofrontal cortex: Neuronal activity in the behaving monkey. Experimental Brain Research 49: 93–115. © Springer Nature.)

sample and delayed response tasks by Joaquin Fuster and colleagues (Rosenkilde, Bauer and Fuster, 1981).

We have also been able to obtain evidence that non-reward used as a signal to reverse behavioral choice is represented in the human orbitofrontal cortex. Kringelbach and Rolls (2003) used the faces of two different people, and if one face was selected then that face smiled, and if the other was selected, the face showed an angry expression. After good performance was acquired, there were repeated reversals of the visual discrimination task (see Fig. 11.15). Kringelbach and Rolls (2003) found that activation of a lateral part of the orbitofrontal cortex in the fMRI study was produced on the error trials, that is when the human chose a face, and did not obtain the expected reward (see Fig. 11.16). Control tasks showed that the response was related to the error, and the mismatch between what was expected and what was obtained, in that just showing an angry face expression did not selectively activate this part of the lateral orbitofrontal cortex. An interesting aspect of this study that makes it relevant to human social behavior is that the conditioned stimuli were faces of particular individuals, and the unconditioned stimuli were face expressions. Moreover, the study reveals that the human orbitofrontal cortex is very sensitive to social feedback when it must be used to change behavior (Kringelbach and Rolls, 2003, 2004).

Further, the right lateral orbitofrontal cortex is strongly activated by non-reward in a one-trial rule-based reward reversal task (Rolls et al., 2020e). In this reversal, after a reward has not been provided when it was expected, on the very next trial that the stimulus formerly associated with punishment is shown, that stimulus is selected (Thorpe, Rolls and Maddison, 1983; Rolls, Vatansever, Li, Cheng and Feng, 2020e). This shows that this is a non-associative, rule-based, process that cannot be accounted for by model-free reinforcement

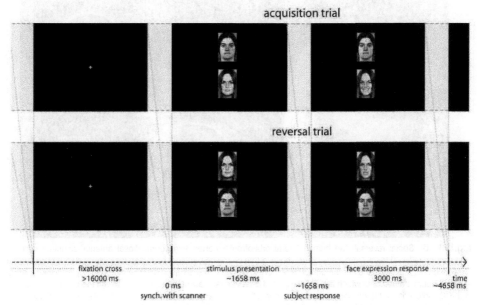

Fig. 11.15 Social reversal task: The trial starts synchronized with the scanner and two people with neutral face expressions are presented to the subject. The subject has to select one of the people by pressing the corresponding button, and the person will then either smile or show an angry face expression for 3000 ms depending on the current mood of the person. The task for the subject is to keep track of the mood of each person and choose the 'happy' person as much as possible (upper row). Over time (after between 4 and 8 correct trials) this will change so that the 'happy' person becomes 'angry' and vice versa, and the subject has to learn to adapt her choices accordingly (bottom row). Randomly intermixed trials with either two men, or two women, were used to control for possible gender and identification effects, and a fixation cross was presented between trials for at least 16000 ms. (Reprinted from Morten L. Kringelbach and Edmund T. Rolls (2003) Neural correlates of rapid reversal learning in a simple model of human social interaction. NeuroImage 20: 1371–83. © Elsevier Inc.)

learning (Rolls et al., 2020e). This is a function of the primate including human orbitofrontal cortex in a type of behavior that is not known to occur in rodents (Hervig et al., 2020), whose orbitofrontal cortex is very different (Rolls, 2019e) (Section 19.10).

One behavioral effect of not receiving reward is that it may be important to stop the behavior. One way to investigate this is in the stop-signal task, in which a signal is delivered on some trials indicating that the response being made should be stopped. In the stop-signal task, the lateral orbitofrontal cortex and the adjoining inferior frontal gyrus are both activated (Deng, Rolls et al (2017)). Impairments in the performance of the stop-signal task, which measures a type of motor impulsiveness, are associated with damage to the right inferior frontal gyrus (Aron, Robbins and Poldrack, 2014). It is proposed that one route by which non-reward can stop behavior is via the pathway from the lateral orbitofrontal cortex to the right inferior frontal gyrus (Rolls, Deco, Huang and Feng, 2023c; Rolls, Cheng, Du, Wei, Qiu, Dai, Zhou, Xie and Feng, 2020b; Du, Rolls, Cheng, Li, Gong, Qiu and Feng, 2020).

The hypotheses about the role of the orbitofrontal cortex in the rapid alteration of stimulus–reinforcer associations, and the functions more generally of the orbitofrontal cortex in human behavior, have been investigated in studies in humans with damage to the orbitofrontal cortex. In a visual discrimination reversal task, patients could learn to obtain points by touching one stimulus when it appeared on a video monitor, but had to withhold a response when a different visual stimulus appeared, otherwise a point was lost. After the subjects had acquired the visual discrimination, the reinforcement contingencies unexpectedly reversed. The patients with orbitofrontal lesions made more errors in the reversal (or in a similar extinction) task, and

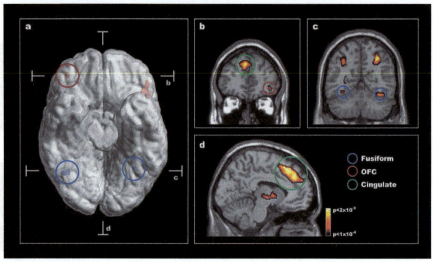

Fig. 11.16 Social reversal: the human lateral orbitofrontal cortex and supracallosal anterior cingulate cortex are activated on reversal trials. Composite figure showing that changing behavior based on face expression is correlated with increased brain activity in the human orbitofrontal cortex. a) The figure is based on two different group statistical contrasts from the neuroimaging data which are superimposed on a ventral view of the human brain with the cerebellum removed, and with indication of the location of the two coronal slices (b,c) and the transverse slice (d). The red activations in the orbitofrontal cortex (denoted OFC, maximal activation: z=4.94 [42 42 −8]; and z=5.51 [−46 30 −8] shown on the rendered brain arise from a comparison of reversal events with stable acquisition events, while the blue activations in the fusiform gyrus (denoted Fusiform, maximal activation: z>8 [36 −60 −20] and z=7.80 [−30 −56 −16]) arise from the main effects of face expression. b) The coronal slice through the frontal part of the brain shows the cluster in the right orbitofrontal cortex across all nine subjects when comparing reversal events with stable acquisition events. Significant activity was also seen in an extended area of the anterior cingulate/paracingulate cortex (denoted Cingulate, maximal activation: z=6.88 [−8 22 52]; green circle). c) The coronal slice through the posterior part of the brain shows the brain response to the main effects of face expression with significant activation in the fusiform gyrus and the cortex in the intraparietal sulcus (maximal activation: z>8 [32 −60 46]; and z>8 [−32 −60 44]). d) The transverse slice shows the extent of the activation in the anterior cingulate/paracingulate cortex when comparing reversal events with stable acquisition events. Group statistical results are superimposed on a ventral view of the human brain with the cerebellum removed, and on coronal and transverse slices of the same template brain (activations are thresholded at p=0.0001 for purposes of illustration to show their extent). (Reprinted from Morten L. Kringelbach and Edmund T. Rolls (2003) Neural correlates of rapid reversal learning in a simple model of human social interaction. NeuroImage 20: 1371–83. © Elsevier Inc.)

completed fewer reversals, than control patients with damage elsewhere in the frontal lobes or in other brain regions (Rolls, Hornak, Wade and McGrath, 1994a) (see Fig. 11.17). A reversal deficit in a similar task in patients with ventromedial prefrontal cortex damage was also reported by Fellows and Farah (2003). In macaques orbitofrontal cortex lesions also impair object reversal learning (Murray and Izquierdo, 2007), with further evaluation of the effects of lesions of the orbitofrontal cortex in macaques provided by Rolls (2019e). Neurotoxic lesions of the macaque orbitofrontal cortex produce effects that are difficult to interpret (Murray and Rudebeck, 2018; Sallet et al., 2020), perhaps because these lesions have not always been based on knowledge of where neurons and activations related to reversal learning are found, and the difficulty of disabling all such orbitofrontal cortex neurons (Rolls, 2023b).

An important aspect of the findings of Rolls, Hornak, Wade and McGrath (1994a) was that the reversal learning impairment correlated highly with the socially inappropriate or disinhibited behavior of the patients (Fig. 11.17), and also with their subjective evaluation of the changes in their emotional state since the brain damage. The patients were not impaired at other types of memory task, such as paired associate learning. It is of interest that the patients can often verbalize the correct response, yet commit the incorrect action. This is consistent with the hypothesis that the orbitofrontal cortex is normally involved in executing behavior when the behavior is performed by evaluating the reinforcement associations of environmental stimuli (see below). The orbitofrontal cortex seems to be involved in this in both humans

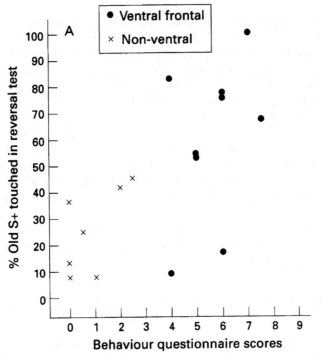

Fig. 11.17 Impaired visual discrimination reversal performance in humans with damage to the ventral part of the frontal lobe (orbitofrontal cortex). The task was to touch the screen when one image, the S+, was shown in order to obtain a point; and to refrain from touching the screen when a different visual stimulus, the S−, was shown in order to obtain a point. The scattergraph shows that during the reversal the group with ventral damage were more likely to touch the previously rewarded stimulus (Old S+), and that this was related to the score on a Behavior Questionnaire. Each point represents one patient in the ventral frontal group or in a control group. The Behavior Questionnaire rating reflected high ratings on at least some of the following: disinhibited or socially inappropriate behavior; misinterpretation of other people's moods; impulsiveness; unconcern about or underestimation of the seriousness of his condition; and lack of initiative. (Reproduced from E. T. Rolls, J.Hornak, D.Wade and J.McGrath (1994) Emotion-related learning in patients with social and emotional changes associated with frontal lobe damage. Journal of Neurology, Neurosurgery and Psychiatry 57: 1518–25. © BMJ Publishing Group Ltd.)

and non-human primates, when the learning must be performed rapidly, in, for example, acquisition, and during reversal.

To seek positive confirmation that effects on stimulus–reinforcer association learning and reversal were related to orbitofrontal cortex damage rather than to any other associated pathology, a different reversal-learning task was used with a group of patients with discrete, surgically produced, lesions of the orbitofrontal cortex. In the new visual discrimination task (the same as that used in our monetary reward functional neuroimaging task, O'Doherty, Kringelbach, Rolls, Hornak and Andrews (2001a)), two stimuli are always present on the video monitor and the patient obtains 'monetary' reward by touching the correct stimulus, and loses 'money' by touching the incorrect stimulus. This design controls for an effect of the lesion in simply increasing the probability that any response will be made (cf. Aron et al. (2003) and Clark et al. (2004)). The task also used probabilistic amounts of reward and punishment on each trial, to make it harder to use a verbal strategy with an explicit rule. It was found that a group of patients with bilateral orbitofrontal cortex lesions were severely impaired at the reversal task, in that they accumulated less money (Hornak, O'Doherty, Bramham, Rolls, Morris, Bullock and Polkey, 2004). These patients often failed to switch their choice of stimulus after a large loss; and often did switch their choice even though they had just received a reward, and this was quantified in a later study (Berlin, Rolls and Kischka, 2004). The importance of the failure to rapidly learn about the value of stimuli from negative feedback has also been described as a critical difficulty for patients with orbitofrontal cortex lesions (Fellows, 2007; Wheeler and Fellows, 2008; Fellows, 2011), and has been contrasted with the effects of lesions to the anterior cingulate cortex which impair the use of feedback to learn about actions (Fellows, 2011; Camille et al., 2011) (see Chapter 12).

We have seen in this section that orbitofrontal cortex non-reward neurons are important in reward-related decision-making, and that damage to this system is associated with impairments in emotion and social behavior in humans. Further analyses of how the orbitofrontal cortex operates during decision-making are described by Rolls (2019e). For example, evidence is described that different rewards (such as flavor and a thermal stimulus applied to the hand) are scaled to the same range in the orbitofrontal cortex (Grabenhorst, D'Souza, Parris, Rolls and Passingham, 2010a), which helps with the decision-making mechanisms implemented in the orbitofrontal cortex / ventromedial prefrontal cortex described below. In Section 18.5 the concepts described here are extended to depression, which is related to the functions of the lateral orbitofrontal cortex in responding to non-reward, which can be associated with depressive feelings.

11.3.5 The human medial orbitofrontal cortex represents rewards, and the lateral orbitofrontal cortex non-reward and punishers

Activations found in functional neuroimaging studies by many types of reward appear to involve relatively medial parts of the human orbitofrontal cortex, and unpleasant stimuli or non-reward more lateral parts of the human orbitofrontal cortex (Grabenhorst and Rolls, 2011; Rolls, 2014a; Kringelbach and Rolls, 2004; Rolls, 2019f; Rolls et al., 2020a; Xie et al., 2021). For example, we have obtained evidence from an experiment using pleasant, painful and neutral somatosensory stimulation that there is some spatial segregation of the representation of rewards and punishers, where the effects of pleasant somatosensory stimulation are spatially dissociable from the effects of painful stimulation in the human orbitofrontal cortex (Rolls, O'Doherty, Kringelbach, Francis, Bowtell and McGlone, 2003d). Further, pleasant odors activate medial, and unpleasant odors lateral, regions of the human orbitofrontal cortex (Rolls, Kringelbach and De Araujo, 2003c). Another example comes from the finding that the administration of amphetamine to naive human subjects activates the orbitofrontal cortex and two regions to which it projects the pregenual cingulate cortex and ventral striatum (Völlm, De Araujo, Cowen, Rolls, Kringelbach, Smith, Jezzard, Heal and Matthews, 2004) (Fig. 11.22). An indication that a rewarding effect is being produced by the amphetamine in part because of an action in the orbitofrontal cortex is that macaques will self-administer amphetamine to the orbitofrontal cortex (Phillips, Mora and Rolls, 1981). A clear indication of a differentiation in function between medial versus lateral areas of the human orbitofrontal cortex was found in our study investigating visual discrimination reversal learning, which showed a clear dissociation between the medial orbitofrontal areas correlating with monetary gain, and the lateral areas correlating with monetary loss (O'Doherty, Kringelbach, Rolls, Hornak and Andrews, 2001a). This result, and some of the other studies included in a meta-analysis (Kringelbach and Rolls, 2004), can be interpreted as evidence for a difference in humans between medial orbitofrontal cortex areas involved in decoding and monitoring the reward value of reinforcers, and lateral areas involved in evaluating punishers that when detected may lead to a change in current behavior. A good example of a study showing the latter involved a visual discrimination reversal task in which face identity was associated with a face expression (Kringelbach and Rolls, 2003). When the face expression associated with one of the faces reversed and the face expression was being interpreted as a punisher and indicated

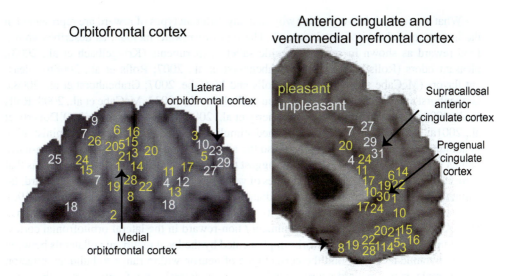

Fig. 11.18 Subjective pleasure is correlated with activations (yellow) in the human medial orbitofrontal cortex and pregenual anterior cingulate and ventromedial prefrontal cortex. Subjective unpleasantness is correlated with activations (white) in the human lateral orbitofrontal cortex and supracallosal anterior cingulate cortex. Yellow: sites where activations correlate with subjective pleasantness. White: sites where activations correlate with subjective unpleasantness. The numbers refer to effects found in specific studies. Taste: 1, 2; odor: 3-10; flavor: 11-16; oral texture: 17, 18; chocolate: 19; water: 20; wine: 21; oral temperature: 22, 23; somatosensory temperature: 24, 25; the sight of touch: 26, 27; facial attractiveness: 28, 29; erotic pictures: 30; laser-induced pain: 31. (Modified from Fabian Grabenhorst and Edmund T. Rolls (2011) Value, pleasure and choice in the ventral prefrontal cortex. Trends in Cognitive Sciences 15: 56–67. © Elsevier Ltd.)

that behavior should change, then lateral parts of the orbitofrontal cortex became activated (Fig. 11.16).

At sites where positive value, produced by a reward, are represented, there are, when they are measured, correlations between the conscious, subjective, state of pleasure and the brain activations, where both are measured on every trial. Similarly, at sites where negative value, produced by a punisher or non-reward, are represented, there are correlations between the subjective state of unpleasantness and the brain activations. Fig. 11.18 shows the peaks of the correlations found in many different investigations related to these subjective states of pleasantness (yellow) and of unpleasantness (white) for both the orbitofrontal and the cingulate and ventromedial prefrontal cortices (see also Chapter 12) (Grabenhorst and Rolls, 2011).

Although our study on abstract reward found that monetary reward and punishment are correlated with activations in different regions of the orbitofrontal cortex (O'Doherty, Kringelbach, Rolls, Hornak and Andrews, 2001a), even this evidence does not show that rewards and punishers have totally separate representations in the human brain. In particular, the medial regions of the orbitofrontal cortex that had activations correlating with the magnitude of monetary reward (area 11) also reflected monetary punishers in the sense that the activations in these medial regions correlated positively with the magnitude of monetary wins and negatively with losses. Similarly, the more lateral regions (area 10) had activations that correlated negatively with the magnitudes of monetary wins and gains, and positively with monetary loss/punishment. This means that in this experiment the medial and lateral regions were apparently coding for both monetary reward and punishment (albeit in opposite ways). An investigation by Xie, Jia, Rolls et al (2021) with 1,877 participants supports this (Fig. 11.9). Further evidence for the same principle, but now for pleasant vs unpleasant odors, is illustrated in Fig. 5.4 (Rolls et al., 2003c).

What account might we give for why so many different types of reward are represented in the human medial orbitofrontal cortex? [The types of reward include, as described above, food reward as shown in sensory-specific satiety experiments (Kringelbach et al., 2003), pleasant odors (Rolls et al., 2003c; Grabenhorst et al., 2007; Rolls et al., 2008b), pleasant flavors (McCabe and Rolls, 2007; Rolls and McCabe, 2007; Grabenhorst et al., 2008a; Grabenhorst and Rolls, 2008), pleasant touch (Rolls et al., 2003d; McCabe et al., 2008; Rolls et al., 2008a), face attractiveness (O'Doherty et al., 2003b), monetary reward (O'Doherty et al., 2001a; Rolls et al., 2008e), conditioned stimuli associated with drug self-administration in addicts (Childress et al., 1999), and also the administration of amphetamine to drug-naive human subjects (Völlm et al., 2004).] I suggest that part of the functional utility of this is that there can be comparison of the magnitudes of what may be quite different types of reward, facilitated by the local lateral inhibition mediated via the inhibitory interneurons (Rolls, 2019e).

I suggest that another part of the utility of functional segregation of reward in the human medial orbitofrontal cortex, and punishment / non-reward in the lateral orbitofrontal cortex, is that this enables attractor networks implemented by the local recurrent collaterals between nearby pyramidal cells to find the correct type of neuron within range to build an attractor, For example, if non-reward neurons tend to be in the lateral orbitofrontal cortex, they may be more likely to find neurons nearby that also respond to non-reward, and then to build a non-reward attractor because of their connections and their co-activity during non-reward. As we have seen, there is evidence for non-reward attractors in the orbitofrontal cortex (Fig. 11.14); and they are likely to be useful because keeping the non-reward state active for at least a few seconds if not longer can help with subsequent behavior on the next few trials; with resetting a rule-based attractor (Section 11.5.4); and with maintaining an emotional state, such as frustrative non-reward, active for at least a short time, which is likely to be evolutionarily adaptive.

In this context, it is interesting that the medial orbitofrontal cortex has strong connectivity with the pregenual anterior cingulate cortex, and that the lateral orbitofrontal cortex has strong connectivity with the supracallosal anterior cingulate cortex (Hsu et al., 2020; Rolls et al., 2019; Du et al., 2020). Perhaps this has the same function, of keeping reward and non-reward systems separate in the anterior cingulate cortex to help in the maintenance of attractors; and to facilitate this by connecting non-reward parts of the orbitofrontal cortex and anterior cingulate together to help the reciprocal connections maintain non-reward attractors. This arrangement may help to make emotional states persist for some time.

11.3.6 Decision-making in the orbitofrontal / ventromedial prefrontal cortex

We have shown that patients with damage to the orbitofrontal cortex are impaired in decision-making tasks, and that a key part of the impairment is that they continue to choose a previously rewarded stimulus when it is no longer rewarded in the reversal of a visual discrimination task (Rolls, Hornak, Wade and McGrath, 1994a). This has been confirmed (Fellows and Farah, 2003). In a probabilistic reversal learning task, patients with surgically induced and therefore localized lesions of the orbitofrontal cortex were impaired, and often failed to switch their choice of stimulus after a large loss; and often did switch their choice even though they had just received a reward (Hornak, O'Doherty, Bramham, Rolls, Morris, Bullock and Polkey, 2004), and this has been further quantified (Berlin, Rolls and Kischka, 2004). The deficit has been related to the inability to respond correctly to non-reward, as described in Section 11.3.4. The importance of the failure to rapidly learn about the value of stimuli from negative feedback as a critical difficulty for patients with orbitofrontal cortex lesions has been confirmed (Fellows, 2007; Wheeler and Fellows, 2008; Fellows, 2011).

Bechara and colleagues also have findings that are consistent with those described above in patients with frontal lobe damage when they perform the Iowa gambling task (Bechara et al., 1994, 1996, 1997; Damasio, 1994; Bechara et al., 2005; Glascher et al., 2012). Fellows and Farah (2005) found that patients with ventromedial prefrontal or with dorsolateral frontal lobe damage were impaired on the Iowa gambling task, yet only the orbitofrontal / ventromedial frontal damage group had a reversal deficit. Moreover the deficit on the gambling task of the orbitofrontal / ventromedial prefrontal patients was related to the fact that in the Iowa gambling task the first few choices of a high-risk deck are rewarded, and that later, when a large loss is received from a high-risk deck, an implicit reversal is required. Thus the deficit of patients with orbitofrontal cortex / ventromedial prefrontal cortex damage in the gambling task may be related at least in part to their failure to perform stimulus–reinforcer association reversal learning, rather than for other reasons. Further, reversal learning may more precisely measure the learning difficulty of patients with orbitofrontal cortex damage than the Iowa gambling task.

In fMRI studies, there is evidence that the orbitofrontal cortex itself represents value on a continuous scale, with the BOLD signal linearly related to pleasantness ratings, whereas a more anterior and medial region, which includes part of medial area 10 and is sometimes termed ventromedial prefrontal cortex, is activated when choices must be made between rewards (Grabenhorst et al., 2008b; Rolls et al., 2010d; Rolls and Grabenhorst, 2008). This was shown in tasks in which decisions were about the pleasantness of olfactory (Rolls, Grabenhorst and Parris, 2010d) or thermal (Grabenhorst, Rolls and Parris, 2008b) stimuli, compared to making ratings of pleasantness about the same stimuli.

Following up on these findings, a biologically plausible integrate-and-fire model of decision-making was used to make predictions of the fMRI signature of decision-making. (The decision-making model is described in Sections 11.5.1 and 11.5.2.) One key prediction was that the fMRI BOLD signal would be linearly related to the difference in magnitude between the decision variables (ΔI) in brain regions where choice decisions were being made. If the difference is large, the decision-making is easy, and participants have confidence in their decision even before the outcome is known.

Figure 11.19 shows experimental data with the fMRI BOLD signal measured on easy and difficult trials of the olfactory affective decision task (left) and the thermal affective decision task (right) (Rolls, Grabenhorst and Deco, 2010b). The upper records are for prefrontal cortex medial area 10 in a region identified by the following criterion as being involved in choice decision-making. The criterion was that a brain region for identical stimuli should show more activity when a choice decision was being made than when a rating on a continuous scale of affective value was being made. Figure 11.19 shows for ventromedial prefrontal cortex area 10 that there is a larger BOLD signal on easy than on difficult trials. The top diagram shows the medial prefrontal area activated in this contrast for decisions about which olfactory stimulus was more pleasant (yellow), and for decisions about whether the thermal stimulus would be chosen in future based on whether it was pleasant or unpleasant (red). Moreover, there was an approximately linear relation between the BOLD signal and ΔI for both the olfactory pleasantness and the thermal pleasantness decision-making tasks, as predicted by the model of decision-making. The neuronal network decision-making model could also predict the BOLD signal on error trials (Rolls, Grabenhorst and Deco, 2010c).

Thus there is evidence both from lesions and from fMRI that decisions between different rewards are made in the ventromedial prefrontal cortex (vmPFC) / anterior orbitofrontal cortex. The theory about how the decisions are made by an attractor decision-making network is described in Section 11.5.1. The finding of the signature of this type of decision-making network in a brain region implicated in the decision-making by larger activations when deci-

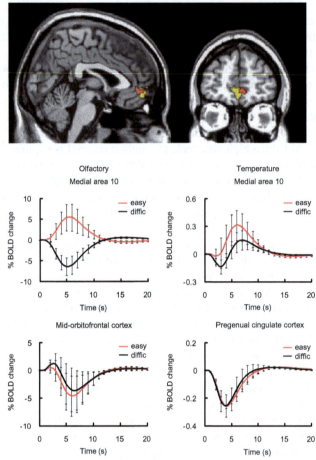

Fig. 11.19 The ventromedial prefrontal cortex area 10 (VMPFC) is implicated in reward-related decision-making. Top: Medial prefrontal cortex area 10 / VMPFC area activated on easy vs difficult trials in the olfactory pleasantness decision task (yellow) and the thermal pleasantness decision task (red). Middle: experimental data showing the BOLD signal in medial area 10 on easy and difficult trials of the olfactory affective decision task (left) and the thermal affective decision task (right). This medial area 10 was a region identified by other criteria (see text) as being involved in choice decision-making. Bottom: The BOLD signal for the same easy and difficult trials, but in parts of the pregenual cingulate and mid-orbitofrontal cortex implicated by other criteria (see text) in representing the subjective reward value of the stimuli on a continuous scale, but not in making choice decisions between the stimuli, or about whether to choose the stimulus in future. (Reprinted from Edmund T. Rolls, Fabian Grabenhorst, and Gustavo Deco (2010) Choice, difficulty, and confidence in the brain. NeuroImage 53: 694–706. © Elsevier Inc.)

sions were being made than when ratings of the identical stimuli were being made provides support for this theory and model of decision-making in the brain (Rolls and Deco, 2010).

11.3.7 The ventromedial prefrontal cortex and memory

Damage to the ventromedial prefrontal cortex (vmPFC) has been found to impair the ability to retrieve vivid autobiographical memories and imagine scenes (McCormick, Ciaramelli, De Luca and Maguire, 2018; Bonnici and Maguire, 2018). These patients are unlike patients with hippocampal damage, who do not have the differences in emotion that are characteristic of patients with damage to the ventromedial prefrontal cortex and orbitofrontal cortex. A characterisation of the difference is that patients with vmPFC damage have an inability to initiate internal reflections, including mental visualizations of extended events, while hippocampal patients seem able to initiate mental events but they are devoid of visual representations of scenes (McCormick et al., 2018). Patients with vmPFC damage show a reduced frequency of mind-wandering and, on the occasions when mind-wandering had occurred, there was a reduced focus on future-oriented thoughts and an increased focus on present-related thought (McCormick et al., 2018).

It has been proposed that part of the reason for difficulties with autobiographical memories in patients with ventromedial prefrontal cortex damage is that the emotional, reward-related, aspects of autobiographical memory will be diminished (Rolls, 2022b). There are connections between the orbitofrontal cortex / vmPFC and the medial temporal lobe and hippocampal system, by both the ventral and dorsal routes, as shown in Figs. 9.1 and 11.28. Given that the emotional context is often part of autobiographical memory, it could be that without this component of autobiographical memory for use in the hippocampal memory system, the hippocampal memory system operates less well in retrieving memories. That would leave as the remaining components scenes, objects and temporal order, as described in Chapter 9. The hippocampal attractor network in CA3 may operate less effectively in recall when one of its major inputs, from the orbitofrontal / ventromedial prefrontal cortex, is absent. Without that input, the hippocampal recall system may receive insufficient input to implement recall properly: the input may be too incomplete to allow for completion by CA3 (Rolls, 2022b).

However, it is also the case that the vmPFC with its inputs from the orbitofrontal cortex may have a special role in memory, because the vmPFC does have strong connections (Morecraft et al., 1992) and connectivity in humans (Rolls et al., 2023c) (see Fig. 11.28) with the posterior cingulate cortex and hippocampal memory system. It has further been proposed (Rolls, 2022b), based on investigations of the connectivity of these regions in humans (Rolls et al., 2023c), that the orbitofrontal cortex and its onward connectivity with the vmPFC and anterior cingulate cortex, play important roles in memory consolidation. These roles include modulation of cholinergic pathways that connect in part via the fornix with the hippocampal system, and with the neocortex; and increasing the depth of processing for episodic memories with some value component, both of which are important in memory consolidation (Rolls, 2022b) (Section 9.2.8.5).

Further, the vmPFC also has connectivity in humans with the posterior cingulate cortex (Rolls et al., 2023c), which is involved in memory (Rolls et al., 2023i) (Chapter 12), and which also receives from the anterior thalamic nuclei, which receive inputs from the mammillo-thalamic tract. The mammillary bodies receive inputs from the hippocampal system via the fornix (and from the vestibular system), and are part of a subcortical system damage to which can impair memory (Bubb, Kinnavane and Aggleton, 2017). That may fit with the observation that neurons in the macaque anterior thalamic nuclei respond to familiar stimuli in a running recognition task (Rolls, Perrett, Caan and Wilson, 1982d). It also fits with the persistent interest in subcortical pathways that include the fornix, mammillary bodies, and anterior thalamic nuclei related to the hippocampal system that somehow relate to the functions of the hippocampal system in memory (Bubb, Kinnavane and Aggleton, 2017; Mathiasen, O'Mara and Aggleton, 2020; Aggleton, Nelson and O'Mara, 2022; Aggleton and O'Mara, 2022). However, the subcortical pathways do not have the network architecture to perform memory-related computations with high memory capacity that cortical regions including the hippocampus do have, as described in Chapter 9 (Rolls, 2018b). For example, thalamic nuclei probably mainly implement a high pass filter because of the local lateral inhibition provided for by the inhibitory interneurons, as in the lateral geniculate nucleus where this is understood (see Chapter 2 and Rolls and Deco (2002)). These subcortical pathways may thus affect how well the memory-related computations are performed in the hippocampal system (Chapter 9), but are most unlikely to perform the memory storage and recall computational operations.

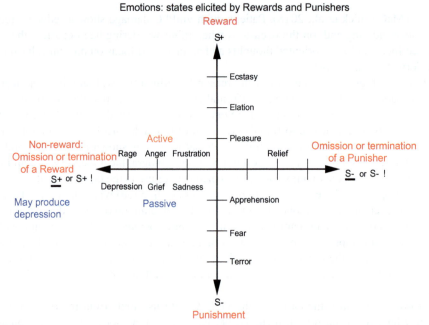

Fig. 11.20 Some of the emotions associated with different reinforcement contingencies are indicated. Intensity increases away from the centre of the diagram, on a continuous scale. The classification scheme created by the different reinforcement contingencies consists with respect to the action of (1) the delivery of a reward (S+), (2) the delivery of a punisher (S−), (3) the omission of a reward (S+) (extinction) or the termination of a reward (S+!) (time out), and (4) the omission of a punisher (S−) (avoidance) or the termination of a punisher (S−!) (escape). Note that the vertical axis describes emotions associated with the delivery of a reward (up) or punisher (down). The horizontal axis describes emotions associated with the non-delivery of an expected reward (left) or the non-delivery of an expected punisher (right). For the contingency of non-reward (horizontal axis, left) different emotions can arise depending on whether an active action is possible to respond to the non-reward, or whether no action is possible, which is labelled as the passive condition. In the passive condition, non-reward may produce depression. The diagram summarizes emotions that might result for one reinforcer as a result of different contingencies. Every separate reinforcer has the potential to operate according to contingencies such as these. This diagram does not imply a dimensional theory of emotion, but shows the types of emotional state that might be produced by a specific reinforcer. Each different reinforcer will produce different emotional states, but the contingencies will operate as shown to produce different specific emotional states for each different reinforcer.

11.3.8 The orbitofrontal cortex and emotion

We have seen that the orbitofrontal cortex is a key brain region involved in representing the reward and punishment value of stimuli. This makes it the key brain region involved in emotion, for emotions can be defined as states elicited by rewards and punishers, that is, by instrumental reinforcers (Rolls, 2014a, 2019e, 2018a, 2013d, 2005a, 1999a).

A reward is anything for which an animal will work. A punisher is anything that an animal will work to escape or avoid, or that will suppress actions on which it is contingent. The force of 'instrumental' in this definition is that the emotional states are seen as defining the goals for arbitrary behavioral actions, made to obtain the instrumental reinforcer. This is very different from classical conditioning, in which a response, typically autonomic, may be elicited to a stimulus, without any need for an intervening state. An important part of the function of emotion is to provide an intervening state, after for example the delivery of a non-reward, in which behavior can be reorganized, with perhaps a new action substituted for what was performed previously, in order to obtain the goal / reward (Rolls, 2014a).

An outline of a classification scheme for how different reinforcement contingencies (delivery of reward, omission or termination of reward, delivery of punishment, omission or termination of punishment) are related to different emotions is shown in Fig. 11.20 (Rolls, 2014a, 2023b). Movement away from the centre of the diagram represents increasing intensity of emotion, on a continuous scale. The diagram shows that emotions associated with the delivery of a reward (S+) include pleasure, elation and ecstasy. Of course, other emotional labels can be included along the same axis. Emotions associated with the delivery of a punisher (S–) include apprehension, fear, and terror (see Fig. 11.20). Emotions associated with the omission of a reward (S+) or the termination of a reward (S+!) include frustration, anger and rage. Emotions associated with the omission of a punisher (S–) or the termination of a punisher (S–!) include relief.

An important point about Fig. 11.20 is that there are a large number of different primary (unlearned, gene-specified) reinforcers, and that for example the reward label S+ shows states that might be elicited by just one type of reward, such as a pleasant touch. There will be a different reward axis (S+) and non-reward axis (S+ and S+!) for each type of reward (e.g. pleasant touch vs sweet taste); and, correspondingly, a different punisher axis (S–) and non-punisher axis (S– and S–!) for each type of punisher (e.g. pain vs bitter taste). Examples of the reinforcers include food reward, water reward, pleasant touch, pain, a potential mate, kin including children, and altruism, with many examples provided in Table 2.1 of *Emotion and Decision-Making Explained* (Rolls, 2014a) (available on line at https://www.oxcns.org) and by Rolls (2023b).

Previously neutral stimuli can become associated by learning with these primary reinforcers, and become secondary reinforcers, which thereby become goals for action. An example is the sight of a new food, which may become a secondary reinforcer by association between its sight and the primary reinforcer of its taste.

It is argued that brains are designed around reward and punishment value systems, because this is the way that genes can build a complex system that will produce appropriate but flexible behavior to increase their fitness (Rolls, 2014a). The way that evolution by natural selection does this is to build us with reward and punishment systems that will direct our behavior towards goals in such a way that survival and in particular reproductive fitness are achieved. By specifying goals, rather than particular responses, genes leave much more open the possible behavioral strategies that might be required to increase their fitness. Specifying particular responses would be inefficient in terms of behavioral flexibility as environments change during evolution, and also would be more genetically costly to specify (in terms of the information to be encoded and the possibility of error). This view of the evolutionary adaptive value for genes to build organisms using reward- and punishment-decoding and action systems in the brain places one squarely in line as a scientist developing ideas from Darwin (1859) onwards (Hamilton, 1964, 1996; Dawkins, 1976), and is a key part of Rolls' theory of emotion and motivation (Rolls, 2014a, 2013d, 2018a, 2019e, 2023b).

The theory helps in understanding much of sensory information processing in the cortex, followed by reward and punishment value encoding, followed by decision-making and action selection to obtain the goals identified by the sensory/reinforcer decoding systems. Value coding systems must be separate from purely sensory or motor systems, and while a goal is being sought, or if a goal is not obtained, the value-related representation must remain to direct further goal-directed behavior, and it is these continuing goal-related states to which emotion is related. The theory is strongly supported by the effects of damage to the orbitofrontal cortex, which impairs emotional feelings and behavior, face and voice expression recognition, and socially appropriate behavior, as well as reward reversal learning (Hornak, Rolls and Wade, 1996; Rolls, 1999b; Rolls, Hornak, Wade and McGrath, 1994a; Hornak, Bramham, Rolls, Morris, O'Doherty, Bullock and Polkey, 2003; Hornak, O'Doherty, Bramham, Rolls, Morris, Bullock and Polkey, 2004; Berlin, Rolls and Kischka, 2004; Berlin, Rolls and Iversen, 2005; Fellows and Farah, 2003; Camille, Tsuchida and Fellows, 2011).

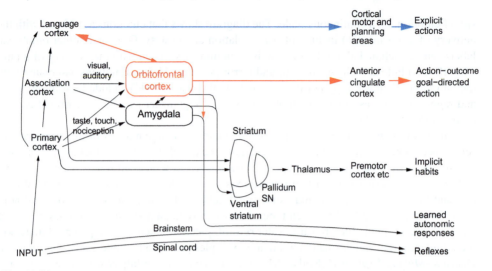

Fig. 11.21 Multiple routes to the initiation of actions and responses to rewarding and punishing stimuli in primates including humans. The lowest (spinal cord and brainstem) levels in the hierarchy are involved in reflexes, including for example reflex withdrawal of a limb to a nociceptive stimulus, and unlearned autonomic responses. The second level in the hierarchy involves associative learning in the amygdala and orbitofrontal cortex between primary reinforcers such as taste, touch and nociceptive stimuli and neutral stimuli such as visual and auditory stimuli from association cortex (e.g. inferior temporal visual cortex) to produce learned autonomic and some other behavioural responses such as approach. The anteroventral viscero-autonomic insula may be one link from the orbitofrontal cortex to autonomic output. A third level in the hierarchy is the route from the orbitofrontal cortex and amygdala via the basal ganglia especially the ventral striatum to produce implicit stimulus-response habits. A fourth level in the hierarchy important in emotion is from the orbitofrontal cortex to the anterior cingulate cortex for actions that depend on the value of the goal in action-outcome learning. For this route, the orbitofrontal cortex implements stimulus-reinforcer association learning, and the anterior cingulate cortex action-outcome learning (where the outcome refers to receiving or not receiving a reward or punisher). A fifth level in the hierarchy is from the orbitofrontal cortex (and much less the amygdala (Rolls et al., 2023b)) via multiple step reasoning systems involving syntax and language. Processing at this fifth level may be related to explicit conscious states. The fifth level may also allow some top-down control of emotion-related states in the orbitofrontal cortex by the explicit processing system. Pallidum / SN - the globus pallidus and substantia nigra. (After Rolls, E. T. 2023b. Emotion, motivation, decision-making, the orbitofrontal cortex, anterior cingulate cortex, and the amygdala. Brain Structure and Function)

A more full description of Rolls' theory of emotion is available in *Emotion and Decision-Making Explained* (Rolls, 2014a), *The Brain, Emotion, and Depression* (Rolls, 2018a), and in Rolls (2023b), all available for free download from https://www.oxcns.org.

11.3.9 Emotional orbitofrontal vs rational routes to action

The evidence in Section 11.3 provides a firm conceptual framework for understanding why the orbitofrontal cortex is so important in emotion, as considered also in Emotion and Decision-Making Explained (Rolls, 2014a). In this section (11.3.9), I show that at least in humans, there are other routes to action that can be invoked in emotion-related situations in which the orbitofrontal cortex may take a role in emotion and action, but not necessarily the whole or only role. Here rational refers to reasoning.

11.3.9.1 Some of the different routes to action produced by emotion-related stimuli

Fig. 11.21 shows several major routes to behavior related to emotional stimuli in primates including humans. An important point made by Fig. 11.21 is that there are multiple routes to output including to action that can be produced by stimuli that produce emotional states. Here emotional states are the states elicited by reward and punishing / non-reward stimuli, as illustrated in Fig. 11.20. The multiple routes are organized in a set of hierarchies, with each level in the system added later in evolution, but with all levels left in operation over the course of evolution (Rolls, 2016b, 2023b). The result of this is that a response such as an autonomic response to a stimulus that happens also to be rewarding might be produced by only the lower levels of the system operating, without necessarily the highest e.g. explicit levels being involved.

The lowest levels in the hierarchy illustrated in Fig. 11.21 are involved in reflexes, including for example reflex withdrawal of a limb to a nociceptive stimulus, and autonomic responses. The second level in the hierarchy can produce learned autonomic and some other behavioural responses to for example a previously neutral visual or auditory stimulus after it has been paired with, for example, a nociceptive or sweet taste stimulus. This route involves classical conditioning (Pavlovian learning) in the amygdala and orbitofrontal cortex. A third level in the hierarchy shown in Fig. 11.21 is the route from the orbitofrontal cortex and amygdala via the basal ganglia especially the ventral striatum to produce implicit stimulus-response habits with dopamine used to facilitate the stimulus-response associations (Chapter 16). A fourth level in the hierarchy that is important in emotion is from the orbitofrontal cortex to the anterior cingulate cortex for actions that depend on the value of the goal (Rolls, 2023b). The orbitofrontal cortex is involved in the stimulus-reward or stimulus-punishment (i.e. stimulus-stimulus) association learning, and the anterior cingulate cortex in the action-outcome learning, where the outcome is the reward or punisher that is or is not delivered. The emotional states implemented at this level may not necessarily be conscious. A fifth level in the hierarchy shown in Fig. 11.21 is from the orbitofrontal cortex (and much less the amygdala (Rolls et al., 2023b)) via multiple step reasoning systems involving syntax and language, which may be related to explicit conscious states (especially I argue if a higher order syntactic thought system for correcting lower order thoughts is involved) (Rolls, 2020a, 2008a, 2014a, 2023a) (see Section 19.6.3). Another route (shown in Fig. 11.28) involves providing goals to the hippocampal and related systems for navigation (Rolls et al., 2023c; Rolls, 2023c).

The route involving a **reasoning system** that may use some form of language with syntax (grammar) to plan several steps ahead is a focus in this Section. This route enables actions to be performed for completely different goals than those specified by genes as primary reinforcers that can use the earlier routes just described for output. This reasoning system is very important for understanding human emotion, because its decisions can be made in a completely different way, and do not necessarily lead to decisions that are consistent with those specified by the gene-defined reinforcers that are important in the first 'emotion-related' route to behavioral output. I argue in this Section that our reasoning system enables us to go beyond what 'Selfish Genes' might encourage (Dawkins, 1976), and that when we use the term 'free will', it is to the rational system that we may wish to refer, together with the non-deterministic, probabilistic, nature of brain computation that is described in Sections 11.5.1 and B.7 – B.8.3 (Rolls and Deco, 2010; Rolls, 2012e, 2014a, 2016b, 2020a). The orbitofrontal cortex has effective connectivity to the language areas via for example Broca's area, and this provides a route for the orbitofrontal cortex, and much less the amygdala, to introduce emotion / reward-related information into the explicit system (Rolls et al., 2023b,f,c).

I will give a simple example to make the point clear. Our genes may predispose us to like foods that are sweet and fatty (with modern supernormal examples ice cream and chocolate), and these may be rewarding to us because of the processes taking place in brain regions such as the orbitofrontal cortex and amygdala. But our reasoning system may know about discoveries in science and medicine that provide evidence that these foods may tend to promote obesity and poor health if eaten in quantity (Rolls, 2016g). So our reasoning system may enable us to override what our gene-based emotional system involving the orbitofrontal cortex urges, and instead to eat the healthy foods, for the potential advantage to the individual person of a healthy and long life.

11.3.9.2 Examples of some complex behaviors that may be performed implicitly

A starting point is that many actions can be performed relatively automatically, without apparent conscious intervention, that is implicitly (Rolls, 2020a).

An example sometimes given is driving a car for a short distance while the person may be thinking about something else.

Another example is the identification of a visual stimulus that can occur without conscious awareness if the stimulus is very short (as in backward masking) or weak (Rolls and Tovee, 1994; Rolls, 2003).

Another example is much of the sensory processing and actions that involve the dorsal stream of visual processing to the parietal cortex, such as a patient posting a letter through a letter box at the correct orientation even when the patient may not be aware of what the object is (Milner and Goodale, 1995; Goodale, 2004; Milner, 2008) because of damage to the ventral visual stream which implements object recognition (Rolls, 2016b).

Another example is blindsight, in which humans with damage to the visual cortex may be able to point to objects even when they are not aware of seeing an object (Weiskrantz, 1997, 1998, 2009).

Similar evidence applies to emotions, some of the processing for which can occur without conscious awareness (De Gelder et al., 1999; Phelps and LeDoux, 2005; LeDoux, 2008; LeDoux and Pine, 2016; LeDoux et al., 2018).

Consistent with the hypothesis of multiple routes to action, only some of which involve conscious awareness, is the evidence that split-brain patients may not be aware of actions being performed by the 'non-dominant' (typically right) hemisphere (Gazzaniga and LeDoux, 1978; Gazzaniga, 1988, 1995). An example is of split brain patients who when the 'non-dominant' right hemisphere was shown a picture of the left side of a house on fire (which would reach the right hemisphere) chose the non-burning house but said 'there is no specific reason for my choice', and 'the two houses are the same anyway'.

Also consistent with multiple, including non-verbal, routes to action, patients with focal brain damage, for example to the orbitofrontal cortex, may perform actions, yet comment verbally that they should not be performing those actions (Rolls, Hornak, Wade and McGrath, 1994a; Hornak, Bramham, Rolls, Morris, O'Doherty, Bullock and Polkey, 2003). In both these types of patient, confabulation may occur, in that a verbal account of why the action was performed may be given, and this may not be related at all to the environmental event that actually triggered the action (Gazzaniga and LeDoux, 1978; Gazzaniga, 1988, 1995; Rolls, Hornak, Wade and McGrath, 1994a).

11.3.9.3 A reasoning, rational, route to action

A reasoning-based, 'explicit', route to action in (at least) humans involves a computation with many 'if ... then' statements, to implement a plan to obtain a reward (Rolls, 2014a, 2019d, 2020a). In this case, the reward may actually be deferred as part of the plan, which might involve working first to obtain one reward, and only then to work for a second more highly valued reward, if this was thought to be overall an optimal strategy in terms of resource usage (e.g. time). In this case, syntax is required, because the many symbols (e.g. names of people) that are part of the plan must be correctly linked or bound. Such linking might be of the form: 'if A does this, then B is likely to do this, and this will cause C to do this ...'. The requirement of syntax for this type of planning implies that involvement of a syntactic system in the brain is required (see Fig. 11.21). **Thus the explicit language system in humans may allow working for deferred rewards by enabling use of a one-off, individual, plan appropriate for each situation.** This explicit system may allow immediate rewards to be deferred, as part of a long-term plan. This ability to defer immediate rewards and plan syntactically in this way for the long term may be an important way in which the explicit system extends the capabilities of the implicit emotion systems that respond more directly to rewards and punishers, or to rewards and punishers with fixed expectancies such as can be learned by reinforcement learning (Sections 19.5 and B.17).

Consistent with the point being made about evolutionarily old emotion-based decision systems vs a recent rational system present in humans (and perhaps other animals with syntactic processing) is that humans trade off immediate costs/benefits against cost/benefits that are delayed by as much as decades, whereas non-human primates have not been observed to engage in unpreprogrammed delay of gratification involving more than a few minutes (Rachlin, 1989; Kagel, Battalio and Green, 1995; McClure, Laibson, Loewenstein and Cohen, 2004; Rosati, 2017).

Another building block for such planning operations in the brain may be the type of short-term memory in which the prefrontal cortex is involved (Chapter 13). This short-term memory may be, for example in non-human primates, of where in space a response has just been made. A development of this type of short-term memory system in humans to enable multiple short-term memories to be held in place correctly, preferably with the temporal order of the different items in the short-term memory coded correctly, may be another building block for the multiple step 'if .... then' type of computation in order to form a multiple step plan. Such short-term memories are implemented in the (dorsolateral and inferior convexity) prefrontal cortex of non-human primates and humans (Goldman-Rakic, 1996; Petrides, 1996; Deco and Rolls, 2003; Rolls, 2016b), and may be part of the reason why prefrontal cortex damage impairs planning and executive function (Gilbert and Burgess, 2008; Shallice and Cipolotti, 2018; Rolls et al., 2023a).

We may examine some of the advantages and behavioral functions that language, present as the most recently added layer to the above system (Fig. 11.21), would confer.

One major advantage would be the ability to plan actions through many potential stages and to evaluate the consequences of those actions without having to perform the actions. For this, the ability to form propositional statements, and to perform syntactic operations on the semantic representations of states in the world, would be important.

Also important in this system would be the ability to have second-order thoughts about the type of thought that I have just described (e.g. I think that she thinks that ..., involving 'theory of mind'), as this would allow much better modelling and prediction of others' behavior, and therefore of planning, particularly planning when it involves others. Second-order thoughts are thoughts about thoughts. Higher-order thoughts refer to second-order, third-order, etc., thoughts about thoughts ... This capability for higher-order thoughts would also enable reflection on past events, which would also be useful in planning [16].

In contrast, non-linguistic behavior would be driven by learned reinforcement associations, learned rules etc., but not by flexible planning for many steps ahead involving a model of the world including others' behavior.

It is important to state that the language ability referred to here is not necessarily human verbal language (though this would be an example). What it is suggested is important to multiple step planning is the syntactic manipulation of symbols, and it is this syntactic

---

[16] A thought may be defined briefly as an intentional mental state, that is a mental state that is about something. Thoughts include beliefs, and are usually described as being propositional (Rosenthal, 2005). An example of a thought is "It is raining". A more detailed definition is as follows. A thought may be defined as an occurrent mental state (or event) that is intentional – that is a mental state that is about something – and also propositional, so that it is evaluable as true or false. Thoughts include occurrent beliefs or judgements. An example of a thought would be an occurrent belief that the earth moves around the sun / that Maurice's boat goes faster with two sails / that it never rains in southern California.

manipulation of symbols that is the sense in which language is defined and used here (Rolls, 2014a, 2004b; Fodor, 1994; Rolls and Deco, 2015a) (see Chapter 14).

Fig. 11.21 shows some direct connections from early cortical visual regions (such as the primary and secondary cortical areas in a hierarchy) to language regions, that bypass association cortical regions (such as the inferior temporal visual cortex). The reason for this suggestion is that explicit, declarative, reports about low-level features of sensory processing that may not be present in association cortical regions (such as the inferior temporal visual cortex where invariant representations with respect to for example position are formed (Rolls, 2021d)), are present in human subjective experience (Rolls, 2004b, 2011b, 2014a, 2020a).

In summary, I understand **reasoning, and rationality**, to involve syntactic manipulations of symbols. Reasoning thus typically may involve multiple steps of 'if ... then' conditional statements, all executed as a one-off or one-time process (see below), and is very different from associatively learned conditional rules typically learned over many trials, such as 'if yellow, a left choice is associated with reward'.

11.3.9.4 The Selfish Gene vs The Selfish Phenotype

I have provided evidence in the earlier part of this section (11.3.9) that there are two main types of route to decision-making and action. The first type of route selects actions by gene-defined goals for action, is closely associated with emotion, and involves brain systems such as the orbitofrontal cortex and cingulate cortex. The second type of route involves multistep planning and reasoning which requires syntactic processing to keep the symbols involved at each step separate from the symbols in different steps. (This second type of route is used by humans and perhaps by closely related animals.) Now the 'interests' of the first and second routes to decision-making and action are different. As argued convincingly by Richard Dawkins in *The Selfish Gene* (Dawkins, 1976, 1989), and by others (Hamilton, 1964; Ridley, 1993; Hamilton, 1996), many behaviors occur in the interests of the survival of the genes, not of the individual (nor of the group), and much behavior can be understood in this way.

I have extended this approach by arguing that an important role for some genes in evolution is to define the goals for actions that will lead to better survival of those genes; that emotions are the states associated with these gene-defined goals; and that the defining of goals for actions rather that actions themselves is an efficient way for genes to operate, as it leaves flexibility of choice of action open until the animal is alive (Rolls, 2014a). This provides great simplification of the genotype, as action details do not need to be specified, just rewarding and punishing stimuli; and also provides flexibility of action in the face of changing environments faced by the genes. Thus the interests that are implied when the first route to action (that typically involves the orbitofrontal and cingulate cortices) is chosen are those of the 'selfish genes', not those of the individual.

However, the second type of route to action allows, by reasoning, decisions to be taken that might not be in the interests of the genes, might be longer term decisions, and might be in the interests of the individual. An example might be a choice not to have children, but instead to devote oneself to science, medicine, music, or literature. The reasoning, rational, system presumably evolved because taking longer-term decisions involving planning rather than choosing a gene-defined goal might be advantageous at least sometimes for genes. But an unforeseen consequence of the evolution of the rational system might be that the decisions would, sometimes, not be to the advantage of any genes in the organism. After all, evolution by natural selection operates utilizing genetic variation like a Blind Watchmaker (Dawkins, 1986). In this sense, the interests when the second route to decision-making is used are at least sometimes those of the 'selfish phenotype'. Hence the decision-making referred to in this Section (11.3.9) is between a first system where the goals are gene-defined, and a second rational system in which the decisions may be made in the interests of the genes, or in the interests of the phenotype and not in the interests of the genes. Thus we may speak of the choice as sometimes being between the 'Selfish Genes' and the 'Selfish Phenes' (Rolls, 2014a).

Now what keeps the decision-making between the 'Selfish Genes' and the 'Selfish Phenes' more or less under control and in balance? If the second, rational, system chose too often for the interests of the 'Selfish Phene', the genes in that phenotype would not survive over generations. Having these two systems in the same individual will only be stable if their potency is approximately equal, so that sometimes decisions are made with the first route, and sometimes with the second route. If the two types of decision-making, then, compete with approximately equal potency, and sometimes one is chosen, and sometimes the other, then this is exactly the scenario in which stochastic processes in the decision-making mechanism are likely to play an important role in the decision that is taken. The same decision, even with the same evidence, may not be taken each time a decision is made, because of noise in the system.

The system itself may have some properties that help to keep the system operating well. One is that if the second, rational, system tends to dominate the decision-making too much, the first, gene-based emotional (orbitofrontal cortex) system might fight back over generations of selection, and enhance the magnitude of the reward value specified by the genes, so that emotions might actually become stronger as a consequence of them having to compete in the interests of the selfish genes with the rational decision-making process.

Another property of the system may be that sometimes the rational system cannot gain all the evidence that would be needed to make a rational choice. Under these circumstances the rational system might fail to make a clear decision, and under these circumstances, basing a decision on the gene-specified emotions involving the orbitofrontal cortex is an alternative. Indeed, Damasio (1994) argued that under circumstances such as this, emotions might take an important role in decision-making. In this respect, I agree with him, basing my reasons on the arguments above. He called the emotional feelings gut feelings, and, in contrast to me (Rolls, 2014a), hypothesized that actual feedback from the gut was involved. His argument seemed to be that if the decision was too complicated for the rational system, then send outputs to the viscera, and whatever is sensed by what the periphery sends back could be used in the decision-making, and would account for the conscious feelings of the emotional states. My reading of the evidence is that the feedback from the periphery is not necessary for the emotional decision-making, or for the feelings, nor would it be computationally efficient to put the viscera and more generally the periphery in the loop given that the information starts from the brain (Rolls, 2014a).

Another property of operation is that the interests of the second, rational, system, although involving a different form of computation, should not be too far from those of the gene-defined emotional system, for the arrangement to be stable in evolution by natural selection. One way that this could be facilitated would be if the gene-based goals felt pleasant or unpleasant in the rational system, and in this way contributed to the operation of the second, rational, system. This is something that I propose is the case. This provides an account of why rewards feel good (Rolls, 2014a).

11.3.9.5 Decision-making between the implicit and explicit systems

The question then arises of how decisions are made in animals such as humans that have both the implicit, direct reward-based, and the explicit, rational, planning systems (see Fig. 11.21). One particular situation in which the first, implicit, system may be especially important is when rapid reactions to stimuli with reward or punishment value must be made, for then the direct connections from structures such as the orbitofrontal cortex to the basal ganglia may allow rapid actions. Another is that when there may be too many factors to be taken into account easily by the explicit, rational, planning, system, then the implicit system may be used to guide action.

In contrast, when the implicit system continually makes errors, it would then be beneficial for the individual to switch from automatic, direct, action based on obtaining what the orbitofrontal cortex system decodes as being the most positively reinforcing choice currently available, to the explicit conscious control system that can evaluate with its long-term planning algorithms what action should be performed next. Indeed, it would be adaptive for the explicit system to be regularly assessing performance by the more automatic system, and to switch itself in to control behavior quite frequently, as otherwise the adaptive value of having the explicit system would be less than optimal.

Another factor that may influence the balance between control by the implicit and explicit systems is the presence of pharmacological agents such as alcohol, which may alter the balance towards control by the implicit system, may allow the implicit system to influence more the explanations made by the explicit system, and may within the explicit system alter the relative value it places on caution and restraint vs commitment to a risky action or plan.

There may also be a flow of influence from the explicit, verbal system to the implicit system, in that the explicit system may decide on a plan of action or strategy, and exert an influence on the implicit system that will alter the reinforcement evaluations made by and the signals produced by the implicit system. An example of this might be that if a pregnant woman feels that she would like to escape a cruel mate, but is aware that she may not survive in the jungle, then it would be adaptive if the explicit system could suppress some aspects of her implicit behavior towards her mate, so that she does not give signals that she is displeased with her situation[17]. Another example might be that the explicit system might, because of its long-term plans, influence the implicit system to increase its response to for example a positive reinforcer. One way in which the explicit system might influence the implicit system is by setting up the conditions in which, for example, when a given stimulus (e.g. person) is present, positive reinforcers are given, to facilitate stimulus–reinforcement association learning by the implicit system of the person receiving the positive reinforcers. Conversely, the implicit system may influence the explicit system, for example by highlighting certain stimuli in the environment that are currently associated with reward, to guide the attention of the explicit system to such stimuli.

However, it may be expected that there is often a conflict between these systems, in that the first, implicit, system is able to guide behavior particularly to obtain the greatest immediate reinforcement, whereas the explicit system can potentially enable immediate rewards to be deferred, and longer-term, multistep, plans to be formed. This type of conflict will occur in animals with a syntactic planning ability, that is in humans and any other animals that have the ability to process a series of 'if ... then' stages of planning. This is a property of the human language system, and the extent to which it is a property of non-human primates is not yet fully clear. In any case, such conflict may be an important aspect of the operation of at least the human mind, because it is so essential for humans to decide correctly, at every moment, whether to invest in a relationship or a group that may offer long-term benefits, or whether to pursue immediate benefits directly (Nesse and Lloyd, 1992).

Decision-making as implemented in neural networks in the brain is now becoming understood, and is described in Sections 11.5.1, B.6.3, B.8.2 and B.8.3. As shown there, two attractor states, each one corresponding to a decision, compete in an attractor single network with the evidence for each of the decisions acting as biases to each of the attractor

---

[17] In the literature on self-deception, it has been suggested that unconscious desires may not be made explicit in consciousness (or actually repressed), so as not to compromise the explicit system in what it produces (Alexander, 1979; Trivers, 1985; Nesse and Lloyd, 1992).

states. The non-linear dynamics, and the way in which noise due to the random spiking of neurons makes the decision-making probabilistic, makes this a biologically plausible model of decision-making consistent with much neurophysiological and fMRI data (Wang, 2002; Rolls and Deco, 2010; Deco, Rolls, Albantakis and Romo, 2013; Rolls, 2016b, 2021b).

I propose (Rolls, 2005a, 2014a) that this model applies to taking decisions between the implicit (unconscious) and explicit (conscious) systems in emotional decision-making, where the two different systems could provide the biasing inputs λ_1 and λ_2 to the model. An implication is that noise will influence with probabilistic outcomes which system takes a decision, depending on the magnitude of the competing inputs from the emotional and rational systems.

An additional way in which this type of decision-making might be influenced is by the reasoning, language-based, system exerting a top-down influence on the emotional system in the orbitofrontal cortex, to perhaps decrease the reward value represented in the orbitofrontal cortex (or perhaps to enhance the emotion-related orbitofrontal cortex representation, when for example listening to opera) (Rolls et al., 2023b,f,c).

When decisions are taken, sometimes confabulation may occur, in that a verbal account of why the action was performed may be given, and this may not be related at all to the environmental event that actually triggered the action (Gazzaniga and LeDoux, 1978; Gazzaniga, 1988, 1995; Rolls, 2014a; LeDoux, 2008; Rolls, 2012e, 2020a). It is accordingly possible that sometimes in normal humans when actions are initiated as a result of processing in a specialized brain region such as the orbitofrontal cortex involved in some types of rewarded behavior, the language system may subsequently elaborate a coherent account of why that action was performed (i.e. confabulate). This would be consistent with a general view of brain evolution in which, as areas of the cortex evolve, they are laid on top of existing circuitry connecting inputs to outputs, and in which each level in this hierarchy of separate input–output pathways may control behavior according to the specialized function it can perform (Rolls, 2016b). This hierarchical overlaying is an important concept for understanding emotion, the different brain systems involved in different aspects of emotion and decision-making, and the relation between the implicit and explicit systems (Rolls, 2014a). When a new layer is added, previous layers may lose some of their importance, as appears to occur in the taste system in which in primates the subcortical processing from the brainstem nucleus of the solitary tract is lost (Section 19.10); when the granular orbitofrontal cortex of primates becomes relatively more important than the amygdala (Rolls et al., 2023b); and when language areas are added on top of existing circuitry (Fig. 11.21) (Rolls, 2016b).

11.3.9.6 The emotional vs rational brain systems, and the strength of emotions in humans

Emotions often seem very intense in humans, indeed sometimes so intense that they produce behavior that does not seem to be adaptive, such as fainting instead of producing an active escape response, or freezing instead of avoiding, or vacillating endlessly about emotional situations and decisions, or falling hopelessly in love even when it can be predicted to be without hope or to bring ruin. The puzzle is not only that the emotion is so intense, but also that even with our rational, reasoning, capacities, humans still find themselves in these situations, and may find it difficult to produce reasonable and effective decisions and behavior for resolving the situation. The reasons for this include, I suggest, the following.

In humans, the reward and punishment brain systems may operate implicitly in comparable ways to those in other animals. But in addition to this, humans have the explicit system, which enables us consciously to look and predict many steps ahead (using language and syntax) the consequences of environmental events, and also to reflect on previous events (Rolls, 2014a, 2018a, 2019d, 2020a). The consequence of this explicit processing is that we can see the full impact of rewarding and punishing events, both looking ahead to see how this will impact us, and reflecting back to previous situations that we can see may never be repeated. For example, in humans grief occurs with the loss of a loved one, and this may be much more intense than might occur simply because of failure to receive a positively reinforcing stimulus, because we can look ahead to see that the person will never be present again, can process all the possible consequences of that, and can remember all the previous occasions with that person. In another example, someone may faint at the sight of blood, and this is more likely to occur in humans because we appreciate the full consequences of major loss of blood, which we all know is life-threatening.

Thus what happens is that reinforcing events may have a very much greater reinforcing value in humans than in other animals, because we have so much cognitive, especially linguistic, processing that leads us to evaluate and appreciate many reinforcing events far more fully than can other animals. Thus humans may decode reinforcers to have supernormal intensity relative to what is usual in other animals, and the supernormal appreciated intensity of the decoded reinforcers leads to super-strong emotions. The emotional states can then be so strong that they are not necessarily adaptive, and indeed language has brought humans out of the environmental conditions under which our emotional systems evolved. For example, the autonomic responses to the sight of blood may be so strong, given that we know the consequences of loss of blood, that we faint rather than helping. Another example is that panic and anxiety states can be exacerbated by feeling the heart pounding, because we are able to use our explicit processing system to think and worry about all the possible causes. One can think of countless other examples from life, and indeed make up other examples, which of course is part of what novelists do (Rolls, 2012e, 2018a).

A second reason for such strong emotions in humans is that the stimuli that produce emotions may be much stronger than those in which our emotional systems evolved. For example, with man-made artefacts (such as cars and guns that may injure many people simultaneously, or a large bus speeding towards one, both of which produce super-normal stimuli), the sights and related stimuli that can be produced in terms of damage to humans are much more intense than those present when our emotional systems evolved. In this way, the things we see can in some cases produce super-strong emotions.

A third reason for the intensely mobilizing, and sometimes immobilizing, effects of emotions in humans is that we can evaluate linguistically, with reasoning, the possible courses of action open to us in emotional situations. Because we can evaluate the possible effects of reinforcers many steps ahead in our plans, and because language enables us to produce flexible one-off plans for actions, and enables us to work for deferred rewards based on one-off plans (Rolls, 2014a, 2018a, 2019d, 2020a), the ways in which reinforcers are used in decision-making becomes much more complex than in those animals that cannot produce similar one-off plans using syntax. The consequence of this is that decision-making can become very difficult, with so many potential but uncertain reinforcement outcomes, that humans may vacillate. They are trying to compute by this explicit method the most favourable outcome of each plan in terms of the net reinforcements received, rather than using reinforcement implicitly to select the highest currently available reinforcer.

A fourth reason for complexity in the human emotional system is that there are, it is suggested, two routes to action for emotions in humans, an implicit (unconscious) and an explicit route. These systems may not always agree. The implicit system may tend to produce one type of behavior, typically for immediately available rewards. The explicit system may tend to produce another planned course of action to produce better deferred rewards. Conflict between these systems can lead to many difficult situations, will involve conscience (what is right as conceived by the explicit system) and the requirement to abide by laws (which assume a rational explicit system responsible for our actions). It appears that the implicit system does often control our behavior, as shown by the effects of frontal lobe damage in humans, which may produce deficits in reward-reversal tasks, even when the human can explicitly state the correct behavior in the situation. (The conflicts that arise between these implicit and explicit systems are again some of the very stuff on which novels in literature often capitalize (Rolls, 2018a)).

A fifth reason for complexity in the human emotional system is that we, as social animals, with major investments in our children who benefit from long-term parental co-operation, and with advantages to be gained from social alliances if the partners can be trusted, may be built to try to estimate the goals and reliability of those we know. For example, it may matter to a woman with children whether her partner has been attracted by / is in love with / a different woman, as this could indicate a reduction of help and provision. Humans may thus be very interested in the emotional lives of each other, as this may impact on their own lives. Indeed, humans will, for this sort of reason, be very interested in who is co-operating with whom, and gossip about this may even have acted as a selective pressure for the evolution of language (Dunbar, 2017). In these circumstances, fascination with unravelling the thoughts and emotions of others (using the capacity described as theory of mind (Frith and Frith, 2012)), and empathy which may facilitate this (Kanske, Bockler and Singer, 2017), would have adaptive value, though it is difficult computationally to model the minds and interactions of groups of other people, and to keep track of who knows what about whom, as this requires many levels of nested syntactical reference. Our resulting fascination with this, and perhaps the value of experience of as wide a range of situations as possible, may then be another reason why human emotions, and guessing others' emotions in complex social situations, may also be part of the stuff of novelists, playwrights, and poets. Indeed, it may be important for us to find it attractive to engage in this type of processing because of its potential adaptive value, and this may be part of the reason why we find drama, novels, and poetry so fascinating (Rolls, 2012e, 2018a).

A sixth reason for complexity in the human emotional system is that high level cognitive processing can reach down in to the emotional systems and influence how they respond. This was demonstrated in the experiment by De Araujo, Rolls et al. (2005) in which it was shown that processing at the linguistic level, in the form of a word label, can influence processing as far down in sensory processing as the secondary olfactory cortex in the orbitofrontal cortex, the first stage in cortical processing at which the reward- or punishment-related (hence affective) significance of stimuli is made explicit in the neuronal representations of stimuli (Section 5.2.7). This emphasizes the importance of cognitive influences on reward value and emotion, and shows how, in situations that might range from enjoying food to a romantic evening, the cognitive top-down influences can play an important role in influencing affective representations in the brain. Indeed, these findings lend support to the hypothesis that an interesting role for cognitive systems in emotion is to help set up the optimal conditions in terms of the reinforcers available and contextual surroundings for reinforcers to produce affective states.

11.3.9.7 The emotional systems in animals, and welfare

An implication of the above approach to emotion and motivation is that when considering animal welfare, it is likely to be important to take into account what value each species places on different rewards and the avoidance of possible aversive stimuli. This can in principle be measured by the choices that animals make between different rewards or avoiding different potential punishers. The procedures are well known in neuroeconomics, in which it is possible to measure for example how many drops of fruit juice A are chosen equally often as two drops of fruit juice B (Kuwabara et al., 2020; Cai and Padoa-Schioppa, 2019; Padoa-Schioppa and Conen, 2017; Rolls, 2014a; Cai and Padoa-Schioppa, 2012; Padoa-Schioppa and Cai, 2011; Padoa-Schioppa, 2011; Padoa-Schioppa and Assad, 2008; Padoa-Schioppa,

2007; Padoa-Schioppa and Assad, 2006; Platt et al., 2016; Yamada et al., 2018; Glimcher and Fehr, 2013; Dawkins, 2021). Similar titration procedures could be used to measure what value, measured by choice, a species places on for example food vs bedding vs having other animals nearby vs overcrowding vs being able to take a swim or shower vs being able to sit on a perch vs being able to reach a branch high above the ground vs being able to perform reproductive behavior, etc. When measuring these choices, it is important to ensure that the choice is being made by the goal-directed reward system for instrumental action, and not by any system involved in a reflex or fixed action pattern, or a learned habit (Rolls, 2023b).

Measuring instrumental goal-directed choices made by particular species may be useful to minimize over-anthropomorphic inferences about the value that a species may place on different 'goods' (the term used in neuroeconomics). Further, even the evidence taken from humans may need to be carefully assessed, for humans are able to provide reasons with their declarative system for their choices made with their syntactic learning system, but may confabulate reasons why they chose a good when the choice has been made by the emotional or by the automatic habit system (Gazzaniga and LeDoux, 1978; Rolls, 2020a, 2011b, 2010c, 2020a).

Another implication is that the taste, olfactory and food texture systems present in different species may result in adequate nutrition in their natural environment, but care may be needed to ensure in other environments that the nutrition being made available is appropriate. In this context, it must be remembered that animals do not have flavor mechanisms built to ensure that every possible nutrient needed is being selected by specific appetites for different nutrients. Instead, in the natural environment animals condition to new foods that provide useful nutrients by physiological effects that may occur some time after the food is ingested (Scott, 2011; Berthoud, Morrison, Ackroff and Sclafani, 2021) (Section 4.2.10).

A set of criteria for achieving good welfare in farm animals, known as the Five Freedoms (Farm Animal Welfare Council (2009)) consist of 1. Freedom from hunger and thirst. 2. Freedom from discomfort. 3. Freedom from pain, injury and disease. 4. Freedom to express normal behavior. 5. Freedom from fear and distress. The present approach suggests that when assessing (4), it will be useful to measure the value of the different types of 'normal behavior' to help assess priorities. The present approach suggests that when assessing (5), farm animals may often be protected from the fears, stressors, and predators that are present in the natural world, but that these provide a scale against which other fear and distress might be calibrated.

11.3.9.8 The orbitofrontal cortex and addiction

Most investigations of the neurobiology of addiction have focussed on habit-related stimulus-response effects mediated by dopamine and fronto-striatal circuitry (Everitt, Giuliano and Belin, 2018; Luscher, Robbins and Everitt, 2020; Compton, Wargo and Volkow, 2022), with opiate drugs also operating via the dopamine pathways (Galaj and Xi, 2021).

However, the administration of amphetamine to naive human participants activates the orbitofrontal cortex and two regions to which it projects, the pregenual anterior cingulate cortex and ventral striatum as illustrated in Fig. 11.22 (Völlm, De Araujo, Cowen, Rolls, Kringelbach, Smith, Jezzard, Heal and Matthews, 2004). An indication that a rewarding effect is being produced by the amphetamine in part because of an action in the orbitofrontal cortex is that macaques will self-administer amphetamine to the orbitofrontal cortex (Phillips, Mora and Rolls, 1981). This indicates that at least part of the reward and pleasure produced by the psychomotor stimulants may be being produced by activation of the medial orbitofrontal and pregenual anterior cingulate cortex, both of which receive dopamine inputs, and in both of which there are neurons and activations produced by natural rewards. Consistently, the orbitofrontal cortex as well as the areas to which it projects such as the ventral striatum are activated in cocaine (another psychomotor stimulant) addicts by exposure to drug-related

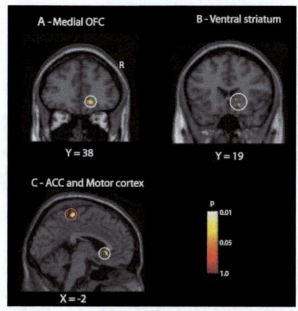

Fig. 11.22 Amphetamine activates the medial orbitofrontal cortex, ventral striatum, and anterior cingulate cortex in drug-naive human participants. The contrast is amphetamine - saline. Activations (shown within the white circles) were found in (a) the medial orbitofrontal cortex (OFC), (b) ventral striatum, and (c) anterior cingulate cortex (ACC), and motor cortex (red circle). The p-values shown are with the small volume correction procedure. (After Völlm, De Araujo, Cowen, Rolls, Kringelbach, Smith, Jezzard, Heal, and Matthews (2004). Methamphetamine activates reward circuitry in drug naive human subjects. Neuropsychopharmacology 29: 1715–1722.)

conditioned stimuli associated with the cocaine (Volkow et al., 2013; Koob and Volkow, 2016; Volkow et al., 2017).

Further, the (Pavlovian) conditioned cues that support addiction and may lead to relapse to addiction by Pavlovian-instrumental transfer (see Cardinal et al. (2002)) may operate in part via the orbitofrontal cortex, for Childress et al. (1999) have shown that cocaine-related cues shown visually in a video to addicts activate the orbitofrontal cortex, and also parts of the anterior cingulate and medial prefrontal cortex. Moreover, the orbitofrontal cortex activation in humans to these drug-conditioned cues can be decreased by baclofen, the GABA-B agonist (Childress et al., 1999). In rodents, cues associated by Pavlovian learning with drug administration also influence the prefrontal and cingulate cortices and related areas (Kelley and Berridge, 2002; Kelley, 2004).

These types of evidence suggest that the primate including human orbitofrontal cortex may play a role in addiction to at least some drugs. The computational hypotheses are as follows. (1) Unconditioned drug reinforcers including the psychomotor stimulants such as amphetamine and cocaine activate the medial orbitofrontal cortex, anterior cingulate cortex, and ventral striatum (Völlm et al., 2004). (2) To-be-conditioned stimuli, such as drug-associated visual stimuli, reach the orbitofrontal cortex via the inferior temporal visual cortex. (3) The visual stimuli become associated with the primary drug-related reinforcer in the orbitofrontal cortex by its stimulus-reinforcer association learning. The mechanism is pattern association learning (Section B.2). (4) When the conditioned visual stimulus is encountered in future, incentive motivation is produced, and this increases the likelihood that the drug will be selected despite what the rational (reasoning) system may be indicating. Incentive motivation is also known as the 'salted nut phenomenon', and was discussed by Hebb (1949). Incentive motivation refers to the fact that delivery of an incentive, e.g. the smell of bread cooking, increases the motivation to obtain bread. Incentive motivation is widely used in advertising, and has

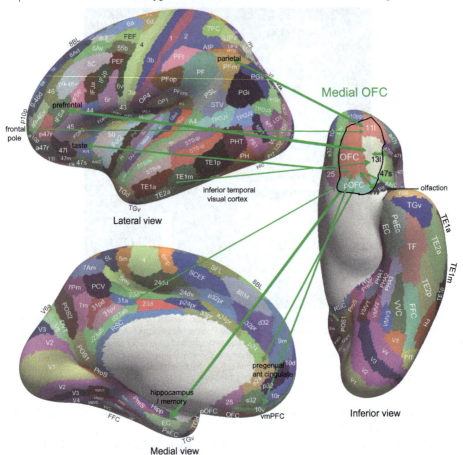

Fig. 11.23 Summary of the effective connectivity of the human medial orbitofrontal cortex. The medial orbitofrontal cortex has taste, olfactory and inferior temporal visual cortex inputs, and connectivity with the hippocampus, pregenual anterior cingulate cortex, ventromedial prefrontal cortex (vmPFC), posterior cingulate cortex (e.g. 31), parietal cortex, inferior prefrontal cortex, and frontal pole. The main regions with which the medial OFC has connectivity are indicated by names with the words in black font. The width of the arrows and the size of the arrow heads in each direction reflects the strength of the effective connectivity. The abbreviations are listed in Section 1.12. (From Rolls, E. T. 2023. Emotion, motivation, decision-making, the orbitofrontal cortex, anterior cingulate cortex, and the amygdala. Brain Structure and Function doi: 10.1007/s00429-023-02644-9)

been banned at the entrances to supermarkets in the UK because it has such a strong effect on choice. The evolutionary value of incentive motivation is that this introduces hysteresis into the reward selection system, which makes the selected actions more efficient by preventing continually switching between almost equal rewards (Rolls, 2014a). Incentive motivation is probably implemented in the orbitofrontal cortex, and occurs before sensory-specific satiety which is implemented in the orbitofrontal cortex (Section 4.2.5) (Rolls, 2014a). (5) Because drugs act on regions beyond where sensory-specific satiety is computed (which is implemented for example in the afferent synapses to the orbitofrontal cortex, Section 4.2.5), drugs are not subject to sensory-specific satiety, and that contributes to their prolonged reward value, because they are a type of reward to which sensory-specific satiety does not apply (Rolls, 2014a). (6) These orbitofrontal cortex processes may be important in the subjective pleasure that can be produced by addictive drugs via the lateral orbitofrontal cortex connectivity with language cortical regions (Rolls et al., 2023b,c), and via connections to the ventral striatum, anterior cingulate cortex, etc (Rolls, 2017c; Rolls et al., 2023b,c).

11.3.10 The connectivity of the human orbitofrontal cortex, and its relation to function

In this section evidence is described on the connectivity of the human orbitofrontal cortex, and its implications for functions (Rolls et al., 2023c,b). The evidence is based on use of the Human Connectome Project - Multimodal cortical Parcellation (HCP-MMP, Section 1.12), and measuring effective connectivity, complemented by functional connectivity and diffusion tractography (Section 1.13) with data from the Human Connectome Project. An example of an effective connectivity map to indicate the underlying measurements is provided in Fig. 12.8 from Rolls et al. (2023c).

11.3.10.1 Human medial orbitofrontal cortex connectivity

The medial orbitofrontal cortex regions defined in the HCP-MMP atlas are 11l, 13l, OFC, pOFC. A summary of the effective connectivity of the human medial orbitofrontal cortex is shown on Fig. 11.23, and the effective connectivity of examples for these regions are shown schematically for region pOFC in Fig. 11.24 and for region 13l in Fig. 11.25 (Rolls et al., 2023c,b).

Parts of the medial orbitofrontal cortex (11l, 13l, OFC and pOFC, which are interconnected) have effective connectivity with the taste/olfactory/visceral anterior agranular insular complex (AAIC); the piriform (olfactory) cortex; the entorhinal cortex (EC); the inferior temporal visual cortex (TE1p, TE2a, TE2p); superior medial parietal 7Pm; inferior parietal PF which is somatosensory (Rolls et al., 2023d); with parts of the posterior cingulate cortex (31pv, 7m, d23ab) related to memory (Rolls et al., 2023i); with the pregenual anterior cingulate cortex (s32, a24, p24, p32, d32) and much less with the supracallosal anterior cingulate cortex (only 33pr); with ventromedial prefrontal 10r, 10d and 9m; with the frontal pole (10pp, p10p, a10p); with lateral orbitofrontal cortex (47m, 47s, a47r); and dorsolateral prefrontal cortex (46 and a9-46v) (Rolls et al., 2023c) (Figs. 11.24 and 11.25). The connectivities are stronger towards the medial orbitofrontal cortex for the inferior temporal visual cortex and frontal pole regions. Medial orbitofrontal cortex regions also have effective connectivity directed towards the caudate nucleus and nucleus accumbens (Rolls et al., 2023c).

Region OFC is remarkable for effective connectivities directed towards more cortical regions than other parts of the medial orbitofrontal cortex, including somatosensory cortex regions 5L and 5m; the fusiform face area (FFC) and some other relatively early visual cortical areas; and some parietal areas including PGp, PGs, and some superior parietal parts of area 7 and intraparietal areas described elsewhere (Rolls et al., 2023d) (Chapter 10). Region OFC also has effective connectivity directed towards the substantia nigra pars compacta (SNpc) and ventral tegmental area (VTA) (Rolls et al., 2023c), which contain dopaminergic neurons.

Regions 11l and 13l have outputs directed to inferior prefrontal areas (IFS and IFJ regions) and to dorsolateral prefrontal areas 46 and a9-46v (Rolls et al., 2023f) both involved in short-term memory (Chapter 13).

pOFC is the only cortical area with effective connectivity directed to the nucleus basalis of Meynert which includes cholinergic neurons that project to the neocortex (Huang et al., 2022; Zaborszky et al., 2018, 2008).

The functional connectivity is generally consistent, adding some evidence for interactions with frontal opercular FOP4 which is probably taste-related, and the somatosensory insula (MI) (Rolls et al., 2023c,f). The diffusion tractography provides evidence that medial orbitofrontal cortex regions have direct connections with the anterior agranular insular complex (AAIC) which is probably taste/olfactory/visceral-related, and with the piriform cortex (Pir); with the hippocampal system; and with temporal pole TGd involved in semantic representations (Rolls et al., 2022b).

522 | The orbitofrontal cortex, amygdala, reward value, emotion, and decision-making

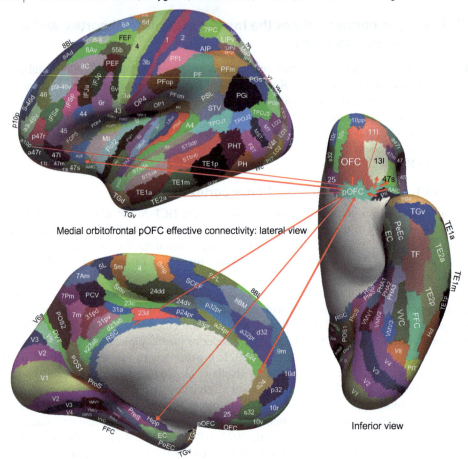

Fig. 11.24 Effective connectivity of the human medial orbitofrontal cortex region pOFC: schematic diagram. The width of the arrows reflects the effective connectivity with the size of the arrowheads reflecting the connectivity in each direction. One arrow in some cases reflects effective connectivity with several related regions: pregenual anterior cingulate a24, p24 and d32; RSC and 23d; frontal pole a10p and p10p. Effective connectivity is shown of pOFC with pyriform (olfactory) cortex Pir, taste cortex AVI and putative visceromotor cortex AAIC, inferior temporal cortex TE2a, pregenual anterior cingulate cortex; and to the hippocampus Hipp. The abbreviations are listed in Section 1.12. (From Rolls,E.T., Deco,G., Huang,C-C. and Feng,J. (2023) Human amygdala compared to orbitofrontal cortex connectivity, and emotion. Progress in Neurobiology 220: 102385.)

To synthesize, with further synthesis below, the medial orbitofrontal cortex is found in humans to have connectivity with regions at the ends of sensory processing hierarchies that provide evidence for 'what' stimulus is present, including taste, olfactory, visual and somatosensory brain systems. This is consistent with the functions described above of representing unlearned rewards; and learning stimulus-reward associations to implement expected value. The medial orbitofrontal cortex also has connectivity that enables it to provide inputs to memory systems, including the hippocampal memory system; and the pregenual cingulate cortex that has onward connectivity to the hippocampal memory system; and parts of the posterior inferior parietal cortex that are related to memory. The medial orbitofrontal cortex also has some connectivity with the supracallosal anterior cingulate cortex implicated in guiding actions to obtain rewards and avoid punishers in action-outcome learning (Chapter 12); and with the lateral orbitofrontal cortex.

What is computed in the orbitofrontal cortex | 523

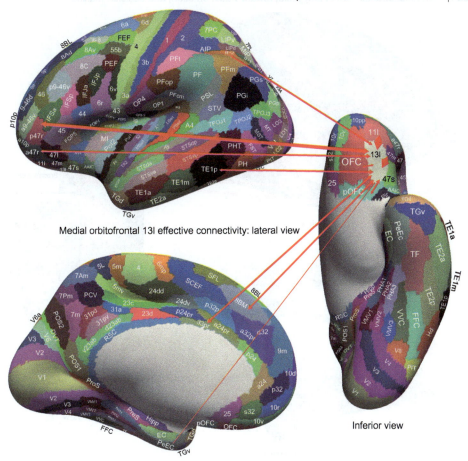

Medial orbitofrontal 13l effective connectivity: lateral view

Medial orbitofrontal 13l effective connectivity: medial view

Inferior view

Fig. 11.25 Effective connectivity of the human medial orbitofrontal cortex region 13l: schematic diagram. The width of the arrows reflects the effective connectivity with the size of the arrowheads reflecting the connectivity in each direction. One arrow reflects effective connectivity with several related regions: IFSa, a9-46v, p9-46v, and p47r. Inputs are shown to 13l from inferior temporal cortex TE1p; with other orbitofrontal cortex regions; with many lateral prefrontal cortex regions; and from 13l to the perirhinal cortex. The abbreviations are listed in Section 1.12. (From Rolls,E.T., Deco,G., Huang,C-C. and Feng,J. (2023) Human amygdala compared to orbitofrontal cortex connectivity, and emotion. Progress in Neurobiology 220: 102385.)

11.3.10.2 Human lateral orbitofrontal cortex connectivity

The lateral orbitofrontal cortex regions defined in the HCP-MMP atlas are 47s, 47l, a47r, p47r and 47m. A summary of the effective connectivity of the human lateral orbitofrontal cortex is shown on Fig. 11.26, and the effective connectivity of an example, 47s, is shown in Fig. 11.27 (Rolls et al., 2023c,b).

The lateral orbitofrontal cortex areas a47r, p47r and 47m share generally similar effective connectivities from the visual inferior temporal cortex (TE areas); from parts of the parietal cortex (PFm which receives visual and auditory object-level information and IP2 which is visuomotor (Rolls et al., 2023d)); from the medial orbitofrontal cortex (11l, 13l, pOFC); from the inferior frontal gyrus regions including IFJ, IFS and BA45; from the dorsolateral prefrontal cortex (8Av, 8BL, a9-46v and p9-46v) implicated in short-term memory (Chapter 13); and from the frontal pole (a10p, p10p, 10pp) (Fig. 11.27) (Rolls et al., 2023c,b). 47m (which is relatively medial in this group) also has effective connectivity with the hippocampal system (Hipp, EC, perirhinal, and TF), and with ventromedial prefrontal region 10r; and

524 | The orbitofrontal cortex, amygdala, reward value, emotion, and decision-making

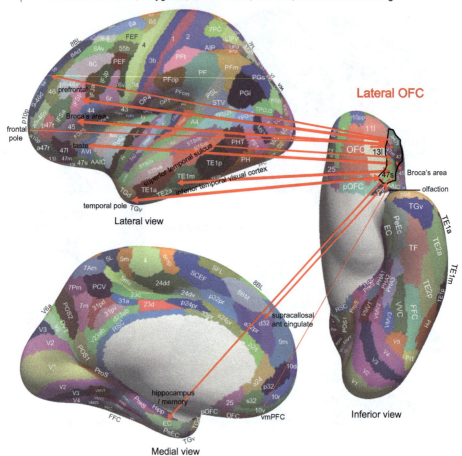

Fig. 11.26 Summary of the effective connectivity of the human lateral orbitofrontal cortex. The lateral orbitofrontal cortex has taste, olfactory and inferior temporal visual cortex inputs, and connectivity with the hippocampus, supracallosal (dorsal) anterior cingulate cortex, inferior and dorsolateral prefrontal cortex, and frontal pole. However, the lateral OFC also has connectivity with language regions (the cortex in the superior temporal sulcus and Broca's area). The main regions with which the lateral OFC has connectivity are indicated by names with the words in black font. The width of the arrows and the size of the arrow heads in each direction reflects the strength of the effective connectivity. The abbreviations are listed in Section 1.12. (From Rolls, E. T. 2023. Emotion, motivation, decision-making, the orbitofrontal cortex, anterior cingulate cortex, and the amygdala. Brain Structure and Function doi: 10.1007/s00429-023-02644-9)

with the frontal pole (10d, and 9m (Rolls et al., 2023a)). Although in most cases there are effective connectivities from a47r, p47r and 47m to these other cortical regions, the effective connectivities are in most cases stronger towards the lateral orbitofrontal, except that the connectivities are stronger from the lateral orbitofrontal cortex towards the set of inferior prefrontal regions including IFJ, IFS, 45 and 44. The functional connectivity is generally consistent. The diffusion tractography provides in addition evidence for connections of these parts of the lateral orbitofrontal cortex with the anterior ventral insular region (AVI) and the frontal opercular areas FOP4 and FOP5 which include the insular taste cortex (Rolls, 2015d, 2016c; Rolls et al., 2023c,b); with the anterior agranular insular complex (AAIC) which may be visceral (Rolls, 2016c) and also has taste-olfactory convergence (De Araujo et al., 2003a); with the middle insular region (MI) which is somatosensory; and with the piriform (olfactory) cortex.

Regions 47s and 47l (which tend to be more posterior, and are close to Broca's region 45) have effective connectivity (Rolls et al., 2023c,b) with regions involved in language (Rolls et al., 2022b). For example, 47s and 47l have effective connectivity with superior temporal

What is computed in the orbitofrontal cortex | 525

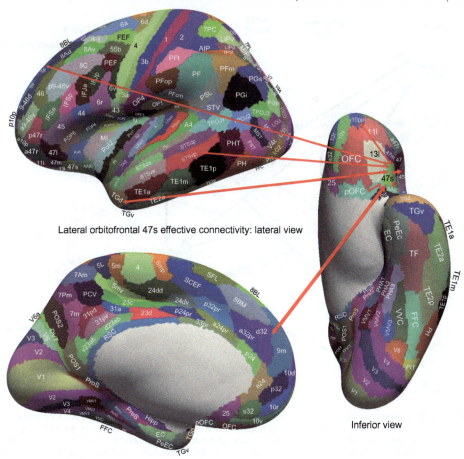

Lateral orbitofrontal 47s effective connectivity: lateral view

Inferior view

Lateral orbitofrontal 47s effective connectivity: medial view

Fig. 11.27 Effective connectivity of the human lateral orbitofrontal cortex region 47s: schematic diagram. The width of the arrows reflects the effective connectivity with the size of the arrowheads reflecting the connectivity in each direction. Some arrows reflect effective connectivity of several related regions: taste cortex AVI and putative visceral cortex AAIC; supracallosal anterior cingulate and medial prefrontal d32 and 9m; dorsal prefrontal 9a, 9p and 8BL; TGv and TGv. The abbreviations are listed in Section 1.12. (From Rolls,E.T., Deco,G., Huang,C-C. and Feng,J. (2023) Human amygdala compared to orbitofrontal cortex connectivity, and emotion. Progress in Neurobiology 220: 102385)

(STS and STG) auditory association / semantic cortical areas; with the temporal pole TG areas implicated in semantic representations; with the PeriSylvian language (PSL), STV and TPOJ regions involved in language (Rolls et al., 2022b); with the superior frontal language area (SFL); and directed to inferior prefrontal regions including IFJ, IFS, 45 and 44 (Broca's area). The connectivity of 47s and 47l with the STS/STG regions is not evident in the diffusion tractography, and may be implemented via the laterally adjacent areas 45 (inferior frontal gyrus pars triangularis) and 44 (inferior frontal gyrus pars opercularis) (both parts of Broca's area), which do have direct connections with these lateral orbitofrontal cortex areas, and towards which 47s and 47l have strong effective connectivity (Rolls et al., 2023c,b). Apart from these language-related connectivities, 47s and 47l have connections with other cortical regions that are similar to those of the other parts of the lateral orbitofrontal cortex (a47r, p47r and 47m) with which they also have connectivity, and it is accordingly proposed that 47s and 47l provide access from the orbitofrontal cortex reward / punishment system to language regions for subjective reports of pleasantness, unpleasantness, and affective value.

The lateral orbitofrontal cortex also has some effective and functional connectivity with

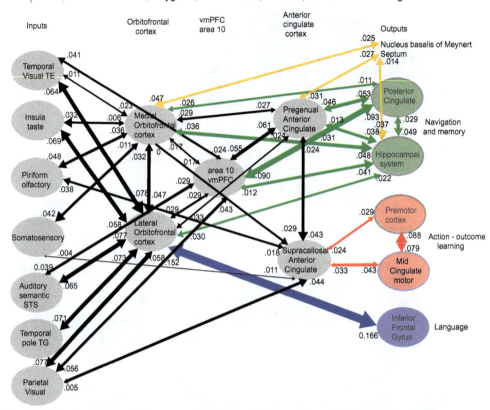

Fig. 11.28 Synthesis of the effective connectivity of the orbitofrontal cortex, vmPFC, and anterior cingulate cortex shown in the middle, with inputs on the left and outputs on the right. The regions included for each of the 5 central ellipses are as defined in the paper cited below. The width of the arrows is proportional to the effective connectivity in the highest direction, and the size of the arrows reflects the strength of the effective connectivity in each direction. The effective connectivities shown are for the strongest link where more than one link between regions applies for a group of brain regions. Effective connectivities with hippocampal memory system regions are shown in green; with premotor / mid-cingulate regions in red; with inferior prefrontal language system in blue; and in yellow to the basal forebrain nuclei of Meynert which contains cholinergic neurons that project to the neocortex and to the septal nuclei which contain cholinergic neurons that project to the hippocampus. The Somatosensory regions include 5 and parietal PF and PFop, which also connect to the pregenual anterior cingulate but are not shown for clarity; the Parietal regions include visual parietal regions 7, PGi and PFm. The connectivity with dorsolateral prefrontal cortex is not included here for clarity. Connectivity is shown for the five groups in the centre of the Figure, and does not include for example connectivity between somatosensory and premotor cortical regions. (From Rolls,E.T., Deco,G., Huang,C-C. and Feng,J. (2023) The human orbitofrontal cortex, vmPFC, and anterior cingulate cortex effective connectome: emotion, memory, and action. Cerebral Cortex 33: 350-356. doi: 10.1093/cercor/bhac070. Copyright © Oxford University Press.)

supracallosal medial prefrontal region 8BM (which is of interest as activations produced by aversive / unpleasant / non-reward stimuli extend into this region (Grabenhorst and Rolls, 2011; Rolls, 2019c; Rolls et al., 2020e)).

A major difference of the connectivity of the lateral orbitofrontal cortex from the other orbitofrontal, ventromedial prefrontal, and anterior cingulate regions (Rolls et al., 2023c,b) is its connectivity with Broca's area (45 and 44) in the inferior frontal gyrus (Rolls et al., 2022b).

A synthesis of the effective connectivity of the human orbitofrontal cortex showing how it has onward connectivity to further regions via the ventromedial prefrontal and anterior cingulate cortex is provided in Fig. 11.28 (Rolls et al., 2023c). Highlights of this human orbitofrontal cortex connectivity, and their implications for function, are considered next.

11.3.10.3 Connectivity of the orbitofrontal cortex to the hippocampal memory system, and memory consolidation

Fig. 11.28 shows how a major output of the human orbitofrontal cortex reaches the hippocampal memory system, both directly, and via the ventromedial prefrontal cortex, and pregenual anterior cingulate cortex and posterior cingulate cortex which are considered further in Chapter 12.

It is proposed in Section 9.2.8.5 that this connectivity enables reward and punishment information that relates to emotion to become a key component of episodic memory, together with 'where' or 'when' and 'what' information. During recall of an episodic memory, the reward / aversive / emotion component can then be recalled back to the orbitofrontal cortex, as described in Chapter 9.

However, even beyond that, it is proposed that the reward / aversive input to the hippocampus provides a 'value' component to each episodic memory, with episodic memories with a 'value' component more likely to be frequently recalled and thought about in humans, and thereby making an important contribution to what becomes consolidated into long-term, typically semantic, memory. This is described further in Section 9.2.8.5 and by Rolls (2022b). This proposal also helps to provide an account of how damage to the orbitofrontal cortex / ventromedial prefrontal cortex / anterior cingulate cortex impairs episodic memory (Section 9.2.8.5, and Rolls (2022b)).

11.3.10.4 Connectivity of the orbitofrontal cortex to the cholinergic basal forebrain nucleus of Meynert, and memory consolidation

Fig. 11.28 shows (in yellow) how another key output of the human orbitofrontal cortex, in particular region pOFC, reaches the cholinergic basal forebrain nucleus of Meynert. This nucleus provides the cholinergic innervation of the neocortex, where acetylcholine is involved in memory consolidation. Accordingly it is proposed that rewarding or punishing stimuli and events, which produce emotion, are decoded by the orbitofrontal cortex, and activate the basal nucleus cholinergic projection to the neocortex. Thus the orbitofrontal cortex plays an important role in this way too in memory consolidation. The evidence for this is presented in Section 9.2.8.5, and by Rolls (2022b). This proposal also helps to provide an account of how damage to the orbitofrontal cortex / ventromedial prefrontal cortex / anterior cingulate cortex impairs episodic memory (Section 9.2.8.5, and Rolls (2022b)).

11.3.10.5 Connectivity of the orbitofrontal cortex to the supracallosal anterior cingulate cortex for action-outcome learning

Fig. 11.28 shows how the human orbitofrontal cortex also has connectivity to the supracallosal anterior cingulate cortex, which is implicated in action-outcome learning. For this type of learning, it is proposed that the orbitofrontal cortex provides the reward or non-reward or punishment outcome that follows an action. The supracallosal anterior cingulate cortex is the part of the anterior cingulate cortex that is proposed to be involved in action-outcome learning, for it has extensive connectivity with premotor cortex regions including the mid-cingulate motor area that are involved in actions, as shown in Fig. 11.28. The evidence for this is described in Chapter 12 and by Rolls et al. (2023c). This is the key output of the orbitofrontal cortex by which it is involved in goal-directed instrumental learning, which is an important aspect of emotion (Rolls, 2014a, 2023b).

The orbitofrontal cortex outputs to language areas (blue in Fig. 11.28) provide one route via which orbitofrontal reward / punishment decoded inputs and thereby emotional states can become incorporated into declarative (experienced) emotion (Rolls et al., 2023b).

11.3.10.6 Connectivity of the orbitofrontal cortex to the basal ganglia and dopaminergic system

The orbitofrontal cortex outputs to the head of the caudate nucleus and ventral striatum provide a route for reinforcers to guide stimulus-response habit learning, as described in Chapter 16.

Very interestingly, in humans orbitofrontal cortex region OFC has effective connectivity to the substantia nigra pars compacta and ventral tegmental area (Rolls et al., 2023c), where the dopamine neurons are located (Rockland et al., 1994). As described in Sections 11.2.2 and 11.4, this is the most likely source of the reward-related information needed if dopamine neurons are to reflect reward prediction error (Schultz, 2016a, 2017), as described further in Chapter 16.

11.3.11 Mental problems associated with the orbitofrontal cortex

The important roles of the orbitofrontal cortex in depression are considered in Section 18.5.

The role in autism of the orbitofrontal cortex and amygdala, and the cortex in the superior temporal sulcus regions that connect to the orbitofrontal cortex and amygdala, is considered in Sections 2.4.9 and 8.2 (Cheng, Rolls, Gu, Zhang and Feng, 2015; Cheng, Rolls, Zhang, Sheng, Ma, Wan, Luo and Feng, 2016b; Rolls, Zhou, Cheng, Gilson, Deco and Feng, 2020f).

The effects of damage to the orbitofrontal cortex and amygdala on emotion in humans are considered earlier in this Chapter 11 (Rolls, 2021h; Rolls et al., 2023b).

However, reduced volume or area or reduced functional connectivity of the orbitofrontal cortex found in a number of neurodevelopmental disorders are associated with emotional and behavioral problems in children and adults, together with cognitive performance reductions associated with reductions in other brain regions. These disorders are of interest not only in neuroscience, but also to clinicians, and are described here.

In one investigation, childhood traumatic events (such as abuse and neglect, and defined by the 'Childhood Trauma' questions in the UK Biobank database) were associated in 9,535 participants aged 45-79 from the UK Biobank with lower functional connectivity involving the medial orbitofrontal cortex and superior temporal sulcus regions that connect to the orbitofrontal cortex conveying social information; the medial temporal cortex memory-related regions; the precuneus (implicated in the sense of self); and the superior, middle and inferior prefrontal cortex (implicated in working memory). These lower functional connectivities significantly mediated the associations between childhood traumatic events and addiction, anxiety, depression and well-being, and cognitive performance (including prospective memory and fluid intelligence) (Wan, Rolls, Cheng and Feng, 2022).

In another investigation, lower parental age, especially in the mother, was associated in the children when 9-11 of 8,709 mothers with lower volume of the anterior cingulate cortex, medial and lateral orbitofrontal cortex and amygdala, parahippocampal gyrus and hippocampus, and temporal lobes. The lower cortical volumes and areas in the children significantly mediated the association between the parental age and the behavioral and cognitive problems in the children. The effects were large, such as the 71% higher depressive problems score, and 28% higher rule-breaking score, in the children of mothers aged 15-19 than the mothers aged 34-35 (Du, Rolls, Gong, Cao, Vatansever, Zhang, Kang, Cheng and Feng, 2022).

In another investigation in 8,756 children aged 9-11 from the Adolescent Brain Cognitive Developmental study, we showed that high family conflict and low parental monitoring scores are associated with the children's behavioral problems, as well as with smaller cortical areas of the orbitofrontal cortex, anterior cingulate cortex, and middle temporal gyrus (Gong, Rolls, Du, Feng and Cheng, 2021).

In another investigation, severe and prolonged nausea and vomiting in pregnancy (extending after the second trimester), was associated in 10,710 children aged 9-11 years with low cortical area and volume, especially of the cingulate cortex, precuneus, and superior medial prefrontal cortex, and with emotional, behavioral, and cognitive problems. The emotional and behavioral problems scores included measures such as anxious/depressed, withdrawn/depressed, somatic complaints, social problems, thought problems, rule-breaking behavior, and aggressive behavior. The cognitive measures were from the NIH Toolbox. The lower cortical volume and area of some brain regions significantly mediated the association between severe and prolonged nausea and vomiting in pregnancy, and the emotional, behavioral and cognitive problems measured in the children when aged 9-11 years (Wang, Rolls, Du, Du, Yang, Li, Li, Cheng and Feng, 2020c).

In another investigation, lower gestational ages were associated in 11,847 adolescents with graded lower cognition and school achievements and with smaller brain volumes of the orbitofrontal and cingulate cortex, fronto-parieto-temporal, fusiform, insula, postcentral, hippocampal, thalamic, and pallidal regions (Ma, Wang, Rolls, Xiang, Li, Li, Zhou, Cheng and Li, 2022b).

It is striking that in these investigations the set of brain regions with reduced volume or area, or reduced functional connectivity, was somewhat similar, and included typically parts of the orbitofrontal and/or anterior cingulate cortex involved in emotion, temporal lobe regions involved in memory, and prefrontal regions involved in executive function. It may be that these regions are particularly susceptible to environmental factors of the type described. However, although many covariates were removed in these investigations (often including the Townsend social deprivation index), the populations involved are complex, and a number of differences including genetic differences may contribute to the associations that have been found. However, that does not at all diminish the fact that there are associations of this type between the orbitofrontal cortex and some other brain regions, and emotional and behavioral problems. Nor does it diminish the clinical relevance of the findings, for it may be useful when assessing problems such as those described to take into account the associated factors such as gestational age, events during pregnancy, and events in the first few years of life. A striking discovery is that the associations described with brain structure and function, and emotional and cognitive measures, lasted into late childhood, early adolescence, and mature adulthood.

11.4 What is computed in the amygdala for emotion

A brain structure that has somewhat similar connections to the orbitofrontal cortex, the amygdala, but is much older in evolution, is described in this section, to help highlight what is special about the orbitofrontal cortex. It will be argued that with the great development of the orbitofrontal cortex in primates including humans, the orbitofrontal cortex becomes much more important in emotion and related functions in humans than the amygdala.

11.4.1 Overview of the functions of the amygdala in emotion

The amygdala is an evolutionarily old subcortical structure with parts of it present in amphibia and reptiles. This is in contrast with the orbitofrontal cortex, which develops greatly in primates including humans as shown in Fig. 11.3 (Passingham, 2021).

The connections of the amygdala are similar to those of the orbitofrontal cortex, as shown in Figs. 11.1 and 11.29, and the amygdala connections do involve many with the orbitofrontal cortex.

The amygdala does have neurons that respond to primary reinforcers such as the taste, flavor, and smell of food; touch; and aversive stimuli. The amygdala also has neurons that learn associations between visual and auditory stimuli, and primary reinforcers. However, this learning does not support rule-based one-trial reversal learning, so the amygdala is less good at this rapid emotion-related learning than the orbitofrontal cortex (Section 11.3.1.2). The primate amygdala also contains a population of neurons specialized to respond to faces, and damage to the human amygdala can alter the ability to discriminate between different facial expressions, though this may be related to how faces are visually fixated.

Classically conditioned responses such as autonomic, freezing, and startle responses to auditory stimuli can depend on outputs from the amygdala to structures such as the hypothalamus and ventral striatum. Bilateral damage to the amygdala can produce a deficit in learning to associate visual and other stimuli with a primary (i.e. unlearned) reward or punisher. For example, monkeys with damage to the amygdala when shown foods and non-foods pick up both and place them in their mouths. When such visual or auditory discrimination learning is tested more formally, it is found that primates including humans with amygdala damage have difficulty in associating the sight or sound of a stimulus with whether it produces a reward, or is noxious and should be avoided. Sensory-specific satiety (the reduced choice of a food devalued by feeding to satiety) is impaired by damage to the amygdala (as is also the case for the orbitofrontal cortex).

In humans and other primates the amygdala does not appear to play such an important role in emotional and social behavior as the orbitofrontal cortex, with the changes to emotion much more subtle after amygdala damage. Further, the deficits described after amygdala damage involve fear conditioning (with classical conditioning of for example autonomic responses and effects on startle especially studied), and somewhat subtle aspects of face expression processing. In evolution, the balance may have moved to the orbitofrontal cortex, which has evolved much more recently, and may allow more powerful computations, such as those involved in rapid reversal learning and rapid correction of behavior, to be implemented.

Indeed, LeDoux, who has performed research on the rodent amygdala, is, with colleagues, now suggesting that the amygdala may have little to do with subjective feelings of emotion (LeDoux et al., 2018); and consistent with this, it has relatively little effective connectivity directed back to neocortical regions (Rolls et al., 2023b). In contrast, the orbitofrontal cortex may be much more closely related to emotional feelings, in that activations in it are linearly related to subjective affective ratings of pleasantness; damage to the orbitofrontal cortex impairs subjective emotional feelings as described earlier in this Chapter and by Rolls (2019e); and the orbitofrontal cortex does have connectivity directed back to many cortical regions, including language areas, providing routes for emotional states to be subjectively reported (Rolls et al., 2023b).

A much fuller analysis of the functions of the amygdala in emotion in primates including humans is provided by Rolls (2014a), with further human studies described in Whalen and Phelps (2009). The rodent literature and how it has focussed on conditioned responses and not on emotional feelings is described more fully elsewhere (Quirk et al., 1996; LeDoux, 2012b; LeDoux and Pine, 2016; LeDoux et al., 2018).

11.4.2 The amygdala and the associative processes involved in emotion-related learning

The amygdala is implicated in some learning processes involved in emotion including some classically conditioned effects, but not in other learning processes involved in emotion. To clarify this, I briefly summarize some of these learning processes, with a much fuller analysis provided elsewhere (Cardinal, Parkinson, Hall and Everitt, 2002; Rolls, 2014a; Balleine, 2019).

When a conditioned stimulus (CS) (such as a tone) is paired with a primary reinforcer or unconditioned stimulus (US) (such as a painful stimulus), then there are opportunities for a number of types of association to be formed.

Some of these involve 'classical conditioning' or 'Pavlovian conditioning', in which no action is performed that affects the contingency between the conditioned stimulus and the unconditioned stimulus. Typically an unconditioned response (UR), for example an alteration of heart rate, is produced by the US, and will come to be elicited by the CS as a conditioned response (CR). These responses are typically autonomic (such as the heart beating faster), or endocrine (for example the release of adrenaline (epinephrine in American usage) by the adrenal gland).

In addition to classical conditioning, the organism may learn to perform an instrumental response with the skeletal muscles in order to alter the probability that the primary reinforcer will be obtained. In our example, the experimenter might alter the contingencies so that when the tone sounded, if the organism performed an action such as pressing a lever, then the painful stimulus could be avoided. This is confirmed to be instrumental learning if the response learned is arbitrary, for example performing the opposite response, such as raising the lever to avoid the painful stimulus.

In the instrumental learning situation there are still opportunities for many classically conditioned responses including emotional states such as fear to occur. For example, in Pavlovian–instrumental transfer, if a stimulus that predicts the arrival of sucrose as a result of Pavlovian conditioning is provided during an instrumental task such as working to obtain sucrose, the responding (e.g. lever pressing) can be enhanced. Further, approach to a food may be under Pavlovian rather than instrumental control. Finally, we must beware of the facts that after overtraining, habits may be formed in which stimuli may become inflexibly linked to responses, with the reward value of the goal no longer directly influencing behavior, as shown by the fact that the response may continue for at least one trial after the goal has been devalued by for example feeding to satiety. This had led to some confusion in the literature (Berridge and Robinson, 1998; Berridge et al., 2009), for when the goal controls the behavior, wanting is driven by liking, and what happens during habits is not an exception, as habits are stimulus-response associations and have little to do with wanting or liking a goal (Rolls, 2014a, 2013d, 2023b).

11.4.3 Connections of the amygdala

The amygdala is a subcortical region in the anterior part of the temporal lobe. It receives massive projections in the primate from the overlying temporal lobe cortex (Van Hoesen, 1981; Amaral et al., 1992; Ghashghaei and Barbas, 2002; Freese and Amaral, 2009) (see Fig. 11.29). Via these inputs, the amygdala receives inputs about objects and faces that could become secondary reinforcers, as a result of pattern association in the amygdala with primary reinforcers. The amygdala also receives inputs that are potentially about primary reinforcers, e.g. taste inputs (from the insula, and from the secondary taste cortex in the orbitofrontal cortex), and somatosensory inputs, potentially about the rewarding or painful aspects of touch (from the somatosensory cortex via the insula). The amygdala receives strong projections from the posterior orbitofrontal cortex (see Fig. 11.29, areas 12 and 13) where there are value representations, and from the anterior cingulate cortex (Carmichael and Price, 1995a; Ghashghaei and Barbas, 2002; Freese and Amaral, 2009).

Although there are some inputs from early on in some sensory pathways, for example auditory inputs from the medial geniculate nucleus (LeDoux, 1992; Pessoa and Adolphs,

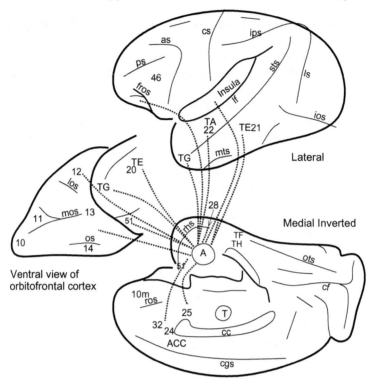

Fig. 11.29 Connections of the amygdala shown on lateral, ventral, and medial inverted views of the monkey brain. Abbreviations: as, arcuate sulcus; cc, corpus callosum; cf, calcarine fissure; cgs, cingulate sulcus; cs, central sulcus; ls, lunate sulcus; ios, inferior occipital sulcus; mos, medial orbital sulcus; os, orbital sulcus; ots, occipito-temporal sulcus; ps, principal sulcus; rhs, rhinal sulcus; sts, superior temporal sulcus; lf, lateral (or Sylvian) fissure (which has been opened to reveal the insula); A, amygdala; ACC, anterior cingulate cortex; INS, insula; T, thalamus; TE (21), inferior temporal visual cortex; TA (22), superior temporal auditory association cortex; TF and TH, parahippocampal cortex; TG, temporal pole cortex; 12, 13, 11, orbitofrontal cortex; 24, 32, parts of the anterior cingulate cortex; 25, subgenual cingulate cortex; 28, entorhinal cortex; 51, olfactory (prepyriform and periamygdaloid) cortex. The cortical connections shown provide afferents to the amygdala, but are reciprocated. (Redrawn and updated from G.W. Van Hoesen (1981) The differential distribution, diversity and sprouting of cortical projections to the amygdala in the rhesus monkey. In Y. Ben-Ari (ed.), The Amygdaloid Complex, pp. 77–90. © Elsevier Inc.)

2010), this route is unlikely to be involved in most emotions, for which cortical analysis of the stimulus is likely to be required. Emotions are usually elicited to environmental stimuli analyzed to the object level (including other organisms), and not to retinal arrays of spots or the frequency (tone) of a sound as represented in the cochlea (Rolls, 2014a).

Some of the outputs of the amygdala relevant to different types of response in rodents are shown in Fig. 11.30, and in addition there are backprojections to the neocortical areas that project to the amygdala.

11.4.4 Effects of amygdala lesions

11.4.5 Amygdala lesions in primates

Bilateral removal of the amygdala in monkeys produces striking behavioral changes which include tameness, a lack of emotional responsiveness, excessive examination of objects, often with the mouth, and eating of previously rejected items such as meat (Weiskrantz, 1956). These behavioral changes comprise much of the Kluver–Bucy syndrome which is produced in monkeys by bilateral anterior temporal lobectomy (Kluver and Bucy, 1939). In analyses of the bases of these behavioral changes, it has been observed that there are deficits in some

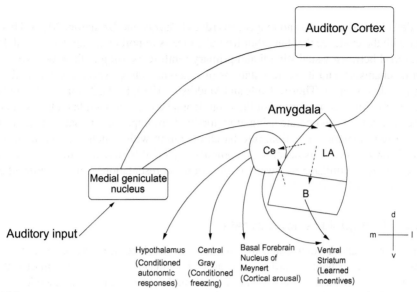

Fig. 11.30 The pathways for fear-conditioning to pure-tone auditory stimuli associated with footshock in the rat. The lateral amygdala (LA) receives auditory information directly from the medial part of the medial geniculate nucleus (the auditory thalamic nucleus), and from the auditory cortex. Intra-amygdala projections (directly and via the basal and basal accessory nuclei, B) end in the central nucleus (Ce) of the amygdala. Different output pathways from the central nucleus and the basal nucleus mediate different conditioned fear-related effects. d, dorsal; v, ventral; m, medial; l, lateral. The 'high road' via the auditory cortex is likely to be important for more complex auditory stimuli than pure tones. (Modified from G.J.Quirk, J.L.Armony, J.C.Repa, X.F.Li, and J.E.LeDoux (1996) Emotional memory: a search for sites of plasticity. Cold Spring Harbor Symposia on Quantitative Biology 61: 247–257. © Cold Spring Harbor Laboratory Press.)

types of learning. For example, Larry Weiskrantz (1956) found that bilateral ablation of the amygdala in the monkey produced a deficit in learning an active avoidance task. The monkeys failed to learn to make a response when a light signalled that shock would follow unless the response was made. He was perhaps the first to suggest that these monkeys had difficulty with forming associations between stimuli and reinforcers, when he suggested that "the effect of amygdalectomy is to make it difficult for reinforcing stimuli, whether positive or negative, to become established or to be recognized as such" (Weiskrantz, 1956). In this avoidance task, associations between a stimulus and punishers were impaired.

It has been confirmed with the more selective type of neurotoxic amygdala lesion that non-foods as well as foods are picked up and eaten, and also that emotional responses to snakes and human intruders are impaired (Murray and Izquierdo, 2007), but there are relatively minor changes in social behavior (Amaral, 2003; Bliss-Moreau, Moadab, Bauman and Amaral, 2013; Bliss-Moreau, Moadab, Santistevan and Amaral, 2017), and this is consistent with the trend for the orbitofrontal cortex to become relatively more important in emotion and social behavior in primates including humans. The amygdala is implicated by lesion studies in learning associations between visual stimuli and rewards, and devaluation by feeding to satiety is impaired too (Murray and Izquierdo, 2007). Interactions between the orbitofrontal cortex and the amygdala may be involved in devaluation of food reward, and interactions between the anterior cingulate cortex and the amygdala may be involved in social valuations (Murray and Fellows, 2022).

A difference between the effects of selective amygdala lesions and orbitofrontal cortex lesions in monkeys is that selective amygdala lesions have no effect on object reversal learning, whereas orbitofrontal cortex lesions do impair object reversal learning (Murray and Izquierdo, 2007). Further, and consistently, orbitofrontal but not selective amygdala lesions impair instrumental extinction (i.e. they showed a large number of choices of the previously rewarded object when it was no longer rewarded) (Murray and Izquierdo, 2007). This is consistent with the evidence that the orbitofrontal cortex is important in rapid, one-trial, learning and reversal between visual stimuli and primary reinforcers using both associative and rule-based mechanisms, and its representations of outcome value, expected value, and negative reward prediction error (Thorpe, Rolls and Maddison, 1983; Rolls, 2014a; Rolls and Grabenhorst, 2008). These contributions of the orbitofrontal cortex are facilitated by its neocortical architecture, which can operate using attractors that are important in many functions including short-term memory, attention, rule-based operation with switching, long-term memory, and decision-making. This neocortical computational ability may help the orbitofrontal cortex to compute and utilize non-reward to reset value representations in the orbitofrontal cortex (Rolls, 2014a, 2016b, 2019e).

11.4.6 Amygdala lesions in rats

In rats, there is also evidence that the amygdala is involved in behavior to stimuli learned as being associated with reward as well as with punishers. We may summarize these investigations in the rat as follows. The central nuclei of the amygdala encode or express Pavlovian S–R (stimulus–response, CS–UR) associations (including conditioned suppression, conditioned orienting, conditioned autonomic and endocrine responses, and Pavlovian–instrumental transfer) (Rolls (2014a) Section 4.6.1; (Cardinal et al., 2002; Balleine, 2019; Burton and Balleine, 2022)); and modulate perhaps by arousal the associability of representations stored elsewhere in the brain (Gallagher and Holland, 1994, 1992; Holland and Gallagher, 1999). In contrast, the basolateral amygdala (BLA) encodes or retrieves the affective value of the predicted US, and can use this to influence action–outcome learning via pathways to brain regions such as the nucleus accumbens and prefrontal cortex including the orbitofrontal cortex (Cardinal et al., 2002). We shall see below that the nucleus accumbens is not involved in action–outcome learning itself, but does allow the affective states retrieved by the BLA to conditioned stimuli to influence instrumental behavior by for example Pavlovian–instrumental transfer, and facilitating locomotor approach to food which appears to be in rats a Pavlovian process (Cardinal, Parkinson, Hall and Everitt, 2002; Cardinal and Everitt, 2004; Everitt and Robbins, 2013; Rolls, 2014a). This leaves parts of the prefrontal and cingulate cortices as strong candidates for action–outcome learning.

In a different model of fear-conditioning in the rat, Davis and colleagues (Davis, 2006), have used the fear-potentiated startle test, in which the amplitude of the acoustic startle reflex is increased when elicited in the presence of a stimulus previously paired with shock. Lesions of either the central nucleus or the lateral and basolateral nuclei of the amygdala block the expression of fear-potentiated startle. These latter amygdala nuclei may be the site of plasticity for fear conditioning, because local infusion of the NMDA (N-methyl-d-aspartate) receptor antagonist AP5 (which blocks long-term potentiation, an index of synaptic plasticity) blocks the acquisition but not the maintenance of fear-potentiated startle (Davis, 2006). These investigations have now been extended to primates, in which similar effects are found, with ibotenic acid-induced lesions of the amygdala preventing the acquisition of fear-potentiated startle, though, remarkably, not the expression of fear-potentiated startle when fear conditioning was carried out prior to the lesion (Davis et al., 2008).

Reconsolidation refers to a process in which after a memory has been stored, it may be weakened or lost if recall is performed during the presence of a protein synthesis inhibitor (Haubrich and Nader, 2018; Debiec, LeDoux and Nader, 2002; Debiec, Doyere, Nader and LeDoux, 2006). The implication that has been drawn is that whenever a memory is recalled, some reconsolidation process requiring protein synthesis may be needed. The computational utility of reconsolidation is considered by Rolls (2016b). Here, it is of interest that this applies to fear association mechanisms in the amygdala (Doyere et al., 2007), and drug-associated memories in the amygdala (Milton et al., 2008). The findings have interesting implications for the treatment of fear-associated memories. For example, in humans old fear memories can be updated with non-fearful information provided during the reconsolidation window. As a consequence, fear responses are no longer expressed, an effect that can last at least a year and is selective only to reactivated memories without affecting other memories (Schiller et al., 2010), although success has so far been limited (Kroes, Schiller, LeDoux and Phelps, 2016; Haubrich and Nader, 2018). Procedures that influence the extinction of fear memory may also be useful in the treatment of fear states (Davis, 2011).

11.4.7 Neuronal activity in the primate amygdala to reinforcing stimuli

There is clear evidence that some neurons in the primate amygdala respond to stimuli that are potentially primary reinforcers. For example, Sanghera, Rolls and Roper-Hall (1979) found some amygdala neurons with taste responses. In an extensive study of 1416 macaque amygdala neurons, Kadohisa, Rolls and Verhagen (2005b) showed that a very rich and detailed representation of the stimulus (such as food) that is in the mouth is provided by neurons that respond to oral stimuli, including taste, viscosity, fat texture, and oral temperature.

Less is known about whether it is the reinforcer value of the stimuli that is represented. It has been shown that satiety produces a rather modest (on average 58%) reduction in the responses of amygdala neurons to taste (Yan and Scott, 1996; Rolls and Scott, 2003), in comparison to the essentially complete reduction of responsiveness found in orbitofrontal cortex taste neurons (Rolls, Sienkiewicz and Yaxley, 1989d). Further, the representation in the amygdala of these oral stimuli does not appear to be on any simple hedonic basis, in that no direction in the multidimensional taste space in Fig. 7 of Kadohisa, Rolls and Verhagen (2005b) reflected the measured preference of the monkeys for the stimuli, nor were the response profiles of the neurons to the set of stimuli closely related to the preferences of the macaques for the stimuli (Kadohisa, Rolls and Verhagen, 2005b). The failure to find very strong effects of satiety on the responsiveness of amygdala taste neurons (Yan and Scott, 1996; Rolls and Scott, 2003) mirrors the earlier finding of Sanghera, Rolls and Roper-Hall (1979) of inconsistent effects of feeding to satiety on the responses of amygdala visual neurons responding to the sight of food.

Recordings from single neurons in the amygdala of the monkey have shown that some neurons do respond to visual stimuli, consistent with the inputs from the temporal lobe visual cortex (Sanghera, Rolls and Roper-Hall, 1979). Other neurons responded to auditory, gustatory, olfactory, or somatosensory stimuli, or in relation to movements. In tests of whether the neurons responded on the basis of the association of stimuli with reinforcers, it was found that approximately 20% of the neurons with visual responses had responses that occurred primarily to stimuli associated with reinforcers, for example to food and to a range of stimuli which the monkey had learned signified food in a visual discrimination task for food reward (Sanghera, Rolls and Roper-Hall, 1979; Rolls, 1981c; Wilson and Rolls, 1993, 2005; Rolls, 2000c). Many of these neurons responded more to the positive discriminative stimulus (S+) than to the negative visual discriminative stimulus (S−) in the Go/NoGo visual discrimination task (Rolls, 2000c; Wilson and Rolls, 2005). However, none of these neurons (in contrast with some neurons in the orbitofrontal cortex) responded exclusively to rewarded stimuli, in that all responded at least partly to one or more neutral, novel, or aversive stimuli.

The degree to which the visual responses of these amygdala neurons are associated with reinforcers has been assessed in learning tasks. When the association between a visual stimulus and an instrumental reinforcer was altered by reversal (so that the visual stimulus formerly associated with juice reward became associated with aversive saline and vice versa), it was found that 10 of 11 neurons did not reverse their responses (and for the other neuron the evidence was not clear) (Sanghera, Rolls and Roper-Hall, 1979; Rolls, 1992b, 2000c).

Although more investigations would be useful, the evidence now available indicates that primate amygdala neurons do not alter their activity flexibly and rapidly (in one or even a few trials) in visual discrimination reversal learning (Rolls, 1992b, 2000c, 2014a). What has been found in contrast is that neurons in the orbitofrontal cortex do show very rapid, often one-trial, reversal of their responses in visual discrimination reversal, and it therefore seems likely that the orbitofrontal cortex is especially involved when repeated relearning and re-assessment of stimulus–reinforcer associations are required, as described above, rather than initial learning, in which the amygdala may be involved. (It is noted that some other studies do not address the issue convincingly of rapid reversal, for they were not studying one-trial reversal with instrumental learning, but instead slow classical conditioning (Paton, Belova, Morrison and Salzman, 2006; Morrison, Saez, Lau and Salzman, 2011). However, more recent studies in that series are in fact consistent with the discoveries we have made that the orbitofrontal cortex updates reward value representations more rapidly and flexibly than the amygdala, in that neural responses to reward-predictive cues updated more rapidly in the orbitofrontal cortex than amygdala, and activity in the orbitofrontal cortex but not the amygdala was modulated by recent reward history (Saez, Saez, Paton, Lau and Salzman, 2017).

Evidence that primate amygdala neurons encode reward value is that while monkeys chose between saving liquid reward with interest and spending the accumulated reward, some of the neurons reflected the accumulating value (Grabenhorst et al., 2012) and reflect whether a macaque will perform economic saving (Hernadi et al., 2015; Grabenhorst et al., 2016). Macaque amygdala neurons can even reflect the value of an object learned by watching the behavior of another monkey (Grabenhorst et al., 2019). Overall, there is thus evidence that some amygdala neurons reflect reward value, yet do not reverse their value-related responses rapidly (in the one trial shown by orbitofrontal cortex neurons), and the evidence from the effects of selective amygdala lesions (Murray and Izquierdo, 2007) is consistent with this.

11.4.8 Neuronal responses in the amygdala to faces

Another interesting group of neurons in the amygdala has been discovered that respond primarily to faces (Rolls, 1981c; Leonard, Rolls, Wilson and Baylis, 1985). Each of these neurons responds to some but not all of a set of faces, and thus across an ensemble could convey information about the identity of the face (see Fig. 11.31). These neurons are found especially in the basal accessory nucleus of the amygdala (Leonard, Rolls, Wilson and Baylis, 1985), a part of the amygdala that develops markedly in primates (Amaral et al., 1992). Similar neurons have been further analyzed (Gothard et al., 2007, 2018), and, as with face-selective neurons in the orbitofrontal cortex (Rolls, Critchley, Browning and Inoue, 2006a), some neurons respond to face identity, some to face expression, and some to combinations of identity and expression. In addition, some neurons in the primate amygdala respond during social interactions, some may respond preferentially to eyes (as do some neurons in the temporal lobe visual cortex (Perrett, Rolls and Caan, 1982)), and their output may influence face expression (Brothers and Ring, 1993; Gothard et al., 2018). Face-selective neurons have also been found now in the human amygdala (Rutishauser et al., 2011, 2015), and some are tuned to fear face expressions, and others to happy face expressions (Wang, Yu, Tyszka, Zhen, Kovach, Sun, Huang, Hurlemann, Ross, Chung, Mamelak, Adolphs and Rutishauser, 2017). In an fMRI investigation, activationof the amygdala predicted rejection of artificial social partners (Rosenthal-von der Putten, Kramer, Maderwald, Brand and Grabenhorst, 2019).

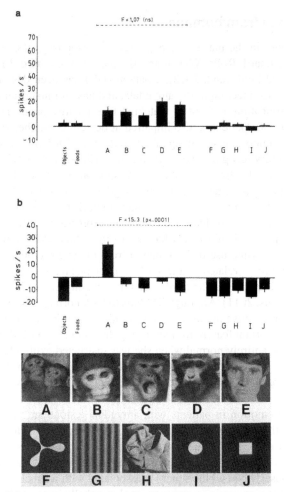

Fig. 11.31 Some amygdala neurons respond to the sight of faces. The responses of two neurons (a,b) in the amygdala to a variety of monkey and human face stimuli (A–E), and to non-face stimuli (F–J, objects, and foods). Each bar represents the mean response above baseline with the standard error calculated over 4 to 10 presentations. The F ratio for an analysis of variance calculated over the face sets indicates that the neurons shown range from very selective between faces (neuron b, Y0809) to relatively non-selective (neuron A, Z0264). Some stimuli produced inhibition below the spontaneous firing rate. (Reprinted from C.M.Leonard, E. T. Rolls, F.A.W.Wilson, and G.C.Baylis (1985) Neurons in the amygdala of the monkey with responses selective for faces. Behavioral Brain Research 15: 159–176. Copyright © Elsevier B.V.)

Neurons that are sensitive to the rank of the individual being viewed in the social hierarchy are found in the macaque amygdala (and also in the closely connected orbitofrontal cortex, and anterior cingulate cortex (Munuera et al., 2018)). In addition, it has been shown in the macaque that amygdala neurons are involved in social, observational learning in a reversal learning task, and that some neurons even predicted the choices of the partner monkey (Grabenhorst et al., 2019). These processes – assessing the social rank of individuals, learning from social partners, anticipating their behavior – are critical for social life. However, the balance may shift from the amygdala towards the orbitofrontal cortex in humans, as described next.

11.4.9 Evidence from humans

In relation to neurons in the macaque amygdala with responses selective for faces and social interactions (Leonard, Rolls, Wilson and Baylis, 1985; Gothard, Mosher, Zimmerman, Putnam, Morrow and Fuglevand, 2018), a patient (DR) has been described who has bilateral damage to or disconnection of the amygdala, and has an impairment of face-expression matching and identification, but not of matching face identity or in discrimination (Young et al., 1995, 1996). This patient is also impaired at detecting whether someone is gazing at the patient, another important social signal (Perrett et al., 1985b). The same patient is also impaired at the auditory recognition of fear and anger (Scott et al., 1997).

Adolphs et al. (1994) also found face expression but not face identity impairments in a patient (SM) with bilateral damage to the amygdala, and extended this to other patients (Adolphs et al., 2002b). The bilateral amygdala patient SM was especially impaired at recognizing the face expression of fear, and also rated expressions of fear, anger, and surprise as less intense than control subjects. It has been shown that SM's impairment stems from an inability to make normal use of information from the eye region of faces when judging emotions, which in turn is related to a lack of spontaneous fixations on the eyes during free viewing of faces (Adolphs et al., 2005), though this is mainly evident just for the first fixation (Kennedy and Adolphs, 2011). Although SM fails to look normally at the eye region in all facial expressions, her selective impairment in recognizing fear is explained by the fact that the eyes are the most important feature for identifying this emotion. Indeed, SM's recognition of fearful faces became entirely normal when she was instructed explicitly to look at the eyes. This finding provides a mechanism to explain the amygdala's role in fear recognition, and points to new approaches for the possible rehabilitation of patients with defective emotion perception.

The changes in emotion in patients with amygdala lesions are much less marked than those in patients with orbitofrontal cortex damage, and special tests, analogous in some cases to those developed in rodent studies, are necessary to reveal deficits (Phelps and LeDoux, 2005). For example, patients with amygdala lesions are impaired at learning conditioned skin conductance responses when a blue square is associated with a shock, and are also impaired in acquiring the same autonomic response to fear by verbally instructed learning or by observational learning (Phelps, 2004; Phelps et al., 2001; Phelps, 2006; Whalen and Phelps, 2009). The human amygdala has been described as being important mainly for some fear responses to some stimuli, such as whether an individual backs off in a social encounter (Adolphs, 2003; Adolphs et al., 2005; Phelps, 2004; Schiller et al., 2010; Feinstein et al., 2011). Interestingly, the amygdala was involved during aversive conditioning with primary reinforcers (electric shock) and less so with a secondary reinforcer (money), as suggested by both an fMRI analysis and a follow-up case study with a patient with bilateral amygdala damage (Delgado et al., 2011).

The important point has been made that the amygdala may be involved in some of the behavioral responses in humans related to emotion, but that the subjective emotional feeling conscious state may be unaltered by treatments that reverse some of these behavioral measures (LeDoux and Pine, 2016; LeDoux et al., 2018). One implication is that the amygdala, at least in humans, may have quite restricted roles in emotional feelings (LeDoux, 2020). In contrast, damage to the orbitofrontal cortex has major effects not only on emotional behavior, but also on subjective, conscious, feelings of emotion in humans as described above (Hornak et al., 2003). Two conclusions follow. First, the orbitofrontal cortex, due to its great development and evolution in primates including humans, may be much more important in emotion than the amygdala (Rolls, 2017b). Second, subjective emotional states are not necessarily closely related to at least some behavioral measures of emotion, consistent with the multiple routes to action concepts developed in Section 11.3.9 and more fully elsewhere (Rolls, 2014a, 2018a). To emphasise what is an important point with many implications: some behavioral measures related to emotion in humans may not reflect or be closely related to subjective emotional state; and vice versa (Rolls et al., 2023b).

An interesting advance conceptually is provided by the finding that personality interacts with whether particular stimuli activate the human amygdala. For example, happy face expressions are more likely to activate the human amygdala in extraverts than in introverts (Canli et al., 2002). In addition, positively affective pictures interact with extraversion to produce activation of the amygdala (Canli et al., 2001). This supports the conceptually important point that part of the basis of personality may be differential sensitivity to different rewards and punishers, and omission and termination of rewards and punishers (Rolls, 2014a). It has additionally been found that negative pictures interact with neuroticism in producing differential activation of the human amygdala (Canli et al., 2001). Further, FFFS and BIS-related personality traits related to an anxiety-related 'Behavioral Inhibition System', and to a fear-related 'Fight, Flight, Freeze System', are positively correlated to activity in the amygdala in response to negative stimuli (Kennis et al., 2013). However, a meta-analysis found that there is over many studies little relation between amygdala structure and function, and psychopathy (Deming et al., 2022).

11.4.10 Connectivity of the human amygdala

To understand better what is computed by the human amygdala, important evidence comes from understanding the inputs to the amygdala, and what it connects to, and the discoveries made in such a study are now described (Rolls et al., 2023b).

The cortical connectivity of the amygdala in humans is shown in Fig. 11.32 (Rolls et al., 2023b). The amygdala's effective connectivity with the cortex is much less than that of the orbitofrontal cortex (cf. Figs. 11.24, 11.25, and 11.27) (Rolls et al., 2023b). The implications of this, and of the connectivities that the amygdala does have with the cortex, and with subcortical structures, are now considered (Rolls et al., 2023b).

The effective connectivity to the human amygdala from the superior anterior parts of the temporal lobe (STSda, STG, TGd and extending back as far as A5) provides a route for auditory and visual information to reach the amygdala (Rolls et al., 2023b) (Fig. 11.32)[18]. The cortex in the macaque superior temporal sulcus (STS) includes neurons that we discovered respond to face expression and to socially relevant head motion such as turning the head or opening or closing the eyes to make or break social contact (Hasselmo, Rolls, Baylis and Nalwa, 1989b; Hasselmo, Rolls and Baylis, 1989a), and there is complementary evidence for humans (Critchley et al., 2000; Yokoyama et al., 2021; Freiwald, 2020) in what has become accepted as a third visual pathway for socially relevant stimuli (Pitcher and Ungerleider, 2021). Consistent with this, neurons in the primate amygdala respond to socially relevant stimuli such as face expression (Leonard, Rolls, Wilson and Baylis, 1985; Rolls, 1984) and the social stimuli produced by others (Grabenhorst and Schultz, 2021; Grabenhorst et al., 2019; Zangemeister et al., 2016; Grabenhorst et al., 2016; Hernadi et al., 2015). Those anterior superior temporal cortical regions receive connectivity from the inferior temporal cortex part of the ventral visual stream so are likely to include representations of objects as well as faces (Rolls et al., 2023e, 2022b). We discovered that these anterior superior temporal cortex regions also contain auditory neurons (Baylis, Rolls and Leonard, 1987), and some

---

[18] The functional connectivity of the amygdala with this set of cortical regions but relatively few others (Rolls et al., 2023b) is supported by another investigation (Klein-Flugge et al., 2022b), though that did not measure effective connectivity nor utilize the helpful categorisation of cortical areas provided by the HCP-MMP atlas (Glasser et al., 2016a; Huang et al., 2022).

540 | The orbitofrontal cortex, amygdala, reward value, emotion, and decision-making

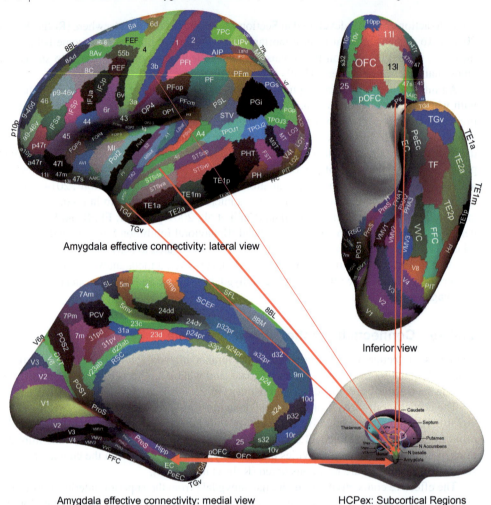

Fig. 11.32 Effective connectivity of the human amygdala: schematic diagram. The width of the arrows reflects the effective connectivity with the size of the arrowheads reflecting the connectivity in each direction. The connectivity from most cortical areas (STGa and TGd, STSda and A5, and pyriform olfactory cortex) is only towards the amygdala. The connectivity with the hippocampal system (Hipp, entorhinal cortex EC, and perirhinal cortex PeEc) is in both directions. The abbreviations are listed in Section 1.12. (From Rolls,E.T., Deco,G., Huang,C-C. and Feng,J. (2023) Human amygdala compared to orbitofrontal cortex connectivity, and emotion. Progress in Neurobiology 220: 102385.)

neurons respond to combinations of auditory and visual stimuli (Khandhadia et al., 2021) which are likely to be important in decoding the meaning of social and related stimuli. Given that there is also connectivity in humans from somatosensory and olfactory cortical regions to the amygdala (Rolls et al., 2023b), these form the inputs needed to associate visual and auditory stimuli with their consequences in the form of primary rewards and punishers such as pleasant or aversive touch and perhaps odor. This system could then be the primate including human equivalent of the auditory to electric shock associative learning investigated in the rodent amygdala (Johansen et al., 2010; LeDoux, 2000; Rogan et al., 1997; Quirk et al., 1996; LeDoux, 1996, 1995, 1994; Killcross et al., 1997).

But the question then arises of what the outputs are of this stimulus-reward or stimulus-punishment associative system in the amygdala. The paucity of the output connectivity of the amygdala directed to the neocortex in humans (Fig. 11.32), with most of the neocortical connectivity being only towards the amygdala without strong backprojections (Rolls et al.,

2023b), and different from the orbitofrontal cortex as illustrated in Figs. 11.24, 11.25, and 11.27, suggests that the amygdala does not have major cortical outputs to lead to actions performed to obtain goals in instrumental learning, which the evidence suggests is implemented by the orbitofrontal cortex outputs to the anterior cingulate cortex (Rushworth et al., 2012, 2011; Rolls et al., 2023c). An alternative, given the paucity of amygdalo-neocortical connectivity for amygdala output, is that much of the amygdala output is directed to brainstem regions in humans as well as rodents (Rolls et al., 2023b; Klein-Flugge et al., 2022b) to elicit responses such as autonomic responses, freezing, conditioned cortical arousal elicited via the cholinergic basal nucleus of Meynert, and incentive effects. That would in fact be consistent with the amygdala outputs identified for the rodent auditory-aversive shock system (Quirk, Armony, Repa, Li and LeDoux, 1996). These effects are conditioned responses, and not instrumental goal-directed actions to obtain reinforcers, and the difference is important for understanding emotional behavior (Cardinal et al., 2002; Rolls, 2014a, 2023b), especially as emotions can be defined as states elicited by instrumental reinforcers (Rolls, 2014a).

In non-human primates, connections are found between the amygdala and the medial orbitofrontal cortex (including pOFC), both directly and via the mediodorsal nucleus of the thalamus pars magnocellularis (Timbie, Garcia-Cabezas, Zikopoulos and Barbas, 2020; Price and Drevets, 2010; Freese and Amaral, 2009). Consistently, in humans anatomical connections were demonstrated with diffusion tractography between the amygdala and medial orbitofrontal cortex region pOFC, and also between the amygdala and pregenual / subgenual anterior cingulate cortex (Rolls et al., 2023b). This is interesting in two ways. First, the amygdala, which is evolutionarily old, has anatomical connections with the human posterior orbitofrontal cortex (region pOFC) which is likely to be the evolutionarily oldest part of the human orbitofrontal cortex (Passingham, 2021). Second, the lack of effective connectivity, and low functional connectivity, provides new evidence that these amygdalo-orbitofrontal connections have relatively low functional effects in humans, and are indeed much lower than the effective connectivity of the orbitofrontal cortex with cortical regions and of the amygdala with subcortical regions including the septum and basal nucleus of Meynert (Rolls et al., 2023b).

The paucity of outputs of the amygdala to the neocortex including language regions in humans (Fig. 11.32) also implies that the human amygdala may not be closely involved in reported human subjective emotions and feelings. That evidence is in fact consistent with what is now believed by those who have worked on the rodent amygdala and auditory to electric shock conditioning, in that interventions such as the use of pharmacological agents that influence amygdala function have little effect on reported human emotions, though they do influence in humans the conditioned responses referred to above that are found in rodents (Taschereau-Dumouchel et al., 2022; Mobbs et al., 2019; LeDoux and Daw, 2018; LeDoux et al., 2018; LeDoux, 2017; LeDoux and Pine, 2016; LeDoux, 2012a, 2020). In addition, damage to the human amygdala may influence some responses, such as which parts of a face are fixated (Adolphs et al., 2005), or learning autonomic responses to a visual stimulus associated an electric shock (Whalen and Phelps, 2009; Phelps, 2006; Delgado et al., 2006; Phelps and LeDoux, 2005; Phelps, 2004; Schiller et al., 2010), but does not lead to severe changes in emotional behavior and reported emotional feelings (Feinstein et al., 2011; Whalen and Phelps, 2009; Young et al., 1995; Aggleton, 1992; Spezio et al., 2007; Adolphs et al., 2005; Young et al., 1996; Calder et al., 1996; Scott et al., 1997; Adolphs et al., 1994, 2002a; Kennedy and Adolphs, 2011; Damasio et al., 2013; LeDoux, 2020) that are comparable to those produced by damage to the orbitofrontal cortex (as described above). Indeed, when patient SM with amygdala damage did fixate faces including the eyes, the reported emotion was not impaired (Adolphs et al., 2005; Kennedy and Adolphs, 2011). That left LeDoux (and colleagues) (LeDoux, 2020; Taschereau-Dumouchel et al., 2022; Mobbs et al.,

2019; LeDoux et al., 2018; LeDoux, 2017; LeDoux and Pine, 2016; LeDoux, 2012a) with the conundrum: if the amygdala is not involved in reported human emotion, what brain systems are?

The answer to that question, of what brain systems are involved in human emotion, is that the orbitofrontal cortex, together with the regions to which its outputs are directed, the ventromedial prefrontal cortex, and anterior cingulate cortex (Rolls et al., 2023c)), are the key brain regions involved in reported (declarative) human emotion (Rolls et al., 2023c; Rolls, 2023b, 2014a, 2019e). For example, damage to the human orbitofrontal cortex impairs not only reward-related reversal learning, and relates to disinhibited emotional behavior (Hornak et al., 2004; Rolls et al., 1994a; Berlin et al., 2005, 2004; Fellows, 2011), and the identification of face and vocal emotional expression (Hornak et al., 2003, 1996; Tsuchida and Fellows, 2012), but also impairs the reported subjective experience of emotion (Hornak et al., 2003; Rolls, 2021h). In addition, activations of the human orbitofrontal cortex occur to many emotion / reward-related and punishment-related stimuli (O'Doherty, Kringelbach, Rolls, Hornak and Andrews, 2001a; O'Doherty, Winston, Critchley, Perrett, Burt and Dolan, 2003b; Grabenhorst and Rolls, 2011; Rolls, O'Doherty, Kringelbach, Francis, Bowtell and McGlone, 2003d; Rolls, 2014a, 2019e), and also linearly track the reported subjective pleasure produced by stimuli (Kringelbach, O'Doherty, Rolls and Andrews, 2003; Grabenhorst, Rolls and Bilderbeck, 2008a; Grabenhorst and Rolls, 2008).

Based on evidence of this type, the human orbitofrontal cortex is the key brain region involved in emotion (including reported, subjectively experienced, emotion) in humans, rather than the amygdala (Rolls, 2014a, 2019e, 2021b), and the evidence on the connectivity of the human amygdala and orbitofrontal cortex described here helps to provide a connectional foundation for this understanding. Further, a new concept proposed (Rolls et al., 2023b) is that given the connectivity of some human lateral orbitofrontal cortex regions (e.g. 47l and 47s) with language regions (Rolls et al., 2022b), some of the impulsiveness of humans with orbitofrontal cortex damage and their focus on immediate rewards rather than long-term planning (Rolls et al., 1994a) may be related to interruption of language-based planning influences of the reasoning system on the orbitofrontal cortex. At the same time, these connectivities from the lateral orbitofrontal cortex to language regions provide a direct route for the orbitofrontal cortex emotion system to gain access to the language systems to make declarations about emotional feelings.

The amygdala is evolutionarily old, and its role may continue to be largely in linking stimuli to responses such as autonomic responses, freezing, cortical arousal, and effects of incentive stimuli. In contrast, the orbitofrontal cortex develops greatly in non-human primates and even further in humans (Rolls, 2019e; Passingham, 2021; Passingham and Wise, 2012), with the extensive cortical connectivity with neocortex described here, and related to this great development and neocortical connectivity, may play a key role in human emotion including reported emotional feelings. Further, it is notable that the amygdala has no effective connectivity directed towards dorsolateral and inferior frontal regions of the prefrontal cortex that are implicated in short-term memory functions (Goldman-Rakic, 1996; Miller et al., 2018) that are even related to language (Rolls et al., 2023f, 2022b); and that prefrontal route (Rolls et al., 2023b) (Fig. 11.32) may be an important route for activity in the human orbitofrontal cortex to become incorporated into experienced and reported emotional feelings (Rolls, 2020a, 2008a; Lau, 2022). The orbitofrontal cortex on the other hand has increasing and strong effective connectivity to these lateral prefrontal cortex regions as one moves forward from pOFC to 13l and to 11l (Rolls et al., 2023b).

A cautionary note is in order here. Sometimes behavioral and autonomic responses such as changes in heart rate and skin conductance, and freezing or other responses, are used as measures of 'emotion'. Given the points just made, we need to be aware that such responses are not closely related to reported human emotion and are mediated by a different brain system, so may not be fully appropriate measures that relate to human subjectively felt and reported emotions. The instrumental choice of stimuli based on reward value may be a better measure of the value of a good to an animal or human (Rolls, 2023b), but even here we cannot be sure that this always reflects reported consciously felt emotions in humans (Rolls, 2021e,g, 2020a). Further, although associations of amygdala functional connectivity with mental disorders have been described (Klein-Flugge et al., 2022b), these are associations, and do not show whether the amygdala functional connectivities are caused by or cause the different mental disorders.

The connectivity of the human amygdala to the basal nucleus of Meynert (Rolls et al., 2023b) which contains cholinergic neurons that provide the cholinergic input to the neocortex (Huang et al., 2022; Zaborszky et al., 2018, 2008) is of considerable interest. Medial orbitofrontal cortex region pOFC is the only cortical area found to have effective connectivity to the nucleus basalis of Meynert (Rolls et al., 2023c). Different magnocellular neurons in the macaque basal nucleus of Meynert which are probably cholinergic respond to reinforcing (reward or punishing), or novel, stimuli (Wilson and Rolls, 1990a,b,c), both represented in the orbitofrontal cortex (Rolls et al., 2005a; Rolls, 2019f,e). It is now proposed that the amygdala, as well as the more recently evolved human orbitofrontal cortex, may both contribute to cortical arousal, attention, and consolidation of memory in the neocortex given that acetylcholine is involved in long-term synaptic potentiation (Zaborszky et al., 2018; Newman et al., 2012; Hasselmo and Sarter, 2011) when aversive or rewarding stimuli are encountered, in ways that are described more fully elsewhere (Rolls, 2022b; Rolls et al., 2023c) (Section 9.2.8.5).

The strong effective connectivity of the human amygdala with the hippocampus, entorhinal, and perirhinal cortex, which is a little stronger towards the hippocampal system (Rolls et al., 2023b), is also of great interest. This connectivity is consistent with what has been described in macaques (Stefanacci et al., 1996). There is corresponding connectivity of the orbitofrontal cortex with the hippocampus (Rolls et al., 2023c,b). It is now proposed here that the amygdala connectivity to the hippocampus implements similar functions to those proposed for the orbitofrontal cortex inputs to the hippocampus, including enabling reward/punishment information to be incorporated into episodic memory, and also enabling any information recalled from episodic memory about rewards and punishers to influence whether that episodic memory is consolidated into neocortical long-term semantic memory, as described in detail elsewhere (Rolls, 2022b) (Section 9.2.8.5). When memories are recalled from the hippocampus to the amygdala, this may enable autonomic and related responses to be produced when memories are retrieved.

In addition to the differences in the connectivity of the human amygdala and orbitofrontal cortex described here, internal differences in their connectivity are likely to contribute to their different computational functions related to emotion. The amygdala has relatively little recurrent collateral excitatory connectivity between its neurons (Millhouse and DeOlmos, 1983)[19], whereas the orbitofrontal cortex, like all neocortex, has highly developed local excitatory recurrent collateral connectivity between its pyramidal cells (Rolls, 2021b, 2016b). These recurrent collaterals are implicated in short-term memory functions, enabling representations to remain active by maintaining the activity of an interconnected set of neurons to continue firing because of the strength of the recurrent collateral synapses of the neurons in each set (Rolls, 2021b, 2016b). An implication is that memory states related to emotion-provoking

---

[19] Nuclei in the brain may in general have much less excitatory recurrent collateral connectivity between their neurons than the neocortex, and this is proposed to be fundamental to understanding computation by the cortex (Rolls, 2021b).

stimuli can be maintained using the orbitofrontal cortex but much less by the amygdala. This orbitofrontal cortex recurrent collateral connectivity not only may enable the memory of rewards and punishers received recently to influence future behavior, but also may enable a mood state to be maintained (e.g. happiness or sadness) that can adaptively influence future behavior (Rolls, 2014a, 2018a). This functionality may become even more developed especially in humans because the orbitofrontal cortex has reciprocal connectivity with areas such as the angular gyrus involved in language that may implement 'long loop' attractors because of the reciprocal connectivity between these two cortical regions, and thereby contribute to the sad ruminating thoughts that can be a feature of human depression (Rolls, 2016e; Cheng, Rolls, Qiu, Liu, Tang, Huang, Wang, Zhang, Lin, Zheng, Pu, Tsai, Yang, Lin, Wang, Xie and Feng, 2016a; Rolls, Cheng and Feng, 2020a; Rolls, 2018a; Zhang, Rolls, Wang, Xie, Cheng and Feng, 2023a).

11.5 How the computations are performed in the orbitofrontal cortex

This section describes current approaches to *how* the orbitofrontal cortex performs some of its key computations.

One of the key computations is decision-making. This is addressed in Sections 11.5.1 and 11.5.2. The context of the description is orbitofrontal cortex computations, but this class of neuronal decision-making network is proposed to apply to decision-making in many cortical areas, each specialized for a different type of decision, so this type of network should be thought of as generic (Rolls and Deco, 2010). Indeed, the application to decision-making in other brain regions is described in Rolls and Deco (2010) and Deco, Rolls, Albantakis and Romo (2013). The description provided in Section 11.5.1 is supplemented by a formal description of the equations in the integrate-and-fire model of decision-making in Sections B.6.2, B.6.3, B.8.2, and B.8.3. Other approaches to decision-making, some much less biologically plausible than the approach described here, such as the drift-diffusion and race models, are described by Deco, Rolls, Albantakis and Romo (2013).

Another key computation performed in the orbitofrontal cortex is association learning between stimuli (such as a visual stimulus) and a reward (such as a taste), and this is probably implemented by pattern association learning of the type described in Section B.2. More generally, this can be described as learning between secondary reinforcers (such as the sight of a food), and primary, unlearned reinforcers, such as the taste of a food (Rolls, 2014a). This is described further in Section 11.5.3

However, when the stimulus-reward association needs to be reversed very rapidly, in one trial, a rule-based system is required that holds in a short-term memory the current rule, which then controls how incoming stimuli are treated, and a model that implements this is described in Section 11.5.3.

Further, when an error is made, and the visual stimulus is no longer associated with the primary reward (in reversal or extinction), then error neurons fire in the orbitofrontal cortex, and a network that can implement this is described in Section 11.5.4.

11.5.1 Decision-making in attractor networks in the brain

11.5.1.1 An attractor decision-making network

Consider the attractor network architecture shown in Fig. 11.33a (with more details in Section B.3). A set of cortical neurons has recurrent collateral excitatory synaptic connections w_{ij} from the other neurons. The evidence for decision 1 is applied via the λ_1 inputs, and for

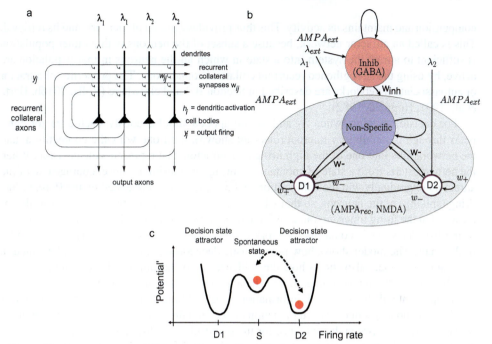

Fig. 11.33 (a) Attractor or autoassociation single network architecture for decision-making. The cell body of each neuron is shown as a triangle (like a cortical pyramidal cell), the dendrite is vertical, and receives recurrent collateral synaptic connections w_{ij} from the other neurons. The evidence for decision 1 is applied via the λ_1 inputs, and for decision 2 via the λ_2 inputs. The synaptic weights w_{ij} have been associatively modified during training in the presence of λ_1 and at a different time of λ_2. When λ_1 and λ_2 are applied, each attractor competes through the inhibitory interneurons (not shown), until one wins the competition, and the network falls into one of the high firing rate attractors that represents the decision. The noise in the network caused by the random spiking times of the neurons (for a given mean rate) means that on some trials, for given inputs, the neurons in the decision 1 (D1) attractor are more likely to win, and on other trials the neurons in the decision 2 (D2) attractor are more likely to win. This makes the decision-making probabilistic, for, as shown in (c), the noise influences when the system will jump out of the spontaneous firing stable (low energy) state S, and whether it jumps into the high firing state for decision 1 (D1) or decision 2 (D2). (b) The architecture of the integrate-and-fire network used to model decision-making (see text). The synaptic weights between the neural populations (decision pools D1 and D2, the non-specific pool, and the inhibitory pool) are 1 except where indicated. In particular, the recurrent weights, indicated by a recurrent arrow, between the neurons within an attractor decision-making pool have strong weights w_+, and between the different pools have the weak strength w_-. (c) A multistable 'effective energy landscape' for decision-making with stable states shown as low 'potential' basins. Even when the inputs are being applied to the network, the spontaneous firing rate state is stable, and noise provokes transitions from the low firing rate spontaneous state S into the high firing rate decision attractor state D1 or D2. If the noise is greater, the escaping time to a decision state, and thus the decision or reaction time, will be shorter. (After Rolls, E. T. and Deco, G. (2010) The Noisy Brain: Stochastic Dynamics as a Principle of Brain Function. Oxford University Press: Oxford; and Rolls, E. T. (2016) Cerebral Cortex: Principles of Operation. Oxford University Press: Oxford.)

decision 2 via the λ_2 inputs. The synaptic weights w_{ij} have been associatively modified during training in the presence of λ_1 and at a different time of λ_2. The Hebbian or associative synaptic modification is such that if the presynaptic terminal and the postsynaptic neuron are simultaneously active, the synaptic connections become stronger. There are inhibitory neurons (not shown in Fig. 11.33a) that keep the total firing in the network within bounds, and in fact implement competition between the neuronal populations. As a result of the associative synaptic modification (specified in Equation B.9), there are strong connections within the set of neurons activated by λ_1, and strong connections within the set of neurons activated by λ_2. These strengthened synapses provide positive feedback, so that if the whole or part of λ_1 is applied, that set of neurons becomes active, and maintains its activity for a long period even when the input λ_1 is removed. The neurons activated by λ_1 if firing inhibit the neurons activated by λ_2 through the inhibitory interneurons, so that just one population wins the competition and maintains its activity. This thus provides a model of memory, and its retrieval. This is called an attractor network, because a subset of the neurons within either population is sufficient to attract the system into a state in which all the neurons in that population are active, by using the strengthened recurrent collateral connections. The properties of attractor or autoassociation networks are described in Section B.3 and elsewhere (Rolls, 2016b; Hertz et al., 1991; Hopfield, 1982).

For decision-making, when λ_1 and λ_2 are applied simultaneously, each attractor competes through the inhibitory interneurons (not shown), until one wins the competition, and the network falls into one of the high firing rate attractors that represents the decision. When the network starts from a state of spontaneous firing, the biasing inputs encourage one of the attractors to gradually win the competition, but this process is influenced by the Poisson-like firing (spiking) of the neurons, so that which attractor wins is probabilistic. (Poisson-like indicates that the firing times are random for a given mean firing rate.) If the evidence in favour of the two decisions is equal, the network chooses each decision probabilistically on 50% of the trials. The model shows how probabilistic decision-making could be implemented in the brain. The model also shows how the evidence can be accumulated over long periods of time because of the integrating action of the attractor short-term memory network, with the recurrent collaterals feeding back information to be combined with the continuing inputs λ_1 and λ_2. The model produces shorter reaction or decision times as a function of the magnitude of the difference between the evidence for the two decisions: difficult decisions take longer, partly because the firing rates take longer to reach a decision threshold if the difference between the inputs is small.

11.5.1.2 An integrate-and-fire implementation of the attractor network for probabilistic decision-making

Because cortical neurons have almost random firing times for a given mean firing rate, i.e. the firing times follow approximately a Poisson distribution (Rolls and Treves, 2011), the mean firing rates over short periods (e.g. 20–100 ms) of all the neurons in one of the decision-making populations may be higher than in the other population. These are referred to as statistical fluctuations. These fluctuations can result in the mean rate of one decision population increasing more than the other on a single trial, and influencing which decision is taken on that trial. To model these neuronal spiking time related fluctuations, we need an implementation of the decision-making network that incorporates spiking times. A simple such model is an integrate-and-fire model, which models the synapses and the membrane potentials as dynamical variables, and then produces a spike (not itself modelled to keep the implementation simple) which is then transmitted to the other neurons.

A leaky integrate-and-fire neuron along the lines just introduced can be modelled as shown schematically in Fig. 11.34. The model describes the depolarization of the membrane potential V (which typically is dynamically changing as a result of the synaptic effects described below between approximately –70 and –50 mV) until threshold V_{thr} (typically –50 mV) is reached when a spike is emitted and the potential is reset to V_{reset} (typically –55 mV). The membrane time constant τ_m is set by the membrane capacitance C_m and the membrane leakage conductance g_m where $\tau_m = C_m/g_m$. Changes in the membrane potential V (see right of Fig. 11.34) are produced by the input spikes operating through the dynamically modelled synapses (left of Fig. 11.34). There are very many such synapses, and the input currents produced from all these synapses result in excitatory postsynaptic potentials (EPSPs) and inhibitory postsynaptic potentials (IPSPs) that are summed by the integrate-and-fire neuron. When the threshold for firing is reached by the membrane potential V, a spike is emitted. The equations for the implementation are given in Section B.6.3.

An attractor network model of decision-making using integrate-and-fire neurons was

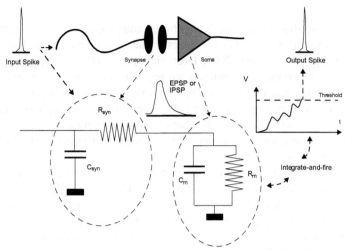

Fig. 11.34 Integrate-and-fire neuron. The basic circuit of an integrate-and-fire model consists of the neuron's membrane capacitance C_m in parallel with the membrane's resistance R_m (the reciprocal of the membrane conductance g_m) driven by a synaptic current with a conductance and time constant determined by the synaptic resistance R_syn (the reciprocal of the synaptic conductance g_j) and capacitance C_syn shown in the figure. These effects produce excitatory or inhibitory postsynaptic potentials, EPSPs or IPSPs. These potentials are integrated by the cell, and if a threshold V_thr is reached a δ-pulse (spike) is fired and transmitted to other neurons, and the membrane potential is reset. (Reproduced from Gustavo Deco and Edmund T. Rolls (2003) Attention and working memory: a dynamical model of neuronal activity in the prefrontal cortex. European Journal of Neuroscience 18: 2374–2390. Copyright © Federation of European Neuroscience Societies and John Wiley and Sons Ltd.)

developed by Wang (2002), based on a neurodynamical model introduced by Brunel and Wang (2001). The model has been extended and successfully applied to several experimental paradigms including attention and short-term memory as well as decision-making (Rolls and Deco, 2002; Deco and Rolls, 2002, 2003, 2004; Deco, Rolls and Horwitz, 2004; Szabo, Almeida, Deco and Stetter, 2004; Deco and Rolls, 2005b, 2006; Wang, 2008; Rolls, Grabenhorst and Deco, 2010b,c; Rolls and Deco, 2010; Smerieri, Rolls and Feng, 2010; Deco, Rolls and Romo, 2010; Rolls and Deco, 2011b; Rolls, 2012c; Martinez-Garcia, Rolls, Deco and Romo, 2011; Rolls, Dempere-Marco and Deco, 2013; Deco, Rolls, Albantakis and Romo, 2013; Rolls and Deco, 2015a,b, 2016; Rolls and Mills, 2019).

In this framework, probabilistic decision-making is modelled by an attractor single network organized into a discrete set of neuronal populations or pools, as illustrated in Fig. 11.33b. The network contains N_E (excitatory) pyramidal cells and N_I inhibitory interneurons. In the simulations, we often use $N_\mathrm{E} = 800$ and $N_\mathrm{I} = 200$, consistent with the neurophysiologically observed proportion of 80% pyramidal cells versus 20% interneurons (Abeles, 1991; Rolls, 2016b) for a network with 1000 neurons, but effects of the number of neurons N in the network can be investigated. The neurons are fully connected (with synaptic strengths that are 1.0 unless specified otherwise). In the network illustrated in Fig. 11.33b, there are two decision-making populations, D1 and D2, each with 10% of the excitatory neurons, but the number of decision populations can be altered as needed. The recurrent synaptic connections within a decision population (indicated by the recurrent arrows in Fig. 11.33b) have a high strength of w_+ (typically 2.1), so that the population is self-sustaining in its activity, once started, and is at a biologically realistic firing rate. The remainder of the excitatory neurons are in a non-specific pool (NS), which represent other neurons in the cortex that are not involved in the particular task but fire spontaneously and contribute to the background noise (randomness) caused by the Poisson-like firing of the integrate-and-fire neurons. Their connections to the decision-making pools and the connections between the different decision-making pools are set to a value w_- which is calculated as a fraction of w_+ to make the total excitation in the network constant so that it balances the inhibition and produces a mean spontaneous firing rate for all the excitatory neurons of 3 spikes/s when no inputs λ_1 etc. have been applied (Brunel and Wang, 2001; Wang, 2002; Deco and Rolls, 2006). A typical value for w_- is 0.86. These synaptic connection strengths are prescribed, but are generally consistent with a Hebbian associative learning process, in which synapses are strengthened when there is both presynaptic and postsynaptic activity (Equation B.9). In this way, the synapses between neurons within a decision-making pool, which tend to be firing at the same time due to the λ inputs, are strong, and the synapses between neurons in different pools, which tend to be active at different times, are weaker.

All the excitatory synapses between the excitatory neurons use glutamate as a transmitter and have short time constant (τ_{AMPA}=10 ms) receptors that open ion channels, and long time constant (τ_{NMDA}=100 ms) receptors that open voltage-dependent ion channels, both of which inject currents into a neuron and produce depolarization in the direction of the firing threshold. (Details are provided in Section B.6.3, and further background to these networks is provided by Rolls (2016b) and Rolls and Deco (2010).) The inclusion of the long time constant NMDA receptors in the model helps to maintain the persistence of the high firing rate attractor state (Wang, 1999), and also prevents gamma oscillations, which arise only if the NMDA receptor contribution is insufficient (Brunel and Wang, 2003; Rolls, Webb and Deco, 2012; Wang, 2010). [I hypothesize that in evolution the NMDA to AMPA channel conductance ratios have been set to a level that minimizes gamma oscillations consistent with the need to allow AMPA to be sufficiently strong to ensure rapid processing into attractor states (Battaglia and Treves, 1998a; Panzeri et al., 2001).] The inhibitory neurons use GABA as a transmitter which hyperpolarizes the neurons, with the strength of w_{inh} typically 1.0 (Fig. 11.33b).

The evidence λ_1 for decision 1 is applied to pool D1 through 800 synapses onto each neuron, and the evidence λ_2 for decision 2 is applied to pool D2 in the same way (Fig. 11.33b). The same sets of 800 synapses on every neuron in the network also receive external inputs at a rate λ_{ext}=3 spikes/s, a typical firing rate for the spontaneous activity of cortical neurons, to reflect background activity from other cortical areas. The distribution of these inputs onto each neuron over time is what would be produced by Poisson spikes trains at 3 spikes/s on each of the 800 externally connected synapses onto each neuron, and this is one of the sources of noise in the network. Another of the sources of noise (randomness) in the network is the almost Poisson distributed spike times of the neurons in the network. As the network becomes larger and approaches an infinite number of neurons, the statistical fluctuations caused by this source of noise in the network become smoothed out and disappear, as described in more detail elsewhere (Rolls, 2016b).

The full model of decision-making is described in Sections B.6–B.8. The parameters for the models were calculated with the mean-field approach described in Sections B.7 – B.8.3, as described by Rolls and Deco (2010). The model of decision-making that we worked with is different from that analyzed by Wang (2002) in that our model is multistable, in that the spontaneous state is stable even when the decision cues are applied, as well as the decision states (see Sections 5.7 and 5.8 of Rolls and Deco (2010)). Thus it is only noise fluctuations in our models that cause the network to jump out of its spontaneous state of firing to move towards a decision. This influences for example the distribution of reaction times. Differences of this integrate-and-fire model of decision-making from the much less biologically plausible drift-diffusion model are set out in Section 5.7 of Rolls and Deco (2010) and by Deco, Rolls, Albantakis and Romo (2013). The book by Rolls and Deco (2010) *The Noisy Brain: Stochastic Dynamics as a Principle of Brain Function* is available for download from https://www.oxcns.org.

11.5.2 Analyses of reward-related decision-making mechanisms in the orbitofrontal cortex

In this Section fMRI evidence to investigate decision-making mechanisms in the orbitofrontal cortex is described. These investigations test whether the decision-making is consistent with the mechanisms described in Section 11.5.1.

The analyses relate to the ways in which probabilistic decision-making is influenced by the easiness vs the difficulty of the decision, and how confidence in a decision emerges as a property of the neuronal attractor network decision-making process.

To address these issues, we first simulated integrate-and-fire models of attractor-based choice decision-making, and predicted from them the neuronal firing rates in the decision attractor populations and the fMRI BOLD signals on easy vs difficult trials (Rolls, Grabenhorst and Deco, 2010b) as described next. We then performed the two fMRI investigations of decision-making described in Section 11.3.6 about the reward value and subjective pleasantness of thermal and olfactory stimuli, and showed that areas implicated by other analyses in decision-making (Rolls and Grabenhorst, 2008; Grabenhorst, Rolls and Parris, 2008b; Rolls, Grabenhorst and Parris, 2010d) do show the predicted difference between activations on easy vs difficult trials in the orbitofrontal cortex (Rolls, Grabenhorst and Deco, 2010b).

11.5.2.1 Neuronal responses on difficult vs easy trials, and decision confidence

Figure 11.35a and e show the mean firing rates of the two neuronal populations D1 and D2 for two trial types, easy trials (ΔI=160 Hz) and difficult trials (ΔI=0) (where ΔI is the difference in spikes/s summed across all synapses to each neuron between the two inputs, λ_1 to population D1, and λ_2 to population D2). The results are shown for correct trials, that is, trials on which the D1 population won the competition and fired with a rate of > 10 spikes/s more than the rate of D2 for the last 1000 ms of the simulation runs. Figure 11.35b shows the mean firing rates of the four populations of neurons on a difficult trial, and Fig. 11.35c shows the rastergrams for the same trial, for which the energy landscape is also shown in Fig. 11.33d. Figure 11.35d shows the firing rates on another difficult trial (ΔI=0) to illustrate the variability shown from trial to trial, with on this trial prolonged competition between the D1 and D2 attractors until the D1 attractor finally won after approximately 1100 ms. Figure 11.35f shows firing rate plots for the four neuronal populations on an example of a single easy trial (ΔI=160), Fig. 11.35g shows the synaptic currents in the four neuronal populations on the same trial, and Fig. 11.35h shows rastergrams for the same trial (Rolls, Grabenhorst and Deco, 2010b).

Three important points are made by the results shown in Fig. 11.35. First, the network falls into its decision attractor faster on easy trials than on difficult trials. We would accordingly expect reaction times to be shorter on easy than on difficult trials. We might also expect the BOLD signal related to the activity of the network to be higher on easy than on difficult trials because it starts sooner on easy trials.

Second, the mean firing rate after the network has settled into the correct decision attractor is higher on easy than on difficult trials. We might therefore expect the BOLD signal related to the activity of the network to be higher on easy than on difficult trials because the maintained activity in the attractor is higher on easy trials. This shows that the exact firing rate in the attractor is a result not only of the internal recurrent collateral effect, but also of the external input to the neurons, which in Fig. 11.35a is 32 Hz to each neuron (summed across all synapses) of D1 and D2, but in Fig. 11.35e is increased by a further 80 Hz to D1, and decreased (from the 32 Hz added) by 80 Hz to D2 (i.e. the total external input to the network is the same, but ΔI=0 for Fig. 11.35a, and ΔI=160 for Fig. 11.35b).

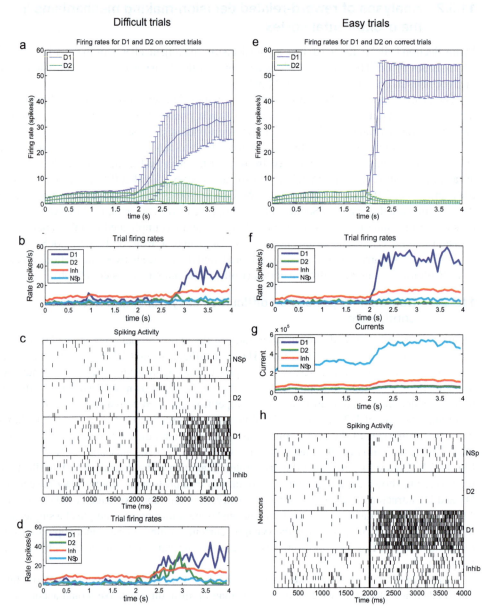

Fig. 11.35 The operation of attractor decision-making networks. (a) and (e) Firing rates (mean ± sd) for difficult (ΔI=0) and easy (ΔI=160) trials. The period 0–2 s is the spontaneous firing, and the decision cues were turned on at time = 2 s. D1: firing rate of the D1 population of neurons on correct trials on which the D1 population won. D2: firing rate of the D2 population of neurons on the correct trials on which the D1 population won. A correct trial was one in which in which the mean rate of the D1 attractor averaged > 10 spikes/s for the last 1000 ms of the simulation runs. (b) The mean firing rates of the four populations of neurons on a difficult trial. Inh is the inhibitory population that uses GABA as a transmitter. NSp is the non-specific population of neurons (see Fig. 11.33). (c) Rastergrams for the trial shown in b. 10 neurons from each of the four pools of neurons are shown. (d) The firing rates on another difficult trial (ΔI=0) showing prolonged competition between the D1 and D2 attractors until the D1 attractor finally wins after approximately 1100 ms. (f) Firing rate plots for the 4 neuronal populations on a single easy trial (ΔI=160). (g) The synaptic currents in the four neuronal populations on the trial shown in f. (h) Rastergrams for the easy trial shown in f and g. 10 neurons from each of the four pools of neurons are shown. (Reproduced from Edmund T. Rolls, Fabian Grabenhorst, and Gustavo Deco (2010) Choice, difficulty, and confidence in the brain. NeuroImage 33: 694–706. © Elsevier Inc.)

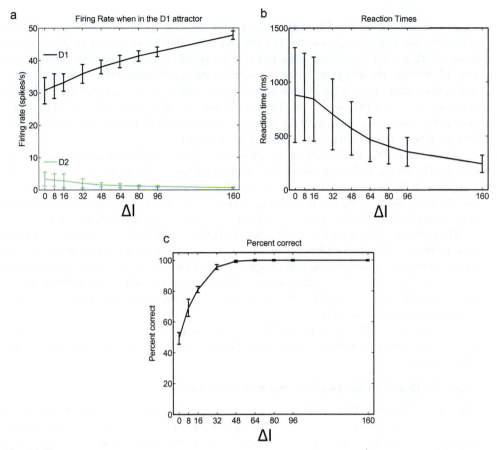

Fig. 11.36 The operation of attractor decision-making networks. (a) Firing rates (mean ± sd) on correct trials when in the D1 attractor as a function of ΔI. $\Delta I=0$ corresponds to difficult, and $\Delta I=160$ spikes/s corresponds to easy. The firing rates for both the winning population D1 and for the losing population D2 are shown for correct trials by thick lines. All the results are for 1000 simulation trials for each parameter value, and all the results shown are statistically highly significant. (b) Reaction times (mean ± sd) for the D1 population to win on correct trials as a function of the difference in inputs ΔI to D1 and D2. (c) Per cent correct performance, i.e. the percentage of trials on which the D1 population won, as a function of the difference in inputs ΔI to D1 and D2. The mean was calculated over 1000 trials, and the standard deviation was estimated by the variation in 10 groups each of 100 trials. (Reproduced from Edmund T. Rolls, Fabian Grabenhorst, and Gustavo Deco (2010) Choice, difficulty, and confidence in the brain. NeuroImage 33: 694–706. © Elsevier Inc.)

Third, the variability of the firing rate is high, with the standard deviations of the mean firing rate calculated in 50 ms epochs indicated in order to quantify the variability. The large standard deviations on difficult trials for the first second after the decision cues are applied at $t=2$ s reflect the fact that on some trials the network has entered an attractor state after 1000 ms, but on other trials it has not yet reached the attractor, although it does so later. This trial by trial variability is indicated by the firing rates on individual trials and the rastergrams in the lower part of Fig. 11.35. The effects evident in Fig. 11.35 are quantified, and elucidated over a range of values for ΔI, next.

Figure 11.36a shows the firing rates (mean ± sd) on correct trials when in the D1 attractor as a function of ΔI. $\Delta I=0$ corresponds to the most difficult decision, and $\Delta I=160$ corresponds to easy. The firing rates for both the winning population D1 and for the losing population D2 are shown. The firing rates were measured in the last 1 s of firing, i.e. between $t=3$ and $t=4$ s. It is clear that the mean firing rate of the winning population increases monotonically as ΔI increases, and interestingly, the increase is approximately linear (Pearson $r = 0.995$, p$< 10^{-6}$). The higher mean firing rates as ΔI increases are due not only to higher peak firing, but also to the fact that the variability becomes less as ΔI increases ($r = -0.95$, p$< 10^{-4}$), reflecting the fact that the system is more noisy and unstable with low ΔI, whereas the firing rate in the attractor is maintained more stably with smaller statistical fluctuations against the Poisson effects of the random spike timings at high ΔI. (The measure of variation indicated in the figure is the standard deviation, and this is shown here unless otherwise stated to quantify the degree of variation, which is a fundamental aspect of the operation of these neuronal decision-making networks.)

As shown in Fig. 11.36a, the firing rates of the losing population decrease as ΔI increases. The decrease of firing rate of the losing population is due in part to feedback inhibition through the inhibitory neurons by the winning population. Thus the difference of firing rates between the winning and losing populations, as well as the firing rate of the winning population D1, both clearly reflect ΔI, and in a sense the confidence in the decision.

The increase of the firing rate when in the D1 attractor (upper thick line) as ΔI increases thus can be related to the confidence in the decision, and, as will be shown next in Fig. 11.36b, the performance as shown by the percentage of correct choices. The firing rate of the losing attractor (D2, lower thick line) decreases as ΔI increases, due to feedback inhibition from the winning D1 attractor, and thus the difference in the firing rates of the two attractors also reflects well the decision confidence.

I emphasize from these findings (Rolls, Grabenhorst and Deco, 2010b) that the firing rate of the winning attractor reflects ΔI, and thus the confidence in the decision which is closely related to ΔI.

11.5.2.2 Decision times of the neuronal responses

The time for the network to reach the correct D1 attractor, i.e. the reaction or decision time of the network, is shown as a function of ΔI in Fig. 11.36b (mean $\pm$ sd). Interestingly, the reaction time continues to decrease ($r = -0.95, p < 10^{-4}$) over a wide range of ΔI, even when as shown in Fig. 11.36c the network is starting to perform at 100% correct. The decreasing reaction time as ΔI increases is attributable to the altered 'effective energy landscape' (Rolls, 2016b): a larger input to D1 tends to produce occasionally higher firing rates, and these statistically are more likely to induce a significant depression in the landscape towards which the network flows sooner than with low ΔI. Correspondingly, the variability (quantified by the standard deviation) of the reaction times is greatest at low ΔI, and decreases as ΔI increases ($r = -0.95, p < 10^{-4}$). This variability would not be found with a deterministic system (i.e. the standard deviations would be 0 throughout, and such systems include those investigated with mean-field analyses), and is entirely due to the random statistical fluctuations caused by the random spiking of the neurons in the integrate-and-fire network.

11.5.2.3 Percentage correct

At $\Delta I=0$, there is no influence on the network to fall more into attractor D1 representing decision 1 than attractor D2 representing decision 2, and its decisions are at chance, with approximately 50% of decisions being for D1. As ΔI increases, the proportion of trials on which D1 is reached increases. The relation between ΔI and percentage correct is shown in Fig. 11.36c. Interestingly, the performance becomes 100% correct with $\Delta I=64$, whereas as shown in Figs. 11.36a and b the firing rates while in the D1 attractor (and therefore potentially the BOLD signal), continue to increase as ΔI increases further, and the reaction times continue to decrease as ΔI increases further. It is a clear prediction for neurophysiological and behavioral measures that the firing rates with decisions made by this attractor process continue to increase as ΔI is increased beyond the level for very good performance as indicated by the percentage of correct decisions, and the neuronal and behavioral reaction times

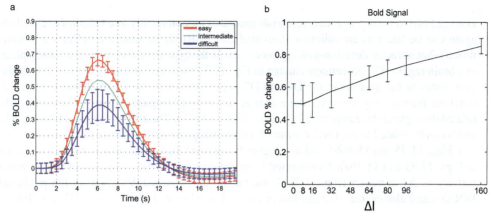

Fig. 11.37 The operation of attractor decision-making networks. (a) The percentage change in the simulated BOLD signal on easy trials (ΔI=160 spikes/s), on intermediate trials (ΔI=80), and on difficult trials (ΔI=0). The mean ± sd are shown for the easy and difficult trials. The percentage change in the BOLD signal was calculated from the firing rates of the D1 and D2 populations, and analogous effects were found with calculation from the synaptic currents averaged for example across all 4 populations of neurons. (b) The percentage change in the BOLD signal (peak mean ± sd) averaged across correct and incorrect trials as a function of ΔI. ΔI=0 corresponds to difficult, and ΔI=160 corresponds to easy. The percent change was measured as the change from the level of activity in a period of 1 s immediately before the decision cues were applied at t=0 s, and was calculated from the firing rates of the neurons in the D1 and D2 populations. The BOLD per cent change scaling is arbitrary, and is set so that the lowest value for the peak of a BOLD response is 0.5%. (Reproduced from Edmund T. Rolls, Fabian Grabenhorst, and Gustavo Deco (2010) Choice, difficulty, and confidence in the brain. NeuroImage 33: 694–706. © Elsevier Inc.)

continue to decrease as ΔI is increased beyond the level for very good performance. Figure 11.36c also shows that the variability in the percentage correct (in this case measured over blocks of 100 trials) is large with ΔI=0, and decreases as ΔI increases. This is consistent with unbiased effects of the noise producing very variable effects in the energy landscape at ΔI=0, but in the external inputs biasing the energy landscape more and more as ΔI increases, so that the flow is much more likely to be towards the D1 attractor.

11.5.2.4 Prediction of the BOLD signals on difficult vs easy decision-making trials

It is now shown how this model makes predictions for the fMRI BOLD signals that would occur in brain areas in which decision-making processing of the type described is taking place. The BOLD signals were predicted from the firing rates of the neurons in the network (or from the synaptic currents flowing in the neurons as described later) by convolving the neuronal activity with the haemodynamic response function.

As shown in Fig. 11.37a, the predicted fMRI response is larger for easy ($\Delta I = 160$ spikes/s) than for difficult trials (ΔI=0), with intermediate trials (ΔI=80) producing an intermediate fMRI response. The difference in the peak response for ΔI=0 and ΔI=160 is highly significant ($p \ll 0.001$). Importantly, the BOLD response is inherently variable from brain regions associated with this type of decision-making process, and this is nothing to do with the noise arising in the measurement of the BOLD response with a scanner. If the system were deterministic, the standard deviations, shown as a measure of the variability in Fig. 11.37a, would be 0. It is the statistical fluctuations caused by the noisy (random) spike timings of the neurons that account for the variability in the BOLD signals in Fig. 11.37a. Interestingly, the variability is larger on the difficult trials (ΔI=0) than on the easy trials (ΔI=160), as shown in Fig. 11.37a, and indeed this also can be taken as an indicator that attractor decision-making processes of the type described here are taking place in a brain region.

Figure 11.37b shows that the percentage change in the BOLD signal (peak mean ± sd) averaged across correct and incorrect trials increases monotonically as a function of ΔI. This again can be taken as an indicator (provided that fMRI signal saturation effects are minimized) that attractor decision-making processes of the type described here are taking place in a brain region. The percentage change in Fig. 11.37b was calculated by convolution of the firing rates of the neurons in the D1 and D2 populations with the haemodynamic response function. Interestingly, the percentage change in the BOLD signal is approximately linearly related throughout this range to ΔI ($r = 0.995, p < 10^{-7}$). The effects shown in Figs. 11.37a and b can be related to the earlier onset of a high firing rate attractor state when ΔI is larger (see Figs. 11.35 and 11.36b), and to a higher firing rate when in the attractor state (as shown in Figs. 11.35 and 11.36a). As expected from the decrease in the variability of the neuronal activity as ΔI increases (Fig. 11.36a), the variability (standard deviation) in the predicted BOLD signal also decreases as ΔI increases, as shown in Fig. 11.37b ($r = 0.955, p < 10^{-4}$).

The description of decision-making implemented by this integrate-and-fire model provided in Sections 11.5.1 and 11.5.2 is supplemented by a formal description of the equations in the model in Sections B.6.2 and B.6.3. As noted above, other approaches to decision-making, including the drift-diffusion and race models, are described by Deco, Rolls, Albantakis and Romo (2013). The application of this approach to decision-making for other brain regions is described in Rolls and Deco (2010) and Deco, Rolls, Albantakis and Romo (2013).

11.5.3 A neurophysiological and computational basis for stimulus–reinforcer association learning and reversal in the orbitofrontal cortex

A possible mechanism for the initial learning of stimulus-reward associations is Hebbian (associative) modification of synapses conveying visual input on to taste-responsive neurons, implementing a pattern-association network (Section B.2). In this model the unconditioned stimulus forcing the output neurons to respond is the (taste) primary reinforcer, and the (visual or olfactory) conditioned stimulus becomes associated with this by associatively modifiable synapses (Fig. B.1 on page 816) (Rolls and Treves, 1998; Rolls, 1999a, 2016b).

A first approach to the reversal is as follows, and can be understood by referring to Fig. B.1. Consider a neuron with unconditioned responses to taste in the orbitofrontal cortex. When a particular visual stimulus, say a triangle, was associated with the taste of glucose, the active synaptic connections for this visual (conditioned) stimulus would have shown long-term synaptic potentiation on to the taste neuron, which would respond to the sight of the triangle. During reversal, the same visual stimulus, the triangle, would again activate the same synaptic afferents to the neuron, but that neuron would be inactive when the taste of saline was given. Active presynaptic inputs and a low level of postsynaptic activation is the condition for homosynaptic long-term synaptic depression (LTD, Fig. 1.5 on page 11, see Rolls (2016b)), which would then occur, resulting in a decline of the response of the neuron to the triangle. At the same time, visual presentation of a square would now be associated with the taste of glucose, which would activate the postsynaptic neuron, leading now to long-term potentiation of afferents on to that neuron made active by the sight of the square.

Although reversal might be implemented in the way just described by having long-term synaptic depression for synapses that represented the reward-associated stimulus before the reversal, and long-term potentiation of the new stimulus that after reversal is associated with reward, this would require one-trial LTP and one-trial homosynaptic LTD to account for one-trial stimulus–reward reversal (Thorpe, Rolls and Maddison, 1983; Rolls, Critchley, Mason and Wakeman, 1996b; Rolls, 2000d). Moreover, the mechanism would not account for rever-

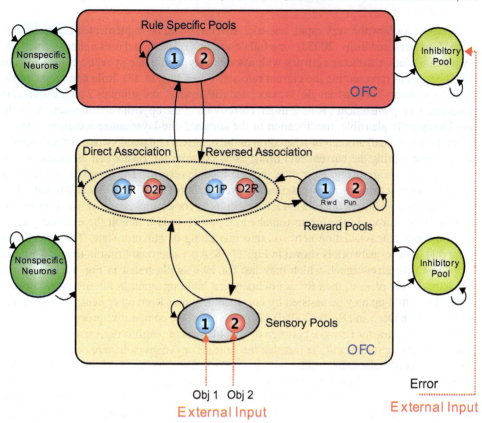

Fig. 11.38 Cortical architecture of the reward reversal computational model. There is a rule module (top) and a sensory – intermediate neuron – reward module (below). Neurons within each module are fully connected, and form attractor states. The sensory – intermediate neuron – reward module consists of three hierarchically organized levels of attractor network, with stronger synaptic connections in the forward than the backprojection direction. The intermediate level of the sensory – intermediate neuron – reward module contains neurons that respond to combinations of an object and its association with reward or punishment, e.g. object 1–reward (O1R, in the direct association set of pools), and object 1–punishment (O1P in the reversed association set of pools). These intermediate level neurons have the properties of 'conditional reward neurons' described in Section 11.3.1.2 and illustrated in Fig. 11.7, and provide a function for such conditional reward neurons. The rule module acts as a biasing input to bias the competition between the object–reward combination neurons at the intermediate level of the sensory – intermediate neuron – reward module. The whole model is implemented with integrate-and-fire neurons. (From G. Deco and E. T. Rolls (2005) Synaptic and spiking dynamics underlying reward reversal in the orbitofrontal cortex. Cerebral Cortex 15: 15–30. © Oxford University Press.)

sal learning set, the process by which during repeated reversal learning, performance gradually improves until reversal can occur in one trial. Even more, the mechanism would not account for the fact that after reversal learning set has been acquired, when the contingency is reversed, the animal makes a response to the current S+ expecting to get reward, but instead obtains the punisher. On the very first subsequent trial on which the pre-reversal S– is shown, the animal will perform a response to it expecting now to get reward, *even though the post-reversal S+ has not since the reversal been associated with reward to produce LTP for the post-reversal S+*. (This is in fact illustrated in Fig. 11.14 on page 496.) To implement this very rapid stimulus–reinforcer association reversal, a different mechanism is therefore needed. The mechanism can not rely on associative processes, but instead on a rule-based (i.e. model-based) process, which requires the current rule to be held in mind, in short-term memory. This, and non-reward neurons that maintain their firing for many seconds as illustrated in Fig. 11.14, may be developments provided for by the evolution of granular orbitofrontal cortex areas in primates (see Section 2.6).

A model for how the very rapid, one-trial, reversal could be implemented has been developed (see Deco and Rolls (2005d) for a full description). The model uses a short-term memory autoassociation attractor network with associatively modifiable synaptic connections to hold the neurons representing the current rule active (see Fig. 11.38). Rule one might correspond to 'stimulus 1 (e.g. a triangle) is associated with reward, and stimulus 2 (e.g. a square) is associated with punishment'. Rule 2 might correspond to the opposite contingency. A small, very biologically plausible, modification of the standard one-layer autoassociation network is that there is a small amount of adaptation in the recurrent collateral synapses that keep the neurons representing the current rule firing. Now consider the case when the neurons representing rule one are firing. How does the rule module reverse? The proposal is that when the non-reward or error neurons described above (Section 11.3.4) fire, this additional set of firing neurons destabilizes the rule attractor module, by for example producing extra firing of the inhibitory neurons in the orbitofrontal cortex, which in turn inhibit the excitatory neurons in the rule autoassociation network, thus quenching its attractor state. This error input to the rule attractor network is shown in Fig. 11.38. After neuronal firing in the network has stopped and the error signal, which may last for 10 s as illustrated in Fig. 11.14 on page 496, is no longer present, then firing gradually can build up again in the rule attractor network. (This build-up may be assisted by non-specific inputs from other neurons in the area, as illustrated in Deco and Rolls (2005d).) However, with the competitive processes operating within the rule attractor network between the populations of neurons representing rule 1 and those representing rule 2, and the fact that the neurons or synapses that are part of the rule 1 attractor are partly adapted, the neurons that win the competition and become active are those representing rule 2, and the rule attractor has reversed its state. This process is illustrated in Fig. 11.39, and takes one trial. Reversal learning set takes a number of reversals to acquire because the correct attractors for the relevant rules, and their connections to other 'mapping' neurons, have to be learned.

To achieve the correct 'mapping' from stimuli to their reinforcer association, and thus emotional state, the rule neurons bias the competition in a mapping module, illustrated in Fig. 11.38. The mapping module has sensory input neurons, intermediate 'conditional reward' neurons (of the type described in Section 11.3.1.2 and illustrated in Fig. 11.7) which respond to combinations of stimuli and whether they are currently associated with reward (or for other neurons to a punisher), and output neurons which represent the reinforcement association of the stimulus currently being viewed. (In the case described there are four populations or pools of neurons at the intermediate level, two for the direct rewarding context: object 1-rewarding, object 2-punishing, and two for the reversal condition: object 1-punishing, object 2-rewarding.) These intermediate pools or populations of neurons respond to combinations of the sensory stimuli and the expected reward, e.g. to object 1 and an expected reward (glucose obtained after licking), and are the conditional reward neurons described in Section 11.3.1.2 and illustrated in Fig. 11.7 on page 487. The sensory – intermediate – reward module thus consists of three hierarchically organized levels of attractor network, with stronger synaptic connections in the forward direction from input to output than the backprojection direction. The rule module acts as a biasing input to bias the competition between the object–reward combination neurons at the intermediate level of the sensory – intermediate – reward module. This biasing is achieved because rule 1 has associatively strengthened connections to object 1–rewarding and object 2–punishing neurons. (The whole network could be set up by simple associative learning operating to strengthen connections made with low probability between different neurons that are conjunctively active during the task in the network – see Deco and Rolls (2005d).)

Thus when object 1, e.g. the triangle, is being presented and rule one for direct mapping is in the rule module and biasing the intermediate neurons of the sensory – intermediate –

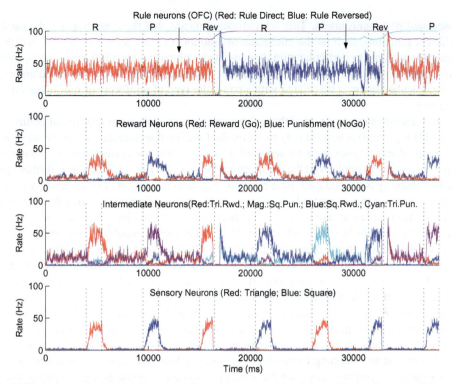

Fig. 11.39 Reward reversal model: Temporal evolution of the averaged population activity for all neural pools (sensory, intermediate (stimulus–reward), and Reward/Punishment) in the stimulus – intermediate – reward module and the rule module, during the execution and the reversal of the Go/NoGo visual discrimination task with a pseudorandom trial sequence after Thorpe, Rolls and Maddison (1983) and Rolls, Critchley, Mason and Wakeman (1996). Bottom row: the sensory neuronal populations, one of which responds to Object 1, a triangle (red), and the other to Object 2, a square (blue). The intermediate conditional stimulus–reward and stimulus–punishment neurons respond to for example Object 1 (Triangle, Tri) when it is associated with reward (Rwd) (e.g. on trial 1, corresponding to O1R in Fig. 11.38), or to Object 2 (Square, Sq) when it is associated with punishment (Pun) (e.g. on trial 2, O2P). The top row shows the firing rate activity in the rule module, with the thin line at the top of this graph showing the mean probability of release P_{rel} of transmitter from the synapses of each population of neurons. The arrows show when the contingencies reversed. R: Reward trial; P: Punishment Trial; Rev: Reversal trial, i.e. the first trial after the reward contingency was reversed when Reward was expected but Punishment was obtained. The intertrial interval was 4 s. The yellow line shows the average activity of the inhibitory neurons. (See text for further details.) (From G. Deco and E. T. Rolls (2005) Synaptic and spiking dynamics underlying reward reversal in the orbitofrontal cortex. Cerebral Cortex 15: 15–30. © Oxford University Press.)

reward module, then the intermediate neurons that fire are the object 1-reward neurons (O1R in Fig. 11.38), and these in turn through associative connections activate the reward neurons (Rwd in Fig. 11.38) at the third, reward/punishment, level of the hierarchy. If on the other hand object 1, e.g. the triangle, is being presented and rule two for reversed mapping is in the rule module and biasing the intermediate neurons of the sensory – intermediate – reward module, then the intermediate neurons that fire are the object 1–punishment (O1P) neurons, and these in turn through associative connections activate the punishment neurons (Pun) at the third, reward/punishment, level of the hierarchy. This model can thus account for one-trial reversal learning, and provides a computationally interesting account for the presence of the conditional reward and conditional punishment neurons found by Thorpe, Rolls and Maddison (1983) and Rolls, Critchley, Mason and Wakeman (1996b) in the orbitofrontal cortex (Section 11.3.1.2).

It is an important part of the architecture that at the intermediate level of the sensory – intermediate – reward module one set of neurons fire if an object being presented is currently associated with reward, and a different set if the object being presented is currently associated with punishment. This representation means that these neurons can be used for different functions, such as the elicitation of emotional or autonomic responses, which can occur for example to particular stimuli associated with particular reinforcers (Rolls, 1999a). For example, particular emotions might arise if a particular cognitively processed input such as a particular person is associated with a particular type of reinforcer or reinforcement contingency.

It is also an interesting part of the architecture that associative synaptic modifiability (LTP, and LTD if present) is needed only to set up the functional architecture of the network while the reversal learning set is being acquired. However, once the correct synaptic connections have been set up to implement the architecture illustrated in Fig. 11.38, then no further synaptic modifiability is needed each time reversal occurs, as reversal is achieved just by the error signal quenching the current rule attractor, and the attractor for the other rule then starting up because its synapses are not adapted. This is an interesting prediction of the model. If tested by NMDA receptor blockers, which can block LTP, then it would be important to ensure that non-specific factors produced by the NMDA blockade such as less overall activity in the network, and the stabilizing effects of the long time constants of NMDA receptors, do not contribute to any result obtained. For this reason, use of a procedure for impairing synaptic modifiability other than NMDA receptor blockade would be useful in testing this prediction.

The network just described uses biased competition from a rule module to bias the mapping from sensory stimuli to the representation of a reward vs a punisher. An analogous rule network reversed in the same way by error signals quenching the current rule attractor, can be used to reverse the mapping from stimuli via intermediate stimulus–response neurons to response neurons, and thus to switch the stimulus-to-motor response being mapped in a model of conditional response learning (Deco and Rolls, 2003, 2005d). While reward rule neurons have not been described yet for the orbitofrontal cortex, neurons that may correspond to stimulus–response rule neurons have been found in the dorsolateral prefrontal cortex (Wallis et al., 2001).

This model also provides a computational account for why the orbitofrontal cortex may play a more important role in rapid reversal learning than the amygdala. The account is based on the fact that a feature of cortical architecture is a highly developed set of local (within 1–2 mm) recurrent collateral excitatory associatively modifiable connections between pyramidal cells (Rolls and Deco, 2002; Rolls and Treves, 1998; Rolls, 2021c). These provide the basis for short-term memory attractor networks, and thus the basis for the rule attractor model which is at the heart of the proposal for how rapid reversal learning is implemented (Deco and Rolls, 2005d). In contrast, the amygdala is thought to have a much less well developed set of recurrent collateral excitatory connections, and thus may not be able to implement rapid reversal learning in the way described using competition biased by a rule module. Instead, the amygdala would need to rely on synaptic relearning as described in the first approach above, and this would be likely to be a slower process, and would certainly not lead to correct choice of the new S+ the first time it is presented after a punishment trial when the reversal contingency changes. Of course, in addition it is possible that the rapidity of LTP, and the efficacy of LTD, both of which would also facilitate rapid reversal, may be enhanced in the orbitofrontal cortex compared to the amygdala. Thus, the cortical neuronal reversal mechanism in the orbitofrontal cortex may be effectively a faster implementation in two ways than what is implemented in the amygdala. The cortical (in this case orbitofrontal cortex) mechanism may have evolved particularly to enable rapid updating by received reinforcers in social and other situations in primates. This hypothesis, that the orbitofrontal cortex, as a rapid learning mechanism, effectively provides an additional route for some of the functions performed by the amygdala, and is very important when this stimulus–reinforcer learning must be rapidly readjusted, has been developed elsewhere (Rolls, 1990c, 1992b, 1996a, 1999a, 2000c, 2005a, 2019e).

Another feature of the rule attractor model of rapid reversal learning (Deco and Rolls, 2005d) is that it does utilize a set of coupled attractor networks in the orbitofrontal cortex. Consistent with this, Hikosaka and Watanabe (2000) have shown that a short-term memory for reward, such as the flavor of a food, is represented by continuing firing in orbitofrontal cortex neurons in a reward delayed match-to-sample short-term memory task. This could be implemented by associatively modified synaptic connections between taste reward neurons in the orbitofrontal cortex.

Although the mechanism has been described so far for visual-to-taste association learning, this is because neurophysiological experiments on this are most direct. It is likely, given the evidence from the effects of lesions, that taste is only one type of primary reinforcer about which such learning occurs in the orbitofrontal cortex, and is likely to be an example of a much more general type of stimulus–reinforcer learning system. Some of the evidence for this is that humans with orbitofrontal cortex damage are impaired at visual discrimination reversal when working for a reward that consists of points (Rolls, Hornak, Wade and McGrath, 1994a) or money (Hornak, Bramham, Rolls, Morris, O'Doherty, Bullock and Polkey, 2003). Moreover, as described above, there is evidence that the representation of the affective aspects of touch are represented in the human orbitofrontal cortex (Rolls, O'Doherty, Kringelbach, Francis, Bowtell and McGlone, 2003d; McCabe, Rolls, Bilderbeck and McGlone, 2008), and learning about what stimuli are associated with this class of primary reinforcer is also likely to be an important aspect of the stimulus–reinforcer association learning performed by the orbitofrontal cortex.

11.5.4 A theory and model of non-reward neural mechanisms in the orbitofrontal cortex

Single neurons in the primate orbitofrontal cortex respond when an expected reward is not obtained, and behavior must change. The human lateral orbitofrontal cortex is activated when non-reward, or loss occurs. The neuronal computation of this negative reward prediction error is fundamental for the emotional changes associated with non-reward, and with changing behavior. A mechanism for this computation has been proposed (Rolls and Deco, 2016), as follows.

A single attractor network has a Reward population (or pool) of neurons that is activated by Expected Reward (Fig. 11.40), and maintain their firing until, after a time, synaptic depression reduces the firing rate in this neuronal population. If a Reward Outcome is not received, the decreasing firing in the Reward neurons releases the inhibition implemented by inhibitory neurons, and this results in a second population of Non-Reward neurons to start and continue firing encouraged by the spiking-related noise in the network. This is illustrated in the integrate-and-fire simulation shown in Fig. 11.41.

If a Reward Outcome is received, this keeps the Reward attractor active, and this through the inhibitory neurons prevents the Non-Reward attractor neurons from being activated. If an Expected Reward has been signalled, and the Reward Attractor neurons are active, their firing can be directly inhibited by a Non-Reward Outcome, and the Non-Reward neurons become activated because the inhibition on them is released (Rolls and Deco, 2016).

The neuronal mechanisms in the orbitofrontal cortex for computing negative reward prediction error are important, for this system may be over-reactive in depression, under-reactive in impulsive behavior, and may influence the dopaminergic 'reward prediction error' neurons.

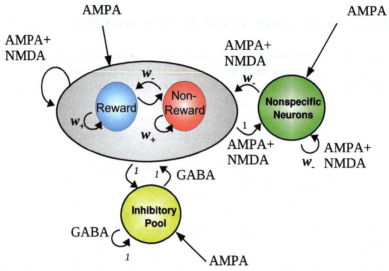

Fig. 11.40 A model for the computation of non-reward in the orbitofrontal cortex. The excitatory neurons are divided into two selective pools S1 (termed the Reward Attractor population of neurons) and S2 (termed the Non-Reward Attractor population of neurons) (with 80 neurons each) with strong intra-pool connection strengths w_+ and one non-selective pool (NS) (with 640 neurons). The value of w_+ for S2 is a little higher than that for S1, so that S2 tends to emerge into a high firing rate if activity is not maintained in S1 after an Expected Reward input has been received. The other connection strengths are 1 or weak w_-. The network contains 1000 neurons, of which 800 are in the excitatory pools and 200 are in the inhibitory pool IH. Every neuron in the network also receives inputs from 800 external neurons, and these neurons increase their firing rates to apply a stimulus to one of the pools S1 or S2. (Modified from Rolls, E. T. and Deco,G. (2016) Non-reward neural mechanisms in the orbitofrontal cortex. Cortex 83: 27–38. © Elsevier Ltd.)

11.6 Highlights: what are the special computational roles of the orbitofrontal cortex in reward, emotion, and decision-making?

It is important in terms of our understanding of brain function to consider what is special about the primate including human orbitofrontal cortex for reward, decision-making, and emotion, compared to other brain regions including the amygdala. This invites an answer about what is special about the computations performed by the orbitofrontal cortex compared to other brain regions.

First, the orbitofrontal cortex, as a neocortical area, has highly developed recurrent collateral connections between its pyramidal cells, which together with associative synaptic plasticity, provide the basis for autoassociation or attractor networks (Rolls, 2021c). (The amygdala in contrast has little recurrent collateral connectivity (Millhouse and DeOlmos, 1983).) These attractor networks provide the basis for short-term memory functions, by maintaining neuronal firing in a stable attractor. These attractor networks can hold on-line which stimuli (and this could be other individuals) are currently rewarding, which is important for social interactions and economic decisions. This memory capability is an important component of rule-based one-trial reversal, in which the current rule must be held in short-term memory (Deco and Rolls, 2005d). Short-term memory is also potentially very useful for holding mood online for some time, so that if for example a reward is not received, the non-reward state of frustration can lead to continuing attempts to regain the reward. Similar short-term memory processes might enable one to remember the recent reinforcement history of individuals, and again can be important in decision-making. The short-term memory aspects of these attractor networks are also important for holding the expected value online, until the reward outcome is received, after which non-reward neurons may be activated in the ways just described (Rolls and Deco, 2016), and such computations may also contribute to reward prediction error, de-

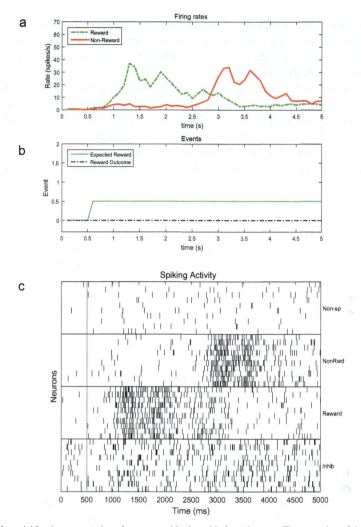

Fig. 11.41 A model for the computation of non-reward in the orbitofrontal cortex. The operation of the network when an Expected Reward is not obtained (extinction). a. The firing rates of the Reward population of neurons and the Non-Reward population of neurons during a 5 s trial. b. After a period of spontaneous activity from 0 until 0.5 s, the Expected Reward input was applied to the reward attractor population of neurons, and maintained at that level for the remainder of the trial. No Reward Outcome input was received. c. Rastergrams showing for each of the four populations of neurons, Non-Specific, Non-Reward, Reward, and Inhibitory, the spiking of ten neurons chosen at random from each population. Each small vertical line represents a spike from a neuron. Each horizontal row shows the spikes of one neuron. The different neurons are from the same trial. (Modified from Rolls, E. T. and Deco,G. (2016) Non-reward neural mechanisms in the orbitofrontal cortex. Cortex 83: 27–38. © Elsevier Ltd.)

fined as the reward outcome value minus the expected reward. The short-term memory also provides the biasing system for top-down attention to reward value (Grabenhorst, Rolls and Bilderbeck, 2008a; Rolls, Grabenhorst, Margot, da Silva and Velazco, 2008b; Grabenhorst and Rolls, 2008; Rolls, 2008f; Ge, Feng, Grabenhorst and Rolls, 2012; Luo, Ge, Grabenhorst, Feng and Rolls, 2013) implemented by biased competition (Sections 2.12 and B.8.4), or by biased activation (Grabenhorst and Rolls, 2010; Rolls, 2013a) (Section 4.3.5).

These attractor networks in the orbitofrontal cortex and ventromedial prefrontal cortex also provide the basis for reward-related decision-making, in which inputs to two competing attractor states in an attractor network lead to a bifurcation and to a decision (Deco, Rolls and Romo, 2009; Rolls and Deco, 2010, 2011b; Deco, Rolls, Albantakis and Romo, 2013).

Part of the utility of this approach to decision-making is that once the decision has been taken in the attractor network, the results of the decision are kept active in the decision-making attractor network to provide the goals for the selection of actions by the cingulate cortex to obtain the rewards (Rolls, 2019e,c).

Second, the primate and human orbitofrontal cortex as a neocortical area is beautifully connected anatomically to receive inputs from representations of 'what' stimulus is present from every sensory modality at the top of each sensory cortical hierarchy, independently of reward value (as shown in Fig. 11.1), and then to compute multimodal representations that are then represented in terms of their reward value. This is very different from the rodent, in which reward is represented throughout the processing systems (Rolls, 2019e) (Section 19.10).

Third, the primate orbitofrontal cortex specializes in reward value, rather than action. This separation allows the value of many stimuli in the high dimensional space of different rewards (Rolls, 2014a) to be represented, and for competition between them to be useful for computing relative reward value (Grabenhorst and Rolls, 2009). Moreover, mood states can be maintained, independently of any actions being performed. In contrast, as described above, the rodent 'orbitofrontal cortex' is also involved in motor responses and actions (Wilson, Takahashi, Schoenbaum and Niv, 2014b), so can be less specialized for representing reward value, and rapidly changing it.

Fourth, the primate orbitofrontal cortex projects reward value representations to the pregenual anterior cingulate cortex, and punishment value representations to the supracallosal anterior cingulate cortex (Hsu et al., 2020; Du et al., 2020; Rolls et al., 2023c), where they can be associated with actions performed recently represented in the supracallosal anterior cingulate cortex (Rolls et al., 2023c), received partly via the posterior cingulate cortex from the parietal cortex, to implement action-outcome learning (Rolls, 2019c). Outputs are then directed from mid-cingulate areas to the premotor cortical areas (Rolls, 2019c; Rolls et al., 2023c). The amygdala does not have similar connectivity.

Fifth, the human lateral orbitofrontal cortex has considerable connectivity with the inferior frontal gyrus areas 45 and 44 which in the left are Broca's area, and this may be part of the route by which the orbitofrontal cortex, especially laterally, becomes functionally connected with language areas in the posterior temporal and parietal areas (Hsu, Rolls, Huang, Chong, Lo, Feng and Lin, 2020; Du, Rolls, Cheng, Li, Gong, Qiu and Feng, 2020; Rolls, Deco, Huang and Feng, 2023c). This provides a route for top-down influences of language-related processing on emotional and social behavior, and indeed is part of the long-loop interactions between attractor networks that are proposed to contribute to increased rumination in depression (Rolls, 2016e; Rolls et al., 2020a) (Section 18.5). This route also enables emotional states represented in the orbitofrontal cortex to gain access to language systems to provide for declarative reports about felt emotional states (Rolls et al., 2023c,b).

To finish this Chapter, it may be interesting to consider the following hypothesis about the evolutionary basis for why the primate including human orbitofrontal cortex has become the part of the cerebral cortex that specialises in reward (and punishment) value decoding, and in emotion. The hypothesis is that the primary taste cortex in the anterior insula projects to the next stage in its hierarchy, which is the orbitofrontal cortex just immediately in front of it (Baylis, Rolls and Baylis, 1995; Rolls, Deco, Huang and Feng, 2023f,c), and that the next computation that needs to be implemented in the taste system after the insular primary taste cortex is reward processing of food, which is rather important for survival. The hypothesis is that the main place to which the primary taste cortex in the anterior insula could project to for reward processing in a hierarchy is the orbitofrontal cortex, for all the cortex posterior to the anterior insula was occupied by body somatosensory insula (see Chapter 6). The hypothesis further is that for the orbitofrontal cortex to implement food reward well, the orbitofrontal cortex needed also olfactory inputs, and somatosensory inputs for the texture of food to build food flavor, and also visual object inputs for the sight of food to be associated with its flavor (which is very important in primates in their ecological niches).

But why did other rewards than food also get built into the orbitofrontal cortex? That is a more open question. But once the orbitofrontal cortex has somatosensory reward for the texture of food, this could be extended to other types of texture, such as the soft gentle touch of skin, with mutual grooming a sign of affiliation and cooperation in primates (Dunbar, 2022). And somatosensory inputs as rewards may also be relevant to reproductive behavior. Again, there is a need for relevant visual inputs to become associated with these primary reinforcers, with it being important to visually recognise the partner in whom you are investing, in part with the evolutionary adaptive value of producing offspring and investing in them to increase their chances of reproduction and maintaining the gene line. That type of reward, and related rewards such as monetary value, may all thereby be computed in the primate including human orbitofrontal cortex, with food reward as an evolutionary origin.

12 The cingulate cortex

12.1 Introduction to and overview of the cingulate cortex

12.1.1 Introduction

A key area included by Broca in his limbic lobe (Broca, 1878) is the cingulate cortex, which hooks around the corpus callosum. The term limbic used by Broca referred to structures that are at the border or edge (the literal meaning of limbic) of the hemispheres (when seen in medial view), and led to the development of the concept of a limbic system (Pessoa and Hof, 2015). Other limbic structures include the hippocampus, and the amygdala (which has major connections with the orbitofrontal cortex). These structures appear to have very different connections and functions. The amygdala and orbitofrontal cortex are key structures involved in emotion and reward value with connections from ventral stream processing areas that decode 'what' the stimulus is (Rolls, 2014a, 2019e) (Chapter 11). The hippocampus is a key structure in episodic memory with 'where' inputs about spatial scenes from the ventromedial visual stream and from the parietal cortex for self-motion update, as well as from the 'what' ventral processing stream and the value system in the orbitofrontal cortex (Kesner and Rolls, 2015; Rolls, 2018b, 2023c) (Chapter 9). Because of the different connectivity and functions of these limbic structures (amygdala, orbitofrontal cortex, and hippocampus) in emotion and in memory, it has been proposed that the concept of a single 'limbic system' is not realistic, and that we should consider separately the connectivity and functions of different limbic structures in emotion and memory (Rolls, 2015b).

However, that leaves the cingulate cortex in an interesting position straddling the emotional and memory domains. The anterior cingulate cortex receives inputs from the orbitofrontal cortex and amygdala which receive from ventral stream areas. Moreover, there is evidence relating the anterior cingulate cortex to action-outcome learning, in which actions are learned to obtain goals based on the outcomes, the rewards and punishers, received for different actions (Rushworth, Kolling, Sallet and Mars, 2012; Kolling, Wittmann, Behrens, Boorman, Mars and Rushworth, 2016; Rolls, 2019c; Klein-Flugge, Bongioanni and Rushworth, 2022a; Rolls, Deco, Huang and Feng, 2023c). The selection of which action to perform to obtain the best reward outcome may involve deciding whether to continue with the present action, termed in the language of foraging 'exploit', or whether to 'explore', that is switch to a different action aimed at a different goal and reward outcome (Klein-Flugge et al., 2022a).

Some parts of the posterior cingulate cortex receive from spatial 'where' systems including via the ventromedial visual stream to the parahippocampal cortex and from the parietal cortex, and other parts from 'what' inferior temporal cortex and related regions, and both connect to the hippocampal memory system.

In this Chapter I provide a framework for understanding the connectivity and functions of the cingulate cortex, and how the cingulate cortex can be involved in at least three important functions, emotion, action-outcome learning, and memory.

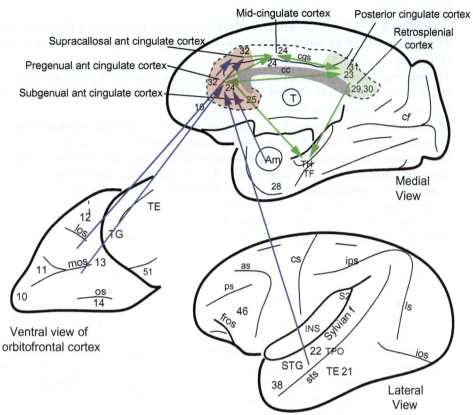

Fig. 12.1 Connections of the anterior cingulate cortex shown on views of the primate brain (see text). The anterior cingulate cortex (including the subgenual cingulate cortex area 25) is shaded in red, the posterior cingulate cortex (areas 23 and 31) and retrosplenial cortex (areas 29 and 30) in green, and the corpus callosum (cc) in grey. The arrows show the main direction of connectivity, but there are connections in both directions. Connections reach the pregenual cingulate cortex especially from the medial/mid-orbitofrontal cortex; and reach the supracallosal anterior cingulate cortex especially from the orbitofrontal cortex as well as premotor cortex regions. Connections to the pregenual anterior cingulate cortex from the temporal lobe are from the (auditory) superior temporal gyrus (STG), from the visual and auditory cortex in the superior temporal sulcus; and from the amygdala. Abbreviations: as – arcuate sulcus; cf – calcarine fissure; cgs – cingulate sulcus; cs – central sulcus; ls – lunate sulcus; ios – inferior occipital sulcus; mos – medial orbital sulcus; os – orbital sulcus; ps – principal sulcus; sts – superior temporal sulcus; Sf – Sylvian (or lateral) fissure (which has been opened to reveal the insula); Am – amygdala; INS – insula; TE (21) – inferior temporal visual cortex; STG (22) – superior temporal gyrus auditory association cortex; TF and TH – parahippocampal cortex; TPO – multimodal cortical area in the superior temporal sulcus; 28 – entorhinal cortex; 38, TG – temporal pole cortex; 13, 11 – medial orbitofrontal cortex; 12 – lateral orbitofrontal cortex; 10 – ventromedial prefrontal cortex; 14 – gyrus rectus; 51 – olfactory (prepyriform and periamygdaloid) cortex.

12.1.2 Overview of what is computed in the cingulate cortex

1. In humans, the pregenual and subgenual anterior cingulate cortex receive information directly and via the ventromedial prefrontal cortex (vmPFC) from the medial orbitofrontal cortex where rewards are represented, and from the lateral orbitofrontal cortex where aversive stimuli are represented. These orbitofrontal cortex areas represent information about value, not about actions or responses, as shown by neuronal recordings in macaques.

2. The pregenual anterior cingulate cortex in humans is activated by many rewards.

3. The pregenual anterior cingulate cortex has onward effective connectivity directed to the hippocampal system, both directly, and via the posterior cingulate cortex. This provides a route for emotional states, and the rewards and punishers that elicit them, to become incorporated into hippocampal episodic memory, and potentially to provide the goals for

navigation. It is appropriate that the reward-related pregenual anterior cingulate cortex should have some of its output directed towards a navigational system, which is set up to find goals.
4. The pregenual anterior cingulate cortex also has effective connectivity directed to the septal nuclei which provide the cholinergic innervation of the hippocampus. This modulation may influence episodic memory consolidation.
5. The memory deficits produced by vmPFC / anterior cingulate cortex damage in humans are probably related to interference with the incorporation of value information into episodic memory, and when the value component is recalled, its effects on memory consolidation by enhancing the depth of processing. In addition, damage to the vmPFC / anterior cingulate regions may impair memory consolidation by interference with the modulation of cholinergic function produced by connectivity from the anterior cingulate cortex to the septal region. This evidence indicates that the vmPFC / anterior cingulate cortex does not implement the computations required for episodic memory, which are performed by the hippocampus.
6. The supracallosal anterior cingulate cortex (also known as the dorsal anterior cingulate cortex dACC) is activated by aversive stimuli and non-reward, receives value-related information about outcomes from the orbitofrontal cortex and pregenual anterior cingulate cortex, and is implicated in action-outcome learning. It has connectivity to premotor cortical regions including the mid-cingulate cortex, which is appropriate for producing actions. If aversive stimuli or non-reward are received, this is likely to lead to a change of actions: in the terminology of foraging, changing from 'exploit' to 'explore'. It is involved in actions directed to obtaining goals, in that devaluation of the goal results in an immediate cessation of the action, even before there has been an opportunity for the action to be made and then not followed by the reward.
7. This is different from stimulus-response habits learned by dopamine-dependent reinforcement learning, which are not driven by the goal, and continue for some time even when the reinforcer is devalued.
8. The anterior cingulate cortex is thereby implicated in emotion, because the pregenual anterior cingulate cortex is involved in processing rewards received from the orbitofrontal cortex and connecting them to navigational systems to obtain rewards; and because the supracallosal anterior cingulate cortex is involved in processing aversive stimuli and non-reward received from the orbitofrontal cortex, and changing actions to 'explore' in order to avoid the punishers and non-reward, and to search for new goals with new actions.
9. The subgenual cingulate cortex (area 25) may link rewards and punishers to autonomic output.
10. The posterior cingulate division postero-ventral regions receive information from the visual inferior temporal cortex and auditory and semantic superior temporal sulcus regions, and from vmPFC and pregenual cingulate reward regions. They have connectivity to the hippocampal system thereby contributing to 'what' information for hippocampal episodic memory.
11. The posterior cingulate division antero-dorsal regions (including the RSC region) receive inputs from the parietal cortex, including areas 7a, VIP and LIP laterally, and area 7m medially, and have effective connectivity to the hippocampal systems thereby contributing to 'where' information for the idiothetic update of scene representations used for hippocampal episodic memory.
12. The retrosplenial scene area is located in DVT the dorsal visual transitional region and in ProS the prostriate cortex region, receives inputs from the occipital scene area, and connects to the parahippocampal scene area (or PPA), providing a ventromedial visual

cortical route for 'where' information about scenes to reach the hippocampal episodic memory system.

12.1.3 Overview of how the computations are performed by the cingulate cortex

1. For action-outcome learning, the system needs to hold active a representation of the action that has just been performed, so that it can be associated with the outcome when it arrives. It may also be useful to hold online evidence about outcomes received from the previously few trials, as this is likely to be useful in probabilistic tasks, that is under uncertainty. Cortical attractor networks in the anterior cingulate cortex are likely to implement this local short-term memory function.

2. The outcomes are in the high dimensional space of many different types of reward that are represented in the orbitofrontal cortex. This enables rapid learning of which actions to perform for which outcomes, because this requires simple associative learning between the particular actions recently performed, and the particular outcomes that have recently been received, with the outcome information provided by the orbitofrontal cortex.

3. This action-outcome learning implemented in the supracallosal anterior cingulate cortex (dACC) is thus much more efficient than stimulus-response habit formation, in which a one-dimensional reinforcer, the dopamine neuron reward prediction error signal, is used to reinforce whatever representations of stimuli and responses throughout the dopamine-influenced basal ganglia system may recently have been active (see Chapter 16).

4. The orbitofrontal cortex–supracallosal anterior cingulate cortex action-outcome learning system is also much more rapid and efficient than the reinforcement learning stimulus-response habit system implemented by dopamine and the basal ganglia, because if the association between the stimulus and the outcome (a stimulus-stimulus association) changes or is reversed, this can be corrected in one trial by the stimulus-reward reversal learning system in the orbitofrontal cortex described in Chapter 11.

5. Error signals generated in the dACC reflect a mismatch between the expected outcome and the action. This is different from the orbitofrontal cortex, in which the error signals reflect a mismatch between the expected value of a stimulus (e.g. the sight of food) and the outcome (e.g. a taste of food).

6. It is proposed that the error signal in the dACC acts to destabilize and reset an attractor network neuronal population that indicates 'exploit' to allow another neuronal population that represents 'explore' to become active in the same attractor network, in order to generate 'explore' behavior when non-reward or a punisher is received from the orbitofrontal cortex. The computational mechanism is similar to that described for reversal of the rule attractor network in Section 11.5.3.

7. The spatial part of the posterior cingulate cortex, together with the retrosplenial cortex, connects information from the parietal lobe which may be at least partly in egocentric coordinates with the hippocampal system via the parahippocampal gyrus which is largely in allocentric coordinates. The posterior cingulate cortex and retrosplenial scene area may be involved in helping to perform these coordinate transforms, in ways that are described in Section 3.4.

12.2 Anterior cingulate cortex

12.2.1 Anterior cingulate cortex anatomy and connections in primates

The anterior cingulate regions occupy approximately the anterior one third of the cingulate cortex (see Fig. 12.1) and are involved in emotion. They may be distinguished from a midcingulate area (i.e. further back than the anterior cingulate regions and occupying approximately the middle third of the cingulate cortex) which has been termed the cingulate motor area (Vogt et al., 1996; Vogt, 2009, 2016, 2019b) and may be involved in action selection (Rushworth et al., 2004, 2011). The anterior cingulate cortex includes parts of area 32 and 24, and comprises the pregenual anterior cingulate cortex, the supracallosal anterior cingulate cortex, and area 25 the subgenual cingulate cortex (Figs. 12.1 and 11.3) (Price, 2006; Ongur, Ferry and Price, 2003; Ongur and Price, 2000; Carmichael and Price, 1996; Vogt, 2009, 2019b). (The midcingulate cortex has been described as having an anterior and a posterior part, with the criteria including cytoarchitecture (Vogt, 2016, 2019b).)

As shown in Figs. 12.1 and 12.2, the anterior cingulate cortex receives strong inputs from the orbitofrontal cortex, and is also characterised by connections with the amygdala (Carmichael and Price, 1995a; Morecraft and Tanji, 2009; Vogt, 2009, 2019b). The anterior cingulate cortex also has connections with some temporal cortical areas involved in memory including the parahippocampal gyrus (which provides via the entorhinal cortex a bridge to the hippocampus); and with the rostral superior temporal gyrus, the auditory superior temporal gyrus, and the dorsal bank of the superior temporal sulcus (Saleem et al., 2008; Vogt, 2009) (see Fig. 12.1). (The cortex in the superior temporal sulcus contains visual neurons that respond to face expression, gesture, and head movement (Hasselmo, Rolls and Baylis, 1989a; Hasselmo, Rolls, Baylis and Nalwa, 1989b).)

In more detail, in macaques a 'medial prefrontal network' (mainly anterior cingulate cortex) selectively involves medial areas 14r, 14c, 24, 25, 32, and 10m, rostral orbital areas 10o and 11m, and agranular insular area Iai in the posterior orbital cortex (Carmichael and Price, 1996). An 'orbital' prefrontal network links most of the areas within the orbital cortex, including areas Iam, Iapm, Ial, 12l, 12m, and 12r in the caudal and lateral parts of the orbital cortex, with areas 13l, 13m, and 13b in the central orbital cortex, which have further onward connections to the rostral orbital area 11l (Carmichael and Price, 1996; Ongur and Price, 2000; Price, 2006). Several orbital areas (including 13a, 12o and 11m) have connections with both the medial and orbital networks. Many of these areas are shown in Figs. 12.1 and 11.2. It is interesting that this macaque medial prefrontal network (anterior cingulate cortex) has connections with the posterior cingulate / retrosplenial cortex, and parahippocampal cortex (Saleem et al., 2008), and has access to the hippocampus in this way; whereas the orbitofrontal cortex has projections to the perirhinal cortex (Saleem et al., 2008), and thus has access to the hippocampus via a more ventral route (Fig. 12.2).

The outputs of the anterior cingulate cortex reach further back in the cingulate cortex towards the mid-cingulate cortex, which includes the cingulate motor area (Vogt et al., 1996; Morecraft and Tanji, 2009; Vogt, 2009, 2016). The anterior cingulate cortex also projects forwards to medial prefrontal cortex area 10 (Price, 2006; Ongur and Price, 2000), and to temporal lobe areas including the parahippocampal gyrus, perirhinal cortex, and entorhinal cortex (Vogt, 2009).

Another route for output is via the projections to the striatum / basal ganglia system.

The anterior cingulate cortex, including the subgenual cingulate cortex area 25, also has outputs that can influence autonomic/visceral function via the hypothalamus, midbrain periaqueductal gray, and insula, as does the orbitofrontal cortex (Rempel-Clower and Barbas, 1998; Price, 2006; Ongur and Price, 2000; Critchley and Harrison, 2013).

The connectivity of the human anterior cingulate cortex (Rolls et al., 2023c) is described in Section 12.2.5, and that has further implications for what is computed in the human anterior cingulate cortex.

12.2.2 Anterior cingulate cortex: A framework

The pregenual anterior cingulate cortex regions can be conceptualized as receiving information from the orbitofrontal cortex about expected rewards and outcomes, and linking to hippocampal systems for navigation towards goals (rewards) and for storage in memory; and linking to the supracallosal anterior cingulate cortex for action-outcome learning; and also linking to the striatum / basal ganglia (see Fig. 12.3 for humans).

The supracallosal anterior cingulate cortex (dACC) can be conceptualized as receiving information from the orbitofrontal cortex about expected punishers and outcomes including non-reward outcomes, and linking these to actions recently performed to implement action-outcome learning. The supracallosal anterior cingulate cortex has much connectivity with premotor and somatosensory systems (Rolls et al., 2023c) (Fig. 12.3), and with the mid-cingulate motor cortex (Vogt, 2016, 2009), to associate recent actions with the outcomes received, in order to optimize the action selected at any given time. If the action involves no change of behavior, this is described as 'exploit'. If behavior changes, perhaps in response to not receiving an expected reward (referred to as 'non-reward'), then behavior changes to 'explore' possible different actions. The mid-cingulate cortex receives inputs about actions from premotor and somatosensory cortical regions and from the parietal cortex directly and via the spatial parts of the posterior cingulate cortex (Rolls et al., 2023i). The learning of action-outcome associations in the supracallosal anterior cingulate cortex enables the correct actions to be selected in future. The connections that provide for this are shown in Figs. 12.1, 12.2, and for humans 12.3.

Bringing together information about specific rewards with information about actions, and the costs associated with actions, is important for associating actions with the value of their outcomes and for selecting the correct action that will lead to a desired reward (Walton et al., 2003; Rushworth et al., 2007b; Rolls, 2009a; Rushworth et al., 2011; Grabenhorst and Rolls, 2011; Rolls, 2014a; Kolling et al., 2016). Indeed, consistent with its strong connections to motor areas (Morecraft and Tanji, 2009), lesions of the anterior cingulate cortex impair reward-guided action selection (Kennerley et al., 2006; Rudebeck et al., 2008), neuroimaging studies have shown that the anterior cingulate cortex is active when outcome information guides choices (Walton et al., 2004), and single neurons in the anterior cingulate cortex encode information about both actions and outcomes including reward prediction errors for actions (Matsumoto et al., 2007; Luk and Wallis, 2009; Kolling et al., 2016; Klein-Flugge et al., 2022a). For example, Luk and Wallis (2009) found that in a task where information about three potential outcomes (three types of juice) had to be associated on a trial-by-trial basis with two different responses (two lever movements), many neurons in the anterior cingulate cortex encoded information about both specific outcomes and specific actions. Action-outcome learning in a pure form to illustrate the concept might involve making an action in the dark (i.e. with no visible stimuli, though perhaps preceded by a 'start' tone to indicate when to start the action), and obtaining a reward outcome or not, and gradually learning the correct action to obtain a reward.

This supracallosal anterior cingulate connectivity with major outputs to premotor cortical areas (green) is compared in Fig. 12.2 with that of the hippocampus, which receives information from the ventral 'what' processing stream (blue) and the dorsal 'where' or 'action' processing stream (red), but then projects back to the neocortical areas from which it receives inputs. The hippocampus receives its inputs via the parahippocampal gyrus (areas TF and TH), and the perirhinal cortex (areas 35 and 36), both of which in turn project to

570 | The cingulate cortex

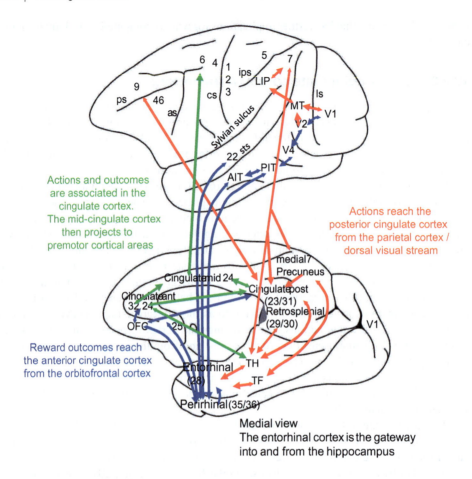

Fig. 12.2 Connections of the anterior, mid- and posterior cingulate cortex with a framework for understanding the functions of the cingulate cortex in action-outcome learning. A medial view of the macaque brain is shown below, and a lateral view is above. The green arrows show the convergence of reward or outcome information from the anterior cingulate cortex (ACC) (red) and of information about actions from the posterior cingulate cortex (red) to the mid-cingulate motor area, which then projects to premotor areas including the premotor cortex area 6 and the supplementary motor area (green). This provides connectivity for action-outcome learning. The ACC receives reward outcome information from the orbitofrontal cortex (OFC) derived from the ventral processing streams (blue). The posterior cingulate cortex receives information about actions from the parietal cortex dorsal processing streams (red). The mid-cingulate cortex projects to premotor areas (green). Abbreviations: as - arcuate sulcus; cs - central sulcus; ips - intraparietal sulcus; ios - inferior occipital sulcus; ls - lunate sulcus; sts - superior temporal sulcus; and see text.

the entorhinal cortex (area 28), send inputs to the hippocampus and receive backprojections from the hippocampus. The forward inputs towards the entorhinal cortex and hippocampus are shown with large arrowheads, and the weaker return backprojections with small arrowheads. The hippocampus receives via the perirhinal cortex areas 35 and 36 which project to the lateral entorhinal cortex area 28 from the ends of the hierarchically organised ventral visual system pathways (V1, V2, V4, PIT, AIT) that represent 'what' object is present (including also faces, and even scenes), from the anterior inferior temporal visual cortex (AIT, BA21, TE) where objects and faces are represented which receives from the posterior inferior temporal cortex (PIT, BA20, TEO); from the reward system in the orbitofrontal cortex (OFC) and amygdala, and from an area to which the OFC projects, the anterior cingulate cortex BA32 and subgenual cingulate cortex (BA25); from the high order auditory cortex (BA22); and from olfactory, taste, and somatosensory 'what' areas (not shown). The hippocampus also receives via the parahippocampal cortex areas TF and TH inputs (shown in red) from the dorsal visual 'where' or 'action' pathways, which reach parietal cortex area 7 via the dorsal visual stream hierarchy, including V1, V2, MT, MST, LIP, and VIP, and from areas to which they are connected, including the dorsolateral prefrontal cortex BA46 and the posterior cingulate (Cingulate post) and retrosplenial cortex. The hippocampus provides a system for all the high-order cortical regions including the reward-related orbitofrontal cortex and pregenual anterior cingulate cortex to converge into a single network in the hippocampal CA3 region, and then for backprojections to reach back to the neocortex (Rolls, 2018b) (see Chapter 9).

12.2.3 Anterior cingulate cortex and action-outcome representations

Some single neuron studies indicating encoding of actions and outcomes have often involved rather dorsal recordings above the pregenual cingulate cortex in the dorsal anterior cingulate cortex (dACC in the dorsal bank of the cingulate sulcus), termed here the supracallosal anterior cingulate cortex (Matsumoto et al., 2007; Luk and Wallis, 2009; Kolling et al., 2016; Klein-Flugge et al., 2022a). In this dACC region, action–outcome associations appear to be represented, in that in tasks in which there were different relations between actions and rewards, it was found that even before a response was made, while the monkey was looking at a visual cue, the activity of anterior cingulate cortex neurons depended on the expectation of reward or non-reward (25%), the intention to move or not (25%), or a combination of movement intention and reward expectation (11%) (Matsumoto et al., 2003). Luk and Wallis (2013) described recordings in the same dorsal anterior cingulate cortex area that reflected the outcomes when monkeys made a choice of a left or right lever response to obtain a reward outcome, and also described a weak dissociation for more stimulus-outcome neurons in the orbitofrontal cortex, that is when monkeys had to choose the reward outcome based on which visual stimulus was shown. In the same dorsal anterior cingulate area neurons were more likely to take into account the costs of the actions required to obtain rewards, as well as the probability of obtaining the reward, than were neurons in the orbitofrontal cortex (Kennerley and Wallis, 2009; Kennerley et al., 2011; Kolling et al., 2016). In the dorsal anterior cingulate cortex, neurons may reflect evidence about the several most recent rewards, and use this to help guide choices (Kolling et al., 2016; Klein-Flugge et al., 2022a).

More ventrally in the pregenual anterior cingulate cortex, neurons are more likely to reflect reward outcome rather than primarily actions, and the outcome representation trailed that in the orbitofrontal cortex (Cai and Padoa-Schioppa, 2012). These findings are consistent with the hypothesis developed here and elsewhere (Rolls, 2019c,b) that the orbitofrontal cortex represents the value of stimuli, and in its more anterior / ventromedial prefrontal area 10 takes decisions about relative reward value (Rolls, Grabenhorst and Deco, 2010b,c; Rolls and Grabenhorst, 2008). That value information is transmitted from the orbitofrontal cortex (in part via the pregenual anterior cingulate cortex, see Fig. 12.3) to the supracallosal anterior cingulate cortex, where there are action-related neurons, and where action-outcome learning takes place. Consistently, in humans the supracallosal anterior cingulate cortex (also referred to as dorsal anterior cingulate cortex dACC) is activated during action-outcome learning (Morris, Dezfouli, Griffiths, Le Pelley and Balleine, 2022; Klein-Flugge, Bongioanni and Rushworth, 2022a).

Foraging studies also implicate the dorsal anterior cingulate cortex in representing value, and in taking into account costs (Klein-Flugge, Bongioanni and Rushworth, 2022a). For example, some neurons responded at higher rates when the monkeys were about to move to another foraging patch, and the threshold amount of this firing before the monkey switched to a new patch depended on the cost of switching (in this case the delay before foraging in the new patch could resume) (Hayden et al., 2011). Consistent with this, the costs of actions can influence reward value representations in the macaque orbitofrontal cortex, even though the actions themselves are not represented in the orbitofrontal cortex (Cai and Padoa-Schioppa, 2019).

In a neuroimaging study that provides evidence that the anterior cingulate cortex is active when outcome information guides choices made by the individual (Walton et al., 2004), the activations were relatively far back in the supracallosal anterior cingulate cortex (y=22, dACC) towards the mid-cingulate cortex. This is consistent with the hypothesis that the reward value information in the pregenual cingulate cortex and the negative value representations in the supracallosal anterior cingulate cortex are being interfaced to action and projected posteriorly to the mid-cingulate motor cortex.

12.2.4 Anterior cingulate cortex lesion effects

Consistent with the points made above and in Chapter 11, lesion studies in monkeys (Rudebeck et al., 2008) and humans (Camille, Tsuchida and Fellows, 2011), have demonstrated a dissociation in the role of the anterior cingulate cortex in action–outcome associations to guide behavior; and of the orbitofrontal cortex in stimulus–outcome associations to update expected value (Rushworth et al., 2012). Lesions of the anterior cingulate cortex in rats impair the ability to take into account the costs of actions, and this is supported by a neuroimaging study in humans (Croxson, Walton, O'Reilly, Behrens and Rushworth, 2009).

An investigation more closely related to the understanding of emotion showed that patients with selective surgical lesions of the antero-ventral part of the anterior cingulate cortex (ACC) and/or medial BA9 were in some cases impaired on voice and face expression identification, had some change in social behavior, such as inappropriateness, and had significant changes in their subjective emotional state (Hornak, Bramham, Rolls, Morris, O'Doherty, Bullock and Polkey, 2003).

There is also neuroimaging evidence that complements the effects of lesions (Hornak et al., 2003) in suggesting a role for certain medial regions in the subjective experience of emotion. In neuroimaging studies with normal human subjects bilateral activations in medial BA9 were found as subjects viewed emotion-laden stimuli, and in both medial BA9 as well as in ventral ACC during self-generated emotional experience (i.e. in the absence of a stimulus) as subjects recalled emotions of sadness or happiness (Lane et al., 1997a,b, 1998; Phillips et al., 2003). On the basis of a review of imaging studies which consistently emphasize the importance of anterior and ventral regions of the anterior cingulate cortex for emotion, Bush et al. (2000) argue that the anterior cingulate cortex can be divided into a ventral 'affective' division (which includes the subcallosal region and the pregenual anterior cingulate cortex), and a dorsal 'cognitive' division (presumably the supracallosal anterior cingulate cortex or dACC), a view strengthened by the demonstration of reciprocally inhibitory interactions between these two regions.

12.2.5 Anterior cingulate cortex and ventromedial prefrontal cortex connectivity and functions in humans

The concepts described above about 'what' computations are performed in different parts of the anterior cingulate cortex can be developed further and elucidated by considering the connectivity of the anterior cingulate cortex and ventromedial prefrontal cortex (vmPFC) in humans (Rolls et al., 2023c) and its implications in Sections 12.2.5 – 12.2.11. To illustrate the points made next, reference to Fig. 12.3 (repeated from earlier) may be helpful.

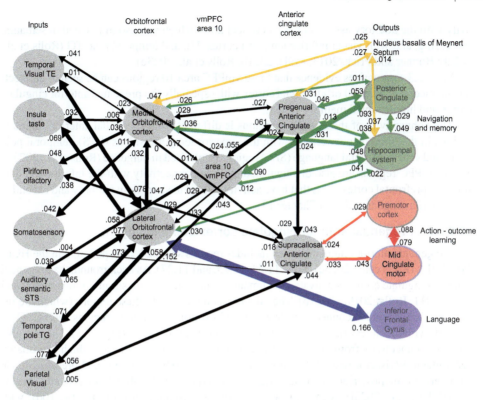

Fig. 12.3 Synthesis of the effective connectivity of the orbitofrontal cortex, vmPFC, and anterior cingulate cortex shown in the middle, with inputs on the left and outputs on the right. The regions included for each of the 5 central ellipses are as defined in the paper cited below. The width of the arrows is proportional to the effective connectivity in the highest direction, and the size of the arrows reflects the strength of the effective connectivity in each direction. The effective connectivities shown are for the strongest link where more than one link between regions applies for a group of brain regions. Effective connectivities with hippocampal memory system regions are shown in green; with premotor / mid-cingulate regions in red; with inferior prefrontal language system in blue; and in yellow to the basal forebrain nuclei of Meynert which contains cholinergic neurons that project to the neocortex and to the septal nuclei which contain cholinergic neurons that project to the hippocampus. The Somatosensory regions include 5 and parietal PF and PFop, which also connect to the pregenual anterior cingulate but are not shown for clarity; the Parietal regions include visual parietal regions 7, PGi and PFm. The connectivity with dorsolateral prefrontal cortex is not included here for clarity. Connectivity is shown for the five groups in the centre of the Figure, and does not include for example connectivity between somatosensory and premotor cortical regions. (From Rolls,E.T., Deco,G., Huang,C-C. and Feng,J. (2023) The human orbitofrontal cortex, vmPFC, and anterior cingulate cortex effective connectome: emotion, memory, and action. Cerebral Cortex 33: 350-356. doi: 10.1093/cercor/bhac270. Copyright © Oxford University Press.)

12.2.5.1 Ventromedial prefrontal cortex connectivity

The connectivity of the human ventromedial prefrontal cortex (vmPFC) regions (10v, 10r, 10d, and 9m in the HCP-MMP atlas) is summarised in Fig. 12.3 and illustrated in Figs. 11.24, 11.25, and 11.27 (Rolls et al., 2023c). These vmPFC regions have effective connectivity with the medial (OFC and pOFC) and lateral (47m, 47s, 47l) orbitofrontal cortex. The vmPFC also has strong effective connectivity with the pregenual anterior cingulate cortex (including especially pregenual areas a24, d32, and p32 to which the effective connectivity is directed). The diffusion tractography indicates direct connections of these area 10 regions with orbitofrontal cortex and with anterior cingulate cortex regions. The vmPFC also has effective connectivity with the hippocampal system and posterior cingulate cortex (including 31pd, 31pv, 7m, d23ab, and v23ab) which are implicated in memory (Rolls et al., 2023i). The vmPFC thus appears to be related in humans to the memory / spatial system and hippocampus as described below for pregenual anterior cingulate cortex. The vmPFC also has some effective connectivity with the auditory association STS cortical areas which are also implicated in semantic processing, and with visual inferior temporal cortex TE, and temporal pole TG (Rolls et al., 2022b; Bonner and Price, 2013; Rolls, 2021b; Rolls et al., 2023e).

Fig. 12.3 summarizes evidence that these vmPFC area 10 regions can be seen as connecting the medial and lateral orbitofrontal cortex with especially the pregenual anterior cingulate cortex and hippocampal memory system.

The connectivity of these vmPFC regions is different from pregenual anterior cingulate regions in that there is connectivity with the superior temporal sulcus (STS), temporal pole (TG), and superior frontal language (SFL) regions implicated in language (Rolls et al., 2022b). These vmPFC regions are also distinguished by little connectivity with the inferior and dorsolateral prefrontal cortex areas that have activity related to short-term memory and executive function (Passingham, 2021) (Chapter 13).

12.2.5.2 Pregenual anterior cingulate cortex connectivity

The pregenual anterior cingulate cortex includes regions s32, a24, p24, p32, d32 in the HCP-MMP atlas (Rolls et al., 2023c) (Figs. 11.24, 11.25, and 11.27). As background, the pregenual anterior cingulate cortex is activated in humans by many rewarding stimuli (Grabenhorst and Rolls, 2011; Rolls, 2019c, 2021b). The effective connectivity to these regions (which are interconnected) includes connectivity from medial orbitofrontal cortex regions (pOFC, OFC and 13l) with much less from lateral orbitofrontal cortex regions 47 (Fig. 12.3). There is also effective connectivity from the anterior agranular insular complex (AAIC) which is probably taste/olfactory/visceral-related; the hippocampal system (Hippocampus and presubiculum); with parts of the posterior cingulate cortex (31pv, 31pd, 7m, d23ab, v23ab) related to memory (Rolls et al., 2023i); with some ventromedial prefrontal regions (10r, 10v, 10d); with prefrontal cortex 8Av, 8Ad, 9a and 9p; and (for d32) with the frontal pole.

Effective connectivities from the pregenual cingulate cortex to the hippocampal system and the memory-related parts of the posterior cingulate are prominent (Fig. 12.3) (Rolls et al., 2023i). Several of the pregenual anterior cingulate cortex regions have bidirectional connectivity with the septum (Rolls et al., 2023c) (Fig. 12.3) which includes cholinergic neurons that project to the hippocampus (Zaborszky et al., 2018, 2008; Rolls et al., 2023i).

12.2.5.3 Subgenual anterior cingulate cortex area 25

Area 25 has relatively similar effective connectivity to the pregenual anterior cingulate cortex regions, except that 25 does not have effective connectivity with the inferior frontal gyrus and dorsolateral prefrontal cortex regions (Rolls et al., 2023i). The connectivity of region 25 is also similar to that of the medially adjacent pOFC. Region 25 also has some connectivity directed to the hippocampus, and interestingly bidirectional connectivity with the septum (Rolls et al., 2023i) which includes cholinergic neurons that project to the hippocampus (Rolls et al., 2023i; Zaborszky et al., 2018, 2008).

12.2.5.4 Supracallosal anterior cingulate cortex

The supracallosal anterior cingulate cortex includes regions a32pr, a24pr, 33pr, p32pr, and p24pr in the HCP-MMP atlas (Rolls et al., 2023c) (Figs. 11.24, 11.25, and 11.27). Part of the context is that this region is activated by aversive stimuli and non-reward in humans (Grabenhorst and Rolls, 2011; Rolls, 2019c, 2021b; Rolls et al., 2020e).

These supracallosal anterior cingulate cortex regions have very similar effective connectivity to each other (Rolls et al., 2023c). There is effective connectivity to supracallosal anterior cingulate cortex regions from somatosensory cortex 5L, 5mv and PFop (Rolls et al., 2023f,d); from superior parietal 7AL and 7Am; from posterior cingulate 23d which is part of the antero-dorsal visuo-motor part (Rolls et al., 2023i); and from the medial orbitofrontal cortex regions 11l, 13l, OFC and pOFC. There is effective connectivity to midcingulate cortex premotor regions 24dd and 24dv; premotor area 6 and the frontal eye fields FEF; frontal opercular FOP and related opercular somatosensory areas; somatosensory insular regions (e.g. MI, PI, AVI, PoI); and to the Peri-Sylvian Language area (PSL). The supracallosal anterior cingulate cortex thus has outputs to cortical areas involved in limb and body movements. The diffusion tractography provides evidence for direct connections with some of the posterior cingulate cortex regions (Rolls et al., 2023c).

This set of connectivities suggests (Rolls et al., 2023c) that the dACC is the key part in humans of the anterior cingulate cortex that is related to learning associations between actions and the rewards or punishers associated with the actions (Rushworth et al., 2012; Noonan et al., 2011), as developed further in Section 12.2.7. As a prelude to that, strong evidence about how reward, punishers, and non-reward are represented in the anterior cingulate cortex is described.

12.2.6 Pregenual anterior cingulate representations of reward value, and supracallosal anterior cingulate representations of punishers and non-reward

Functional magnetic resonance neuroimaging (fMRI) studies show that there are rather separate representations of positively affective, pleasant, stimuli in the pregenual anterior cingulate cortex (yellow in Fig. 11.18); and of negative, unpleasant, stimuli just posterior to this above the corpus callosum in the supracallosal anterior cingulate cortex (white in Fig. 11.18) (Rolls, 2009a; Grabenhorst and Rolls, 2011).

The regions involved can be illustrated by the pregenual cingulate activations produced by the pleasant taste of glucose (Fig. 4.6 top right image), and the supracallosal anterior cingulate cortex region activated by the much less pleasant taste of inosine monophosphate (Fig. 4.6 second image down on the right) (De Araujo, Kringelbach, Rolls and Hobden, 2003b). In this investigation, small amounts of the taste solutions were delivered into the mouth, and the participants just rated the intensity of the tastes, so there is no particular change of action necessary that depended on the particular taste that was delivered.

The area activated by pain is typically 10–30 mm behind and above the most anterior (i.e. pregenual) part of the anterior cingulate cortex (see e.g. Rolls, O'Doherty, Kringelbach, Francis, Bowtell and McGlone (2003d), Fig. 11.18, Vogt and Sikes (2000) and Vogt et al. (1996)). Pleasant touch was found to activate the most anterior part of the anterior cingulate cortex, just in front of the genu (or knee) of the corpus callosum (i.e. pregenual anterior cingulate cortex) (Rolls, O'Doherty, Kringelbach, Francis, Bowtell and McGlone, 2003d; McCabe, Rolls, Bilderbeck and McGlone, 2008) (Fig. 11.18). Pleasant temperature applied to the hand also produces a linear activation related to the degree of subjective pleasantness in the pregenual cingulate cortex (Grabenhorst, Rolls and Parris, 2008b). Oral somatosensory stimuli such as viscosity and the pleasantness of fat texture also activate this pregenual part of the anterior cingulate cortex (De Araujo and Rolls, 2004; Grabenhorst, Rolls, Parris and D'Souza, 2010b). Not only does pleasant taste activate the pregenual anterior cingulate cortex (De Araujo and Rolls, 2004; De Araujo, Kringelbach, Rolls and Hobden, 2003b), but in addition attention to pleasantness (Grabenhorst and Rolls, 2008) and cognitive modulation of pleasantness (Grabenhorst, Rolls and Bilderbeck, 2008a) also enhance activations. The same is found for pleasant odors in the pregenual anterior cingulate cortex (Rolls, Kringelbach and De Araujo, 2003c) (Fig. 5.5), and effects are found here too for cognitive inputs that influence the pleasantness of odors (De Araujo et al., 2005), and also top-down inputs that produce selective attention to odor pleasantness (Rolls, Grabenhorst, Margot, da Silva and Velazco, 2008b). Unpleasant odors activate the supracallosal anterior cingulate cortex (Rolls,

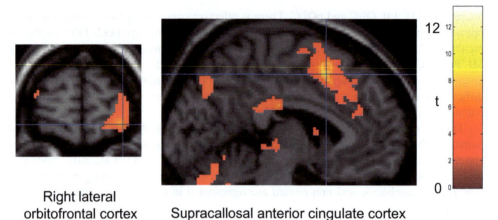

Right lateral orbitofrontal cortex   Supracallosal anterior cingulate cortex

Fig. 12.4 Brain regions activated on reward reversal trials in a deterministic Go/NoGo visual discrimination task for points reward. The supracallosal anterior cingulate cortex and the right lateral orbitofrontal cortex and adjoining part of the inferior frontal gyrus were activated on the reversal trials when an expected large reward was not obtained, and the human participants changed their behavior to select the other visual stimulus in this one-trial rule-based reversal. (After Rolls, Vatansever, Li, Cheng and Feng. (2020) Rapid rule-based reward reversal and the lateral orbitofrontal cortex. Cerebral Cortex Communications 1: tgaa087. Copyright © Oxford University Press.)

Kringelbach and De Araujo, 2003c) (Fig. 5.5). Activations in the pregenual cingulate cortex are also produced by the taste of water when it is rewarding because of thirst (De Araujo, Kringelbach, Rolls and McGlone, 2003c), by the flavor of food (Kringelbach, O'Doherty, Rolls and Andrews, 2003), and by monetary reward (O'Doherty, Kringelbach, Rolls, Hornak and Andrews, 2001a). Moreover, the pregenual anterior cingulate cortex is activated by both the outcome value and the expected value of monetary reward (Rolls, McCabe and Redoute, 2008e). The locations of some of these activations are shown in Fig. 11.18.

In these studies, the anterior cingulate activations were linearly related to the subjective pleasantness or unpleasantness of the stimuli, providing evidence that the pregenual anterior cingulate cortex provides a representation of value on a continuous scale (Fig. 11.18). Moreover, evidence was found that there is a common scale of value in the pregenual anterior cingulate cortex, with the affective pleasantness of taste stimuli and of thermal stimuli applied to the hand producing identically scaled BOLD activations (Grabenhorst, D'Souza, Parris, Rolls and Passingham, 2010a). The implication is that the pregenual anterior cingulate cortex contains a value representation used in decision-making, but that the decision itself may be made elsewhere. Decisions about actions that reflect the outcomes represented in the pregenual anterior cingulate cortex may be made in the supracallosal (i.e. dorsal) anterior cingulate cortex which is further posterior towards the mid-cingulate cortex. Decisions about the value of stimuli may be made in the medial prefrontal cortex area 10 (or ventromedial prefrontal cortex, vmPFC) (Rolls et al., 2010b,c), which receives inputs from the orbitofrontal cortex and also from the anterior cingulate cortex. Consistent with this, in macaques single neurons in the ventromedial prefrontal cortex rapidly come to signal the value of the chosen offer, suggesting that the circuit serves to produce a choice (Strait et al., 2014), and consistent with the attractor model of decision-making (Rolls and Deco, 2010; Rolls, 2016b) (Sections 11.5.1 and 11.5.2).

Value representations in the pregenual anterior cingulate cortex are confirmed by recording studies in monkeys (Rolls, 2008c, 2009a; Kolling et al., 2016). For example, Gabbott, Verhagen, Kadohisa and Rolls found neurons (see Rolls (2008c)) in the pregenual anterior

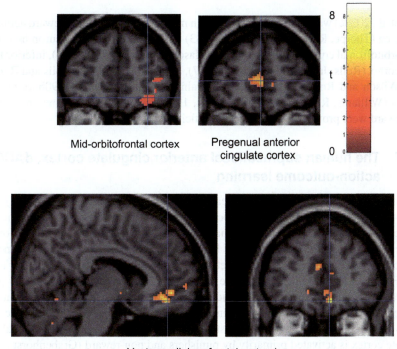

Fig. 12.5 Brain regions activated by reward, winning 25 points, in a deterministic Go/NoGo visual discrimination task for points reward. Activations to the reward outcome were found in the medial/mid-orbitofrontal cortex, ventromedial prefrontal cortex, and pregenual anterior cingulate cortex. (After Rolls, Vatansever, Li, Cheng and Feng. (2020) Rapid rule-based reward reversal and the lateral orbitofrontal cortex. Cerebral Cortex Communications 1: tgaa087. Copyright © Oxford University Press.)

cingulate cortex that respond to taste and it was demonstrated that the representation is of reward value, for devaluation by feeding to satiety selectively decreased neuronal responses to the food with which the animal was satiated. The supracallosal part of the anterior cingulate cortex is proposed to use these value representations in action-outcome learning, as considered in Section 12.2.5.4 (Rolls et al., 2023c; Rolls, 2022b). The functions of the pregenual anterior cingulate cortex are considered further below.

Evidence that the supracallosal anterior cingulate cortex is activated by non-reward is shown in Fig. 11.16 for reward reversal in a probabilistic task using face expressions as the stimuli (Kringelbach and Rolls, 2003).

In a one-trial deterministic visual reversal task for points, the supracallosal anterior cingulate cortex, and the right lateral orbitofrontal cortex and adjoining part of the inferior frontal gyrus, were activated on the reversal trials, as shown in Fig. 12.4 (Rolls, Vatansever, Li, Cheng and Feng, 2020e). This shows that the supracallosal anterior cingulate cortex is activated when an expected reward was not received, that is, to non-reward. This type of non-reward computation is likely to be important in action-outcome learning, and in changing behavior in foraging tasks, from 'exploit', to 'explore'.

Obtaining a reward outcome (+25 points) on reward (Go) trials produced (as expected) reward-related activations in the medial/mid orbitofrontal cortex, pregenual anterior cingulate cortex, and ventromedial prefrontal cortex (Fig. 12.5). On NoGo trials, on which there was a small loss of 5 points, activations were found in the lateral orbitofrontal cortex, with a small loss-related activation in the supracallosal anterior cingulate cortex (Rolls et al., 2020e). The one-trial rule-based Go/NoGo visual discrimination reversal task used in this investigation

(Rolls et al., 2020e) was the same as that used in macaques in which non-reward neurons were discovered (Thorpe, Rolls and Maddison, 1983) (and in further single-neuron investigations in the orbitofrontal cortex (Rolls, Critchley, Mason and Wakeman, 1996b), inferior temporal visual cortex (Rolls, Judge and Sanghera, 1977), amygdala (Sanghera, Rolls and Roper-Hall, 1979; Wilson and Rolls, 2005), basal forebrain (Wilson and Rolls, 1990b,a), and ventral striatum (Williams, Rolls, Leonard and Stern, 1993; Rolls, 1994c). (Points instead of fruit juice reward were provided for the human participants.)

12.2.7 The human supracallosal anterior cingulate cortex, dACC, and action-outcome learning

The connectivities of the human supracallosal anterior cingulate cortex (dACC) (Section 12.2.5.4), and the other evidence described above (including in Sections 12.2.2 and 12.2.3), provide evidence (Rolls et al., 2023c) that the dACC is the key part in humans of the anterior cingulate cortex that is related to learning associations between actions and the rewards or punishers associated with the actions (Rushworth et al., 2012; Noonan et al., 2011; Klein-Flugge et al., 2022a). For this, the orbitofrontal cortex inputs provide it is proposed the reward/punishment representation, and the connectivity of the dACC with somatosensory and premotor regions the required evidence about actions just performed, and the required outputs to especially limb and body systems. The findings that the supracallosal anterior cingulate cortex is activated primarily by punishers and non-reward (Grabenhorst and Rolls, 2011; Rolls, 2019c, 2021b; Rolls et al., 2020e) (Section 12.2.6) may relate to the limb and body movements that utilise premotor cortical output regions often made to avoid aversive stimuli. However, reward information is also likely to reach the supracallosal anterior cingulate cortex, in part via the pregenual anterior cingulate cortex (Fig. 12.3) (Rolls et al., 2023c).

If aversive stimuli or non-reward are received, this is likely to lead to a change of actions: in the terminology of foraging, changing from 'exploit' to 'explore' (Klein-Flugge et al., 2022a). Error signals generated in the dACC reflect a mismatch between the expected reward outcome for the action and the actual outcome (Klein-Flugge et al., 2022a). The computational mechanism proposed for 'how' this system operates is that the error signal in the dACC activates a neuronal population that represents 'explore' to become active in a single attractor network with 'explore' vs 'exploit' neuronal populations in competition with each other. The computational mechanism is similar to that described for reversal of the rule attractor network in Section 11.5.3. In 'explore' mode, actions can be made to test whether the outcomes are better than previously, and if so the 'exploit' attractor neuronal population is activated by the higher reward rate than previously, and the behavior becomes stable in 'exploit' mode.

In summary, the proposed computational mechanism is that non-reward or punishment resets the 'exploit' neuronal population to fall out of its attractor in the exploit/explore rule attractor network, thereby releasing the 'explore' population from inhibition by the inhibitory neurons. This could be achieved by non-reward or punishment directly activating the 'explore' attractor to produce exploratory behavior. Then while exploring, rewards that are better than previously activate the 'exploit' attractor neuronal population, which quench the 'explore' neuronal population through the inhibitory neurons in the exploit/explore rule attractor single network. The actual location of this exploit/explore rule attractor single network could be in the dACC, but another interesting possibility is that it is in the frontal pole, from where it can control the whole of the dorsolateral prefrontal cortex, as described in Section 13.5 (Rolls et al., 2023a).

12.2.8 Reward value outputs from the orbitofrontal and pregenual anterior cortex, and vmPFC, to the hippocampal memory system

It is indicated in green in Fig. 9.19, and in Fig. 12.3 (Rolls et al., 2023c), that the human medial and lateral orbitofrontal cortex have effective connectivity directed to the hippocampal system (hippocampus, entorhinal cortex, perirhinal cortex) both directly, and via the vmPFC, via the pregenual anterior cingulate cortex, and via the memory-related (posterior) parts of the posterior cingulate cortex (Rolls et al., 2023i). These are the routes by which value / emotion-related information can reach the human hippocampal memory system from the orbitofrontal cortex. The information does reach the hippocampus and is incorporated into memory in that some primate hippocampal spatial view cells (Georges-François et al., 1999; Rolls et al., 1997a; Rolls and Wirth, 2018; Rolls, 2021f,b; Rolls et al., 1998b; Robertson et al., 1998; Rolls et al., 2005c; Wirth et al., 2017; Rolls, 2023c) respond to the reward value of a location viewed in space in a reward-spatial location memory task (Rolls and Xiang, 2005, 2006).

A considerable part of the output of the human medial and lateral orbitofrontal cortex value / emotion system is thus directed towards the hippocampal system for memory (Fig. 12.3) (Rolls et al., 2023c; Rolls, 2022b). It is proposed that this connectivity provides a key input about reward / punishment value for the hippocampal episodic memory system, adding to the 'what, 'where', and 'when' information that are also key components of episodic memory. Damage to the vmPFC / anterior cingulate cortex system is likely to contribute to episodic memory impairments produced by damage to these OFC/ vmPFC / anterior cingulate cortex regions by impairing a key component of episodic memory, the reward / punishment / emotional value component. Such damage would impair the value information reaching the hippocampal system for storage, and also for later retrieval. Indeed, if one of the possible inputs such as the reward input used for hippocampal memory retrieval by completion in the CA3 attractor network was missing, that would be expected to impair memory retrieval (Treves and Rolls, 1994; Rolls, 2018b; Treves and Rolls, 1991; Rolls, 2021b). That is one mechanism that is proposed (Rolls, 2022b) to contribute to the episodic memory impairments produced by damage in humans to the anterior cingulate cortex and vmPFC (Ciaramelli et al., 2019; McCormick et al., 2018) (Section 9.2.8.5).

12.2.9 The pregenual anterior cingulate cortex has connectivity with the septal cholinergic system that is involved in memory consolidation

The human pregenual anterior cingulate cortex (with subgenual 25 and vmPFC 10r) in humans has effective connectivity directed to the septal nuclei (yellow in Fig. 12.3 (Rolls et al., 2023c)), which contains cholinergic neurons that project to the hippocampus in humans (Mesulam, 1990; Zaborszky et al., 2018, 2008). These pregenual anterior cingulate regions are likely to be important influences on septal neurons, for the only other cortical regions found with substantial effective connectivity to the human septal region (Rolls et al., 2023c) are the hippocampus, subiculum, and v23ab which is part of the posterior cingulate cortex also implicated in episodic memory (Rolls et al., 2023i). In accordance with this, it is proposed (Rolls, 2022b) that the damage in humans to the orbitofrontal and anterior cingulate cortex regions that impairs episodic memory (Ciaramelli et al., 2019; McCormick et al., 2018) arises in part because of the reduced release of acetylcholine to reward / punishing / salient stimuli, which may impair long-term synaptic potentiation and thus memory storage in both the hippocampus and neocortex (Zaborszky et al., 2018; Newman et al., 2012; Hasselmo and

Sarter, 2011; Giocomo and Hasselmo, 2007; Hasselmo and Giocomo, 2006; Rolls, 2021b) (Section 9.2.8.5).

There are thus three memory-related influences of the orbitofrontal and pregenual anterior cingulate cortex uncovered by the effective connectivity in humans (Fig. 12.3): (1) reward as a component of hippocampal episodic memory; and cholinergic influences both on (2) the neocortex and (3) on the hippocampus driven by the orbitofrontal and pregenual anterior cingulate cortex (Rolls et al., 2023c; Rolls, 2022b) (Section 9.2.8.5). Together, these three processes are it is proposed likely to make major contributions to the memory deficits reported to follow ventromedial prefrontal cortex damage in humans (McCormick and Maguire, 2021; McCormick et al., 2020; Ciaramelli et al., 2019; McCormick et al., 2018; Bonnici and Maguire, 2018; Ciaramelli and Treves, 2019). Although it has been suggested that scene processing types of computation are affected by ventromedial prefrontal cortex damage (De Luca, McCormick, Ciaramelli and Maguire, 2019), this might be expected given that the hippocampus with its spatial view neurons (Georges-François et al., 1999; Robertson et al., 1998; Rolls et al., 1997a; Rolls and Xiang, 2006; Rolls et al., 2005c; Rolls and Xiang, 2005; Rolls and Wirth, 2018; Wirth et al., 2017; Tsitsiklis et al., 2020; Rolls, 2023c) is involved in scene processing (Rolls, 2021f); and given that the cholinergic influence on the hippocampus is likely to be very important in hippocampal functioning including memory storage (because acetylcholine facilitates synaptic long-term potentiation and reduces at the same time the relative efficacy of the CA3 recurrent collateral synapses to help emphasise new rather than existing memories) (Zaborszky et al., 2018; Newman et al., 2012; Hasselmo and Sarter, 2011; Giocomo and Hasselmo, 2007; Hasselmo and Giocomo, 2006; Rolls, 2021b).

These new discoveries provide a new approach to understanding how memory is consolidated in the human brain (Rolls, 2022b) (Section 9.2.8.5).

12.2.10 Reward value outputs from the orbitofrontal and pregenual anterior cortex, and vmPFC, to the hippocampal system to provide the goals for navigation

The hippocampus is also implicated in navigation (O'Keefe and Nadel, 1978; Burgess and O'Keefe, 1996; Ekstrom et al., 2014; Miller et al., 2013; Tsitsiklis et al., 2020; McNaughton et al., 2006; Bellmund et al., 2018; Ekstrom and Isham, 2017; Clark et al., 2019; Nau et al., 2018a; Rolls and Wirth, 2018; Rolls, 2021f). It is proposed that the reward value input from the orbitofrontal / vmPFC / pregenual anterior cortex to the hippocampal and memory-related posterior cingulate cortex (green in Fig. 9.19 (Rolls et al., 2023c)) provides important connectivity also required for navigation, and indeed it is a key feature of navigation that it is generally towards goals, usually rewards (Rolls et al., 2023c; Rolls, 2023c). Supporting this, neurons in the primate hippocampus encode the locations in viewed scenes at which rewards are located (Rolls and Xiang, 2005), including the goals for navigation (Wirth et al., 2017; Rolls and Wirth, 2018). The information transmitted from the orbitofrontal cortex is about which particular of many possible rewards represented in the orbitofrontal cortex (Rolls, 2014a, 2016g, 2019e,f) is the current goal for navigation, so is a high-dimensional vector on neuronal firing.

The navigation in humans and other primates is proposed to frequently involve navigation from viewed landmark to viewed landmark using spatial view cells (Rolls, 2021f). This is in contrast to what is frequently proposed to be used in rodents, which is path integration from place to place performed by the hippocampus (McNaughton, Barnes, Gerrard, Gothard, Jung, Knierim, Kudrimoti, Qin, Skaggs, Suster and Weaver, 1996; Burgess and O'Keefe, 1996; Hartley, Lever, Burgess and O'Keefe, 2014; Edvardsen, Bicanski and Burgess, 2020). Humans might wish to try some navigation themselves with the eyes closed to help to confirm the greatly utility of landmarks in views of spatial scenes in navigation in humans, which are encoded by hippocampal and parahippocampal spatial view cells (Rolls, 2023c).

12.2.11 Subgenual cingulate cortex

The subgenual part (area 25) of the anterior cingulate cortex is, via its outputs to the hypothalamus and brainstem autonomic regions, involved in at least the autonomic component of emotion (Koski and Paus, 2000; Barbas and Pandya, 1989; Ongur and Price, 2000; Gabbott et al., 2003; Vogt, 2009; Alexander et al., 2019). The anterior cingulate cortex is also activated in relation to autonomic events, and Nagai, Critchley, Featherstone, Trimble and Dolan (2004) have shown that there is a correlation with skin conductance, a measure of autonomic activity related to sympathetic activation, in the anterior cingulate cortex and related areas. The dorsal anterior and mid-cingulate cortical areas may be especially related to blood pressure, pupil size, heart rate, and electrodermal activity, whereas the subgenual cingulate cortex, with ventromedial prefrontal cortex, appears antisympathetic (and parasympathetic) (Critchley and Harrison, 2013). The subgenual cingulate cortex is connected with the ventromedial prefrontal cortical areas (Johansen-Berg et al., 2008; Hsu et al., 2020).

Evidence implicating the subgenual and more generally the subcallosal cingulate cortex in depression (Hamani et al., 2011; Laxton et al., 2013; Price and Drevets, 2012; Drevets et al., 2008; Holtzheimer et al., 2017) is described in Section 18.5.4.4. Interestingly, neurons in the human subcallosal cingulate cortex responded to emotion categories present in visual stimuli, with more neurons responding to negatively valenced than positively valenced emotion categories (Laxton, Neimat, Davis, Womelsdorf, Hutchison, Dostrovsky, Hamani, Mayberg and Lozano, 2013).

12.3 Posterior cingulate cortex

12.3.1 Introduction and overview

The human posterior cingulate cortex (PCC) includes Brodmann areas 23 and 31, is also present in macaques, and is absent in rodents (Vogt, 2009). The retrosplenial cortex (RSC) Brodmann area 29/30 in humans is a small region wrapped round the splenium of the corpus callosum (Vogt, 2019a, 2009; Vogt et al., 1995) (see Figs. 12.6 and 12.7). The HCP-MMP (Section 1.12) 'Posterior Cingulate Division' (PCD) includes also some medial parietal cortex regions such as 7m, and some transitional regions with earlier cortical visual regions (DVT and ProS where the retrosplenial scene area is located (Sulpizio et al., 2020; Rolls, 2023c), Section 9.2.8.1).

The research described in this section (Rolls, Wirth, Deco, Huang and Feng, 2023i) shows that the postero-ventral parts of the PCD (31pd, 31pv, 7m, d23ab and v23ab) have effective connectivity with the temporal pole, inferior temporal visual cortex, cortex in the superior temporal sulcus implicated in auditory and semantic processing, with the reward-related vmPFC and pregenual anterior cingulate cortex, with the inferior parietal cortex, and with the hippocampal system (Fig. 12.6). This connectivity implicates it in hippocampal episodic memory, providing routes for 'what', reward and semantic schema-related information to access the hippocampus.

The antero-dorsal parts of the PCD (especially 31a and 23d, the precuneus visual region PCV, and also RSC) have connectivity with early visual cortical areas including those that represent spatial scenes, with the superior parietal cortex, with the pregenual anterior cingulate cortex, and with the hippocampal system (Fig. 12.7). This connectivity implicates it in the 'where' component for hippocampal episodic memory and for spatial navigation (Rolls, Wirth, Deco, Huang and Feng, 2023i).

The transitional regions Dorsal-Transitional-Visual (DVT) and ProStriate where the retrosplenial scene area is located (Sulpizio et al., 2020) (see Fig. 9.18) have connectivity from early visual cortical areas to the parahippocampal scene area, providing a ventromedial route for spatial scene information to reach the hippocampus (Rolls et al., 2023i,e).

These groups of human posterior cingulate division regions are based on the connectivities and functions of the different regions, as described by Rolls, Wirth, Deco, Huang and Feng (2023i).

These connectivities of the posterior cingulate division regions provide important routes for 'what', reward, and 'where' scene-related information for human hippocampal episodic memory and navigation (Rolls et al., 2023i).

A hypothesis less based on this connectivity evidence has suggested that the dorsal Posterior Cingulate Cortex is involved in executive function, that the ventral Posterior Cingulate Cortex is involved in memory, and that the retrosplenial cortex is involved in spatial processing (Foster et al., 2023).

12.3.2 Postero-ventral posterior cingulate and medial parietal regions 31pd, 31pv, d23ab, v23ab and 7m, and their relation to episodic memory

This group of posterior cingulate division (PCD) regions has connectivity illustrated in Fig. 12.6 (Rolls, Wirth, Deco, Huang and Feng, 2023i):

with ventral stream high-order visual (TE) and auditory (STS) association cortical areas that represent what object or person is present as shown by discoveries in macaques (Perrett, Rolls and Caan, 1982; Booth and Rolls, 1998; Rolls, 2021d,b; Arcaro and Livingstone, 2021; Freiwald, 2020; Lehky and Tanaka, 2016; Rolls, Deco, Huang and Feng, 2023e) with complementary evidence in humans (Kanwisher et al., 1997; Finzi et al., 2021; Collins and Olson, 2014);

with the pregenual anterior cingulate cortex (9m, a24, d32, p32 and 10d) and vmPFC (10r and 10v) where reward value and emotion are represented (Grabenhorst and Rolls, 2011; Rolls et al., 2023c; Rolls, 2019c, 2022b) (Section 12.2.6);

with some inferior parietal cortex regions (PGi and PGs, which are in the angular gyrus BA 39 and are implicated in memory and semantic processing (Davis et al., 2018; Papagno, 2018; Rolls et al., 2023d), Section 10.5);

with temporal pole (TG) regions implicated in semantic memory (Bonner and Price, 2013; Rolls et al., 2022b);

with frontal pole regions (10pp, p10p) (Rolls et al., 2023a);

and with the hippocampal system which is involved in episodic memory (Squire and Wixted, 2011; Dere et al., 2008; Moscovitch et al., 2016; Ekstrom and Ranganath, 2018; Rolls, 2018b, 2021b).

The connections to this set of brain regions (Rolls, Wirth, Deco, Huang and Feng, 2023i) suggest that this ventral and posterior part of the PCD is involved in hippocampal episodic memory, providing routes for the relevant 'what', reward and semantic schema-related information to gain access to the hippocampus during storage; and to be on the route back to these cortical areas during hippocampal episodic memory retrieval (Rolls, 2022b, 2021b). The regions in this group are thus especially related to ventral stream 'what' processing (Ungerleider and Haxby, 1994; Rolls, 2021d), and allow many widely separated brain regions at the top of processing streams to provide 'what', 'when' and reward inputs to the hippocampal system. Consistent with involvement of these PCD regions in linking reward and emotion

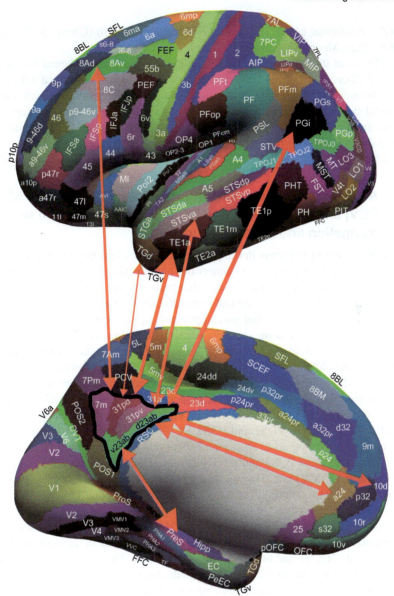

Posteroventral part of Posterior Cingulate Cortex Division

Fig. 12.6 Effective connectivity of the posteroventral part of the posterior cingulate cortex division shown on medial (below) and lateral (above) views of the human brain, with the sulci expanded to show regions inside the sulci. These regions (within the black boundary) are v23ab and d23ab, 31pd and 31pv, and 7m. The width of the lines reflects the effective connectivity in the strongest direction, and the size of the arrow heads reflects the effective connectivity in each direction. These regions have effective connectivity with the hippocampal system (presubiculum, subiculum, entorhinal cortex and hippocampus); anterior cingulate cortex (a24); frontal pole 10d; inferior parietal cortex PGi and PGs; the auditory cortex in the superior temporal sulcus (STS); the anterior inferior temporal cortex (TE1a); the dorsolateral prefrontal cortex 8Ad; and the temporal pole TGi. The abbreviations are listed in Section 1.12. (From Rolls,E.T., Wirth,S., Deco,G., Huang,C-C. and Feng,J. (2023) The human posterior cingulate, retrosplenial and medial parietal cortex effective connectome, and implications for memory and navigation. Human Brain Mapping 44: 629-655. doi: 10.1002/HBM.26089.)

systems to memory, the precuneus has increased functional connectivity in depression with the lateral orbitofrontal cortex non-reward / punishment system (Cheng, Rolls, Qiu, Yang, Ruan, Wei, Zhao, Meng, Xie and Feng, 2018c).

The relation of this group of PCD regions to memory is strengthened by the evidence (Rolls, Wirth, Deco, Huang and Feng, 2023i) that these regions associated with hippocampal function receive effective connectivity from the mammillary bodies which are part of a hippocampal circuit involved in episodic memory (Bubb et al., 2017), and the septum (which projects to the hippocampal system) and adjoining basal nucleus of Meynert both of which contain cholinergic neurons that are implicated in memory (Hasselmo and Giocomo, 2006; Rolls and Deco, 2015b; Rolls, 2022b).

12.3.3 Antero-dorsal Posterior Cingulate Division regions 23d, 31a, PCV; and RSC, POS2, and POS1; and their relation to navigation and executive function

POS1 and POS2 are visual areas in the parieto-occipital sulcus close to the primary visual cortex V1 (Fig. 12.7), have extensive connections and functional connectivity with early visual cortical areas, and provide inputs to the other brain regions in this group, 23d, 31a, PCV, and RSC (Rolls, Wirth, Deco, Huang and Feng, 2023i). Further, POS1 and POS2 also have effective connectivity to the medial parahippocampal gyrus PHA1-3 regions (corresponding to macaque TH)) where scenes are represented (Sulpizio et al., 2020; Natu et al., 2021; Kamps et al., 2016; Epstein and Kanwisher, 1998; Epstein and Baker, 2019; Epstein and Julian, 2013; Epstein, 2008, 2005; Rolls, 2023c), and with the hippocampal system. POS1 and POS2 may thus be involved in scene representations reaching the hippocampal system, and are likely to contribute to the activation of hippocampal spatial view cells, and thereby be involved in providing information important in episodic memory and navigation (Rolls and Wirth, 2018; Rolls, 2023c). POS1 and POS2 are also likely to be involved in memory and navigation by providing inputs to other members of this group of regions as follows.

Anterior to POS1 and POS2 and receiving visual inputs from these regions are the precuneus visual area (PCV) and 31a and 23d which are dorsal and extend anteriorly in the Posterior Cingulate Division (Fig. 12.7) and have connectivity (Fig. 12.7, Rolls, Wirth, Deco, Huang and Feng (2023i)) directed to the hippocampal system (hippocampus, entorhinal cortex, and presubiculum), to the parahippocampal PHA1-3 regions with visual scene representations (Sulpizio et al., 2020; Natu et al., 2021; Kamps et al., 2016; Epstein and Kanwisher, 1998; Rolls et al., 2023e), and to the mid-cingulate cortex. They receive effective connectivity not only from POS1 and POS2, but also from the temporo-parietal junction (a multimodal region implicated in social behavior and language (Patel et al., 2019; Coslett and Schwartz, 2018; DiNicola et al., 2020; Buckner and DiNicola, 2019; Quesque and Brass, 2019; Rolls et al., 2022b)); the superior parietal cortex (7Pm and 7Am) (Rolls et al., 2023d); frontal pole regions p10p and a10p implicated in planning and sequencing (Shallice and Cipolotti, 2018; Shallice and Burgess, 1996; Gilbert and Burgess, 2008), 'exploit' vs 'explore' (Rolls et al., 2023a) (Section 13.5), and prospective as well as retrospective memory (Underwood et al., 2015); the pregenual anterior cingulate including d32, p24, and p32 implicated in reward (Grabenhorst and Rolls, 2011; Rolls et al., 2023c; Rolls, 2022b); and dorsolateral prefrontal cortex 8Ad, 9a, 9p involved in short-term memory and thereby top-down attention (Germann and Petrides, 2020b; Deco and Rolls, 2005a; Rolls et al., 2023f) (Chapter 13). This part of the Posterior Cingulate Division is special in its strong connectivity from p10p which is part of the frontal pole cortex (Rolls et al., 2023a) (Section 13.5); the reward-related pregenual anterior cingulate d32, p24, p32 and medial orbitofrontal cortex (regions 11l, 13l and OFC) (Rolls et al., 2023c); and the midcingulate premotor cortex.

This connectivity including the connectivity to the parahippocampal scene or place area

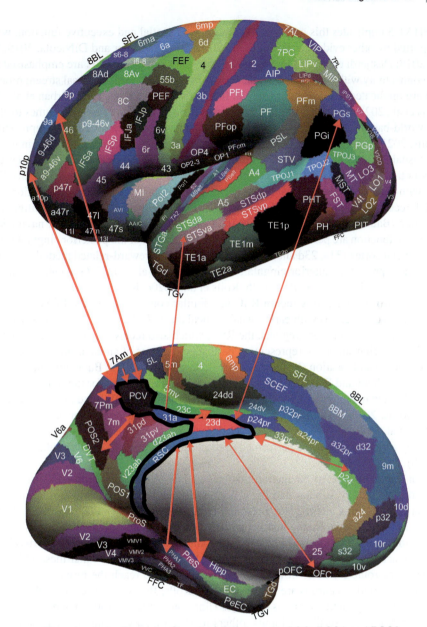

Dorsal anterior Posterior Cingulate Division with RSC, POS1 and POS2

Fig. 12.7 Effective connectivity of the anterior and dorsal parts of the posterior cingulate cortex and related regions shown on medial (below) and lateral (above) views of the human brain, with the sulci expanded to show regions inside the sulci. The brain regions include POS1 and POS2 (early visual cortical areas), which provide inputs to the other members of the group (surrounded by a black boundary), PCV, 31a, 23d, and the retrosplenial cortex (RSC). The width of the lines reflects the effective connectivity in the strongest direction, and the size of the arrow heads reflects the effective connectivity in each direction. Visuo-spatial inputs are also received from medial parietal cortex areas 7Pm and 7Am. These regions also have connectivity with the pregenual anterior cingulate cortex p24 and d32, with region OFC, with parietal PGs, with frontal pole p10p, and with dorsolateral prefrontal cortex 9p. Outputs of these regions are directed to the hippocampal system, including the hippocampus, presubiculum and parahippocampal TH (PHA1-3); and to the midcingulate motor cortex 23c. The abbreviations are listed in Section 1.12. (From Rolls,E.T., Wirth,S., Deco,G., Huang,C-C. and Feng,J. (2023) The human posterior cingulate, retrosplenial and medial parietal cortex effective connectome, and implications for memory and navigation. Human Brain Mapping 44: 629-655. doi: 10.1002/HBM.26089.)

in PHA1-3 implicates this group of PCD regions in spatial and executive function, which is supported by other evidence (Foster et al., 2013, 2012; Buckner and DiNicola, 2019; Fox et al., 2018; Dastjerdi et al., 2011). Spatial roles for this part of the PCC are emphasised too by the connectivity with superior parietal areas 7Am and 7Pm, parts of dorsal stream processing that are implicated in visuo-motor spatial functions (Snyder et al., 1998; Orban et al., 2021b; Rolls et al., 2023e,d) and coordinate transforms from egocentric eye-based frames to allocentric world-based frames suitable for idiothetic update of hippocampal spatial representations (Rolls, 2021f, 2020b; Snyder et al., 1998; Rolls, 2023c). Consistent with this, a cingulate sulcus visual area has been described that responds selectively to visual and vestibular cues to self-motion (Smith et al., 2018), and this may be in or near 23d (Rolls et al., 2023i). Consistent with the above evidence that this group of PCD regions is involved in navigation, area 31 which receives from POS1 and POS2 is implicated by neuroimaging in representing heading direction (Baumann and Mattingley, 2021). Consistent with the concept that navigation and executive function are performed to achieve goals, this part of the posterior cingulate and medial parietal cortex (31a, 23d and PCV) receives from the reward-related medial orbitofrontal cortex and pregenual anterior cingulate cortex (Rolls et al., 2023i; Grabenhorst and Rolls, 2011; Rolls et al., 2023c; Rolls, 2022b; Rolls et al., 2020e; Rolls, 2023c).

The retrosplenial cortex region RSC has similar connectivity to the PCV, 31a and 23d, but also has connections with early visual cortical areas (Rolls et al., 2023i). Consistent with visuo-spatial roles for these regions, the RSC, which also receives from POS2, is implicated by neuroimaging studies in representing permanent features of an environment such as landmark identity and location (Rolls et al., 2023i; Auger et al., 2012; Baumann and Mattingley, 2021; Persichetti and Dilks, 2019). However care is needed here, for the retrosplenial scene area is located in humans not in RSC, but just posterior to it in DVT and ProS (Sulpizio et al., 2020; Rolls, 2023c). The input from the reward-related pregenual anterior cingulate cortex and medial orbitofrontal cortex (p24, p32, 11l) to region RSC is of interest, for it provides a pathway for navigation to be performed to reach rewards or goals (Rolls et al., 2023c; Rolls, 2022b).

An important type of navigation involves update of location based on self-motion, and one area in which vestibular and optic flow information is represented is macaque area 7a (Avila et al., 2019; Cullen, 2019; Bremmer et al., 2000; Wurtz and Duffy, 1992). As shown by Rolls, Wirth, Deco, Huang and Feng (2023i), there is connectivity of area 7 regions with the regions in this PCD group, which in turn connect to the parahippocampal gyrus (PHA1-3, TH in macaques) / hippocampal system (Fig. 12.7). It is proposed that these PCD regions provide one route for optic flow and vestibular signals to reach the hippocampus in which whole body motion neurons are found (O'Mara, Rolls, Berthoz and Kesner, 1994). Some of these whole body motion neurons respond to linear and others to rotational motion, and some of them respond to vestibular inputs, others to visual inputs for motion, and some to both (O'Mara et al., 1994). These neurons are probably involved in navigation especially when the view details are obscured, that is, idiothetic (self-motion updated) navigation (O'Mara et al., 1994; Rolls, 2020b, 2021f). (The rodent equivalent is probably 'speed cells' (Kropff et al., 2015; Spalla et al., 2022).) Consistent with this proposal, in macaques there are neurons in a dorsal posterior cingulate region (and to a smaller extent in the RSC) that respond to vestibular inputs (Liu et al., 2021). Additional egomotion areas in the human brain as shown by neuroimaging include intraparietal sulcus area 1 (IPS1) and V3A in the occipital region; and V6 (Sulpizio et al., 2020); and all of these regions connect to DVT and ProS, which in turn connect to the PCD regions in the present antero-dorsal group, which in turn connect to parietal 7 (7Pm and 7Am) (Rolls, Wirth, Deco, Huang and Feng, 2023i). These connectivities help to show how self-motion information can reach hippocampal whole body motion cells

(O'Mara et al., 1994) for use in idiothetic navigational updating (Rolls, 2020b, 2021f; Rolls et al., 2023e; Rolls, 2023c).

It is therefore proposed that the regions in this antero-dorsal PCD group by virtue of the connectivity described here support spatial functions including navigation, and executive function, consistent with human neuroimaging and brain lesion evidence (Foster et al., 2013, 2012; Buckner and DiNicola, 2019; Fox et al., 2018; Dastjerdi et al., 2011; Ekstrom et al., 2017; Teghil et al., 2021).

12.3.4 Dorsal Visual Transitional area and ProStriate region: the retrosplenial scene area

The ProStriate region (ProS) is adjacent to V1, and the Dorsal Transitional Visual Area (DVT) is an area posterior to most of the Posterior Cingulate Division, found just lateral to POS2 (Fig. 12.7). Importantly, the retrosplenial cortex scene area is located in the dorsal visual transitional region (DVT) and prostriate region (ProS) with some extension into parieto-occipital sulcus region 1 (POS1) (Sulpizio et al., 2020; Rolls et al., 2023i) (Fig. 9.18). The ProS and DVT regions have connectivity with early cortical visual regions, with areas representing visual scenes (PHA1-3 and VMV regions (Rolls et al., 2023i; Sulpizio et al., 2020)), with the parietal cortex, with hippocampal system regions (hippocampus and presubiculum), and with the premotor mid-cingulate cortex and associated somatosensory area 5 (Rolls et al., 2023i). Unlike the postero-ventral DVD regions (Section 12.3.2), ProS and DVT do not have connectivity as a hub-like region useful for episodic memory, in that they have no connectivity with the inferior temporal visual cortex (TE) or superior temporal auditory association cortex, with the dorsolateral prefrontal cortex, or with the postero-ventral PCD regions (Section 12.3.2). Unlike the antero-dorsal regions, the DVT and ProS regions have connectivity with somatosensory cortex (5), and have no connectivity with the frontal cortex (Rolls et al., 2023i). The DVT and ProS regions thus appear to be involved in relatively low-level visual processing, with connectivity with the superior parietal cortex area 7 which suggests that these regions are involved in visuo-motor control appropriate for motor actions in visual space (Andersen, 1995b; Huang and Sereno, 2018; Urgen and Orban, 2021; Orban et al., 2021b; Rolls et al., 2023e,d), and perhaps in the necessary spatial coordinate transforms (Salinas and Sejnowski, 2001; Rolls, 2020b). Indeed, spatial coordinate transforms are also necessary for idiothetic update of spatial representations useful for hippocampal function including navigation when the spatial view is obscured (Snyder et al., 1998; Rolls, 2020b, 2021f; Dean and Platt, 2006; Vedder et al., 2017; Rolls, 2023c).

The DVT receives input from V6 and V6A (Rolls, Wirth, Deco, Huang and Feng, 2023i). Area V6A in the macaque is a visual-somatosensory area which occupies the posterior part of the dorsal precuneate cortex (Gamberini et al., 2021, 2020; Rolls et al., 2023e). It represents the upper limbs and is involved in the control of goal-directed arm movements (Fattori et al., 2017). Macaque V6A hosts the so called 'real-position cells', that is visual cells that encode spatial position in head-based (craniotopic) coordinates not in retinotopic coordinates (Galletti et al., 1993). Area V6A is strongly connected with prestriate visual areas, with superior parietal areas, and with the premotor frontal cortex representing arm movement (Gamberini et al., 2021; Rolls et al., 2023e). Macaque V6A is divided into two subareas that together are involved in the visual and somatosensory aspects of 'reach-to-grasp': V6Av which is more visual and V6Ad which is more somatosensory (Gamberini et al., 2018). The human homolog of V6Av has been identified in the posterior, dorsal-most part of precuneate cortex (Pitzalis et al., 2013), in a territory probably included in the DVT region of the HCP-MMP1 atlas (Glasser et al., 2016a) and which (like macaque V6Av) is activated by optic flow (Pitzalis et al., 2013). Another part of the macaque dorsal precuneate region includes the medial portion of area PEc (Gamberini et al., 2020). Area PEc is a visual-somatosensory area which represents both upper and lower limbs and is probably involved in locomotion and in the analysis of related optic flow (Gamberini et al., 2020; Raffi et al., 2011). Area PEc is strongly connected with part of posterior cingulate cortex 31, area 7m and retrosplenial cortex (Bakola et al., 2010). The human homolog of PEc has been identified in the dorsal-most part of the precuneate cortex (Pitzalis et al., 2019).

DVT and ProS (in addition to POS1, POS2 and the RSC in the anterodorsal group) may provide a route for scene information to be represented in the VMV regions (Sulpizio et al., 2020) and thus to reach the parahippocampal cortex PHA1-3 (TH) and hippocampal system, and thereby to provide a key input to drive spatial view cells (Rolls and Wirth, 2018; Georges-François et al., 1999; Rolls et al., 1998b; Robertson et al., 1998; Rolls et al., 1997a; Tsitsiklis et al., 2020; Wirth et al., 2017; Rolls, 2023c). These spatial view cells provide a component of primate (including human) episodic memory by enabling objects, people, or rewards to be associated with their location in visual scenes (Rolls and Xiang, 2006; Rolls et al., 2005c; Rolls and Xiang, 2005), and are likely to be useful in navigation from viewed landmark to viewed landmark too (Rolls, 2021f). This is part of a ventromedial visual cortical stream that is proposed to encode scene information to provide 'where' inputs to the hippocampal spatial and memory system (Rolls et al., 2023e). In this context, the dorsal visual transitional region (DVT) and prostriate region (ProS) are key parts of the retrosplenial scene area (Sulpizio et al., 2020), which connect earlier visual cortex ventral stream regions to the parahippocampal scene area (or PPA) in the VMV and PHA1-3 regions (Rolls et al., 2023e; Rolls, 2023c) (Fig. 9.18).

DVT and ProS may also provide a route for vestibular and optic flow information useful in navigation to reach hippocampal whole body motion neurons, for they receive inputs from VIP and V6A in which optic flow is represented (Duhamel et al., 1997; Sherrill et al., 2015; Delle Monache et al., 2021).

12.4 Mid-cingulate cortex, the cingulate motor area, and action–outcome learning

The anterior cingulate area may be distinguished from a mid-cingulate area (i.e. further back than the perigenual cingulate region and occupying approximately the middle third of the cingulate cortex), which has been termed the cingulate motor area (Vogt et al., 1996, 2003; Vogt, 2009, 2016, 2019b). The mid-cingulate area may be divided into an anterior or rostral cingulate motor area (24c' and 24a') concerned with skeletomotor control which may be required in avoidance and fear tasks, and a posterior or caudal cingulate motor area (24d and p24') which may be more involved in skeletomotor orientation (Vogt et al., 2003; Vogt, 2016). (As has been noted above, what has been termed the anterior mid-cingulate cortex (Vogt, 2016) may overlap with or be similar to what is described as the supracallosal part of the anterior cingulate cortex in this Chapter.)

This midcingulate cortex is activated by pain but, because this area is also activated in response selection tasks such as divided attention and Stroop tasks (which involve cues that cause conflict such as the word red written in green when the task is to make a response to the green color), it was suggested that activation of this mid-cingulate area by painful stimuli is related to the response selection processes initiated by painful stimuli (Vogt et al., 1996; Derbyshire et al., 1998). Both the anterior cingulate and the mid-cingulate areas may be activated in functional neuroimaging studies not only by physical pain, but also by social pain, for example being excluded from a social group (Eisenberger and Lieberman, 2004).

In human imaging studies it has been found that the anterior/mid-cingulate cortex is activated when there is a change in response set or when there is conflict between possible responses, but it is not activated when only stimulus selection is at issue (van Veen et al., 2001; Rushworth et al., 2002).

Some anterior/mid-cingulate neurons respond when errors are made (Niki and Watanabe, 1979; Kolling et al., 2016; Procyk et al., 2016), or when rewards are reduced (Shima and Tanji, 1998) (and activations are found in corresponding imaging studies (Bush et al., 2002; Procyk et al., 2016)). In humans, an event-related potential (ERP), called the error related negativity (ERN), may originate in the area 24c′ (Ullsperger and von Cramon, 2001), and many studies provide evidence that errors made in many tasks activate the anterior/mid-cingulate cortex, whereas tasks with response conflict activate the superior frontal gyrus (Rushworth et al., 2004; Kolling et al., 2016; Procyk et al., 2016).

Correspondingly, in rodents a part of the medial prefrontal / anterior cingulate cortex termed the prelimbic cortex is involved in learning relations between behavioral responses and reinforcers, that is between actions and outcomes (Balleine and Dickinson, 1998; Cardinal et al., 2002; Killcross and Coutureau, 2003). Balleine and Dickinson (1998) showed that the sensitivity of instrumental behavior to whether a particular action was followed by a reward was impaired by prelimbic cortex lesions. When making decisions about actions, it is important to take into account the costs as well as the benefits. There is some evidence implicating the rodent anterior cingulate cortex (prelimbic cortex) in this, in that rats with prelimbic cortex lesions were impaired in a task that required decisions about an action with a large reward but a high barrier to climb, vs an action with a lower reward but no barrier (Walton et al., 2002, 2003; Klein-Flugge et al., 2022a).

The concept has been advanced (Rolls, 2019c) that the midcingulate cortex may be part of a cingulate system that enables reward outcome information from the orbitofrontal cortex to be associated with action information from the posterior cingulate cortex, with the output directed to premotor cortical areas, as described in this Chapter.

12.5 How the computations are performed by the cingulate cortex

12.5.1 The anterior cingulate cortex and emotion

The anterior cingulate cortex receives information from its topologically nearby neocortical area, the orbitofrontal cortex (most of which is neocortical in primates, and which receives from ventral stream 'what' areas), and also the amygdala (also a recipient of ventral stream projections), and projects this information to a number of areas, including autonomic areas in the brainstem as well as in the insula, to the midcingulate cortex, and to the striatum. Because reward value is important in producing emotions, the anterior cingulate cortex becomes involved in emotion (Rolls, 2014a, 2019e), and damage to it in humans can impair emotions (Hornak, Bramham, Rolls, Morris, O'Doherty, Bullock and Polkey, 2003). This provides for an emotion-related function of the cingulate cortex.

The reciprocal connections between the reward-related medial orbitofrontal cortex and the pregenual and subgenual anterior cingulate cortex (Du et al., 2020; Hsu et al., 2020; Rolls et al., 2023c), and the local topology for reward representations in these areas (Grabenhorst and Rolls, 2011), may help in the formation of attractor networks for positive emotions, because within each of these cortical areas connections are likely to be made onto reward neurons, without dilution caused by intermingling of punishment neurons. The attractor potentiality is likely to be facilitated by associative synaptic modifiability of the forward and

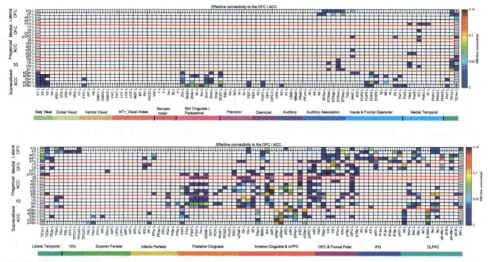

Fig. 12.8 Effective connectivity to the orbitofrontal cortex (OFC) and anterior cingulate cortex (ACC) from all 180 cortical regions in the left hemisphere of the human brain. The area 10 group consists of 10v, 10r, 10d and 9m, and are included here because they are close to and have somewhat similar connectivity to the pregenual ACC group, and are part of what is sometimes termed the ventromedial prefrontal cortex. The effective connectivity is read from column to row. All effective connectivities greater than 0 are shown, and effective connectivities of 0 are shown as a blank. The connectivities from the first set of cortical regions are shown above, and from the second set below. All effective connectivity maps are scaled to show 0.15 as the maximum, as this is the highest effective connectivity found between this set of brain regions. The effective connectivity algorithm for the whole brain is set to have a maximum of 0.2, and this was for connectivity between V1 and V2. The abbreviations are listed in Section 1.12, and the brain regions are illustrated in Fig. 11.24. (From Rolls,E.T., Deco,G., Huang,C-C. and Feng,J. (2023) The human orbitofrontal cortex, vmPFC, and anterior cingulate cortex effective connectome: emotion, memory, and action. Cerebral Cortex 33: 350-356. doi: 10.1093/cercor/bhac270. Copyright © Oxford University Press.)

backconnections, which also help to build an attractor network. This may help mood related attractors to be stable and enduring, which is likely to be evolutionarily adaptive.

The anterior cingulate cortex may also provide an important route for value representations in the orbitofrontal cortex to produce goal-related actions, as described above. For example, sensation-seeking behavior in humans can be predicted from the strength of the functional connectivity between the medial orbitofrontal cortex and the anterior cingulate cortex (Wan, Rolls, Cheng and Feng, 2020), and so can risk-taking behavior (Rolls et al., 2022c). Our hypothesis is that because some rewards have high value to particular individuals, the orbitofrontal representation of this may strongly drive the action system in the anterior cingulate cortex to perform actions to obtain these rewards. Part of the interest here is that risk-taking may be being driven by strong effects from the reward system, rather than problems with responding to non-reward or failing to inhibit behavior because of less functionality of the lateral orbitofrontal cortex / inferior frontal gyrus, which may be a different type of impulsivity (Aron et al., 2014; Deng et al., 2017).

12.5.2 Action-outcome learning in the supracallosal anterior cingulate cortex (dACC)

An important function of the supracallosal anterior cingulate cortex (or dACC) is to associate actions with outcomes, as indicated by the connections shown in green in Fig. 12.2 and in red in Fig. 12.3. My hypotheses are as follows. As shown by effective connectivity analyses in humans, the supracallosal anterior cingulate cortex receives information about recent actions from the premotor cortical area 6 and midcingulate cortex; somatosensory cortical regions including area 5, frontal opercular (FOP) regions and the insula; from parietal area 7 and inferior parietal region PF; and from the posterior cingulate cortex (23d and 31a) (Rolls et al., 2023c) (see Fig. 12.8). The supracallosal anterior cingulate cortex also receives effective connectivity from reward-related regions that provide evidence about reward outcome, the medial orbitofrontal cortex (pOFC, OFC, 13l and 11l) and pregenual anterior cingulate cortex (d32, p24) (Rolls et al., 2023c). The same analyses show that the supracallosal anterior cingulate cortex has connectivity with the dorsolateral prefrontal cortex regions 46 and 9-46d (Rolls et al., 2023c), and these prefrontal regions implicated in short-term memory may help to maintain a memory trace of recent actions and outcomes, so that an average can be made that is useful in probabilistic tasks and situations. Computationally, this enables the high dimensional space of many possible actions, and any relevant spatial information from the parietal cortex or some object information from the inferior temporal visual cortex (regions PIT and TE2p in Fig. 12.8) to be associated with the high dimensional space of many possible reward/punishment/non-reward outcomes received from the orbitofrontal cortex and anterior cingulate cortex, to enable the outcomes of each possible action to become associated. The type of action-outcome learning involved could be as simple as pattern association between the action input and the reward outcome output, with previous actions and their associated outcomes taken into account using the neocortical short-term memory capability.

The computational issue then arises about how to choose the action that leads to best outcome currently available. Part of the selection involved it is proposed takes place at the level of the reward value as implemented in the orbitofrontal cortex, using mechanisms such as sensory-specific satiety, long-term sensory specific satiety, homeostatic reward modulation by internal state, etc (Chapter 11). But an important part of the mechanism for the action to select to obtain the best reward currently available may be using an 'exploit' vs 'explore' mechanism. As described above, the proposed computational mechanism is that non-reward or punishment resets an 'exploit' neuronal population to fall out of its attractor in an exploit/explore rule attractor network, thereby releasing the 'explore' population from inhibition by the inhibitory neurons. This could be achieved by non-reward or punishment directly activating the 'explore' attractor to produce exploratory behavior. Then while exploring, rewards that are better than previously received activate the 'exploit' attractor neuronal population, which quenches the 'explore' neuronal population through the inhibitory neurons in the exploit/explore rule single attractor network. The computational mechanism is similar to that described for reversal of the rule attractor network in Section 11.5.3. The actual location of this exploit/explore rule attractor single network could be in the dACC, but another interesting possibility is that it is in the frontal pole, from where it can control the whole of the dorsolateral prefrontal cortex, as described in Section 13.5 (Rolls et al., 2023a).

A useful computational property of the exploit/explore network would be some adaptation over time in its synapses. That would enable the system if in 'exploit' mode to gradually reduce its tendency to exploit, so that eventually the 'explore' attractor population of neurons would jump up out of the noise (see Section 11.5.1 and Rolls and Deco (2002)), and exploration would occur behaviorally to investigate whether different rewards were available. Correspondingly, adaptation in the 'explore' population of neurons would ensure that if exploration had been proceeding for a long time, the 'exploit' neuronal population in the exploit/explore single attractor network should jump up out of the noise, so that behaviorally the individual would settle on the exploitation of whatever resource was currently available.

The outcomes are in the high dimensional space of many different types of reward that are represented in the orbitofrontal cortex. This enables rapid learning of which actions to perform for which outcomes, because this requires simple associative learning between the particular action that has just been performed, and the particular outcome that has just been received and is signalled by the orbitofrontal cortex. It also seem likely that the cingulate cortex has a repertoire of previously learned actions, which can rapidly be associated with new different outcomes by rapid associative learning between actions and outcomes.

This cingulate action-outcome learning is thus much more efficient than stimulus-response habit formation, in which a one-dimensional reinforcer, the dopamine neuron reward prediction error signal, is used to reinforce whatever representations of stimuli and responses throughout the dopamine-influenced system in for example the basal ganglia may recently have been active (see Section 19.5 and Chapter 16).

The orbitofrontal cortex–cingulate cortex action-outcome learning system is also much more rapid and efficient than the reinforcement learning stimulus-response habit system implemented by dopamine and the basal ganglia, because if the association between the stimulus and the outcome (a stimulus-stimulus association) changes or is reversed, this can be corrected in one trial by the stimulus-reward reversal learning system in the orbitofrontal cortex described in Chapter 11.

Error signals generated reflect a mismatch between the expected outcome and the action. This is different from the orbitofrontal cortex, in which the error signals reflect a mismatch between the expected value of a stimulus (e.g. the sight of food) and the outcome (e.g. a taste of food).

12.5.3 Connectivity of the posterior cingulate cortex with the hippocampal memory system

Another important function of the cingulate cortex is related to the hippocampal memory system (Rolls, 2018b), as shown in Figs. 12.2 and Fig. 12.3. The connectivity shown in these Figures indicate two routes for reward-related information to reach the hippocampal memory system. The first, more direct, route is from the orbitofrontal cortex, vmPFC, anterior cingulate cortex and amygdala to the perirhinal cortex with information derived from the ventral visual and auditory 'what' processing streams (blue in Fig. 12.2). A second route for reward-related information is via the orbitofrontal cortex / vmPFC / pregenual anterior cingulate cortex to the posterior cingulate cortex and thereby to the hippocampal system (Fig. 12.3). These concepts are further elaborated elsewhere (Rolls, 2019c,b; Rolls et al., 2023i; Rolls, 2022b).

The posterior cingulate cortex appears to have three main groups of region. A posterior ventral group provides a path for 'what' information to reach the hippocampal memory system (Section 12.3.2). An anterodorsal group provides a path of 'where' information to reach the hippocampal memory system (Section 12.3.3). The retrosplenial scene area in DVT and PRoS provides a route for ventral visual stream information to reach the parahippocampal scene area (Section 12.3.4). The coordinates in the parahippocampal scene area and hippocampus are at least for many neurons in allocentric coordinates (Chapter 9 including Section 9.6). Humans often describe scenes in a perhaps partly egocentric view-based framework, as the view of a scene from where they are located, though in practice exactly where they are located on one side of the scene often makes little difference (see Section 9.6). Hippocampal spatial view cells could also be involved in this type of episodic / autobiographical memory. However, of course the information at earlier stages of the visual system is in egocentric coordinates, so transforms from retinal through to allocentric coordinates are needed. Possible mechanisms for these spatial coordinate transforms are described in Section 3.4. The retrosplenial cortical regions, and perhaps the antero-dorsal posterior cingulate division regions, connect information from the parietal lobe which may be at least partly in egocentric coordinates with the hippocampal system via the parahippocampal gyrus. The posterior cingulate and retrosplenial cortex may be involved in helping to perform these coordinate transforms, in the ways that are described in Section 3.4.

12.6 Synthesis and conclusions

The conceptualization provided here of the cingulate cortex, a key brain region with proisocortical structure, shows how its connections are related to both the ventral and the dorsal cortical processing streams; how its functions are important in emotion, episodic memory, and action-outcome learning; and how its functions are related to those of other limbic structures including the hippocampus, and to the functions of different neocortical areas. Some of the key points that are made (Rolls, 2019c; Rolls et al., 2023c,i) are as follows, and relate to what is shown in Figs. 12.2, 12.3, 12.6, 12.7, and 9.18.

1. The cingulate cortex has several different functions, which can be related to the connections of its different parts. As an area of proisocortex (a type of neocortex) it forms a connectional bridge between neocortical areas and areas such as the hippocampus (which is archicortex, a type of allocortex) (Pandya et al., 2015; Rolls, 2019c). The connections of the cingulate cortex can in this way be related to its evolutionary history as a proisocortical structure, and the topological position of its different parts.

2. In this framework, the posterior cingulate cortex in its anterodorsal part (including 23d, 31a, and retrosplenial regions, Fig. 12.7) receives information from the nearby neocortical areas such as the parietal cortex about spatial representations, and projects this onwards via the PHA1-3 medial parahippocampal cortex to the hippocampus, where it provides a spatial component related to idiothetic update for object-space episodic memories. This provides for a 'where' memory-related contribution of the cingulate cortex.

3. The posterior cingulate in its posteroventral part (most of regions 31 and 23, Fig. 12.6) has connectivity with 'what' regions including the inferior temporal visual cortex and cortex in the superior temporal sulcus involved in auditory and semantic representations, and with reward / value / emotion-related regions including the vmPFC and pregenual anterior cingulate cortex. The onward connectivity to the hippocampal system (Fig. 12.6, (Rolls et al., 2023i)) provides for a 'what' and reward memory-related function of the cingulate cortex.

4. The retrosplenial regions DVT and PRos are where the retrosplenial scene area is located, and may be involved in coordinate transforms from egocentric to allocentric representations.

5. The pregenual anterior cingulate cortex receives from the orbitofrontal cortex and the vmPFC, and has connectivity directly with the hippocampal system and via the posteroventral part of the posterior cingulate cortex to provide reward / value / emotion-related information to the hippocampus (Fig. 12.3). The hippocampus can use this as a key component of episodic memory, and to set the goals for navigation.

6. The pregenual anterior cingulate cortex has connectivity to the septal nuclei which contain cholinergic neurons that project to the hippocampus. This enables the pregenual anterior cingulate cortex to influence memory consolidation. This complements the functions of the medial orbitofrontal cortex region pOFC which has effective connectivity to the basal forebrain nuclei of Meynert which contain cholinergic neurons that project to the neocortex, and also thereby can influence memory consolidation.

7. The effects of damage to the human anterior cingulate cortex and vmPFC and orbitofrontal cortex which produce memory impairments therefore probably do so largely by disconnecting reward value inputs from the hippocampal system and by impairing the roles of the choliner-

gic systems in memory consolidation (Rolls, 2022b) (Section 9.2.8.5), rather than by implementing the computational functions required for episodic memory, which are performed by the hippocampus (Chapter 9).

8. The supracallosal anterior cingulate cortex has strong connectivity with somatosensory, premotor, and midcingulate motor areas, and also receives reward outcome information from the orbitofrontal cortex and pregenual anterior cingulate cortex (Fig. 12.3). This provides a foundation for its involvement in goal-related action-outcome learning which is a key output system for the orbitofrontal cortex to implement actions in relation to emotion-provoking stimuli, i.e. rewards and punishers.

The further conclusions described next add detail to the framework just described.

9. The orbitofrontal cortex, which represents value and not actions, projects reward value information from the medial orbitofrontal cortex, and punishment and non-reward information from the lateral orbitofrontal cortex, to the anterior cingulate cortex. The pregenual anterior cingulate cortex is activated by rewards, and the supracallosal anterior cingulate cortex by punishers and non-reward (Grabenhorst and Rolls, 2011; Rolls, 2019e).

10. A source of information about actions reaches the posterior cingulate cortex from the parietal cortex (Vogt, 2009). The parietal cortex represents actions in terms of body and eye movements in space (lateral parietal cortex), and of the self in a spatial context (medial parietal cortex including the precuneus) (Rolls and Wirth, 2018; Rolls, 2020b) (Chapter 10).

11. After storage of information in the hippocampus, the information needs to be retrieved from the hippocampus, and utilizes backprojections originating in hippocampal CA1 back to neocortex, through the whole series of backprojections involving the lateral entorhinal cortex, and perirhinal cortex to the ventral stream areas, and orbitofrontal cortex, for the ventral route shown in blue in Fig. 12.2; and involving the medial entorhinal cortex, parahippocampal gyrus, posterior cingulate cortex, to the parietal cortex areas, for the dorsal route shown in red in Fig. 12.2.

This backprojection system enables the object information from an episodic memory to be recalled to the ventral stream areas, the reward information to the orbitofrontal cortex, and the spatial information to the parietal cortex (Kesner and Rolls, 2015; Rolls, 2016b, 2018b).

12. These functions related to different connectivity of the different parts of the cingulate cortex provide further evidence that we should no longer think of a single limbic system, but instead of multiple limbic systems (Rolls, 2015b).

One limbic system may involve the amygdala, orbitofrontal cortex, and anterior cingulate cortex for emotion.

A second limbic system may involve the hippocampus, perirhinal and parahippocampal cortex, and posterior cingulate cortex for episodic memory, including object-spatial associations, and object or spatial associations with temporal order. Reward information can also enter this hippocampal episodic memory system from the orbitofrontal cortex and anterior cingulate cortex so that reward value information can be included in an episodic memory (Kesner and Rolls, 2015; Rolls, 2016b, 2018b; Rolls and Wirth, 2018; Rolls, 2022b, 2023c).

A third limbic system may involve associations with the cingulate cortex for action-outcome learning, with the action information entering via the posterior cingulate cortex, the reward value outcome information via the anterior cingulate cortex, and the resulting association directed from the midcingulate cortex to premotor cortical areas.

The cingulate cortex is of interest within this context, as a limbic structure that is involved in all three of these functions, and this is related to the different connectivity of the different parts of this proisocortical structure.

13. It is useful to note that spatial scene representations are built along a pathway from early visual areas to the occipital scene area, then to the retrosplenial scene area in DVT and ProS, and then to the parahippocampal scene area in VMV1-3 and PHA1-3, and then to the hippocampus (Fig. 9.18, (Rolls et al., 2023e)).

14. The overall computational role of the posterior cingulate and related regions in the HCP-MMP posterior cingulate division can be conceptualised as now proposed. The cortical regions can be thought of as transitional in structure and evolutionary history between the hippocampal type of archicortex, and the neocortex or isocortex (Pandya, Seltzer, Petrides and Cipolloni, 2015). Parts of the posterior cingulate division are likely to have arisen in evolution after the hippocampal archicortex, and before the neocortex become highly developed. The posterior cingulate cortex can be thought of as interfacing neocortical regions involved in 'what', 'where' and reward representations to the hippocampal memory and navigation system. In another example, the pregenual anterior cingulate cortex connects the orbitofrontal cortex with the hippocampus to enable reward value information to enter the hippocampal memory system. The supracallosal anterior cingulate cortex can be thought of as interfacing neocortical somatosensory and premotor cortex regions with reward systems including the orbitofrontal cortex. Thus a conceptual framework for understanding the cingulate cortex is in terms of its transitional role in structure and evolutionary history for connectivity between later neocortex and earlier structures involved in memory such as the hippocampus and with reward systems.

13 The prefrontal cortex

13.1 Introduction and overview

The prefrontal cortex is the part of the frontal lobe anterior to motor area 4 and premotor area 6, and is approximately the cortex in and anterior to the arcuate sulcus, as shown in Fig. 13.1. It comprises architectonic areas 46 in and close to the principal sulcus; 45 and 44 inferiorly (the inferior frontal gyrus in humans); 8A, which includes the frontal eye field posterior to the principal sulcus and anterior to the arcuate sulcus; area 8B superiorly (which continues onto the medial wall); and areas 9 and 10 anteriorly. The prefrontal cortex also includes the orbitofrontal cortex, and that is considered in Chapter 11. Fig. 13.2 compares the prefrontal areas in macaques and humans. The prefrontal cortex also includes the anterior cingulate cortex, and that is considered in Chapter 12.

Fig. 13.1 provides a foundation for understanding the computational architecture of the prefrontal cortex. The occipital cortex is dominated by visual sensory input. The temporal lobe is dominated by hierarchical levels of analysis of ventral stream visual and auditory inputs. The parietal lobe is dominated by spatial dorsal visual stream and somatosensory processing (and their combination). All of these processing systems must devote their resources to sensory processing, and must remain continuously dedicated to this, otherwise we would be blind or deaf to what was happening in the world, which would be in evolutionary terms at great risk. The motor and premotor cortex (areas 4 and 6) must remain continuously devoted to and ready for action. That leaves the prefrontal cortex in a position to perform 'off-line' processing, including holding items in a short-term memory when the items are no longer present in the input processing streams. This off-line capacity develops into a capability of manipulating and rearranging items in short-term memory, and this is called working memory, which is also implemented in the prefrontal cortex. This ability in humans develops into systems that can plan ahead, and then can control behavior according to such plans, which is referred to as 'executive function' (Rosati, 2017; Fiske and Holmboe, 2019; Shallice and Cipolotti, 2018).

This concept, that computationally the posterior cortical regions including the temporal and parietal cortex must be devoted to incoming sensory inputs from the world, and that the prefrontal cortex therefore can specialise in short-term memory for previous states using inputs from posterior cortical regions, provides a key computational basis for understanding the prefrontal cortex. This concept was missed in some earlier descriptions of the functions of the prefrontal cortex as being involved in 'voluntary action' (Passingham and Wise, 2012; Passingham, 2021), which is difficult to define and measure (Rolls et al., 2023f). A more precise approach to the functions of the prefrontal cortex is to take a computational approach that the prefrontal cortex is involved when actions are generated from short-term or working memory. This type of computation provides an approach to planning ahead, for which keeping several steps of a plan active in working memory is needed (Rolls et al., 2023f). This foundation for understanding the functions of the prefrontal cortex emphasises that it is involved when actions are internally generated (from short term and working memory), rather than being in response to an incoming stimulus from the world processed by posterior cortical, temporal and parietal, regions (Rolls et al., 2023f). Working memory refers here to the ability to ma-

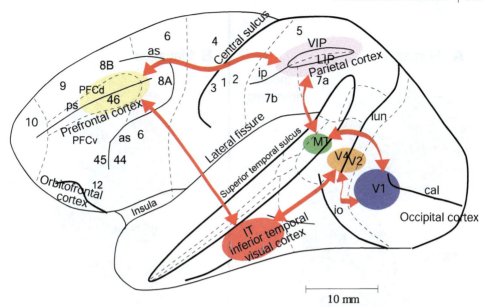

Fig. 13.1 Lateral view of the macaque brain showing some connections to the prefrontal cortex. The ventral visual stream projects to the temporal lobe visual cortical areas which in turn project to ventral parts of the prefrontal cortex. The dorsal visual stream projects to parietal cortex areas which in turn project to dorsal parts of the prefrontal cortex. There are backprojections from the prefrontal cortex. V1, primary visual area; V2, V4, extrastriate visual areas; IT, inferior temporal visual cortex; LIP, lateral intraparietal cortex visual area; PP, posterior parietal cortex; PFCv, ventrolateral prefrontal cortex; PFCd, dorsolateral prefrontal cortex; VIP, ventral intraparietal cortex visual area; as, arcuate sulcus; cal, calcarine sulcus; io, inferior occipital sulcus; ip, intraparietal sulcus; lun, lunate sulcus; ps, principal sulcus. (Modified from Gustavo Deco and Edmund T. Rolls (2005) Attention, short-term memory, and action selection: A unifying theory. *Progress in Neurobiology* 76: 236–256. © Elsevier Ltd.)

nipulate items held in short-term memory, and provides a basis for planning (Baddeley, 2007, 2012; Baddeley et al., 2019; Baddeley, 2021).

In order to operate in this way, the prefrontal cortex needs material to work on in its short-term or working memory. As indicated in Fig. 13.1, the prefrontal cortex receives visual, auditory and somatosensory information from the temporal and parietal lobes. The prefrontal cortex also receives taste and olfactory and reward value information from the orbitofrontal cortex. To then control behavior based on what is in its short-term or working memory, the prefrontal cortex then needs routes to motor output, and it is well placed for this, as it is placed close to, and sends projections to, premotor cortical areas including area 6. For the computations performed by the prefrontal cortex to be useful, it must be able to influence behavioral output, via for example its connections to premotor cortical areas.

But the prefrontal cortex can do more than this. Because it can hold items in short-term memory, and because it has top-down backprojections to the temporal and parietal areas from which it receives inputs, it can implement top-down attentional control, again by the pathways shown in Fig. 13.1. This enables the prefrontal cortex to gently bias incoming sensory inputs using top-down biased competition (see Section 2.12) and top-down biased activation (see Section 4.3.5) to give preference to whatever sensory and other inputs and processing may be relevant to the goal that may be being implemented by what is held in the prefrontal cortex short-term memory / planning system.

Thus the prefrontal cortex can influence behavioral output both by its connections to nearby premotor cortex areas, and also by top-down biassing of inputs in the temporal and parietal sensory processing streams.

Different parts of the prefrontal cortex are organised to implement these functions by connections to different parts of the temporal and parietal cortex. For example, the dorsal

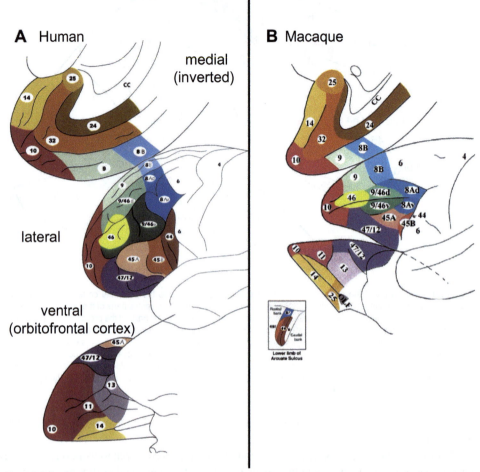

Fig. 13.2 Cytoarchitectonic maps of the lateral, medial, and orbital surfaces of the frontal lobe of the human (A) and the macaque monkey (B) brains as parcellated by Petrides and Pandya (1994). In B, the inset diagram displays the region within the lower limb of the arcuate sulcus to show the cytoarchitectonic areas lying within its banks. (Modified from Michael Petrides, Francesco Tomaiuolo, Edward H. Yeterian, and Deepak N. Pandya (2012) The prefrontal cortex: Comparative architectonic organization in the human and the macaque monkey brains. *Cortex* 48: 46–57. © Elsevier Srl.)

parts of area 46 in the dorsal bank of the principal sulcus are involved especially in spatial ('where') short-term memory, because they tend to receive projections from the dorsal parts of the sensory processing systems, the parietal cortex (as indicated in Fig. 13.1). Conversely, the ventral parts of area 46 in the ventral bank of the principal sulcus are involved especially in object ('what') spatial short-term memory, because they tend to receive projections from the ventral parts of the sensory processing systems, the temporal cortex. In addition, the frontal eye field in area 8A is involved in spatial working memory for eye position, with connections to the parts of the parietal lobe involved in eye position control such as LIP and VIP.

The computational ability to hold items in a short-term memory, and even better to rearrange them in a working memory and to plan ahead, has clear evolutionary adaptive value, by enabling behavior to extend beyond the current sensory input. This computational capability was driven by the development of the cortex, which by implementing associatively modifiable synaptic connections between nearby pyramidal cells, enables autoassociation or attractor networks to be implemented, which are the building blocks of short-term memory (see Section B.3) (Rolls, 2016b). However, having attractor networks in the sensory processing areas in the temporal and parietal cortex is not sufficient to overcome the issue that the next sensory input must drive these areas into the next state. The great evolutionary advantage of the prefrontal cortex is that it provides computationally separate attractor networks from what is happening in the sensory processing cortical areas. The prefrontal networks are sufficiently connected to sensory areas that the prefrontal networks can receive information, and can go into an attractor state that represents the inputs from posterior brain regions. But once in that attractor state, the prefrontal autoassociation networks must be sufficiently stable that they can remain in their short-term memory attractor state, and be independent of the changing sensory processing in the sensory processing streams. This requires the correct degree of coupling between the prefrontal and the posterior networks: if too weak, the prefrontal networks will never be activated by the sensory input; and if too strong, then the sensory input will dominate the prefrontal attractor networks, which will not be independent. This is an important computational issue for understanding the functions of the prefrontal cortex, and we have therefore investigated this considerably, and have identified the quantitative regimes within which the correct operation occurs, as described in Sections B.9 and 13.6.2.2 (Renart, Parga and Rolls, 1999b,a). Further, if the stability of this prefrontal processing is too great, then this may lead to malfunction in behavior, and indeed a number of mental disorders including obsessive-compulsive disorder, depression and attention deficit hyperactivity disorder (ADHD) are likely to reflect overstability or at least altered stability of some prefrontal and related processing modules, and some other disorders such as some aspects of schizophrenia and over-impulsivity may reflect too little stability (see Chapter 18).

The mechanisms that implement the short-term memory in the prefrontal cortex are autoassociation or attractor networks, as described in this Chapter, with the operation of this type of network described in Section B.3.

This computational approach to understanding the functions of the prefrontal cortex can be contrasted with the more neuropsychological approach based considerably on the effects of lesions to different parts of the prefrontal cortex (Passingham and Wise, 2012; Passingham, 2021). The approach there was to list the many tasks in monkeys that are impaired by lesions of the prefrontal cortex, and to infer a function from those. Many of the tasks were described as involving "flexibility". This led to the proposal that "The granular prefrontal cortex generates goals that are appropriate to the current context and current needs, and it can do so based on a single event." In terms of the evolutionary advantage, it was proposed that "the granular prefrontal cortex evolved in primates as an adaptation to reducing the number of unproductive, risky, or costly foraging choices that phylogenetically older learning mechanisms produce. ... The new mechanism that primates evolved brings single events – conjunctions of contexts, goals, actions, and outcomes – to bear on the choice of foraging goals" (Passingham and Wise, 2012).

That is an interesting contrast to the more computational description provided above of the functions of the prefrontal cortex and its adaptive value. The computational account recognises a unifying function of the prefrontal cortex, as an offline buffer store that can hold items in a short-term and working memory; and of course must be able to influence actions based on what is in the memory or plan, which must in that sense provide goals for actions. Of course the fractionation of the prefrontal cortex based on the connectivity of its different parts, the effects of lesions to its different parts, and the neuronal activity and neuroimaging activations in its different parts, together with computational neuroscience approaches are key to understanding exactly how the system operates, and it is to what has been learned with these approaches that we now turn.

Some of the background evidence on the neuroscience of the prefrontal cortex is available elsewhere (Fuster, 2015; Passingham and Wise, 2012; Passingham, 2021). Here the focus is on what computations are performed by the prefrontal cortex (Sections 13.2–13.4), and how they are performed (Section 13.6).

13.2 Divisions of the lateral prefrontal cortex

Some parts of the prefrontal cortex are described elsewhere in this book. The orbitofrontal cortex is considered in Chapter 11. The anterior cingulate cortex is considered in Chapter 12. The left inferior frontal gyrus, which includes Broca's area and is involved in language production, is described in Chapter 14 and Section 8.3.

Here we consider other parts of the prefrontal cortex, which are those mainly on the lateral surface as shown in Figs. 13.1 and 13.2. The computations in which these areas are involved include short-term memory (Sections 13.2.1–13.2.3), and top-down attentional control (Section 13.4). The connectional and computational organisation of the human prefrontal cortex is described in Section 13.3. How these computations for short-term memory and for attention are performed are described in Section 13.6.

13.2.1 The dorsolateral prefrontal cortex

This is area 46, the cortex in and close to the principal sulcus. The dorsal part has strong connectivity with parietal cortex areas, as shown in Fig. 13.1. It is involved in spatial short-term memory, for example remembering where in space a response should be made. A prototypical task is a delayed spatial response task (Goldman-Rakic, 1996; Fuster, 2015). In such a task performed by a monkey, a light beside one of two response keys illuminates briefly, there is then a delay of several seconds, and then the monkey must touch the appropriate key in order to obtain a food reward. The monkey must not initiate the response until the end of the delay period, and must hold a central key continuously in the delay period. Lesions of the prefrontal cortex in the region of the principal sulcus impair the performance of this task if there is a delay, but not if there is no delay. Some neurons in this region fire in the delay period, while the response is being remembered (Fuster, 1973, 1989; Goldman-Rakic, 1996; Fuster, 2015). Different neurons fire for the two different responses.

In pioneering research, Patricia Goldman-Rakic and colleagues had shown that lesions of the cortex in the principal sulcus impaired such spatial tasks, but only if there was a delay involved, showing that this is a system needed for short-term memory (Goldman et al., 1971; Goldman-Rakic, 1996).

The ventral part of the lateral prefrontal cortex has strong connectivity with temporal cortical areas including the inferior temporal cortex, as shown in Fig. 13.1. It is involved in object short-term memory, for example in a delayed match to sample task. For example, neuronal firing is found in the delay period in an object short-term memory task (delayed match to sample) in the inferior frontal convexity cortex, in a region connected to the ventral temporal cortex (Fuster, 1989; Wilson, Scalaidhe and Goldman-Rakic, 1993).

Some neurons in the principal sulcus region area 46 may be involved in both spatial and object short-term memory tasks (Rao, Rainer and Miller, 1997). Heterogeneous populations of neurons, some with more spatial input, others with more object input, and top-down attentional modulation of the different subpopulations depending on the task, start to provide an explanation for these findings (Kadohisa et al., 2023).

Given that inputs from the parietal cortex, involved in spatial computation, project more to the dorsolateral prefrontal cortex, for example to the cortex in the principal sulcus, and that inputs from the temporal lobe visual cortex, involved in computations about objects, project ventrolaterally to the prefrontal cortex (see Figs. 2.1, 3.1, and 2.3), it could be that the dorsolateral prefrontal cortex is especially involved in spatial short-term memory, and the inferior convexity prefrontal cortex more in object short-term memory (Goldman-Rakic, 1996, 1987; Fuster et al., 1982). This organization-by-stimulus-domain hypothesis (Miller, 2000) holds that spatial ('where') working memory is supported by the dorsolateral PFC in the neighborhood of the principal sulcus (Brodmann's area (BA) 46/9 in the middle frontal gyrus (MFG)); and object ('what') working memory is supported by the ventrolateral PFC on the lateral/inferior convexity (BA 45 in the inferior frontal gyrus (IFG)). Consistent with this, lesions of the cortex in the principal sulcus impair delayed spatial response memory, and lesions of the inferior convexity can impair delayed (object) matching to sample short-term memory (Goldman-Rakic, 1996) (especially when there are intervening stimuli between the sample and the matching object, as described above). Further, Wilson, Scalaidhe and Goldman-Rakic (1993) found that neurons dorsolaterally in the prefrontal cortex were more likely to be related to spatial working memory, and in the inferior convexity to object working memory. Some fMRI studies in humans support this topographical organization (Leung et al., 2002), and some do not (Postle and D'Esposito, 2000, 1999). Rao, Rainer and Miller (1997) found in a task that had a spatial short-term memory component and an object short-term memory component that some prefrontal cortex neurons are involved in both, and thus questioned whether there is segregation of spatial and object short-term memory in the prefrontal cortex. Some segregation does seem likely, in that for example the neurons with activity related to delayed oculomotor saccades are in the frontal eye field (Funahashi, Bruce and Goldman-Rakic, 1989) (see Fig. 13.3), and this area has not been implicated in object working memory. Further, neurons in the dorsolateral prefrontal cortex are more likely to be involved in spatial processing in a delay task, and neurons in the inferior prefrontal convexity (ventrolateral prefrontal cortex) and more likely to be involved in object and spatial coding (Kadohisa et al., 2023).

Part of the conceptual resolution of the discussion about segregation of functions in the lateral prefrontal cortex is that sometimes combinations of objects and places must be held in short-term memory. For example, in one such task, a *conditional object–response (associative) task* with a delay, a monkey was shown one of two stimulus objects (O1 or O2), and after a delay had to make either a rightward or leftward oculomotor saccade response depending on which stimulus was shown. In another such task, a *delayed spatial response task*, the same stimuli were used, but the rule required was different, namely to respond after the delay towards the left or right location where the stimulus object had been shown (Asaad, Rainer and Miller, 2000). The tasks could be run on some trial blocks with the mappings reversed. Thus the monkey had to remember in any trial block the particular object–place mapping that was required in the delay period. In this task, neurons were found that responded to combinations of the object and the spatial position (Asaad et al., 2000). This bringing together of the spatial and object components of the task is important in how the short-term memory task was solved, as described in the computational model of these functions in Section 13.6.3. Mixed object and spatial coding in a more complex foraging task with a short-term memory component was also found (Kadohisa et al., 2023). However, this makes the conceptual point that at least some mixing of the spatial and object representations in the lateral prefrontal cortex is needed in order for some short-term memory tasks to be solved, and thus total segregation of 'what' and 'where' processing in the lateral prefrontal cortex should not be expected.

The maintenance of a short-term memory by the continuing firing of neurons in a delay period is a fundamental aspect of the operation of the prefrontal cortex, but there has been discussion of whether the neuronal firing is maintained sufficiently well in the short-term memory period (Miller et al., 2018). Part of the resolution to this is that we have shown that if even a few neurons in the population maintain some firing in the delay period, then at the end of the delay period the firing of the whole population can be reinstated from those few neur-

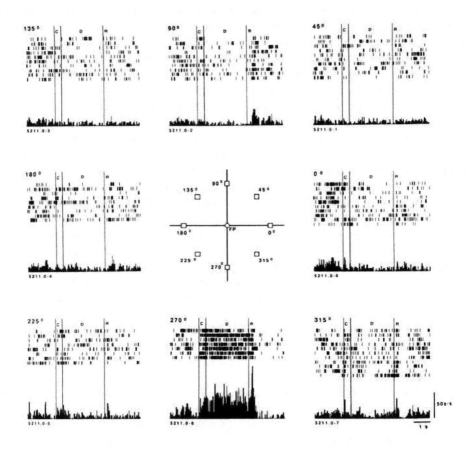

Fig. 13.3 The activity of a single neuron in the dorsolateral prefrontal cortical area involved in remembered saccades. Each row is a single trial, with each spike shown by a vertical line. A cue is shown in the cue (C) period, there is then a delay (D) period without the cue in which the cue position must be remembered, then there is a response (R) period. The monkey fixates the central fixation point (FP) during the cue and delay periods, and saccades to the position where the cue was shown, in one of the eight positions indicated, in the response period. The neuron increased its activity primarily for saccades to position 270°. The increase of activity was in the cue, delay, and response period while the response was made. The time calibration is 1 s. (Reproduced from Funahashi,S., Bruce,C. and Goldman-Rakic,P. (1989) Mnemonic coding of visual space in monkey dorsolateral prefrontal cortex. Journal of Neurophysiology 61: 331–349. © American Physiological Society.)

ons that are still active by a non-specific retrieval cue such as a cue that the delay period has ended (Martinez-Garcia, Rolls, Deco and Romo, 2011; Deco, Rolls and Romo, 2010). Another possible computational mechanism is short-term synaptic plasticity (Martinez-Garcia, Rolls, Deco and Romo, 2011).

The dorsolateral prefrontal cortex is also involved in temporal order / sequence memory, which is evident in the recall of items from short-term memory in the original order, and in neuronal firing (Naya, Chen, Yang and Suzuki, 2017; Tiganj, Cromer, Roy, Miller and Howard, 2018). The recall of the last few items in short-term memory is in the correct order, and this is a property of the 'recency' effect in short-term memory (Baddeley, 2012, 2021).

13.2.2 The caudal prefrontal cortex

The caudal prefrontal cortex is area 8A shown in Fig. 13.1. It is known as the frontal eye field, and is involved in eye movement related tasks that require a short-term memory, such as a delayed saccade task. This area is strongly connected with parietal areas involved in eye movement control, including VIP and LIP.

An example of a neuron responding in this dorsal and posterior part of the prefrontal cortex involved in remembering the position in visual space to which an eye movement (a saccade) should be made is illustrated in Fig. 13.3 (Funahashi, Bruce and Goldman-Rakic, 1989; Goldman-Rakic, 1996). In this case, the monkey was asked to remember which of eight lights appeared, and, after the delay, to move his eyes to the light that was briefly illuminated. The short-term memory function is topographically organized, in that lesions in small parts of the system impair remembered eye movements only to that eye position. Moreover, neurons in the appropriate part of the topographic map respond to eye movements in one but not in other directions (see Fig. 13.3). As shown below, such a memory system could be easily implemented in such a topographically organized system by having local cortical connections between nearby pyramidal cells which implement an attractor network (Fig. 13.9). Then triggering activity in one part of the topographically organized system would lead to sustained activity in that part of the map, thus implementing a short-term or working memory for delayed eye movements to that position in space.

13.2.3 The ventrolateral prefrontal cortex

The ventrolateral prefrontal cortex includes area 45, which on the left with 44 is Broca's area in the human inferior frontal gyrus. It has strong connections with the superior (auditory) and inferior (visual) temporal cortex. One of its functions in macaques may be to map visual and auditory inputs to motor responses, for damage to this region impairs conditional visual–spatial response learning, that is, when a visual stimulus must be mapped to a particular spatial response (Passingham, 2021). In macaques, the ventrolateral prefrontal cortex contains neurons that respond to auditory stimuli and that process both face and vocal stimuli, supporting the hypothesis that this may be an essential brain region for both auditory and audiovisual working memory (Plakke and Romanski, 2016).

In humans, this may be a key region in mapping semantic representations in the anterior temporal lobe to motor responses that include the generation of speech, as considered in more detail in Section 14.5. There is strong connectivity in humans between areas 45 and 44 and the temporal pole as well as other anterior parts of the temporal lobe (Rolls, Deco, Huang and Feng, 2022b; Hsu, Rolls, Huang, Chong, Lo, Feng and Lin, 2020).

On the inferior prefrontal convexity there is a part that in humans is termed the inferior frontal gyrus pars orbitalis, and which has similarities both with the lateral orbitofrontal cortex (area 12), and with the inferior frontal gyrus (see Section 13.3.1 and Chapters 14, 11 and 18), including in its connectivity (Rolls, Deco, Huang and Feng, 2022b; Du, Rolls, Cheng, Li, Gong, Qiu and Feng, 2020; Hsu, Rolls, Huang, Chong, Lo, Feng and Lin, 2020).

13.3 The connectivity and computational organisation of the human prefrontal cortex

The organisation of the human prefrontal cortex using the Human Connectome Project - Multimodal cortical Parcellation (HCP-MMP, Section 1.12), and measuring effective connectivity, complemented by functional connectivity and diffusion tractography (Section 1.13) with data from the Human Connectome Project, is described next (Rolls et al., 2023f).

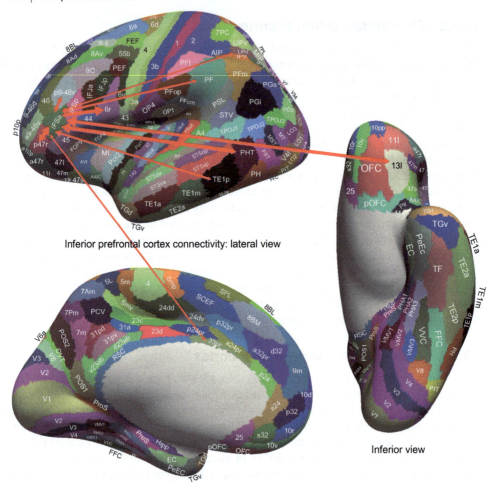

Fig. 13.4 Inferior prefrontal cortex effective connectivity. The connectivity of IFSa is shown as an example of the connectivity of IFja, IFJp, IFSa and IFSp. The width of the arrows reflects the effective connectivity with the size of the arrowheads reflecting the connectivity in each direction. The effective connectivity with the inferior temporal visual cortex (TE1p, TE2p and PHT); and with the medial orbitofrontal cortex 13l and 11l, and the lateral orbitofrontal cortex p47r and a47r are notable. IFSa has moderate effective connectivity with the other IF regions. (From Rolls,E.T., Deco,G., Huang,C-C. and Feng,J. (2023) Prefrontal and somatosensory-motor cortex effective connectivity in humans. Cerebral Cortex doi: 10.1093/cercor/bhac391. Copyright © Oxford University Press.)

13.3.1 Inferior frontal gyrus

The inferior frontal gyrus regions include 44, 45, 47l, a47r, IFJa, IFJp, IFSa, IFSp and p47r (Fig. 13.4).

The three inferior frontal gyrus regions 44, 45 and 47l are considered first, and are considered further in Chapter 14 and elsewhere (Rolls et al., 2022b) (Fig. 14.3). Areas 44 and 45 are brain regions normally considered as Broca's area (Sprung-Much et al., 2022; Weiller et al., 2021; Petrides, 2014; Sprung-Much et al., 2022; Weiller et al., 2021; Rauschecker, 2018a; Milton et al., 2021; Friederici et al., 2017), but 47l at least in the left hemisphere has very similar connectivity to them. These regions receive from two semantic systems (Rolls et al., 2023f, 2022b). One semantic system is in the ventral part of the superior temporal sulcus (STSva and STSvp) connected with the inferior temporal visual cortical TE regions and parietal PGi and PGs involved in visual representations of objects (Rolls et al., 2022b).

A second semantic system is in the STSda and STSdp, STGa, auditory A5, TPOJ1, the STV and the PeriSylvian Language area (PSL) and has effective connectivity with auditory areas (A1, A4, A5, Pbelt); with relatively early visual areas involved in motion e.g. MT and MST, and faces/words (FFC); with somatosensory regions (frontal opercular FOP, insula and parietal PF); with other TPOJ regions; and with the inferior frontal gyrus regions (IFJa and IFSp) (Rolls et al., 2022b, 2023f,h). In macaques, area 45 has connectivity with the cortex in the superior temporal sulcus (Petrides and Pandya, 2002). Of relevance to the findings described here, the somatosensory 'ventral what stream' regions (frontal opercular FOP, insula and parietal PF) are incorporated into the second semantic system (Rolls et al., 2022b, 2023f), and the somatosensory 'dorsal action' stream is less incorporated into language-related semantic processing.

Of especial interest is that Broca's area 44 and 45 at least in the left hemisphere involves much surrounding cortex as shown by the connectivity, including 47l which is part of the lateral orbitofrontal cortex, and whole swathes of the inferior frontal gyrus, including IFJa, IFsp and IFsa which are strongly interconnected (Rolls et al., 2023f). Area 44 is implicated in syntax (Friederici, Chomsky, Berwick, Moro and Bolhuis, 2017), but the close interconnections of 44, 45 47l, IFJa, IFsp and IFsa are consistent with the hypothesis that inferior frontal gyrus sequentially linked attractor networks could provide an implementation of the sequential syntactic operations involved in speech production, but would need many such linked attractor systems to deal with the different sequential processing needed for the active vs the passive tense, and for different languages (Rolls and Deco, 2015a) (Section 14.5).

The connectivity of inferior frontal regions IFJa, IFJp, IFSa, IFSp is considered next, with Fig. 13.4 providing a schematic overview of the effective connectivity of IFSa, chosen as typical of this set of interconnected regions (Rolls et al., 2023f). A feature of the connectivity of the IFJ and IFS regions is that they receive from inferior temporal visual cortical regions (e.g. TE1p, TE2a, TE2p and PHT) involved in object representations (Rolls, 2021d,b; Rolls et al., 2023e). This makes it likely that in humans these IFJ and IFS regions specialize in the short-term memory of visual object-based 'what' representations. The connectivity of some of these regions with language-related regions 44, 45, 47l, TPOJ1, STV, 55b and some STS regions also provides a route for this visual object and face related information to gain access to these language-related regions (Rolls et al., 2022b). There are also some inputs from intraparietal visual motion/grasp-related regions (Rolls et al., 2023d) such as AIP, LIPd, MIP and IP0-2, so that some aspects of the motion of objects, also represented in the superior temporal sulcus (STS) regions (Rolls et al., 2023e) are utilised in the inferior frontal regions. Interestingly, there are also inputs from the orbitofrontal cortex (e.g. 11l and 13l) (Rolls et al., 2023f) involved in reward / punishment value representations and thereby in emotion (Rolls, 2019e,f; Rolls et al., 2023c). The IFS and IFJ regions may therefore be involved in maintaining information about visual objects, visual motion, and emotional value and mood in short-term memory by maintaining firing in attractor networks in these inferior frontal gyrus regions (Fuster, 2015; Constantinidis et al., 2018; Martinez-Garcia et al., 2011; Rolls, 2021b). These IFS and IFJ regions also provide a route for these types of input to access language systems, and may also provide additional attractor networks that can be involved with Broca's area regions in syntax (Rolls and Deco, 2015a; Rolls et al., 2022b) (Section 14.5). Conversely, these IFS and IFJ regions may provide a route for language-related rational thought systems to have a top-down influence on the emotion-related processing system in the orbitofrontal cortex.

a47r and p47r are anterolateral parts of the orbitofrontal cortex considered by (Rolls et al., 2023c) (Chapter 11). They have connectivity with other orbitofrontal cortex regions (13l, 11l, OFC, 47m), inferior temporal cortex (TE1p, TE2a, TE1m and PHT), medial prefrontal 8BM,

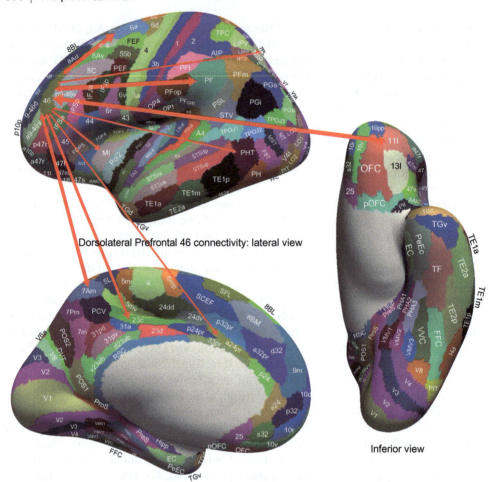

Dorsolateral Prefrontal 46 connectivity: lateral view

Inferior view

Dorsolateral Prefrontal 46 connectivity: medial view

Fig. 13.5 Dorsolateral prefrontal cortex effective connectivity. The connectivity of region 46 is shown as an example of the connectivity of regions 46, 9-46d, a9-46v and p9-46v. The width of the arrows reflects the effective connectivity with the size of the arrowheads reflecting the connectivity in each direction. The effective connectivity with the superior parietal cortex 7Am and 7PL, the strong connectivity with inferior parietal PF, and with the medial orbitofrontal cortex 11l are notable. 46 has moderate effective connectivity with the other DLPFC regions 9-46d, a9-46v and p9-46v. (From Rolls,E.T., Deco,G., Huang,C-C. and Feng,J. (2023) Prefrontal and somatosensory-motor cortex effective connectivity in humans. Cerebral Cortex doi: 10.1093/cercor/bhac391. Copyright © Oxford University Press.)

and inferior parietal visual region PFm, and are involved in value/emotion-related processing (Rolls et al., 2023c; Rolls, 2019e,f; Rolls et al., 2020a, 2023b).

13.3.2 Dorsolateral prefrontal cortex division

The effective connectivity of the regions in the dorsolateral prefrontal cortex division (46, 8Ad, 8Av, 8BL, 8C, 9-46d, 9a, 9p, a9-46v, i6-8, p9-46v and s6-8) is illustrated in Fig. 13.5 (Rolls et al., 2023f).

A first group of regions comprises dorsolateral prefrontal cortex (DLPFC) regions 46, 9-46d, a9-46v and p9-46v, with the connectivity of region 46 a key example illustrated schematically in Fig. 13.5. These regions have connectivity with superior parietal cortex regions in area 7 and intraparietal regions involved in actions in space ('where'), and with inferior parietal PF and PFm and the insula which can be considered as in the somatosensory 'what' hierarchy (Rolls et al., 2023f,d) (Chapter 6). Interestingly, these regions also receive inputs from the orbitofrontal cortex (11l, 13l, Fig. 13.5). These DLPFC regions are thus classic dorsolateral prefrontal cortex regions, and are probably involved in limb/body-related spatial working memory functions probably in egocentric space (rather than eye movement-related) (Passingham, 2021). There is connectivity directed towards premotor 6ma, 6a and 6r and the midcingulate motor region 23c, and to the supracallosal anterior cingulate a24pr, p24pr, a32pr, p32pr, and 33pr. The latter connectivity could be useful it is proposed for action-outcome learning implemented in the supracallosal anterior cingulate cortex (Rolls et al., 2023c), by providing a memory-related input about recent actions until a reward or punishment outcome is received (Chapter 12).

A second group of regions that is more dorsal (superior) in the prefrontal cortex comprises 8Ad, 8Av, 8BL, 9p, i6-8 and s6-8, with the connectivity of region 8Ad as an example illustrated schematically in Fig. 13.6 (Rolls et al., 2023f). The effective connectivity of this 'dorsal prefrontal' group with the inferior parietal visual regions PFm, PGs and PGi is notable. There is also connectivity with the entorhinal cortex (EC) and parahippocampal gyrus regions PHA1-2, and with the memory-related parts of the posterior cingulate division (31pd, 31pv, v23ab), and 7m (Rolls et al., 2023i). This group also has some connectivity with visual inferior temporal TE1m, TE1p and TE2a; and with STSvp; and with the frontal pole a10p and p10p. 8BL, 9a and 9p have connectivity with temporal pole TGd and TGv. 8Ad also has some connectivity with reward-related regions the ventromedial prefrontal cortex 10d and 10r, and the pregenual anterior cingulate cortex d32 and p32 (Rolls et al., 2023c). 8Ad has moderate effective connectivity with other dorsal prefrontal regions 8Av, 9p, i6-8 and s6-8. There is connectivity directed towards language regions: the superior frontal language area SFL, 44, 45, 47l and 55b; and to the premotor eye field PEF. These dorsal frontal regions in front of the eye fields may be involved in visual and auditory attention (Germann and Petrides, 2020a,b; Passingham, 2021), and their connectivity with inferior parietal visual/multimodal cortical regions may be part of the implementation of top-down attention (Deco and Rolls, 2005b,a; Rolls, 2021b).

The computational functions of these dorsolateral and dorsal prefrontal cortex regions are likely to be to maintain information in short-term/working memory by maintaining firing in attractor networks (Fuster, 2015; Constantinidis et al., 2018; Martinez-Garcia et al., 2011; Rolls, 2021b; Goldman-Rakic, 1996; Funahashi et al., 1989). The dorsolateral prefrontal cortex could thereby implement some aspects of executive function (Funahashi, 2017), with those aspects perhaps being described better not as 'voluntary action' (Passingham and Wise, 2012; Passingham, 2021) which is difficult to define and measure, but I suggest instead as 'internally generated from for example memory'. But other key aspects of the dorsolateral and dorsal prefrontal cortex include top-down attention implemented by providing the biassing source held in short-term memory, which can also bias action selection (Deco and Rolls, 2005a, 2004, 2003; Rolls, 2021b). Another key property of prefrontal cortex attractor networks may be not only holding information in a short-term memory, but also transferring information using linked attractor networks from for example a short-term memory attractor network for sensory stimuli to another attractor network in which actions are represented (Deco, Ledberg, Almeida and Fuster, 2005), thereby implementing stimulus-delay-response tasks.

In macaques the connections and neuronal recordings suggest the following subregions of the dorsolateral prefrontal cortex (Petrides and Pandya, 1999; Passingham, 2021; Goulas et al., 2017; Pandya et al., 2015; Petrides, 2014; Yeterian et al., 2012; Petrides et al., 2012; Kelly et al., 2010). The posterior part near the arcuate sulcus contains a frontal eye field FEF. A dorsal part, FEFd is closely associated with the immediately anterior 8Ad which has connectivity with dorsal stream intraparietal regions, and a ventral part FEFv is closely

608 | The prefrontal cortex

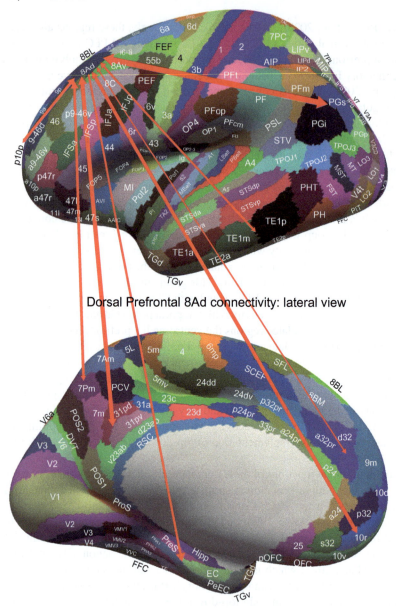

Fig. 13.6 Dorsal prefrontal cortex effective connectivity. The effective connectivity of region 8Ad is shown as an example of the connectivity of regions 8Ad, 8Av, 9p, i6-8 and s6-8. The width of the arrows reflects the effective connectivity with the size of the arrowheads reflecting the connectivity in each direction. The effective connectivity with the inferior parietal PGs and PGi, and with 7Pm are notable. There is also connectivity with the entorhinal cortex (EC) and parahippocampal gyrus regions PHA1-2, and with the memory-related parts of the posterior cingulate division (31pd, 31pv, v23ab), and 7m. 8Ad also has some connectivity with TE1m and TE1p. 8Ad also has some connectivity with reward-related regions the ventromedial prefrontal cortex 10d and 10r, and the pregenual anterior cingulate cortex d32, p32 (Rolls et al., 2023c). 8Ad has moderate effective connectivity with the other dorsal prefrontal regions 8Av, 9p, i6-8 and s6-8. (From Rolls,E.T., Deco,G., Huang,C-C. and Feng,J. (2023) Prefrontal and somatosensory-motor cortex effective connectivity in humans. Cerebral Cortex doi: 10.1093/cercor/bhac391. Copyright © Oxford University Press.)

associated with the immediately anterior 8Av which has connectivity with ventral stream inferior temporal visual cortex regions (Petrides and Pandya, 1999; Passingham, 2021). The FEF and the adjacent area 46 cortex in the posterior part of the principal sulcus is especially implicated in eye movements to visual stimuli remembered over a short delay (Funahashi et al., 1989, 1993; Goldman-Rakic, 1996), consistent with short-term memory functions of the dorsolateral prefrontal regions. The more mid and anterior parts of area 46 in the macaque principal sulcus are involved more in remembered limb movements (Passingham, 2021). In humans, area 46 is far anterior (Sallet et al., 2013), and probably includes some of 46 and a9-46v in the HCP-MMP atlas (Glasser et al., 2016a; Huang et al., 2022).

13.4 The lateral prefrontal cortex and top-down attention

The lateral prefrontal cortex is a region implicated in top-down attentional control (Corbetta and Shulman, 2002; Bressler et al., 2008; Pessoa, 2009; Rolls, 2008d, 2016b, 2014a; Fiebelkorn and Kastner, 2020).

In an example of this, we have found that with taste and flavor stimuli (Grabenhorst and Rolls, 2008), and olfactory stimuli (Rolls, Grabenhorst, Margot, da Silva and Velazco, 2008b), selective attention to pleasantness modulates representations in the orbitofrontal cortex, whereas selective attention to intensity modulates activations in areas such as the insular primary taste cortex (Fig. 13.7).

In a study using psychophysiological interaction (PPI) analysis (Friston, Buechel, Fink, Morris, Rolls and Dolan, 1997), we found that two sites where selective attention to pleasantness increased the activation to taste, the orbitofrontal cortex and a region to which it is connected, the pregenual anterior cingulate cortex, both had functional connectivity with a quite anterior (mean $Y \approx 50$) part of the lateral prefrontal cortex (Grabenhorst and Rolls, 2008), illustrated in Grabenhorst and Rolls (2010) (Fig. 13.8). These parts of the orbitofrontal cortex and pregenual anterior cingulate cortex are a functionally appropriate target site for a top-down attentional modulation, in that their activations are correlated with the subjectively rated pleasantness of the taste (Grabenhorst and Rolls, 2008). Moreover, the lateral prefrontal cortex has been shown to represent current task sets and attentional demands for different types of tasks (Passingham and Wise, 2012; Passingham, 2021).

The implication of these findings is therefore that a part of the lateral prefrontal cortex, not a site normally implicated in affective value and emotion, may be able to modulate emotion-related / affect-related processing in the brain by a top-down attentional influence. This may be one way in which higher cognitive functions, such as a reasoning-based strategy and route to action, or verbal instruction to direct processing towards or away from emotion-related brain processing, or conscious volition, can influence the degree to which the affect-related parts of the brain process incoming (or potentially remembered) stimuli that can produce emotional responses. This is thus a part of the way in which cognition can influence, and control, emotion (Rolls, 2014a, 2018a, 2023b).

We also found that two sites where selective attention to intensity increased the activation to the taste delivery into the mouth, the anterior and mid insula, both had functional connectivity with a less anterior (mean $Y \approx 37$) part of the lateral prefrontal cortex (Grabenhorst and Rolls, 2010) (Fig. 13.8). These parts of the insula are a functionally appropriate site for a top-down attentional modulation, in that their activations are correlated with the subjectively rated intensity of the taste (Grabenhorst and Rolls, 2008; Grabenhorst et al., 2008a). The anterior insular site may be the primary taste cortex (Pritchard, Hamilton, Morse and Norgren, 1986; Yaxley, Rolls and Sienkiewicz, 1990; De Araujo, Kringelbach, Rolls and Hobden, 2003b; De Araujo and Rolls, 2004; Rolls, 2008c, 2016c), and the mid-insular site a region activated by other oral including somatosensory and fat texture inputs from the oral cavity (De Araujo, Kringelbach, Rolls and McGlone, 2003c; De Araujo and Rolls, 2004) and perhaps by taste

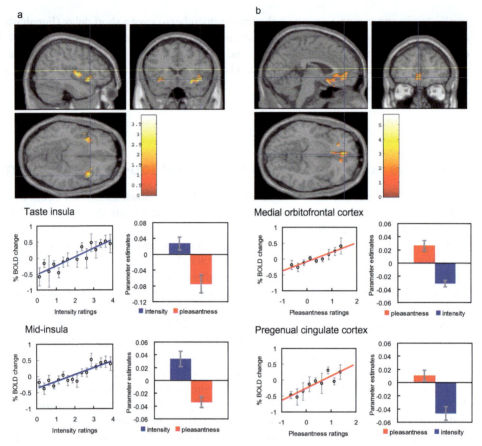

Fig. 13.7 Effect of paying attention to the pleasantness vs the intensity of a taste stimulus. a. Top: A significant difference related to the taste period was found in the taste insula at [42 18 -14] (indicated by the cursor) and in the mid insula at [40 -2 4]. Middle: Taste Insula. Right: The parameter estimates (mean ± sem) for the activation at the specified coordinate for the conditions of paying attention to pleasantness or to intensity. The parameter estimates were significantly different for the taste insula p=0.001. Left: The correlation between the intensity ratings and the activation (% BOLD change) at the specified coordinate (r=0.91, p<0.001). Bottom: Mid Insula. Right: The parameter estimates for the activation at the specified coordinate for the conditions of paying attention to pleasantness or to intensity. The parameter estimates were significantly different for the mid insula p=0.001. Left: The correlation between the intensity ratings and the activation at the specified coordinate (r=0.89, p<<0.001). The taste stimulus, monosodium glutamate, was identical on all trials. b. Top: A significant difference related to the taste period was found in the medial orbitofrontal cortex at [-6 14 -20] (towards the back of the area of activation shown) and in the pregenual cingulate cortex at [-4 46 -8] (at the cursor). Middle: Medial orbitofrontal cortex. Right: The parameter estimates for the activation at the specified coordinate for the conditions of paying attention to pleasantness or to intensity. The parameter estimates were significantly different for the orbitofrontal cortex p< 10^{-4}. Left: The correlation between the pleasantness ratings and the activation at the specified coordinate (r=0.94, p<0.001). Bottom: Pregenual cingulate cortex. Conventions as above. Right: The parameter estimates were significantly different for the pregenual cingulate cortex p< 10^{-5}. Left: The correlation between the pleasantness ratings and the activation at the specified coordinate (r=0.89, p=0.001). The taste stimulus, 0.1 M monosodium glutamate, was identical on all trials. (Reproduced from Fabian Grabenhorst and Edmund T. Rolls (2008) Selective attention to affective value alters how the brain processes taste stimuli. European Journal of Neuroscience 27: 723–729.)

per se (Small, 2010; Rolls, 2016c), in that the activations there were correlated with the trial-by-trial subjective ratings of the taste intensity made during the scanning (Grabenhorst and Rolls, 2008). In the analyses described here, such somatosensory inputs could contribute to the attention-dependent correlations found between the mid insula and other areas.

The statistics used in the calculation of PPI effects (Friston, Buechel, Fink, Morris, Rolls and Dolan, 1997) do not reveal the directionality of the connectivity, for they are based on correlations. However, the directionality in this case is likely to be from the prefrontal cor-

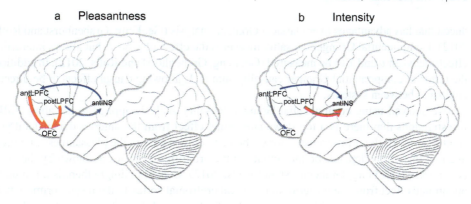

Fig. 13.8 Componential Granger causality analysis of top-down effects on taste processing from different lateral prefrontal cortex areas during attention to either the pleasantness (a) or to the intensity (b) of a taste. Significant causal influences from t tests with a Bonferroni correction are marked by blue arrows (i.e. cross-componential Granger causality is greater than 0). Red arrows indicate where significant top-down effects exist in addition to significant causal influences (i.e. a significant cross-componential Granger causality that is different in the two directions). The areas are anterior (mean Y≈50) and posterior (mean Y≈37) lateral prefrontal cortex (antLPFC, postLPFC); orbitofrontal cortex secondary cortical taste area (OFC); and anterior insular cortex primary cortical taste area (antINS). (Reprinted from Tian Ge, Jianfeng Feng, Fabian Grabenhorst, and Edmund T. Rolls (2012) Componential Granger causality, and its application to identifying the source and mechanisms of the top-down biased activation that controls attention to affective vs sensory processing. NeuroImage 59: 1846–58. © Elsevier Inc.)

tex to the orbitofrontal and pregenual cingulate cortices, for the following reasons. First, the prefrontal cortex has a powerfully developed recurrent collateral system (Elston et al., 2006), which provides the basis for the short-term memory that is needed to hold the subject of attention active, providing the source of the bias for top-down biased competition. Second, prefrontal cortex lesions impair attention (Beck and Kastner, 2009; Rossi et al., 2009; Passingham, 2021). Third, activations in areas of the lateral prefrontal cortex are related to task set, attentional instructions, and remembering rules that guide task performance (Beck and Kastner, 2009; Rossi et al., 2009; Passingham and Wise, 2012; Passingham, 2021). Fourth, direct anatomical connections have been shown in macaques between the lateral prefrontal cortex and the orbitofrontal and pregenual anterior cingulate cortices (Price, 2006).

Given that PPI analysis is based on correlations, it is helpful to go beyond this. Understanding how one brain area may influence another, for example by providing it with inputs, or by top-down modulation, is fundamental to understanding how the brain functions. Hence, inferring causal influences from time series data has been attracting intense interest. Granger causality has become popular due to its easy implementation and many successful applications to econometrics, neuroscience, etc., and in particular, the study of brain function (Bressler and Seth, 2011; Ding et al., 2006). The application of Granger causality analysis to BOLD fMRI signals which are inherently slow has been discussed elsewhere (Stephan and Roebroeck, 2012). The use of this approach is described next, though effective connectivity measured with the Hopf algorithm is providing a very useful alternative (Rolls et al., 2022a, 2023c,i,d, 2022b, 2023e,h,f,a).

Granger causality is based on precedence and predictability. Originally proposed by Wiener (1956) and further formalized by Granger (1969), it states that given two times series x and y, if the inclusion of the past history of y helps to predict the future states of x in some plausible statistical sense, then y is a cause of x in the Granger sense. In spite of the wide acceptance of this definition, classical Granger causality is not tailored to measure the effects of interactions between time series x and y on the causal influences, and cannot measure systematically the effects of the past history of x on x (Ge, Feng, Grabenhorst and Rolls, 2012). In this situation, a componential form of Granger causality analysis has been introduced that has advantages over classical Granger analysis (Ge, Feng, Grabenhorst and Rolls, 2012). Componential Granger causality measures the effect of y on x, but allows interaction effects between y and x to be measured (Ge, Feng, Grabenhorst and Rolls, 2012). In addition, the terms in componential Granger causality sum to 1, allowing causal effects to be directly compared between systems.

We showed using componential Granger causality analysis applied to the above fMRI investigations that there is a top-down attentional effect from the anterior dorsolateral prefrontal cortex to the orbitofrontal cortex when attention is paid to the pleasantness of a taste, and that this effect depends on the activity in the orbitofrontal cortex as shown by the interaction term (Ge, Feng, Grabenhorst and Rolls, 2012). Correspondingly there is a top-down attentional effect from the posterior dorsolateral prefrontal cortex to the insular primary taste cortex when attention is paid to the intensity of a taste, and this effect depends on the activity of the insular primary taste cortex as shown by the interaction term. The prefrontal cortex sites are those identified by the PPI analysis (Grabenhorst and Rolls, 2010) and the effects are shown schematically in Fig. 13.8. Componential Granger causality thus not only can reveal the directionality of effects between areas (and these can be bidirectional), but also allows the mechanisms to be understood in terms of whether the causal influence of one system on another depends on the state of the system being causally influenced. Componential Granger causality measures the full effects of second order statistics by including variance and covariance effects between each time series, thus allowing interaction effects to be measured, and also provides a systematic framework within which to measure the effects of cross, self, and noise contributions to causality (Ge, Feng, Grabenhorst and Rolls, 2012).

These findings reveal some of the mechanisms involved in a biased activation theory of selective attention, which is summarized in Section 4.3.5. The top-down biased competition approach is summarized in Section 2.12.

13.5 The frontal pole cortex

The connectivity and functions of the human frontal polar cortex, Area 10, are being explored. Shallice and colleagues found that patients with frontal pole damage had problems optimising a plan to visit many shops in an efficient order, and more generally had disorganized behavior (Shallice and Cipolotti, 2018; Shallice and Burgess, 1991). These patients also have deficits in tasks that require abstract reasoning, problem-solving, or multitasking (Hogeveen, Medalla, Ainsworth, Galeazzi, Hanlon, Mansouri and Costa, 2022a). In humans, the frontal pole is activated by tasks that require cognitive branching, value-based decision-making, and metacognition (Hogeveen et al., 2022a). These are tasks that require appropriate action to two or more competing goals (Mansouri et al., 2017b; Hogeveen et al., 2022b,a; Mansouri et al., 2017a; Averbeck, 2015). The frontal pole in humans is activated by counterfactual choice tasks with the frontal pole sensitive to the value of unchosen or alternative options during decision-making (Hogeveen et al., 2022a). Consistent with this, in a foraging task, the frontal pole cortex is implicated in whether to exploit what is currently available, or to explore other options in case greater rewards might be available (Hogeveen et al., 2022b). However, relatively little is known of the connectivity of the frontal pole cortex. In macaques, connections from superior temporal cortex auditory regions, from dorsolateral prefrontal cortex (Areas 9 and 46), and orbitofrontal cortex have been described (Barbas, 2015; Yeterian et al., 2012; Petrides et al., 2012; Markov et al., 2014a; Medalla and Barbas, 2010, 2014; Hogeveen et al., 2022a).

Give this background, the connectivity of the human frontal pole cortex, regions 10d, 10pp, a10p, and p10p in the HCP-MMP atlas, with also the two regions 10r and 10v that extend more posteriorly, has been investigated (Rolls et al., 2023a). Unlike dorsolateral prefrontal cortex regions implicated in working memory with which the frontal pole regions were compared, the frontal pole does not have connectivity to premotor and related regions via which behavior can be controlled. However, the frontal pole regions have surprisingly stronger connectivity directed to than from the dorsolateral prefrontal cortex regions, and inferior temporal, inferior parietal, posterior cingulate, and orbitofrontal cortex (Rolls et al., 2023a).

With this evidence and the known effects of damage to and the activations of the frontal pole cortex, it is proposed that the frontal pole contains autoassociation networks with attractor dynamics that are normally stable in a short-term memory state, and maintain stability in dorsolateral prefrontal networks, temporal and parietal networks when stable exploitation of goals and strategies is useful. However, if an input is received from regions such as the orbitofrontal or anterior cingulate cortex that non-reward or punishment is being received, this input destabilises the frontal pole networks to enable exploration of competing alternative goals and strategies. The frontal pole thus in the context of this connectivity is proposed to provide a control over brain resources to influence whether to exploit or explore (Rolls et al., 2023a).

13.6 How the computations are performed in the prefrontal cortex

13.6.1 Cortical short-term memory systems and attractor networks

There are a number of different prefrontal cortex short-term memory systems, each implemented in a different cortical area. The particular systems considered here each implement short-term memory by subpopulations of neurons that show maintained activity in a delay period, while a stimulus or event is being remembered. These memories may operate as autoassociative attractor networks, the operation of which is described in Section B.3. The actual autoassociation could be implemented by associatively modifiable synapses between connected pyramidal cells within an area, or by the forward and backward connections between adjacent cortical areas in a hierarchy.

An example of how this could be implemented to account for the delayed saccade type of neuronal firing illustrated in Fig. 13.3 is shown in Fig. 13.9. The short-term memory function is topographically organized, in that lesions in small parts of the system impair remembered eye movements only to that eye position. Moreover, neurons in the appropriate part of the topographic map respond to eye movements in one but not in other directions (see Fig. 13.3). Such a memory system could be easily implemented in such a topographically organized system by having local cortical connections between nearby pyramidal cells which implement an attractor network (Fig. 13.9). Then triggering activity in one part of the topographically organized system would lead to sustained activity in that part of the map, thus implementing a short-term or working memory for eye movements to that position in space.

Another short-term memory system is implemented in the inferior temporal visual cortex, especially more ventrally towards the perirhinal cortex (see Section 9.2.7). This memory is for whether a particular visual stimulus (such as a face) has been seen recently. This is implemented in two ways. One way is that some neurons respond more to a novel than to a familiar visual stimulus in such tasks, or in other cases respond to the familiar, selected, stimulus (Baylis and Rolls, 1987; Miller and Desimone, 1994) (see Section 9.2.7). The other way is that some neurons, especially more ventrally, continue to fire in the delay period of a delayed match to sample task (Fahy et al., 1993; Miyashita, 1993), and fire for several

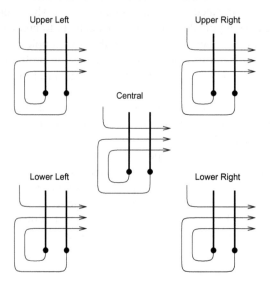

Fig. 13.9 A possible cortical model of a topographically organized set of attractor networks in the prefrontal cortex that could be used to remember the position to which saccades should be made. Excitatory local recurrent collateral Hebb-modifiable connections would enable a set of separate attractors to operate. The input that would trigger one of the attractors into continuing activity in a memory delay period would come from the parietal cortex, and topology of the inputs would result in separate attractors for remembering different positions in space. (For example inputs for the Upper Left of space would trigger an attractor that would remember the upper left of space.) Neurons in different parts of this cortical area would have activity related to remembering one part of space; and damage to a part of this cortical area concerned with one part of space would result in impairments in remembering targets to which to saccade for only one part of space.

hundred milliseconds after a 16 ms visual stimulus has been presented (Rolls and Tovee, 1994) (see Fig. C.19). These neurons can be considered to reflect the implementation of an attractor network between the pyramidal cells in this region (Amit, 1995; Rolls, 2016b). A cortical syndrome that may reflect loss of such a short-term visual memory system is simultanagnosia, in which more than one visual stimulus cannot be remembered for more than a few seconds (Warrington and Weiskrantz, 1973; Kolb and Whishaw, 2021).

Continuing firing of neurons in short-term memory tasks in the delay period is also found in other cortical areas. It is found in the parietal cortex when monkeys are remembering a target to which a saccade should be made (Andersen, 1995a); and in the motor cortex when a monkey is remembering a direction in which to reach with the arm (Georgopoulos, 1995).

Another short-term memory system is human auditory–verbal short-term memory, which appears to be implemented in the left hemisphere at the junction of the temporal, parietal, and occipital lobes. Patients with damage to this system are described clinically as showing conduction aphasia, in that they cannot repeat a heard string of words (cannot conduct the input to the output) (Warrington and Weiskrantz, 1973; Kolb and Whishaw, 2021).

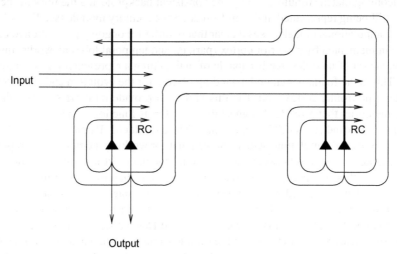

Fig. 13.10 Role of the prefrontal cortex in short-term memory. A short-term memory autoassociation network in the prefrontal cortex could hold active a working memory representation by maintaining its firing in an attractor state. The prefrontal module would be loaded with the to-be-remembered stimulus by the posterior module (in the temporal or parietal cortex) in which the incoming stimuli are represented. Backprojections from the prefrontal short-term memory module to the posterior module would enable the working memory to be unloaded, to for example influence on-going perception (see text). RC, recurrent collateral connections.

13.6.2 Prefrontal cortex short-term memory networks, and their relation to temporal and parietal perceptual networks

13.6.2.1 A prefrontal short-term memory network supporting a temporal lobe perceptual system

As described in Section 13.6.1, a common way that the brain uses to implement a short-term memory is to maintain the firing of neurons during a short memory period after the end of a stimulus (see Rolls (2016b) and Fuster (2015)). In the inferior temporal cortex this firing may be maintained for a few hundred milliseconds even when the monkey is not performing a memory task (Rolls and Tovee, 1994; Rolls, Tovee, Purcell, Stewart and Azzopardi, 1994b; Rolls, Tovee and Panzeri, 1999b; Desimone, 1996) (see Fig. C.19). In more ventral temporal cortical areas such as the entorhinal cortex the firing may be maintained for longer periods in delayed match to sample tasks (Suzuki, Miller and Desimone, 1997), and in the prefrontal cortex for even tens of seconds (Fuster, 1997, 2015).

For the short-term memory to be maintained during periods in which new stimuli are to be perceived, there must be separate networks for the perceptual and short-term memory functions, and indeed two coupled networks, one in the inferior temporal visual cortex for perceptual functions, and another in the prefrontal cortex for maintaining the short-term memory during intervening stimuli, provide a precise model of the interaction of perceptual and short-term memory systems (Renart, Parga and Rolls, 2000; Renart, Moreno, Rocha, Parga and Rolls, 2001) (see Fig. 13.10). In particular, this model shows how a prefrontal cortex attractor (autoassociation) network could be triggered by a sample visual stimulus represented in the inferior temporal visual cortex in a delayed match to sample task, and could keep this attractor active during a memory interval in which intervening stimuli are shown. Then when the sample stimulus reappears in the task as a match stimulus, the inferior temporal cortex module shows a large response to the match stimulus, because it is activated both by the visual incoming match stimulus, and by the consistent backprojected memory of the sample stimulus still being represented in the prefrontal cortex memory module (see Fig. 13.10).

This computational model makes it clear that in order for ongoing perception to occur unhindered implemented by posterior cortex (parietal and temporal lobe) networks, there must be a separate set of modules that is capable of maintaining a representation over intervening stimuli. This is the fundamental understanding offered for the evolution and functions of the dorsolateral prefrontal cortex, and it is this ability to provide multiple separate short-term attractor memories that provides I suggest the basis for its functions in planning.

Renart, Parga and Rolls (2000) and Renart, Moreno, Rocha, Parga and Rolls (2001) performed analyses and simulations which showed that for working memory to be implemented in this way, the connections between the perceptual and the short-term memory modules (see Fig. 13.10) must be relatively weak. As a starting point, they used the neurophysiological data showing that in delayed match to sample tasks with intervening stimuli, the neuronal activity in the inferior temporal visual cortex (IT) is driven by each new incoming visual stimulus (Miller, Li and Desimone, 1993; Miller and Desimone, 1994), whereas in the prefrontal cortex, neurons start to fire when the sample stimulus is shown, and continue the firing that represents the sample stimulus even when the potential match stimuli are being shown (Miller, Erickson and Desimone, 1996).

The architecture studied by Renart, Parga and Rolls (2000) is as shown in Fig. 13.10, with both the intramodular (recurrent collateral) and the intermodular (forward IT to PF, and backward PF to IT) connections trained on the set of patterns with an associative synaptic modification rule. A crucial parameter is the strength of the intermodular connections, g, which indicates the relative strength of the intermodular to the intramodular connections. (This parameter measures effectively the relative strengths of the currents injected into the neurons by the inter-modular relative to the intra-modular connections, and the importance of setting this parameter to relatively weak values for useful interactions between coupled attractor networks was highlighted by Renart, Parga and Rolls (1999b) and Renart, Parga and Rolls (1999a), as shown in Sections B.9 and 13.6.2.2.) The patterns themselves were sets of random numbers, and the simulation utilized a dynamical approach with neurons with continuous (hyperbolic tangent) activation functions (see Section 13.6.2.2) (Shiino and Fukai, 1990; Kuhn, 1990; Kuhn, Bos and van Hemmen, 1991; Amit and Tsodyks, 1991). The external current injected into IT by the incoming visual stimuli was sufficiently strong to trigger the IT module into a state representing the incoming stimulus. When the sample was shown, the initially silent PF module was triggered into activity by the weak ($g > 0.002$) intermodular connections. The PF module remained firing to the sample stimulus even when IT was responding to potential match stimuli later in the trial, provided that g was less than 0.024, because then the intramodular recurrent connections could dominate the firing (see Fig. 13.11). If g was higher than this, then the PF module was pushed out of the attractor state produced by the sample stimulus. The IT module responded to each incoming potentially matching stimulus provided that g was not greater than approximately 0.024. Moreover, this value of g was sufficiently large that a larger response of the IT module was found when the stimulus matched the sample stimulus (the match enhancement effect found neurophysiologically, and a mechanism by which the matching stimulus can be identified). This simple model thus shows that the operation of the prefrontal cortex in short-term memory tasks such as delayed match to sample with intervening stimuli, and its relation to posterior perceptual networks, can be understood by the interaction of two weakly coupled attractor networks, as shown in Figs. 13.10 and 13.11.

The same network can also be used to illustrate the interaction between the prefrontal cortex short-term memory system and the posterior (IT or PP) perceptual regions in visual search tasks, as illustrated in Fig. 13.12.

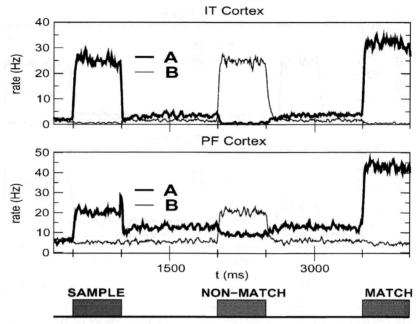

Fig. 13.11 Role of the prefrontal cortex in short-term memory. Interaction between the prefrontal cortex (PF) and the inferior temporal cortex (IT) in a delayed match to sample task with intervening stimuli with the architecture illustrated in Fig. 13.10. Above: activity in the IT attractor module. Below: activity in the PF attractor module. The thick lines show the firing rates of the set of neurons with activity selective for the sample stimulus (which is also shown as the match stimulus, and is labelled **A**), and the thin lines the activity of the neurons with activity selective for the non-match stimulus, which is shown as an intervening stimulus between the sample and match stimulus, and is labelled **B**. A trial is illustrated in which **A** is the sample (and match) stimulus. The prefrontal cortex module is pushed into an attractor state for the sample stimulus by the IT activity induced by the sample stimulus. Because of the weak coupling to the PF module from the IT module, the PF module remains in this sample-related attractor state during the delay periods, and even while the IT module is responding to the non-match stimulus. The PF module remains in its sample-related state even during the non-match stimulus because once a module is in an attractor state, it is relatively stable. When the sample stimulus reappears as the match stimulus, the PF module shows higher sample stimulus-related firing, because the incoming input from IT is now adding to the activity in the PF attractor network. This in turn also produces a match enhancement effect in the IT neurons with sample stimulus-related selectivity, because the backprojected activity from the PF module matches the incoming activity to the IT module. (From Renart, A., Moreno, R., de la Rocha, J., Parga, N. and Rolls, E. T. (2001) A model of the IT-PF network in object working memory which includes balanced persistent activity and tuned inhibition. Neurocomputing 38–40: 1525–1531. © Elsevier B.V.)

13.6.2.2 Computational details of the prefrontal–inferior temporal model of short-term memory

The model network of Renart, Parga and Rolls (2000) and Renart, Moreno, Rocha, Parga and Rolls (2001) consists of a large number of (excitatory) neurons arranged in two modules with the architecture shown in Fig. 13.10. Following Kuhn (1990) and Amit and Tsodyks (1991), each neuron is assumed to be a dynamical element which transforms an incoming afferent current into an output spike rate according to a given transduction function. A given afferent current I_{ai} to neuron i $(i = 1, \ldots, N)$ in module a $(a = \mathbf{IT}, \mathbf{PF})$ decays with a characteristic time constant τ but increases proportionally to the spike rates of the rest of the neurons in the network (from both inside and outside its module) connected to it, the contribution of each presynaptic neuron, e.g. neuron j from module b, and in proportion to the synaptic efficacy J_{ij}^{ab} between the two[20]. This can be expressed through the following equation

---

[20]On this occasion we vert to the theoretical physicists' usual notation for synaptic weights or couplings, J_{ij} instead of w_{ij}.

618 | The prefrontal cortex

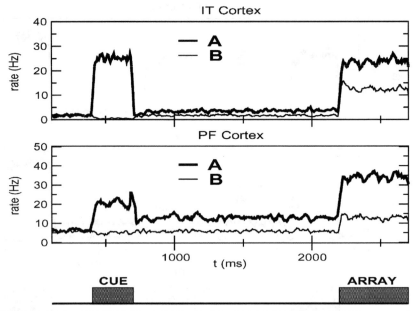

Fig. 13.12 Role of the prefrontal cortex in short-term memory. Interaction between the prefrontal cortex (PF) and the inferior temporal cortex (IT) in a visual search task with the architecture illustrated in Fig. 13.10. Above: activity in the IT attractor module. Below: activity in the PF attractor module. The thick lines show the firing rates of the set of neurons with activity selective for search stimulus **A**, and the thin lines the activity of the neurons with activity selective for stimulus **B**. During the cue period either **A** or **B** is shown, to indicate to the monkey which stimulus to select when an array containing both **A** and **B** is shown after a delay period. The trial shown is for the case when **A** is the cue stimulus. When stimulus **A** is shown as a cue, then via the IT module, the PF module is pushed into an attractor state **A**, and the PF module remembers this state during the delay period. When the array **A** + **B** is shown later, there is more activity in the PF module for the neurons selective for **A**, because they have inputs both from the continuing attractor state held in the PF module and from the forward activity from the IT module which now contains both **A** and **B**. This PF firing to **A** in turn also produces greater firing of the population of IT neurons selective for **A** than in the IT neurons selective for **B**, because the IT neurons selective for **A** are receiving both **A**-related visual inputs, and **A**-related backprojected inputs from the PF module. (From Renart,A., Moreno,R., de la Rocha,J., Parga,N. and Rolls, E. T. (2001) A model of the IT-PF network in object working memory which includes balanced persistent activity and tuned inhibition. Neurocomputing 38–40: 1525–1531. © Elsevier B.V.)

$$\frac{dI_{ai}(t)}{dt} = -\frac{I_{ai}(t)}{\tau} + \sum_{b,j} J_{ij}^{(a,b)} \nu_{bj} + h_{ai}^{(\text{ext})} \;. \tag{13.1}$$

An external current $h_{ai}^{(\text{ext})}$ from outside the network, representing the stimuli, can also be imposed on every neuron. Selective stimuli are modelled as proportional to the stored patterns, i.e. $h_{ai}^{\mu(\text{ext})} = h_a \eta_{ai}^\mu$, where h_a is the intensity of the external current to module a.

The transduction function of the neurons transforming currents into rates was chosen as a threshold hyperbolic tangent of gain G and threshold θ. Thus, when the current is very large the firing rates saturate to an arbitrary value of 1.

The synaptic efficacies between the neurons of each module and between the neurons in different modules are respectively

$$J_{ij}^{(a,a)} = \frac{J_0}{f(1-f)N_t} \sum_{\mu=1}^{P} (\eta_{ai}^\mu - f)(\eta_{aj}^\mu - f) \quad i \neq j \;; \; a = \mathbf{IT}, \mathbf{PF} \tag{13.2}$$

$$J_{ij}^{(a,b)} = \frac{g}{f(1-f)N_t} \sum_{\mu=1}^{P} (\eta_{ai}^\mu - f)(\eta_{bj}^\mu - f) \quad \forall \; i,j \;; \; a \neq b \;. \tag{13.3}$$

The intra-modular connections are such that a number P of sparse independent configurations of neural activity are dynamically stable, constituting the possible sustained activity states in each module. This is expressed by saying that each module has learned P binary patterns $\{\eta_{ai}^{\mu} = 0, 1, \ \mu = 1, \ldots, P\}$, each of them signalling which neurons are active in each of the sustained activity configurations. Each variable η_{ai}^{μ} is allowed to take the values 1 and 0 with probabilities f and $(1-f)$ respectively, independently across neurons and across patterns. The inter-modular connections reflect the temporal associations between the sustained activity states of each module. In this way, every stored pattern μ in the IT module has an associated pattern in the PF module which is labelled by the same index. The normalization constant $N_t = N(J_0 + g)$ was chosen so that the sum of the magnitudes of the inter- and the intra-modular connections remains constant and equal to 1 while their relative values are varied. When this constraint is imposed the strength of the connections can be expressed in terms of a single independent parameter g measuring the relative intensity of the inter- vs the intra-modular connections (J_0 can be set equal to 1 everywhere).

Both modules implicitly include an inhibitory population of neurons receiving and sending signals to the excitatory neurons through uniform synapses. In this case the inhibitory population can be treated as a single inhibitory neuron with an activity dependent only on the mean activity of the excitatory population. We chose the transduction function of the inhibitory neuron to be linear with slope γ.

Since the number of neurons in a typical network one may be interested in is very large, e.g. $\sim 10^5 - 10^6$, the analytical treatment of the set of coupled differential equations (13.1) becomes untractable. On the other hand, when the number of neurons is large, a reliable description of the asymptotic solutions of these equations can be found using the techniques of statistical mechanics (Kuhn, 1990). In this framework, instead of characterizing the states of the system by the state of every neuron, this characterization is performed in terms of *macroscopic* quantities called *order parameters* which measure and quantify some global properties of the network as a whole. The relevant order parameters appearing in the description of the system are the overlap of the state of each module with each of the stored patterns m_a^{μ} and the average activity of each module x_a, defined respectively as:

$$m_a^{\mu} = \frac{1}{\chi N} \ll \sum_i (\eta_{ai}^{\mu} - f) \nu_{ai} \gg_{\eta} \ ; \ x_a = \frac{1}{N} \ll \sum_i \nu_{ai} \gg_{\eta} \ , \quad (13.4)$$

where the symbol $\ll \ldots \gg_{\eta}$ stands for an average over the stored patterns.

Using the free energy per neuron of the system at zero temperature $\mathcal{F}$ (which is not written explicitly to reduce the technicalities to a minimum), Renart, Parga and Rolls (2000) and Renart, Moreno, Rocha, Parga and Rolls (2001) modelled the experiments by giving the order parameters the following dynamics:

$$\tau \frac{\partial m_a^{\mu}}{\partial t} = -\frac{\partial \mathcal{F}}{\partial m_a^{\mu}} \ ; \ \tau \frac{\partial x_a}{\partial t} = -\frac{\partial \mathcal{F}}{\partial x_a} \ . \quad (13.5)$$

These dynamics ensure that the stationary solutions, corresponding to the values of the order parameters at the attractors, correspond also to minima of the free energy, and that, as the system evolves, the free energy is always minimized through its gradient. The time constant of the macroscopical dynamics was chosen to be equal to the time constant of the individual neurons, which reflects the assumption that neurons operate in parallel. Equations (13.5) were solved by a simple discretizing procedure (first order Runge–Kutta method). An appropriate value for the time interval corresponding to one computer iteration was found to be $\tau/10$ and the time constant was the value $\tau = 10$ ms.

Since not all neurons in the network receive the same inputs, not all of them behave in the same way, i.e. have the same firing rates. In fact, the neurons in each of the modules can be split into different subpopulations according to their state of activity in each of the stored patterns. The mean firing rate of the neurons in each subpopulation depends on the particular state realized by the network (characterized by the values of the order parameters). Associated with each pattern there are two large subpopulations denoted as foreground (all active neurons) and background (all inactive neurons) for that pattern. The overlap with a given pattern can be expressed as the difference between the mean firing rate of the neurons in its foreground and its background. The average was calculated over all other subpopulations to which each neuron in the foreground (background) belonged, where the probability of a given subpopulation is equal to the fraction of neurons in the module belonging to it (determined by the probability distribution of the stored patterns as given above). This partition of the neurons into subpopulations is appealing since, in neurophysiological experiments, cells are usually classified in terms of their response properties to a set of fixed stimuli, i.e. whether each stimulus is effective or ineffective in driving their response.

The modelling of the different experiments proceeded according to the macroscopic dynamics (13.5), where each stimulus was implemented as an extra current into free energy for a desired period of time.

Using this model, results of the type described in Section 13.6.2 were found (Renart, Parga and Rolls, 2000; Renart, Moreno, Rocha, Parga and Rolls, 2001). The paper by Renart, Moreno, Rocha, Parga and Rolls (2001) extended the earlier findings of Renart, Parga and Rolls (2000) to integrate-and-fire neurons, and it is results from the integrate-and-fire simulations that are shown in Figs. 13.11 and 13.12.

13.6.3 Mapping from one representation to another in short-term memory

Short-term memory attractor dynamics helps us to understand the underlying mechanisms that implement mappings from one representation to another, for example from sensory to motor, and where short-term memory is required. For example, Deco and Rolls (2003) investigated the 3-level integrate-and-fire hierarchical model of the prefrontal cortex, with sensory neurons, intermediate neurons, and premotor neurons illustrated in Fig. 13.13, in a model of the neuronal activity recorded in the prefrontal cortex during such tasks (Asaad, Rainer and Miller, 2000). The hierarchical structure of the populations (or pools) of neurons is to ensure that the mapping is from the sensory pools to the intermediate pools and then to the premotor pools, and is achieved by setting the synaptic weights to be stronger in the forward than in the reverse direction between the thus hierarchically organized 3 levels of attractor networks. In this particular investigation, a top-down rule bias could be applied to the intermediate level neurons, so that the mapping could be selected to be for example according to an object-response or a spatial-response mapping rule. The attractor dynamics of each population of neurons enables the task to be performed when there are delays between the stimuli and the responses.

This concept of a set of attractor networks that are hierarchically organized in this way is formally somewhat similar to the interacting attractors used to solve short-term memory with intervening stimuli described in Section 13.6.2, and the interacting attractors used to describe attentional processing (Rolls and Deco, 2002; Rolls, 2016b).

Another application of this concept that shows the temporal organization that can be involved is in delayed response tasks in which there may be separate attractors for the sensory stimuli and for the responses. The sensory attractors may be started by sensory cues, may hold the cue for a time, but there may then be a gradual transition to premotor neuron attractors, so that some pools gradually become quiescent, and others start up, during a delay period (Deco et al., 2005) (see Fig. 13.14). For this, the forward coupling between the sensory and

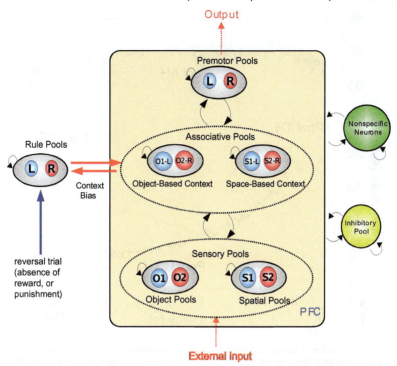

Fig. 13.13 Network architecture of the prefrontal cortex unified model of attention, working memory, and decision-making. There are sensory neuronal populations or pools for object type (O1 or O2) and spatial position (S1 or S2). These connect hierarchically (with stronger forward than backward connections) to the intermediate or 'associative' pools in which neurons may respond to combinations of the inputs received from the sensory pools for some types of mapping such as reversal, as described by Deco and Rolls (2003). For the simulation of the neurophysiological data of Asaad, Rainer and Miller (2000) these intermediate pools respond to O1–L, O2–R, S1–L, or S2–R. These intermediate pools receive an attentional bias from the Rule Pools, which in the case of this particular simulation biases either the object-based context pools or the spatial-based context pools. The Rule Pools are reset by an error to bias the opposite set of associative pools, so that the rule attentional context switches from favouring mapping through the object-based context pools to through the spatial-based context pools, or vice versa. The intermediate pools are connected hierarchically to the premotor pools, which in this case code for a Left or Right response. Each of the pools is an attractor network in which there are stronger associatively modified synaptic weights between the neurons that represent the same state (e.g. object type for a sensory pool, or response for a premotor pool) than between neurons in the other pools or populations. However, all the neurons in the network are associatively connected by at least weak synaptic weights. The attractor properties, the competition implemented by the inhibitory interneurons, and the biasing inputs result in the same network implementing both short-term memory and biased competition, and the stronger feed forward than feedback connections between the sensory, intermediate, and premotor pools results in the hierarchical property by which sensory inputs can be mapped to motor outputs in a way that depends on the biasing contextual or rule input. (After Deco,G. and Rolls, E. T. (2003) Attention and working memory: a dynamical model of neuronal activity in the prefrontal cortex. European Journal of Neuroscience 18: 2374–2390.)

motor attractors must be weak (Rolls, 2016b). This whole process will be stochastic, with the transition times, especially of individual neurons in each of the attractors, being probabilistic from trial to trial because the process is being influenced by noise. The activity of the different populations of neurons shown in Fig. 13.14 matches those recorded in the prefrontal cortex (Fuster, Bodner and Kroger, 2000).

13.6.4 The mechanisms of top-down attention

The top-down biased competition approach is summarized in Section 2.12. Some of the mechanisms involved in a biased activation theory of selective attention are summarized in Section 4.3.5. Similar mechanisms are likely to apply to the top-down effects that cognition has on earlier processing. The process and mechanisms of top-down attention are considered

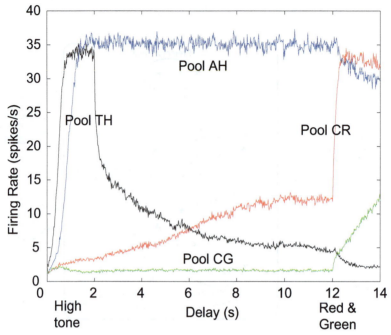

Fig. 13.14 Paired-associate / temporal order memory using stronger forward than reverse connections between attractors. In this spiking network model, input attractor network neuronal pools tone high (TH) and tone low (TL) have stronger forward than reverse synaptic connections to output attractor network neuronal pools color red (CR) and color green (CG) respectively. (In addition, there are associative attractor populations of neurons AH and AL that receive stronger forward inputs from TH and TL respectively, and have stronger forward than reverse weights to CR and CG respectively. These associative pools help to keep a short-term memory state initiated by one of the stimuli active throughout a trial.) The mean firing rate of some of these pools is shown in the figure on a trial on which the TH stimulus was shown at time 0–2 s, there was then a delay from 2–12 s, and then red and green stimuli were shown from time 12–14 s, with red being the correct paired associate. On average across trials there is a gradual transition from the stimulus input pool of neurons (in this case TH) to the associated output pool of neurons (in this case CR), which is frequently found in the dorsolateral prefrontal cortex during paired associate tasks. On individual trials the dynamics are noisy, with different time courses averaged across neurons for the transition from the input to the output neuronal population, and in addition somewhat different time courses for different neurons within a pool within a trial. (After Deco,G., Ledberg,A., Almeida,R. and Fuster,J. (2005) Neural dynamics of crossmodal and crosstemporal associations. Experimental Brain Research 166: 325–336.)

much further elsewhere (Desimone and Duncan, 1995; Deco and Rolls, 2003, 2004; Fletcher et al., 1998; Deco and Rolls, 2005a; Rolls, 2008f,d, 2013a; Luo et al., 2013; Rolls, 2014a, 2016b).

13.6.5 Computational necessity for a separate, prefrontal cortex, short-term memory system

This approach emphasizes that in order to provide a useful brain lesion test of prefrontal cortex short-term memory functions, the task set should require a short-term memory for stimuli over an interval in which other stimuli are being processed, because otherwise the posterior cortex perceptual modules could implement the short-term memory function by their own recurrent collateral connections. This approach also emphasizes that there are many at least partially independent modules for short-term memory functions in the prefrontal cortex (e.g. several modules for delayed saccades; one or more for delayed spatial (body) responses in the dorsolateral prefrontal cortex; one or more for remembering visual stimuli in the more ventral prefrontal cortex; and at least one in the left prefrontal cortex used for remembering the words produced in a verbal fluency task – see Section 13.6.1; and Section 10.3 of Rolls and Treves (1998)).

This computational approach thus provides a clear understanding of why a separate (prefrontal) mechanism is needed for working memory functions, as elaborated in Section 13.6.2. It may also be commented that if a prefrontal cortex module is to control behavior in a working memory task, then it must be capable of assuming some type of executive control. There may be no need to have a single central executive additional to the control that must be capable of being exerted by every short-term memory module. This is in contrast to what has traditionally been assumed for the prefrontal cortex (Shallice and Burgess, 1996).

13.6.6 Synaptic modification is needed to set up but not to reuse short-term memory systems

To set up a new short-term memory attractor, synaptic modification is needed to form the new stable attractor. Once the attractor is set up, it may be used repeatedly when triggered by an appropriate cue to hold the short-term memory state active by continued neuronal firing even without any further synaptic modification (see Section B.3 and Kesner and Rolls (2001)). Thus manipulations that impair the long term potentiation of synapses (LTP) may impair the formation of new short-term memory states, but not the use of previously learned short-term memory states. Kesner and Rolls (2001) analyzed many studies of the effects of blockade of LTP in the hippocampus on spatial working memory tasks, and found evidence consistent with this prediction. Interestingly, it was found that if there was a large change in the delay interval over which the spatial information had to be remembered, then the task became susceptible, during the transition to the new delay interval, to the effects of blockade of LTP. The implication is that some new learning is required when the rat must learn the strategy of retaining information for longer periods when the retention interval is changed.

13.6.7 Sequence memory

The hippocampus has a mechanism for implementing temporal sequence memory using time cells (Section 9.3.4). The dorsolateral prefrontal cortex is also involved in temporal order / sequence memory, which is evident from impairment in the recall of the order of items from short-term memory after prefrontal cortex damage, and in neuronal firing (Naya, Chen, Yang and Suzuki, 2017; Tiganj, Cromer, Roy, Miller and Howard, 2018). Neurons in the prefrontal cortex can respond to combinations of temporal order and object, and can maintain their activity in a delay period (Naya, Chen, Yang and Suzuki, 2017). The hippocampal time cells described in Section 9.3.4 may contribute to the temporal order encoding of the prefrontal cortex, by providing temporal order information.

13.6.8 Working memory, and planning

Baddeley (2007; 2012; 2019) has argued that a key type of human memory is working memory, the ability to manipulate items in short-term memory. An example of such a task might be to repeat a set of numbers backwards. This is probably implemented in the prefrontal cortex, but the computational mechanisms involved in rearranging the order of items in working memory are not known. This ability is likely to be a component of planning, which is also implemented in the prefrontal cortex. For example, people with damage to the anterior part of area 10 are impaired in a planning task, in which they have to plan the optimal route to a number of shops, but again the mechanisms are not yet known (Shallice and Burgess, 1991; Shallice and Cipolotti, 2018; Gilbert and Burgess, 2008; Spiers and Gilbert, 2015).

14 Language and syntax in the brain

14.1 Introduction and overview

14.1.1 Introduction

When considering the computational processes underlying language, it is helpful to analyze the rules being followed (Chomsky, 1965; Pinker, 1995; Jackendoff, 2002). From this, it is tempting to see what one can infer about how the computations are implemented, using for example logical operations within a rule-based system, and switches turned on during development. [The wider issue of whether there is a universal grammar with innate rules raised by these approaches has many critics (e.g. Evans (2014)).]

In this Chapter, instead the approach is to take what has been learned from a great deal of the neuropsychology of language based on the types of language deficit occurring after damage to different regions of the brain (Kemmerer, 2015), and now supplemented by neuroimaging studies of language (Kemmerer, 2015), neurolinguistics (Brennan, 2022), and language modelling investigations (Reichle, 2021), to build an understanding of what computations may be being performed by different brain regions. This is complemented by a computational neuroscience approach in which we take some of the key principles of the operation of the cerebral cortex (Rolls, 2016b), and how information is encoded in the brain (Appendix C), and then set up hypotheses that are then tested in computational models about how some of these computational mechanisms might be useful and used in the implementation of language in the brain (e.g. Rolls and Deco (2015a)).

However, language is perhaps the last major frontier where we do not yet have a good set of computational ideas for how the computations are implemented in the brain, so what is described here is intended to provide a foundation of ideas for future research, rather than proposals for how the brain approaches this computational problem. This is a contrast with many other brain systems, as described in this book.

Some of the brain regions involved in different aspects of language and speech are shown in Figs. 14.1 and 14.2.

14.1.2 Overview

1. Semantic representations are in the anterior temporal lobe as described in Section 8.3, with the possible computational mechanisms involved considered in Sections 8.5 and 14.4. It is suggested that the parietal lobe provides inputs to the semantic system when information about the body and actions needs to be part of the semantic representation (Section 14.2.6).
2. Effective connectivity identifies a semantic system that includes cortex in the inferior bank of the superior temporal sulcus (STS) that extends from the temporal pole, includes the inferior temporal visual cortex, extends up into parietal region PGi, and is involved in the visual representation of objects and people. Another semantic system includes cortex in the superior bank of the STS and some auditory regions, and extends from the frontal pole to the temporo-parieto-occipital junction. This system is involved in semantic representations of auditory and especially moving visual stimuli including heads and faces. Both semantic systems connect to Broca's area regions 44 and 45 and the nearby inferior frontal

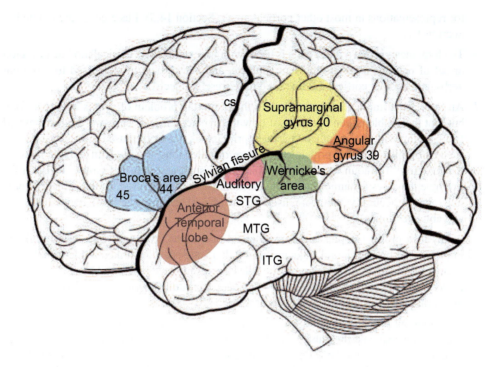

Fig. 14.1 Brain structures implicated in language are shown on a lateral view of the left hemisphere of the human brain. Broca's area, a traditional term, refers to the Inferior Frontal Gyrus pars triangularis area 45, and the Inferior Frontal Gyrus pars opercularis area 44. It is implicated in syntactic manipulations of semantic information for speech production. The Anterior Temporal Lobe is involved in semantic representations, as described in Section 8.3. Wernicke's area, a traditional term, refers to the posterior part of the superior temporal gyrus area, part of area 22, and a part of the supramarginal gyrus area 40. It is involved in phonological processing but not in language comprehension. The angular gyrus, area 39 in the parietal cortex, may be involved in providing and combining attributes for semantic representations. The Auditory cortex is also shown. cs–central sulcus; ITG–Inferior temporal Gyrus; MTG–Middle Temporal Gyrus; STG–Superior Temporal Gyrus.

gyrus regions which are proposed to use linked attractor networks to implement the serial nature of language (Rolls et al., 2022b) (Section 14.3).

3. The dual-stream model (Section 14.2.2) holds that a ventral stream, which involves the temporal lobe, is involved in processing speech signals for comprehension. A dorsal stream, which involves structures at the left parietal-temporal junction and the left inferior frontal gyrus ('Broca's area'), is involved in translating acoustic-based representations of speech signals into articulatory representations essential for speech production.

4. A fundamental computational issue is how the cortex implements binding of elements such as words or features with the correct relationship between the elements. The problem in the context of language might arise if we have neuronal populations each firing to represent a subject, a verb, and an object of a sentence. If all we had were three populations of neurons firing, how would we know which was the subject, which the verb, and which the object? How would we know that the subject was related to the verb, and that the verb operated on the object? How these relations are encoded is part of the problem of syntactic binding (Sections 14.2.5 and 14.5).

5. One possible solution that is described in this Chapter is that a place code is used to solve syntax, which would simply bringing syntax into the same framework as is used

for representations in most other cortical areas (Section 14.5). Place codes are defined in Section 1.7.

6. The hypothesis is that a place code is used, with for example one cortical module or region or set of neurons used to represent subjects, another cortical module used to represent verbs, and another cortical module used to represent objects.

7. An interesting implication is that within the brain, the problem of syntax is then solved, but that the problem then becomes of how the syntactic role of each word is transmitted from one individual to another. One such principle is word order used in some languages such as English. Another principle is the use of inflections, usually suffixes, that indicate the function of a noun, used in other languages such as Latin and Greek. In Latin for example the cases for amica, a friend, are nominative (amica, used for the subject), vocative (amica), accusative (amicam, used for the object), genitive (amicae), dative (amicae), and ablative (amica).

8. A key idea in this Chapter is that syntactical operations involving word order might be implemented by a temporal trajectory through a state space of linked attractor networks each specializing in different syntactic roles, for example subject, verb, and object, with each attractor network being activated by the appropriate semantic representation from the temporal lobe (Section 14.5 and Rolls and Deco (2015a)).

9. An important property of this system is that the actual trajectory through the system, the order of for example the subject, verb, and object, would be learned for each language by experience with that language, using mechanisms such as stronger forward than backward connections between coupled cortical attractor networks, and spike-timing dependent plasticity. This is thus not an innate system. In the situation where word order is important in syntax, the subject and object are essentially defined by where they occur in the temporal trajectory through the state space (e.g. subject > verb > object in English).

10. Simulations of a set of linked cortical attractor networks with stronger forward than backward interconnections between the networks show how a temporal trajectory could be made through a state space of grammatical entities to generate appropriate sequences of word orders. It is also shown how a recipient could decode such a word order sequence, and assign the words to activate the correct cortical modules (Section 14.5) (Rolls and Deco, 2015a).

14.2 What is computed in different brain systems to implement language

14.2.1 The Wernicke-Lichtheim-Geschwind hypothesis

The classical Wernicke-Lichtheim-Geschwind model of the neural architecture of language held that language comprehension involves Wernicke's area, and language production involves Broca's area. Conduction aphasia, the inability to repeat a spoken phrase, was described as a disconnection between these two (Geschwind, 1970; Coslett and Schwartz, 2018). It has now become clear that comprehension and production are not as clearly separated as once thought (Hagoort and Indefrey, 2014; Binder, 2015). Further, the region known as Wernicke's area, in the posterior superior temporal gyrus and part of the supramarginal gyrus area 40, is involved in phonological processing, but not in language comprehension (Binder, 2015). Damage to 'Wernicke's area' results in conduction aphasia and in phonemic paraphasias, providing evidence that this region is involved in phonemic retrieval (Binder, 2015).

14.2.2 The dual-stream hypothesis of speech comprehension

The dual-stream model (Fig. 14.2) (Hickok, 2022) holds that a ventral stream, which involves structures bilaterally in the superior and middle portions of the temporal lobe, is involved in processing speech signals for comprehension. The evidence that this is bilateral is that it is bilateral not unilateral lesions of the superior temporal cortex that have a major effect on auditory language comprehension, evident as word deafness (Hickok and Poeppel, 2015).

A dorsal stream, which involves structures at the left parietal-temporal junction and in the left inferior frontal gyrus, is involved in translating acoustic-based representations of speech signals into articulatory representations essential for speech production (Hickok and Poeppel, 2007, 2015; Bornkessel-Schlesewsky et al., 2015; Kemmerer, 2015; Hickok, 2022). Monitoring self-produced speech and motor control are associated with the posterior Superior Temporal Gyrus, part of the auditory dorsal stream (DeWitt and Rauschecker, 2013). The functional role of the dorsal stream in the model is to subserve speech production by computing a mapping between phonological representations of speech in the STG/STS and motor-based speech codes in the frontal lobe. This mapping is mediated by a cortical auditory-motor transformation zone in the posterior Sylvian region at the temporal–parietal boundary (termed Spt) (Hickok, 2022).

For the ventral stream (Hickok and Poeppel, 2007, 2015; Bornkessel-Schlesewsky et al., 2015; Kemmerer, 2015; Hickok, 2022), one area involved in speech comprehension is the posterior part of the middle temporal gyrus, and this is also implicated in lexical-semantic access (Hickok and Poeppel, 2015). This is of course not far from the primary auditory cortex (Fig. 14.1). Anterior temporal lobe regions are implicated in sentence-level processing (syntactic and/or semantic integration processes), and more generally in semantic processing (Hickok and Poeppel, 2015; Patterson et al., 2007). Indeed, the anterior Superior Temporal Gyrus (STG), part of the auditory ventral stream, is involved in the recognition of species-specific vocalizations in non-human primates and word-form recognition in humans (DeWitt and Rauschecker, 2013). Auditory object formation is a form of categorization, in which spectrotemporal properties are grouped into perceptual and, at higher hierarchical levels, conceptual units. Thus, it provides the computational basis for a mapping from spectrotemporal patterns to concepts (DeWitt and Rauschecker, 2013). Consistent with this hierarchical model, damage to the anterior parts of the temporal lobes, as in semantic variant primary progressive aphasia, provides evidence for the anterior part of the temporal lobe as being a main centre for semantic representations (DeWitt and Rauschecker, 2013). It may be that the attributes or properties of objects are represented in the anterior part of the temporal lobe which operates as a hub area with associative connections to modality-specific cortical areas that encode for example the visual properties of objects (visual inferior temporal lobe areas), their auditory properties (superior temporal auditory areas), their reward value (orbitofrontal cortex), and/or actions that can be performed on or by the objects (parietal cortex), etc.

It is suggested that sequence-based processing in which the order of the items is important in the syntax, as in English, is supported by the dorsal stream; and that case-based processing (for example nominative vs accusative), which are order insensitive (as in German), is supported by the ventral cortical stream (DeWitt and Rauschecker, 2013).

14.2.3 Reading requires different brain systems to hearing speech

It has been proposed that a mechanism very much like the hierarchical feature combination VisNet model of object recognition described in Chapter 2 (Wallis and Rolls, 1997; Rolls, 2012d, 2021d) is used for building visually-evoked representations of individual letters, and then low-order combinations of letters, and then whole words, in the occipito-temporal cortex (Dehaene et al., 2005). The mechanism was described as a Local Combination Detector

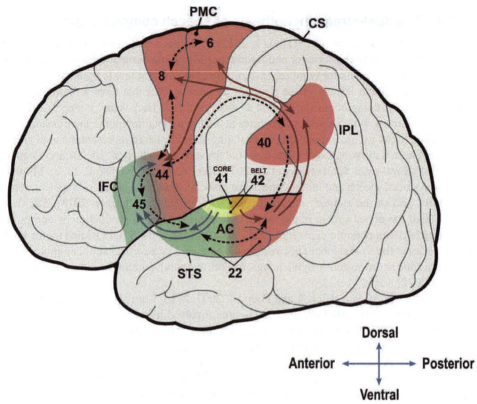

Fig. 14.2 Dual streams supporting language processing in the human brain. A left (postero-)dorsal (red) stream is involved in translating acoustic-based representations of speech signals into articulatory representations essential for speech production. An (antero-)ventral (green) stream is involved in processing speech signals for comprehension. Cross-stream integration in the inferior frontal gyrus is depicted by the transition from red to green. Black broken arrows denote feedback connections. Inferior Frontal Gyrus pars triangularis area 45, and the Inferior Frontal Gyrus pars opercularis area 44 are Broca's area. It is implicated in syntactic manipulations of semantic information for speech production. The posterior part of the superior temporal gyrus area, part of area 22, and a part of the supramarginal gyrus area 40 is traditionally referred to as Wernicke's area. It is involved in phonological processing but not in language comprehension. Abbreviations: AC, auditory cortex; CS, central sulcus; IFC, inferior frontal cortex; IPL, inferior parietal lobule; PMC, premotor cortex; STS, superior temporal sulcus. Numbers denote Brodmann areas (Section 1.11). (From Ina Bornkessel-Schlesewsky, Matthias Schlesewsky, Steven L. Small, and Josef P. Rauschecker (2014) Neurobiological roots of language in primate audition: common computational properties. Trends in Cognitive Sciences 19: 142–150. © Elsevier Ltd.)

Model of visual word recognition (Dehaene et al., 2005; Kemmerer, 2015; Hannagan et al., 2021). Indeed, in the macaque inferior temporal visual cortex, neurons are found to respond to combinations of letters that have been visually presented previously (Rajalingham et al., 2020), heightening the likelihood that the mechanisms utilised in VisNet (Rolls, 2021d) are used for letter combination recognition. fMRI evidence in humans suggested that this letter combination mechanism was implemented in the ventral visual system up to a region in the left occipito-temporal sulcus at y=-48 (Vinckier et al., 2007) leading to the Visual Word Form Area for orthographic representations, in the left mid-fusiform cortex (Dehaene and Cohen, 2011; Hannagan et al., 2021). Activations in the Visual Word Form Area are visual and prelexical, yet invariant for the location and the upper vs lower case of the stimulus words, but not for mirror reflection of letters (as required for reading to distinguish between for example b and d). Lesions affecting the Visual Word Form Area cause pure alexia, a selective deficit in word recognition (Dehaene and Cohen, 2011).

For processing beyond the Visual Word Form Area, a dual-route model of reading is described next, one involving phoneme-to-grapheme conversion, and the other a whole-word route (Coltheart et al., 1993; Pritchard et al., 2018).

The indirect, or sublexical, or grapho-phonological, route goes via grapheme-to-phoneme conversion to a phonological word representation and from there to word meaning. According to this hypothesis, the relay stations of the indirect route are located in the left superior and middle temporal gyrus, the supramarginal gyrus and the inferior frontal gyrus pars opercularis (area 44), while the regions involved in processing meaning are located in the left basal temporal area, posterior middle temporal gyrus, and inferior frontal gyrus pars triangularis (area 45) (Jobard et al., 2003).

The direct, or lexical, or lexico-semantic, route is based on whole-word recognition, maps the written word form directly onto the meaning, and goes directly from the visual word form area to the regions involved in processing meaning including the medial temporal gyrus (Jobard et al., 2003; Liuzzi et al., 2019).

14.2.4 Semantic representations

Semantics refers to the meanings that language expresses (Jackendoff, 2002; Kemmerer, 2015). We have already seen in Sections 8.3 and 14.2.2 that the anterior part of the temporal lobe is involved in semantic representations. Further, I suggest in Section 14.2.6 that the angular gyrus area 39 provides semantic attributes derived from processing in the dorsal processing stream about for example actions performed by or on objects, whereas the ventral stream anterior temporal lobe system provides semantic attributes related to the visual, auditory, tactile, and olfactory descriptors of objects. Approaches to brain systems involved in semantics are considered further here. At a more general level, a 'Hub and Spoke Model' postulates that there is a semantic hub in the anterior temporal lobe, with associative links to modality-specific cortical areas involved in processing different attributes of objects such as their visual appearance, odor, sound, etc (Kemmerer, 2015).

Comprehending speech involves the rapid and optimally efficient mapping from sound to meaning. A cohort model for lexical representations produced by spoken words proposes that the onset of a spoken word initiates a continuous process of activation of the lexical and semantic properties of the word candidates matching the speech input, and competition between them, which continues until the point at which the word is differentiated from all other cohort candidates (the uniqueness point, UP) (Marslen-Wilson and Welsh, 1978). At this point, the word is recognized uniquely and only the target word's semantics are active. Using magnetoencephalograhy (MEG), early transient effects approximately 400 ms before the UP of lexical competition were found in the left supramarginal gyrus, left superior temporal gyrus, left middle temporal gyrus (MTG) which is associated with processing the semantic properties of words, and left inferior frontal gyrus (IFG). Evidence was found of semantic competition in the MTG, left angular gyrus, and IFG. After the UP, target-specific semantic effects were found in the middle temporal gyrus (Kocagoncu, Clarke, Devereux and Tyler, 2017).

The use of semantic models in neuroimaging has confirmed that the anterior part of the temporal lobe is involved in semantics, but has pointed in addition to a more medial part of the temporal lobe, the perirhinal cortex (Bruffaerts et al., 2019; Liuzzi et al., 2019). The perirhinal cortex is increasingly engaged for objects that are more semantically confusable, suggesting that object-specific semantic information is represented in the perirhinal cortex (Clarke and Tyler, 2015, 2014).

Object representations, such as those found in the inferior temporal visual cortex, enable an object or face to be identified, as described in Chapter 2. Semantic representations involve in addition information about the attributes of an object, for example for a bicycle that it has two wheels, handlebars, a saddle, and usually but not always a chain, and just sometimes a second saddle. The suggestion therefore is that the individual object, person, etc needs to be associated with a set of attributes to provide a semantic representation. Those attributes can be learned, at least to some extent, by associative learning. The hypothesis is that this is implemented in the anterior temporal lobe. A well-known connectionist model, *interactive activation*, that captures this, has been described (McClelland, 1981; McClelland, Rumelhart and Hinton, 1986), and has been made available for tutorial use (McClelland and Rumelhart, 1989). This approach has been continued, with an example described in Section 14.4 (Devereux, Clarke and Tyler, 2018).

Further evidence for semantic representations is that some single neurons in the human medial temporal lobe cortex respond not only to the sight of an individual person, such as Jennifer Aniston, but also to her associates, such as people in the same movie, and the places associated with Jennifer Aniston (Quian Quiroga, 2012, 2013; Ison et al., 2015; De Falco et al., 2016; Bausch et al., 2021). These have been termed 'concept cells'. Although it has been argued that concept cells, in responding to for example the sight of a person, or to places associated with that person, may be specially present in humans (Quian Quiroga, 2012, 2013; Ison et al., 2015; De Falco et al., 2016; Quian Quiroga, 2023), it has been pointed out (Rolls, 2023c,d) that single neurons in the macaque medial temporal lobe might on these bases be described as 'concept cells', in that they respond to the sight or an object, or to the place associated with that object (Rolls, Xiang and Franco, 2005c; Rolls and Xiang, 2006; Rolls, 2023d).

14.2.5 Syntactic processing

A good introduction to the many rules of syntactic processing, and the many exceptions to them, is provided by Kemmerer (2015). The proposal made in this Chapter is that one way that syntax may be implemented in the brain is by a temporal trajectory through a state space of attractor networks (Section 14.5). This provides a system that can operate according to what appear to be a series of learned rules, and at the same time can deal with exceptions, which again are learned.

A long history of neuropsychological research places language function within a primarily left-lateralized frontotemporal system (Kemmerer, 2015). However, neuroimaging results appear to extend this language network to include a number of regions (Kemmerer, 2015) traditionally thought of as 'domain-general'. These include dorsal frontal, parietal, and medial temporal lobe regions known to underpin cognitive functions such as attention and memory. However, it has been argued that these domain-general systems are not required for language processing and are instead an artefact of the tasks typically used to study language. Recent work shows that when syntactic processing – arguably the only domain-specific language function – is measured in a task-free, naturalistic manner, only the left-lateralized frontotemporal syntax system and auditory network are activated. When syntax is measured within the context of a task, several other domain-general networks come online and are functionally connected to the frontotemporal system. Thus syntax appears to be implemented in a domain-specific frontotemporal syntax system (Campbell and Tyler, 2018).

An example of such syntactic processing measured within the context of natural listening is when there is temporary syntactic ambiguity such as: 'bullying teenagers' in the sentence 'The newspaper reported that bullying teenagers are a problem for the local school'). The region involved in this syntactic processing was primarily the left inferior frontal gyrus, with a smaller area in the left superior part of the temporal lobe (Campbell and Tyler, 2018).

There are hypotheses about how syntax is implemented in the brain by a number of different linked processes that perform operations such as mapping participant roles (e.g. actor or undergoer) to grammatical relations, like subject and object, and then implementing word ordering or case marking (as e.g. subject vs object) (Kemmerer, 2015). However, these have generally not reached the stage of neurobiologically plausible models.

14.2.6 The parietal cortex: supramarginal and angular gyri

Parts of the parietal cortex (especially the angular and supramarginal gyri) were at one time thought to be a major part of the language system (Binder, 2015). The role, at least for the supramarginal gyrus, is now thought to be more limited: phonological processing can activate the parietal cortex, particularly when sound-based representations are transformed into representations that can drive the action system (Coslett and Schwartz, 2018). In addition, the parietal cortex may contribute to auditory-verbal short term memory, with damage there impairing auditory rehearsal. This parietal system is incorporated into the dual-stream hypothesis, and is included in Fig. 14.2. In contrast, the inferior frontal gyrus is implicated more in articulatory rehearsal (Coslett and Schwartz, 2018).

Thus the supramarginal gyrus area 40 appears to support retrieval of phonological forms (mental representations of phoneme sequences), which are used for speech output and short-term memory tasks. Focal damage to this region produces phonemic paraphasia without impairing word comprehension, i.e., conduction aphasia. Phonologic processing does also activate cortex in the superior temporal sulcus (Hickok and Poeppel, 2015).

The angular gyrus area 39, as a multimodal region in the parietal cortex, has been implicated in semantic processing (Seghier, 2013), perhaps, it has been suggested, in combining the different attributes required for semantic representations (Price et al., 2015). I propose that one way in which the angular gyrus is involved in semantic processing is that it provides semantic attributes derived from processing in the dorsal processing stream about for example actions performed by or on objects. I propose that in contrast, the ventral stream anterior temporal lobe system provides semantic attributes related to the visual, auditory, tactile, olfactory and even taste descriptors of objects. It is an interesting issue about whether the parietal information reaches the temporal lobe semantic representations and the combination of the action and object information occurs in the temporal lobe; or whether the parietal action and temporal lobe object information have separate projections to the inferior frontal gyrus.

14.3 Cortical regions for language and their connectivity in humans

The connectivity between brain regions involved in language is a topic of importance for understanding human brain function and in order to minimize language impairments during neurosurgery (Milton et al., 2021; Ding et al., 2016; Hickok and Poeppel, 2015, 2007; Hickok, 2022; Bornkessel-Schlesewsky et al., 2015; DeWitt and Rauschecker, 2013; Rauschecker, 2012; Chang et al., 2015; Bouchard et al., 2013; Battistella et al., 2020). Part of the background is research on the auditory cortex in non-human primates (Kaas and Hackett, 2000; Rauschecker, 1998a; Rauschecker et al., 1995), and the connectivity of auditory cortical regions in humans (Rolls et al., 2023h) (Chapter 7). In research utilising the Human Connectome Project multimodal parcellation (HCP-MMP) atlas (Glasser et al., 2016a), 157 task-based fMRI studies were analyzed to identify brain regions in the HCP-MMP atlas related to semantics based on categorization of visual words and objects, and auditory words and stories, and the following regions were identified as part of the semantic network: 44,

45, 55b, IFJa, 8C, p32pr, SFL, SCEF, 8BM, STSdp, STSvp, TE1p, PHT and PBelt, and were shown to be interconnected with tractography (Milton et al., 2021).

In research on the connectivity of cortical regions involved in language, community analysis was performed on the 360x360 effective connectivity data for both hemispheres, and a community of 26 cortical regions was identified (Rolls et al., 2022b) that included most of those or very similar regions noted above (Milton et al., 2021) related to language. We then performed analyses on the connections, functional connectivity, and effective connectivity of these 26 left hemisphere cortical regions with the 360 cortical regions in the HCP-MMP atlas (Rolls et al., 2022b). Having identified 26 cortical regions related to language in the left hemisphere, a further community analysis (Rubinov and Sporns, 2010) was performed on the effective connectivities of the 26 language-related ROIs from all 180 cortical areas in the left hemisphere, to investigate whether any grouping could be made. It was found that three communities were formed, as follows: Group 1: STSva STSvp TE1a TGd PGi 10v 9m 10pp 47s 8Av 8BL 9a 9p. Group 2: TGv 44 45 47l SFL 55b. Group 3: A5 STGa STSda STSdp PSL STV TPOJ1. The connectivity of these three groups of language-related cortical regions (Rolls et al., 2022b) is described next.

14.3.1 A semantic system that includes the inferior bank of the superior temporal sulcus including object representations

The regions in Group 1 (STSva STSvp TE1a TGd PGi 10v 9m 10pp 47s 8Av 8BL 9a 9p), are considered next. The connectivities of regions in the ventral bank of the superior temporal sulcus, STSva and STSvp, are illustrated in Fig. 2.24, and of another region in this group, PGi, in Fig. 8.3 (Section 8.4.1). The regions involving cortical inferior regions of the superior temporal sulcus (STS) have effective connectivity with the adjacent inferior temporal visual cortex TE1a and temporal pole TG. The connected parietal PGi region has effective connectivity with inferior temporal visual cortex (TE) regions, with parietal PFm which also has connectivity with visual regions, with posterior cingulate cortex and parahippocampal TF memory-related regions, with the frontal pole, with the medial orbitofrontal cortex and related ventromedial prefrontal cortex reward-related regions, with the dorsolateral prefrontal cortex, and with 44 and 45 ('Broca's area') for output regions. PGi also receives inputs from PGs which includes visuo-motor as well as visual object system connectivity (Rolls et al., 2023d). This inferior STS semantic network is likely to be more involved in invariant object and face identity representations for static visual stimuli of the type represented in the inferior temporal visual cortex, whereas the superior (/ dorsal) STS regions are more likely to be involved in responses to face expression and visual motion including that which can be combined with auditory stimuli such as the sight and sound of a vocalization (Baylis et al., 1987; Hasselmo et al., 1989b,a; Rolls, 2021b).

As described in Section 8.4.1, the connectivity of these Group 1 semantic regions with inferior temporal visual cortex TE regions provides for transform-invariant visual representations of objects and faces as shown by discoveries in macaques (Rolls, 2021d,b; Perrett, Rolls and Caan, 1982; Booth and Rolls, 1998; Arcaro and Livingstone, 2021; Freiwald, 2020; Lehky and Tanaka, 2016) with complementary evidence from human neuroimaging (Kanwisher et al., 1997; Finzi et al., 2021; Collins and Olson, 2014) to be incorporated into semantic representations provided by this network of semantic cortical regions.

The connectivity with inferior parietal cortex PGi and to a smaller extent PGs regions may allow information about the visual motion of objects, such as a head turning away, or the eyes closing, or the lips moving, to convey a social signal such as a greeting (lip-smack) or threat, or when vocalizing, to reach STS areas (Rolls et al., 2023d).

Effective connectivity of the Group 1 regions with the frontal pole (10pp, 9m, 9a, 9p) regions implicated in planning and sequencing (Shallice and Cipolotti, 2018; Shallice and Burgess, 1996; Gilbert and Burgess, 2008) and prospective as well as retrospective memory (Underwood et al., 2015) is likely to provide information about the temporal order / sequence of events, which is important in interpreting causal interactions in the world (Rolls, 2021e).

Similarly, the connectivity via the parahippocampal TF region Fig. 8.3 with the hippocampal system implicated in episodic memory (Dere et al., 2008; Ekstrom and Ranganath, 2018; Rolls, 2018b, 2021b; Moscovitch et al., 2016) is likely to be important in building semantic information about the semantic meaning of events by enabling the memory of particular past events to be taken into account. The connectivity of the Group 1 regions with the posteroventral parts of the posterior cingulate cortex which are implicated in episodic memory (Vann et al., 2009; Leech and Smallwood, 2019; Leech and Sharp, 2014; Rolls et al., 2023i) by providing a route to the hippocampal system may in a similar way be important in enabling the Group 1 regions, especially those in the temporal lobe but also in the inferior parietal cortex (Davis et al., 2018; Papagno, 2018), to build semantic representations by taking particular previous episodes into account. Consistent with this, increasing activation of the angular gyrus and decreasing activation of the hippocampus occurs when episodic memories become incorporated into schemas (van der Linden et al., 2017).

The connectivity of the Group 1 regions with the orbitofrontal cortex (regions OFC and pOFC), pregenual anterior cingulate cortex (d32) and some ventromedial prefrontal cortex regions where reward value and emotion are represented (Grabenhorst and Rolls, 2011; Rolls et al., 2023c; Rolls, 2019c,e; Rolls et al., 2020a; Rolls, 2014a; Padoa-Schioppa and Conen, 2017; Cai and Padoa-Schioppa, 2012; Reber et al., 2017; Rolls, 2021h) provides another fundamental type of input, reward / emotion related, for building semantic representations about people and objects.

This ventral STS Group 1 semantic system also receives information from the top of the somatosensory hierarchy, parietal cortex region PF (Rolls et al., 2023d,f, 2022b) (Section 10.2). PF has effective connectivity directed towards language-related regions - the PeriSylvian language area (PSL), TPOJ2, STSvp (Rolls et al., 2022b) (and to prefrontal cortex areas involved in short-term memory related functions IFsa and 46 (Rolls et al., 2023d)). The diffusion tractography (Rolls et al., 2023d) further emphasizes connections of region PF with language-related areas 44, 45 and PSL (Rolls et al., 2023d). PF may on this connectivity evidence (Fig. 10.1) be the top of a somatosensory hierarchy which adds visual to somatosensory inputs to form semantic representations of felt objects, which can then gain access to language systems, as well as having outputs to superior parietal and intraparietal areas involved in performing actions such as reach and grasping for felt or seen objects. PF may thus build a multimodal, semantic, representation of felt objects. The PeriSylvian Language region (PSL) is very interesting, because it receives somatosensory inputs from the adjacent PF (Fig. 8.4), and has connections to STS semantic areas, so PSL may be a route for tactile inputs to become part of object representations (Rolls et al., 2022b).

The extensive connectivity of the Group 1 regions with the lateral prefrontal cortex which is implicated in working memory and planning (Goldman-Rakic, 1996; Baddeley, 2021) is likely to enable semantic representations to be held online to facilitate planning, reasoning, and rearrangement of the order of components if a task fails (Rolls, 2020a).

Regions in the more inferior part of the STS and linked with inferior temporal cortex visual regions in Group 1 are implicated in 'semantic representations involved in speech, reading, and visual and supra-modal mental objects that are linked to word forms' (Hertrich et al., 2020). The temporo-parietal junction and angular gyrus regions in Group 1 are implicated in 'pragmatic processing, context integration, words with multiple meanings, perspective taking, and social cognition' (Hertrich et al., 2020), consistent with some of the points made above about the regions in the Group 1 network.

Overall, this evidence shows that there is a network of brain regions that includes regions in the ventral bank of the superior temporal sulcus that combines evidence from its strongly interconnected brain regions to build multimodal representations of objects, including visual and somatosensory information. The human connectivity described here shows that this is a remarkable system extending from the temporal pole TG regions through the inferior temporal visual cortex and the ventral bank of the superior temporal sulcus through to PGi as illustrated in Fig. 8.3, and which also has connectivity with some dorsal prefrontal cortex regions 9a, 9b and 9m (Fig. 8.3). This semantic system also has connectivity with the hippocampal memory system, in part through the posterior cingulate cortex postero-ventral 'what' memory-related regions (Fig. 8.3, (Rolls et al., 2023i)), and this connectivity is likely to be important in how episodic memory is used to help build semantic representations, as described in Section 9.2.8.5 (Rolls, 2022b).

14.3.2 A semantic system that includes the superior bank of the superior temporal sulcus including visual motion, auditory, somatosensory and social information

The regions in Group 3 (A5 STGa STSda STSdp PSL STV TPOJ1), are considered next, with their connectivities illustrated in Figs. 2.25 and 8.4, with introductions in Sections 2.5.3 and 8.4.2.

In the superior (or dorsal) bank of the cortex in the Superior Temporal Sulcus (STS), regions STSda and STSdp were identified by a community analysis as part of a superior temporal lobe semantic system involved in language (Rolls et al., 2022b). Visual inputs to regions STSda and STSdp in this superior STS semantic system come from PGi (Fig. 2.25), and provide a route for moving visual stimuli / objects analyzed in the parietal cortex to reach STS regions (Rolls et al., 2023d). Visual inputs also reach STSdp from the Superior Temporal Visual (STV) region which receives from both MT and FFC (Fig. 2.25), and which could contribute to the neuronal activity in the cortex in the STS which has been shown to respond to moving heads, faces and objects in macaques (Hasselmo et al., 1989b,a), as described in Section 2.5.3. STSda and STSdp also have connectivity from STSva and STSvp which have strong connectivity with the Ventrolateral Visual Stream (Figs. 2.23 and 2.25). STSda and STSdp also receive auditory effective connectivity from A5 (Fig. 2.25). STSdp has connectivity directed towards Broca's area 44 and 45, and related areas (47l), and to the PeriSylvian Language region PSL and to the Superior Frontal Language region SFL (Rolls et al., 2022b).

It was proposed that this dorsal bank of the STS region is a third visual system that combines inputs from dorsal and ventral visual streams (Hasselmo et al., 1989b,a; Baylis et al., 1987), and this has recently received support (Pitcher and Ungerleider, 2021). Moreover, the same STS regions also contain neurons that respond to auditory stimuli including in some cases vocalization (Baylis, Rolls and Leonard, 1987). It is likely that neurons in these STS regions respond to combinations of auditory and synchronized visual stimuli such as vocalization and moving lips and are important in speech analysis by the viewer/hearer not only in noisy environments, but also to confirm who is speaking, and to learn associations between the sight of a person's face and the sound of their voice, which is part of what is required for the semantic representation of a person. Neurons of these types, including responsiveness to face expression, underlie the importance of this region in interpreting the social meaning of visual and auditory stimuli, which is a key part of semantic representations implemented in these STS regions, and that contribute to theory of mind, that is, of another individual's intentions and even thoughts. Consistent with this, individual STS cortex neurons have now been reported in macaques to respond to both visual face stimuli and to auditory stimuli (Khandhadia, Murphy, Romanski, Bizley and Leopold, 2021).

Region TPOJ1 has robust effective connectivity with auditory association cortex, including A5, A4 and to some extent LBelt, PBelt and TA2 (Fig. 8.4). The visual input to TPOJ1 is not from inferior temporal visual cortex (TE regions), but instead with some earlier visual cortical regions involved in motion processing (MST, MT, especially to STV and TPOJ1) and in face processing (the fusiform face cortex FFC and posterior inferior temporal cortex PIT). This is proposed to contribute to the responsiveness of neurons in this region, and in the dorsal bank of the STS, to moving heads and face movements important in social behavior as described in Section 8.4 (Rolls et al., 2023e, 2022b).

Another type of influence on these Group 3 regions comes from somatosensory cortical areas, as is especially evident in the functional connectivity (Rolls et al., 2022b). The functional connectivity of Group 3 regions is not only with 1-3b and 5, but also with frontal opercular and insular cortex, and there is some evidence for this too in the effective connectivity, including with parietal PF which can be considered as the top of the somatosensory hierarchy (Rolls et al., 2023d). This may contribute to semantic representations of body image and the sense of self (Rolls et al., 2023d).

This 'superior STS cortex semantic system' thus enables multimodal representations including visual, auditory, and probably also somatosensory via PGi and earlier somatosensory cortex regions, to gain access to the language system (Rolls et al., 2022b). There is also a link via TF to the hippocampal memory system (Fig. 2.25), which is likely to be important in how episodic memory is used to help build semantic representations, as described in Section 9.2.8.5 (Rolls, 2022b).

Although the description of a region around the temporo-parieto-occipital junction as Wernicke's area involved in language comprehension is now much less clear than previously thought (Section 14.2.1), what is clear based on the evidence described here (Rolls et al., 2022b) is that regions in this general area of the brain in what are parts of the dorsal and ventral STS semantic streams are very strongly implicated now as having key roles in semantic representations, and with communicating with Broca's area as described in Section 14.3.4.

An anterior part of the superior temporal lobe (in Group 3) is identified as an auditory word form area (Hertrich et al., 2020; DeWitt and Rauschecker, 2013; Binder, 2017, 2015). A more posterior part of the superior temporal lobe in the superior temporal gyrus is involved in auditory-phonological processing (Hertrich et al., 2020), consistent with the auditory connectivity described here. Just inferior to that in posterior parts of the superior temporal gyrus, superior temporal sulcus, and middle temporal gyrus is a region implicated in 'syntax and semantics' (Hertrich et al., 2020). This is probably close to the temporo-parieto-occipital junction region (part of Group 3) the connectivity of which is shown in Fig. 8.4.

14.3.3 Multimodal semantic representations

So far, the emphasis has been on visual and auditory semantic representations, partly because 'what' visual and auditory processing, which is primarily about the external world, is performed in the temporal lobes. However, some neurons in the cortex in the macaque superior temporal sulcus do respond to somatosensory stimuli (Baylis, Rolls and Leonard, 1987). Even the parietal PGi system is at least dominated by visual system connectivity (Rolls et al., 2023d), and what seems to be missing so far in the PGi part of this system, is information about the somatosensory properties of objects, and how the objects can be manipulated, perhaps as tools, under somatosensory as well as visual control. Now of course any information from the somatosensory system is quite different in kind from what is represented in the temporal lobes, for the somatosensory system involves touch to the body or the position of the body, which is not a property that needs to be taken into account by the temporal lobe analysis of objects 'out there' in the world. The way is which somatosensory information is incorporated into semantic systems appears to be implemented using the Group 3 regions that have effective connectivity with somatosensory regions (frontal opercular FOP, insula and parietal PF). Consistent with this, the Group 3 regions such as STV receive inputs from posterior cingulate cortex region PCV (precuneus visual region) (Rolls et al., 2023i), and this may provide for visual inputs relating to visually-guided reaching to grasp for objects, to be incorporated into semantic representations of objects.

A key region for multimodal convergence is the set of temporo-parieto-occipital junction regions TPOJ1-3, which are highly connected with each other, and which between them have effective connectivities with all the major systems just described involved in language, including visual, auditory, STS, PF, and PGi (Rolls et al., 2023d). The implication is that in terms of connectivity the TPOJ2 and TPOJ3 regions both of which have connectivity with the Group 3 regions (Rolls et al., 2023d) contribute to bringing together semantic representations involving all of these types of representation in the brain. Further, the Group 3 region PSL, the Peri-Sylvian Language region, receives effective connectivity from PF which can be considered as the top of the somatosensory hierarchy (Rolls et al., 2023d). Another input to the TPOJ regions comes from the cortex just lateral to the fusiform face area, which is the visual word-form area (VWFA) (Yeatman and White, 2021; Dehaene et al., 2005; Dehaene and Cohen, 2011; Caffarra et al., 2021). Disruption of the connectivity of the VWFA is likely to account for problems such as alexia and dyslexia in which the visual analysis required for reading cannot reach the semantic TPOJ regions (Pritchard et al., 2018; Liuzzi et al., 2019). Indeed, the FFC has effective connectivity to TPOJ1 and TPOJ2 and to the superior temporal visual area (STV) which in turn connects strongly with the nearby TPOJ regions. Further, PHT, lateral to the FFC, projects to TPOJ2.

The reward value is also an important semantic property of people, objects, places, etc, and this also can be incorporated into semantic representations by inputs to these semantic systems, especially Group 1, from the orbitofrontal cortex, ventromedial prefrontal cortex, and anterior cingulate cortex (Rolls et al., 2022b).

The temporal pole TG regions of the cortex are also likely to form multimodal 'semantic' representations, but primarily based on visual and auditory properties of objects, which is what are represented in the temporal lobes.

The ways in which inputs reach these semantic brain regions in the temporal lobes and temporo-parieto-occipital junction regions from different specialized areas, and the subtypes of sensory modality in which each part of the semantic system appears to specialize as described here in terms of connectivity, not only provides a connectomic basis for the semantic maps that can be visualized using natural speech as inputs (Huth et al., 2016), but also provides a connectional basis for understanding the many dissociations between syndromes found in neuropsychology, including phonological vs visual-based impairments of language processing. Indeed, the connectivity described here is consistent with evidence that the inferior parietal cortex is involved in language-based semantic processing and phonological operations (Coslett and Schwartz, 2018). In this context, it has been suggested that the parietal cortex is involved in the transcoding of sound-based representations into a format that can drive action systems (Coslett and Schwartz, 2018). Although there is much debate about how different language functions may map to different brain regions, one recent study tested patients with strokes in different brain regions, and found some evidence that damage to the posterior middle temporal gyrus is associated with syntactic comprehension deficits; that damage to the posterior inferior frontal gyrus is associated with expressive agrammatism; and that damage to the inferior angular gyrus is associated with semantic category word fluency deficits (Matchin et al., 2022), consistent with a theoretical proposal (Matchin and Hickok, 2020; Hickok, 2022).

In another approach to brain regions involved in different aspects of language, the long-lasting effects of brain damage on different aspects of language have been described using voxel-based lesion-symptom mapping (VLSM) as follows (Dronkers et al., 2017; Baldo et al., 2018; Turken and Dronkers, 2011). Damage to the middle temporal gyrus (and its underlying white matter) results in difficulty in comprehending sentences, the symptoms of which are those of Wernicke's aphasia. Damage more anteriorly, to the superior temporal gyrus, produces morphosyntactic problems. Damage to the lateral part of BA 47 (the lateral part of the orbitofrontal cortex / inferior prefrontal convexity cortex where it adjoins 'Broca's area' region BA 45) produces complex morphosyntactic problems, for example with sentences such as 'The girl who the man chased'. (This region is likely to include 47l in the HCP-MMP1 parcellation which has connectivity with 45 and 44 and other language regions (Rolls et al., 2022b). This region is likely to be involved in setting up the grammatically appropriate positions of items in sentences.) A region in the posterior superior temporal sulcus BA39 extending up into parietal cortex is described as being involved in auditory memory, and not specifically in language.

14.3.4 Broca's area and related regions (TGv 44 45 47l SFL 55b)

The Group 2 language-related regions are indicated in bold italic font and are outlined in black in Fig. 14.3, and are: TGv 44 45 47l SFL 55b (Rolls et al., 2022b). Effective connectivity of region 45 is chosen as an example of the effective connectivity of a Group 2 region (Fig. 14.3). There is connectivity with the superior STS auditory-visual semantic stream (e.g. STSdp and STGa), with the inferior STS visual semantic stream (e.g. STSvp and TG), with the Peri Sylvian Language area and TPOJ1, with nearby inferior frontal gyrus regions 44, IFSp, 47l and 47s. Probable output regions for 45 include premotor 55b and the (supplementary area) Superior Frontal Language region (SFL). There is some effective connectivity too with the frontal pole, dorsolateral prefrontal 9a and 8BL.

The Group 2 regions and network are likely to be involved in speech processing (Rolls et al., 2022b). One region in Group 2 is 55b, which is situated in the premotor cortex sandwiched between the frontal eye fields FEF and PEF. 55b is likely to be an output region for 44 and 45, and it was proposed that it is involved in vocalization (Rolls et al., 2022b) given the importance of vocal cord control in speech production (Ekert et al., 2021b). Consistent with this proposal, it has now been found that 55b (a 'dorsal precentral speech area') codes voice pitch during vocalisation, and may be involved in the prosody of speech (Hickok et al., 2023). Similarly, the Superior Frontal Language area (SFL) also part of Group 2 may be a supplementary premotor cortical area involved in speech production. The involvement of 47l and 47s in the inferior frontal gyrus regions linked by effective connectivity with language systems is found here in the context of left hemisphere functions. These orbital parts of the language system may be involved in retrieving articulatory plans from semantic stimuli (i.e. semantic-to-articulatory recoding) (Ekert et al., 2021b). The left inferior frontal sulcus (IFS) regions found here to have connectivity with the Group 2 regions may be involved in similar functions (Ekert et al., 2021b). In the right hemisphere the corresponding 47l and 47s regions may be able to function more as lateral orbitofrontal areas involved in non-reward, punishment, and emotion, and consistent with this, functional connectivities and activations related to emotion computations are more prominent in the right hemisphere (Cheng et al., 2016a; Rolls et al., 2020a,b,e).

The connectivity of Broca's region (Rolls et al., 2022b) extends previous concepts about

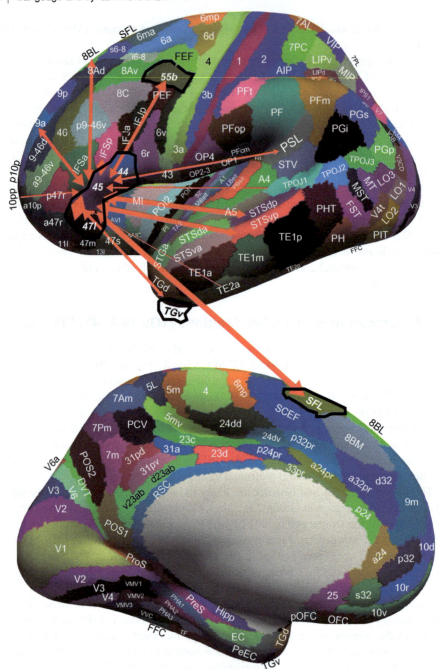

Fig. 14.3 Effective connectivity of region 45 chosen as an example of the effective connectivity of a Group 2 language-related region. The Group 2 regions are indicated in bold italic font and are outlined in black, and are: TGv 44 45 47l SFL 55b. There is connectivity with the superior STS auditory-visual stream (e.g. STSdp and STGa), with the inferior STS visual stream (e.g. STSvp and TG), with the Peri Sylvian Language area and TPOJ1, with nearby inferior frontal gyrus regions 44, IFSp, 47l and 47s. Probable output regions for 45 include premotor 55b and the (supplementary area) Superior Frontal Language region (SFL). There is some effective connectivity too with the frontal pole, dorsolateral prefrontal 9a and 8BL. The widths of the lines and the size of the arrowheads indicate the magnitude and direction of the effective connectivity. The abbreviations are listed in Section 1.12. (From Rolls,E.T., Deco,G., Huang,C-C. and Feng,J. (2022) The human language effective connectome. Neuroimage 258: 119352.)

Broca's area (Clos et al., 2013; Amunts and Zilles, 2012), by showing that there is a whole group of interconnected areas in the frontal lobe of the left hemisphere that are implicated in language, not only regions 44 and 45 in the HCP-MMP atlas (which may not correspond exactly to BA44 and BA45), but also IFSp and IFJa, and 47l and 47s. Similarly, the concept of a Wernicke's area involved in speech comprehension at the temporo-parietal junction is no longer accepted (DeWitt and Rauschecker, 2013; Binder, 2017), but the concept here is that there is a semantic system that extends from the temporal pole to PGi (and PF for body including somatosensory representations (Rolls et al., 2023d)) in the parietal lobe, which in the temporal lobe has an inferior more visual and object-related part (Group 1), and a more superior auditory/visual motion/somatosensory related part (Group 3). Region 45 has more effective connectivity with (especially anterior) STS regions than does region 44 (Rolls et al., 2023h). Parts of the supramarginal part of the parietal lobe (which include PF regions) are implicated in auditory short-term memory and articulatory sequencing (Oberhuber et al., 2016). Parts of the angular gyrus of the parietal lobe (which include PG regions) are implicated in semantic processing involved for example in comprehension when reading (Seghier et al., 2010). It should be noted that the inferior STS (Group 1) and superior STS (Group 3) temporal lobe semantic systems identified here by their connectivity do not correspond to the ventral and dorsal auditory pathways in which a ventral pathway is involved in 'what' and a dorsal pathway in 'where' or action processing (DeWitt and Rauschecker, 2013; Rauschecker, 2018b; Rauschecker and Scott, 2009; Tian et al., 2001; Archakov et al., 2020; Rolls et al., 2023h).

It is noted that Broca's area, BA44 and BA45, is no longer thought to be essential for speech production in terms of articulation as shown by the analysis of effects of damage to it (Gajardo-Vidal et al., 2021), but is implicated in some aspects of language, such as the timing of speech items (Long et al., 2016), and syntax as described next (Friederici et al., 2017; Flinker et al., 2015; Matchin and Hickok, 2020; Hickok, 2022).

The Group 2 network described here involving outputs from other language regions to areas 44, 45 and a closely connected inferior frontal gyrus region including IFja and IFSp, and extending into left orbitofrontal 47s and 47l is suggested here to be involved in syntax (Rolls et al., 2022b), with the syntactic processing (Rolls and Deco, 2015a) being driven by semantic inputs from the Group 1 inferior STS temporal lobe visual object 'what' semantic network and the Group 3 superior STS temporal lobe visual motion / auditory / somatosensory semantic network. Consistent with this, there is evidence from neuroimaging and related neuropsychological studies that implicates area 44 in syntax processing, manipulating and detecting structures above the word level (Hertrich et al., 2020; Friederici et al., 2017). In more detail, area 44 is seen as the key region for syntactic processing by implementing the 'merge' operation that is key for understanding syntax (Friederici, Chomsky, Berwick, Moro and Bolhuis, 2017). Merge is an operation that takes exactly two (syntactic) elements – call them x and y – and puts them together to form the unordered set[x,y] (Friederici et al., 2017). The elements x and y can be word-like building blocks that are drawn from the lexicon or previously constructed phrases that are assembled into an unbounded array of hierarchically structured internal representations (phrases and, ultimately, sentences) (Friederici, Chomsky, Berwick, Moro and Bolhuis, 2017). Merge is a recursive operation, but as analyzed by Treves and Rolls (1994), in the brain recurrent processing could be implemented by an equivalent series of linked networks. Area 45 is described as a lexical-semantic core area linking phonological codes to lexical meanings (Hertrich et al., 2020; Friederici et al., 2017).

From a study using direct cortical recordings during vocal repetition of written and spoken words, it was found that Broca's area mediates a cascade of activation from sensory representations of words in temporal cortex to their corresponding articulatory gestures in motor cortex, but is quiescent during articulation (Flinker, Korzeniewska, Shestyuk, Franaszczuk,

Dronkers, Knight and Crone, 2015). It was proposed that Broca's area does not participate in the production of individual words, but coordinates the transformation of information processing across large-scale cortical networks involved in spoken word production, prior to articulation. It has also been proposed that Broca's area is involved in lexical selection / sequencing (Hickok et al., 2023).

It has been remarked (Rolls et al., 2022b) that if neuroimaging studies could be mapped into a single atlas such as the HCP-MMP atlas using the tools that are available (Dickie et al., 2019; Glasser et al., 2016a; Huang et al., 2022), this would help in the development of our understanding of language systems, especially now that the connectivity between these language-related regions is becoming better understood, as described here.

14.4 Hypotheses about how semantic representations are computed

Object representations, such as those found in the inferior temporal visual cortex, enable an object or face to be identified, as described in Chapter 2. Semantic representations involve in addition information about all the attributes of an object, for example for a bicycle that it has two wheels, handlebars, a saddle, and usually but not always a chain, and just sometimes a second saddle, as described in Sections 8.3 and 14.2.4. Those attributes are part of what ventral stream processing helps to define. Further, I suggested in Section 14.2.6 that the angular gyrus area 39 provides semantic attributes derived from processing in the dorsal processing streams about for example actions performed by or on objects, that are also important in building semantic representations. For example, a property of a hammer is that it is to hit the head of a nail; and of the head of a nail that it is that part of the nail that is to be hit. An implication is that damage to the left parietal cortex would impair especially action-related attributes of objects; that damage to the left anterior temporal lobe cortex would impair especially use of the physical properties of objects such as their shape, color, odor, sound, tactile qualities etc as semantic descriptors; and that both types of descriptor would need to be connected to the left inferior frontal gyrus for syntactic processing to produce speech. Consistent with this hypothesis, in humans parietal areas such as the angular gyrus, as well as the anterior temporal lobe, have direct connections with the inferior frontal gyrus language-related areas as shown with diffusion tractography imaging (Hsu, Rolls, Huang, Chong, Lo, Feng and Lin, 2020), with the interactions evident with functional connectivity (Du, Rolls, Cheng, Li, Gong, Qiu and Feng, 2020).

The suggestion therefore is that to form a semantic representation, the individual object, person, etc needs to be associated with a set of attributes. The attributes of objects etc can be learned, at least to a considerable extent, by associative learning. The hypothesis is that this is implemented in the anterior temporal lobe, and may include information from the angular gyrus. A well-known connectionist model, interactive activation, that captures the operation of a semantic system with attributes associated with each individual, has been described (McClelland, 1981; McClelland et al., 1986), and was made available for tutorial use (McClelland and Rumelhart, 1989).

A model that illustrates such a system for semantic representations (Devereux, Clarke and Tyler, 2018) is now considered. The first part of the model involved an artificial deep convolutional neural network to categorise visual inputs. This was followed by an attractor network model of semantics, in which each visual object was associated with a set of attributes or 'semantic features'. There were 2,469 semantic attributes, such as 'has wheels', 'has skin/peel', 'is sweet', selected as appropriate to represent the 629 objects. The synaptic weights between the object nodes and the semantic attribute nodes were trained using continuous recurrent back-propagation through time, in such a way that correct semantic features were produced when each object was presented. This type of learning is not biologically plausible, so this was an artificial model. The activity in the semantic part of the model was described as similar to fMRI activations that had been found in the perirhinal cortex (Devereux et al., 2018).

These interactive activation approaches to semantic representations do make the useful point that once an object has been recognised by for example the visual system, its semantic attributes then need to be learned.

14.5 A neurodynamical hypothesis about how syntax is computed

14.5.1 Binding by synchrony?

A fundamental computational issue is how the brain implements binding of elements such as features with the correct relationship between the elements. The problem in the context of language might arise if we have neuronal populations each firing to represent a subject, a verb, and an object of a sentence. If all we had were three populations of neurons firing, how would we know which was the subject, which the verb, and which the object? How would we know that the subject was related to the verb, and that the verb operated on the object? How these relations are encoded is part of the problem of binding.

Von der Malsburg (1990) considered this computational problem, and suggested a dynamical link architecture in which neuronal populations might be bound together temporarily by increased synaptic strength which brought them into temporary synchrony. This led to a great deal of research into whether arbitrary relinking of features in different combinations is implemented in visual cortical areas using synchrony (Singer, Gray, Engel, Konig, Artola and Brocher, 1990; Engel, Konig, Kreiter, Schillen and Singer, 1992; Singer and Gray, 1995; Singer, 1999; Abeles, 1991; Fries, 2009), and this has been modelled (Hummel and Biederman, 1992). However, although this approach could specify that two elements are bound, it does not specify the relation (Rolls, 2016b). For example, in vision, we might know that a triangle and a square are part of the same object because of synchrony between the neurons, but we would not know the spatial relation, for example whether the circle was inside the triangle, or above, below it, etc. Similarly for language, we might know that a subject and an object were part of the same sentence, but we would not know which was the subject and which the object, that the subject operated (via a verb) on the object, etc, that is, the syntactic relations would not be encoded just by synchrony. Indeed, neurophysiological recordings show that although synchrony can occur in a dynamical system such as the brain, synchrony *per se* between neurons in high order visual cortical areas conveys little information about which objects are being represented, with 95% of the information present in the number of spikes being emitted by each of the neurons in the population, i.e. a firing rate code (Rolls, 2016b; Rolls and Treves, 2011) (Appendix C).

Instead, in high order visual cortical areas, the spatial relations between features to form objects are implemented by feature combinations neurons (Chapter 2), and this feature/place coding scheme is computationally feasible (Elliffe, Rolls and Stringer, 2002) (Section 2.8.5). The spatial relations between objects are encoded by neurons that have spatially biased receptive fields relative to the fovea (Aggelopoulos and Rolls, 2005; Rolls, 2016b, 2012d). Further, temporal synchrony measured by coherence does not appear to be well suited for information transmission, for in quantitative neuronal network simulations, it is found that information is transmitted between neuronal populations at much lower values of synaptic strength than those needed to achieve coherence (Rolls, Webb and Deco, 2012) (Section 2.8.5.1).

In this situation, I now make alternative proposals for how syntactic relations are encoded in the cortex, as described next (see Rolls and Deco (2015a)). Approaches used in neurolinguistics to syntax are described elsewhere (Kemmerer, 2015, 2019).

14.5.2 Syntax using a place code

The overview of encoding in the cortex in Appendix C (Rolls, 2016b; Rolls and Treves, 2011) leads to a hypothesis about how syntax, or the relations between the parts of a sentence, is encoded for language. My hypothesis is that a place code is used, with for example one cortical module or region used to represent subjects, another cortical module used to represent verbs, and another cortical module used to represent objects (see Rolls and Deco (2015a)).

The size of any such neocortical module need not be large. An attractor network in the cortex need occupy no more than a local cortical area perhaps 2–3 mm in diameter within which there are anatomically dense recurrent collateral associatively modifiable connections between the neurons (Rolls, 2016b). This cortical computational attractor network module would thus be about the size of a cortical column. It is an attractor network module in the sense that neurons more than a few mm away would not be sufficiently strongly activated to form part of the same attractor network (Rolls, 2016b). An attractor network of this type with sparse distributed representations can store and encode approximately as many items are there are synaptic connections onto each cortical neuron from the nearby neurons (Treves and Rolls, 1991; Rolls and Treves, 1998; Rolls, 2016b). The implication for language is that of order 10,000 nouns could be stored in a single cortical attractor network with 10,000 recurrent collateral connections on to each neuron. This capacity is only realized if there is only a low probability of more than one recurrent collateral connection between any pair of the neurons in a module, and this has been proposed as one of the underlying reasons for why cortical connectivity is diluted, with a probability in the order of 0.1 for connections between any pair of nearby neurons in the neocortex, and 0.02 for CA3 neurons in the rodent hippocampus (Rolls, 2012b).

The hypothesis is further that some local cortical modules encode the nouns that are the subjects of sentences, and that these are different from the cortical modules that encode the objects of sentences. A prediction is thus that there will be single neurons in a human cortical language area that respond to a noun when it is the subject but not the object of a sentence, and vice versa. Consistent with the hypothesis, evidence was found in an fMRI study that the agent (or actor, the subject of an active sentence) is localised separately from the patient (or object of an active sentence) in the left mid-superior temporal cortex (Frankland and Greene, 2015).

Clearly the full details of the system would be more complicated, but the general hypothesis is that adjectives and adjectival phrases that are related to the subject of a sentence will have strong connections to the subject module or modules; that adverbs and adverbial phrases that are related to the verbs of sentence will have strong connections to the verb module or modules; and that adjectives and adjectival phrases that are related to the object of a sentence will have strong connections to the object module or modules.

14.5.3 Temporal trajectories through a state space of attractors

To represent syntactical structure *within* the brain, what has been proposed already might be along lines that are consistent with the principles of cortical computation (Rolls, 2016b). The high representational capacity would be provided for by the high capacity of a local cortical attractor network, and syntactic binding within a brain would be implemented by using a place code in which the syntactic role would be defined by which neurons are firing – for example, subjects in one cortical module or modules, and objects in another cortical module or modules.

However, a problem arises if we wish to communicate this representation to another person, for the neural implementation described so far could not be transferred to another person without transferring which neurons in the language areas were currently active, and having a well trained person as the decoder!

To transfer or communicate what is encoded in the representations to another person, and the relations or syntax, it is proposed that a number of mechanisms might be used. One might be a temporal order encoding, for example the subject–verb–object encoding that is usual in English, and which has the advantage of following the temporal order that usually underlies causality in the world. Another mechanism might be the use of inflections (usually suffixes) to words to indicate their place in the syntax, such as cases for nouns (e.g. nominative for the subject or agent, and accusative for the object or patient, dative, and genitive), and person for verbs (e.g. first, second, and third person singular and plural, to specify I, you, he/she/it, we, you, they) used to help disambiguate which noun or nouns operate on the verb. Another mechanism is the use of qualifying prepositions to indicate syntactic role of a temporally related word, with examples being 'with', 'to', and 'from'. This mechanism is used in combination with temporal order in English.

In this Section, I focus on temporal order as an encoder of syntactical relations, and next set out hypotheses on how this could be implemented in the cerebral cortex based on the above computational neuroscience background (Rolls and Deco, 2015a).

14.5.4 Hypotheses about the implementation of language in the cerebral cortex

In what follows, the Deep Network models semantic representations in the anterior temporal lobe; and the Word network models syntactic operations in the inferior frontal gyrus.

1. Subjects, verbs, and objects are encoded using sparse distributed representations (Rolls, 2016b; Rolls and Treves, 2011) in localised cortical attractor networks. One cortical module with a diameter of 2–3 mm and 10,000 recurrent collateral connections per neuron could encode in the order of 10,000 items (e.g. subjects or verbs or objects) (Rolls, 2016b; Treves and Rolls, 1991) (Appendix B). One cortical module would thus be sufficient to encode all the objects, all the verbs, or all the objects (depending on the module) in most people's working vocabulary, which is of the order to several thousand nouns, or verbs.

This follows from the analysis that the capacity of an attractor network with sparse encoding a (where for binary networks a is the proportion of neurons active for any one memory pattern) is as follows, and from the fact that there are in the order of 10,000 recurrent collateral connections on each neuron (Rolls, 2016b). The capacity is measured by the number of patterns p that can be stored and correctly retrieved from the attractor network

$$p \approx \frac{C}{a \ln(\frac{1}{a})} k \tag{14.1}$$

where C is the number of synapses on the dendrites of each neuron devoted to the recurrent collaterals from other neurons in the network, and k is a factor that depends weakly on the detailed structure of the rate distribution, on the connectivity pattern, etc., but is roughly in the order of 0.2–0.3 (Treves and Rolls, 1991; Rolls, 2016b, 2012b) (Appendix B).

The use of attractor networks for language-based functions is itself important. Cortical computation operates at the neuronal level by computing the similarity or dot product or correlation between an input vector of neuronal firing rates and the synaptic weights that connect the inputs to the neurons (Rolls, 2016b, 2012e) (Appendix B). The output of the neuron is a firing rate, usually between 0 and 100 spikes/s. Cortical computation at the neuronal level is thus largely analogue. This is inherently not well suited to language, in which precise, frequently apparently logical, rules are followed on symbolic representations. This gap may be bridged by attractor or autoassociation networks in the brain, which can enter discrete attractor high firing rate states that can provide for error correction in the analogue computation, and to the robustness to noise, that are often associated with the processing of discrete symbols (Treves, 2005; Rolls, 2016b, 2012e). These discrete attractor states are network properties, not the properties of single neurons, and this capability is at the heart of much cortical computation including long-term memory, short-term memory, and decision-making (Rolls, 2016b, 2014a), as elucidated in this book.

2. Place coding with sparse distributed representations is used in these attractors. The result is that the module that is active specifies the syntactic role of what is represented in it. One cortical module would be for subjects, another for verbs, another for objects, etc.

3. The presence of these weakly coupled attractors would enable linguistic operations of a certain type to be performed within the brain, but the information with the syntax could not be communicated in this form to other people. In this statement, 'weakly coupled' is clearly and quantitatively defined by attractors that have weak interconnections so that they can have different basins of attraction, yet can influence each other (Rolls, 2016b) (Section B.9). The computations involved in these interactions might instantiate a 'language of thought' that would be below the level of written or spoken speech, and would involve for example constraint satisfaction within coupled attractors, and the types of brain-style computation described by Rolls (2012e) (see Section 19.3 on brain computation vs computation in a digital computer). The cortical computational processes could be usefully influenced and made creative by the stochastic dynamics of neuronal networks in the brain that are due to the 'noisy' Poisson-like firing of neurons (Rolls, 2016b; Rolls and Deco, 2010). When someone has a hunch that they have solved a problem, this may be the computational system involved in the processing. This might be termed a 'deep' structure or layer of linguistic processing.

4. To enable these computations that involve syntactical relations to be communicated to another person or written down to be elaborated into an extended argument, the process considered is one involving weakly forward-coupled attractor networks. One such system would be to have weak forward coupling between subject–verb–object attractor networks. The exact trajectories followed (from subject to verb to object) could be set up during early language learning, by forming during such learning stronger forward than reverse connections between the attractors, by for example spike-timing dependent plasticity (Markram et al., 1997; Bi and Poo, 1998; Feldman, 2012) and experience with the order of items that is provided during language learning. Which trajectory was followed would be biased by which subject, which verb, and which object representation was currently active in the deep layer. These temporal trajectories through the word attractors would enable the syntactical relations to be encoded in the temporal order of the words.

With this relatively weak coupling between attractors implemented with integrate-and-fire neurons and low firing rates, the transition from one active attractor to the next can be relatively slow, taking 100–400 or more ms (Deco and Rolls, 2005c). This property of the system adapts it well to the production of speech, in which words are produced sequentially with a spacing in the order of 300–500 ms, a rate that is influenced by the mechanics and therefore dynamics of the speech production muscles and apparatus.

A simulation testing this system and making the details of the operation of the system and their biological plausibility clear is described in the Methods and Results sections of Rolls and Deco (2015a).

5. The system for enabling the syntax to be communicated to other people or written down would have some computational advantages apart from purely the communication. In particular, once the syntax can be formally expressed in written statements, it becomes easier to perform logical operations on the statements, which become propositional, and can be tested. These logical operations, and reasoning, may not be the style of computation utilized in general by computational processes within the brain (see Rolls (2012e) Section 2.15), but may become algorithms that can be followed to achieve quantitatively precise and accurate results, as in long division, or by learning logic. Thus the importance of communication using syntax may allow other environmental tools to be applied to enable reasoning and logic that is not the natural style of neural computation (see Section 19.3).

6. To enable the system to produce words in the correct temporal order, and also to remember with a lower level of neuronal firing what has just been said for monitoring in case it needs correcting, a mechanism such as spike frequency adaptation may be used, as described next.

A property of cortical neurons is that they tend to adapt with repeated input (Abbott et al., 1997; Fuhrmann et al., 2002a). The mechanism is understood as follows. The afterpolarization (AHP) that follows the generation of a spike in a neuron is primarily mediated by two calcium-activated potassium currents, I_{AHP} and the sI_{AHP} (Sah and Faber, 2002), which are activated by calcium influx during action potentials. The I_{AHP} current is mediated by small conductance calcium-activated potassium (SK) channels, and its time course primarily follows cytosolic calcium, rising rapidly after action potentials and decaying with a time constant of 50 to several hundred milliseconds (Sah and Faber, 2002). In contrast, the kinetics of the sI_{AHP} are slower, exhibiting a distinct rising phase and decaying with a time constant of 1–2 s (Sah, 1996). A variety of neuromodulators, including acetylcholine (ACh) acting via a muscarinic receptor, noradrenaline, and glutamate acting via G-protein-coupled receptors, suppress the sI_{AHP} and thus reduce spike-frequency adaptation (Nicoll, 1988).

When recordings are made from single neurons operating in physiological conditions in the awake behaving monkey, peristimulus time histograms of inferior temporal cortex neurons to visual stimuli show only limited adaptation. There is typically an onset of the neuronal response at 80–100 ms after the stimulus, followed within 50 ms by the highest firing rate. There is after that some reduction in the firing rate, but the firing rate is still typically more than half-maximal 500 ms later (see example in Tovee, Rolls, Treves and Bellis (1993); Fig. 2.16). Thus under normal physiological conditions, firing rate adaptation can occur.

This adaptation can be studied by including a time–varying intrinsic (potassium-like) conductance in the cell membrane (Brown, Gähwiler, Griffith and Halliwell, 1990a; Treves, 1993; Rolls, 2016b). This can be done by specifying that this conductance, which if open tends to shunt the membrane and thus to prevent firing, opens by a fixed amount with the potential excursion associated with each spike, and then relaxes exponentially to its closed state. In this manner sustained firing driven by a constant input current occurs at lower rates after the first few spikes, in a way similar, if the relevant parameters are set appropriately, to the behavior observed in vitro of many pyramidal cells (for example, Lanthorn, Storm and Andersen (1984), Mason and Larkman (1990)). The details of the implementation used are described by Rolls and Deco (2015a).

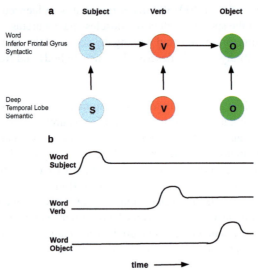

Fig. 14.4 Schematic diagram of a model of syntactic processing. a. Each circle indicates a local cortical attractor network capable of storing 10,000 items. The Deep layer local cortical attractor networks use place coding to encode the syntactic role of the sematic representation in the Deep layer. That is, the syntactic role of each attractor network for semantic representations uses a place code to define its syntactic role. The possible syntactic roles are Subject (S), Verb (V), and Object (O). The deep layer nodes model semantic representations in the anterior temporal lobe. In this implementation there are separate Subject (S), Verb (V), and Object (O) syntactic networks in the inferior frontal gyrus, labelled 'Word'. Syntax within the brain is implemented by place encoding. For communication, the deep representation must be converted into a sequence of words. To implement this, the Deep attractor networks provide a weak selective bias to the Word attractor networks, which have weak non-selective forward coupling S to V to O. b. The operation in time of the system. The Deep networks fire continuously, and the syntax is implemented using place encoding. The Deep networks apply a weak selective bias to the Word networks, which is insufficient to make a word attractor fire, but is sufficiently strong to bias it later into the correct one of its 10,000 possible attractor states, each corresponding to a word. Sentence production is started by a small extra input to the Subject Word network. This with the selective bias from the Deep subject network make the Word subject network fall into an attractor, the peak firing of which is sufficient to elicit production of the subject word. Adaptation in the subject network makes its firing rate decrease, but still remain in a moderate firing rate attractor state to provide a short-term memory for the words uttered in a sentence, in case they need to be corrected or repeated. The high and moderate firing rate in the Subject Word network provides non-selective forward bias to the whole of the Object Word network, which falls into a particular attractor produced by the selective bias from the Deep Verb network, and the verb is uttered. Similar processes then lead to the correct object being uttered next. The sentence can be seen as a trajectory through a high dimensional state space of words in which the particular words in the sentence are due to the selective bias from the Deep networks, and the temporal order is determined by the weak forward non-selective connections between the networks, i.e. connections from subject-to-verb, and verb-to-object networks. The simulations show dynamical network principles by which this type of sentence encoding and also decoding could be implemented. The overall concept is that syntax within the brain can be solved by the place coding used in most other representations in the brain; and that the problems with syntax arise when this place-coded information must be transmitted to another individual, when one solution is to encode the role in syntax of a word by its temporal order in a sentence. (After Rolls, E. T. and Deco,G. (2015) Networks for memory, perception, and decision-making, and beyond to how the syntax for language might be implemented in the brain. Brain Research 1621: 316–334. © Elsevier B.V.)

14.5.5 Tests of the hypotheses – a model

14.5.5.1 An integrate-and-fire network with three attractor network modules connected by stronger forward than backward connections

The computational neuroscience aspects of the hypotheses described above were investigated with an integrate-and-fire network with three attractor network modules connected by stronger forward than backward connections, the operation of which is illustrated conceptually in Figs. 14.4 and 14.5, and the architecture of which is illustrated in Fig. 14.6. Each module is an integrate-and-fire attractor network with n possible attractor states. For the simulations described (Rolls and Deco, 2015a) there were $n=10$ orthogonal attractor states in

A neurodynamical hypothesis about how syntax is computed | 647

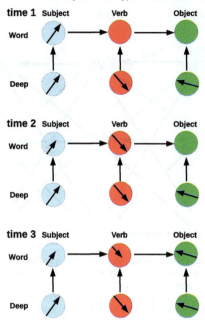

Fig. 14.5 A model of syntactic processing. The operation of the model, illustrated at three different time steps. Time 1 is during the production of the subject work, time 2 during the verb word, and time 3 during the object word. Each circle represents an attractor network that can fall into one of 10,000 possible states indicated by the direction of the arrow vector, each state corresponding to a word (for the Word-level networks) or a semantic concept (for the Deep-level networks). The length of the arrow vector indicates the firing rate of the selected attractor. The Deep attractor networks fire continuously, with the syntactic role indicated by the particular network using place coding. The Deep networks, which represent semantics or meaning, provide a weak selective bias continuously to the Word attractor networks. The sequential operation of the Subject then Verb then Object Word networks is produced by the weak non-selective forward connections between the networks. After its initial high firing rate, a Word attractor network remains active at a lower firing rate as a result of adaptation, to provide a short-term memory for the words uttered in a sentence, in case they need to be corrected or repeated. (After Rolls, E. T. and Deco,G. (2015) Networks for memory, perception, and decision-making, and beyond to how the syntax for language might be implemented in the brain. Brain Research 1621: 316–334. © Elsevier B.V.)

each module, each implemented by a population of neurons with strong excitatory connections between the neurons with value $w_+ = 2.1$ for the NMDA and AMPA synapses. There were $N=8000$ neurons in each module, of which 0.8 (i.e. 6400) were excitatory, and 1600 were inhibitory. The first module could represent one of 10 subjects (S), the second module one of 10 verbs (V), and the third module one of 10 objects (O). In the cerebral cortex, each module might be expected to be able to encode up to 10,000 items using sparse distributed representations, and assuming of order 10,000 excitatory recurrent collateral connection onto each neuron (Treves and Rolls, 1991, 1994; Rolls, 2016b). The parameters in each module were set so that the spontaneous firing state with no input applied was stable, and so that only one of its n possible attractor states was active at any time when inputs were applied (Rolls, 2016b; Rolls and Deco, 2010; Deco, Rolls, Albantakis and Romo, 2013).

In the model, there are forward connections from all excitatory neurons in one module to all excitatory neurons in the next module, with uniform strength w_{ff}. The role of these forward connections is to produce some non-specific input to the next module of the network when the previous module enters an attractor state with one of its neuronal pools. The role of this forward input is to encourage the next module in the series to start firing with some small delay after the previous module, to enable a temporal trajectory through a state space of an active attractor pool in one module to an active attractor pool in the next module. In the cerebral cortex, there are typically both stronger forward than backward connections between modules in different cortical areas, and connections in both directions between modules in

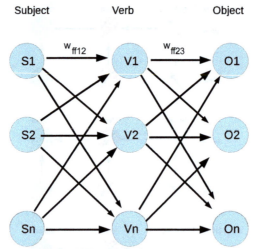

Fig. 14.6 The attractor network model of syntactic processing. There are three Word-level modules, Subject (S), Verb (V), and Object (O). Each module is a fully connected attractor network with $n=10$ pools of excitatory neurons. The ten excitatory pools each have 640 excitatory neurons, and each module has 1600 inhibitory neurons using GABA as the transmitter. Each excitatory pool has recurrent connections with strength $w_+ = 2.1$ to other neurons in the same pool implemented with AMPA and NMDA receptors. There are forward connections with strength w_{ff12} from all excitatory neurons in module 1 (S) to all excitatory neurons in module 2 (V). There are forward connections with strength w_{ff23} from all excitatory neurons in module 2 (V) to all excitatory neurons in module 3 (O). An external bias from a deep, semantic, temporal lobe, pool can be applied to any one or more of the Word-level attractor pools in each of the modules. In operation for production, a stronger bias is applied to one pool in module 1 to start the process, and then an attractor emerges sequentially in time in each of the following modules. The particular Wold-level pool that emerges in each of the later modules depends on which pool in that module is receiving a weak bias from the Deep, semantic, temporal lobe, structure that selects the semantic items to be included in a sentence. The syntax of the sentence, encoded in the order of the items, is determined by the connectivity and dynamics of the Word-level network shown in this figure. The same network can be used for decoding (see text). (After Rolls, E. T. and Deco,G. (2015) Networks for memory, perception, and decision-making, and beyond to how the syntax for language might be implemented in the brain. Brain Research 1621: 316–334. © Elsevier B.V.)

the same cortical area (Rolls, 2016b). In the latter case, the hypothesis is that the stronger connections in one direction than the reverse between nearby modules might be set up by spike-timing dependent plasticity (Markram et al., 1997; Bi and Poo, 1998; Feldman, 2012) based on the temporal order in which the relevant modules were normally activated during a stage when a language was being learned. For the simulations, only weak forward connections were implemented for simplicity.

During operation, one attractor pool in each module receives a continuous bias throughout a trial from a Deep network (see Figs. 14.4 and 14.5). The Deep Network models semantic representations in the anterior temporal lobe. The Word network models syntactic operations in the inferior frontal gyrus. For example the Subject Word module might receive bias from a Deep attractor pool representing 'James', the Verb Word module might receive bias from an attractor pool representing 'chased', and the Object Word module might receive bias from an attractor pool representing 'John'. These biases would represent the deep structure of the sentence, what it is intended to say, but not the generation of the sentence, which is the function of the network shown in Fig. 14.6. The biases in all the modules apart from the first are insufficient to push any attractor pool in a Word module into an attractor state. In the first (or head) Word module, the bias is sufficiently strong to make the attractor pool being biased enter a high firing rate attractor state. The concept is that because of the forward connections to all neurons in the second (Verb Word) module, the attractor pool in the second module receiving a steady bias from the Deep, Verb, pool (in our example, the 'chased' pool) then has sufficient input for it to gradually enter an attractor. The same process is then repeated for the biased attractor in Word module 3 which is being biased by the Deep, semantic, temporal lobe, Object pool, which then enters a high firing rate state. Due to the slow stochastic dynamics of the network, there are delays between the firing in each of the Word modules. It is this that provides the sequentiality to the process that generates the words in the sentence in the correct order.

In addition, a concept of the cortical dynamics of this system is that each module should maintain a level of continuing firing in its winning attractor for the remainder of the sentence, and even for a few seconds afterwards. The purpose of this is to enable correction of the process (by for example a higher order thought or monitoring process, see Rolls (2014a) and Rolls (2020a)) if the process needs to be corrected. The maintenance of the attractors in a continuing state of firing enables monitoring of exactly which attractors did occur in the trajectory through the state space, in case there was a slip of the tongue. (Indeed, 'slips of the tongue' or speech production errors are accounted for in this framework by the somewhat noisy trajectory through the state space that is likely to occur because of the close to Poisson spiking times of the neurons for a given mean rate, which introduces noise into the system (Rolls, 2016b; Rolls and Deco, 2010; Rolls, 2014a)). The main parameters of each module that enable this to be achieved are w_+, and the external bias entering each attractor pool.

However, although it is desired to have a short-term memory trace of previous activity during and for a short time after a sentence, it is also important that each word is uttered at its correct time in the sentence, for this carries the syntactic relations in this system. To achieve the production of the word at the correct time, the firing of each attractor has a mechanism to produce high firing initially for perhaps 200–300 ms, and then lower firing later to maintain an active memory trace of previous neuronal activity. The mechanism used to achieve this initial high firing when a neuronal pool enters a high firing rate state, was spike frequency adaptation, and which has been implemented and utilized previously (Liu and Wang, 2001; Deco and Rolls, 2005c; Rolls and Deco, 2015a).

14.5.5.2 The operation of a single attractor network module

The aim is to investigate the operation of the system in a biophysically realistic attractor framework, so that the properties of receptors, synaptic currents and the statistical effects related to the probabilistic spiking of the neurons can be part of the model. We use a minimal architecture, a single attractor or autoassociation network (Hopfield, 1982; Amit, 1989; Hertz et al., 1991; Rolls and Treves, 1998; Rolls and Deco, 2002; Rolls, 2016b) for each module. A recurrent (attractor) integrate-and-fire network model which includes synaptic channels for AMPA, NMDA and $GABA_A$ receptors (Brunel and Wang, 2001; Rolls and Deco, 2010) was used.

Each Word attractor network contains 6400 excitatory, and 1600 inhibitory neurons, which is consistent with the observed proportions of pyramidal cells and interneurons in the cerebral cortex (Abeles, 1991; Braitenberg and Schüz, 1991). The connection strengths are adjusted using mean-field analysis (Brunel and Wang, 2001; Deco and Rolls, 2006; Rolls and Deco, 2010), so that the excitatory and inhibitory neurons exhibit a spontaneous activity of 3 Hz and 9 Hz, respectively (Wilson et al., 1994b; Koch and Fuster, 1989). The recurrent excitation mediated by the AMPA and NMDA receptors is dominated by the NMDA current to avoid instabilities during delay periods (Wang, 2002).

The architecture of the Word-level cortical attractor network module illustrated in Fig. 14.7 has 10 selective pools each with 640 neurons. The connection weights between the neurons within each pool or population are called the intra-pool connection strengths w_+, which were set to 2.1 for the simulations described. All other weights including w_{inh} were set to 1.

All the excitatory neurons in each Word-level attractor pool S1, S2 ... SN receive an external bias input $\lambda_1, \lambda_2 \ldots \lambda_N$. This external input consists of Poisson external input spikes via AMPA receptors which are envisioned to originate from 800 external neurons. One com-

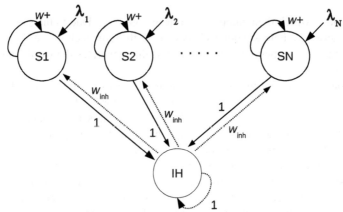

Fig. 14.7 A model of syntactic processing. The architecture of one Word-level module containing one fully connected attractor network. The excitatory neurons are divided into N=10 selective pools or neuronal populations S1–SN of which three are shown, S1, S2 and SN. The synaptic connections have strengths that are consistent with associative learning. In particular, there are strong intra-pool connection strengths w_+. The excitatory neurons receive inputs from the inhibitory neurons with synaptic connection strength w_{inh}=1. The other connection strengths are 1. The integrate-and-fire spiking module contained 8000 neurons, with 640 in each of the 10 non-overlapping excitatory pools, and 1600 in the inhibitory pool IH. Each neuron in the network receives external Poisson inputs λ from 800 external neurons at a typical rate of 3 Hz/synapse to simulate the effect of inputs coming from Deep, semantic, pools. The biasing inputs remain constant during the operation of the whole network to produce an ordered Word-level output sequence. The Word-level module illustrated is similar for the Subject, Verb, and Object Word-level modules. (After Rolls, E. T. and Deco,G. (2015) Networks for memory, perception, and decision-making, and beyond to how the syntax for language might be implemented in the brain. Brain Research 1621: 316–334. © Elsevier B.V.)

ponent of this bias which is present by default arrives at an average spontaneous firing rate of 3 Hz from each external neuron onto each of the 800 synapses for external inputs, consistent with the spontaneous activity observed in the cerebral cortex (Wilson et al., 1994b; Rolls and Treves, 1998; Rolls, 2016b). The second component is a selective bias from a deep structure system which provides a bias present throughout a trial to one of the attractor pools in each module, corresponding to the subject, verb, or object (depending on the module) to be used in the sentence being generated. This bias makes it more likely that the attractor pool will become active if there are other inputs, but is not sufficiently strong (except in the first module) to initiate a high firing rate attractor state. (This selective bias might be set up by associative synaptic modification between the Deep and the Word modules.) In addition, all excitatory neurons in a module receive inputs with a uniform synaptic strength of w_{ff} from all the excitatory neurons in the preceding module, as illustrated in Fig. 14.6.

Both excitatory and inhibitory neurons are represented by a leaky integrate-and-fire model (Tuckwell, 1988). The basic state variable of a single model neuron is the membrane potential. It decays in time when the neurons receive no synaptic input down to a resting potential. When synaptic input causes the membrane potential to reach a threshold, a spike is emitted and the neuron is set to the reset potential at which it is kept for the refractory period. The emitted action potential is propagated to the other neurons in the network. The excitatory neurons transmit their action potentials via the glutamatergic receptors AMPA and NMDA which are both modeled by their effect in producing exponentially decaying currents in the postsynaptic neuron. The rise time of the AMPA current is neglected, because it is typically very short. The NMDA channel is modeled with an alpha function including both a rise and a decay term. In addition, the synaptic function of the NMDA current includes a voltage dependence controlled by the extracellular magnesium concentration (Jahr and Stevens, 1990). The inhibitory postsynaptic potential is mediated by a $GABA_A$ receptor model and is described by a decay term. A detailed mathematical description is provided by Rolls and Deco (2015a).

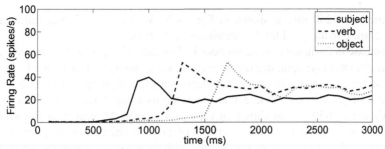

Fig. 14.8 A model of syntactic processing. Firing rates of the biased pools in the Subject–Verb–Object modules as a function of time. (After Rolls, E. T. and Deco,G. (2015) Networks for memory, perception, and decision-making, and beyond to how the syntax for language might be implemented in the brain. Brain Research 1621: 316–334. © Elsevier B.V.)

14.5.5.3 Spike frequency adaptation mechanism

A specific implementation of the spike-frequency adaptation mechanism using Ca^{2+}-activated K^+ hyper-polarizing currents (Liu and Wang, 2001) was implemented. Its parameters were chosen to produce spike frequency adaptation similar in timecourse to that found in the inferior temporal visual cortex of the behaving macaque (Tovee, Rolls, Treves and Bellis, 1993) (Fig. 2.16). In particular, $[Ca^{2+}]$ is initially set to be 0 μM, $\tau_{Ca} = 300$ ms, $\alpha = 0.002$, $V_K = -80$ mV and g_{AHP}=200 nS. (I note that there are a number of other biological mechanisms that might implement the slow transitions from one attractor state to another, some investigated by Deco and Rolls (2005c), and that we use the spike frequency adaptation mechanism to illustrate the principles of operation of the networks.)

14.5.6 Tests of the hypotheses – findings with the model

14.5.6.1 A production system

The operation of the integrate-and-fire system illustrated in Fig. 14.6 is shown in Fig. 14.8 when it is producing a subject – verb – object sequence. The firing rates of attractor pools 1 in Word modules 1 (subject), 2 (verb), and 3 (object) are shown. No other pool had any increase of its firing rate above baseline. The attractor pools 1 in modules 2 and 3 received an increase above the baseline rate of 3.00 Hz per synapse (or 2400 spikes/s per neuron given that each neuron receives these inputs through 800 synapses) to 3.03 Hz per synapse throughout the trial. This itself was insufficient to move any attractor pool in modules 2 and 3 into a high firing rate state, as illustrated, until one of the attractor pools in a preceding module had entered a high firing rate attractor state. At time = 500 ms, the external input into attractor pool 1 of module 1 (subject) was increased to 3.20 Hz per synapse, and maintained at this value for the rest of the trial. This produced after a little delay due to the stochastic recurrent dynamics an increase in the firing of pool 1 in module 1, which peaked at approximately 1000 ms. The initial peak firing rate of approximately 40 spikes/s was followed by a reduction due to the spike frequency adaptation to approximately 25 spikes/s, and this level was maintained for the remainder of the trial, as shown in Fig. 14.8. The parameters for the spike frequency adaptation for all the excitatory neurons in the network were V_k=-80 mV, g_{AHP}=200 nS, α_{Ca}=0.002, and $\tau_{Ca} = 300$ ms.

The increase in the firing in attractor pool 1 of module 1 influenced the neurons in module 2 via the feedforward synaptic strength of w_{ff12}=0.55, and, because attractor pool 1 in module 2 already had a weak external bias from the Deep, semantic, Verb level to help it be selected, it was attractor pool 1 in module 2 that increased its firing, with the peak rate occurring at approximately 1250 ms, as shown in Fig. 14.8. Again, the peak was followed by low maintained firing in this pool for the remainder of the trial.

The increase in the firing in attractor pool 1 of module 2 influenced the neurons in module 3 via the feedforward synaptic strength of w_{ff23}=0.4, and, because attractor pool 1 in module 3 already had a weak external bias from the Deep, semantic, object pool to help it be selected, it was attractor pool 1 in module 3 that increased its firing, with the peak rate occurring at approximately 1650 ms, as shown in Fig. 14.8. Again, the peak was followed by low maintained firing in this pool for the remainder of the trial. The value of w_{ff23} was optimally a little lower than that of w_{ff12}, probably because with the parameters used the firing in module 2 was somewhat higher than that in module 1. All subsequent stages would be expected to operate with w_{ff}=0.4.

The network thus shows that the whole system can reliably perform a trajectory that is sequential and delayed at each step through the state space, with the item selected in each module determined by the steady bias being received from a deep structure containing the semantic items to be included in the sentence. However, the order in which the items were produced and which specified the syntax was determined by the connectivity and dynamics of the Word network. In this particular example, the resulting sentence might correspond to 'James chased John', which has a completely different syntax and meaning to 'John chased James', 'chased John James', etc. The peak of firing in each module could be used to produce the appropriate word in the correct order. The lower rate of ongoing firing in each module provided the basis for the items produced in the sentence to be remembered and used for monitoring, with the role of each item in the sentence made explicit by the module in which the attractor pool was still active.

14.5.6.2 A decoding system

In Section 14.5.6.1 the operation of the system when it is operating to produce a subject–verb–object sequence in which the temporal sequence encodes syntactic information is described. In this section, the operation of the system when it decodes a Subject–Verb–Object sentence is considered. The aim is to receive as input the temporal sequence, and to activate the correct attractor in the Subject, Verb, and Object Word attractor modules. The syntactic information in the sequence allows correct decoding of the subject and object nouns in the sentence, when the position in the sequence is the only information that enables a noun to activate a noun attractor in the subject or the object module. The deep semantic attractor modules could then be activated from the Word attractor modules, using selective, associatively modifiable, synaptic connections.

The operation of the system in decoding mode is illustrated in Fig. 14.9. The architecture of the network is the same as that already described. The baseline input to each of the 800 external synapses is maintained at 3 Hz per synapse in all pools in all modules throughout the sentence except where stated. Throughout the trial all pools in module 1 receive a bias of 0.24 Hz on each of the 800 external input synapses. (This corresponds to an extra 192 spikes/s received by every neuron in each of attractor pools.) The aim of this is to prepare all the attractors in module 1, the subject attractor, to respond if an input cue, a word, is received. This bias essentially sets the system into a mode where it is waiting for an input stream to arrive in module 1. All the attractors in module 1 are stable with low firing rates while only this bias is being applied.

At time 500–1000 ms module 1 pool 1 and module 3 pool 1 receive a noun recall cue as an additional input on the external synapses at an additional 0.08 Hz per synapse. (This corresponds to an extra 64 spikes/s received by every neuron in these two pools of neurons.) Module 1 pool 1 goes into an attractor, as illustrated in Fig. 14.9, because it is receiving a noun recall cue and the bias. Module 3 pool 1 does not enter a high firing rate attractor state,

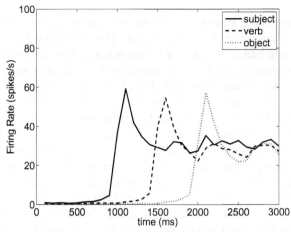

Fig. 14.9 A model of syntactic processing. Decoding the Subject–Verb–Object sequence to produce activation in the Subject (module 1), Verb (module 2), and Object (module 3) modules. A weak bias was applied to all pools in module 1 throughout the trial (see text). Noun 1, the subject, was applied to module 1 pool 1 and module 3 pool 1 during the period 500–1000 ms. Verb 2, was applied to module 2 pool 2 during the period 1000–1500 ms. Noun 3, the object, was applied to module 1 pool 3 and module 3 pool 3 during the period 1500–2000 ms. The firing of module 1 attractor 1 neurons that reflect the decoded subject, of module 2 attractor 2 neurons that reflect the decoded verb, and of module 3 attractor 3 neurons that reflect the decoded object, are shown. None of the other 30 attractor neural populations became active. (After Rolls, E. T. and Deco,G. (2015) Networks for memory, perception, and decision-making, and beyond to how the syntax for language might be implemented in the brain. Brain Research 1621: 316–334. © Elsevier B.V.)

even though the word recall cue for its attractor 1 is being applied, because it is not receiving a bias. This shows how the system can decode correctly a noun due to its position in the sequence as a subject or as an object. In the simulations the bias to pool 1 can be left on, or turned off at this stage in the trial, for once an attractor state has been reached by a pool in module 1, it remains with a stable high firing rate for the remainder of the sentence. The continuing firing is implemented to ensure that the subject remains decoded in the system while the rest of the sentence is decoded, and for use even after the end of the sentence. At time 1000 ms, the noun applied to attractor pools 1 in modules 1 and 3 is removed, as it is no longer present in the environment.

At time 1000–1500 ms the verb recall cue is applied to module 2 pool 2, which enters an attractor. The strength of this recall cue alone (the same as before, an additional 0.08 Hz per synapse) is insufficient to cause this pool in module 2 to enter an attractor. However, all pools in module 2 are receiving now via the feed-forward connections w_{ff12} a priming input from the firing now occurring in module 1, and when the verb recall cue is applied to module 2 pool 2, the combined effects of the recall cue and the feedforward inputs cause module 2 pool 2 to enter its correct attractor state to indicate the presence of this verb in the sentence. The intention of the priming forward input from the preceding module is to provide for future expansion of the system, to allow for example correct decoding of two verbs at different positions within the sequence of words in a sentence. Module 2 pool 2 has the Verb recall cue removed at time 1500 ms as it is no longer present in the environment. Module 2 pool 2 however keeps firing in its stable high firing rate attractor state to ensure that the verb remains decoded in the system while the rest of the sentence is decoded, and for use even after the end of the sentence.

At time 1500–2000 ms the object recall cue is applied to module 3 pool 3, and, as a control and test of the syntactic operation of the system, simultaneously also to module 1 pool 3. Module 3 pool 3 enters its correct object attractor, utilising the feedforward priming inputs w_{ff23}. These priming inputs again provide for further expansion of the system, in case there is another object in the sentence in a later clause. Meanwhile module 1 remains in its pool 1 subject attractor state which is now stable in the face of interfering noun inputs because of its deep low energy basin of attraction. This shows how this noun is forced by its order in the sequence into the Object pool, demonstrating how the system is able to decode information about syntactic role that is present from the position of the item in the sequence. Module 3 pool 3 keeps firing in its stable high firing rate attractor state to ensure that the object remains decoded in the system for use even after the end of the sentence.

As noted, the architecture and overall dynamical principles of operation of the system used for decoding were the same as for encoding. The firing rate adaption was left to operate as before, though it is less useful for the decoding. The only parameters that were adjusted a little for the decoding system were $w_+ = 2.3$ (to help stability of the high firing rate attractor state in the face of for example interfering nouns); $w_{ff12} = w_{ff23} = 0.2$; bias for all pools in module 1 $= 0.24$ Hz per synapse; and recall cue $= 0.08$ Hz per synapse.

The results just described and illustrated in Fig. 14.9 illustrate some of the principles of operation of the functional architecture when decoding sentences. Further results were as follows. If during the application of the noun for the subject (time 500–1000 ms in the simulations) an input effective for an attractor in module 2 was also applied, then a pool in module 2 tends to enter a high firing rate attractor state, for it is receiving both a recall cue and the forward bias from the high firing starting in module 1 and applied to module 2 via w_{ff12}. An implication is that only nouns should be applied to Subject and Object attractor modules. Having attractors for verbs that respond to different recall cues (words that are verbs) helps the system to decode the input stream into the correct modules and pools. Thus the semantics, the words being applied to the network, are important in enabling the system to respond correctly.

14.5.7 Evaluation of the hypotheses

The system described here shows how a word production system might operate using neuronal architecture of the type found in the cerebral cortex.

One possible objection to such a computational implementation is how to deal with the passive form. What I propose is that temporal order could again be used, but with different coupling between the attractors appropriate for implementing the passive voice that is again learned by early experience, and is selected instead of the active voice by top-down bias in the general way that we have described elsewhere (Deco and Rolls, 2003, 2005d). The hypothesis is thus that operation of the system for passive sentences would require a different set of connections to be used to generate the correct temporal trajectory through these or possible different modules, with the head of the sentence no longer being (in English) the subject (e.g. James in 'James chased John'), but instead the object (e.g. 'John was chased by James').

In a similar way, it is proposed that different languages are implemented by different forward connectivity between the different modules representing subjects, verbs, and objects in that language, with the connectivity for each language learned by repeated experience and forced trajectories during learning using for example spike-timing-dependent plasticity. Separate neuronal implementation of different languages is consistent with neurological evidence that after brain damage one language but not another may be impaired.

The system would require considerable elaboration to provide for adjectives and adjectival phrases qualifying the subject or the object, and for adverbs or adverbial phrases qualifying the verbs, but a possible principle is stronger synaptic connectivity between the modules in which the qualifiers are represented. To be specific, one type of implementation might have adjectives in modules that qualify subjects connected with relatively stronger synapses to subject modules than to object modules. This should be feasible given that any one attractor network capable of encoding thousands of words need occupy only 2–3 mm of neocortical area.

In such a system, the problem does arise of how the nouns in the subject attractor module can refer to the same object in the word as the nouns in the object attractor, and of the extent to which when one representation (e.g. in the subject module) is updated by modifying its properties (encoded by which neurons are active in the sparse distributed representation within a module), the representation of the same object in another module (e.g. in the object module) is updated to correspond.

The results on the operation of the system when it is decoding a sentence illustrated in Fig. 14.9 illustrate how the temporal sequence of the words can be used to place them into the appropriate module, for example to place a noun into a subject or an object module. Interestingly, if during the application of the noun for the subject (time 500–1000 ms in the simulations) an input effective for an attractor in module 2 (the verb module) was also applied, then a pool in module 2 tended to enter a high firing rate attractor state, for it was receiving both a recall cue and the forward bias from the high firing starting in module 1 and applied to module 2 via w_{ff12}. An implication is that only nouns should be applied to Subject and Object attractors. Having attractors for verbs that respond to different input cue (words that are verbs) helps the system to decode the input stream into the correct modules and pools. Thus the semantics, the words being applied to the network, are important in enabling the system to respond correctly.

Indeed, overall the system might be thought of as having different modules and pools for different types of word (subject noun, object noun, verb, adverb, adjective, etc) and using the match of the incoming word to the word defined in a module to provide an important cue to which module should have an attractor activated, and then adding to this the temporal sequence sensitivity also considered here to help disambiguate the syntax, for example whether a noun is a subject or an object. Thus the semantics, the word as a noun, verb, or potentially adjective or adverb, help the dynamics because the cue details (adverb, noun, verb, adjective etc) provides constraints on the trajectories and dynamics of the system, and thus on how it decodes input sequences.

Language would thus be brittle if there were not subject-noun, object-noun, verb, adjective, adverb etc pools. It is proposed that the inflections in an inflected language help words to activate the correct pools. For example, if an inflection was present in a word that indicated it was the subject of the sentence, then the inflection suffix acting as a bias on the Word-level Subject attractor network could encourage the Subject attractor network to be activated by and enter an attractor state for that word. If inflections are lost or not present in a language, then the order in a sequence can compensate to some extent, but the system still relies on the words activating selective pools, with the temporal dynamics used for example to disambiguate matters if a noun might otherwise be a subject or an object, or an adjective might qualify a subject vs an object, etc. Moreover, because language is often irregular, particular words must also favour particular dynamics / relations.

In such a stochastic dynamical system (Rolls, 2016b; Rolls and Deco, 2010), speech or writing errors such as words appearing in the incorrect order, word substitution, and repetition of the same word, could be easily accounted for by failures in the stochastically influenced (Rolls, 2016b; Rolls and Deco, 2010) transitions from one attractor to the next, and in the word selected in each attractor. This supports the proposed account of the cortical implementation of language.

Overall, in this Section the coding and dynamical principles of the operation of the cerebral cortex have been considered in the context of how they may be relevant to the implementation of language in the cerebral cortex. It has been proposed that the high capacity of local attractor networks in the neocortex would provide a useful substrate for representations of words with different syntactical roles, for example subject noun, object noun, adjective modifying a subject, adjective modifying an object, verb, and adverb. With this as a principle of operation, in an inflected language the words produced can have the appropriate suffix (typically) added to specify the module from which it originated and therefore its syntactic role in the sentence. In an inflected language, the inflections added to words can indicate case, person etc, and during decoding of the sentence (when listening or reading) these inflections can be used to help the word to activate attractors in the correct module. In a language without inflections, or that is losing inflections, the order in the sequence can be used to supplement the information present in the word to help activate a representation in the correct attractor. Examples of how cortical dynamics might help in this process both during production and during decoding are provided in the simulations in this Chapter (Rolls and Deco, 2015a).

Interestingly, at least during decoding, temporal dynamics alone was found to be brittle in enabling words to be decoded by the correct module, and the system was found to work much more robustly if words find matches only in different specialized modules, for example with nouns being decodable by only subject noun or object noun modules, verbs only by verb modules, etc. The actual decoding is of course a great strength of the type of attractor neuronal network approach described here, for attractor networks are beautifully suited to performing such decoding based on the vector dot product similarity of the recall cue to what is stored in the network (Rolls, 2016b; Hopfield, 1982; Amit, 1989). The implication is that content addressable specialized word attractor cortical modules are important in the implementation of language, and that temporal dynamics utilizing the order of a word in the sequence can be used to help disambiguate the syntactic role of a word being received by enabling it to activate a representation in the correct module, using mechanisms of the general type described.

This raises the interesting point that in the present proposal, the syntactic role of a representation is encoded in the brain by the particular cortical module that is active, with different cortical modules for different parts of speech. An implication is that for the internal operations of this syntactical system, the syntax is encoded by the module within which the representation is active, and this is a form of place coding. Much may be computed internally by such a system based on this specification of the syntactic role of each module in the thought process. The problem arises when these thoughts must be communicated to others. Then a production system is needed, and in this system the syntactic role of which module the representation arises from can be specified partly by the word itself (with noun words indicating that they arise from a subject or object noun representations, verb words indicating that they arise from a verb module); and this specification is supported by inflection and/or by temporal order information to help disambiguate the module from which the word originates. Then during decoding of a sentence, the word again allows it to match only certain modules, with inflection and/or order in the sequence being used to disambiguate the module that should be activated by the word.

Thus an internal language of thought may be implemented by allocating different cortical modules to different syntactic roles, and using place encoding. However, when language becomes externalized in the process of communication, the way in which language can be used as a computational mechanism may be enhanced. Once a language has the rules that allow syntactic role to be expressed in for example written form, this enables formal syntactic operations including logic to be checked in an extended argument or algorithm or proof, and this then provides language with much greater power, providing a basis for formal reasoned extended argument, which may not be a general property of neuronal network operations (Rolls, 2016b), and which facilitates the use of the reasoned route to action (Rolls, 2014a).

One of the hypotheses considered here is that place coding in quite small cortical modules approximately the size of a cortical column (i.e. a region within which there is a high density of local recurrent collaterals to support attractor functionality, and within which local inhibitory neurons operate) may be used to encode the syntactic role of a word might not easily reveal itself at the brain lesion or functional neuroimaging levels, which generally operate with less resolution than this. For example, such studies of the effects of brain damage and of activations do not provide clear evidence for segregation by syntactic role, such as noun-selective vs verb-selective areas (Vigliocco et al., 2011). Although effects produced by nouns vs verbs do segregate to some extent into the temporal and frontal lobes, this may be because the semantic associations of nouns with objects, and verbs with actions, will tend to activate different cortical areas because of the semantic not purely because of the syntactic difference (Vigliocco et al., 2011). One of the hypotheses developed here is that nouns as subjects and nouns as objects may use different place coding, and one way that this might become evident in future is if single neuron recordings from language areas support this. Indeed, it is a specific and testable prediction of the approach described here that some neurons in language-related cortical areas will have responses to words that depend on the syntactic role of the word. For example, such a neuron might respond preferentially to a noun word when it is a subject compared to when it is an object.

It will be interesting in future to investigate whether this approach based on known principles of cortical computation can be extended to show whether it could provide at least a part of the biological foundation for the implementation of language in the brain. Because of its use of place coding, the system would not be recursive. But language may not be recursive, and indeed some of the interesting properties but also limitations of language may be understood in future as arising from the limitations of its biological implementation.

I note that there are a number of biological mechanisms that might implement the slow transitions from one attractor state to another, some investigated by Deco and Rolls (2005c), and that we are not wedded to any particular mechanism. The speed with which the trajectory through the state space of attractors is executed will depend on factors such as the magnitude of the inputs including the biassing inputs, the strengths of the synapses between the modules, the NMDA dynamics, the effects of finite size noise which will be influenced by the number of spiking neurons, the dilution of the connectivity, and the graded nature of the firing (Rolls and Deco, 2010; Webb et al., 2011; Rolls and Webb, 2012). An implication is that the speed of speech production might be influenced by factors that influence for example NMDA receptors, such as dopamine via D1 receptors (Rolls and Deco, 2010).

One such extension in the future of the approach taken in this Chapter would be to extend the implementation from a single cortical attractor network for each linguistic type (subject nouns, object nouns, verbs, etc) to a set of attractor networks for each linguistic type. If each single local cortical attractor network could store say S patterns (the p referred to above), then how would the system operate with M such attractor nets or modules? There would be two types of connection in such a system. One would be the synaptic connections between the neurons in each attractor network or module. The other connections would be the typically weaker connections between cortical modules (see Rolls (2016b)). The whole system of coupled interacting attractor nets is known as a Potts attractor (Treves, 2005; Kropff and Treves, 2005; Akrami, Russo and Treves, 2012; Song, Yao and Treves, 2014; Ryom, Stendardi, Ciaramelli and Treves, 2023). In a language system representing for example nouns, one attractor net or 'unit' in Potts terminology might contain properties such as shape, another color, another texture, etc, and the full semantic description of the object might be represented by which attractors in which of the M modules are active, that is in a high firing rate state. One advantage of such a system is that all of the properties of an object could be encoded in this way, so we could specify whether the hat is round, red, smooth in texture, etc. Associated with this advantage, the total capacity of the system, that is the number of possible objects that could be represented, is now proportional to S^2. Thus if a single attractor network could store $S=10,000$ items (10^4), a Potts system with 5 such modules might be able to represent of order 5×10^8 such objects. In more detail, the number of patterns P_c that can be represented over the Potts attractor is

$$P_c \approx c_M S^2 / a_M \tag{14.2}$$

where c_M is the number of other modules on average with which a module is connected, S is the number of different attractor states within any one module, and a_M is the proportion of the attractor modules in which there is an active attractor, i.e. a high firing rate attractor state (Treves, 2005; Kropff and Treves, 2005). Such a Potts system only works well if (1) long-range connections between the different modules are non-uniformly distributed and (2) only a sparse set of the modules (measured by a_M) is in a high firing rate attractor state (Treves, 2005). In principle, the dynamical system described here could be replaced by substituting each cortical word type module (e.g. that for subject nouns) with a Potts attractor system each with several attractor network modules coding for different properties of features such as shape, color, texture, etc.

An overview at present is that such a Potts system might be useful for a semantic network (Treves, 2005; Ryom et al., 2023), which might correspond to the deep network that biases the word modules in the architecture described in this Chapter. That semantic system would then bias the word modules (with one cortical module for each type of word, subject noun etc), and this architecture might have the advantage that word representations may be more uncorrelated than are semantic representations, which would keep the word representation capacity high. However, in the Potts system simulated so far to model language, the units corresponded to semantic features not to words; and place coding was not used, with instead the syntactic roles of the semantic representations requiring further Potts units to specify the syntactic roles of the semantic units (Pirmoradian and Treves, 2013).

Treves (2005) also considered how such a Potts system might have dynamics that might display some of the properties of language. Adaptation was introduced into each of the attractor networks. After a population of neurons had been active in a high firing rate state in one attractor module for a short time, due to adaptation in that neuronal population, the system then jumped to another attractor state in the same module, or in another connected module a jump might occur to another attractor state, because its inputs had changed due to the adaptation in the other module. The result was a latching process that resulted in complex dynamics of the overall system (Treves, 2005; Song et al., 2014). Whether that complex dynamics is how language is produced has not been proven yet. My view here is that there are sensory inputs from the world, or remembered states that enter short-term memory, and that these states in the deep, semantic, networks then bias the word networks to produce the sequential stream of language. That keeps the processing not a random trajectory through a state space perhaps biased by the statistics of the correlations within a language, but instead a trajectory useful for communication that reflects the states produced by the world or recalled into memory and that can then be communicated to others as a stream of words.

14.5.8 Further approaches

It has been argued that connectionist approaches to language that rely on Elman-style discrete step recurrent networks (Elman, 1990), which take account only of word sequence and have no representation of global structure, cannot capture typical syntax (Jackendoff, 2002, 2003, 2007).

Jackendoff has proposed a Parallel Architecture approach to the structure of grammar that contrasts with mainstream generative grammar in that (a) it treats phonology, syntax, and semantics as independent generative components whose structures are linked by interface rules; (b) it uses a parallel constraint-based formalism that is non-directional; and (c) it treats words and rules alike as pieces of linguistic structure stored in long-term memory (Jackendoff, 2002,

2003, 2007). He proposes that the following processes are involved, but does not take them as far as to propose how they are implemented in the brain:

1. Phonetic processing provides strings of phonemes in phonological working memory.
2. The phonemic strings initiate a call to the lexicon in long-term memory, seeking candidate words that match parts of the strings.
3. Activated lexical items set up candidate phonological parsings, often in multiple drafts, each draft linked to a lexical item or sequence of lexical items.
4. Activated lexical items also set up corresponding strings of syntactic units and collections of semantic units in the relevant departments of working memory.
5. Syntactic integration proceeds right away, by activating and binding to treelets stored in the lexicon.
6. When semantic integration depends on syntactic constituency, it cannot begin until syntactic integration of the relevant constituents is complete. (However, semantic integration does not have to wait for the entire sentence to be syntactically integrated–only for local constituents.)
7. Semantic disambiguation among multiple drafts requires semantic integration with the context (linguistic or non-linguistic). In general semantic disambiguation will therefore be slower than syntactic disambiguation.
8. The last step in disambiguation is the suppression of phonological candidates by feedback.

Models of reading, mainly at the computational not neuroscience level, are described by Reichle (2021). Neurocomputational models of language processing are reviewed by Hale, Campanelli, Li, Bhattasali, Pallier and Brennan (2022).

In conclusion, I have described new hypotheses in this Chapter about how some of the principles of cortical computation used to implement episodic memory, short-term memory, perception, attention, and decision-making (Rolls, 2016b; Rolls and Deco, 2015a) might contribute to the implementation of language including syntax in the cortex. What I have proposed is quite different in its implementation to the systems that follow formal syntactic rules in many neurolinguistic approaches to syntax and language. My proposal is that a series of linked cortical attractors learn what regularities there are in the use of language to which the listener is exposed; and that such attractor networks can also learn the exceptions to the syntactic rules which apply when perhaps particular keywords trigger the system into a trajectory through a different set of Word-level modules. Thus the system I propose is a mechanism for how the syntactic rules of language could be learned by a set of coupled attractor networks, that is, by a dynamical system.

This is a major frontier in neuroscience, and much remains to be done on how language and syntax may be implemented in the cerebral cortex.

15 The motor cortical areas

15.1 Introduction and overview

Some of the main cortical areas involved in the initiation and control of movement are shown in Fig. 15.1 (Rizzolatti and Kalaska, 2013; Scott and Kalaska, 2021; Giarrocco and Averbeck, 2021). A key feature is the hierarchical organisation, with inputs from parietal cortex areas projecting to premotor cortical areas in BA 6, which project to the primary motor cortex. Although the organisation is hierarchical, motor neurons for output descend to subcortical and spinal cord regions from all of these areas. Area 4 is special in its motor outputs, which make direct connections to spinal cord motor neurons for fine control of the hands. Further, although the organization is overall hierarchical, there is specialization of different parietal and premotor areas for different functions as described in this Chapter. In addition there are separate pathways for the control of eye movements (Goldberg and Walker, 2021).

The somatosensory areas 1, 2, and 3 (described in Section 6.1.2) and area PE provide somatosensory input (including touch and proprioceptive information) to M1 (F1) (area 4). Area M1 (or F1) contains a large sector that controls the fingers, hand, and wrist. The precentral motor cortical areas include the primary motor cortex (M1, F1); F5, a subdivision of PMv; and the ventral premotor cortex (Fig. 15.1).

In terms of processing streams, the visuomotor transformation necessary for reaching is mediated by the parietofrontal network shown in Fig. 15.1 (Rizzolatti and Kalaska, 2013; Scott and Kalaska, 2021; Giarrocco and Averbeck, 2021). The areas located within the intraparietal sulcus are shown in an unfolded view of the sulcus. Two serial pathways are involved in the organization of reaching movements. The ventral stream has its principal nodes in the ventral intraparietal area (VIP) and area F4 of the ventral premotor cortex, whereas the dorsal stream has synaptic relays in the superior parietal lobe (MIP, V6A) and the dorsal premotor cortex (PMd), which includes area F2. (The parietal areas include AIP, anterior intraparietal area; LIP, lateral intraparietal area; and V6A, the parietal portion of the parieto-occipital area.)

The visuomotor transformation necessary for grasping is mediated by the parietofrontal network shown in Fig. 15.1 (Rizzolatti and Kalaska, 2013; Scott and Kalaska, 2021; Giarrocco and Averbeck, 2021). The AIP and PFG areas are concerned mostly with hand movements, whereas area PF is concerned with mouth movements. Area F5 in PMv is concerned with both hand and mouth motor acts. Some grasping neurons have been found in F2, the ventral part of PMd.

The representations in these cortical areas provide evidence about what is computed in these areas, and are described next.

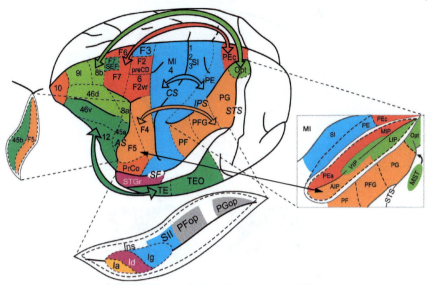

Fig. 15.1 Motor and premotor cortical areas in the macaque and some of their connections. The motor cortex area 4, M1, is anterior to the central sulcus (CS), and is part of the precentral cortex. The premotor cortex area 6 is the area just anterior to this, with subdivisions F2, F4, F5, etc. There are major inputs to premotor cortical areas from the parietal cortex, from areas within the intraparietal sulcus (IPS, opened, right) for reaching, and from more ventral parietal areas such as PF and PFG for grasping. AS, arcuate sulcus; CS, central sulcus; IPS, intraparietal sulcus; SF, Sylvian fissure (opened, below); STS, superior temporal sulcus; F3, supplementary motor cortex; F6, pre-SMA; S1, 1,2,3 - primary somatosensory cortex; Ins, insula; Opt, parietal region Opt. (Adapted from Giarrocco,F. and Averbeck,B.B. 2021. Organization of parieto-prefrontal and temporo-prefrontal networks in the macaque. Journal of Neurophysiology 126: 1289-1309.)

15.2 What is computed in different cortical motor-related areas

15.2.1 Ventral parietal and ventral premotor cortex F4

One of the ventral parietal areas, the ventral intraparietal cortex (VIP) (Fig. 15.1A), receives projections from MT (medial temporal) and MST (medial superior temporal) (see Chapter 3). Neurons in VIP respond to visual stimuli moving in peripersonal space, and some neurons combine this with tactile somatosensory responses to stimuli in a corresponding part of peripersonal space. The tactile receptive fields are often on the face or hands or arms. These neurons may respond for example to a visual stimulus moving towards a tactile receptive field. This type of visual-tactile responsiveness could be set up by associative learning from much previous experience. There are strong connections from VIP to ventral premotor area F4, in which most of the neurons respond to tactile stimuli, and about half to corresponding visual stimuli. The implication is that the spatial reference frame for these visual neurons might be parts of the body.

15.2.2 Superior parietal areas with activity related to reaching

Neurons in superior parietal areas such as PEc, V6 and MIP (Fig. 15.1) often respond to visual stimuli involved in reaching, and the coordinate frame reflects not only retinal and eye position but also arm posture and hand position. In PEip the neurons are more related to arm posture and hand position. The dorsal premotor neurons to which these parietal areas project are strongly influenced by the direction of movement to the target, rather than by visual stimuli. Some of these neurons respond to the shape of the object depending on how the object can be grasped. These cortical regions are described further in Section 3.6.

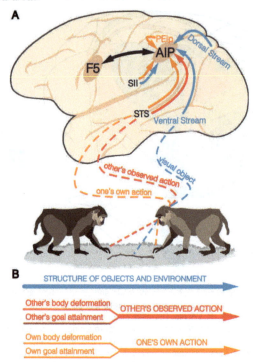

Fig. 15.2 Convergence of visual objects, observed actions, and own hand visual and proprioceptive signals in Posterior Parietal Cortex territories devoted to manipulative actions. A Own action planning benefits from (1) motor affordances provided by the 3D structure of objects and the environment (blue), (2) social affordances provided by others' observed actions (red), (3) own actions' visual and somatosensory/proprioceptive feedback from the subject's body (orange). Distinct anatomo-functional visual components of observed actions can be identified in the goal-attainment signals (rostral STS) and body movement signals (middle STS) concerning the observed actions of others, which are paralleled by the analysis of visual/proprioceptive feedback from the subject's own actions (conveyed by the STS, PEip, SII, and F5, particularly concerning haptic information about the manipulated object). B Schematic view of the different signals that contribute to the encoding of the physical properties of objects and the environment, the subject's own actions, and others' actions. PEip intraparietal area PE; SII secondary somatosensory cortex; STS superior temporal sulcus. (From Orban,G.A., Sepe,A. and Bonini,L. 2021. Parietal maps of visual signals for bodily action planning. Brain Structure and Function 226: 2967-2988.)

15.2.3 Inferior parietal areas with activity related to grasping, and ventral premotor cortex F5

Neurons in inferior parietal areas such as AIP and PFG (Fig. 15.1) frequently respond when looking at an object and/or when grasping it, and were made famous by the pioneering studies of Mountcastle, Sakata and colleagues (Mountcastle, Lynch, Georgopoulos, Sakata and Acuna, 1975). These areas project to ventral premotor cortex area F5, where neurons can encode the nature of the grasp needed to grip objects with different shapes (Murata et al., 1997). The pathways implicated in manipulative actions are illustrated in Fig. 15.2 (Orban et al., 2021b,a; Urgen and Orban, 2021).

These cortical regions are described further in Section 3.6.

15.3 The mirror neuron system

Neurons with movement-related activity in for example premotor cortex area F5 and in the parietal cortex respond to the sight of grasping an object, as well as to actually grasping an object, in the mirror neuron system shown in Fig. 15.3 (Rizzolatti and Craighero, 2004; Rizzolatti and Sinigaglia, 2016; Rizzolatti and Rozzi, 2018). It has been suggested that the mirror

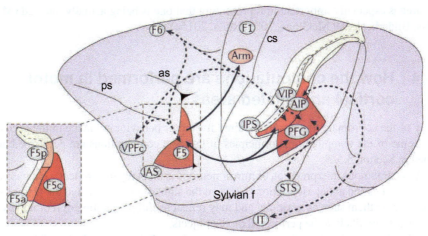

Fig. 15.3 The monkey parietofrontal mirror network for hand-grasping actions. Lateral view of the macaque monkey brain localizing the main areas that are involved in action observation with mirror neurons: the ventral premotor cortex (area F5), area PFG, and the anterior intraparietal area (AIP). The intraparietal sulcus (IPS) has been opened to show the areas inside. The parietofrontal network receives high-order visual information from areas that are located inside the superior temporal sulcus (STS) and inferior temporal lobule (IT). Neither of these temporal regions has mirror properties. Area F5 is connected with area F1, which also contains mirror neurons. The parietofrontal circuit is under the control of the frontal lobe (area F6 or pre-supplementary motor area and ventral prefrontal cortex (vPFC)). The inset shows an enlarged view of area F5, displaying its sectors buried inside the arcuate sulcus. The label 'Arm' indicates the area where the arm is represented. IAS, inferior limb of the arcuate sulcus; VIP, ventral intraparietal area; as, arcuate sulcus; cs, central sulcus; ps, principal sulcus; Sf, Sylvian fissure. (Reproduced from Rizzolatti,G. and Sinigaglia,C. (2016) The mirror mechanism: a basic principle of brain function. Nature Reviews Neuroscience 17: 757–765. © Springer Nature.)

mechanism transforms sensory representations of others' actions into motor representations of the same actions in the brain of the observer (Rizzolatti and Rozzi, 2018). The implication is that this is useful for observational learning. It has also been suggested that the mirror mechanism plays an important role in understanding actions of others (Rizzolatti and Rozzi, 2018).

As shown in Section 6.1.6 mirror-neuron-like effects are not restricted to systems in which visual and motor representations are found, but can also be produced even in the human primary somatosensory cortex S1 by the sight of touch to the arm, as well as by touch to the arm (McCabe, Rolls, Bilderbeck and McGlone, 2008). Comparison of the sight of an arm being rubbed with cream to a visual control with no contact revealed effects in the inferior frontal gyrus (corresponding probably to F5 in the monkey, a mirror neuron area in which neurons respond to motor actions and to the sight of the action being performed (Rizzolatti and Craighero, 2004)), area 7, and even the primary somatosensory cortex S1, implicating these regions in the imagined or intentional aspects of touch (McCabe et al., 2008). Although neurons in S1 are not activated by most visual or auditory stimuli, effects can be found if these stimuli are relevant to somatosensory processing, such as the sound of a stimulus rubbing the skin (Delhaye et al., 2018). Thus the construct that mirror neurons are present especially for the sight of movements such as grasping and the actual movement of grasping does not seem to be supported by what happens in the somatosensory system. We may be dealing more with anatomical convergence that allows such affects to be learned by association, and that includes the evidence that backprojections in the cortex can learn the correct associations to recall activity in early cortical processing areas (Rolls, 2016b). It was found that the sight of touch did not activate somatosensory regions in the insula, and it was therefore proposed that this area is especially important in representing that one is being actually touched (McCabe, Rolls, Bilderbeck and McGlone, 2008; Rolls, 2016a).

15.4 How the computations are performed in motor cortical and related areas

Many of the coordinate transforms required for motor behavior are made in the parietal cortex. Some of the computational principles of how the computations are performed are described in Section 3.5.

A parsimonious interpretation of mirror neurons is that they may reflect what has been associatively learned about associations between the sight of objects etc and the actions needed to operate on them such as grasping, and may reflect useful preparation of motor systems for actions that are likely to be performed on the objects.

'Visual fixation' and similar neurons in parietal area 7 that respond when objects are visually fixated and when movements are made for the objects were described as 'command neurons' (Mountcastle, Lynch, Georgopoulos, Sakata and Acuna, 1975) that reflected goals and motivation. However, when compared with orbitofrontal cortex neurons, the parietal neurons do not reflect reward value, in that they respond as much when a non-reward object is fixated as a reward object, and do not decrease their responses when the value is reduced by feeding to satiety (Rolls, Perrett, Thorpe, Puerto, Roper-Hall and Maddison, 1979a) (Section 6.1.4). The neurons reflect instead whether an action is likely to be performed on the object, independently of its reward value. Actions may be made for example to reject aversive objects, and then parietal neurons are active. Thus many parietal neurons appear to be involved in action rather than reward value.

16 The basal ganglia

16.1 Introduction and overview

1. The basal ganglia provides an evolutionarily old system that receives from many of whatever higher parts of the brain are present, and helps to produce a single output stream of behavior.
2. In mammals, the layer 5 neurons of every part of the neocortex provide the main excitatory inputs to the striatum, which is stage 1 of the computation.
   Each part of the cortex projects primarily to its own part of the striatum.
   The striatum then sends its outputs to the globus pallidus and substantia nigra pars reticularis, where there is convergence to produce what is largely a single output stream with further selection performed by the mutual inhibition between the principal neurons.
   Although earlier in evolution the outputs may have been directed to lower brain output systems, in mammals the outputs return via the thalamus to the cortex.
   The probable role in mammals is still to select a single output stream, but for this to exert its effects through influences on the cerebral cortex.
   These anatomical pathways are shown schematically Fig. 16.1, with the location of the parts of the basal ganglia shown in Fig. 16.2. These diagrams show the connectivity in primates (including humans), and the treatment here is for primate including human brains, as rodents appear to have such less well developed and computationally separate cortical regions, and because reward processing is so different in rodents, with reward influencing even early sensory processing (see Section 19.10).
3. The response selection is performed by mutual inhibition between the principal neurons in both the striatum and the globus pallidus using the inhibitory transmitter GABA (gamma-amino-butyric acid). There is no recurrent excitation as in the cortex, so short-term memory and planning are beyond the computational capabilities of the basal ganglia.
4. Instead, the functions of the basal ganglia include learning of stimulus-response combinations to produce habits, which are well-learned responses.
5. The learning is facilitated by reinforcement learning in which a third term, dopamine neuron firing, which provides a reward prediction error signal, increases the learning rate for whatever stimulus-response combinations are present just before the reinforcer is received.
6. Because this is stimulus-response learning, and actions are not being produced in order to obtain rewards, the stimulus-response habit continues for some time even when the original reinforcer is devalued, for example by feeding to satiety.
7. At least in primates including humans, the orbitofrontal cortex provides some of the reward-related information to the dopamine neurons, via several routes, including via the ventral striatum, and via the habenula (Fig. 11.4) (Rolls, 2017c).
8. Although some of the dopamine neurons do appear to encode a reward prediction error signal, it has become evident that the signal is more complicated than that, with phasic and sustained or tonic components that the striatum is supposed to understand, and with many dopamine neurons responding to quite different events, including aversive stimuli,

the long-term reward value of stimuli (in contrast to reward prediction error), and movements. The dopamine neurons appear to convey little evidence about the particular reward that has been obtained, making it a somewhat impoverished learning system compared to the orbitofrontal cortex – anterior cingulate cortex system. If there is insufficiency of dopamine, then the transmission through the basal ganglia is impaired and Parkinson's disease occurs, in which there is great difficulty in initiating movements.

9. Computationally, it is proposed that the basal ganglia are a two-stage system with convergence occurring in each stage so that by the second stage, the globus pallidus and substantia nigra, there is sufficient convergence for all the cortical areas that project into the striatum for all these inputs to be combined (see Fig. 16.9). The selection by mutual inhibition at each stage of this two stage process is safe, as there is no danger of runaway excitation and epilepsy as there are no excitatory connections between the principal neurons.

10. The basal ganglia are thus a great contrast with the orbitofrontal cortex to anterior cingulate cortex system, which is much more powerful than the basal ganglia, because it learns associations between actions and outcomes (with the outcome a reward or punisher). For reinforcement learning, the reinforcer is just a modulator of activity that happens to be present when the reinforcement error signal arrives, rather than a direct association between a particular reward outcome and a particular action. This much greater computational power of the orbitofrontal cortex reward to anterior cingulate action learning system than reinforcement learning is brought out further in Section 19.5.

We first consider the anatomical connectivity of the basal ganglia; then what is computed in the basal ganglia as shown by neuronal recording and by the effects of damage to it; and then how the basal ganglia perform their computations, including the role of dopamine in reinforcement learning.

16.2 Systems-level architecture of the basal ganglia

The point-to-point connectivity of the basal ganglia as shown by experimental anterograde and retrograde neuroanatomical path tracing techniques in the primate is indicated in Figs. 16.1 and 16.2. The general connectivity is for cortical or limbic inputs to reach the striatum, which then projects to the globus pallidus and substantia nigra pars reticulata, which in turn project via the thalamus back to the cerebral cortex (DeLong and Wichmann, 2010; Gerfen and Surmeier, 2011; Buot and Yelnik, 2012; Haber, 2016). Within this overall scheme, there is a set of at least partially segregated parallel processing streams, as illustrated in Figs. 16.1 and 16.2 (Rolls and Johnstone, 1992; Rolls, 2014a, 2016b; Haber, 2016; Bostan, Dum and Strick, 2018; Heilbronner, Rodriguez-Romaguera, Quirk, Groenewegen and Haber, 2016).

First, the motor cortex (area 4) and somatosensory cortex (areas 3, 1, and 2) project somatotopically to the putamen, which has connections through the globus pallidus and substantia nigra to the ventral anterior thalamic nuclei and thus to the supplementary motor cortex. Experiments with a virus transneuronal pathway tracing technique have shown that there might be at least partial segregation within this stream, with different parts of the globus pallidus projecting via different parts of the ventrolateral (VL) thalamic nuclei to the supplementary motor area, the primary motor cortex (area 4), and to the ventral premotor area on the lateral surface of the hemisphere (Middleton and Strick, 1996a).

Second, there is an oculomotor circuit (see Fig. 16.1).

Third, the dorsolateral prefrontal and the parietal cortices project to the head and body of the caudate nucleus, which has connections through parts of the globus pallidus and substantia

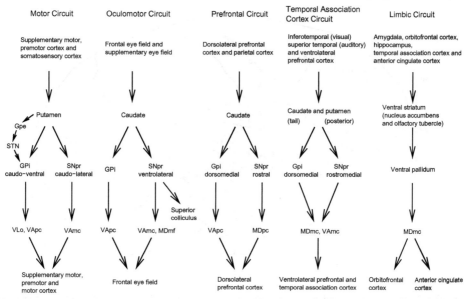

Fig. 16.1 A synthesis of some of the anatomical studies (see text) of the connections of the basal ganglia. GPe, Globus Pallidus, external segment; GPi, Globus Pallidus, internal segment; MD, nucleus medialis dorsalis; SNpr, Substantia Nigra, pars reticulata; VAmc, n. ventralis anterior pars magnocellularis of the thalamus; VApc, n. ventralis anterior pars compacta; VLo, n. ventralis lateralis pars oralis; VLm, n. ventralis pars medialis. An indirect pathway from the striatum via the external segment of the globus pallidus and the subthalamic nucleus (STN) to the internal segment of the globus pallidus is present for the first four circuits (left to right in the figure) of the basal ganglia.

nigra to the ventral anterior group of thalamic nuclei and thus to the dorsolateral prefrontal cortex.

Fourth, the inferior temporal visual cortex and the ventrolateral (inferior convexity) prefrontal cortex to which it is connected project to the posterior and ventral parts of the putamen and the tail of the caudate nucleus (Kemp and Powell, 1970; Saint-Cyr, Ungerleider and Desimone, 1990; Graybiel and Kimura, 1995). Moreover, part of the globus pallidus, perhaps the part influenced by the temporal lobe visual cortex, area TE, may project back (via the thalamus) to area TE (Middleton and Strick, 1996b).

Fifth, and of especial interest in the context of reward mechanisms in the brain, limbic and related structures such as the amygdala, orbitofrontal cortex, and hippocampus project to the ventral striatum (which includes the nucleus accumbens and olfactory tubercle), which has connections through the ventral pallidum to the mediodorsal nucleus of the thalamus and thus to the prefrontal and cingulate cortices (Buot and Yelnik, 2012; Julian et al., 2018; Haber, 2016; Heilbronner et al., 2016, 2018). It is notable that the projections from the amygdala and orbitofrontal cortex are not restricted to the nucleus accumbens, but also reach the adjacent ventral part of the head of the caudate nucleus (Amaral and Price, 1984; Seleman and Goldman-Rakic, 1985; Haber, 2016; Heilbronner, Rodriguez-Romaguera, Quirk, Groenewegen and Haber, 2016). A broadly similar organization is found in humans (Morris et al., 2016). These same reward and memory-related regions may also project to the striosomes or patches (in for example the head of the caudate nucleus), which are set in the matrix formed by the other cortico-striatal systems (Bloem, Huda, Sur and Graybiel, 2017; Friedman, Homma, Gibb, Amemori, Rubin, Hood, Riad and Graybiel, 2015). The striosomes in turn project directly to the dopamine neurons, and via the globus pallidus to the lateral habenula, which in turn projects to the dopamine neurons. As described in Section 11.2.2 and Fig. 11.4, this provides a route for reward-related information from the orbitofrontal cortex and amygdala to influence the dopamine neurons (Rolls, 2017c). But more than that, **these con-**

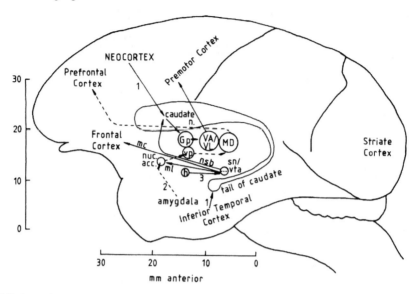

Fig. 16.2 Some of the striatal and connected regions in which the activity of single neurons is described shown on a lateral view of the brain of the macaque monkey. Gp, globus pallidus; h, hypothalamus; sn, substantia nigra, pars compacta (A9 cell group), which gives rise to the nigrostriatal dopaminergic pathway, or nigrostriatal bundle (nsb); vta, ventral tegmental area, containing the A10 cell group, which gives rise to the mesocortical dopamine pathway (mc) projecting to the frontal and cingulate cortices and to the mesolimbic dopamine pathway (ml), which projects to the nucleus accumbens (nuc acc). There is a route from the nucleus accumbens to the ventral pallidum (vp) which then projects to the mediodorsal nucleus of the thalamus (MD) which in turn projects to the prefrontal cortex. Correspondingly, the globus pallidus projects via the ventral anterior and ventrolateral (VA/VL) thalamic nuclei to cortical areas such as the premotor cortex.

nections to the striosomes or patches allow reward-related information from the orbitofrontal cortex and amygdala to influence the striatum *even independently of dopamine inputs*.

The striatum then projects to the globus pallidus (including the ventral pallidum) and substantia nigra, where again the principal neurons are mutually directly inhibitory. The globus pallidus and substantia nigra have many fewer neurons, and as shown below, there is an anatomical basis for convergence (see Fig. 16.8). At striatal neurons of the direct pathway (from the striatum directly to the globus pallidus internal segment), dopamine has excitatory effects via the D1 receptor by eliciting or prolonging glutamate excitatory inputs. At striatal neurons in the indirect pathway (from the striatum via the external segment of the globus pallidus via the subthalamic nucleus to the internal segment of the globus pallidus, see Fig. 16.1), D2 receptor activation has inhibitory effects by reducing glutamate release and prolonging membrane down states (hyperpolarization). Both effects of dopamine tend to promote behavioral output (Gerfen and Surmeier, 2011). The pallidal and nigral neurons then project to the thalamus, which in turn projects back to the neocortex (Fig. 16.1). Although the connections return to the separate cortical areas, a key concept developed below is that the basal ganglia enable information from different parts of the cortex to form combinations and also to compete in the basal ganglia, to enable learning of stimulus-response combinations, and to focus on a single stream of output (Fig. 16.9).

16.3 What computations are performed by the basal ganglia?

16.3.1 Effects of striatal lesions

16.3.1.1 Ventral striatum including nucleus accumbens

There is evidence linking the ventral striatum and its dopamine input to reward, for manipulations of this system alter the incentive effects that learned rewarding stimuli have on behavior in the rat (Robbins, Cador, Taylor and Everitt, 1989; Everitt and Robbins, 1992, 2013). The type of task affected is one in which a visual or auditory stimulus is delivered at or just before the delivery of food for which an animal is working. The tone or light becomes associated by learning with the food. Its effects can be measured by whether the rat learns a new operant response to obtain the conditioned reinforcer (the tone or light). This effect in rats is probably produced via the inputs of the amygdala to the ventral striatum, for the effect is abolished by dopamine-depleting lesions of the nucleus accumbens, and amphetamine injections to the nucleus accumbens (which increase the release of dopamine) increase the effects that these learned or secondary reinforcers have on behavior (Robbins et al., 1989).

In primates, neurotoxic lesions of the ventral striatum produced some changes in emotionality, including increased activity and violent and aggressive behavior when reward was no longer available during extinction (frustrative non-reward); but some of the changes found in rats were not apparent, perhaps because the lesions in primates were small (Stern and Passingham, 1995, 1996), and in any case in primates the amygdala projects not only to the ventral striatum, but also to the adjoining part of the caudate nucleus.

In addition to this role in reward related probably to inputs to the ventral striatum from the amygdala and orbitofrontal cortex (see Chapter 11), the ventral striatum is also implicated in effects that could be mediated by the hippocampal inputs to the ventral striatum. For example, spatial learning (Schacter et al., 1989) and locomotor activity elicited by novel stimuli (Iversen, 1984), are influenced by manipulations of the nucleus accumbens.

The nucleus accumbens may not be involved in action–outcome learning, but does allow the affective states retrieved by the basolateral amygdala (BLA) to conditioned stimuli to influence instrumental behavior by for example Pavlovian-instrumental transfer, and facilitating locomotor approach to food which appears to be in rats a Pavlovian process (Cardinal et al., 2002; Cardinal and Everitt, 2004).

16.3.1.2 Dorsal striatum

In humans, depletion of dopamine in the striatum is found in Parkinson's disease, in which there is akinesia, that is a lack of voluntary movement, bradykinesia (slow movement), rigidity, and tremor (Hornykiewicz, 1973; Braak, Ghebremedhin, Rub, Bratzke and Del Tredici, 2004; Armstrong and Okun, 2020; Wang, Cheng, Rolls, Dai, Gong, Du, Zhang, Wang, Liu, Wang, Brown and Feng, 2020d). However, consistent with the anatomical evidence, the effects of damage to different regions of the striatum also suggest that there is functional specialization within the striatum (Divac and Oberg, 1979; Oberg and Divac, 1979). The selective effects may be related to the function of the cortex or limbic structure from which a region of the striatum receives inputs. For example, in the monkey, lesions of the anterodorsal part of the head of the caudate nucleus disrupted delayed spatial alternation performance, a task that requires spatial short-term memory, which is also impaired by lesions of the corresponding cortical region, the dorsolateral prefrontal cortex. Lesions of the ventrolateral part of the head of the caudate nucleus (as of the orbitofrontal cortex which projects to it) impaired object reversal performance, which measures the ability to reverse stimulus–reinforcer associations. Lesions of the tail of the caudate nucleus (as of the inferior temporal visual cortex which projects to this part of the caudate) produced a visual pattern discrimination deficit (Divac, Rosvold and Szwarcbart, 1967; Iversen, 1979). Analogously, in the rat, lesions of the anteromedial head of the caudate nucleus (or of the medial prefrontal cortex, which projects to it) impaired spatial habit reversal, while lesions of the ventrolateral part of the head of the caudate nucleus (or of the orbital prefrontal cortex from which it receives) impaired the withholding of responses in a Go/No-Go task or in extinction (Dunnett and Iversen, 1982b; Iversen, 1984). Further, in the rat a sensori-motor orientation deficit was produced by damage to a part of the dorsal striatum which receives inputs from lateral cortical areas (Dunnett and Iversen, 1982a; Iversen, 1984). Similar deficits are produced by selective depletion of dopamine using 6-hydroxydopamine in each of these areas (Dunnett and Iversen, 1982b,a; Iversen, 1984).

In rats, the dorsomedial striatum (the equivalent of the primate caudate nucleus) may with its inputs from prelimbic (cingulate) areas be involved in action–outcome learning; the dorsolateral striatum (the equivalent of the primate putamen) with its inputs from sensorimotor cortex in stimulus-response habit behavior; and the ventral striatum may be involved in some effects of rewards and predicted rewards on both directed behavior and habits (Balleine et al., 2009; Balleine and O'Doherty, 2010).

16.3.2 Neuronal activity in different parts of the striatum

Neuronal recording studies in primates and neuroimaging studies in humans show that very different type of information are represented in different parts of the striatum, and reflect the inputs from the cortex to each part of the striatum. We will focus first on neuronal activity in the ventral striatum, because it is particularly relevant to the processing of rewards by the basal ganglia. We again focus on neuronal research in monkeys and activations in neuroimaging studies in humans, because the rodent orbitofrontal cortex (Rolls (2019e) Chapter 8) and brain systems-level organisation (Section19.10; Rolls (2019e) Chapter 8) are so different.

16.3.2.1 Ventral striatum

To analyze the functions of the ventral striatum, the responses of more than 1000 single neurons were recorded (Rolls and Williams, 1987a; Williams, Rolls, Leonard and Stern, 1993) in a region that included the nucleus accumbens and olfactory tubercle in five macaque monkeys in test situations in which lesions of the orbitofrontal cortex, amygdala, hippocampus, and inferior temporal cortex produce deficits, and in which neurons in these structures respond (Rolls, 2014a, 2016b, 2019e).

One population of ventral striatal neurons was found to respond differently in a visual discrimination task to visual stimuli that indicate that if a lick response is made, the taste of glucose reward will be obtained, and to other visual stimuli that indicate that if a lick response is made, the taste of aversive saline will be obtained (Rolls and Williams, 1987a; Williams, Rolls, Leonard and Stern, 1993). Responses of an example of a neuron of this type are shown in Fig. 16.3. The neuron increased its firing rate to the visual stimulus that indicated that saline would be obtained if a lick was made (the S–), and decreased its firing rate to the visual stimulus that indicated that a response could be made to obtain a taste of glucose (the S+). The differential response latency of this neuron to the reward-related and to the saline-related visual stimulus was approximately 150 ms (see Fig. 16.3), and this value was typical. This neuron thus coded for the valence of the visual stimuli (i.e. whether the visual stimulus was associated with a reward vs a punisher).

Of the neurons that responded to visual stimuli that were rewarding, relatively few responded to all the rewarding stimuli used. That is, only few (1.8%) ventral striatal neurons responded both when food was shown and to the positive discriminative visual stimulus, the

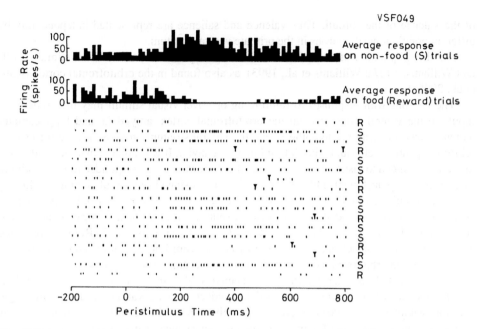

Fig. 16.3 Responses of a ventral striatal neuron in a visual discrimination task. The neuron reduced its firing rate to the visual discriminative stimulus S+ on food reward trials (R), and increased its firing rate to the S− on non-food trials (S) on which aversive saline was obtained if a lick was made. Rastergrams and peristimulus time histograms are shown. The inverted triangles show where lick responses were made on the food reward (R) trials. (Reprinted from Graham V. Williams, Edmund T. Rolls, Christiana M. Leonard, and Chantal Stern (1993) Neuronal responses in the ventral striatum of the behaving macaque. *Behavioural Brain Research* 55: 243–252. © Elsevier B.V.)

S+ (e.g. a triangle shown on a video monitor), in a visual discrimination task. Instead, the reward-related neuronal responses were typically more context or stimulus-dependent, responding for example to the sight of food but not to the S+ which signified food (4.3%), differentially to the S+ or S− but not to food (4.0%), or to food if shown in one context but not in another context. Some neurons were classified as having taste or olfactory responses to food (Williams, Rolls, Leonard and Stern, 1993; Rolls and Williams, 1987a). Some other neurons (1.4%) responded to aversive stimuli. These neurons did not respond simply in relation to arousal, which was produced in control tests by inputs from different modalities, for example by touch of the leg. Thus 13.9% of primate ventral striatal neurons encoded the valence of visual stimuli (Rolls and Williams, 1987a; Williams et al., 1993). Neurons in the ventral striatum (and orbitofrontal cortex) with activity related to the expectation of reward have been confirmed (Schultz, Apicella, Scarnati and Ljungberg, 1992; Schultz, Tremblay and Hollerman, 2000), and as described above reflect inputs from the orbitofrontal cortex (Simmons, Ravel, Shidara and Richmond, 2007). Even ventral striatal interneurons, the activity of which is produced by the principal neurons in the ventral striatum, reflect reward value (Falcone et al., 2019).

Other ventral striatal neurons responded to faces; to other visual stimuli than discriminative stimuli and faces; in relation to somatosensory stimulation and movement; or to cues that signalled the start of a task (Rolls and Williams, 1987a; Williams, Rolls, Leonard and Stern, 1993). The cue-related neurons in the ventral striatum were similar to those found in the head of the caudate nucleus (see Section 16.3.2.4), in that they responded to warning cues that signalled the start of a trial, and stopped responding to the cue if it no longer signalled the start of a trial (see example in Fig. 16.5). 15.9% of ventral striatal neurons had cue-related responses. These can thus be described as encoding the salience of stimuli, and respond independently of the valence of the stimuli. Thus valence and salience are represented independently by different populations of neurons in the primate ventral striatum.

Another population of ventral striatal neurons responded to novel visual stimuli (Rolls and Williams, 1987a; Williams et al., 1993), as also found in the orbitofrontal cortex (Rolls et al., 2005a).

The neurons with responses to reinforcing or novel visual stimuli may thus reflect the inputs to the ventral striatum from the orbitofrontal cortex, amygdala, and hippocampus, and are consistent with the hypothesis that the ventral striatum provides a route for learned reinforcing and novel visual stimuli to influence behavior. It was notable that although some neurons responded to visual stimuli associated with reward, 1.4% responded to visual stimuli associated with punishment, and 12% responded to arousing visual stimuli or non-specifically to visual stimuli. It was also notable that these neurons were not restricted to the nucleus accumbens, but were found also in the adjacent ventral part of the head of the caudate nucleus (Rolls and Williams, 1987a; Williams, Rolls, Leonard and Stern, 1993; Rolls, Thorpe and Maddison, 1983b), which also receives projections from both the amygdala (Amaral and Price, 1984) and orbitofrontal cortex (Seleman and Goldman-Rakic, 1985).

In human fMRI studies, activations have been described in the ventral striatum that reflect whether monetary rewards can be obtained, and indeed more activation is found for the larger rewards (Knutson et al., 2001). Interestingly, activations in the ventral striatum are not only correlated with the amount of money won in a monetary incentive delay task, but also reflect activations in the medial orbitofrontal cortex (Xie, Jia, Rolls, Robbins, Sahakian, Zhang, Liu, Cheng, Luo, Zac Lo, Wang, Banaschewski, Barker, Bodke, Buchel, Quinlan, Desrivieres, Flor, Grigis, Garavan, Gowland, Heinz, Hohmann, Ittermann, Martinot, Martinot, Nees, Papadopoulos Orfanos, Paus, Poustka, Frohner, Smolka, Walter, Whelan, Schumann, Feng and IMAGEN, 2021). One of the strongest activations that is found in the ventral striatum is produced by reward/punishment prediction errors in Pavlovian (i.e. classical conditioning) tasks (O'Doherty et al., 2003a; McClure et al., 2003; Seymour et al., 2004) and in instrumental decision-making tasks (Hare et al., 2008; Kim et al., 2006). For example, in a classical conditioning task, a first visual stimulus probabilistically predicted high vs low pain, and a second visual stimulus perfectly predicted whether the pain would be high or low on that trial. Activation of the ventral striatum and a part of the insula was related to the temporal difference error, which arose for example at the transition between the first and second visual stimulus if the first visual stimulus had predicted low pain, but the second informed the subject that the pain would be high (Seymour et al., 2004).

The ventral striatum activations may reflect the operation of a 'critic' in reinforcement learning, in that activations in it are related to temporal difference errors in Pavlovian conditions in which actions are not made (O'Doherty et al., 2004). In contrast, activation in the dorsal striatum may be closely related to temporal difference prediction errors used to correct an actor, as these activations occurred during an instrumental version of the task in which the subjects had to choose between two stimuli associated with a high probability or low probability of obtaining juice reward (O'Doherty et al., 2004). (The distinction between a 'critic' and an 'actor' in reinforcement learning is described in Section B.17.3.)

Activations in the ventral striatum related to temporal difference reward/punishment prediction errors in a monetary reward *decision* task are exemplified in the study by Rolls, McCabe and Redoute (2008e). The design of the task meant that sometimes the participants were expecting a low probability of a high reward of 30 pence, and unexpectedly obtained a high reward value of 30 pence. On these trials, the temporal difference prediction error from the expected value part of the trial to the reward value part of the trial when subjects were informed whether they would obtain the large reward was positive. On other trials when the expected value was high but probabilistically no reward was obtained, the temporal differ-

TD error signal in the ventral striatum in a probabilistic monetary decision-making task

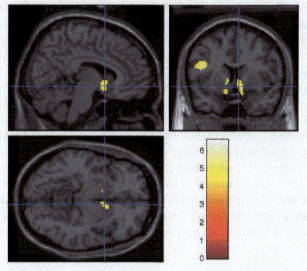

Fig. 16.4 Temporal Difference (TD) error signal in the ventral striatum in a probabilistic monetary decision-making task. The correlation between the TD error and the activation in the nucleus accumbens was significant in a group random effects analysis fully corrected at the cluster level with $p<0.048$ (voxel $z=3.84$) at MNI coordinates [8 8 –8]. (Reproduced from E. T. Rolls, C. McCabe, and J. Redoute. (2008) Expected value, reward outcome, and temporal difference error representations in a probabilistic decision task. *Cerebral Cortex* 18: 652–663. © Oxford University Press.)

ence prediction error from the expected value part of the trial to the reward value part of the trial was negative. (Temporal difference (TD) errors are described in Section B.17.3.) It was found that the fMRI BOLD signal in the nucleus accumbens reflected this temporal difference error signal, calculated at the part of the trial when the reward prediction changed from the expected value for that trial block to the actual reward available on that trial, as shown in Fig. 16.4.

Further analyses showed that the activation in the ventral striatum was positively correlated with the reward actually obtained on that trial but not with the expected value. Thus the TD error correlation arose in the nucleus accumbens because at the time that the expected value period ended and the subject was informed about how much reward had been obtained on that trial, the BOLD signal changed to a higher value for large rewards, and to a lower value for low or no reward, from a value that was not a function of the expected value on that trial. A TD error correlation was also found in left cortical area 44 (Broca's area) (as shown in Fig. 16.4), but here the TD correlation arose because the activation became low when the subject was informed that no reward was obtained on a trial, and it appeared that the area was activated especially when the decision was difficult, between two approximately equal values of the expected value. In a part of the midbrain near the dopamine neurons at [14 –20 –16], there was also a correlation with the TD error, but here this was related to a negative correlation between the BOLD signal in the expected value period of each trial and the expected value. (The TD error was thus positive for example whatever reward became available if it was a low expected value trial block, and the TD error was negative if it was a high expected value trial block.) This shows that TD error regressions with functional neuroimaging can arise for a number of different reasons. In this investigation, the reward value on a trial was correlated with the activation in parts of the orbitofrontal cortex, and the expected value was negatively correlated with activations in the anterior insula [–38 24 16], and these cortical areas may be the origins of some of the signals found on other brain areas.

These findings do exemplify the fact that activation of the ventral striatum does reflect the changing expectations of reward (see Appendix 1, Section B.17.3) during the trials of a task, and indeed this is what is illustrated at the neuronal level in Fig. 16.3, where the neuron altered its firing rate within 170 ms of the monkey being shown a visual stimulus that indicated whether reward or saline was available on that trial. Given that ventral striatal neurons of the type illustrated in Fig. 16.3 alter their activity when the visual stimulus is shown informing the macaque about whether reward is available on that trial, it is in fact not surprising that the fMRI correlation analyses do pick up signals during trials that can be interpreted as temporal difference error signals. Whether these fMRI correlations with a temporal difference error reflect more than the activity of single neurons that respond as shown in Fig. 16.3 to the predicted reward value ($\hat{v}$ of Section B.17.3) rather that the phasic temporal difference error (Δ) will be interesting to examine in future neuronal recordings.

Activations of the ventral striatum that reflect the inputs that it receives from the orbitofrontal cortex and amygdala are commonly reported in functional neuroimaging studies, but it will be important to examine the mechanisms at the neuronal level in the ventral striatum to understand better the exact signals represented by neurons, and exactly what computations the ventral striatum performs using its inputs.

16.3.2.2 Tail of the caudate nucleus, and posteroventral putamen

The projections from the inferior temporal cortex and the prestriate cortex to the striatum arrive mainly, although not exclusively, in the tail (and genu) of the caudate nucleus and in the posteroventral portions of the putamen (Kemp and Powell, 1970; Saint-Cyr et al., 1990). The activity of single neurons was analyzed in the tail of the caudate nucleus and adjoining part of the ventral putamen by Caan, Perrett and Rolls (1984). Of 195 neurons analyzed in two macaque monkeys, 109 (56%) responded to visual stimuli, with latencies of 90–150 ms for the majority of the neurons. The neurons responded to a limited range of complex visual stimuli, and in some cases responded to simpler stimuli such as bars and edges. Typically (for 75% of neurons tested) the neurons habituated rapidly, within 1–8 exposures, to each visual stimulus, but remained responsive to other visual stimuli with a different pattern. This habituation was orientation-specific, in that the neurons responded to the same pattern shown at an orthogonal orientation. The habituation was also relatively short term, in that at least partial dishabituation to one stimulus could be produced by a single intervening presentation of a different visual stimulus. These neurons were relatively unresponsive in a visual discrimination task, having habituated to the discriminative stimuli that had been presented in the task on many previous trials. Consistent findings were obtained by Brown et al. (1995).

Given these responses, it may be suggested that these neurons are involved in short-term pattern-specific habituation to visual stimuli. This system would be distinguishable from other habituation systems (involved, for example, in habituation to spots of light) in that it is specialized for patterned visual stimuli that have been highly processed through visual cortical analysis mechanisms, as shown not only by the nature of the neuronal responses, but also by the fact that this system receives inputs from the inferior temporal visual cortex. It may also be suggested that this sensitivity to visual pattern change may have a role in alerting the monkey's attention to new stimuli. This suggestion is consistent with the changes in attention and orientation to stimuli produced by damage to the striatum.

In view of these neurophysiological findings, and the finding that in a visual discrimination task neurons that reflected the reinforcement contingencies of the stimuli were not found, Caan, Perrett and Rolls (1984) suggested that the tail of the caudate nucleus is not directly involved in the development and maintenance of reward or punishment associations to stimuli (and therefore is not closely involved in emotion-related processing), but may aid visual discrimination performance by its sensitivity to change in visual stimuli. Neurons in some other parts of the striatum may, however, be involved in connecting visual stimuli to appropriate motor responses. For example, in the putamen some neurons have early movement-related firing during the performance of a visual discrimination task (Rolls, Thorpe, Boytim, Szabo and Perrett, 1984); and some neurons in the head of the caudate nucleus respond to environmental cues that signal that reward may be obtained (Rolls, Thorpe and Maddison, 1983b).

If there are long-term differences over several days in the associations of visual stimuli with rewards, it has been found that some tail of caudate neurons respond more to the sight of an object with a high and stable reward value, but these neurons do not reverse rapidly during reversals, so do not reflect the current reward value, nor reward prediction error, but a stable longer term bias to look at highly rewarded objects (Yamamoto, Kim and Hikosaka, 2013; Greve and Fischl, 2009). They may thus reflect habit-based stimulus–response associations, and not stimulus–value associations. These neurons in the tail of the caudate nucleus appear to encode long-term value memories of visual objects and to guide gaze automatically to stably valued objects (Kim, Ghazizadeh and Hikosaka, 2015a; Kim and Hikosaka, 2015; Hikosaka, Ghazizadeh, Griggs and Amita, 2018). A type of dopamine neuron in the monkey caudolateral part of the substantia nigra pars compacta that project to the tail of the caudate nucleus retain past learned reward values stably, and continue to respond differentially to the objects, even when reward is not expected. These dopamine neurons may provide a training signal for the tail of the caudate nucleus (Kim, Ghazizadeh and Hikosaka, 2015a).

16.3.2.3 Postero-ventral putamen

Following these investigations on the caudal striatum which implicated it in visual functions related to a short-term habituation or memory process, a further study was performed to investigate the role of the posterior putamen in visual short-term memory tasks (Johnstone and Rolls, 1990; Rolls and Johnstone, 1992). Both the inferior temporal visual cortex and the prefrontal cortex project to the posterior ventral parts of the putamen (Goldman and Nauta, 1977; Van Hoesen et al., 1981) and these cortical areas are known to subserve a variety of complex functions, including functions related to memory. For example, cells in both areas respond in a variety of short-term memory tasks (Fuster, 1973, 2008; Fuster and Jervey, 1982; Baylis and Rolls, 1987; Miyashita and Chang, 1988).

Two main groups of neurons with memory-related activity were found in the postero-ventral putamen in a delayed match-to-sample (DMS) task. In the task, the monkey was shown a sample stimulus, and had to remember it during a 2–5 s delay period, after which if a matching stimulus was shown he could make one response, but if a non-matching stimulus was shown he had to make no response (Johnstone and Rolls, 1990; Rolls and Johnstone, 1992).

First, 11% of the 621 neurons studied responded to the test stimulus which followed the sample stimulus, but did not respond to the sample stimulus. Of these neurons, 43% responded only on non-match trials (test different from sample), 16% only on match trials (test same as the sample), and 41% to the test stimulus irrespective of whether it was the same or different from the sample. These neuronal responses were not related to the licking motor responses since (i) the neurons did not respond in other tasks in which a lick response was required (for example, in an auditory delayed match-to-sample task which was identical to the visual delayed match-to-sample task except that auditory short-term memory rather than visual short-term memory was required; in a serial recognition memory task; or in a visual discrimination task), and (ii) a periresponse time spike-density function indicated that the stimulus onset better predicted neuronal activity.

Second, 9.5% of the neurons responded in the delay period after the sample stimulus, during which the sample was being remembered. These neurons did not respond in the auditory version of the task, indicating that the responses were visual modality-specific (as were the

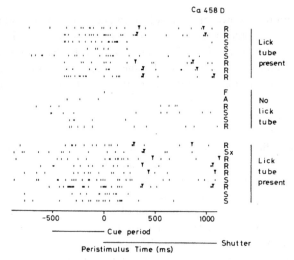

Fig. 16.5 Responses of a cue-related neuron in the head of the caudate nucleus in a Go/NoGo visual discrimination task in which the visual stimulus was presented at time 0. Each trial is a single row of the rastergram, each action potential is represented by a single dot, and a lick made to obtain fruit juice is represented by an inverted triangle. R, Reward trials on which fruit juice was obtained. S, Salt trials on which if a lick was made, a small drop of saline was obtained. Tone and light emitting diode cues were provided starting 500 ms before the visual stimulus was shown. Top set of trials: normal performance of the task with the lick tube close to the mouth. Middle set of trials: the lick tube was removed out of reach, but the tone/LED cue, and discriminative visual stimuli, were still provided. Bottom set of trials: normal performance of the task with the lick tube close to the mouth. F, food reward was shown. A, an aversive visual stimulus was shown. (Reprinted from E. T. Rolls, S.J.Thorpe, and S.P.Maddison (1983) Responses of striatal neurons in the behaving monkey. 1. Head of the caudate nucleus. *Behavioural Brain Research* 7:179–210. © Elsevier B.V.)

responses of all other neurons in this part of the putamen with activity related to the delayed match-to-sample task). Given that the visual and auditory tasks were very similar apart from the modality of the input stimuli, this suggests that the activity of the neurons was not related to movements, or to rewards or punishers obtained in the tasks (and is thus not closely linked to emotion-related processing), but instead to modality-specific short-term memory-related processing.

In recordings made from pallidal neurons it was found that some responded in both visual and auditory versions of the task (Johnstone and Rolls, 1990; Rolls and Johnstone, 1992). Of 37 neurons responsive in the visual DMS task that were also tested in the auditory version, seven (19%) responded also in the auditory DMS task. The finding that some of the pallidal neurons active in the DMS task were not modality-specific, whereas only visual modality-specific DMS units were located in the postero-ventral part of the striatum, provides evidence that **the globus pallidus may represent a further stage in information processing in which information from different parts of the striatum can converge.**

16.3.2.4 Head of the caudate nucleus

The activity of 394 neurons in the head of the caudate nucleus and most anterior part of the putamen was analyzed in three behaving rhesus monkeys (Rolls, Thorpe and Maddison, 1983b). Of these neurons, 64.2% had responses related to environmental stimuli, movements, the performance of a visual discrimination task, or eating. However, only relatively small proportions of these neurons had responses that were unconditionally related to visual (9.6%), auditory (3.5%), or gustatory (0.5%) stimuli, or to movements (4.1%). Instead, the majority of the neurons had responses that occurred conditionally in relation to stimuli or movements, in that the responses occurred in only some test situations, *and were often dependent on the performance of a task by the monkeys.* Thus, it was found that in a visual discrimination task

14.5% of the neurons responded during a 0.5 s tone/light cue that signalled the start of each trial (cue-related neurons); 31.1% responded in the period in which the discriminative visual stimuli were shown, with 24.3% of these responding more either to the visual stimulus that predicted food reward or to a stimulus that predicted punishment (by a taste of saline) (reward prediction neurons); and 6.2% responded in relation to lick responses.

An example of a *cue-related* neuron in the head of the caudate nucleus that started responding as soon as a tone/light-emitting diode (LED) cue was presented indicating that a trial was about to start is shown in Fig. 16.5. At time 0 a discriminative visual stimulus was shown, which indicated if for example it was a triangle that reward could be obtained, or if it was a square that saline would be obtained if a lick was made. The reward trials (R) on which a lick could be made to obtain fruit juice, and saline (S) trials on which a lick should not be made otherwise a drop of aversive saline was obtained, each occurred with probability 0.5. This cue-related neuron stopped responding soon after the visual stimulus appeared, and did not discriminate between reward (R) and punishment (S) trials. It was thus a cue neuron and not a reward-predicting neuron. It could be described as encoding *salience* but not valence. Further evidence that the neuron was not reward or punishment related is that it did not respond on trials on which a food reward was shown (F), or an aversive visual stimulus was shown (A).

If the lick tube was moved away from the lips by a few mm so that juice reward could not be obtained (but the tone/LED still sounded, and was followed by a discriminative visual stimulus), the neuron stopped responding to the tone/LED cue, providing evidence that it was only when the tone/LED cue predicted the start of a trial in the visual discrimination task that the head of caudate neuron responded to the cue. This is shown by the middle set of trials in Fig. 16.5.

Approximately half of the cue-related neurons tested showed this learning whereby they only responded to a warning cue normally used to start a trial if it actually did signal the start a trial. It typically took just a few trials for this trial predicting effect of a tone/LED cue to be learned and unlearned by these neurons.

Most of these cue-related neurons learned to respond to whichever cue, either a 500 Hz tone, or a light-emitting diode, signalled the start of a trial (see example in Fig. 16.6).

An example of a *reward-predicting* neuron in the head of the caudate nucleus that started responding as soon as a cue was available that a trial was about to start, and which continued firing after a visual stimulus was shown which indicated that a lick response could be made to obtain juice reward (R), but which stopped firing after a visual stimulus was shown that indicated that if a lick response was made, aversive saline (S) would be obtained, is shown in Fig. 16.7. The reward (R) and saline (S) trials each occurred with probability 0.5. This type of neuron, common in the head of the primate caudate nucleus, thus increased its firing as soon as the probability of reward increased at the start of a trial to 0.5, learned to respond to the first cue that signalled the start of a trial, and stopped responding as soon as the probability of reward decreased to 0 on punishment (S) trials. These neurons typically did not respond in relation to the cue stimuli, to the visual stimuli, or to movements, when these occurred independently of the task or performance of the task was prevented, for example by withdrawing the lick tube from which fruit juice could be obtained (Rolls, Thorpe and Maddison, 1983b) (as illustrated for a cue-related neuron in Fig. 16.5). That is, the responses of these neurons reflected whether reward would be obtained, and more generally, reflect how much reward will be obtained (Cromwell and Schultz, 2003). Similar neurons in the head of the caudate nucleus responded to punishment-predicting stimuli, and indeed approximately as many neurons responded to the saline punishment-associated visual stimulus in the Go/NoGo visual discrimination task as to the juice reward-predicting stimulus (Rolls, Thorpe and Maddison, 1983b; Rolls, Thorpe, Maddison, Roper-Hall, Puerto and Perrett, 1979c; Rolls, 1984).

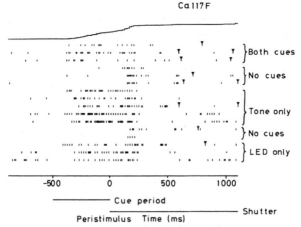

Fig. 16.6 Responses of a cue-related neuron in the head of the caudate nucleus in a Go/NoGo visual discrimination task in which the visual stimulus was presented at time 0, when a mechanical shutter opened to reveal the discriminative stimulus. Each trial is a single row of the rastergram, each action potential is represented by a single dot, and a lick made to obtain fruit juice on Reward trials only is represented by an inverted triangle. Tone and/or light emitting diode (LED) cues were provided starting 500 ms before the visual stimulus was shown. If no 500 ms warning cue was given for the start of a trial, the neuron responded to the first indication that a trial was beginning, the sound of the shutter opening at time 0. The neuron did not predict whether reward would or would not be obtained, in that there was no differential neuronal response on Reward trials (on which licks were made), compared to non-reward trials (on which licks were correctly not made). The line at the top shows the cusum (cumulative sum) statistic. (Reprinted from E. T. Rolls, S.J.Thorpe, and S.P.Maddison (1983) Responses of striatal neurons in the behaving monkey. 1. Head of the caudate nucleus. *Behavioural Brain Research* 7:179–210. © Elsevier B.V.)

Thus some neurons in the head of the caudate nucleus encode the *valence* of visual stimuli. Consistently, Watanabe, Lauwereyns and Hikosaka (2003) have found that one population of neurons in the primate caudate nucleus responds to rewarded eye movements, and a separate population to unrewarded eye movements.

Similar types of response were found when the neurons were tested outside the visual discrimination task, during feeding. Of the neurons tested during feeding, 25.8% responded when the food was seen by the monkey, 6.2% when he tasted it, and 22.4% during a cue given by the experimenter that a food or non-food object was about to be presented. Further evidence on the nature of these neuronal responses was that many of the neurons with cue-related responses only responded to the tone/light cue stimuli when they were cues for the performance of the task or the presentation of food as described above, and some responded to the different cues used in the task (tone/LED) and feeding test (an arm movement made by the experimenter to reach behind a screen to obtain a food or non-food object) situations (Rolls, Thorpe and Maddison, 1983b).

Similar neurons have been described by Hikosaka and colleagues, who emphasise that head of caudate neurons rapidly change their responses to reflect the current value of a reward stimulus when it changes, and are thus suitable for flexible reward-related behavior when the reward contingencies change (Kim and Hikosaka, 2015; Hikosaka et al., 2018). This is in contrast to tail of caudate neurons that respond to the long-term value of visual stimuli such as objects, even when the contingencies flexibly reverse. These tail of caudate neurons are thus implicated in habitual behavioral responses to objects based on their long-term reward value (Kim and Hikosaka, 2015; Hikosaka et al., 2018).

The finding that such head of caudate neurons may respond to environmental stimuli only when they are significant in predicting for example the onset of a trial (a cue neuron), or the delivery of reward (a reward-predicting neuron) (Rolls, Thorpe, Maddison, Roper-Hall, Puerto and Perrett, 1979c; Rolls, Thorpe and Maddison, 1983b), was confirmed by Evarts and his colleagues. They showed that some neurons in the putamen only responded to the

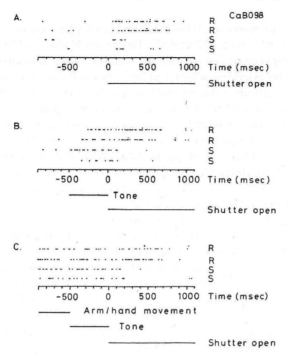

Fig. 16.7 Responses of a reward-predicting neuron in the head of the caudate nucleus in a Go/NoGo visual discrimination task in which the visual stimulus was presented at time 0. Each trial is a single row of the rastergram, each action potential is represented by a single dot, and a lick made to obtain fruit juice is represented by a vertical pair of dots. R, Reward trials on which fruit juice was obtained. S, Salt trials on which if a lick was made, a small drop of saline was obtained. (A) The neuron started to respond approximately 80 ms after the start of the trial when a shutter opened to reveal the discriminative stimulus, continued to respond on reward trials until after the fruit juice was obtained, and stopped responding at approximately 160 ms on trials on which the punisher-related stimulus (S) was shown. (B) The neuron started responding soon after a cue tone sounded indicating the start of a trial. (C) The neuron started responding at the earliest indication that the trial would start, an arm movement made by the macaque to press a button to start the trial. (Reprinted from E. T. Rolls, S.J.Thorpe, and S.P.Maddison (1983) Responses of striatal neurons in the behaving monkey. 1. Head of the caudate nucleus. *Behavioural Brain Research* 7:179–210. © Elsevier B.V.)

click of a solenoid when it indicated that a fruit juice reward could be obtained (Evarts and Wise, 1984). The findings have also been confirmed by Tremblay and Schultz (1998) (see also Schultz, Tremblay and Hollerman (2003)), who reported that macaque caudate neurons come to respond during learning to cues related to the preparation of movement or expectation of reward, and do not respond to cues that do not predict such events.

We have found that this decoding of the significance of environmental events that are signals for the preparation for or initiation of a behavioral response is represented in the firing of a population of neurons in the dorsolateral prefrontal cortex, which projects into the head of the caudate nucleus (E. T. Rolls and G. C. Baylis, unpublished observations 1984). These neurons only respond to the tone cue if it signals the start of a trial of the visual discrimination task, just as do the corresponding population of neurons in the head of the caudate nucleus. The indication that the decoding of significance is performed by the prefrontal cortex, and that the striatum receives only the results of the cortical computation, is considered below and elsewhere (Rolls and Williams, 1987b).

These findings indicate that the head of the caudate nucleus and most anterior part of the putamen contain populations of neurons that respond to predictive sensory cues that enable preparation for the performance of tasks such as feeding and tasks in which movements must be initiated, and others that respond during the performance of such tasks in relation to sensory cue that predict reward, and that the majority of these neurons have no unconditional sensory or motor responses. It has therefore been suggested (Rolls, Thorpe, Maddison, Roper-Hall, Puerto and Perrett, 1979c; Rolls, Thorpe and Maddison, 1983b) that the anterior neostriatum contains neurons that are important for the utilization of environmental cues for the preparation for behavioral responses, and for particular behavioral responses made in particular situations to particular environmental stimuli, that is in stimulus–motor response habit formation. Different neurons in the cue-related group often respond to different subsets of environmentally significant events, and thus convey some information that would be useful in switching behavior, in preparing to make responses, and in connecting inputs to particular responses (Rolls, Thorpe, Maddison, Roper-Hall, Puerto and Perrett, 1979c; Rolls, Thorpe and Maddison, 1983b; Rolls, 1984). Striatal neurons with similar types of response have also been recorded by Wolfram Schultz and colleagues (Schultz, Apicella, Romo and Scarnati, 1995a; Tremblay and Schultz, 1998; Cromwell and Schultz, 2003; Schultz, Tremblay and Hollerman, 2003). Striatal tonically active interneurons (TANs) which have high spontaneous firing rates and respond by decreasing their firing rates may respond to similar cue-predicting and reward-predicting events (Graybiel and Kimura, 1995), presumably by receiving inhibitory inputs from the principal striatal neurons described above, the medium spiny neurons.

It is of interest, and just as expected, that some dopamine neurons respond to these cue-related inputs, and other salient including novel and aversive stimuli (Bromberg-Martin, Matsumoto and Hikosaka, 2010a) as described in Section 16.4.3, that are found in the head of the caudate nucleus and ventral striatum, for these parts of the striatum provide inputs to the dopamine neurons (Haber and Knutson, 2009).

In a habit-learning, sequential saccade, task, neurons in the head of the caudate nucleus reflected the learning of the task, and the cost-benefit signals that would be consistent with reinforcement learning (Desrochers et al., 2015; Graybiel and Grafton, 2015).

In human fMRI studies, activations have been described in the striatum that reflect whether monetary rewards can be obtained, that is they reflect expected reward value (Delgado, Nystrom, Fissell, Noll and Fiez, 2000; Knutson, Adams, Fong and Hommer, 2001; Haber and Knutson, 2009; Knutson, Delgado and Phillips, 2009; Wu, Sacchet and Knutson, 2012) and also reward outcome value (Rolls, McCabe and Redoute, 2008e). These activations presumably reflect the activity of the reward-predicting striatal neurons (Rolls, Thorpe, Maddison, Roper-Hall, Puerto and Perrett, 1979c; Rolls, Thorpe and Maddison, 1983b; Rolls, 1984). Activations to monetary reward only if it is being worked for instrumentally (Zink et al., 2004) may reflect the type of task dependence illustrated for a cue-related neuron in Fig. 16.5. Human striatal fMRI activations to non-rewarding but salient stimuli (Zink et al., 2003) may reflect the types of trial-predicting (i.e. cue-related) neurons shown in Figs. 16.5 and 16.6 but not reward-predicting neurons of the type shown in Fig. 16.7.

One would expect human striatal activations also to be demonstrable to punishment-predicting stimuli, given that approximately half of the striatal reward/punishment-predicting neurons respond to punishment-predicting stimuli (Rolls, Thorpe, Maddison, Roper-Hall, Puerto and Perrett, 1979c; Rolls, Thorpe and Maddison, 1983b; Rolls, 1984), and there is some human fMRI evidence for this (Seymour et al., 2004). It is a difficulty (Bromberg-Martin, Matsumoto and Hikosaka, 2010a) for the dopamine reward prediction error hypothesis (Schultz et al., 1995b, 1997; Waelti et al., 2001; Schultz, 2004, 2013) that it cannot account for the formation of striatal neurons that fire to predict punishment. [In particular, if dopamine neurons decrease their firing rate if an expected reward is not received or a punishment is received (Mirenowicz and Schultz, 1996; Waelti, Dickinson and Schultz, 2001; Tobler, Dickinson and Schultz, 2003), then this would not promote learning in the striatum whereby striatal neurons might respond more to the stimulus (e.g. a discriminative stimulus in a visual discrimination task) that predicted punishment.] However, such reward and punisher predicting information is reflected in the firing of orbitofrontal cortex neurons, some of which predict reward, and others of which predict punishment (see Chapter 11), and it is presumably by this orbitofrontal cortex route that punishment-predicting neurons in the head of the caudate nucleus receive this information (rather than being reinforced into this type of firing by a dopamine reward error prediction signal).

It is very interesting that the type of head of caudate neuron shown in Fig. 16.7 has certain similarities to the midbrain dopamine neurons described by Schultz and colleagues (Schultz et al., 1995b; Mirenowicz and Schultz, 1996; Waelti et al., 2001), except that the dopamine neurons respond to the transitions in reward probabilities, rather than the reward probabilities themselves which is what appears to be encoded by the type of head of caudate neuron shown in Fig. 16.7. Thus an alternative to the hypothesis that the dopamine neurons provide a reward-prediction error teaching signal (see Section 16.4.3) is that the firing of the dopamine neurons may reflect feedback connections from these striatal regions to the dopamine neurons in the substantia nigra, pars compacta, and ventral tegmental area. These feedback connections would then influence the dopamine neurons for short periods primarily when the firing of the striatal neurons changed, implemented by a high-pass filtering effect. This would leave much more open what the functions of the dopamine neurons are (see Section 16.4.3), in that a simple feedback effect might be being implemented (from striatum to the dopamine neurons and back), perhaps to dynamically reset thresholds or gains in the striatum.

16.3.2.5 Anterior putamen

It is clear that the activity of many neurons in the putamen is related to movements (Anderson, 1978; Crutcher and DeLong, 1984a,b; DeLong et al., 1984; DeLong and Wichmann, 2010). There is a somatotopic organization of neurons in the putamen, with separate areas containing neurons responding to arm, leg, or orofacial movements. Some of these neurons respond only to active movements, and others to active and to passive movements. Some of these neurons respond to somatosensory stimulation, with multiple clusters of neurons responding, for example, to the movement of each joint. Some neurons in the putamen have been shown in experiments in which the arm has been given assisting and opposing loads to respond in relation to the direction of an intended movement, rather than in relation to the muscle forces required to execute the movement (Crutcher and DeLong, 1984b). Also, the firing rate of neurons in the putamen tends to be linearly related to the amplitude of movements (Crutcher and DeLong, 1984b), and this is of potential clinical relevance, since patients with basal ganglia disease frequently have difficulty in controlling the amplitude of their limb movements.

In order to obtain further evidence on specialization of function within the striatum, the activity of neurons in the putamen has been compared with the activity of neurons recorded in different parts of the striatum in the same tasks (Rolls, Thorpe, Boytim, Szabo and Perrett, 1984). Of 234 neurons recorded in the putamen of two macaque monkeys during the performance of a visual discrimination task and the other tests in which other striatal neurons have been shown to respond (Rolls, Thorpe and Maddison, 1983b; Caan, Perrett and Rolls, 1984), 68 (29%) had activity that was phasically related to movements (Rolls, Thorpe, Boytim, Szabo and Perrett, 1984). Many of these responded in relation to mouth movements such as licking. Similar neurons were found in the substantia nigra, pars reticulata, to which the putamen projects (Mora, Mogenson and Rolls, 1977). The neurons did not have activity related to taste, in that they responded, for example, during tongue protrusion made to a food or non-food object. Some of these neurons responded in relation to the licking mouth movements made in the visual discrimination task, and always also responded when mouth movements were made during clinical testing when a food or non-food object was brought close to the mouth. Their responses were thus unconditionally related to movements, in that they responded in whichever testing situation was used, and were therefore different from the responses of neurons in the head of the caudate nucleus (Rolls, Thorpe and Maddison, 1983b).

Of the 68 neurons in the putamen with movement-related activity in these tests, 61 had activity related to mouth movements, and seven had activity related to movements of the body. Of the remaining neurons, 24 (10%) had activity that was task-related in that some change of firing rate associated with the presentation of the tone cue or the opening of the shutter occurred on each trial (Rolls, Thorpe, Boytim, Szabo and Perrett, 1984), four had auditory responses, one responded to environmental stimuli (Rolls, Thorpe and Maddison, 1983b), and 137 were not responsive in these test situations.

These findings (Rolls, Thorpe, Boytim, Szabo and Perrett, 1984) provide further evidence that differences between neuronal activity in different regions of the striatum are found even in the same testing situations, and also that the inputs that activate these neurons are derived functionally from the cortex which projects into a particular region of the striatum (in this case sensori-motor cortex, areas 3, 1, 2, 4, and 6).

In these four parts of the striatum in which a comparison can be made of processing in the striatum with that in the cortical area that projects to that part of the striatum, it thus appears that the full information represented in the cortex does not reach the striatum, but that rather the striatum receives the output of the computation being performed by a cortical area, and could use this to initiate, switch, or alter behavior.

The hypothesis arises from these findings that some parts of the striatum, particularly the caudate nucleus, ventral striatum, and posterior putamen, receive the output of these cortical memory-related and cognitive computations, but do not themselves perform them. Instead, on receiving the cortical and limbic outputs, the striatum may be involved in switching behavior as appropriate as determined by the different, sometimes conflicting, information received from these cortical and limbic areas. On this view, the striatum would be particularly involved in the selection of behavioral responses, and in producing one coherent stream of behavioral output, with the possibility to switch if a higher priority input was received. This process may be achieved by a laterally spreading competitive interaction between striatal or pallidal neurons, which might be implemented by the direct inhibitory connections between neurons that are close together in the striatum and globus pallidus. In addition, the inhibitory interneurons within the striatum, the dendrites of which in the striatum may cross the boundary between the matrix and striosomes, may play a part in this interaction between striatal processing streams (Groves, 1983; Graybiel and Kimura, 1995; Groves et al., 1995).

Dopamine could play an important role in setting the sensitivity of this response selection function, as suggested by direct iontophoresis of dopamine on to single striatal neurons, which produces a similar decrease in the response of the neuron and in its spontaneous activity in the behaving macaque (Rolls, Thorpe, Boytim, Szabo and Perrett, 1984; Rolls and Williams, 1987b). Consistent with dopamine playing an important role of this type, dopamine acting via D1 receptors in the direct pathway, and via D2 receptors in the indirect pathway, promotes behavioral output (Gerfen and Surmeier, 2011).

In addition to this response selection function by competition, the basal ganglia may, by the convergence discussed, enable signals originating from non-motor parts of the cerebral cortex to be mapped into motor signals to produce behavioral output. In this way, stimulus-response habit learning could be implemented. Indeed, there is considerable agreement that the basal ganglia are involved in stimulus-response habit learning (Graybiel and Grafton, 2015; Robbins and Costa, 2017). The ways in which these computations might be performed are considered next.

16.4 How do the basal ganglia perform their computations?

16.4.1 Interaction between neurons and selection of output

On the hypothesis just raised, different regions of the striatum, or at least the outputs of such regions, would need to interact. Is there within the striatum the possibility for different regions to interact, and is the partial functional segregation seen within the striatum maintained in processing beyond the striatum? For example, is the segregation maintained throughout the globus pallidus and thalamus with projections to different premotor and even prefrontal regions reached by different regions of the striatum, or is there convergence or the possibility for interaction at some stage during this post-striatal processing?

Given the anatomy of the basal ganglia, interactions between signals reaching the basal ganglia could happen in a number of different ways. One would be for each part of the striatum to receive at least some input from a number of different cortical regions. As discussed above, there is evidence for patches of input from different sources to be brought adjacent to each other in the striatum (Van Hoesen et al., 1981; Seleman and Goldman-Rakic, 1985; Graybiel and Kimura, 1995). For example, in the caudate nucleus, different regions of association cortex project to adjacent longitudinal strips (Seleman and Goldman-Rakic, 1985). Now, the dendrites of striatal neurons have the shape of large plates that lie at right angles to the incoming cortico-striatal fibres (Percheron, Yelnik and François, 1984b,a; Percheron, Yelnik, François, Fenelon and Talbi, 1994; Yelnik, 2002; Buot and Yelnik, 2012) (see Figs. 16.8 and 16.9). Thus one way in which interaction may start in the basal ganglia is by virtue of the same striatal neuron receiving inputs on its dendrites from more than just a limited area of the cerebral cortex. This convergence may provide a first level of integration over limited sets of cortico-striatal fibres. The large number of cortical inputs received by each striatal neuron, in the order of 10,000 (Wilson, 1995), is consistent with the hypothesis that convergence of inputs carrying different signals is an important aspect of the function of the basal ganglia. The computation that could be performed by this architecture is discussed below for the inputs to the globus pallidus, where the connectivity pattern is comparable.

The regional segregation of neuronal response types in the striatum described above is consistent with mainly local integration over limited, adjacent sets of cortico-striatal inputs, as suggested by this anatomy. Short-range integration or interactions within the striatum may also be produced by the short length (for example 0.5 mm) of the intra-striatal axons of striatal neurons. These could produce a more widespread influence if the effect of a strong input to one part of the striatum spread like a lateral competition signal (cf. Groves (1983), Groves et al. (1995)). Such a mechanism could contribute to behavioral response selection in the face of different competing input signals to the striatum. The lateral inhibition could operate, for example, between the striatal principal (that is medium spiny) neurons by their direct connections, to inhibit each other. (These neurons receive excitatory connections from the cortex, respond by increasing their firing rates, and could inhibit each other by their local axonal arborizations, which spread in an area as large as their dendritic trees, and which utilize GABA as their inhibitory transmitter to enable the principal neurons of the striatum to directly inhibit each other.) Further lateral inhibition could operate in the pallidum and substantia nigra (see Fig. 16.9). Here again there are local axon collaterals, as widespread as the very large pallidal and nigral dendritic fields. The lateral competition could again operate by direct inhibitory connections between the neurons.

[Note that pallidal and nigral cells have high spontaneous firing rates (often 25–50 spikes/s), and respond (to their inhibitory striatal inputs) by reducing their firing rates below this high spontaneous rate. Such a decrease in the firing rate of one neuron would release inhibition

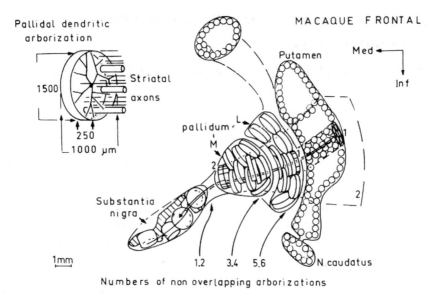

Fig. 16.8 Semi-schematic spatial diagram of the striato-pallido-nigral system (see text). The numbers represent the numbers of non-overlapping arborizations of dendrites in the plane shown. L, lateral or external segment of the globus pallidus; M, medial or internal segment of the globus pallidus. The inserted diagram in the upper left shows the geometry of the dendrites of a typical pallidal neuron, and how the flat dendritic arborization is pierced at right angles by the striatal axons, which make occasional synapses en passage. (Reproduced from Gerard Percheron, Jerome Yelnik, and Chantal Francois (1984) A Golgi analysis of the primate globus pallidus. III. Spatial organization of the striatopallidal complex. Journal of Comparative Neurology 227: 214–227. Copyright © Alan R. Liss, Inc.)

on nearby neurons, causing them to increase their firing rates, equivalent to responding less. It is very interesting that direct inhibitory connections between the neurons can implement selection, even though at the striatal level the neurons have low spontaneous firing rates and respond by increasing their firing rates, whereas in the globus pallidus and substantia nigra pars reticulata the neurons have a high spontaneous firing rate, and respond by decreasing their firing rate.]

A selection function of this type between processing streams in the basal ganglia, even without any convergence anatomically between the processing streams implemented by feedforward inputs, might provide an important computational raison d'être for the basal ganglia. As noted, the direct inhibitory local connectivity between the principal neurons within the striatum and globus pallidus would seem to provide a simple, and perhaps evolutionarily old, way in which to implement competition between neurons and processing streams. This might even be a primitive design principle that characterizes the basal ganglia. A system such as the basal ganglia with direct inhibitory recurrent collaterals may have evolved easily because it is easier to make stable than architectures such as the cerebral cortex with recurrent excitatory connections. The basal ganglia architecture may have been especially appropriate in motor systems in which instability could produce movement and co-ordination difficulties (Rolls and Treves, 1998; Rolls, 2014a). Equations that describe the way in which this mutual inhibition between the principal neurons can result in contrast enhancement of neuronal activity in the different competing neurons, and thus selection, are provided by Grossberg (1988), Gurney et al. (2001a), Gurney et al. (2001b), and Grossberg (2021).

This hypothesis of lateral competition between the neurons of the basal ganglia can be sketched simply (see Fig. 16.9 and Rolls and Treves (1998) and Rolls (2014a), where a more detailed neuronal network theory of the operation of the basal ganglia is presented). The inputs from the cortex to the striatum are excitatory, and competition between striatal neurons

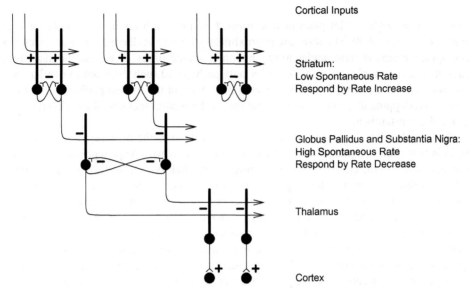

Fig. 16.9 Schematic hypothesis of basal ganglia network architecture. A key aspect is that in both the striatum, and in the globus pallidus and substantia nigra pars reticulata, there are direct inhibitory connections (–) between the principal neurons, as shown. These synapses use GABA as a transmitter. Excitatory inputs to the striatum are shown as +. (Reproduced from E. T. Rolls and A. Treves. (1998) Neural Networks and Brain Function. Oxford University Press.)

is implemented by the use of an inhibitory transmitter (GABA), and direct connections between striatal neurons, within an area which is approximately co-extensive with the dendritic arborization. Given that the lateral connections between the striatal neurons are collaterals of the output axons, the output must be inhibitory on to pallidal and nigral neurons. This means that to transmit signals usefully, and in contrast with striatal neurons, the neurons in the globus pallidus and substantia nigra (pars reticulata) must have high spontaneous firing rates, and respond by reducing their firing rates. These pallidal and nigral neurons then repeat the simple scheme for lateral competition between output neurons by having direct lateral inhibitory connections to the other pallidal and nigral neurons. When nigral and pallidal neurons respond by reducing their firing rates, the reduced inhibition through the recurrent collaterals allows the connected pallidal and nigral neurons to fire faster, and also at the same time the main output of the pallidal and nigral neurons allows the thalamic neurons to fire faster. The thalamic neurons then have the standard excitatory influence on their cortical targets.

The simple, and perhaps evolutionarily early, aspect of this basal ganglia architecture is that the striatal, pallidal, and nigral neurons implement competition (for selection) by direct inhibitory recurrent lateral connections of the main output neurons on to other output neurons, with the inputs to each stage of processing (e.g. striatum, globus pallidus) synapsing directly on to the output neurons that inhibit each other (see Fig. 16.9).

Another possible mechanism for interaction within the striatum is provided by the dopaminergic pathway, through which a signal that has descended from, for example, the orbitofrontal cortex via the ventral striatum and habenula to the dopamine neurons in the midbrain (Fig. 11.4, (Rolls, 2017c)) might thereby influence other parts of the striatum. Because of the slow conduction speed of the dopaminergic neurons, this latter system would probably not be suitable for rapid switching of behavior, but only for more tonic, long-term adjustments of connectivity and sensitivity.

Further levels for integration within the basal ganglia are provided by the striato-pallidal and striato-nigral projections (Percheron, Yelnik and François, 1984b,a; Percheron, Yelnik, François, Fenelon and Talbi, 1994; Yelnik, 2002). The afferent fibres from the striatum again cross at right angles a flat plate or disc formed by the dendrites of the pallidal or nigral neurons (see Fig. 16.8). The discs are approximately 1.5 mm in diameter, and are stacked up one upon the next at right angles to the incoming striatal fibres. The dendritic discs are so large that in the monkey there is room for only perhaps 50 such discs not to overlap in the external pallidal segment, for 10 non-overlapping discs in the medial pallidal segment, and for one overlapping disc in the most medial part of the medial segment of the globus pallidus and in the substantia nigra.

One result of this convergence achieved by this stage of the medial pallidum/substantia nigra is that even if inputs from different cortical regions were kept segregated by specific wiring rules on to different neurons, there might nevertheless well be the possibility for mutual competition between different pallidal neurons, implemented by their mutual inhibitory connections. Given the relatively small number of neurons into which the cortical signals had now been compressed, it would be feasible to have competition (the same effect as lateral inhibition implemented by inhibitory neurons would achieve elsewhere) implemented between the relatively small population of neurons, now all collected into a relatively restricted space, so that the competition could spread widely within these nuclei. This could allow selection by competition between these pathways, that is effectively between information processing originating in different cortical areas. This could be important in allowing each cortical area to control output when appropriate (depending on the task being performed). Even if full segregation were maintained in the return paths to the cerebral cortex, the return paths could influence each cortical area, allowing it to continue processing if it had the strongest 'call'. Each cortical area on a fully segregated hypothesis might thus have its own non-basal ganglia output routes, but might according to the current suggestion utilize the basal ganglia as a system to select a cortical area or set of areas, depending on how strongly each cortical area is calling for output. The thalamic outputs from the basal ganglia (nuclei VA and VLo of the thalamus) might according to this hypothesis have to some extent an activity or gain-controlling function on a cortical area (such as might be mediated by diffuse terminals in superficial cortical layers), rather than the strong and selective inputs implemented by a specific thalamic nucleus such as the lateral geniculate.

16.4.2 Convergence within the basal ganglia, useful for stimulus-response habit learning

In addition to this selection function, it is also useful to consider the further hypothesis that there is some convergent mapping achieved by the basal ganglia. This could allow for example a stimulus reflecting an input or event from any part of the cerebral cortex to be associated together with for example a response of the type represented in the putamen. The anatomical arrangement just described provides a possibility for some convergence on to single striatal neurons of cortical input, and on to single pallidal and nigral (pars reticulata) neurons of signals from relatively different parts of the striatum. For what computation might such anatomy provide a structural basis? Within the pallidum, each dendritic disc is flat, is orthogonal to the input fibres that pierce it, but is not filled with dendritic arborizations. Instead, each dendrite typically consists of 4–5 branches that are spread out to occupy only a small part of the surface area of the dendritic disc (see Fig. 16.8). There are thousands of such sparsely populated plates stacked on top of one another. Each pallidal neuron is contacted by a number of the mass of fibres from the striatum that pass it, and given the relatively small collecting area of each pallidal or nigral neuron (4 or 5 dendritic branches in a plane), each such neuron is thus likely to receive a random combination of inputs from different striatal neurons within its collection field. The thinness of the dendritic sheet may help to ensure that each axon does not make more than a few synapses with each dendrite, and that the combinations of inputs received by each dendrite are approximately random. This architecture thus appears to be appropriate for bringing together at random on to single pallidal and nigral neurons, inputs that originate from quite diverse parts of the cerebral cortex. (This is a two-stage process, cortex to striatum, and striatum to pallidum and substantia nigra). By the stage of the medial pallidum and substantia nigra, there is the opportunity for the input field of a single neuron to effectively become very wide. Empirical evidence that convergence does occur functionally from striatum to pallidum is the finding that some of the pallidal neurons active in the delayed match to sample task described in Section 16.3.2.3 were not modality-specific, whereas only visual or auditory modality-specific delayed match to sample neurons were located in the postero-ventral part of the striatum (Johnstone and Rolls, 1990; Rolls and Johnstone, 1992).

Given that this architecture could allow individual pallidal and nigral neurons to receive random combinations of inputs from different striatal neurons, the following functional implications arise. Simple associative (Hebbian) learning in the striatum would enable strongly firing striatal neurons to increase the strength of the synapses from the active cortical inputs in what would operate as a competitive network. (Descriptions of competitive networks are provided in Section B.4.) This could enable associations between, for example, stimuli and responses, to be learned. That learning could be made more efficient if a third input increased the associative plasticity, and dopamine could provide that modulating input (Nakahara et al., 2002). The evidence that the firing of dopamine neurons could reflect a reward prediction error (Schultz, 2013; Jiao et al., 2022) could in this reinforcement learning scenario (Schultz, 2016a; Fremaux and Gerstner, 2015) help to enable co-active stimulus and response inputs to striatal neurons that increase the firing of the striatal neurons to be strengthened by the receipt of a reinforcer such as food.

Consistent with this hypothesis (Rolls, 1999a), long-term potentiation (LTP) used to measure an increase of synaptic strength has been demonstrated in at least some parts of the basal ganglia. For example, Pennartz et al. (1993) demonstrated LTP of limbic inputs to the nucleus accumbens, and were able to show that such LTP is facilitated by dopamine. Further, it was shown that coincident cortical input and depolarization in a striatal neuron can induce long-term depression (LTD) of the cortico-striatal synapse if some dopamine is present (Calabresi et al., 1992), and LTP if there is a phasic release of dopamine (Wickens and Kotter, 1995; Wickens et al., 1996; Reynolds and Wickens, 2002). Dopamine can have diverse effects on striatal circuitry (Cox and Witten, 2019; Schultz, 2019; Bamford et al., 2018).

The system just described would not be very efficient, because the dopamine is broadcast throughout the striatum, and so must enable striatal neurons that have just been active to have their input synapses strengthened. The use of a reward prediction error signal would though be useful, for the stimulus-response connections would only be stamped in harder to make the habit stronger if the reward received (the outcome) was better than expected, as described further below in Section 16.4.3.

I suggest that this associative learning in the striatum may not rely only on the dopamine neuron firing: inputs from the orbitofrontal cortex and amygdala that will reflect rewards do reach the striosomes or patches within the striatal matrix (Bloem, Huda, Sur and Graybiel, 2017; Friedman, Homma, Gibb, Amemori, Rubin, Hood, Riad and Graybiel, 2015), and could provide an additional mechanism for guiding learning in the striatum.

In the pallidum, if additional conjunctive learning of coactive inputs occurs, it would be more complex, requiring, for example, a strongly inhibited pallidal neuron to show synaptic strengthening from strongly firing but inhibitory inputs from the striatum. Then, if a particular pallidal or nigral neuron received inputs by chance from striatal neurons that responded to an environmental cue signal that something significant was about to happen, and from striatal neurons that fired because the animal was making a postural adjustment, this conjunction of events might make that pallidal or nigral neuron become inhibited by (that is respond to) either input alone. Then, in the future, the occurrence of only one of the inputs, for example only the environmental cue, would result in a decrease of firing of that pallidal or nigral neuron, and thus in the appropriate postural adjustment being made by virtue of the output connections of that pallidal or nigral neuron.

This is a proposal that the basal ganglia are able to detect combinations of conjunctively active inputs from quite widespread regions of the cerebral cortex using their combinatorial architecture and a property of synaptic modifiability. In this way it would be possible to trigger any complex pattern of behavioral responses by any complex pattern of environmental inputs, using what is effectively an associative network (operating as a competitive network or pattern associator) to link by learning an antecedent input (for example the environmental salient cue inputs to the striatum) with the succeeding activity (for example a motor signal driving motor responses), especially if these are followed by a reinforcement signal.

It may be noted that the input events need not include only those from environmental stimuli represented in the caudate nucleus and ventral striatum, but also, if the overlapping properties of the dendrites described above provide sufficient opportunity for convergence, of the context of the movement, provided by inputs via the putamen from sensorimotor cortex. This would then make a system appropriate for triggering an appropriate motor response (learned by trial and error, with the final solution becoming associated with the triggering input events) to any environmental input state. As such, this hypothesis provides a suggested neural basis for 'habit' learning in which the basal ganglia have been implicated (Phillips et al., 1988; Petri and Mishkin, 1994; Balleine et al., 2009; Graybiel and Grafton, 2015; Robbins and Costa, 2017). The hypothesis could be said to provide a basis for the storage of motor plans in the basal ganglia, which would be instantiated as a series of look-ups of the appropriate motor output pattern to an evolving sequence of input information.

An interesting aspect of this hypothesis is that other parts of the motor system, such as the anterior cingulate cortex action-outcome learning system (Chapter 12), may mediate the control of action in a voluntary, goal-directed, way in the early stages of learning. The input context for the movement and the appropriate motor signals (originating during learning from motor cortical areas) could then be learned by the basal ganglia, until after many trials the basal ganglia can perform the required look-up of the correct motor output in an automated, 'habit', or 'stimulus–response', mode. In this sense, the cingulate and other cortical learning systems would set up the conditions, which because of their continuing repetition would be learned by the basal ganglia.

The hypothesis introduced above also may provide a basis for the switching between different types of behavior proposed as a function of the basal ganglia, for if a strong new pattern of inputs was received by the basal ganglia, this would result in a different pattern of outputs being associatively 'looked up' than that currently in progress.

16.4.3 Dopamine as a reward prediction error signal for reinforcement learning in the striatum

There is considerable evidence that some dopamine neurons (which are located in the midbrain substantia nigra pars compacta (A9) and ventral tegmental area (A10)) respond to reward prediction error, and project that information to the striatum (Mirenowicz and Schultz, 1996; Schultz, 1998; Glimcher, 2011b; Schultz, 2013, 2016a,b,c, 2017, 2019). Reward prediction error is the reward outcome value minus the expected value, and is illustrated for a midbrain dopamine neuron in Fig. 16.10. Reward prediction error is a key part of the teaching signal in reinforcement learning, which is described in Sections B.17 and 19.5.

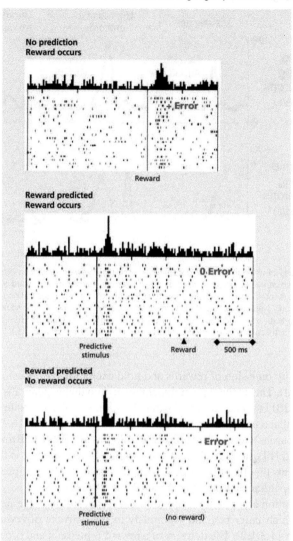

Fig. 16.10 A reward prediction error neuron. The reward outcome is delivered at the time indicated by 'Reward', and is a taste of juice. The Expected Value is signalled by the 'Predictive stimulus'. The neuron fires faster if the reward outcome is larger than expected (top, + Error); does not respond to the reward outcome if it is expected (middle, 0 Error); and fires less if the reward outcome is less than expected (bottom, - Error). The firing is shown on different trials in the rows; and the sum of the firing is represented in the histogram above. (After Schultz, W. 1998. Predictive reward signal of dopamine neurons. Journal of Neurophysiology 80: 1–27.)

One type of positive reward prediction error neuron, illustrated in Fig. 16.11A (Matsumoto and Hikosaka, 2009), increases its firing rate to a visual cue that predicts that reward (juice) will be delivered, and decreases its rate to a visual cue that predicts that an aversive stimulus (an air puff) will be delivered (left); and is not activated when a predicted reward is obtained, that is when the juice is delivered (not illustrated in Fig. 16.11A). This type of neuron increases its firing rate to an unpredicted reward outcome, and this is termed a positive reward prediction error response, for the reward outcome is greater than was predicted. This type of neuron decreases its firing if an expected reward stimulus is not received (Fig. 16.11A right), suggesting that it encodes the sign of the prediction error by whether it increases or decreases its firing rate. These neurons encode an accurate prediction error signal, including

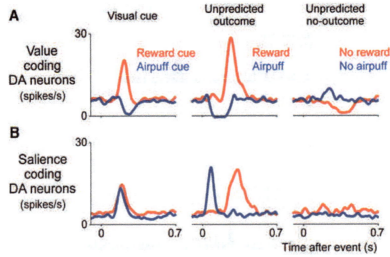

Fig. 16.11 Responses of different types of dopamine neuron. (A) A reward prediction error neuron (see text). The neuron responds to a visual cue that predicts reward (left). It does not respond to the reward outcome if it is as predicted (not illustrated). It does respond if an unpredicted reward is given (middle). It decreases its firing rate if an expected reward is not delivered (right). (B) Neurons activated by aversive and also by rewarding stimuli, sometimes called motivational salience neurons (see text). (Reproduced from Masayuki Matsumoto and Okihide Hikosaka (2009) Two types of dopamine neuron distinctly convey positive and negative motivational signals. *Nature* 459: 7248. © Springer Nature.)

strong inhibition by omission of rewards and mild excitation by omission of aversive events (Fig. 16.11A right). This is the type of dopamine neuron that is generally discussed (Schultz, 2013; Glimcher, 2011a). The neuron illustrated responds in the opposite direction to a visual cue that indicate that a mildly aversive airpuff will be delivered Fig. 16.11A.

Dopamine neurons can perform one-trial rule based reversal (Bromberg-Martin, Matsumoto, Hong and Hikosaka, 2010b), and the origin of this I suggest is the orbitofrontal cortex, which performs this function as described in Section 11.3.4 and projects via the ventral striatum to the dopamine neurons (Fig. 11.4, (Rolls, 2017c)).

Reward prediction error neurons are different to reward outcome neurons in the orbitofrontal cortex, which latter respond vigorously to the delivery of reward, even when it is expected (Section 11.3.1.2). The delivery of a reward is pleasant and produces emotions even when expected, so the dopamine neurons are not related to emotions associated with reward delivery. The reward prediction error signal instead seems more suitable for a learning signal. Moreover, the orbitofrontal cortex reward outcome neurons specify exactly what type of reward has been delivered (taste, oral texture, touch, temperature etc), whereas the reward signal conveyed by dopamine neurons appears to be one-dimensional, that a positive reward prediction error has occurred, but not what the type of reward was.

It should also be noted that these dopamine neurons are completely different to the negative reward prediction error neurons found in the orbitofrontal cortex, which increase their firing rate when an expected reward is not obtained (Thorpe, Rolls and Maddison (1983); see Section 11.3.4) and which has never been found for dopamine neurons.

Dopamine neurons respond not only to the phasic reward prediction error signals just described, but also their firing rate increases steadily during a 2 s period in which another conditioned stimulus is being shown that predicts that reward will be obtained with a probability P of 0.5 (Fiorillo, Tobler and Schultz, 2003). This tonic firing was lower for lower and higher probabilities of reward than 0.5, and so reflects reward uncertainty (see Fig. 16.12). These results are difficult to reconcile with the previously hypothesized (Waelti, Dickinson and Schultz, 2001; Dayan and Abbott, 2001) 'reward prediction error' training signal funct-

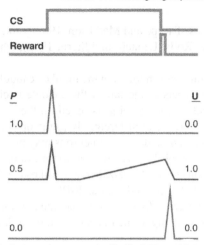

Fig. 16.12 Recordings from midbrain dopamine neurons by Fiorillo, Tobler and Schultz (2003) in a task in which different visual conditioned stimuli (CS) predicted different probabilities P of juice reward after a delay period when the stimulus switched off. The intertrial interval was variable, so that the conditioned stimulus provided information about reward delivery even when $P = 1.0$. When $P = 1.0$, the neurons responded phasically at the onset of the CS, and did not respond to the delivery of the taste reward. When $P = 0.0$, there was no response to the CS, and no response at the end of the CS unless reward was unexpectedly given (as illustrated). However, when $P = 0.5$, the dopamine neurons responded with gradually increasing and sustained firing during the CS. U indicates the uncertainty of reward. (Reproduced from P. Shizgal and A. Arvanitogiannis (2003) Gambling on dopamine. *Science* 299: 1856–1858. © The American Association for the Advancement of Science.)

ion of the firing of dopamine neurons, for it is difficult to understand how any brain system receiving the phasic ('prediction error') and tonic ('uncertainty of reward') dopamine signals by the same set of neurons could disentangle them and use them for different functions (Shizgal and Arvanitogiannis, 2003).

It is also an issue that there is an asymmetry in the errors that could be conveyed by dopamine neurons, given their low spontaneous firing rate of a few spikes/s (Niv et al., 2005). As a result of this asymmetry, positive prediction errors could be represented by dopamine neurons by firing rates of ≈270% above baseline, while negative errors could be represented by a decrease of only ≈55% below baseline (see Fig. 16.11). This asymmetry in prediction errors remains a potential problem for the dopamine error hypothesis.

Another potential problem with the dopamine reward prediction error hypothesis is that there are other types of dopamine neuron, some of which have been studied (Matsumoto and Hikosaka, 2009; Bromberg-Martin, Matsumoto and Hikosaka, 2010a). These neurons, illustrated in Fig. 16.11B, respond to both rewarding and to aversive stimuli, and could not therefore signal reward prediction error. In more detail, these dopamine neurons increase their firing rate to stimuli predicting reward and to stimuli predicting aversive events (left); and also respond when either an unpredicted reward outcome or an unpredicted aversive stimulus is obtained (middle). These are called 'motivational salience' neurons (Matsumoto and Hikosaka, 2009; Bromberg-Martin et al., 2010a), in that they encode something about both positive and negative reinforcers, but not a reward prediction error signal. Another type of dopamine neuron responds only to a cue predicting an aversive stimulus, or to an unpredicted aversive outcome.

Another type of dopamine neuron responds to novel stimuli (see Bromberg-Martin et al. (2010a)).

Another type of dopamine neuron responds to alerting cues, for example to the first cue in a trial that indicates that a trial is beginning (Bromberg-Martin et al., 2010a; Horvitz, 2000; Redgrave et al., 1999). These responses are very similar to those that we recorded in the head of the caudate nucleus (Rolls, Thorpe and Maddison, 1983b) and ventral striatum (Rolls and Williams, 1987a; Williams, Rolls, Leonard and Stern, 1993), which send projections to the dopamine neurons.

Another type of dopamine neuron found in the monkey caudolateral part of the substantia nigra pars compacta that projects to the tail of the caudate nucleus respond not to reward prediction error, but instead respond to objects based on their stable long-term association with rewards and continue to respond differentially to the objects, even when reward is not expected (Kim et al., 2015a). These dopamine neurons may provide a training signal for the tail of the caudate nucleus for habit-based responses, to for example look at objects with stable long-term reward associations (Kim, Ghazizadeh and Hikosaka, 2015a; Kim and Hikosaka, 2015; Hikosaka, Ghazizadeh, Griggs and Amita, 2018).

In rodents, there is also a great diversity of dopamine neuron response types, with some other dopamine neurons responding to the distance to a reward, or to movements (Cox and Witten, 2019).

However, activation of the dopamine neurons projecting to the ventral striatum can induce cue approach and lead the cue to become reinforcing, so it may be that dopamine neurons projecting to different regions have different functions, and some may function to implement a reward prediction error signal for reinforcement learning in the basal ganglia (Cox and Witten, 2019; Schultz, 2019). Indeed, it is now clear that dopamine neurons have far more diverse types of response than signalling reward prediction errors (Schultz, 2019).

Further discussion of the effects of dopamine on behavior is provided in Rolls (2014a). The dopamine system is also implicated in addiction to several types of drug (Everitt et al., 2008; Everitt and Robbins, 2013; Everitt et al., 2018; Luscher et al., 2020), and the habit, stimulus-response functions in habit of the basal ganglia have been related to the addictive properties of drugs that activate the dopamine system (Wise and Jordan, 2021).

Reinforcement learning models (Sections B.17 and 19.5) have been used to model in fMRI studies where reward prediction error may be represented in the brain, with one area in which reward prediction error is represented the ventral striatum (Hare et al., 2008; Colas et al., 2017; O'Doherty et al., 2017).

16.5 Comparison of computations for selection in the basal ganglia and cerebral cortex

The basal ganglia architecture is that the striatal, pallidal, and nigral neurons implement competition (for selection) by direct inhibitory recurrent lateral connections of the main output neurons on to other output neurons. The inputs to each stage of processing (e.g. striatum, globus pallidus) synapse directly on to the output neurons that inhibit each other (see Fig. 16.9). This is a simple and evolutionarily early design in that the basal ganglia were present in the brain before the neocortex evolved. A system such as the basal ganglia with direct inhibitory recurrent collaterals may have evolved easily because it is easier to make stable than architectures such as the cerebral cortex with recurrent excitatory connections. As noted above, the basal ganglia architecture may have been especially appropriate in motor systems in which instability could produce movement and co-ordination difficulties (Rolls and Treves, 1998; Rolls, 2014a, 2016b), and it is important to select motor responses before sending any output to muscles so that the muscles do not oppose each other. Thus a major advantage of this method of selecting outputs is that it is safe, with direct mutual inhibition of neurons, and no excitatory recurrent collaterals as in the neocortex.

This selection performed by the basal ganglia is then fed back to the cortex via the thalamus, and the selection performed in the basal ganglia may help to control many parts of the cerebral cortex to reflect the selection being performed in the basal ganglia, and also its stimulus-response habit learning.

In contrast, the neocortex with its excitatory recurrent collaterals, can also implement selection, by falling into a basin of attraction in which one mutually excitatory subpopulation of neurons ends up with high firing rates, as described in Section B.3. In this circuitry, the inhibitory neurons perform feedback inhibition to try to keep the system stable, with the very dangerous risk of runaway excitation always present. Indeed, epilepsy may be viewed as the price that is paid for this type of architecture (which applies to neocortex, hippocampal cortex, and pyriform cortex). So what in these circumstances are the advantages of performing the selection using cortical architecture with excitatory recurrent collaterals?

Perhaps the major advantage is that the recurrent collaterals allow a subset of the neurons in the network, once activated, to maintain their activity for some time, in a stable attractor, as described in Section B.3 (Rolls and Deco, 2010; Rolls, 2016b). This allows short-term memory, which has a major advantage of allowing animals to remember what has happened recently, and just as much, to even plan ahead by holding a number of items active simultaneously to form a plan. Thus attractor networks allow both retrospective and prospective memory.

Another major property of the cortical attractor approach is that when used for memory functions, it can complete a memory given a partial retrieval cue (Section B.3). This of course has major adaptive advantages, such as being able to remember where a food was located in response to a food cue or memory of a food (Chapter 9).

Another important property of the cortical attractor approach is that it can be used as a long-term memory system, with quite a high capacity if sparse representations are used (Section B.3). Indeed, in the order of 10,000 memories might be stored in a small cortical region with a diameter of 1–2 mm with 10,000 excitatory recurrent collateral synapses onto each neuron.

Another advantage of the cortical attractor approach is that when used as a decision-making system, the results of the decision can be kept 'on-line', by continuing firing of the attractor, to guide actions which may take some time to performed, or which may need to be delayed.

Another advantage of the cortical attractor approach is that when used for long-term memory, the system can, when influenced by the spiking-related noise, make jumps in different directions on different occasions, and thus implement such important functions as creativity and predator avoidance (Section B.3, Rolls and Deco (2010)).

Another advantage of the cortical attractor approach is that it allows weak interactions between attractors to implement many important cognitive functions, including top-down attention (Chapter 13).

Another advantage of the selection performed by the cerebral cortex is that for action-outcome learning, the exact nature of the outcome provided by the orbitofrontal cortex can be associated with the action that was performed to try to obtain the outcome, and this is likely to be much more powerful than reinforcement learning of stimulus-response associations for habits, as described in Section 19.5.

Given the advantages of attractor networks in the cerebral cortex, it is important to consider further disadvantages than the risk of epilepsy. It appears that variation of the stability of cortical attractor networks is being maintained for natural selection because having relatively low or relatively high stability might confer advantages to some individuals (see Chapter 18). In this context, we must remember that there are many different attractor networks in different cortical areas, and that the stability of every one may be being explored by natural selection, to find combinations that may have high fitness in different environments. For example, having low stability in some cortical attractor networks may contribute to creativity by facilitating the tendency to jump to new parts of the high-dimensional space (see Section B.3), but if the stability is too low, the low stability may contribute to the cognitive symptoms in schizophrenia such as difficulty in maintaining attention, and also to the positive symptoms in schizophrenia (Loh, Rolls and Deco, 2007a; Rolls, Loh, Deco and Winterer, 2008d; Rolls, 2012c). At the other end of what I see as a continuum, relatively high stability in some networks may help attention to remain focussed on a task (because of the high stability of the controlling attractor network providing the top-down input), but too much stability is some cortical systems may contribute to obsessive compulsive disorders (Rolls, Loh and Deco, 2008c; Rolls, 2012c). In the lateral orbitofrontal cortex, too little stability may contribute to impulsivity, and too much to depression (Rolls, 2016e) (see Chapter 18).

Thus a comparison of the cerebral cortex with the basal ganglia helps to draw out the advantages and disadvantages of these two types of architecture, and highlights the advantages of many of the operational principles of the cerebral cortex that are implemented by its excitatory recurrent collateral connections which can support attractors, which are almost a defining feature of the architecture of the cerebral cortex.

17 Cerebellar cortex

17.1 Introduction

The cerebellar cortex is not cerebral cortex, as it is part of the hindbrain, but its cortical structure is exquisitely developed, and is quite different to that of the cerebral cortex. It is thus very useful to compare its architecture and computational principles of operation to those of the cerebral cortex, for this helps to highlight some of the very different computations performed by different brain areas, that can be related to the major differences in their neuronal network architectures.

In this Chapter, the focus is on the structure of the cerebellar cortex, on the insights this provides into *how* it performs its computations, and on comparing the computational style of the cerebellar cortex with that of the cerebral neocortex.

A comparison with the cerebral cortex also shows how important the architecture and connectivity of a neural system, for example a type of cortex, are to understanding its principles of operation, that is its principles of computation. This goes far beyond trying to produce an arrow diagram to show the flow of information through a set of neurons (Shepherd and Grillner, 2010), which though the fine structure is crucially important, may do little to elucidate our understanding of the function of a type of cortex, as in some canonical microcircuit approaches (see e.g. Figs. 1.15, 1.16, and Rolls (2016b)). The pioneer in taking evidence from the quantitative aspects of the fine structure of the cortex forward to help formulate possible computational principles of operation of the cortex was David Marr (the Cambridge mathematician who came to learn from Giles Brindley in the Physiological Laboratory at Cambridge, when I was a medical student), who produced papers on the cerebellum (Marr, 1969), neocortex (Marr, 1970), and hippocampal cortex (Marr, 1971). My research has followed that pioneering approach, though I have gone beyond the combination of quantitative anatomical and mathematical approaches pioneered by Marr, to include also direct evidence on the neuronal activity at each connected stage of the system, evidence on neuronal encoding, evidence from fMRI in humans, evidence on the effects of damage to the system, and in addition also the approaches of theoretical physics, in collaborations with Alessandro Treves, Gustavo Deco, and many other theoretical physicists (Rolls and Treves, 1998; Rolls, 2008d; Rolls and Deco, 2010; Rolls, 2014a, 2016b).

The cerebellum is involved in the accurate control of movements. If the cerebellum is damaged, movements can still be initiated, but the movements are not directed accurately at the target, and frequently oscillate on the way to the target (Lisberger and Thach, 2013). There is insufficient time during rapid movements for feedback control to operate, and the computational hypothesis is that the cerebellum performs feedforward control by learning to control the motor commands to the limbs and body in such a way that movements are smooth and precise. The cerebellum is thus described as a system for adaptive feedforward motor control (Ito, 1984, 2010). Network theories of cerebellar function are directed at showing how it learns to take the context for a movement, which might consist of a desired movement from the cerebral neocortex and the starting position of the limbs and body, and produce the appropriate output signals. The appropriate output signals are learned as a result of the errors that have occurred on previous trials.

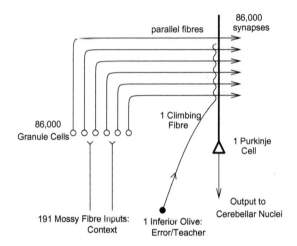

Fig. 17.1 Overall architecture of the cerebellum. Inputs relayed from the pontine nuclei form the mossy fibres which synapse onto dentate granule cells. The dentate granule cells via their parallel fibres form modifiable synapses on the Purkinje cells, from which outputs leave the cerebellar cortex. Each Purkinje cell receives one climbing fibre input. The numbers indicate the approximate numbers of cells of different types, relative to one Purkinje cell (see Ito, 1984). The numbers indicate expansion recoding of the mossy fibre inputs to the parallel fibres. A working hypothesis is that the context for a movement (for example limb state and motor command) reaches the Purkinje cells via the parallel fibres, and that the effect that this input has on the Purkinje cell output is learned through synaptic modification taught by the climbing fibre, so that the cerebellar output produces smooth error-free movements.

However, the human cerebellum is also involved in other functions, including cognitive, emotional, and social functions, as described in Section 17.5.

Much of the fundamental anatomy and physiology of the cerebellum are described by Masao Ito (1984; 2010) with classical neuroanatomy provided by Eccles, Ito and Szentagothai (1967), and pioneering computational neuroscience approaches provided by Marr (1969) and Albus (1971).

Some additional cell types and local circuitry in the cerebellum have been described more recently (Hull and Regehr, 2022). One example is that Purkinje cells have recurrent collaterals that inhibit other Purkinje cells and other cell types, and this may be part of a mechanism to keep the output of the cerebellum under feedback control (Hull and Regehr, 2022). But another possible function is that the mutual inhibition by Purkinje cells may act as a form of competitive interaction to sharpen the tuning of the neurons, in a similar way that is proposed for the striatal neurons and for the pallidal neurons in the basal ganglia (Chapter 16). It is interesting that both of these evolutionarily old brain systems (the basal ganglia and cerebellum) appear to use the same mutual inhibition of the output neurons, which is a safe way to compute, compared to the neocortex with its excitatory recurrent collateral connections between the pyramidal cells that are set up to maintain neuronal activity for functions such as short-term memory. Because there is a risk of runaway self-excitation in the neocortex, extra neuronal types to implement inhibition to keep the activity of the pyramidal cells under control are needed.

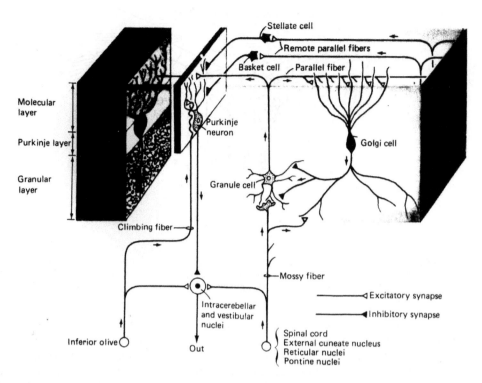

Fig. 17.2 Schematic diagram providing a 3D impression of the connectivity of a small part of the cerebellar cortex. Some of the inhibitory interneurons (Golgi, stellate, and basket cells) are shown.

17.2 Architecture of the cerebellum

The overall architecture of the cerebellum and the main hypothesis about the functions of the different inputs it receives are shown schematically in Fig. 17.1. The mossy fibres convey the context or to-be-modified input which is applied, after expansion recoding implemented via the granule cells, via modifiable parallel fibre synapses onto the Purkinje cells, which provide the output of the network. There is a climbing fibre input to each Purkinje cell, and this is thought to carry the teacher or error signal that is used during learning to modify the strength of the parallel fibre synapses onto each Purkinje cell. This network architecture is implemented beautifully in the very regular cerebellar cortex. As cortex, it is a layered system. The cerebellar cortex has great regularity and precision, and this has helped analysis of its network connectivity.

17.2.1 The connections of the parallel fibres onto the Purkinje cells

A small part of the anatomy of the cerebellum is shown schematically in Fig. 17.2. Large numbers of parallel fibres course at right angles over the dendritic trees of Purkinje cells. The dendritic tree of each Purkinje cell has the shape of a flat fan approximately 250 μm by 250 μm by 6 μm thick. The dendrites of different Purkinje cells are lined up as a series of flat plates (see Fig. 17.3). As the parallel fibres cross the Purkinje cell dendrites, each fibre makes one synapse with approximately every fifth Purkinje cell (Ito, 1984). Each parallel fibre runs for approximately 2 mm, in the course of which it makes synapses with approximately 45 Purkinje cells. Each Purkinje cell receives approximately 80,000 synapses, each from a different parallel fibre. The great regularity of this cerebellar anatomy thus beautifully provides for a simple connectivity matrix, with even sampling by the Purkinje cells of the

698 | Cerebellar cortex

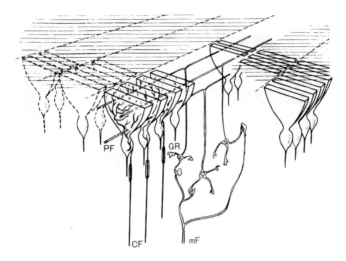

Fig. 17.3 The connections of the parallel fibres (PF) onto the Purkinje cells. Five rows of Purkinje cells with their fan-shaped dendritic trees are shown. CF, climbing fibre; GR, granule cell; mF, mossy fibre. (Reproduced from Szentagothai, J. (1968) Structuro-functional considerations of the cerebellar network. Proceedings of the IEEE 56: 960–968. © IEEE.)

parallel fibre input. This architecture provides for only one synapse from any parallel fibre to any one Purkinje cell, and not 2 or 3 synapses occasionally. The significance of this, it is suggested, is that in a perceptron (Section B.11), just as in a pattern association network as analyzed by Rolls (2015a), this maximizes the number of input patterns that can be correctly associated with outputs. The concept here is that if there are any double or triple connections from any input axon (a parallel fibre) to an output neuron (a Purkinje cell), this creates effectively double or triple strength connections between some neurons, which distorts the pattern association computation by emphasizing the contributions of some input neurons more than others (Rolls, 2015a).

17.2.2 The climbing fibre input to the Purkinje cell

The other main input to the Purkinje cell is the climbing fibre. There is one climbing fibre to each Purkinje cell, and this climbing fibre spreads to reach every part of the dendritic tree of the Purkinje cell. (Although the climbing fibre does not reach quite to the end of every dendrite, the effects of it on the Purkinje cell will reach to the apical extremity of every dendrite.) Although each Purkinje cell has an input from only one climbing fibre, each climbing fibre does branch and innervate approximately 10–15 different Purkinje cells in different parts of the cerebellum. The climbing fibres have their cell bodies in the inferior olive.

17.2.3 The mossy fibre to granule cell connectivity

The parallel fibres do not arise directly from the neurons in the pontine and vestibular nuclei (see Fig. 17.1). Instead, axons of the pontine and vestibular cells become the mossy fibres of the cerebellum, which synapse onto the granule cells, the axons of which form the parallel fibres (see Fig. 17.2). There are approximately 450 times as many granule cells (and thus parallel fibres) as mossy fibres (see Ito (1984), p. 116). In the human cerebellum, it is estimated that there are $10^{10} - 10^{11}$ granule cells (see Ito (1984), p. 76), which makes them the most numerous cell type in the brain. What is the significance of this architecture? It was suggested by Marr (1969) that the expansion recoding achieved by the remapping onto granule cells is to decorrelate or orthogonalize the representation before it is applied to the modifiable synapses onto the Purkinje cells. It is shown in Section B.2.7.3 how such expansion recoding can maximize capacity, reduce interference, and allow arbitrary mappings through a simple associative or similar network.

The granule cells of the cerebellum can therefore be regarded as analogous computationally to the dentate granule cells of the hippocampus, and to the granule / stellate cells in layer 4 of the neocortex, both of which perform pattern separation (Rolls, 2016b). The use again of granule cells for pattern separation in the cerebellum as well as in the hippocampus and neocortex is additional evidence for some of the fundamental computational principles of operation of the cortex described in this book and by Rolls (2016b).

As implied by the numbers given above, and as summarized in Fig. 17.1 in which I show (by extracting numbers from Ito (1984)) estimates of the relative numbers of the cells discussed so far in the cerebellum, there is a massive expansion in the number of cells used to code the same amount of information, in that the ratio of granule cells to mossy fibres is approximately 450. This provides a system comparable to a binary decoder. Consider an 8 bit binary number representation system, which can be used to represent the numbers 0–255 (decimal) (that is 2^8 numbers). Now, the bits that represent these numbers are often highly correlated with each other. For example, the bits that are set in the binary representations of the numbers 127 and 255 are identical apart from the highest order bit. (127 is 01111111 in binary and 255 is 11111111.) These two numbers would thus appear very similar in an associative memory system, such as that described in Section B.2, so there would be great interference between the two numbers in such a memory system. However, if the numbers 0–255 were each represented by a different active axon synapsing onto the output cell, then there would be no interference between the different numbers, that is the representations would be orthogonalized by binary decoding. The 450-fold increase in the number of fibres as information passes from mossy to parallel fibres potentially allows this expansion recoding to take place to implement pattern separation.

This architecture of the brain provides an interesting contrast with that of conventional digital computers. The type of information storage device that has evolved in the brain uses a distributed representation over a large number of input connections to a neuron, and gains from this the useful properties of generalization, graceful degradation, and the capacity to function with low information capacity stores (that is synapses), but pays the penalty that some decorrelation of the inputs is required. The brain apparently has evolved a number of specialized mechanisms to do this. One is exemplified by the granule cell system of the cerebellum, with its enormous expansion recoding. In effect, the brain provides an enormous number of what may be low resolution storage locations, which in the cerebellum are the vast number of parallel fibre to Purkinje cell synapses. It is astounding that the number of storage locations in the (human) cerebellum would thus be approximately 3×10^{10} parallel fibres with every parallel fibre making approximately 300 synapses, or approximately 10^{13} modifiable storage locations. (10 Terabits of storage.)

The recoding that could be performed by the mossy fibre to granule cell system can be understood more precisely by considering the quantitative aspects of the recoding. Each mossy fibre ends in several hundred rosettes, where excitatory contact is made with the dendrites of granule cells. Each granule cell has dendrites in 1–7 mossy rosettes, with an average of four. Thus, on average, each granule cell receives from four mossy fibres. Due to the spacing of the mossy fibres, in almost all cases the four inputs to a granule cell will be from different mossy fibres. Approximately 28 granule cell dendrites contact each rosette. There are approximately 450 times as many granule cells as mossy fibres. The result of this architecture is that the probability that any given granule cell has all its C inputs active, and is therefore likely to fire, is low. It is in fact P^C, where P is the probability that any mossy fibre is active.

Thus if the probability that a mossy fibre is active is 0.1, the probability that all of the average four inputs to a granule cell are active is 0.1^4 or 0.0001. The probability that three of the four inputs to a given granule cell are active would be 0.001. Given that each mossy fibre forms rosettes over a rather wide area of the cerebellum, that is over several folia, cells with three or four active inputs would be dotted randomly, with a low probability, within any one area.

One further aspect of this recoding must be considered. The output of the parallel fibres is sampled by the Golgi cells of the cerebellum via synapses with parallel fibres. Each Golgi cell feeds back inhibitory influences to about 5,000–10,000 granule cells. Neighbouring Golgi cells overlap somewhat in their dendritic fields, which are approximately 300 μm across, and in their axon arborization. Every granule cell is inhibited by at least one Golgi cell. The Golgi cells terminate directly on the mossy rosettes, inhibiting the granule cells at this point. This very broad inhibitory feedback system suggests the function of an automatic gain control. Thus Albus (1971) argued that the Golgi cells serve to maintain granule cell, and hence parallel fibre, activity at a constant rate. If few parallel fibres are active, Golgi inhibitory feedback decreases, allowing granule cells with lower numbers (for example 3 instead of 4) of excitatory inputs to fire. If many parallel fibres become active, Golgi feedback increases, allowing only those few granule cells with many (for example 5 or 6) active mossy inputs to fire. In addition to this feedback inhibitory control of granule cell activity, there is also a feedforward inhibitory control implemented by endings of the mossy fibres directly on Golgi cells. This feedforward inhibition probably serves a speed-up function, to make the overall inhibitory effect produced by the Golgi cells more smooth in time. The net effect of this inhibitory control is probably thus to maintain a relatively low proportion, perhaps 1%, of parallel fibres active at any one time. This relatively low proportion of active input fibres to the Purkinje cell learning mechanism optimizes information storage in the synaptic storage matrix, in that the sparse representation enables many different patterns to be learned by the parallel fibre to Purkinje cell system (see Section B.2).

17.3 Modifiable synapses of parallel fibres onto Purkinje cell dendrites

The climbing fibres take part in determining the modifiability of the parallel fibre to Purkinje cell synapses (Ito et al., 2014). In particular, the parallel fibre to Purkinje cell synapses decrease in strength, that is, they show long-term depression (LTD), when the climbing fibre to a Purkinje cell fires, if the parallel fibre is active (Ito, 1984; Ito et al., 2014). Thus the associative learning is between the parallel fibre and the Purkinje cell, but the 'teacher' is the climbing fibre, which produces a plateau potential in the Purkinje cell. This can be thought of as a type of error learning (Ito, 1984, 2013). If a parallel fibre is firing and tending to activate the Purkinje cell when is should not, then firing of the climbing fibre to indicate an error would reduce the strength of the synapse from that parallel fibre. If the climbing fibre does carry an error signal (which is a systems-level question (Ito, 2013), see below), then this would make the computation performed by the cerebellar cortex that of a one-layer perceptron (Ito, 1984, 2006, 2010) (see Section B.11). If the climbing fibre is on average not firing when a parallel fibre is firing, then that parallel fibre to Purkinje cell synapse will become stronger (i.e. show associative long-term potentiation, LTP).

It is interesting to note that despite an early theory that predicted modifiability of the parallel fibre to Purkinje cell synapses (Marr, 1969), experimental evidence for modifiability was only obtained in the 1980s (Ito, 1984). Part of the reason for this was that it was only when the physiology of the inferior olive was understood better, by making recordings from single neurons, that it was found that inferior olive neurons, which give rise to the climbing fibres, rarely fire at more than a few spikes per second. It was not until such relatively low-frequency stimulation (at 4 Hz) was used by Ito and his colleagues (see Ito (1984)) that the synaptic modifiability was demonstrated. (David Marr had tried with Jack Eccles to obtain evidence for synaptic modification, but they did not know the normally low firing rates of inferior olive neurons. Possibly as a result, David Marr felt that neuroscience methods were not yet available to test his theories on the principles of operation of cortical circuitry, and moved into more abstract theoretical work on vision (Marr, 1982; Rolls, 2011c).)

17.4 The cerebellar cortex as a perceptron

The overall concept that the work of Marr (1969), Albus (1971), and Ito (1984; 2006; 2013) has led towards is that the cerebellum acts as an adaptive feedforward controller with the general form shown in Fig. 17.2. The command for the movement and its context given by the current state of the limbs, trunk, etc., signalled by proprioceptive input would be fed to the intracerebellar (deep cerebellar) nuclei to produce a motor output ('Out' in Fig. 17.2). But in addition the input would be fed via the mossy fibres and then via the granule cells to the parallel fibres. There the appropriate firing of the Purkinje cells to enable the movement to be controlled smoothly would be produced via the parallel fibre to Purkinje cell synapses. These synapses would be set to the appropriate values by error signals received on many previous trials and projected via the climbing fibres to provide the teaching input for modifying the synapses utilizing LTD. The proposal described by Ito (1984) is thus that the cerebellum would be in a sideloop, with the overall gain or output of the system resulting from the direct, relatively unmodifiable output produced through the deep cerebellar nuclei, and the variable gain output contributed by the cerebellar sideloop.

This is a generic model of cerebellar function. Different parts of the cerebellum are concerned with different types of motor output (Ito, 1984; Lisberger and Thach, 2013). One part, the flocculus, is involved in the control of eye movements, and in particular with the way in which eye movements compensate for head movements, helping the images on the retina to remain steady during head movement. This is called the vestibulo-ocular reflex (VOR). Another part of the cerebellum is concerned with the accurate and smooth control of limb movements. Another part is implicated in the classical conditioning of skeletal responses, in which a sensory input such as a tone comes by learning to produce learned reflex responses. In order to assess how the generic circuitry of the cerebellum contributes to these types of adaptive control of motor output, evidence on how the cerebellum contributes to each of these types of motor learning is relevant, and is considered elsewhere (Ito, 1984, 2006, 2013; Lisberger and Thach, 2013).

A proposal that the cerebellum performs a predictive computation to produce an internal forward model for what the cortex is trying to achieve in terms for example of movement fits with earlier concepts, but does yet have any learning mechanism that uses for example the climbing fibres (Tanaka et al., 2020). Further, although the cerebellum is usually considered to implement supervised learning, there is recent interest in the possibility that the climbing fibres carry a signal that would be useful in temporal difference reinforcement learning (Hull, 2020). There is also increasing interest in how the cerebellum is involved in cognitive function, and on its relations with the basal ganglia and cerebral cortex (Sokolov et al., 2017; Caligiore et al., 2017).

One point about the theory that has always intrigued me is how a climbing fibre 'knows' which Purkinje cell to connect to, and therefore to provide the correct error or teaching input for that neuron. Or perhaps it is the other way round: the climbing fibre may determine what functions are being performed by a Purkinje cell, and some connections on the output side of the cerebellum need to be set up for that Purkinje cell's outputs (via the deep cerebellar nuclei) to act appropriately.

According to the Marr-Albus hypothesis, the cerebellar cortex is a supervised system, with a single teacher (the climbing fibre) for each Purkinje cell. In contrast, the basal ganglia is held to implement reinforcement learning, with a single teaching signal, dopamine release, broadcast to the whole of the striatum (Chapter 16). Neurons that signal reward delivery, expected reward, and non-reward, have now been found in the rodent cerebellum (Kostadinov and Hausser, 2022). Perhaps we should not be surprised, if all parts of the neocortex have connections to the cerebellum, for exactly these signals are found in the orbitofrontal cortex (Thorpe, Rolls and Maddison, 1983; Rolls, 2019f,e). However, this finding has led to the suggestion that the cerebellum may operate not just as a supervised system, but may also make use of reinforcement learning (Kostadinov and Hausser, 2022). However, the cerebellar system is odd, in that some climbing fibers signal violations in reward expectation with an increase in firing, regardless of whether the quality of reward was better or worse than expected – i.e., an unsigned prediction error (Kostadinov and Hausser, 2022). Perhaps the cerebellar error signal is used in the early stages of learning a task where a general reinforcement signal might be useful to guide the system to the correct part of the decision space, and then supervised learning is used to refine the details of the output required from the cerebellum (for example to touch a particular position).

The point of this brief survey has been not only to highlight some of the quantitatively remarkable and precise aspects of the design of the cerebellar cortex, but also to use the differences of its design from that of the cerebral cortex (neocortex, hippocampal cortex, and pyriform cortex) to illuminate the principles of operation and computation of all these types of cortex.

17.5 Cognitive functions of the cerebellum

Although traditionally the cerebellum has been viewed as a brain region with primarily motor functions and with connections with neocortical motor and premotor regions, evidence has started to accumulate that the cerebellum is also involved in cognitive, emotional, and social functions, as described next (Schmahmann et al., 2019; Schmahmann, 2021; Van Overwalle et al., 2020; Guell and Schmahmann, 2020; Stoodley and Tsai, 2021).

17.5.1 Anatomical connections from most neocortical regions

Connections from all neocortical regions via the pontine nuclei in the brainstem reach different parts of the cerebellar cortex (Schmahmann et al., 2019). The return pathways from the cerebellum connect mainly via the ventrolateral thalamic nuclei (VL) but also by the mediodorsal thalamic nuclei (MD) and intralaminar nuclei to all neocortical regions, and the paths are segregated throughout this whole connectivity (Schmahmann et al., 2019). For example, the primary motor cortex connectivity is with cerebellar lobules III–VI and VIII; and the dorsolateral prefrontal cortex area 46 connections are with cerebellar crus II and lobule X (Schmahmann et al., 2019). The cingulate cortex has connectivity that relates it to cerebellar lobule IX, the ventral paraflocculus (Schmahmann, 2021).

17.5.2 Functional connectivity of different cortical systems with different parts of the cerebellum

Different neocortical networks (central executive, default mode, dorsal attention, salience) have resting state functional connectivity with different parts of the cerebellar cortex (Habas, 2021). The polymodal neocerebellum (lobules VII, VIII, and IX) is massively interconnected with associative cortices, as well as with the striatum and amygdala (Habas, 2021). Fig. 17.5a provides further evidence on the parts of the human cerebellum with functional connectivity with different resting state networks in humans.

17.5.3 Activation of different cerebellar cortical regions in different tasks

Task-based fMRI meta-analysis has shown involvement of the neocerebellum, including lobules VI, VII, and VIII, in executive, linguistic, and emotional functions (Schmahmann et al., 2019; Stoodley and Tsai, 2021; Stoodley et al., 2012). Fig. 17.4a shows that different parts of the cerebellar cortex are activated by finger tapping (red), working memory (purple), verb generation (blue), and mental rotation (green) (Stoodley et al., 2010). Fig. 17.4b shows that for lobule VIIB which relates to the neocortical dorsal attention network, in a working memory task the locus of spatial attention encoding is medially situated, and the attentional load content is more laterally situated (Schmahmann et al., 2019). Fig. 17.4d shows that both task activations and changes in task-related functional connectivity provide evidence that several different parts of the cerebellar cortex are activated during three different tasks, a motor task, story listening, and working memory (Schmahmann et al., 2019). Fig. 17.5a shows activations produced in the cerebellum by different types of task.

17.5.4 Damage to different parts of the cerebellum can produce different cognitive, emotional, and motor impairments

In patients with stroke, lesions of different parts of the cerebellar cortex can produce symptoms that may include ataxia or cognitive/emotional deficits. Fig. 17.4c shows that lesions of lobules IV–V of the anterior lobe extending into adjacent lobule VI produce the cerebellar motor syndrome of ataxia. Lesions confined to posterior lobe lobules crus II through lobule IX produce the cerebellar cognitive affective/Schmahmann syndrome but no motor ataxia (Schmahmann et al., 2019; Schmahmann, 2021). The symptoms of the cerebellar cognitive affective/Schmahmann syndrome include impaired executive function (planning, set-shifting, abstract reasoning, verbal fluency, working memory), often with perseveration, distractibility or inattention; visual–spatial disorganization and impaired visual–spatial memory; personality change with blunting of affect or disinhibited and inappropriate behavior; and difficulties with language production including dysprosodia, agrammatism, and mild anomia (Schmahmann, 2021).

17.5.5 Neocortical–cerebellar cortical computations for cognition

One approach is that the cerebellum implements an internal forward model that analyses the causal relationship between a command and the outcomes of that command, predicting the outcome of the performed action given the current context (Stoodley and Tsai, 2021; Ito, 1984). The mossy fiber input may introduce information about the motor command and the present context into the cerebellar circuit, and the climbing fibres need to provide the correct prediction error (Stoodley and Tsai, 2021; Hull, 2020).

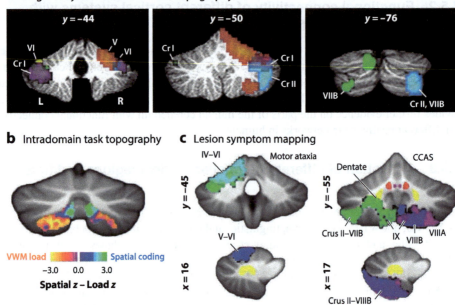

Fig. 17.4 Cerebellar functional topography in humans. (a) Intraindividual topography of task-based activations in the cerebellum for finger tapping (red), working memory (purple), verb generation (blue), and mental rotation (green) (Stoodley et al., 2010). (b) Spatial gradients within the dorsal attention network in lobule VIIB on a working memory task. The locus of spatial attention encoding is medially situated; attentional load content is more lateral. Panel b adapted from Brissenden et al. (2018). (c) In patients with stroke, lesions of lobules IV-V of the anterior lobe extending into adjacent lobule VI produce the cerebellar motor syndrome of ataxia. Lesions confined to posterior lobe lobules crus II through lobule IX produce the cerebellar cognitive affective/Schmahmann syndrome but no motor ataxia. Panel c adapted from Stoodley et al. (2016). (d) Task and resting-state activation topography in motor and nonmotor domains. Task activation (top row) reveals a pattern of two motor (first column) and three nonmotor representations (second and third columns). An overlapping pattern was observed when calculating resting-state functional connectivity from cerebral cortical activation peaks for each corresponding task activity contrast (bottom row). First motor (lobules I-VI) or first nonmotor representation (VI/crus I) (green arrows), second motor (VIII) or second nonmotor representation (crus II/lobule VIIB) (yellow arrows), and third nonmotor representation (IX/X) (red arrows) are shown. First and second nonmotor representations can be contiguous (as in story listening) or separate (as in working memory). Panel d adapted from Guell et al. (2018a). Abbreviations: CCAS, cerebellar cognitive affective syndrome; Cr, crus; L, left; R, right; VWM, verbal working memory. (From Schmahmann,J.D., Guell,X., Stoodley,C.J. and Halko,M.A. 2019. The theory and neuroscience of cerebellar cognition. Ann Rev Neurosci 42:337-364.)

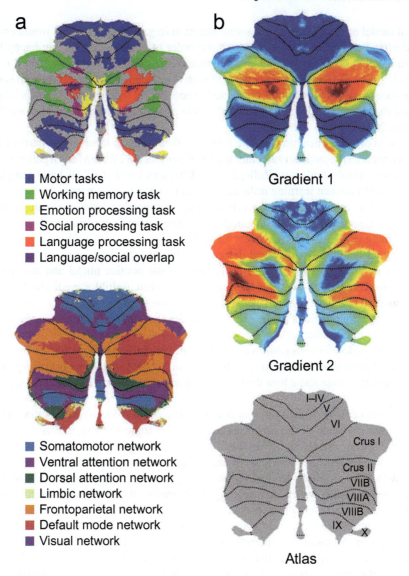

Fig. 17.5 Cerebellar functional topography in humans. (a) Discrete task activity maps (adapted from Guell et al. (2018a)); and resting-state functional connectivity maps (adapted from Buckner et al. (2011)). (b) Cerebellar gradients 1 and 2 and the cerebellum flatmap atlas. Gradient 1 extends from the language task/default mode network to motor regions, and gradient 2 isolates working memory/frontoparietal network areas. Panel b adapted from Guell et al. (2018b). (Modified from Schmahmann,J.D., Guell,X., Stoodley,C.J. and Halko,M.A. 2019. The theory and neuroscience of cerebellar cognition. Ann Rev Neurosci 42:337-364.)

With this background, it has been suggested that the cerebellum provides the circuit properties to generate, update, and automatize predictions using both supervised and reinforcement learning (Stoodley and Tsai, 2021). These predictive and adaptive internal models may enable precise performance, timing, and learning of complex behaviors, including those relevant to social interactions. The suggestion is that 'cerebellar circuits, acting at the implicit level and using social information conveyed through extensive cerebrocerebellar connections, could build internal models of complex behaviors, allowing for automatic information processing and appropriate behaviors in a range of socially relevant processes ranging from perception of biological motion to understanding the mental states of others. For example, an internal model of the dynamics of a social situation (e.g., a birthday party) would enable one to understand and accurately predict both the order of events (e.g., singing happy birthday prior to cake) and their emotional consequences (e.g., child excited to eat cake)' (Stoodley and Tsai, 2021). This approach is consistent with the evidence that the cerebellum is engaged during social tasks, is functionally connected to neocortical regions critical for social processing, and that cerebellar disruption can be associated with altered social behaviors (Stoodley and Tsai, 2021).

In terms of neocortical design, one feature is that the deep layers of all parts of the neocortex connect to the striatum and enter the basal ganglia circuit with return pathways back to the neocortex via the thalamus (Rolls, 2016b) (Chapters 1 and 16). This basal ganglia circuit may use reinforcement learning utilising dopamine neuron firing reward prediction error to create complex combinations of neocortical inputs that together define a stimulus/context that can be then associated in the basal ganglia with a response to implement stimulus-response habit learning (Rolls, 2016b) (Chapters 1 and 16).

A second feature of neocortical design may be that the deep layers of all parts of the neocortex may be specified to send projections to the pontine nuclei and thereby to gain access to the cerebellum. In evolution, this may have been useful for predictive feed-forward motor control, but given that this genetic specification of this connectivity was once set up between some brain regions (Rolls and Stringer, 2000), it may have been a useful strategy in evolution not to interfere with the genetic specification of connectivity as other neocortical regions were added. The suggestion then is that the cerebellum may perform some predictive feedforward input that is useful to cognitive, emotional, and social neocortical regions. If so, it is an important issue about how the correct training signal is provided to the climbing fibres (Hull, 2020).

These concepts may shed light on neocortical design. A key feature is that outputs are taken from every stage of the neocortex and used for some purpose, and are not just taken from the ends of processing hierarchies (Rolls and Stringer, 2000). It is possible that the deep layers (5,6) of the neocortex are of earlier evolutionary origin than the superficial layers (2, 3), with 2,3 specialised for feedforward computations up hierarchies to build new representations at each stage of the hierarchy. That implies that the design constraints for the superficial and deep layers of the neocortex may be different, and may include more continuous representations for the deep layers (Rolls and Mills, 2017). Another difference may be that the representations in the superficial layers of the neocortex may need to be sparse to facilitate the competitive learning that takes place from cortical stage to stage in a hierarchy. In contrast, in the deep layers of the neocortex the representations might be less sparse, because these layers provide backprojections for memory recall and top-down attentional modulation, and less sparse representations may be useful for these functions in the context of the diluted connectivity of the neocortex (Rolls, 2023e). Possible specialisations of the deep layers of the neocortex that make them appropriate for providing signals for computations to be performed by the cerebellum is a topic of interest.

Another interesting difference is how rewards are used computationally by the cerebellum, basal ganglia, and neocortex. As described above, the cerebellum may operate as a supervised system with a separate teacher for each Purkinje cell, with perhaps some influence by reward-related errors in a type of reinforcement-related learning. This may be appropriate for refining the details of output using predictive feedforward control. The basal ganglia is held to implement reinforcement learning, with a single teaching signal, dopamine release, broadcast to the whole of the striatum to implement stimulus-response habit learning (Chapter 16). This may be appropriate for setting up fixed responses that take into account the activity of all cortical areas channelled through the striatum, and therefore a very large set of possible inputs. In contrast, the neocortex in the orbitofrontal cortex – anterior cingulate cortex system sends details of the exact reward or punisher received in terms of its value (Chapter 11) to the anterior cingulate cortex where it can be associated with the particular goal-directed action that will obtain the best outcome in terms of its reward-punishment value in action-outcome learning (Chapter 12). This type of action-outcome learning implemented by these neocortical areas is very effective because the actions are always under control of the current value of the goal as received from the orbitofrontal cortex (as shown by devaluing the goal), because the full details of the goal value are specified (e.g. is it this type of food, or that type of food, and is there any sensory-specific satiety for that particular goal), and because the neocortex with its short-term memory capability implemented by recurrent collateral attractor networks can take into account the action-outcome results for the previous few trials.

17.6 Highlights: differences between cerebral and cerebellar cortex microcircuitry

1. First, this comparison does highlight how the design of different types of cortex is very different, and at the same time how precisely types of cortex are designed. The implication is that the quantitative details of the connectivity are important, a point understood by Marr, but hardly emphasized in most 'canonical models' of the microcircuitry of the cerebral cortex, most of which may not even show recurrent collateral connections between classes of pyramidal cells, let alone consider their number, and what the computational significance may be (see e.g. Figs. 1.15 and 1.16, but compare Fig. 1.17 and Rolls (2016b)).

2. Second, the cerebellar cortex does not have excitatory recurrent collaterals, and the cerebral cortex does. This helps to make excitatory recurrent collaterals what is probably the most fundamental aspect of the design of the cerebral cortex, which provides the ability to maintain information by positive excitatory feedback, to enable short-term memory, long-term memory, decision-making, top-down attention, etc, as described throughout this book and by Rolls (2016b).

3. Third, analysis of the cerebellum shows how important the quantitative aspects of the connectivity are for brain computation, with large numbers of parallel fibre synapses for example onto each Purkinje cell. The importance of this is that the number of synapses onto each neuron is the leading factor in the number of memories that can be stored in pattern associators, perceptrons, and autoassociation networks, so these numbers are just as important for the cerebral cortex (Appendix B).

4. Fourth, analysis of the cerebellum shows how important it is for associative memories to have relatively orthogonal patterns presented to the network, with this being implemented by the 10^{10} or more granule cells in the cerebellum. In the same way, the hippocampus has granule cells in the dentate gyrus to perform pattern separation, and the neocortex has stellate cells in layer 4 to do the same, especially where it appears that much orthogonalization is required, in primary sensory cortical areas such as the primary visual cortex, V1 (see Rolls (2016b)).

5. Fifth, a major difference from the cerebral cortex is that each Purkinje cell has its own teacher, its climbing fibre. There appears to be nothing like this in the cerebral cortex. Instead, the hypothesis developed by Rolls (2016b) and in this book is that in the neocortex the correct neocortical pyramidal cells are selected by which ones win in an unsupervised, competitive network, style of computation for any given input pattern. Further, the hypothesis is that in the hippocampus, the selection of which CA3 cells should be activated is performed by random selection, using the mossy fibres, as described in Chapter 9. The

difference from the neocortex is that the computation performed by the hippocampal CA3 network is to store large numbers of memories separately, and for this, picking neurons at random to be part of each memory is appropriate. In contrast, in the neocortex, the aim of the computation is much more sophisticated, to build useful representations for categorising complex inputs, and for this purpose competitive learning is used to produce neocortical neurons that respond to different non-linear combinations of their inputs (Section B.4 and Rolls (2016b)).

6. Sixth, the human cerebellum is also involved in other functions, including cognitive, emotional, and social functions, as described in Section 17.5. Different neocortical regions have connectivity with different parts of the cerebellum, and the different parts of the human cerebellum are activated during the performance of different tasks. Moreover, damage to some parts of the human cerebellum can produce clinically relevant cognitive, emotional, or social problems. It has been suggested that cerebellar circuits could build internal models of complex behaviors that facilitate predictions, allowing for automatic information processing and appropriate behaviors in a range of processes ranging from perception of biological motion to understanding the mental states of others (Stoodley and Tsai, 2021).

18 Cortical attractor dynamics and connectivity, stochasticity, psychiatric disorders, and aging

18.1 Introduction and overview

18.1.1 Introduction

The cerebral neocortex has highly developed local recurrent collateral connections allowing neurons within 2–3 mm to have a probability of approximately 0.1 of connecting with each other, and given associative synaptic modifiability, these can form local attractor networks (Section B.3) (Rolls, 2016b). These attractor networks provide a foundation for *what* is computed in many cortical systems, including short-term memory (Section 13.6.1), decision-making (Section 11.5.1), language (Section 14.5), episodic memory (Chapter 9), and visual perception by contributing to a trace of previous neuronal firing (Chapter 2). The operation of attractor or autoassociation networks is described in Sections B.3 and 11.5.1.

In this chapter we consider *how* the operation of attractor networks in the brain is influenced by noise in the brain produced by the random firing times of neurons for a given mean firing rate; how this can in fact be beneficial to the operation of the brain; and how the stability of these systems and how they are influenced by noise in the brain is relevant to understanding a number of mental disorders. These concepts can inform understanding of the brain that is relevant not only to its operation in health, but also in disease, and how it may be possible to ameliorate some of the effects found in these mental and other disorders, which is a key aim of this book.

18.1.2 Overview

1. The stability of attractor networks in the face of the random spiking times of neurons for a given mean neuronal firing rate is analyzed. The stability of attractor networks is increased if the receptor conductances, or at a different level the synaptic weights, or at another level the functional connectivity, is increased. Such networks with this higher stability can have more persistent short-term memory, and are less distractible.
2. Hypotheses are described about how increased or decreased stability of different cortical networks may contribute to psychiatric disorders and to the memory changes in normal aging.
3. In schizophrenia, the positive symptoms such as hallucinations and intrusive thoughts may be associated with too little stability of attractor networks caused by reduced inhibition (and/or increased glutamatergic function) in the temporal lobe cortex and related areas. The reduction of stability results in some networks entering high firing rate attractor states even with no or little input.
4. In schizophrenia, the cognitive symptoms such as impaired attention and working memory may be related to reduced efficacy of NMDA glutamate receptors and/or decreased numbers of spines introducing excitatory input to neurons in the prefrontal cortex involved in

short-term memory and attention. The reduced firing rate would decrease the stability of high firing rate attractor network states involved in maintaining stable working memory and attention.

5. In schizophrenia, the same changes as in (4) in the orbitofrontal cortex would decrease the firing rates of neurons involved in reward, punishment, emotion, and motivation, and thus produce the negative symptoms of decreased mood and motivation.

6. Going beyond the disconnectivity hypothesis of schizophrenia, it is shown using effective connectivity that although the forward (stronger) connections between cortical areas are decreased, the backprojections are much less reduced. This produces an imbalance, with internally generated states becoming more prevalent compared to states elicited by bottom-up inputs from the world.

7. In addition, in schizophrenia there is reduced functional connectivity and therefore increased temporal variability of the thalamic inputs for visual and auditory stimuli, which is related to decreased efficacy of inputs from the world relative to internally generated processing related to increased backprojections from the precuneus and posterior cingulate gyrus which have been identified in schizophrenia.

8. In obsessive-compulsive disorder, enhanced glutamatergic activity may make a number of different cortical attractor networks overstable. The details of which attractor networks are overstable may be different in different patients. Overactivity of some frontal cortical attractor networks might produce over-stability and perseveration of plans. Overstability of other frontal cortical attractor networks might produce obsessive actions.

9. In depression, oversensitivity, overactivity and increased functional connectivity of a lateral orbitofrontal cortex network involved in non-reward and punishment may lead it to enter too often and remain too long in high firing rate attractor states, leading to the symptoms of persistent sadness that can be produced by non-reward. This higher connectivity is normalised by conventional antidepressant drugs (e.g. SSRIs). In depression, the medial orbitofrontal cortex reward system has reduced sensitivity to reward and reduced functional connectivity with medial temporal lobe memory systems, resulting in anhedonia and fewer happy memory states (see *The Brain, Emotion, and Depression* (Rolls, 2018a) and Zhang, Rolls et al (2023a)). The medial orbitofrontal cortex is a site where ketamine acting as an antidepressant may act (Zhang et al., 2023a).

10. In normal aging, reduced neuronal firing rates in attractor memory networks may contribute to the reduced working memory. The reduction of firing rates may be related to decreased synaptic efficacy and learning, and to increased cortical adaptation. Decreasing cholinergic function in aging may contribute to the memory problems in normal aging by reducing long-term synaptic modification, and by increasing neuronal adaptation thereby decreasing the firing rates in attractor networks used in memory. The orbitofrontal cortex has connectivity to the cholinergic systems, and may also thereby be involved in the memory problems that can occur in normal aging. This applies to both hippocampal episodic memory and to prefrontal cortex short-term / working memory.

11. All these hypotheses have implications for potential treatments, and provide a new way to conceptualize some psychiatric disorders, and the effects of normal aging on memory.

12. Part of the value of the approach is that it links changes at the neuronal and synaptic level, and how they are influenced by treatments, to the symptoms, through understanding the computational principles of operation of neuronal networks in the cerebral cortex.

18.2 The noisy cortex: stochastic dynamics, decisions, and memory

The spiking of the neurons in the brain is almost random in time for a given mean firing rate, i.e. the spiking is approximately Poissonian, and this randomness introduces noise into the system, which makes the system behave stochastically. The effect that this stochasticity has on a neural system, and more generally the dynamics of the system, for example how long it takes to respond, and how long it remains in a given state, can be investigated using integrate-and-fire neuronal network simulations, which model how the currents through the different synaptic receptor-activated ion channels are integrated to produce the membrane potential of a neuron, which fires an action potential when the threshold is reached. The integrate-and-fire neuronal network approach is described in Section B.6, and as used here dynamically models the membrane potential of point neurons, and the dynamics of the opening and closing of different receptor-activated ion channels. Each of the simulated neurons shows spiking that is very much like that of neurons recorded in the brain. From such integrate-and-fire models it is possible to make predictions not only about synaptic and neuronal activity, but also about the signals recorded in functional neuroimaging experiments, and the behavior of the system, in terms for example of its probabilistic choices, its reaction times, and its stability. This makes a close link with human behavior possible (Rolls, Grabenhorst and Deco, 2010b,c). The theory as to how networks operate stochastically (Rolls and Deco, 2010; Deco et al., 2013) has implications throughout the cortex, some of which are described in this chapter.

First we consider the sources of the noise in the cortex (Section 18.2.1). Then we consider how the spiking-related noise influences the stability of short-term memory mechanisms in the cortex (Section 18.2.2). How the spiking-related noise influences decision-making mechanisms in the cortex has been described in Section 11.5.1. Some advantages of noise in the brain, and how these play out in some different ways in the cortex, are described in Sections 18.2.5–18.2.8. Fundamental approaches to stochastic dynamics in the cortex, including equations, are provided in Sections B.6–B.8.

18.2.1 Reasons why the brain is inherently noisy and stochastic

Why is the spiking activity of neurons probabilistic, and what are the advantages that this may confer? The answer suggested (see Rolls (2016b) and Rolls and Deco (2010)) is that the spiking activity is approximately Poisson-like (as if generated by a random process with a given mean rate, both in the brain and in the integrate-and-fire simulations I describe), because the neurons are held close to (just slightly below) their firing threshold, so that any incoming input can rapidly cause sufficient further depolarization to produce a spike. It is this ability to respond rapidly to an input, rather than having to charge up the cell membrane from the resting potential to the threshold, a slow process determined by the time constant of the neuron and influenced by that of the synapses, that enables neuronal networks in the brain, including attractor networks, to operate and retrieve information so rapidly (Treves, 1993; Rolls and Treves, 1998; Battaglia and Treves, 1998a; Rolls, 2016b; Panzeri, Rolls, Battaglia and Lavis, 2001; Rolls and Deco, 2010). The spike trains are essentially Poisson-like because the cell potential hovers noisily close to the threshold for firing (Dayan and Abbott, 2001), the noise being generated in part by the Poisson-like firing of the other neurons in the network (Jackson, 2004). The noise and spontaneous firing help to ensure that when a stimulus arrives, there are always some neurons very close to threshold that respond rapidly, and then communicate their firing to other neurons through the modified synaptic weights, so that an attractor process can take place very rapidly (Rolls, 2016b; Rolls and Deco, 2010).

The implication of these concepts is that the operation of networks in the brain is inherently noisy because of the Poisson-like timing of the spikes of the neurons, which itself is related to the mechanisms that enable neurons to respond rapidly to their inputs (Rolls, 2016b). However, the consequence of the Poisson-like firing is that, even with quite large attractor networks of thousands of neurons with hundreds of neurons representing each pattern or memory, the network inevitably settles probabilistically to a given attractor state. This results, *inter alia*, in decision-making being probabilistic. Factors that influence the probabilistic behavior of the network include the strength of the inputs (with the difference in the inputs / the magnitude of the inputs being relevant to decision-making and Weber's Law as described in Section 11.5.1); the depth and position of the basins of attraction, which if shallow or correlated with other basins will tend to slow the network; noise in the synapses due to probabilistic release of transmitters (Koch, 1999; Abbott and Regehr, 2004); and the mean firing rates of the neurons during the decision-making itself, the firing rate distribution (Webb, Rolls, Deco and Feng, 2011), and the dilution of the connectivity (Rolls and Webb, 2012). In terms of synaptic noise, if the probability of release, p, is constant, then the only effect is that the releases in response to a Poisson presynaptic train at rate r are described by a Poisson process with rate pr, rather than r. However, if the synapse has short-term depression or facilitation, the statistics change (Fuhrmann et al., 2002b; Abbott and Regehr, 2004). A combination of these factors contributes to the probabilistic behavior of the network becoming poorer and slower as the difference between the inputs divided by the base frequency is decreased (Deco and Rolls, 2006).

In signal-detection theory, behavioral indeterminacy is accounted for in terms of noisy input (Green and Swets, 1966). In the present approach, indeterminacy is accounted for in part in terms of internal noise inherent to the operation of spiking neuronal circuitry (Rolls, 2016b; Rolls and Deco, 2010) (see also Wang (2008) and Faisal, Selen and Wolpert (2008)).

In fact, there are many sources of noise, both external to the brain and internal (Faisal, Selen and Wolpert, 2008). A simple measure of the variability of neuronal responses is the Fano factor, which is the ratio of the variance to the mean. A Poisson process has a Fano factor of 1, and neurons often have Fano factors close to one, though in some systems and for some neurons they can be lower (less variable than a Poisson process), or higher (Faisal et al., 2008). The sources of noise include the following, with citations to original findings provided by Faisal et al. (2008).

First, there is sensory noise, arising external to the brain. Thermodynamic noise is present for example in chemical sensing (including smell and gustation) because molecules arrive at the receptor at random rates owing to diffusion. Quantum noise can also be a factor, with photons arriving at the photoreceptor at a rate governed by a Poisson process. The peripheral nervous system (e.g. the retina, and in the olfactory bulb the glomeruli) often sums inputs over many receptors in order to limit this type of noise. In addition to these processes inherent in the transduction and subsequent amplification of the signals, there may of course be variation in the signal itself arriving from the world.

Second, there is cellular or neuronal noise arising even in the absence of variation in synaptic input. This cellular noise arises from the stochastic opening and closing of voltage or ligand-gated ion channels, the fusing of synaptic vesicles, and the diffusion and binding of signalling molecules to the receptors. The channel noise becomes appreciable in small axons and cell bodies (where the number of channels and molecules involved becomes relatively small). This channel noise can affect not only the membrane potential of the cell body and the initiation of spikes, but also spike propagation in thin axons. There may also be some cross-talk between neurons, caused by processes such as ephaptic coupling, changes in extracellular ion concentration after electrical signalling, and spillover of neurotransmitters between adjacent unrelated synapses.

Third, there is synaptic noise evident for example as spontaneous miniature postsynaptic currents (mPSCs) that are generated by the 'quantal' (discrete) nature of released neurotransmitter vesicles (Fatt and Katz, 1950; Manwani and Koch, 2001). This synaptic noise can be produced by processes that include spontaneous opening of intracellular Ca^{2+} stores, synaptic Ca^{2+}-channel noise, spontaneous triggering of the vesicle-release pathway, and spontaneous fusion of a vesicle with the membrane. In addition, at the synapses there is variation in the number of transmitter molecules in a released vesicle, and there are random diffusion processes of the molecules (Franks et al., 2003). In addition, there is randomness in whether an action potential releases a vesicle, with the probability sometimes being low, and being influenced by factors such as synaptic plasticity and synaptic adaptation (Faisal et al., 2008; Abbott and Regehr, 2004; Manwani and Koch, 2001).

The sources of noise in the brain arise from the effects described earlier that make the firing properties of neurons very often close to Poisson-like. If the system were infinitely large (as the mean field approach described here assumes) then the Poisson firing would average out to produce a steady average firing rate averaged across all the neurons. However, if the system has a finite number of neurons, then the Poisson or semirandom effects will not average out, and the average firing rate of the population will fluctuate statistically. These effects are referred to as coherent fluctuations. The magnitude of these fluctuations decreases with the square root of the size of the network (the number of neurons in the population in a fully connected network, and the number of connections per neuron in a network with diluted connectivity) (Mattia and Del Giudice, 2002). The magnitude of these fluctuations is described by the standard deviation of the firing rates divided by the mean rate, and this can be used to measure the noise in the network. These effects are described in detail in the Appendix of *The Noisy Brain: Stochastic Dynamics as a Principle of Brain Function* (Rolls and Deco, 2010) (available for download at https://www.oxcns.org).

The signal-to-noise ratio can be measured in a network by the average firing rate change produced by the signal in the neuronal population divided by the standard deviation of the firing rates. Non-linearities in the system will affect how the signal-to-noise ratio described in this way is reflected in the output of the system. Another type of measure that reflects the signal-to-noise ratio is the stability of the system as described by its trial to trial variability, as described in Sections 18.2.2 and 18.2.4 and by Rolls, Loh, Deco and Winterer (2008d).

Although many approaches have seen noise as a problem in the brain that needs to be averaged out or resolved (Faisal, Selen and Wolpert, 2008), and this is certainly important in sensory systems, the thrust of *The Noisy Brain* (Rolls and Deco, 2010) is to show that in fact noise inherent in brain activity has a number of advantages by making the dynamics stochastic, which allows for many remarkable features of the brain, including creativity, probabilistic decision-making, stochastic resonance, unpredictability, conflict resolution, symmetry breaking, allocation to discrete categories, and many other important properties described later in this Chapter.

The size of a network is an important factor in influencing how noisy the network is in relation to the statistical fluctuations related to the Poisson nature of the neuronal spiking. An infinite size network would have no noise, and its performance can be calculated analytically using mean field methods and checked with numerical simulations (Hopfield, 1982; Amit, 1989; Treves and Rolls, 1991; Treves, 1991b, 1990; Rolls, Treves, Foster and Perez-Vicente, 1997c; Rolls, 2012b) (Section B.3.3.7). In terms of relevance to cortical function, attractor networks with even thousands of neurons show probabilistic behavior, showing that the spiking-related noise of neurons does influence cortical networks of biologically relevant size. For example, even when a fully connected recurrent attractor network has 4,000 neurons, the operation of the network is still probabilistic (Deco and Rolls, 2006). Under these conditions, the probabilistic spiking of the excitatory (pyramidal) cells in the recurrent collateral firing, rather than variability in the external inputs to the network, is what makes the major contribution to the noise in the network (Deco and Rolls, 2006). Thus, once the firing in the recurrent collaterals is spike-implemented by integrate-and-fire neurons, the probabilistic behavior seems inevitable, even up to quite large attractor network sizes.

The graded nature of the sparse distributed representations in the cortex tends to increase the noise (Webb, Rolls, Deco and Feng, 2011). Representations in the cortex are often distributed with graded firing rates in the neuronal populations. The firing rate probability distribution of each neuron to a set of stimuli is often exponential or gamma (see Section C.3.1.1) (Webb et al., 2011). In integrate-and-fire simulations of an attractor decision-making network, we showed that the noise is indeed greater for a given sparseness of the representation for graded, exponential, than for binary firing rate distributions. The greater noise was measured by faster escaping times from the spontaneous firing rate state when the decision cues are applied, and this corresponds to faster decision or reaction times. The greater noise was also evident as less stability of the spontaneous firing state before the decision cues are applied. The implication is that spiking-related noise will continue to be a factor that influences processes such as decision-making, signal detection, short-term memory, and memory recall even with the quite large networks found in the cerebral cortex. In these networks there are several thousand recurrent collateral synapses onto each neuron. The greater noise with graded firing rate distributions has the advantage that it can increase the speed of operation of cortical circuitry (Webb, Rolls, Deco and Feng, 2011).

Dilution of the connectivity within an attractor network can have the effect of decreasing the noise compared to a fully connected network with the same number of connections onto each neuron and therefore the same memory capacity (Rolls and Webb, 2012). The connectivity of the cerebral cortex is diluted, with the probability of excitatory connections between even nearby pyramidal cells rarely more than 0.1, and in the hippocampus 0.04 (Chapter 9 and Rolls (2016b)). To investigate the extent to which this diluted connectivity affects the dynamics of attractor networks in the cerebral cortex, we simulated an integrate-and-fire attractor network taking decisions between competing inputs with diluted connectivity of 0.25 or 0.1, and with the same number of synaptic connections per neuron for the recurrent collateral synapses within an attractor population as for full connectivity. The results indicated that there was less spiking-related noise with the diluted connectivity, in that the stability of the network when in the spontaneous state of firing increased, and the accuracy of the correct decisions increased. The decision times were a little slower with diluted than with complete connectivity. Given that the capacity of the network is set by the number of recurrent collateral synaptic connections per neuron, on which there is a biological limit, the findings indicate that the stability of cortical networks, and the accuracy of their correct decisions or memory recall operations, can be increased by utilizing diluted connectivity and correspondingly increasing the number of neurons in the network, with little impact on the speed of processing of the cortex (Rolls and Webb, 2012).

18.2.2 Attractor networks, energy landscapes, and stochastic neurodynamics

Attractor networks can be used for short-term memory and long-term memory, and for decision making (Section B.3). This section considers approaches to the stability of these networks. This section can be thought of as explaining the stability of memory networks, though the principles apply just as much to the decision-making networks considered in Section 11.5.1.

Autoassociation attractor systems (described in Section B.3) can have two types of stable fixed points: a spontaneous state with a low firing rate, and one or more attractor states with

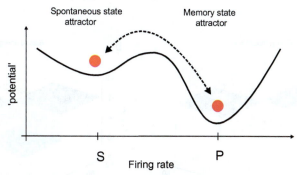

Fig. 18.1 Stability and noise in an attractor network: an energy landscape. The noise influences when the system will jump out of the spontaneous firing stable (low energy) state S, and whether it jumps into the high firing rate state labelled P (with persistent or continuing firing in a state which is even more stable with even lower energy), which might correspond to a short-term memory, or to a decision.

high firing rates in which the positive feedback implemented by the recurrent collateral connections maintains a high firing rate. We sometimes refer to this latter state as the persistent state, because the high firing normally persists to maintain a set of neurons active, which might implement a short-term memory, or the recall of a long-term memory that persists for a short time.

The stable points of the system can be visualized in an energy landscape (see Fig. 18.1). The area in the energy landscape within which the system will move to a stable attractor state is called its basin of attraction. The attractor dynamics can be pictured by energy landscapes, which indicate the basins of attraction by valleys, and the attractor states or fixed points by the bottom of the valleys (see Fig. 18.1).

The stability of an attractor is characterized by the average time in which the system stays in the basin of attraction under the influence of noise. The noise provokes transitions to other attractor states. One source of noise results from the interplay between the Poissonian character of the spikes and the finite-size effect due to the limited number of neurons in the network.

Two factors determine the stability. First, if the depths of the attractors are shallow (as in the left compared to the right valley in Figure 18.1), then less force is needed to move a ball from one valley to the next. Second, high noise will make it more likely that the system will jump over an energy boundary from one state to another. We envision that the brain as a dynamical system has characteristics of such an attractor system including statistical fluctuations (see further Rolls and Deco (2010), where the effects of noise are defined quantitatively). The noise could arise not only from the probabilistic spiking of the neurons which has significant effects in finite size integrate-and-fire networks (Deco and Rolls, 2006), but also from any other source of noise in the brain or the environment (Faisal et al., 2008), including the effects of distracting stimuli.

In an attractor network in which a retrieval cue is provided to initiate recall but then removed, a landscape can be defined in terms of the synaptic weights. An example is shown in Fig. 18.2a. The basins in the landscape can be defined by the strengths of the synaptic weights which describe the stable operating points of the system, where the depth of the basins can be defined in terms of the synaptic weight space, in terms defined by an associative rule operating on the firing rates of pairs of neurons during the learning as follows

$$w_{ij} = y_i y_j \tag{18.1}$$

where y_i is the firing rate of the postsynaptic neuron, y_j is the firing rate of the presynaptic neuron, and w_{ij} is the strength of the synapses connecting these neurons.

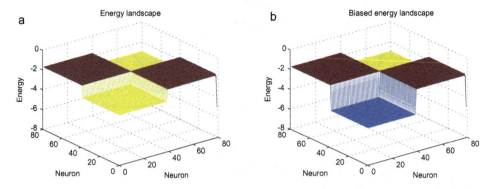

Fig. 18.2 Stability and noise in an attractor network. (a) Energy landscape without any differential bias applied. The landscape is for a network with neurons 1–40 connected by strengthened synapses so that they form attractor 1, and neurons 41–80 connected by synapses strengthened (by the same amount) so that they form attractor 2. The energy basins in the two-dimensional landscape are calculated by Equation 18.2. In this two-dimensional landscape, there are two stable attractors, and each will be reached equally probably under the influence of noise. This scenario might correspond to decision-making where the input λ_1 to attractor 1 has the same value as the input λ_2 to attractor 2, and the network is equally likely under the influence of the noise to fall into attractor 1 representing decision 1 as into attractor 2 representing decision 2. (b) Energy landscape with bias applied to neurons 1–40. This make the basin of attraction deeper for attractor 1, as calculated with Equation 18.2. Thus, under the influence of noise caused by the randomness in the firing of the neurons, the network will reach attractor 1 more probably than it will reach attractor 2. This scenario might correspond to decision-making, where the evidence for decision 1 is stronger than for decision 2, so that a higher firing rate is applied as λ_1 to neurons 1–40. The scenario might also correspond to memory recall, in which memory 1 might be probabilistically more likely to be recalled than memory 2 if the evidence for memory 1 is stronger. Nevertheless, memory 2 will be recalled sometimes in what operates as a non-deterministic system. (From Rolls, E. T. and Deco, G. (2010) The Noisy Brain: Stochastic Dynamics as a Principle of Brain Function. Oxford University Press: Oxford.)

Hopfield (1982) showed how many stable states a simple attractor system might contain, and this is the capacity of the network described in Section B.3.3.7. He showed that the recall process in his attractor network can be conceptualized as movement towards basins of attraction, and his equation defines the energy at a given point in time as being a function of the synaptic weights and the current firing rates as follows

$$E = -\frac{1}{2} \sum_{i,j} w_{ij}(y_i - <y>)(y_j - <y>). \tag{18.2}$$

where y_i is the firing rate of the postsynaptic neuron, y_j is the firing rate of the presynaptic neuron, w_{ij} is the strength of the synapse connecting them, and $<y>$ is the mean firing rate of the neurons. I note that the system defined by Hopfield had an energy function, in that the neurons were connected by symmetric synaptic weights (produced for example by associative synaptic modification of the recurrent collateral synapses) and there was no self-coupling (Hertz, Krogh and Palmer, 1991; Moreno-Bote, Rinzel and Rubin, 2007; Hopfield and Herz, 1995). (Equation 18.2 can be understood as showing that the system will be stable if high firing rate neurons are connected by strong synaptic weights, and a stable fixed point can be thought of as having low energy so that the system does not jump somewhere else in the energy landscape.)

The situation is more complicated in an attractor network if it does not have a formal energy function. One such condition is when the connectivity is randomly diluted, for then the synaptic weights between pairs of neurons will not be symmetric. Indeed, in general, neuronal systems do not admit such an energy function. (This is the case in that it is not in general possible to define the flow in terms of the gradient of an energy function. Hopfield defined first an energy function, and from there derived dynamics.) However, such diluted connectivity systems can still operate as attractor systems (Treves, 1993, 1991a,b; Treves and Rolls, 1991; Treves, Rolls and Simmen, 1997; Rolls and Treves, 1998; Battaglia and Treves, 1998a), and the concept of an energy function and landscape is useful for discussion purposes. In practice, a Lyapunov function can be used to prove analytically that there is a stable fixed point such as an attractor basin (Khalil, 1996), and even in systems where this can not be proved analytically, it may still be possible to show numerically that there are stable fixed points, to measure the flow towards those fixed points which describes the depth of the attractor basin as we have done for this type of network (Loh, Rolls and Deco, 2007a), and to use the concept of energy or potential landscapes to help visualize the properties of the system (Rolls and Deco, 2010).

If an external input remains on during the retrieval process, this will influence the energy function of such a network, and its stable points, as implied by Equation 18.2, and as illustrated in Fig. 18.2b. In this situation, the external inputs bias the stable points of the system. Indeed, in this situation, a landscape, though not necessarily formally an energy landscape, can be specified by a combination of the synaptic weights and external inputs that bias the firing rates. The noise introduced into the network by for example the random neuronal spiking can be conceptualized as influencing the way that the system flows across this fixed landscape shaped by the synaptic weights, and by the external inputs if they remain on during operation of the network, in what is referred to as a 'clamped' condition, the normal condition that applies during decision-making (see Section 11.5.1).

In more detail, the flow, which is the time derivative of the neuronal activity, specifies the landscape in an attractor system. The flow is defined in the mean field analysis in terms of the effects of the synaptic weights between the neurons and the external inputs (Loh, Rolls and Deco, 2007a; Rolls and Deco, 2010). The flow is the force that drives the system towards the attractor given a parameter value in phase space, i.e. the firing rates of the pools (populations) of neurons. This is measured by fixing the value of the firing rate of the selective pool and letting the other values converge to their fixed point. The flow can then be computed with this configuration (Mascaro and Amit, 1999). This landscape is thus fixed by the synaptic and the external inputs. The noise, produced for example by the almost Poissonian spiking of the neurons, can be conceptualized as influencing the way that the system flows across this fixed landscape. Moreover, the noise can enable the system to jump over a barrier in this fixed landscape, as illustrated in Figs. 18.1 and 11.33.

In Fig. 18.2a (and in Fig. 11.33) the decision basins of attraction are equally deep, because the inputs λ_1 and λ_2 to the decision-making network are equal, that is, ΔI the difference between them is zero. If λ_1 is greater than λ_2, the basin will be deeper for λ_1. The shape of the landscape is thus a function of the synaptic weights and the biassing inputs to the system. This is illustrated in Fig. 18.2b. Noise can be thought of as provoking movements across the 'effective energy landscape' conceptualized in this way.

The way in which we conceptualise the operation of an attractor network used for noise-driven stochastic decision-making, stimulus detection, etc, is as follows. The noise in the system (caused for example by statistical fluctuations produced by the Poisson-like neuronal firing in a finite-sized system as described in Section 18.2.1) produces changes in neuronal firing. These changes may accumulate stochastically, and eventually may become sufficiently large that the firing is sufficient to produce energy to cause the system to jump over an energy barrier (see Fig. 18.3). Opposing this noise-driven fluctuation will be the flow being caused by the shape and depth of the fixed energy landscape defined by the synaptic weights and the applied external input bias or biases. The noisy statistical fluctuation is a diffusion-like process. If the spontaneous firing rate state is stable with the decision cues applied (see Fig. 18.4 middle), eventually the noise may provoke a transition over the energy barrier in an escaping time, and the system will drop, again noisily, down the valley on the other side of the hill.

718 | Cortical attractor dynamics and connectivity, stochasticity, psychiatric disorders, and aging

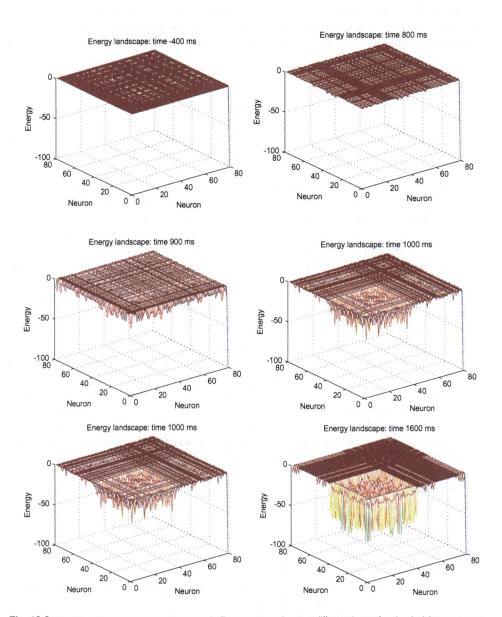

Fig. 18.3 Stability and noise in an attractor network. Energy states shown at different times after the decision cues were applied. Neurons 1–40 are in attractor 1 and are connected by strong weights with each other; and neurons 41–80 are in attractor 2 and are connected by strong weights with each other. The energy state is defined in Equation 18.2, and the energy between any pair of neurons is a product of the firing rates of each neuron and the synaptic weight that connects them. These are the energy states for the trial shown in Fig. 11.35b and c on page 550. Time 0 is the time when the decision stimuli were applied (and this corresponds to time 2 s in Fig. 11.35). (From Rolls, E. T. and Deco, G. (2010) The Noisy Brain: Stochastic Dynamics as a Principle of Brain Function. Oxford University Press: Oxford.)

The rate of change of the firing rate is again measured by the flow, and is influenced by the synaptic weights and applied biases, and by the statistical fluctuations. In this scenario, the reaction times will depend on the amount of noise, influenced by the size of the network, and by the fixed 'effective energy landscape' as determined by the synaptic weights and applied biasing inputs λ, which will produce an escaping time as defined further in the Appendix of Rolls and Deco (2010).

If the spontaneous state is not stable (see Fig. 18.4 right), the reaction times will be influenced primarily by the flow as influenced by the gradient of the energy landscape, and by the noise caused by the random neuronal firings. A noise-produced escaping time from a stable spontaneous state attractor will not in this situation contribute to the reaction times.

The noise-driven escaping time from the stable spontaneous state is important in understanding long and variable reaction times, and such reaction times are present primarily in the scenario when the parameters make the spontaneous state stable, as described further by Marti et al. (2008). While in a spontaneous stable state the system may be thought of as being driven by the noise, and it is primarily when the system has reached a ridge at the edge of the spontaneous valley and the system is close to a bifurcation point into a high firing rate close to the ridge that the attractor system can be thought of as accumulating evidence from the input stimuli (Deco et al., 2007). While in the spontaneous state valley (see Fig. 18.4 middle), the inputs can be thought of as biasing the 'effective energy landscape' across which the noise is driving the system stochastically.

An interesting aspect of the model is that the recurrent connectivity, and the relatively long time constant of the NMDA receptors (Wang, 2002), may together enable the attractor network to accumulate evidence over a long time period of several hundred milliseconds. Important aspects of the functionality of attractor networks are that they can accumulate and maintain information.

18.2.3 A multistable system with noise

In the situation illustrated in Figs. 18.1 and 11.33, there is multistability, in that the spontaneous state and a large number of high firing rate persistent states are stable. More generally, and depending on the network parameters including the strengths of the inputs, a number of different scenarios can occur. These are illustrated in Fig. 18.4. Let us consider the activity of a given neuronal population while inputs are being applied.

In Fig. 18.4 (left) we see a situation in which only the spontaneous state S is stable. This might occur if the external inputs λ_1 and λ_2 are weak.

On the right we have a situation in which our neuronal population is either in a high firing rate stable state C2, or in a low firing rate state C1 because another population is firing fast and inhibiting our neuronal population. There is no stable spontaneous state.

In the middle of Fig. 18.4 we see a situation in which our population may be either in C1, or in C2, or in a spontaneous state of firing S when no population has won the competition. We emphasize that this can be a scenario even when the decision cues λ_1 and λ_2 are being applied during the decision-making period. We refer to this system as a multistable system.

The differences between these scenarios are of interest in relation to how noise influences the decision-making. In the scenario shown in the middle of Fig. 18.4 we see that there are three stable states when the inputs λ_1 and λ_2 are being applied, and that it is the stochastic noise that influences whether the system jumps from the initial spontaneous state to a high firing rate state in which one of the decision-state populations fires fast, producing either C2 if our population wins, or C1 if our population loses. The statistical properties of the noise (including its amplitude and frequency spectrum), and the shape of the different basins in the energy landscape, influence whether a decision will be taken, the time when it will be

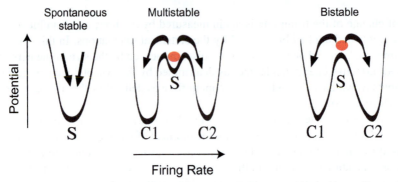

Fig. 18.4 Computational principles underlying the different dynamical regimes of the decision-making attractor network (see text). The x-axis represents the neuronal activity of one of the populations (ν_i) and the landscape represents an energy landscape ('potential') regulating the evolution of the system. S is a stable state of spontaneous activity, C2 is a high firing rate state of this neuronal population corresponding to the decision implemented by this population, and C1 is a low firing rate state present when the other population wins the competition.

taken, and which high firing rate decision attractor wins. In contrast, in the scenario shown in Fig. 18.4 (right) the energy landscape when the stimuli are being applied is such that there is no stable spontaneous state, so the system moves to one of the high firing rate decision attractors without requiring noise. In this case, the noise, and the shape of the energy landscape, influence which high firing rate decision state attractor will win.

A more detailed analysis suggests that there are two scenarios that are needed to understand the time course of processes such as decision-making and memory retrieval (which are very similar processes involving an attractor network driven by one input, or by several inputs) (Marti, Deco, Mattia, Gigante and Del Giudice, 2008).

First, in the scenario investigated by Wang (2002), the spontaneous state is unstable when the decision cues are applied. The network, initially in the spontaneous state, is driven to a competition regime by an increase of the external input (that is, upon stimulus presentation) that destabilizes the initial state. The decision process can then be seen as the relaxation from an unstable stationary state towards either of the two stable decision states (Fig. 18.4 (right)). When the system is completely symmetric (i.e. when there is no bias in the external inputs that favours one choice over the other), this destabilization occurs because the system undergoes a pitchfork bifurcation for sufficiently high inputs. The time spent by the system to evolve from the initial state to either of the two decision states is determined by the actual stochastic trajectory of the system in the phase space. In particular, the transition time increases significantly when the system wanders in the vicinity of the saddle that appears when the spontaneous state becomes unstable. Reaction times in the order of hundreds of ms may be produced in this way, and are strongly influenced by the long time constants of the NMDA receptors (Wang, 2002). The transition can be further slowed down by setting the external input slightly above the bifurcation value. This tuning can be exploited to obtain realistic decision times.

Second, there is a scenario in which the stimuli do not destabilize the spontaneous state, but rather increase the probability for a noise-driven transition from a stable spontaneous state to one of the decision states (see Fig. 18.4 (centre) and Section 18.2.3). Due to the presence of finite-size noise in the system there is a nonzero probability that this transition occurs and hence a finite mean transition rate between the spontaneous and the decision states. It has been shown that in this scenario mean decision times tend to the Van't Hoff-Arrhenius exponential dependence on the amplitude of noise in the limit of infinitely large networks. As a consequence, in this limit, mean decision times increase exponentially with the size of the network (Marti, Deco, Mattia, Gigante and Del Giudice, 2008). Further, the decision events become Poissonian in the limit of vanishing noise, leading to an exponential distribution of decision times. For small noise a decrease in the mean input to the network leads to an increase of the positive skewness of decision-time distributions.

These results suggest that noise-driven decision models as in this second scenario provide an alternative dynamical mechanism for the variability and wide range of decision times observed, which span from a few hundred milliseconds to more than one second (Marti et al., 2008). In this scenario, there is an escaping time from the spontaneous firing state (Rolls and Deco, 2010). In this time the information can be thought of as accumulating in the sense that the stochastic noise may slowly drive the firing rates in a diffusion-like way such than an energy barrier is jumped over and escaped (see Fig. 18.1 on page 715 and Fig. 18.2). In this situation, a landscape can be specified by a combination of the synaptic weights and external decision-related input evidence that biases the firing rates of the decision attractors, as described in Section 18.2.2. The noise introduced into the network by for example the random neuronal spiking can be conceptualized as influencing the way that the system flows across this fixed landscape shaped by the synaptic weights, and by the external inputs if they remain on during operation of the network.

The model for the second scenario, with a stable spontaneous state even when the decision cues are being applied, makes specific predictions about reaction times. The analysis shows that there will be a gamma-like distribution with an exponential tail of long reaction times in the reaction time distribution with this second scenario (Marti et al., 2008).

For the reasons just described, all of the research that I have performed with integrate-and-fire networks has been with the second scenario, termed a multistable system, in which the spontaneous firing state is stable even when the decision cues (or recall cue) are being applied, and shown in 18.4 (centre). This is in contrast to the situation studied by Wang (2002), which corresponds to the bistable system shown in the right of Fig. 18.4.

18.2.4 Stochastic dynamics and the stability of short-term memory

I now introduce concepts on how noise produced by neuronal spiking, or noise from other sources, influences short-term memory, with illustrations drawn from Loh, Rolls and Deco (2007a) and Rolls, Loh and Deco (2008c).

The noise caused by the probabilistic firing of neurons can influence the stability of short-term memory. To investigate this, it is necessary to use a model of short-term memory which is a biophysically realistic integrate-and-fire attractor network with spiking of the neurons, so that the properties of receptors, synaptic currents and the statistical effects related to the noisy probabilistic spiking of the neurons can be analyzed. Loh, Rolls and Deco (2007a) and Rolls, Loh and Deco (2008c) used a minimal architecture, a single attractor or autoassociation network (Hopfield, 1982; Amit, 1989; Hertz et al., 1991; Rolls and Treves, 1998; Rolls, 2016b) (see Section B.3), to investigate how spiking-related stochastic noise influences the stability of short-term memory. They chose a recurrent (attractor) integrate-and-fire network model which includes synaptic channels for AMPA, NMDA and $GABA_A$ receptors (Brunel and Wang, 2001). The integrate-and-fire model was necessary to characterize and exploit the effects of the spiking noise produced by the neurons in a finite-sized network. However, to initialize the parameters of the integrate-and-fire model such as the synaptic connection strengths to produce stable attractors, and to ensure that the spontaneous activity is in the correct range, they used a mean-field approximation consistent with the integrate-and-fire network, as described in Section B.8.2. Both excitatory and inhibitory neurons were represented by a leaky integrate-and-fire model (Tuckwell, 1988) described in detail in Section B.6.3.

The single attractor network contained 400 excitatory and 100 inhibitory neurons, which

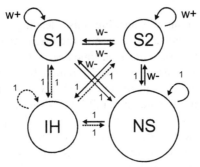

Fig. 18.5 The attractor network model for short-term memory, attention, and decision-making. The excitatory neurons are divided into two selective pools S1 and S2 (with 40 neurons each) with strong intra-pool connection strengths w_+, and one non-selective pool (NS) (with 320 neurons). The other connection strengths are 1 or weak w_-. The network contains 500 neurons, of which 400 are in the excitatory pools and 100 are in the inhibitory pool IH. Each neuron in the network also receives inputs from 800 external neurons, and these neurons increase their firing rates to apply a stimulus or distracter to one of the pools S1 or S2. The synaptic connection matrices are shown in Tables 18.1 and 18.2. (Reproduced from Loh,M., Rolls, E. T. and Deco,G. (2007) A Dynamical Systems hypothesis of Schizophrenia. *PLoS Computational Biology* 3: e228.)

is consistent with the observed proportions of pyramidal cells and interneurons in the cerebral cortex (Abeles, 1991; Braitenberg and Schüz, 1991). The connection strengths were adjusted using mean-field analysis (see Brunel and Wang (2001) and Section B.8.2), so that the excitatory and inhibitory neurons exhibited a spontaneous activity of 3 Hz and 9 Hz respectively (Koch and Fuster, 1989; Wilson et al., 1994a). The recurrent excitation mediated by the AMPA and NMDA receptors is dominated by the long time constant NMDA currents to avoid instabilities during the delay periods (Wang, 1999, 2002).

The cortical network model featured a minimal architecture to investigate stability (and also distractibility), and consisted of two selective pools (or populations of neurons) S1 and S2, as shown in Fig. 18.5. Pool S1 is used for the short-term memory item to be remembered, sometimes called the target; and pool S2 is used for a distracter stimulus. The non-selective pool NS modelled the spiking of other cortical neurons and served to generate an approximately Poisson spiking dynamics in the model (Brunel and Wang, 2001), which is what is observed in the cortex. The inhibitory pool IH contained 100 inhibitory neurons. There were thus four populations or pools of neurons in the network, and the connection weights were set up using a mean-field analysis to make S1 and S2 have stable attractor properties. The connection weights between the neurons within each selective pool or population were called the intra-pool connection strengths w_+. The increased strength of the intra-pool connections was counterbalanced by the other excitatory connections (w_-) to keep the average input to a neuron constant. The actual synaptic strengths are shown in Tables 18.1 and 18.2 where $w_- = \frac{0.8 - f_{S1}w_+}{0.8 - f_{S1}}$, and f_{S1} is the fraction of the total number of excitatory neurons in pool S1. For these investigations, $w_+ = 2.1$ was selected, because with the default values of the NMDA and GABA conductances this yielded relatively stable dynamics with some effect of the noise being apparent, that is, a relatively stable spontaneous state if no retrieval cue was applied, and a relatively stable state of persistent firing after a retrieval cue had been applied and removed.

Each neuron in the network received Poisson input spikes via AMPA receptors which are envisioned to originate from 800 external neurons at an average spontaneous firing rate of 3 Hz from each external neuron, consistent with the spontaneous activity observed in the cerebral cortex (Wilson et al., 1994a; Rolls and Treves, 1998; Rolls, 2016b) (see Section B.6.3).

Table 18.1 The attractor network model: Connection matrix for AMPA and NMDA – [from, to]

	S1	S2	NS	IH
S1	w_+	w_-	1	1
S2	w_-	w_+	1	1
NS	w_-	w_-	1	1
IH	0	0	0	0

Table 18.2 The attractor network model: Connection matrix for GABA – [from, to]

	S1	S2	NS	IH
S1	0	0	0	0
S2	0	0	0	0
NS	0	0	0	0
IH	1	1	1	1

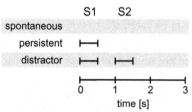

Fig. 18.6 The attractor network model for the stability of short-term memory and attention: The simulation protocols. Stimuli to either S1 or S2 are applied at different times depending on the type of simulations. The spontaneous simulations include no input. The 'persistent' simulations assess how stably a stimulus is retained in short-term memory by the network. The distracter simulations add a distracter stimulus to further address the stability of the network activity in the face of a distracting stimulus, and thus both the stability of attention, and the shifting of attention. (Reproduced from Loh,M., Rolls, E. T. and Deco,G. (2007) A Dynamical Systems hypothesis of Schizophrenia. *PLoS Computational Biology* 3: e228.)

18.2.4.1 Analysis of the stability of short-term memory

The analyses (Loh, Rolls and Deco, 2007a; Rolls, Loh and Deco, 2008c) aimed to investigate the stability of the short-term memory implemented by the attractor network. Simulations were performed for many separate trials, each run with a different random seed to analyze the statistical variability of the network as the noise varied from trial to trial. We focussed on simulations of two different conditions: the spontaneous, and persistent, conditions.

In spontaneous simulations (see Fig. 18.6), we ran spiking simulations for 3 s without any extra external input. The aim of this condition was to test whether the network was stable in maintaining a low average firing rate in the absence of any inputs, or whether it fell into one of its attractor states without any external input.

In persistent simulations, an external cue of 120 Hz above the background firing rate of 2400 Hz was applied to each neuron in pool S1 during the first 500 ms to induce a high activity state and then the system was run without the additional external cue of 120 Hz for another 2.5 s, which was a short-term memory period. The 2400 Hz was distributed across the 800 synapses of each S1 neuron for the external inputs, with the spontaneous Poisson spike trains received by each synapse thus having a mean rate of 3 Hz. The aim of this condition was to investigate whether once in an attractor short-term memory state, the network can maintain its activity stably, or whether it fell out of its attractor, which might correspond to an inability to maintain short-term memory.

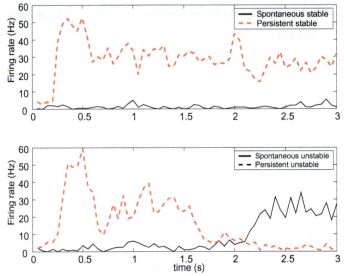

Fig. 18.7 The attractor network model for the stability of short-term memory. Example trials of the Integrate-and-Fire attractor network simulations of short-term memory. The average firing rate of all the neurons in the S1 pool is shown. Top. Normal operation. On a trial in which a recall stimulus was applied to S1 at 0–500 ms, firing continued normally until the end of the trial in the 'persistent' simulation condition. On a trial on which no recall stimulus was applied to S1, spontaneous firing continued until the end of the trial in the 'spontaneous' simulation condition. Bottom: Unstable operation. On this persistent condition trial, the firing decreased during the trial as the network fell out of the attractor because of the statistical fluctuations caused by the spiking dynamics. On the spontaneous condition trial, the firing increased during the trial because of the statistical fluctuations. In these simulations the network parameter was w_+=2.1. (After Rolls, E. T., Loh,M. and Deco,G. (2008) An attractor hypothesis of obsessive-compulsive disorder. European Journal of Neuroscience 28: 782–793. © Federation of European Neuroscience Societies.)

18.2.4.2 Stability and noise in a model of short-term memory

To clarify the concept of stability, we show examples of trials of spontaneous and persistent simulations in which the statistical fluctuations have different impacts on the temporal dynamics. Fig. 18.7 shows the possibilities, as follows.

In the spontaneous state simulations, no cue was applied, and we are interested in whether the network remains stably in the spontaneous firing state, or whether it is unstable and on some trials due to statistical fluctuations entered one of the attractors, thus falsely retrieving a memory. Figure 18.7 (top) shows an example of a trial on which the network correctly stayed in the low spontaneous firing rate regime, and (bottom) another trial (labelled spontaneous unstable) in which statistical spiking-related fluctuations in the network caused it to enter a high activity state, moving into one of the attractors even without a stimulus.

In the persistent state simulations (in which the short-term memory was implemented by the continuing neuronal firing), a strong excitatory input was given to the S1 neuronal population between 0 and 500 ms. Two such trials are shown in Fig. 18.7. In Fig. 18.7 (top), the S1 neurons (correctly) keep firing at approximately 30 Hz after the retrieval cue is removed at 500 ms. However, due to statistical fluctuations in the network related to the spiking activity, on the trial labelled persistent unstable the high firing rate in the attractor for S1 was not stable, and the firing decreased back towards the spontaneous level, in the example shown starting after 1.5 s (Fig. 18.7 bottom). This trial illustrates a failure to maintain a stable short-term memory state.

When an average was taken over many trials, for the persistent run simulations, in which the cue triggered the attractor into the high firing rate attractor state, the network was still in the high firing rate attractor state in the baseline condition on 88% of the runs. The noise had thus caused the network to fail to maintain the short-term memory on 12% of the runs.

The spontaneous state was unstable on approximately 10% of the trials, that is, on 10% of the trials the spiking noise in the network caused the network run in the condition without any initial retrieval cue to end up in a high firing rate attractor state. This is of course an error that is related to the spiking noise in the network.

We emphasise that the transitions to the incorrect activity states illustrated in Fig. 18.7 are caused by statistical fluctuations (noise) in the spiking activity of the integrate-and-fire neurons. Indeed, we used a mean-field approach with an equivalent network with the same parameters but without noise to establish parameter values where the spontaneous state and the high firing rate short-term memory ('persistent') state would be stable without the spiking noise, and then in integrate-and-fire simulations with the same parameter values examined the effects of the spiking noise (Loh, Rolls and Deco, 2007a; Rolls, Loh and Deco, 2008c). The mean-field approach used to calculate the stationary attractor states of the network for the delay period (Brunel and Wang, 2001) is described in Section B.7. These attractor states are independent of any simulation protocol of the spiking simulations and represent the behavior of the network by mean firing rates to which the system would converge in the absence of statistical fluctuations caused by the spiking of the neurons and by external changes. Therefore the mean-field technique is suitable for tasks in which temporal dynamics and fluctuations are negligible. It also allows a first assessment of the attractor landscape and the depths of the basin of attraction which then need to be investigated in detail with stochastical spiking simulations. Part of the utility of the mean-field approach is that it allows the parameter region for the synaptic strengths to be investigated to determine which synaptic strengths will on average produce stable activity in the network, for example of persistent activity in a delay period after the removal of a stimulus. For the spontaneous state, the initial conditions for numerical simulations of the mean-field method were set to 3 Hz for all excitatory pools and 9 Hz for the inhibitory pool. These values correspond to the approximate values of the spontaneous attractors when the network is not driven by stimulus-specific inputs. For the persistent state, the network parameters resulted in a selective pool having a high firing rate value of approximately 30 Hz when in its attractor state (Loh, Rolls and Deco, 2007a; Rolls, Loh and Deco, 2008c).

I note that there are two sources of noise in the simulated integrate-and-fire spiking networks that cause the statistical fluctuations: the randomly arriving external Poisson spike trains, and the statistical fluctuations caused by the spiking of the neurons in the finite sized network. Some of the evidence that the statistical fluctuations caused by the neuronal spiking do provide an important source of noise in attractor networks in the brain is that factors that affect the noise in the network such as the number of neurons in the network have clear effects on the operation of integrate-and-fire attractor networks, as considered further in Section 11.5.1. Indeed, the magnitude of these fluctuations increases as the number of neurons in the network becomes smaller (Mattia and Del Giudice, 2004).

The ways in which alterations in the inputs to the different synapse types in the different neurons in the network influence the stability of the network, and their applications to understanding psychiatric disorders and normal aging, are described next.

18.2.5 Stochastic dynamics in decision-making, and the evolutionary utility of probabilistic choice

Attractor decision-making networks are described in Sections 11.5.1 and B.6–B.8. Here we consider some advantages of the stochastic dynamics in the decision-making process (see further Rolls and Deco (2010)).

Probabilistic decision-making can be evolutionarily advantageous in that sometimes taking a decision that is not optimal based on previous history may provide information that is useful, and that may contribute to learning. Consider for example a probabilistic decision task in which choice 1 provides rewards on 80% of the occasions, and choice 2 on 20% of the occasions. A deterministic system with knowledge of the previous reinforcement history would always make choice 1. But this is not how animals including humans behave. Instead (especially when the overall probabilities are low and the situation involves random probabilistic baiting, and there is a penalty for changing the choice), the proportion of choices made approximately matches the outcomes that are available, in what is called the matching law (Sugrue, Corrado and Newsome, 2005; Corrado, Sugrue, Seung and Newsome, 2005; Rolls, McCabe and Redoute, 2008e). By making the less favoured choice sometimes, the organism can keep obtaining evidence on whether the environment is changing (for example on whether the probability of a reward for choice 2 has increased), and by doing this approximately according to the matching law minimizes the cost of the disadvantageous choices in obtaining information about the environment.

This probabilistic exploration of the environment is very important in trial-and-error learning, and indeed has been incorporated into a simple reinforcement algorithm in which noise is added to the system, and if this improves outcomes above the expected value, then changes are made to the synaptic weights in the correct direction (in the associative reward-penalty algorithm) (Sutton and Barto, 1981; Barto, 1985; Rolls, 2016b).

In perceptual learning, probabilistic exploratory behavior may be part of the mechanism by which perceptual representations can be shaped to have appropriate selectivities for the behavioral categorization being performed (Sigala and Logothetis, 2002; Szabo et al., 2006).

Another example is in food foraging, which probabilistically may reflect the outcomes (Krebs and Davies, 1991; Kacelnik and Brito e Abreu, 1998), and is a way to keep sampling the environment and exploring the space of possible choices. Foraging can be performed optimally in terms of the costs and benefits of staying, or of moving on to forage elsewhere. Some noise in the system may help the amount of foraging to be optimally adjusted.

Another sense in which probabilistic decision-making may be evolutionarily advantageous is with respect to detecting signals that are close to threshold in the process termed stochastic resonance (Rolls and Deco, 2010; Deco, Rolls, Albantakis and Romo, 2013).

Intrinsic indeterminacy may be essential for unpredictable behavior (Glimcher, 2005). For example, in interactive games like matching pennies or rock–paper–scissors, any trend that deviates from random choice by an agent could be exploited to his or her opponent's advantage.

18.2.6 Selection between conscious vs unconscious decision-making, and free will

Another application of this type of model of stochastic decision-making is to taking decisions between the implicit (unconscious) and explicit (conscious) systems in emotional decision-making (see Rolls (2014a), Rolls (2016b) and Rolls (2020a)), where again the two different systems could provide the biasing inputs λ_1 and λ_2 to the model. An implication is that noise will influence with probabilistic outcomes which system, the implicit or the conscious reasoning system, takes a decision (Rolls, 2016b, 2020a).

When decisions are taken, sometimes confabulation may occur, in that a verbal account of why the action was performed may be given, and this may not be related at all to the environmental event that actually triggered the action (Gazzaniga and LeDoux, 1978; Gazzaniga, 1988, 1995; Rolls, 2014a; LeDoux, 2008). It is accordingly possible that sometimes in normal humans when actions are initiated as a result of processing in a specialized brain region such as those involved in some types of rewarded behavior, the language system may subsequently elaborate a coherent account of why that action was performed (i.e. confabulate)

(Rolls, 2020a). This would be consistent with a general view of brain evolution in which, as areas of the cortex evolve, they are laid on top of existing circuitry connecting inputs to outputs, and in which each level in this hierarchy of separate input–output pathways may control behavior according to the specialized function it can perform.

This raises the issue of free will in decision-making (Rolls, 2016b, 2020a).

First, we can note that in so far as the brain operates with some degree of randomness due to the statistical fluctuations produced by the random spiking times of neurons, brain function is to some extent non-deterministic, as defined in terms of these statistical fluctuations. That is, the behavior of the system, and of the individual, can vary from trial to trial based on these statistical fluctuations, in ways that are described in this book. Indeed, given that each neuron has this randomness, and that there are sufficiently small numbers of synapses on the neurons in each network (between a few thousand and 20,000) that these statistical fluctuations are not smoothed out, and that there are a number of different networks involved in typical thoughts and actions each one of which may behave probabilistically, and with 10^{11} neurons in the brain each with the number of synapses noted above, the system has so many degrees of freedom that it operates effectively as a non-deterministic system. (Philosophers may wish to argue about different senses of the term deterministic, but it is being used here in a precise, scientific, and quantitative way, which has been clearly defined.)

Second, do we have free will when both the implicit and the explicit systems have made the choice? Free will would in Rolls' view (Rolls, 2014a, 2008a, 2016b, 2010c, 2011b, 2020a) involve the use of language to check many moves ahead on a number of possible series of actions and their outcomes, and then with this information to make a choice from the likely outcomes of different possible series of actions. (If, in contrast, choices were made only on the basis of the reinforcement value of immediately available stimuli, without the arbitrary syntactic symbol manipulation made possible by language, then the choice strategy would be much more limited, and we might not want to use the term free will, as all the consequences of those actions would not have been computed.) It is suggested that when this type of reflective, conscious, information processing is occurring and leading to action (see Section 19.6.3), the system performing this processing and producing the action would have to believe that it could cause the action, for otherwise inconsistencies would arise, and the system might no longer try to initiate action. This belief held by the system may partly underlie the feeling of free will. At other times, when other brain modules are initiating actions (in the implicit systems), the conscious processor (the explicit system) may confabulate and believe that it caused the action, or at least give an account (possibly wrong) of why the action was initiated. The fact that the conscious processor may have the belief even in these circumstances that it initiated the action may arise as a property of it being inconsistent for a system that can take overall control using conscious verbal processing to believe that it was overridden by another system. This may be the underlying computational reason why confabulation occurs (Rolls, 2020a).

The interesting view we are led to is thus that when probabilistic choices influenced by stochastic dynamics are made between the implicit and explicit systems, we may not be aware of which system made the choice. Further, when the stochastic noise has made us choose with the implicit system, we may confabulate and say that we made the choice of our own free will, and provide a guess at why the decision was taken. In this scenario, the stochastic dynamics of the brain plays a role even in how we understand free will (Rolls, 2010c, 2016b, 2020a).

18.2.7 Stochastic dynamics and creative thought

Another way in which probabilistic decision-making may be evolutionarily advantageous is in creative thought, which is influenced in part by associations between one memory, representation, or thought, and another. If the system were deterministic, i.e. for the present purposes without noise, then the trajectory through a set of thoughts would be deterministic and would tend to follow the same furrow each time. However, if the recall of one memory or thought from another were influenced by the statistical noise due to the random spiking of neurons, then the trajectory through the state space would be different on different occasions, and we might be led in different directions on different occasions, facilitating creative thought (Rolls, 2016b; Rolls and Deco, 2010).

Of course, if the basins of attraction of each thought were too shallow, then the statistical noise might lead one to have very unstable thoughts that were too loosely and even bizarrely associated to each other, and to have a short-term memory and attentional system that is unstable and distractible, and indeed this is an account that we have proposed for some of the symptoms of schizophrenia (Rolls, 2014a, 2016b; Loh, Rolls and Deco, 2007a,b; Rolls, Loh, Deco and Winterer, 2008d) (see Section 18.3).

The stochastic noise caused by the probabilistic neuronal spiking plays an important role in these hypotheses, because it is the noise that destabilizes the attractors when the depth of the basins of attraction is reduced. If the basins of attraction were too deep, then the noise might be insufficient to destabilize attractors, and this leads to an approach to understanding obsessive-compulsive disorders (Rolls, Loh and Deco, 2008c) (see Section 18.4).

It is key to this hypothesis of an important mechanism of human creativity that the noise promotes a jump in an associative semantic (or similar) network, so that the jump is to a location in the attractor network that is associated with the starting point, and is thus not just to a random point in the space. This promotes finding solutions similar to some that may have been useful before and are not too far away within the associative space. This is a very different use to the noise that is sometimes used in artificial neural networks to avoid becoming stuck in a local minimum during gradient descent using error correction. It is proposed that use of noise in associative semantic networks to influence jumps to nearby locations in the energy landscape is likely to be useful in increasing creativity in Artificial Intelligence networks.

In an fMRI investigation of these hypotheses, the starting point was that creative individuals exhibit the ability to switch between different modes of thinking and shift their mental focus (Sun, Liu, Rolls, Chen, Yao, Yang, Wei, Zhang, Zhang, Feng and Qiu, 2019b). This suggests a connection between creativity and dynamic interactions of brain networks. We found that individuals' verbal creativity correlates with the temporal variability of the functional connectivity patterns of the lateral prefrontal cortex, the precuneus, and the parahippocampal gyrus. High variability of these regions indicates flexible connectivity patterns which may facilitate executive functions. In addition, verbal creativity was correlated with the temporal variability of functional connectivity patterns within the default mode network (DMN), between the DMN and attention/sensorimotor network, and between control and sensory networks. High variability of flexible connectivity patterns between the DMN and attention networks may characterize frequent adjustments of attention. This investigation (Sun et al., 2019b) revealed that there is a close relationship between verbal creativity and high variability of cortical networks involved in spontaneous thought, attention and cognitive control, consistent with the stochastic dynamics approach described here.

18.2.8 Stochastic dynamics and unpredictable behavior

An area where the spiking-related noise in the decision-making process may be evolutionarily advantageous is in the generation of unpredictable behavior, which can be advantageous in a number of situations, for example when a prey is trying to escape from a predator, and perhaps in some social and economic situations in which organisms may not wish to reveal their intentions (Maynard Smith, 1982, 1984; Dawkins, 1995). I note that such probabilistic decisions may have long-term consequences. For example, a probabilistic decision in a 'war of attrition' such as staring down a competitor e.g. in dominance hierarchy formation, may fix the relative status of the two individual animals involved, who then tend to maintain that relationship stably for a considerable period of weeks or more (Maynard Smith, 1982, 1984; Dawkins, 1995).

Thus intrinsic indeterminacy may be essential for unpredictable behavior. I also note the example provided by Glimcher (2005): in interactive games like matching pennies or rock–paper–scissors, any trend that deviates from random choice by an agent could be exploited to his or her opponent's advantage.

18.3 Attractor dynamics and schizophrenia

18.3.1 Introduction

Schizophrenia is a major mental illness, which has a great impact on patients and their environment. One of the difficulties in proposing models for schizophrenia is the complexity and heterogeneity of the illness. We propose that part of the reason for the inconsistent symptoms may be a reduced signal-to-noise ratio and increased statistical fluctuations in different cortical brain networks. The novelty of the approach described here is that instead of basing our hypothesis purely on biological mechanisms, we develop a top-down approach based on the different types of symptoms and relate them to instabilities in attractor neural networks (Rolls, 2005a; Loh, Rolls and Deco, 2007a,b; Rolls, Loh, Deco and Winterer, 2008d; Rolls, 2016b; Deco, Rolls and Romo, 2009; Rolls and Deco, 2011a; Rolls, 2012c, 2014a, 2016b, 2021a).

The main assumption of our hypothesis is that attractor dynamics are important in cognitive processes. Our hypothesis is based on the concept of attractor dynamics in a network of interconnected neurons which in their associatively modified synaptic connections store a set of patterns, which could be memories, perceptual representations, or thoughts (Hopfield, 1982; Amit, 1989; Rolls, 2016b; Rolls and Deco, 2010). The attractor states are important in cognitive processes such as short-term memory, attention, and action selection (Deco and Rolls, 2005a; Rolls, 2016b). The network may be in a state of spontaneous activity, or one set of neurons may have a high firing rate, each set representing a different memory state, normally recalled in response to a retrieval stimulus. Each of the states is an attractor in the sense that retrieval stimuli cause the network to fall into the closest attractor state, and thus to recall a complete memory in response to a partial or incorrect cue. Each attractor state can produce stable and continuing or persistent firing of the relevant neurons. The concept of an energy landscape (Hopfield, 1982) is that each pattern has a basin of attraction, and each is stable if the basins are far apart, and also if each basin is deep, caused for example by high firing rates and strong synaptic connections between the neurons representing each pattern, which together make the attractor state resistant to distraction by a different stimulus (Section 18.2). The spontaneous firing state, before a retrieval cue is applied, should also be stable. Noise in the network caused by statistical fluctuations in the stochastic spiking of different neurons can contribute to making the network transition from one state to another, and we take this into account by performing integrate-and-fire simulations with spiking activity, and relate this to the concept of an altered signal-to-noise ratio in schizophrenia (Winterer et al., 2000, 2004, 2006).

Schizophrenia is characterized by three main types of symptom: cognitive dysfunction, negative symptoms, and positive symptoms (Liddle, 1987; Baxter and Liddle, 1998; Mueser and McGurk, 2004; Owen, Sawa and Mortensen, 2016; Rolls, Lu, Wan, Yan, Wang, Yang, Tan, Li, Chinese-Schizophrenia-Collaboration, Yu, Liddle, Palaniyappan, Zhang, Yue and Feng, 2017). We consider how the basic characteristics of these three categories might be produced in a neurodynamical system, as follows.

Dysfunction of working memory, the core of the cognitive symptoms, may be related to instabilities of persistent attractor states (Durstewitz et al., 2000b; Wang, 2001) which we show can be produced by reduced firing rates in attractor networks, in brain regions such as the prefrontal cortex.

The negative symptoms such as flattening of affect or reduction of emotions may be caused by a consistent reduction in firing rates of neurons in regions associated with emotion such as the orbitofrontal cortex (Rolls, 2014a, 2016b, 2019e,f, 2023b). These hypotheses are supported by the frequently observed hypofrontality, a reduced activity in frontal brain regions in schizophrenic patients during cognitive tasks (Ingvar and Franzen, 1974; Kircher and Thienel, 2005; Scheuerecker et al., 2008).

The positive symptoms are characterized by phenomenologically overactive perceptions or thoughts such as hallucinations or delusions which are reflected for example by higher activity in the temporal lobes (Shergill et al., 2000; Scheuerecker et al., 2008). We relate this category of symptoms to a spontaneous appearance of activity in attractor networks in the brain and more generally to instability of both the spontaneous and persistent attractor states (Loh, Rolls and Deco, 2007a; Rolls, 2021a).

18.3.2 A dynamical systems hypothesis of the symptoms of schizophrenia

There is evidence on GABA-mediated inhibition impairments in schizophrenia, and also of decreased spine density that would reduce excitatory transmission in attractor networks (Lewis, 2014; Gonzalez-Burgos, Hashimoto and Lewis, 2010; Gonzalez-Burgos and Lewis, 2012; Glausier and Lewis, 2018; MacDonald, Alhassan, Newman, Richard, Gu, Kelly, Sampson, Fish, Penzes, Wills, Lewis and Sweet, 2017; Hoftman, Datta and Lewis, 2017; Dienel, Schoonover and Lewis, 2022; Smucny, Dienel, Lewis and Carter, 2022). This is an indication that the stability of cortical circuits is likely to be impaired in schizophrenia. In this section, models are described that show some of the effects that would be produced by altered levels of excitatory and inhibitory transmission on the stability of cortical circuitry, and how this might influence processes such as working memory and attention and lead to some of the symptoms of schizophrenia.

We relate the three types of symptoms of schizophrenia to the dynamical systems attractor framework described earlier as follows (Loh, Rolls and Deco, 2007a,b; Rolls, Loh, Deco and Winterer, 2008d; Rolls, 2016b; Deco, Rolls and Romo, 2009; Rolls and Deco, 2011a; Rolls, 2012c, 2014a).

The *cognitive symptoms* of schizophrenia include distractibility, poor attention, and the dysexecutive syndrome (Liddle, 1987; Green, 1996; Mueser and McGurk, 2004; Owen et al., 2016). The core of the cognitive symptoms is a working memory deficit in which there is a difficulty in maintaining items in short-term memory (Goldman-Rakic, 1994, 1999; Glausier and Lewis, 2018; Dienel, Schoonover and Lewis, 2022; Smucny, Dienel, Lewis and Carter, 2022), which could directly or indirectly account for a wide range of the cognitive symptoms.

We propose that these symptoms may be related to instabilities of persistent states in attractor neural networks, consistent with the body of theoretical research on network models of working memory (Durstewitz, Seamans and Sejnowski, 2000b). The neurons are firing at a lower rate, leading to shallower basins of attraction of the persistent states, and thus a difficulty in maintaining a stable short-term memory, normally the source of the bias in biased competition models of attention (Rolls and Deco, 2002; Deco and Rolls, 2005a; Rolls, 2008d, 2016b). The shallower basins of attraction would thus result in working memory deficits, poor attention, distractibility, and problems with executive function and action selection (Deco and Rolls, 2003, 2005a; Rolls, 2016b).

The *negative symptoms* refer to the flattening of affect and a reduction in emotion. Behavioral indicators are blunted affect, emotional and passive withdrawal, poor rapport, lack of spontaneity, motor retardation, and disturbance of volition (Liddle, 1987; Mueser and McGurk, 2004; Owen et al., 2016). The negative symptoms are a major source of difference between schizophrenic patients, and show a continuous gradation in magnitude between different people with schizophrenia (Rolls, Lu, Wan, Yan, Wang, Yang, Tan, Li, Chinese-Schizophrenia-Collaboration, Yu, Liddle, Palaniyappan, Zhang, Yue and Feng, 2017). Moreover, we have found in a large-scale study that the negative symptoms, as well as the positive and general symptoms, are reduced by treatment with antipsychotic drugs (Rolls et al., 2017). We propose that the negative symptoms are related to decreases in firing rates in the orbitofrontal cortex and/or anterior cingulate cortex (Rolls, 2014a, 2016b), where neuronal firing rates and activations in fMRI investigations are correlated with reward value and pleasure (Rolls, 2014a, 2006b, 2007f; Rolls and Grabenhorst, 2008; Rolls, 2008c, 2019e,c). Consistent with this, imaging studies have identified a relationship between negative symptoms and prefrontal hypometabolism, i.e. a reduced activation of frontal areas (Wolkin et al., 1992; Aleman and Kahn, 2005).

The *positive symptoms* of schizophrenia include bizarre (psychotic) trains of thoughts, hallucinations, and (paranoid) delusions (Liddle, 1987; Mueser and McGurk, 2004; Owen, Sawa and Mortensen, 2016; Rolls, Lu, Wan, Yan, Wang, Yang, Tan, Li, Chinese-Schizophrenia-Collaboration, Yu, Liddle, Palaniyappan, Zhang, Yue and Feng, 2017). We propose that these symptoms are related to shallow basins of attraction of both the spontaneous and persistent states in the temporal lobe semantic memory networks and to the statistical fluctuations caused by the probabilistic spiking of the neurons. This could result in activations arising spontaneously, and thoughts moving too freely round the energy landscape, loosely from thought to weakly associated thought, leading to bizarre thoughts and associations, which may eventually over time be associated together in semantic memory to lead to false beliefs and delusions. Consistent with this, neuroimaging studies suggest higher activation especially in areas of the temporal lobe (Weiss and Heckers, 1999; Shergill et al., 2000; Scheuerecker et al., 2008).

To further investigate our hypothesis, we used an attractor network, as this is likely to be implemented in many parts of the cerebral cortex by the recurrent collateral connections between pyramidal cells, and has short-term memory properties with basins of attraction which allow systematic investigation of stability and distractibility. The particular neural network implementation we adopted includes channels activated by AMPA, NMDA and $GABA_A$ receptors and allows not only the spiking activity to be simulated, but also a consistent mean-field approach to be used (Brunel and Wang, 2001). The network, and some of the simulations performed with it, are described in Section 18.2 and Section B.6.

The main findings were as follows, and are summarized in Fig. 18.8 (Loh, Rolls and Deco, 2007a,b; Rolls, Loh, Deco and Winterer, 2008d).

A reduction of the NMDA receptor activated synaptic conductances (−NMDA) reduces

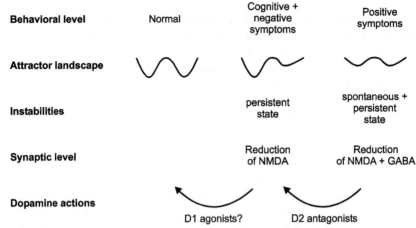

Fig. 18.8 Summary of attractor hypothesis of schizophrenic symptoms and simulation results (see text). The first basin (from the left) in each energy landscape is the spontaneous state, and the second basin is the persistent attractor state. The vertical axis of each landscape is the energy potential. (After Loh,M., Rolls, E. T. and Deco,G. (2007) A dynamical systems hypothesis of schizophrenia. PLoS Computational Biology 3: e228.)

the stability of the persistent state drastically. We hypothesized that this type of change might be related to the cognitive symptoms, since it shows a reduced stability of the working memory properties. The network was also more sensitive to a weak external stimulus, and we related this to increased distractibility. Consistent with this, there is a reduced spine density on excitatory neurons in the prefrontal cortex (Glausier and Lewis, 2013; Konopaske et al., 2014; Glantz and Lewis, 2000; Dienel et al., 2022). If present also in the orbitofrontal and anterior cingulate cortex, this could reduce the firing rates of these cortical neurons, and thus produce the negative symptoms of schizophrenia. This simulation relates directly to the glutamate hypothesis of schizophrenia, and particularly to hypofunction of the NMDA receptor (Uno and Coyle, 2019; Coyle, Ruzicka and Balu, 2020).

When both NMDA and GABA synaptic conductances are reduced, the stability of the high firing rate attractor state was reduced, and so was the stability of the spontaneous low firing rate state. We relate this pattern to the positive symptoms of schizophrenia, in which both the spontaneous and attractor states are shallow, and the system by the influence of statistical fluctuations wanders between the different (spontaneous and high firing rate attractor) states, as illustrated in Fig. 18.9.

The positive symptoms (Fig. 18.8, right column) of schizophrenia include delusions, hallucinations, thought disorder, and bizarre behavior. Examples of delusions are beliefs that others are trying to harm the person, impressions that others control the person's thoughts, and delusions of grandeur. Hallucinations are perceptual experiences, which are not shared by others, and are frequently auditory but can affect any sensory modality. These symptoms may be related to activity in the temporal lobes (Liddle, 1987; Epstein et al., 1999; Mueser and McGurk, 2004). The attractor framework approach taken here hypothesizes that the basins of attraction of both spontaneous and persistent states are shallow (Fig. 18.8). Due to the shallowness of the spontaneous state, the system can jump spontaneously up to a high activity state causing hallucinations to arise and leading to bizarre thoughts and associations. This might be the cause for the higher activations in schizophrenics in temporal lobe areas which are identified in imaging experiments (Shergill et al., 2000; Scheuerecker et al., 2008).

We relate the positive symptoms to not only a reduction in NMDA conductance (cf. Coyle, Ruzicka and Balu (2020)), but especially also to a reduction in what we modelled as GABA conductance, but more generally to any reduction of inhibitory neuron efficacy that might lead to higher firing rates of cortical excitatory neurons (Loh, Rolls and Deco, 2007a,b; Rolls,

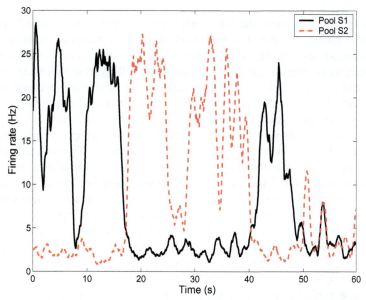

Fig. 18.9 Wandering between attractor states by virtue of statistical fluctuations caused by the randomness of the spiking activity. We simulated a single long trial (60 s) in the spontaneous test condition for the synaptic modification (−NMDA, −GABA). The two curves show the activity of the two selective pools over time smoothed with a 1 s sliding averaging window. The activity moves noisily between the attractor for the spontaneous state and the two persistent states S1 and S2. (After Loh,M., Rolls, E. T. and Deco,G. (2007) A dynamical systems hypothesis of schizophrenia. PLoS Computational Biology 3: e228.)

Loh, Deco and Winterer, 2008d). This is consistent with the fact that the positive symptoms usually follow the cognitive and negative ones and represent a qualitative worsening of the illness (Mueser and McGurk, 2004). Alterations in GABA receptors have been identified in schizophrenia (Lewis, 2014; Gonzalez-Burgos et al., 2010; Gonzalez-Burgos and Lewis, 2012; Glausier and Lewis, 2018), and the hippocampus has increased metabolism and activity in schizophrenia (Wegrzyn, Juckel and Faissner, 2022).

The evidence on GABA-mediated inhibition impairments in schizophrenia, and also of decreased spine density that would reduce excitatory transmission (Lewis, 2014; Gonzalez-Burgos et al., 2010; Gonzalez-Burgos and Lewis, 2012; MacDonald et al., 2017; Hoftman et al., 2017; Glausier and Lewis, 2018; Rolls, 2021a; Dienel et al., 2022), is an indication that the stability of cortical attractor networks is likely to be impaired in schizophrenia. The models described here have shown some of the effects that would be produced by altered levels of excitatory and inhibitory transmission on the stability of cortical circuitry, and how this might influence processes such as working memory and attention, and produce some of the symptoms of schizophrenia.

18.3.3 Reduced functional connectivity of some brain regions in schizophrenia

One way to investigate further the hypothesis that some networks in the brain are less stable in schizophrenia is to measure whether the functional connectivity between some brain regions is lower in schizophrenia. Functional connectivity can be measured by the Pearson correlation between the BOLD signal for each pair of brain regions over a time period of several minutes. A higher correlation is interpreted as showing that the nodes (the brain regions) are more strongly connected, in that they are influencing each other's BOLD signals, or have a common input.

In one such investigation, the functional connectivity in a group of 123 patients with chronic schizophrenia compared to 136 matched healthy controls is shown in Fig. 18.10B (Rolls, Cheng and Feng, 2021b). The matrix shows the functional connectivity differences for pairs of brain areas from the automated anatomical labelling atlas 3 (AAL3) (Rolls, Huang, Lin, Feng and Joliot, 2020d). First, it is evident that many of the functional connectivities are significantly lower in schizophrenia. This is consistent with the hypothesis that the level of excitation between cortical areas is lower in schizophrenia, which is equivalent in the simulations described above to a reduction in the NMDA synaptic conductances. This is consistent with the disconnectivity hypothesis of schizophrenia (Friston and Frith, 1995).

Moving beyond the disconnectivity hypothesis, the reduced functional connectivities evident in Fig. 18.10B might lead us to expect that there might be signs of less stability in the BOLD signal in schizophrenia. This was shown to be the case, in that the temporal variability of the functional connectivities of many of the brain regions was higher in schizophrenia, as shown in Fig. 18.10A[21]. The higher temporal variability was especially clear for some early visual cortical areas (Inferior Occipital and Fusiform), the temporal lobe areas connected to these, and the orbitofrontal cortex. This is an indication of increased instability of these brain regions in schizophrenia (Rolls, Cheng and Feng, 2021b,a).

Very interestingly, this higher temporal variability reflecting instability of some early visual cortical areas, the temporal lobe areas connected to these, and the orbitofrontal cortex could be related to lower functional connectivities of especially these areas, as shown in Fig. 18.10B. Especially interesting was that the functional connectivities of the thalamic sensory visual relay, the lateral geniculate nucleus, and the thalamic sensory auditory relay, the medial geniculate nucleus, were lower in schizophrenia (Fig. 18.10B). This was in interesting contrast to the association thalamic nuclei, which had increased functional connectivity in schizophrenia. This finding was cross-validated in a different set of patients with first-episode schizophrenia, who had similar though somewhat smaller differences from controls (Rolls et al., 2021b).

These findings are consistent with the hypothesis that a factor in schizophrenia is a reduction in the connectivity and therefore excitability of some brain regions, which destabilizes attractor networks in these regions because the firing rates are insufficient to maintain the networks in a high firing rate state. In particular, we propose that in schizophrenia these differences bias processing away from external visual and auditory inputs, and towards internal cognitive processing in associative cortical areas such as the prefrontal and temporal cortical areas. We relate this to the tendency for people with schizophrenia to be disconnected from the world, and to be unable to maintain attention (Rolls, Cheng and Feng, 2021b).

18.3.4 Beyond the disconnectivity hypothesis of schizophrenia: reduced forward but not backward connectivity

It has been possible to go beyond the disconnectivity hypothesis of schizophrenia (Friston and Frith, 1995), not only in terms of reduced dynamical stability of early visual cortical and

---

[21] The temporal variability measures how much the functional connectivity of a brain region k with other brain regions changes across time. The temporal variability of a given brain region was obtained as follows. We first segmented all BOLD signals into n non-overlapping windows with length l. The whole-brain FC network F_i (an $m*m$ matrix, with $m = 132$ nodes) in the ith time window was then constructed, with the Pearson correlation being the measure of Functional Connectivity. The Functional Connectivity profile of region k at time window i is denoted by $F_i(k,:)$ (shortened as $F_{i,k}$, which is an m-dimensional vector that represents all the functional connections of region k. The variability of a region k is defined as:

$$V_k = 1 - (\text{corrcoef}(F_{(i,k)}, F_{(j,k)})) \qquad i,j = 1, 2, 3, \ldots, n, i \neq j \qquad (18.3)$$

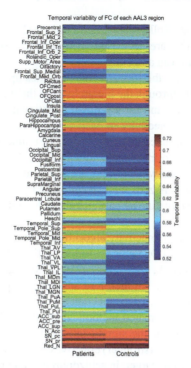

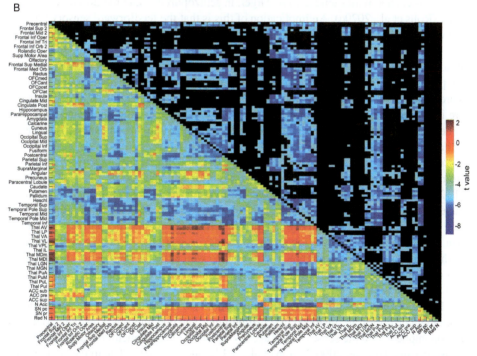

Fig. 18.10 A) The temporal variability of different AAL3 regions in the chronic schizophrenic and control groups. B) The functional connectivity of AAL3 regions for the chronic schizophrenic group minus controls. The lower left shows the t value for the difference in functional connectivity of patients - controls; the upper right shows the significance after Bonferroni correction. (After Rolls, E. T., Cheng, W. and Feng, J. (2021) Brain dynamics: the temporal variability of connectivity, and differences in schizophrenia and ADHD. Translational Psychiatry 11: 70.)

related areas as described above (Rolls, Cheng and Feng, 2021b), but also in terms of the direction of the connectivities that are decreased, as described next (Rolls, Cheng, Gilson, Gong, Deco, Lo, Yang, Tsai, Liu, Lin and Feng, 2020c).

In hierarchical cortical systems, the forward connectivities up through the hierarchy are strong, to drive the processing up through the hierarchy; and the backprojections are weaker, as they are used for memory recall and for top-down attentional bias (Rolls, 2016b). Measurements can be made of the connectivity in each of these directions, by making use of differences in the signals between successive timesteps. The connectivity in each direction is termed the *effective connectivity*. To investigate how the directed or effective connectivities are different in schizophrenia, to see whether they are different for particular brain areas, or in particular directions, we have analyzed effective connectivity in schizophrenia, comparing the resting state effective connectivity in 181 participants with schizophrenia and 208 controls (Rolls et al., 2020c).

It is difficult to apply directed connectivity algorithms to the fMRI BOLD signal, which is fairly slow, but an approach called Dynamic Causal Modelling (DCM) has been developed (Marreiros et al., 2008; Stephan et al., 2010). However, DCM is generally limited to a relatively small number of brain regions. We therefore adopted an approach (Gilson, Moreno-Bote, Ponce-Alvarez, Ritter and Deco, 2016) that can allow effective connectivity measurements between the 94 areas in the automated anatomical labelling atlas 2 (Rolls et al., 2015a).

The first key finding was that for the significantly different effective connectivities in schizophrenia, on average the forward (stronger) effective connectivities were smaller, but the backward connectivities tended to be larger, in schizophrenia, and the difference was significant (Rolls et al., 2020c). An implication of this is that the feedforward sensory inputs from the world are less effective in schizophrenia; and that the top-down backward connectivities that mediate the effects of memory recall and attention (Rolls, 2016b) show little difference in schizophrenia. This would tend to disconnect the individual from the world; and enclose the patient in an imaginary world too dominated by internal representations not corrected towards reality by sensory information from the world. Put in another way, if top-down signals are increased relative to bottom-up signals this would increase the importance of priors, ie, beliefs, at the cost of sensory signals, representing a possible mechanism for the emergence of hallucinations and delusions (Tschacher et al., 2017).

A second key finding in schizophrenia was the high effective connectivity directed away from the precuneus and the closely related posterior cingulate cortex (Fig. 18.11) (Rolls et al., 2020c). The connectivity in the strong (or forward) direction in schizophrenia to the precuneus is similar to that in the healthy controls, and it is in the weaker (backprojection) direction that the effective connectivity is higher in schizophrenia than in controls. It is suggested that by influencing other areas too much by its backprojections, the precuneus may contribute to the symptoms of schizophrenia. The regions to which the backprojections from the posterior cingulate cortex are higher in schizophrenia than in controls include the parahippocampal and temporal cortices (Rolls et al., 2020c).

I therefore consider how these differences in the connectivity of the precuneus and posterior cingulate cortex are involved in schizophrenia. The precuneus is a medial parietal cortex region implicated in the sense of self, agency, autobiographical memory, and spatial function (Cavanna and Trimble, 2006; Freton et al., 2014), and this may relate to the altered sense of self that is a feature of schizophrenia. The precuneus and the adjoining retrosplenial cortex (areas 29 and 30) (Kobayashi and Amaral, 2007) are key regions related to spatial function, memory, and navigation (Bubb et al., 2017; Cavanna and Trimble, 2006; Freton et al., 2014; Rolls and Wirth, 2018; Rolls, 2020b, 2021f; Rolls et al., 2023i; Rolls, 2023c) (Chapters 10 and 9). The retrosplenial cortex provides connections to and receives connections from the hippocampal system, connecting especially with the parahippocampal gyrus areas TF and

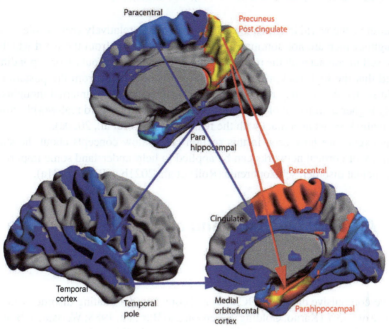

Fig. 18.11 Differences in effective connectivity in schizophrenia. The source regions (Region 1) are shown in the upper view of the brain, and the target regions (Region 2) in the two lower views of the brain. The Automated Anatomical Labelling atlas 2 regions with these differences show higher effective connectivity in red to yellow; and lower effective connectivity in blue. (After Rolls, E. T., Cheng,W., Gilson,M., Gong,W., Deco,G., Zac Lo,C-Y., Yang,A.C., Tsai,S-J., Liu,M-E., Lin,C-P. and Feng,J. (2020) Beyond the disconnectivity hypothesis of schizophrenia. Cerebral Cortex 30: 1213–1233. © Oxford University Press.)

TH, and with the subiculum (Bubb et al., 2017; Kobayashi and Amaral, 2007; Rolls et al., 2023i; Rolls, 2023c) (Fig. 9.1). The precuneus can be conceptualized as providing access to the hippocampus for spatial and related information from the parietal cortex (given the rich connections between the precuneus and parietal cortex (Vogt, 2009; Kobayashi and Amaral, 2007; Rolls et al., 2023i,d). This increased effective connectivity from the precuneus to the hippocampal system is of special interest as it may contribute to the overactivity of the hippocampus in schizophrenia (Wegrzyn et al., 2022), which is consistent with the high Sigma parameter reflecting signal variance in schizophrenia also found for the hippocampus (Rolls, Cheng, Gilson, Gong, Deco, Lo, Yang, Tsai, Liu, Lin and Feng, 2020c). Further, the precuneus has rich connectivity with the posterior cingulate cortex (Vogt, 2009; Rolls et al., 2023i), which provides a pathway into the hippocampal memory system (Rolls and Wirth, 2018; Rolls, 2019c, 2020b, 2021f; Rolls et al., 2023i; Rolls, 2023c). The precuneus is part of the default mode network, which becomes more active when tasks are not being performed in the world, and instead internal thoughts and processing are occurring.

The posterior cingulate cortex is also a key region of the default mode network with strong connectivity in primates with the entorhinal cortex and parahippocampal gyrus, and thus with the hippocampal memory system (Bubb et al., 2017; Vogt, 2009; Rolls, 2019c; Rolls et al., 2023i). The posterior cingulate region (including the retrosplenial cortex) is consistently engaged by a range of tasks that examine episodic memory including autobiographical memory, and imagining the future; and also spatial navigation and scene processing (Auger and Maguire, 2013; Leech and Sharp, 2014; Rolls, 2019c; Rolls et al., 2023i; Rolls, 2022b).

The proposal made based on the findings described here and the evidence about the functions of the precuneus and posterior cingulate cortex is that the high backprojection effective connectivities from the precuneus may relate to increased internal thoughts about the self in schizophrenia, the world in which the self exists, and the relatively greater role of these internal thoughts which are not dominated by the sensory inputs from the word which normally keep the self in contact with the real world and with real-word inputs. Correspondingly, it was proposed that the high backprojection effective connectivities from the posterior cingulate cortex in schizophrenia may relate to increased memory-related internal thoughts involving relatively higher dominance of memories over the normal forward real-world sensory inputs that normally keep us in contact with the real world (Rolls et al., 2020c).

Thus overall we have seen in this section (18.3) how concepts about the stability and connectivity of cortical networks can be applied to help understand some important aspects of a key mental disorder, schizophrenia (Rolls et al., 2021b,a; Rolls, 2021a).

18.4 Attractor dynamics and obsessive-compulsive disorder

18.4.1 Introduction

Obsessive-compulsive disorder (OCD) is a chronically debilitating disorder with a lifetime prevalence of 2–3% (Karno, Golding, Sorenson and Burnam, 1988; Weissman, Bland, Canino, Greenwald, Hwu, Lee, Newman, Oakley-Browne, Rubio-Stipec, Wickramaratne et al., 1994; Pauls, Abramovitch, Rauch and Geller, 2014; Stein, Kogan, Atmaca, Fineberg, Fontenelle, Grant, Matsunaga, Reddy, Simpson, Thomsen, van den Heuvel, Veale, Woods and Reed, 2016; Robbins, Vaghi and Banca, 2019; Fineberg and Robbins, 2021). It is characterized by two sets of symptoms, obsessive and compulsive. Obsessions are unwanted, intrusive, recurrent thoughts or impulses that are often concerned with themes of contamination and 'germs', checking household items in case of fire or burglary, order and symmetry of objects, or fears of harming oneself or others (Chamberlain, Solly, Hook, Vaghi and Robbins, 2021). Compulsions are ritualistic, repetitive behaviors or mental acts carried out in relation to these obsessions e.g. washing, household safety checks, counting, rearrangement of objects in symmetrical arrays or constant checking of oneself and others to ensure no harm has occurred (Menzies et al., 2008; Stein et al., 2016; Robbins et al., 2019). Patients with OCD experience the persistent intrusion of thoughts that they generally perceive as foreign and irrational but which cannot be dismissed. The anxiety associated with these unwanted and disturbing thoughts can be extremely intense; it is often described as a feeling that something is incomplete or wrong, or that terrible consequences will ensue if specific actions are not taken. Many patients engage in repetitive, compulsive behaviors that aim to discharge the anxieties associated with these obsessional thoughts. Severely affected patients can spend many hours each day in their obsessional thinking and resultant compulsive behaviors, leading to marked disability (Pittenger et al., 2006; Stein et al., 2016). While patients with OCD and related disorders exhibit a wide variety of obsessions and compulsions, the symptoms tend to fall into specific clusters. Common patterns include obsessions of contamination, with accompanying cleaning compulsions; obsessions with symmetry or order, with accompanying ordering behaviors; obsessions of saving, with accompanying hoarding; somatic obsessions; aggressive obsessions with checking compulsions; and sexual and religious obsessions (Pittenger et al., 2006; Stein et al., 2016; van den Heuvel et al., 2016; Grant and Chamberlain, 2019; Robbins et al., 2019; Fineberg and Robbins, 2021).

In this section a theory is described of how obsessive-compulsive disorders arise, and of the different symptoms. The theory (Rolls, Loh and Deco, 2008c; Rolls, 2012c) is based on the proposal that there is overstability of attractor neuronal networks in some cortical and related areas in obsessive-compulsive disorders.

18.4.2 A hypothesis about the increased stability of attractor networks and the symptoms of obsessive-compulsive disorder

We hypothesized (Rolls, Loh and Deco, 2008c) that cortical and related attractor networks become too stable in obsessive-compulsive disorder, so that once in an attractor state, the networks tend to remain there too long (Rolls, Loh and Deco, 2008c; Rolls, 2012c). The hypothesis is that the depths of the basins of attraction become deeper, and that this is what makes the attractor networks more stable. We further hypothesize that part of the mechanism for the increased depth of the basins of attraction is increased glutamatergic transmission, which increases the depth of the basins of attraction by increasing the firing rates of the neurons, and by increasing the effective value of the synaptic weights between the associatively modified synapses that define the attractor, as is made evident in Equation B.12. The synaptic strength is effectively increased if more glutamate is released per action potential at the synapse, or if in other ways the currents injected into the neurons through the NMDA (N-methyl-d-aspartate) and/or AMPA synapses are larger. In addition, if NMDA receptor function is increased, this could also increase the stability of the system because of the temporal smoothing effect of the long time constant of the NMDA receptors (Wang, 1999). This increased stability of cortical and related attractor networks, and the associated higher neuronal firing rates, could occur in different brain regions, and thereby produce different symptoms, as follows. If these effects occurred in high order motor areas, the symptoms could include inability to move out of one motor pattern, resulting for example in repeated movements or actions. In parts of the cingulate cortex and dorsal medial prefrontal cortex, this could result in difficulty in switching between actions or strategies (Rushworth et al., 2007a,b), as the system would be locked into one action or strategy. If an action was locked into a high order motor area due to increased stability of an attractor network, then lower order motor areas might thereby not be able to escape easily what they implement, such as a sequence of movements, so that the sequence would be repeated.

A similar account, of becoming locked in one action and having difficulty in switching to another action, can be provided for response inhibition deficits, which have been found in OCD. The response inhibition deficit has been found in tasks such as go/no-go and stop-signal reaction time (SSRT) which examine motor inhibitory processes, and also the Stroop task, a putative test of cognitive inhibition (Hartston and Swerdlow, 1999; Bannon et al., 2002; Penades et al., 2005; Bannon et al., 2006; Chamberlain et al., 2006, 2007; Penades et al., 2007; Robbins et al., 2019). For example, response inhibition deficits have been reported in OCD patients when performing the SSRT, which measures the time taken to internally suppress pre-potent motor responses (Chamberlain et al., 2006). Unaffected first-degree relatives of OCD patients are also impaired on this task compared with unrelated healthy controls, suggesting that response inhibition may be an endophenotype (or intermediate phenotype) for OCD (Chamberlain et al., 2007; Menzies et al., 2008).

If occurring in the lateral prefrontal cortex (including the dorsolateral and ventrolateral parts), the increased stability of attractor networks could produce symptoms that include a difficulty in shifting attention and in cognitive set shifting. These are in fact important symptoms that can be found in obsessive-compulsive disorder (Menzies, Chamberlain, Laird, Thelen, Sahakian and Bullmore, 2008; Chamberlain, Solly, Hook, Vaghi and Robbins, 2021). Two different forms of shifting have been investigated: affective set shifting, where the affective or reward value of a stimulus changes over time (e.g. a rewarded stimulus is no longer rewarded) (intradimensional or ID set shifting); and attentional set shifting, where the stimulus dimension (e.g. shapes or colors) to which the subject must attend is changed (extradimensional or ED set shifting). Deficits of attentional set shifting in OCD have been found in several neurocognitive studies using the CANTAB ID/ED set shifting task (Veale, Sahakian,

Owen and Marks, 1996; Watkins, Sahakian, Robertson, Veale, Rogers, Pickard, Aitken and Robbins, 2005; Chamberlain, Fineberg, Blackwell, Robbins and Sahakian, 2006; Chamberlain, Fineberg, Menzies, Blackwell, Bullmore, Robbins and Sahakian, 2007; Robbins, Vaghi and Banca, 2019; Chamberlain, Solly, Hook, Vaghi and Robbins, 2021). This deficit is most consistently reported at the ED stage (in which the stimulus dimension, e.g. shape, color or number, alters and subjects have to inhibit their attention to this dimension and attend to a new, previously irrelevant dimension). The ED stage is analogous to the stage in the Wisconsin Card Sorting Task where a previously correct rule for card sorting is changed and the subject has to respond to the new rule (Berg, 1948; Chamberlain et al., 2021). This ED shift impairment in OCD patients is considered to reflect a lack of cognitive or attentional flexibility and may be related to the repetitive nature of OCD symptoms and behaviors(Chamberlain et al., 2021). Deficits in attentional set shifting are considered to be more dependent upon dorsolateral and ventrolateral prefrontal regions than the orbital prefrontal regions included in the orbitofronto-striatal model of OCD (Pantelis et al., 1999; Rogers et al., 2000; Nagahama et al., 2001; Hampshire and Owen, 2006; Robbins et al., 2019; Chamberlain et al., 2021), suggesting that cognitive deficits in OCD may not be underpinned exclusively by orbitofrontal cortex pathology. Indeed, intradimensional or affective set shifting may not be consistently impaired in OCD (Menzies et al., 2008; Chamberlain et al., 2021).

Planning may also be impaired in patients with OCD (Menzies et al., 2008), and this could arise because there is too much stability of attractor networks in the dorsolateral prefrontal cortex concerned with holding in mind the different short-term memory representations that encode the different steps of a plan (Rolls, 2016b). Indeed, there is evidence for dorsolateral prefrontal cortex (DLPFC) dysfunction in patients with OCD, in conjunction with impairment on a version of the Tower of London, a task often used to probe planning aspects of executive function (van den Heuvel et al., 2005). Impairment on the Tower of London task has also been demonstrated in healthy first-degree relatives of OCD patients (Delorme et al., 2007).

An increased firing rate of neurons in the orbitofrontal cortex, and anterior cingulate cortex, produced by hyperactivity of glutamatergic transmitter systems, would increase emotionality, which is frequently found in obsessive-compulsive disorder. Part of the increased anxiety found in obsessive-compulsive disorder could be related to an inability to complete tasks or actions in which one is locked. But part of our unifying proposal is that part of the increased emotionality in OCD may be directly related to increased firing produced by the increased glutamatergic activity in brain areas such as the orbitofrontal and anterior cingulate cortex. The orbitofrontal cortex and anterior cingulate cortex are involved in emotion, in that they are activated by primary and secondary reinforcers that produce affective states (Rolls, 2004a, 2014a, 2016b; Rolls and Grabenhorst, 2008; Rolls, 2019e, 2023b), and in that damage to these regions alters emotional behavior and emotional experience (Rolls, Hornak, Wade and McGrath, 1994a; Hornak, Rolls and Wade, 1996; Hornak, Bramham, Rolls, Morris, O'Doherty, Bullock and Polkey, 2003; Hornak, O'Doherty, Bramham, Rolls, Morris, Bullock and Polkey, 2004; Berlin, Rolls and Kischka, 2004; Berlin, Rolls and Iversen, 2005; Rolls, 2019e, 2021h) (Chapter 11). Indeed, negative emotions as well as positive emotions activate the orbitofrontal cortex, with the emotional states produced by negative events tending to be represented in the lateral orbitofrontal cortex and dorsal part of the anterior cingulate cortex (Kringelbach and Rolls, 2004; Rolls, 2014a, 2016b, 2009a; Grabenhorst and Rolls, 2011; Rolls, 2019e; Rolls et al., 2020a; Zhang et al., 2023a; Rolls et al., 2023b). We may note that stimulus-reinforcer reversal tasks (also known as intra-dimensional shifts or affective reversal) are not generally impaired in patients with OCD (Menzies et al., 2008), and this is as predicted, for the machinery for the reversal including the detection of non-reward (Rolls, 2014a, 2019e) (Chapter 11) is present even if the system is hyperglutamatergic.

If the increased stability of attractor networks occurred in temporal lobe semantic memory networks, then this would result in a difficulty in moving from one thought to another, and possibly in stereotyped thoughts, which again may be a symptom of obsessive-compulsive disorder (Menzies et al., 2008; Robbins et al., 2019; Fineberg and Robbins, 2021). The obsessional states are thus proposed to arise because cortical areas concerned with cognitive functions have states that become too stable. The compulsive states are proposed to arise partly in response to the obsessional states, but also partly because cortical areas concerned with actions have states that become too stable. The theory provides a unifying computational account of both the obsessional and compulsive symptoms, in that both arise due to increased stability of cortical attractor networks, with the different symptoms related to overstability in different cortical areas. The theory is also unifying in that a similar increase in glutamatergic activity in the orbitofrontal and anterior cingulate cortex could increase emotionality, as described earlier.

18.4.3 Glutamate and increased depth of the basins of attraction of attractor networks

To demonstrate how alterations of glutamate as a transmitter for the connections between the neurons may influence the stability of attractor networks, Rolls, Loh and Deco (2008c) performed integrate-and-fire simulations of the stability of a short-term memory attractor network of the type described in Section 13.6.1 and Section 18.3. A feature of these simulations is that we simulated the currents produced by activation of NMDA and AMPA receptors in the recurrent collateral synapses, and took into account the effects of the spiking-related noise, which is an important factor in determining whether the attractor stays in a basin of attraction, or jumps over an energy barrier into another basin (Loh, Rolls and Deco, 2007a; Rolls, Loh, Deco and Winterer, 2008d; Deco, Rolls and Romo, 2009).

We found that increasing the NMDA receptor-activated synaptic currents by 3% or the AMPA by 10% increased the stability of the high firing rate short-term memory state of the network. Thinking about possible treatments, we showed that increasing the inhibition in the network by increasing the GABA receptor-mediated currents by 10% could ameliorate the overstability produced by increased glutamate-related effects. We also showed that the increased NMDA-receptor mediated effects produced less distractibility of the short-term memory state by another stimulus, which is a further sign of overstability.

This provides a new approach to the symptoms of obsessive-compulsive disorder, for it deals with the symptoms in terms of overstability of attractor networks in the cerebral cortex (Rolls, Loh and Deco, 2008c; Rolls, 2012c). Consistent with this approach, hyperactivity of the lateral orbitofrontal cortex is found during symptom provocation, and this normalized over the course of behavioral therapy for OCD (Robbins et al., 2019). If the same generic change in activity and therefore in stability were produced in different cortical areas, then we have indicated how different symptoms might arise. Of course, if these changes were more evident in some areas than in others in different patients, this would help to account for the different symptoms in different patients. Having proposed a generic hypothesis for the disorder, we recognize of course that the exact symptoms that arise if stability in some systems is increased will be subject to the exact effects that these will have in an individual patient, who may react to these effects, and produce explanatory accounts for the effects, and ways to deal with them, that may be quite different from individual to individual.

This simulation evidence, that an increase of glutamatergic synaptic efficacy can increase the stability of attractor networks and thus potentially provide an account for some of the symptoms of obsessive-compulsive disorder, is consistent with evidence that glutamatergic function may be increased in some brain systems in obsessive-compulsive disorder (Rosenberg et al., 2000, 2001, 2004; Pittenger et al., 2006; Rolls, 2012c; Pittenger et al., 2011; Pittenger, 2015; Karthik et al., 2020) and that cerebro-spinal-fluid glutamate levels are elevated (Chakrabarty et al., 2005), though the evidence is still tentative (Pittenger, 2021). Consistent with this, agents with antiglutamatergic activity such as memantine and riluzole, which can decrease glutamate transmitter release, may be efficacious in obsessive-compulsive disorder (Pittenger et al., 2006; Bhattacharyya and Chakraborty, 2007; Pittenger et al., 2011; Pittenger, 2015, 2021).

Further evidence for a link between glutamate as a neurotransmitter and OCD comes from genetic studies. There is evidence for a significant association between the SLC glutamate transporter genes and OCD (Stewart et al., 2007; Pauls et al., 2014). These transporters are crucial in terminating the action of glutamate as an excitatory neurotransmitter and in maintaining extracellular glutamate concentrations within a normal range (Bhattacharyya and Chakraborty, 2007; Pauls et al., 2014). In addition, it has been postulated that N-methyl-d-aspartate (NMDA) receptors are involved in OCD, and specifically that polymorphisms in the 3′ untranslated region of GRIN2B (glutamate receptor, ionotropic, N-methyl-d-aspartate 2B) were associated with OCD in affected families (Arnold et al., 2004; Pittenger et al., 2011), and more recent evidence has also found some association to glutamate-related genes (Pauls et al., 2014). However, genetic studies of OCD have not yet produced robust conclusions (Fernandez, Leckman and Pittenger, 2018; Pittenger, 2021).

18.5 Depression and attractor dynamics

18.5.1 Introduction

Major depressive disorder is ranked by the World Health Organization as the leading cause of years-of-life lived with disability, with more than 300 million people having major depressive disorder (Drevets, 2007; Gotlib and Hammen, 2009; Hamilton et al., 2013; WHO, 2017). Major depressive episodes, found in both major depressive disorder and bipolar disorder are pathological mood states characterized by persistently sad or depressed mood. Major depressive disorders are generally accompanied by: (1) altered incentive and reward processing, evidenced by amotivation, apathy, and anhedonia; (2) impaired modulation of anxiety and worry, manifested by generalized, social and panic anxiety, and oversensitivity to negative feedback; (3) inflexibility of thought and behavior in association with changing reinforcement contingencies, apparent as ruminative thoughts of self-reproach, pessimism, and guilt, and inertia toward initiating goal-directed behavior; (4) altered integration of sensory and social information, as evidenced by mood-congruent processing biases; (5) impaired attention and memory, shown as performance deficits on tests of attention set-shifting and maintenance, and autobiographical and short-term memory; and 6) visceral disturbances, including altered weight, appetite, sleep, and endocrine and autonomic function (Drevets, 2007; Gotlib and Hammen, 2009; Rolls, 2018a; Thapar et al., 2022). This section describes an attractor-based theory of some of the brain mechanisms that are related to depression (Rolls, 2016e), and tests of the theory (Rolls, Cheng and Feng, 2020a; Zhang, Rolls, Wang, Xie, Cheng and Feng, 2023a).

The attractor theory of depression starts with the evidence that the orbitofrontal cortex contains a population of error neurons that respond to non-reward and maintain their firing for many seconds after the non-reward, providing evidence that they have entered an attractor state that maintains a memory of the non-reward (Thorpe, Rolls and Maddison, 1983; Rosenkilde, Bauer and Fuster, 1981; Rolls, 2014a, 2018a, 2019e) (Section 11.3.4). An example of such a neuron is shown in Fig. 11.14. The human lateral orbitofrontal cortex is activated by non-reward during reward reversal (Kringelbach and Rolls, 2003) (Fig. 11.16), by losing money (O'Doherty et al., 2001a) or not winning (Xie et al., 2021) (Fig. 11.9), and by many other aversive stimuli (Grabenhorst and Rolls, 2011) (Fig. 11.18). Further evidence that the orbitofrontal cortex is involved in changing rewarded behavior when non-reward is detected is that damage to the human orbitofrontal cortex impairs reward reversal learning, in that the previously rewarded stimulus is still chosen during reversal even when no reward is being obtained (Rolls, Hornak, Wade and McGrath, 1994a; Hornak, O'Doherty, Bramham, Rolls, Morris, Bullock and Polkey, 2004; Fellows and Farah, 2003; Fellows, 2011). Further, the right lateral orbitofrontal cortex is strongly activated by non-reward in a one-trial rule-based reward reversal task (Rolls, Vatansever, Li, Cheng and Feng, 2020e), which is the same brain region with increased functional connectivity in depression as described below.

Now it is well established that not receiving expected reward, or receiving unpleasant stimuli or events, can produce feelings of depression (Beck, 2008; Drevets, 2007; Harmer and Cowen, 2013; Price and Drevets, 2012; Pryce et al., 2011; Eshel and Roiser, 2010; Rolls, 2018a). A clear example is that if a member of the family dies, then this is the removal of reward (in that we would work to try to avoid this), and the result of the removal of the reward can be depression. More formally, in terms of learning theory, the omission or termination of a reward can give rise to sadness or depression, depending on the magnitude of the reward that is lost, if there is no action that can be taken to restore the reward (Rolls, 2005a, 2013d, 2014a, 2018a) (Fig. 11.20). If an action can be taken, then frustration and anger may arise to the same reinforcement contingency (Rolls, 2014a, 2018a, 2019e,f, 2023b) (Section 11.3.8). This relates the current approach to the learned helplessness approach to depression, in which depression arises because no actions are being taken to restore rewards (Forgeard et al., 2011; Pryce et al., 2011; Maier and Seligman, 2016).

18.5.2 A non-reward attractor theory of depression

The theory has been proposed that in depression, the lateral orbitofrontal cortex non-reward / punishment attractor network system is more easily triggered, and maintains its attractor-related firing for longer (Rolls, 2016e, 2017c, 2019f, 2018a). The greater attractor-related firing of the non-reward / punishment system triggers negative cognitive states held on-line in other cortical systems such as the language system and in the dorsolateral prefrontal cortex which is implicated in attentional control. These other cortical systems then in turn have top-down effects on the orbitofrontal non-reward system that bias it in a negative direction (Rolls, 2013a) (see Section 4.3.5 and Fig. 4.16), and thus increase the sensitivity of the lateral orbitofrontal cortex to non-reward and maintain its overactivity (Rolls, 2016e) (Fig. 18.12). It is proposed that the interaction of non-reward and language / attentional brain systems of these types accounts for the ruminating and continuing depressive thoughts, which occur as a result of a positive feedback cycle between these types of brain system (Rolls, 2016e).

Indeed, we have shown that cognitive states can have 'top-down' effects on affective representations in the orbitofrontal cortex (De Araujo, Rolls, Velazco, Margot and Cayeux, 2005; Grabenhorst, Rolls and Bilderbeck, 2008a; McCabe, Rolls, Bilderbeck and McGlone, 2008; Rolls, 2013a). Further, top-down selective attention can also influence affective representations in the orbitofrontal cortex (Rolls et al., 2008b; Grabenhorst and Rolls, 2008; Ge et al., 2012; Luo et al., 2013; Rolls, 2013a), and paying attention to depressive symptoms when depressed may in this way exacerbate the problems in a positive feedback way.

More generally, the presence of the cognitive ability that is afforded by language to think ahead and see the implications of recent events may be a computational development in the brain that exacerbates the vulnerability of the human brain to depression (Rolls, 2014a, 2018a). For example, with language we can think ahead and see that perhaps the loss of an

Interaction of non-reward and language networks in depression

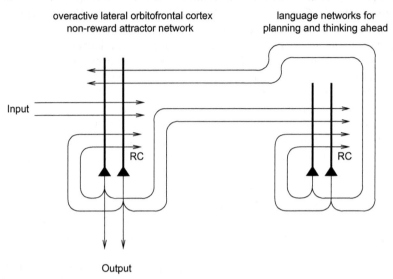

Fig. 18.12 Interaction of orbitofrontal cortex non-reward networks with language networks in depression. Illustration of how an overactive non-reward attractor network in the lateral orbitofrontal cortex could send excitatory information forward to networks for language and planning ahead; which could in turn send excitatory 'top-down' feedback back down to the orbitofrontal non-reward network to maintain its over-activity. It is suggested that such a system with mutual 'long loop' re-excitation contributes to the persistent ruminating thoughts in depression. (After Rolls, E. T. (2016) A non-reward attractor theory of depression. Neuroscience and Biobehavioral Reviews 68: 47–58. © Elsevier.)

individual in one's life may be long-term, and this thought and its consequences for our future can become fully evident.

The theory is that one way in which depression could result from over-activity in this lateral orbitofrontal cortex system is if there is a major negatively reinforcing life event that produces reactive depression and activates this system, which then becomes self-re-exciting based on the cycle between the lateral orbitofrontal cortex non-reward / punishment attractor system and the cognitive / language system, which together operate as a systems-level attractor (Fig. 18.12). (The generic cortical architecture for such reciprocal feedforward and feedback excitatory effects is illustrated by Rolls (2016b).)

The theory is that a second way in which depression might arise is if this lateral orbitofrontal cortex non-reward / punishment system is especially sensitive in some individuals. This might be related for example to genetic predisposition, or to the effects of stress (Gold, 2015). In this case, the orbitofrontal system would over-react to normal levels of non-reward or punishment, and start the local attractor circuit in the lateral orbitofrontal cortex (Section 11.3.4) (Rolls, 2016e; Rolls and Deco, 2016), which in turn would activate the cognitive system, which would feed back to the over-reactive lateral orbitofrontal cortex system to maintain now a systems-level attractor with ruminating thoughts. This is described as a 'systems-level' attractor because it includes mutual excitations between different brain areas.

Given that the activations of the lateral and medial orbitofrontal cortex often appear to be reciprocally oppositely related (O'Doherty, Kringelbach, Rolls, Hornak and Andrews, 2001a; Rolls, Kringelbach and De Araujo, 2003c; Xie, Jia, Rolls, Robbins, Sahakian, Zhang, Liu, Cheng, Luo, Zac Lo, Wang, Banaschewski, Barker, Bodke, Buchel, Quinlan, Desrivieres, Flor, Grigis, Garavan, Gowland, Heinz, Hohmann, Ittermann, Martinot, Martinot, Nees, Papadopoulos Orfanos, Paus, Poustka, Frohner, Smolka, Walter, Whelan, Schumann, Feng and IMAGEN, 2021; Zhang, Rolls, Wang, Xie, Cheng and Feng, 2023a), the other part of the theory of depression is that in depression there may be underactivity, under-sensitivity, or

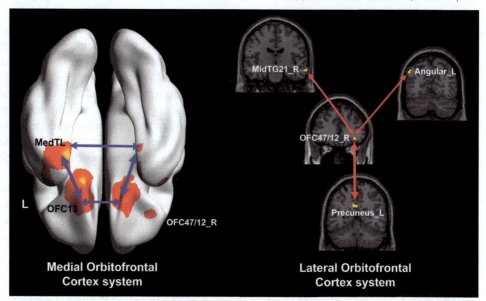

Fig. 18.13 Resting state functional connectivity in depression. The medial orbitofrontal cortex has reduced functional connectivity (blue) in depression with medial temporal lobe memory systems. The lateral orbitofrontal cortex has increased functional connectivity (red) in depression with the angular gyrus, precuneus, and middle temporal gyrus. MedTL – medial temporal lobe from the parahippocampal gyrus to the temporal pole; MidTG21R – middle temporal gyrus area 21 right; OFC13 – medial orbitofrontal cortex area 13; OFC12/47R – lateral orbitofrontal cortex area 12/47 right. The lateral orbitofrontal cortex cluster in OFC12/47 is visible on the ventral view of the brain anterior and lateral to the OFC13 clusters. (After Cheng,W., Rolls,E.T., Qiu,J., Liu,W., Tang,Y., Huang,C-C., Wang,XF., Zhang,J., Lin,W., Zheng,L., Pu,JC., Tsai,S-J., Yang,AC., Lin,C-P., Wang,F., Xie,P. and Feng,J. (2016) Medial reward and lateral non-reward orbitofrontal cortex circuits change in opposite directions in depression. Brain 139: 3296–3309. © Oxford University Press.)

under-connectivity of the (reward-related) medial orbitofrontal cortex in depression (Rolls, 2016e, 2018a; Uran et al., 2022). The theory is further that under-responsiveness of the medial orbitofrontal cortex could contribute to other aspects of depression, such as anhedonia.

18.5.3 The orbitofrontal cortex, and the theory of depression

There is some evidence for altered structure and function of the lateral orbitofrontal cortex in depression (Drevets, 2007; Ma, 2015; Price and Drevets, 2012; Zhang, Rolls, Wang, Xie, Cheng and Feng, 2023a). For example, reductions of grey-matter volume and cortex thickness have been demonstrated in the posterolateral OFC (BA 12/47, caudal BA 11 and the adjoining BA 45), and also in the subgenual cingulate cortex (BA 24, 25) (Drevets, 2007; Nugent et al., 2006; Schmaal et al., 2017), and in the medial orbitofrontal cortex (Schmaal et al., 2017). In depression, there is increased cerebral blood flow in areas that include the ventrolateral orbitofrontal cortex (which is a prediction of the theory), and also in regions such as the subgenual cingulate cortex and amygdala, and these increases appear to be related to the mood change, in that they become more normal when the mood state remits (Drevets, 2007; Lally, Nugent, Luckenbaugh, Niciu, Roiser and Zarate, 2015; Zhang, Rolls, Wang, Xie, Cheng and Feng, 2023a).

In the first brain-wide voxel-level resting state functional connectivity neuroimaging analysis of depression (with 421 patients with major depressive disorder and 488 controls), we have found that one major circuit with altered functional connectivity involved the medial orbitofrontal cortex BA 13, which had reduced functional connectivity in depression with memory systems in the parahippocampal gyrus and medial temporal lobe (Cheng, Rolls, Qiu, Liu, Tang, Huang, Wang, Zhang, Lin, Zheng, Pu, Tsai, Yang, Lin, Wang, Xie and Feng,

2016a) (Fig. 18.13). The lateral orbitofrontal cortex BA 12/47, involved in non-reward and punishing events, did not have this reduced functional connectivity with memory systems, so that there is an imbalance in depression towards decreased reward-related memory system functionality.

A second major circuit change was that the lateral orbitofrontal cortex area BA 12/47 had increased functional connectivity with the precuneus, the angular gyrus, and the temporal visual cortex BA 21 (Cheng et al., 2016a) (Fig. 18.13). This enhanced functional connectivity of the non-reward/punishment system (BA 12/47) with the precuneus (involved in the sense of self and agency), and the angular gyrus (involved in language) is thus related to the explicit affectively negative sense of the self, and of self-esteem, in depression.

The differences in orbitofrontal connectivity with these brain regions were related to the depression by evidence that the symptoms of depression were correlated with these differences of functional connectivity; and that the lateral orbitofrontal cortex functional connectivity links described were less high if the patients were receiving antidepressant medication (Cheng et al., 2016a).

The reduced functional connectivity of the medial orbitofrontal cortex, implicated in reward, with memory systems provides a new way of understanding how memory systems may be biased away from pleasant events in depression. The increased functional connectivity of the lateral orbitofrontal cortex, implicated in non-reward and punishment, with areas of the brain implicated in representing the self, language, and inputs from face and related perceptual systems provides a new way of understanding how unpleasant events and thoughts, and lowered self-esteem, may be exacerbated in depression (Cheng et al., 2016a; Rolls et al., 2018a).

These differences of functional connectivity are related to the orbitofrontal cortex attractor theory of depression, because increased functional connectivity of the non-reward lateral orbitofrontal cortex would increase the stability and persistence of its negative attractor mood-related states; and decreased functional connectivity of the reward-related medial orbitofrontal cortex would decrease the stability and persistence of its positive mood states (Rolls, 2018a).

These advances have stimulated many other large-scale voxel-level investigations of functional connectivity in depression, described in Section 18.5.4. A recent large-scale activation investigation of the role of the orbitofrontal cortex in depressive symptoms is described in Section 18.5.5. Implications for treatments are considered in Section 18.5.6.

18.5.4 Altered connectivity of the orbitofrontal cortex in depression

Further investigations have provided more evidence for different functional connectivity of the orbitofrontal cortex in depression, as described next, with a summary of some of the differences shown in Fig. 18.14 (Rolls, Cheng and Feng, 2020a). **These differences of functional connectivity all relate to altered stability of the circuits involved, which help to account for some of the symptoms of depression.**

18.5.4.1 Precuneus: higher connectivity with the lateral orbitofrontal cortex

The precuneus is a medial parietal cortex region implicated in the sense of self and agency, autobiographical memory, spatial function, and navigation (Cavanna and Trimble, 2006; Freton et al., 2014). The retrosplenial cortex provides connections to and receives connections from the hippocampal system, connecting especially with the parahippocampal gyrus areas TF and TH, and with the subiculum (Bubb et al., 2017; Kobayashi and Amaral, 2007; Rolls et al., 2023i) (Fig. 9.1). The precuneus can be conceptualized as providing access to the hippo-

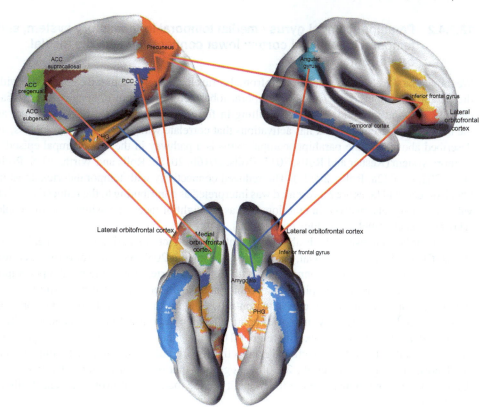

Fig. 18.14 Functional connectivity (FC) differences of the medial and lateral orbitofrontal cortex in major depressive disorder. Higher functional connectivity in depression is shown in red, and includes higher functional connectivity of the non-reward / punishment-related lateral orbitofrontal cortex with the precuneus, posterior cingulate cortex (PCC), subgenual anterior cingulate cortex (ACC subgenual), angular gyrus, and inferior frontal gyrus. Lower functional connectivity in depression is shown in blue, and includes lower functional connectivity of the medial orbitofrontal cortex with the parahippocampal gyrus memory system (PHG), amygdala, and temporal cortex. The part of the medial orbitofrontal cortex in which voxels were found with lower functional connectivity in depression is indicated in green. The areas apart from the medial orbitofrontal cortex shown are as defined in the automated anatomical labelling atlas 2 (Rolls, Joliot and Tzourio-Mazoyer, 2015), although the investigations that form the basis for the summary were at the voxel level. (After Rolls, E. T., Cheng, W. and Feng, J. (2020) The orbitofrontal cortex: reward, emotion, and depression. Brain Communications 2: fcaa196.)

campus for spatial and related information from the parietal cortex (given the rich connections between the precuneus and parietal cortex) (Rolls, 2018a; Rolls et al., 2023i).

To further analyze the functioning of the precuneus in depression, resting state functional connectivity was measured in 282 patients with major depressive disorder and 254 controls (Cheng, Rolls, Qiu, Yang, Ruan, Wei, Zhao, Meng, Xie and Feng, 2018c). In 125 patients not receiving medication, voxels in the precuneus had significantly higher functional connectivity with the lateral orbitofrontal cortex (Fig. 18.14). In patients receiving medication, the functional connectivity between the lateral orbitofrontal cortex and precuneus was decreased back towards that in the controls (Cheng et al., 2018c).

These findings support the theory that the non-reward system in the lateral orbitofrontal cortex has increased effects on areas in which the self is represented including the precuneus, which could relate to the low self-esteem in depressed patients (Rolls, 2016e, 2018a; Rolls et al., 2020a).

18.5.4.2 Parahippocampal gyrus / medial temporal lobe memory system, and temporal lobe visual cortex: lower connectivity with the medial orbitofrontal cortex

We found that voxels in the medial orbitofrontal cortex had lower functional connectivity with the parahippocampal gyrus / medial temporal lobe memory system (Cheng et al., 2016a) (Fig. 18.13), and interpreted this as resulting in fewer happy memories being recalled, as the medial orbitofrontal cortex has activations that correlate with subjective pleasantness, as described above, and the parahippocampal gyrus is a pathway in the hippocampal episodic memory system (Kesner and Rolls, 2015; Rolls, 2016b, 2018b; Rolls and Wirth, 2018; Rolls et al., 2023e, 2022a; Rolls, 2023c). The reduced connectivity with temporal cortex areas in which objects and faces are represented was interpreted as contributing to the reduced positive valuation of signals involved in emotion such as the sight of face expressions, and of people (Hasselmo et al., 1989a; Critchley et al., 2000).

In a further analysis, which also investigated the effects of antidepressant medication (Rolls, Cheng, Du, Wei, Qiu, Dai, Zhou, Xie and Feng, 2020b), medial orbitofrontal cortex voxels had lower functional connectivity with temporal cortex areas, the parahippocampal gyrus, fusiform gyrus, and supplementary motor area, and medication did not result in these functional connectivities being closer to controls. This is consistent with the anhedonia of depression and reduced happy memories being related to these low functional connectivities of the medial orbitofrontal cortex with temporal lobe and memory systems. What is especially interesting is that these low functional connectivities are not normalized by treatment with antidepressant drugs (Rolls et al., 2020b), suggesting that one goal of future treatment for depression might be to increase the functionality of the medial orbitofrontal cortex (Rolls et al., 2020a).

18.5.4.3 Posterior cingulate cortex: higher functional connectivity with the lateral orbitofrontal cortex in depression

The posterior cingulate cortex is a region with strong connectivity in primates with the entorhinal cortex and parahippocampal gyrus (areas TF and TH), and thus with the hippocampal memory system (Vogt, 2009; Bubb et al., 2017; Rolls and Wirth, 2018; Rolls, 2019c) (Fig. 9.1). The posterior cingulate cortex also has connections with the orbitofrontal cortex (Vogt and Pandya, 1987; Vogt, 2009; Hsu et al., 2020), and the posterior cingulate cortex has high functional connectivity with the parahippocampal regions that are involved in memory (Cheng et al., 2018b; Rolls, 2019c). The posterior cingulate region (including the retrosplenial cortex) is consistently engaged by a range of tasks that examine episodic memory including autobiographical memory, and imagining the future; and also spatial navigation and scene processing (Leech and Sharp, 2014; Auger and Maguire, 2013). Self-reflection and self-imagery activate the ventral part of the posterior cingulate cortex (vPCC, the part with which we will be mainly concerned here) (Kircher et al., 2002, 2000; Johnson et al., 2002; Sugiura et al., 2005; Rolls, 2019c; Rolls et al., 2023i).

To analyze the functioning of the posterior cingulate cortex in depression, we performed a fully voxel-level resting-state functional connectivity neuroimaging analysis of depression of the posterior cingulate cortex, with 336 patients with major depressive disorder and 350 controls (Cheng, Rolls, Qiu, Xie, Wei, Huang, Yang, Tsai, Li, Meng, Lin, Xie and Feng, 2018b). In depression, the posterior cingulate cortex had significantly higher functional connectivity with the lateral orbitofrontal cortex (Fig. 18.14). In patients receiving medication, the functional connectivity between the lateral orbitofrontal cortex and the posterior cingulate cortex was decreased back towards that in the controls.

These findings are consistent with the hypothesis that the non-reward system in the lateral orbitofrontal cortex has increased effects on memory systems, which contribute to the rumination about sad memories and events in depression (Cheng et al., 2018b).

18.5.4.4 Anterior cingulate cortex: higher connectivity with the orbitofrontal cortex in depression

The orbitofrontal cortex projects to the anterior cingulate cortex (Vogt, 2009; Bubb et al., 2017; Rolls, 2019c; Vogt, 2019b; Rolls et al., 2023c; Zhang et al., 2023a). As shown in Chapter 12, the supracallosal anterior cingulate cortex is activated by many aversive stimuli, and has strong connectivity with the lateral orbitofrontal cortex (Rolls, Cheng, Gong, Qiu, Zhou, Zhang, Lv, Ruan, Wei, Cheng, Meng, Xie and Feng, 2019; Hsu, Rolls, Huang, Chong, Lo, Feng and Lin, 2020; Du, Rolls, Cheng, Li, Gong, Qiu and Feng, 2020). The pregenual anterior cingulate cortex is activated by many pleasant, rewarding, stimuli, and has strong functional connectivity with the medial orbitofrontal cortex (Rolls et al., 2019; Hsu et al., 2020; Du et al., 2020; Rolls et al., 2023c). However, the dorsal or supracallosal anterior cingulate cortex appears to be involved in learning actions to obtain rewards (action-outcome learning), where the outcome refers to the reward or punisher for which an action is being learned (Rolls, 2019c). In contrast, the medial orbitofrontal cortex is implicated in reward-related processing and learning, and the lateral orbitofrontal cortex in non-reward and punishment-related processing and learning. These involve stimulus-stimulus associations, where the second stimulus is a reward (or its omission), or a punisher (Rolls, 2019f,e). Now given that emotions can be considered as states elicited by rewarding and punishing stimuli, and that moods such as depression can arise from prolonged non-reward or punishment (see above and Chapter 11), the part of the brain that processes these stimulus-reward associations, the orbitofrontal cortex, is more likely to be involved in depression than the action-related parts of the cingulate cortex, although the anterior cingulate cortex and other regions related to action such as the right inferior frontal gyrus could contribute to depression as it is an output region for the orbitofrontal cortex (Rolls et al., 2023c,b).

However, the subgenual (or subcallosal) cingulate cortex has been implicated in depression, and electrical stimulation in that region may relieve depression (Lujan et al., 2013; Laxton et al., 2013; Lozano et al., 2012; Hamani et al., 2011, 2009; Mayberg, 2003) (although it has not been possible to confirm this in a double-blind study (Holtzheimer et al., 2017)). The subgenual cingulate cortex is also implicated in autonomic function (Gabbott et al., 2003), and this could be related to some of the effects found in this area that are related to depression. Whether the subgenual cingulate cortex is activated because of inputs from the orbitofrontal cortex, or performs separate computations is not yet clear. Further, the possibility is considered that electrical stimulation of the subcallosal region, which includes parts of the ventromedial prefrontal cortex (Laxton et al., 2013), that may relieve depression, may do so at least in part by activating connections involving the orbitofrontal cortex, other parts of the anterior cingulate cortex, and the striatum (Lujan et al., 2013; Hamani et al., 2009; Johansen-Berg et al., 2008; Elias et al., 2022a; Zhang et al., 2023a).

In a study of depression, overall the anterior cingulate cortex (ACC) had significantly higher functional connectivity with the orbitofrontal cortex, inferior frontal gyrus, superior parietal lobule, and with early cortical visual areas (Fig. 18.14) (Rolls, Cheng, Gong, Qiu, Zhou, Zhang, Lv, Ruan, Wei, Cheng, Meng, Xie and Feng, 2019). A pregenual ACC subdivision had high functional connectivity with medial orbitofrontal cortex areas, and a supracallosal ACC subdivision had high functional connectivity with the lateral orbitofrontal cortex and inferior frontal gyrus. The high FC in depression between the lateral orbitofrontal cortex and the subcallosal (subgenual) parts of the ACC may provide a mechanism for more non-reward information transmission to the ACC, contributing to depression. The high functional connectivity between the medial orbitofrontal cortex and supracallosal ACC in depression may also contribute to depressive symptoms. These higher functional connectivities in unmedicated patients were ameliorated by treatment with antidepressants (Rolls et al., 2019).

18.5.4.5 Inferior frontal gyrus: increased connectivity with the lateral orbitofrontal cortex in depression

The lateral orbitofrontal cortex projects to the inferior frontal gyrus (Hsu et al., 2020; Rolls et al., 2023c,b), and very interestingly higher functional connectivity was found in depression of voxels in the right inferior frontal gyrus with voxels in the lateral and medial orbitofrontal cortex, cingulate cortex, inferior and middle temporal gyrus and temporal pole, the angular gyrus, precuneus, hippocampus and mid- and superior frontal gyrus connectivity with the orbitofrontal cortex, temporal lobe areas, the parahippocampal gyrus and hippocampus, and motor areas (Fig. 18.14) (Rolls, Cheng, Du, Wei, Qiu, Dai, Zhou, Xie and Feng, 2020b). In medicated patients these functional connectivities of the inferior frontal gyrus were lower and towards those in controls.

The hypothesis was proposed (Rolls et al., 2020b,a) that one way in which the orbitofrontal cortex influences behavior in depression is via the right inferior frontal gyrus, which projects in turn to premotor cortical areas (Du, Rolls, Cheng, Li, Gong, Qiu and Feng, 2020; Rolls, Deco, Huang and Feng, 2023f). Consistent with the consequent hypothesis that the inferior frontal gyrus route may allow non-reward signals to have too great an effect to inhibit behavior in depression, lesions of the right inferior frontal gyrus impair stopping in the stop-signal task, and produce impulsiveness (Aron, Robbins and Poldrack, 2014; Dalley and Robbins, 2017). Also consistent with the hypothesis, successful stopping in the stop-signal task is associated with high activation of the inferior frontal gyrus and lateral orbitofrontal cortex (Deng, Rolls et al (2017)).

18.5.4.6 Amygdala: reduced connectivity with the orbitofrontal cortex in depression

The amygdala is involved in emotion, though as shown in Chapter 11, it may be overshadowed in humans by the orbitofrontal cortex (LeDoux and Pine, 2016; Rolls, 2019e; Rolls et al., 2023b). In a large scale study of depression, amygdala voxels had decreased functional connectivity with the medial orbitofrontal cortex (involved in reward); the lateral orbitofrontal cortex (involved in non-reward and punishment); temporal lobe areas (involved in visual and auditory perception including face expression analysis (Perrett, Rolls and Caan, 1982; Rolls, 2011d, 2012d; Leonard, Rolls, Wilson and Baylis, 1985); and the parahippocampal gyrus (involved in memory) (Fig. 18.14) (Cheng, Rolls, Qiu, Xie, Lyu, Li, Huang, Yang, Tsai, Lyu, Zhuang, Lin, Xie and Feng, 2018a). This disconnectivity of the amygdala may contribute to particularly some of the changed behavioral and autonomic responses in depression, and perhaps not to the depressed subjective feelings (Rolls et al., 2023b).

18.5.4.7 Sleep, depression, and increased lateral orbitofrontal cortex connectivity

Sleep is frequently impaired in depression (Becker et al., 2017). To advance understanding of the brain regions involved in sleep and depression, the relation between functional connectivity, depressive symptoms (the Adult Self-Report Depressive Problems scores), and poor sleep quality was measured in 1017 participants from the general population in the Human Connectome Project (Cheng, Rolls, Ruan and Feng, 2018d). The brain areas with increased functional connectivity of these common links related to both sleep and depressive scores included the lateral orbitofrontal cortex; the dorsolateral prefrontal cortex; the anterior and posterior cingulate cortex; the insula; the parahippocampal gyrus and hippocampus; the amygdala; the temporal cortex; and the precuneus. A mediation analysis showed that these functional connectivities in the brain contribute to the relation between depression and poor sleep quality.

Evidence was also found in this general population that the Depressive Problems scores were correlated with functional connectivities between areas that included the lateral orbitofrontal cortex, cingulate cortex, precuneus, angular gyrus, and temporal cortex (Cheng, Rolls, Ruan and Feng, 2018d). Part of the importance of this is that it provides strong support for a role of the lateral orbitofrontal cortex in depression in a general population in the U.S.A. in which a tendency to have depressive problems could be assessed. This cross-validation in a completely different population and in people not selected to have depression (Cheng et al., 2018d) provides support for the theory that the lateral orbitofrontal cortex is a key brain area that might be targeted in the search for treatments for depression (Rolls, 2016e). (Further validation is provided by a European cohort of 1,877 adolescents (Xie et al., 2021).) Low sleep duration and high depressive scores are also related to lower cortical area of the orbitofrontal cortex in a sample of 11,067 participants (Cheng, Rolls, Gong, Du, Zhang, Zhang, Li and Feng, 2021).

18.5.4.8 Effective connectivity in depression

Effective connectivity measures the effect of one brain region on another in a particular direction, and can in principle therefore provide information related to the causal processes that operate in brain function, that is, how one brain region influences another.

In a resting state fMRI investigation, effective connectivity directed to the medial orbitofrontal cortex from areas including the parahippocampal gyrus, temporal pole, inferior temporal gyrus, and amygdala was decreased in depression (Rolls, Cheng, Gilson, Qiu, Hu, Ruan, Li, Huang, Yang, Tsai, Zhang, Zhuang, Lin, Deco, Xie and Feng, 2018a). This implies less strong positive driving influences of these input regions on the medial and middle orbitofrontal cortex, regions implicated in reward, and thus helps to elucidate part of the decreased feelings of happy states in depression (Rolls, 2016e). The links from temporal cortical areas to the precuneus were increased in depression, and this may relate to representations of the sense of self (Cavanna and Trimble, 2006), which become more negative in depression (Rolls, 2016e; Cheng et al., 2016a). The lateral orbitofrontal cortex, implicated in non-reward and punishment, had an increased level of activity as reflected in the analysis in the depressed group. In addition, activity in the analysis was also higher in the right and left hippocampus of patients with depression, implying heightened memory-related processing (Rolls et al., 2018a).

18.5.5 Increased activations to non-reward of the lateral orbitofrontal cortex, and decreased sensitivity to reward of the medial orbitofrontal cortex, are related to depression scores

In 1140 adolescents at age 19 and 1877 at age 14 in the monetary incentive delay task, we found that the medial orbitofrontal cortex had graded increases in activation as the reward (Win) value increased (Xie, Jia, Rolls et al (2021)). The lateral orbitofrontal cortex had graded increases of activation as the reward value dropped to zero (the No-Win condition) (Fig. 11.9).

In a subgroup with a high score on the Adolescent Depression Rating Scale at age 19 and 14, the medial orbitofrontal cortex activations had reduced sensitivity to the different reward conditions; and the lateral orbitofrontal cortex activation showed high activation to the No-Win (i.e. Non-reward) condition (Xie et al., 2021) (Fig. 18.15). These new findings provide support for the hypothesis that those with symptoms of depression have increased sensitivity to non-reward in the lateral orbitofrontal cortex, and decreased sensitivity for differences

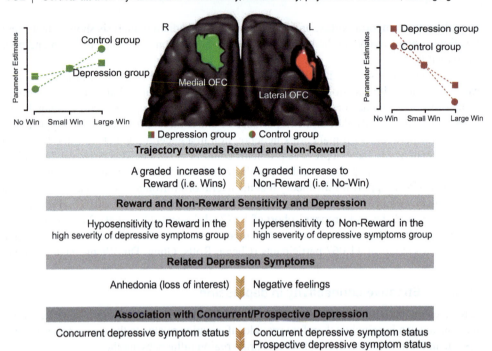

Fig. 18.15 Reduced sensitivity to reward of the medial orbitofrontal cortex, and increased sensitivity of the lateral orbitofrontal cortex to non-reward (No Win) in individuals with high scores on the Adolescent Depression Rating Scale (squares) compared to a control group (circles) in the Monetary Incentive Delay task. The summary is based on findings in 1140 adolescents at age 19 and 1877 at age 14. L, left; R, right. (After Xie,C., Jia,T., Rolls, E. T. et al (2021) Reward versus Nonreward sensitivity of the Medial versus Lateral Orbitofrontal Cortex relates to the severity of depressive symptoms. Biological Psychiatry: Cognitive Neuroscience and Neuroimaging 6: 259-269.)

in reward of the medial orbitofrontal cortex. Moreover, these differences are evident at an age as early as 14 years old (Xie et al., 2021). This increase in Non-reward sensitivity of the lateral orbitofrontal cortex in depression, and decreased Reward sensitivity of the medial orbitofrontal cortex, may act together with the altered functional connectivity of these regions just described, to make some individuals susceptible to depression (Rolls et al., 2020a; Zhang et al., 2023a).

It is hypothesized that as part of the process of evolution, variation of the sensitivity of individuals to specific types of Reward and Non-Reward may be present (Rolls, 2014a). Individuals with high sensitivity to Non-Reward may be susceptible to depression, and individuals with low sensitivity to Non-Reward may be impulsive because they are little affected by non-reward (Rolls, 2014a, 2018a). Individuals with high sensitivity to Reward may be sensation-seekers (Wan, Rolls, Cheng and Feng, 2020) and risk-takers (Rolls, Wan, Cheng and Feng, 2022c) (with increased functional connectivity of the medial orbitofrontal cortex with for example the anterior cingulate cortex, and for that reason also impulsive (Wan, Rolls, Cheng and Feng, 2020; Rolls, Wan, Cheng and Feng, 2022c)); and individuals with low sensitivity to Reward may have reduced goal-seeking behavior and reduced motivation (Rolls, 2014a, 2018a; Zhang, Rolls, Wang, Xie, Cheng and Feng, 2023a). These types of natural variation may be important foundations for different types of personality (Rolls, 2014a, 2012e, 2023b).

18.5.6 Implications, and possible treatments, and subtypes of depression

The differences of functional connectivity described in this section (18.5) all relate to altered stability of the circuits involved, which help to account for some of the symptoms of depression. I now consider some of the implications of these advances (Rolls, Cheng and Feng, 2020a; Zhang, Rolls, Wang, Xie, Cheng and Feng, 2023a).

Because the lateral orbitofrontal cortex responds to many punishing and non-rewarding stimuli (Grabenhorst and Rolls, 2011; Rolls, 2014a,b, 2019e; Zhang et al., 2023a; Rolls, 2023b) that are likely to elicit autonomic/visceral responses, as does the supracallosal anterior cingulate cortex, and in view of connections from these areas to the anterior insula which is implicated in autonomic/visceral function (Critchley and Harrison, 2013; Rolls, 2016c), the anterior insula would also be expected to be overactive in depression, which it is (Drevets, 2007; Hamilton et al., 2013; Ma, 2015).

A notable discovery is that ketamine, a N-methyl-D-aspartate (NMDA) receptor antagonist, in subanaesthetic doses, produces rapid (within hours) antidepressant responses in patients who are resistant to typical antidepressants, and that the effects may last for two weeks or longer (Zanos and Gould, 2018; Iadarola et al., 2015; Maltbie et al., 2017; Zanos et al., 2016; Wilkinson et al., 2018; Rhee et al., 2022). Clinically, ketamine may be useful with a single dose, or doses may be repeated (Rhee et al., 2022). The short-term effects of ketamine include blocking excitatory NMDA receptors on cortical pyramidal cells which reduces the excitatory effect produced by the excitatory transmitter glutamate; and blocking excitatory receptors on GABA inhibitory neurons, which will tend to decrease GABAergic neuron firing, resulting in a potential increase in pyramidal cell firing. However, ketamine produces further effects, such as inducing synaptogenesis on excitatory neurons, increased glutamate transmission, reversing the synaptic deficits caused by chronic stress, and effects mediated by a ketamine metabolite hydroxynorketamine (Duman and Aghajanian, 2012; Ghasemi et al., 2017; Zorumski et al., 2016; Abdallah et al., 2016; Aleksandrova et al., 2017; Zanos and Gould, 2018; Zhang et al., 2023a). Another way in which ketamine may be effective in depression is by reducing inflammatory processes, which are sometimes related to depression (Ghasemi et al., 2017).

Ketamine may act in part by quashing the attractor state in the lateral orbitofrontal cortex at least for a number of days. Evidence consistent with this is that the activity (metabolism) of the inferior frontal gyrus and orbitofrontal cortex was decreased by a single dose of ketamine, which reduced the anhedonia of depression (see further below) (Lally et al., 2015). This NMDA receptor blocker may act at least in part by decreasing the high firing rate state of attractor networks by reducing transmission in the recurrent collateral excitatory connections between the neurons (Rolls, 2016b; Rolls, Loh, Deco and Winterer, 2008d; Rolls and Deco, 2010; Rolls, 2012c; Deco, Rolls, Albantakis and Romo, 2013; Rolls and Deco, 2015b). Treatment with conventional antidepressant drugs (e.g. SSRIs) decreases the activity and connectivity of this lateral orbitofrontal cortex system (Ma, 2015; Rolls et al., 2020a; Rolls, 2018a; Rolls et al., 2020a). Electroconvulsive therapy may have antidepressant effects, may and might knock the non-reward system out of its attractor state.

Given that a ketamine metabolite, hydroxynorketamine, may be related to the antidepressant effects of ketamine and may act via facilitating effects mediated by AMPA receptors (Zanos et al., 2016), the effects of ketamine might be mediated by increasing the activity of the medial orbitofrontal cortex reward-related system (which tends to be reciprocally inversely related to the lateral orbitofrontal cortex non-reward system), or the functional connectivity of the medial orbitofrontal cortex reward system with the hippocampal system which is reduced in depression (Fig. 18.13). There is now some evidence for an action of ketamine to increase activity or connectivity in the medial orbitofrontal cortex, as follows (Zhang, Rolls, Wang, Xie, Cheng and Feng, 2023a).

A pharmacological investigation tested 10 treatment resistant depression (TRD) patients with a monetary incentive delay task before and after ketamine infusions. The study showed that ketamine administration induced a sustained increase in medial orbitofrontal cortex and nucleus accumbens activation during both the anticipation of positive reward cues and during the receipt of positive feedback (the outcome phase). The enhanced reactivity of the medial orbitofrontal cortex and nucleus accumbens was accompanied by decreased depression symptoms and better behavioral performance to positive items (Sterpenich et al., 2019). Consistent with this, in one of the first clinical studies to investigate the anti-anhedonic mechanisms of ketamine in depression, 52 TRD patients received a single ketamine infusion. The primary outcome indicated that ketamine rapidly reduced levels of anhedonia, with a substantial effect within 40 minutes which lasted up to 3 days post-infusion (Lally et al., 2015). Importantly, in a subgroup of patients who received PET scans, the single ketamine infusion decreased glucose metabolism within medial orbitofrontal cortex regions, and the reduced magnitude of the orbitofrontal cortex metabolism was positively correlated with the changes in the anhedonia symptoms (i.e., changes in SHAPS scores) (Lally et al., 2015). In addition, a double-blind, placebo-controlled, crossover trial in TRD and healthy controls also showed that ketamine infusion increased the functional connectivity between the right medial orbitofrontal cortex and ventral rostral putamen for the TRD patients toward the levels observed in healthy controls, and the increased magnitude of orbitofrontal cortex-putamen connectivity was correlated with improved levels of anhedonia symptoms (i.e., reductions in SHAPS scores) (Mkrtchian, Evans, Kraus, Yuan, Kadriu, Nugent, Roiser and Zarate, 2021). Taken together, these findings provide evidence that ketamine has acute and chronic anti-anhedonic effects in major depressive disorder by acting in part to restore activity and sensitivity to reward, and increasing functional connectivity, of the medial orbitofrontal cortex.

A very interesting possibility arises. Ketamine may act at least in part to increase sensitivity to reward and connectivity of the medial orbitofrontal cortex, and thereby ameliorate the anhedonia and motivational symptoms of depression (Zhang, Rolls, Wang, Xie, Cheng and Feng, 2023a). Conventional antidepressants such as the selective serotonin reuptake inhibitors may act in part on the non-reward-related lateral orbitofrontal cortex to decrease its elevated sensitivity to non-reward and connectivity in depression, and thereby treat the symptoms of sadness related to non-reward over-efficacy (Rolls et al., 2020a; Zhang et al., 2023a). It is suggested that low doses of both types of treatment would be useful to explore.

Deep brain stimulation of the orbitofrontal cortex may be useful in the treatment of mood disorders and depression. The macaque orbitofrontal cortex is a key brain site at which deep brain electrical stimulation is rewarding (Rolls et al., 1980b; Rolls, 2005a, 2019e). Electrical stimulation of the human orbitofrontal cortex can also produce reward and raise mood (Rao et al., 2018), and many of the sites were in the middle part of the orbitofrontal cortex, areas 13 and 11, which are categorised as medial orbitofrontal cortex, the area activated by rewards (Rolls, 2019e). It is likely that these medial orbitofrontal cortex sites will produce better reward in humans than stimulation in the lateral orbitofrontal cortex BA12/47, for these lateral sites are activated by unpleasant stimuli and by not obtaining expected rewards. The medial (/middle) orbitofrontal cortex may for the reasons described here and elsewhere (Rolls, 2019e) be a key area of interest for deep brain stimulation to help relieve depression (Rolls et al., 2020a).

The anterior cingulate cortex, including the subcallosal cingulate cortex, is a key brain region to which the orbitofrontal cortex projects (Hsu et al., 2020; Du et al., 2020; Rolls et al., 2019; Rolls, 2019e; Rolls et al., 2023c). It is possible that brain stimulation of the subcallosal cingulate cortex might be useful in the treatment of at least some patients with depression (Riva-Posse et al., 2018; Holtzheimer et al., 2017; Dunlop et al., 2017; Lujan et al., 2013; Johansen-Berg et al., 2008), and it is possible that the subcallosal cingulate stimulation affects pathways that connect with the orbitofrontal cortex (Riva-Posse et al., 2018; Dunlop et al., 2017; Lujan et al., 2013; Johansen-Berg et al., 2008; Elias et al., 2022b,a). Given that the anterior cingulate cortex is an output region of the orbitofrontal cortex, it may be that treatments of the orbitofrontal cortex, where emotion-related processing is implemented, may be a better target for potential treatments for depression (Rolls et al., 2020a).

This non-reward / punishment attractor network sensitivity theory of depression has implications for treatments. These implications can be understood and further explored in the context of investigations of the factors that influence the stability of attractor neuronal networks with integrate-and-fire neurons with noise introduced by the close to Poisson spiking times of the neurons (Section 18.2) (Wang, 2002; Rolls, 2016b; Deco et al., 2009; Rolls and Deco, 2010; Deco et al., 2013; Loh et al., 2007a; Rolls and Deco, 2015b; Rolls, 2016b).

One implication is that antianxiety drugs, by increasing inhibition, might reduce the stability of the high firing rate state of the non-reward attractor, thus acting to quash the depression-related attractor state.

A second implication is that it might be possible to produce agents that decrease the efficacy of NMDA receptors in the lateral orbitofrontal cortex, thereby reducing the stability of the depression-related attractor state. The evidence that there are genes that are selective for NMDA receptors for the neurons in different populations is that there are separate knockouts for NMDA receptors in the CA3 and CA1 regions of the hippocampus (Nakazawa et al., 2002; Tonegawa et al., 2003; Nakazawa et al., 2003, 2004). The present theory suggests that searching for ways to influence the attractor networks in the lateral orbitofrontal cortex by decreasing excitatory or increasing inhibitory transmission in this region may be of considerable interest. It should be noted that the present theory is a theory specifically of non-reward and punishment-related attractor networks in the lateral orbitofrontal cortex and related areas in relation to depression, and of reduced efficacy of the medial orbitofrontal cortex, and that alterations of attractor networks in other cortical areas may be related to other psychiatric disorders (Rolls, 2012c).

In terms of the implications of the attractor-based aspect of the present theory, an important point is that the attractor dynamics must be kept stable in the face of the randomness or noise introduced into the system by the almost Poisson firing times of neurons for a given mean firing rate. Moreover, the spontaneous firing rate state of the non-reward attractor must be maintained stable when no non-reward inputs are present (or otherwise the non-reward attractor would jump into a high firing rate non-reward state for no external reason, contributing to depression). The inhibitory transmitter GABA may be important in maintaining this type of stability (Rolls and Deco, 2010). Moreover, the high firing rate state produced by non-reward must not reach too high a firing rate, as this would cause overstability of the non-reward / depression state. In a complementary way, if the high firing rate attractor state is insufficiently high, then that attractor state might be unstable, and the individual might be relatively insensitive to non-reward, not depressed, and impulsive because of not responding sufficiently to non-reward or punishment. The excitatory transmitter glutamate acting at NMDA or AMPA receptors may be important in setting the stability of the high firing rate attractor state. In this respect and in this sense, the tendency to become depressed or to be impulsive may be reciprocally related to each other. Predictions for treatments follow from understanding these noisy attractor-based dynamics (Rolls and Deco, 2010; Rolls, 2012c).

There is growing interest in possible subtypes of depression, for it may be possible to treat different subtypes differently, for example by targeting different brain systems, or by different types of cognitive therapy (Drysdale et al., 2017). In one investigation, the subtypes appeared to reflect different combinations of depression and anxiety (Drysdale et al., 2017).

A subtype with anxiety may be especially helped by repetitive transcranial stimulation of the right lateral orbitofrontal cortex (Feffer, Fettes, Giacobbe, Daskalakis, Blumberger and Downar, 2018).

The approach to understanding depression does suggest that differences in depression in different people could relate to the different systems described here (Rolls, 2019e; Drysdale et al., 2017; Fettes et al., 2017; Rolls et al., 2020a). One subtype may relate to reduced functioning of the reward-related medial orbitofrontal cortex and related brain systems such as the ventral striatum, and could be related to anhedonia, a reduction in pleasure, and a reduction in reward-related learning.

A second subtype may relate to increased sensitivity of networks in the lateral orbitofrontal cortex non-reward / punishment system, and may related to prominent and persistent (almost compulsive) negative thoughts, and to increased anxiety and neuroticism, and to suicidal ideation.

A third subtype may relate to relate to decreased connectivity of the orbitofrontal cortex with the anterior cingulate cortex, which by breaking the link between value / outcome representations in the orbitofrontal cortex and the action-outcome learning system in the anterior cingulate cortex (Rolls, 2019c) could lead to reduced motivation to perform actions, and to reduced learning by receiving reward outcomes for actions. Consistent with the way in which this subsystem may operate is that the functional connectivity between only the reward-related orbitofrontal cortex and the anterior cingulate cortex can be used to predict sensation-seeking in a large population of individuals (Wan, Rolls, Cheng and Feng, 2020), showing how important the connectivity between these two brain regions is likely to be in how individuals respond to rewards in the world.

Strengths of the approach to understanding depression described here are that it has its foundations in an understanding of the brain systems involved in normal emotions and mood states (Rolls, 2014a, 2018a, 2019f; Rolls et al., 2020a; Rolls, 2023b); and that it incorporates concepts of the stability of attractor networks in the cortex, which are a key feature of cortical design (Rolls and Deco, 2010; Rolls, 2016b).

18.5.7 Mania and bipolar disorder

So far in this Section 18.5, we have been considering unipolar depression.

Bipolar disorder includes periods of mania in addition to periods of depression (Kato, 2019). The severity of the mania is greatest in bipolar I disorder, moderate in bipolar II disorder, and lower in cyclothymia. During depression, people feel helplessness, reduced energy, and risk aversion, while with mania behaviors include grandiosity, increased energy, less sleep, and risk preference / impulsivity.

What is the relation between mania and depression? Could it be that in mania, there is something that in terms of reward/non-reward systems, is almost the opposite of depression? Might there be in mania *increased sensitivity to reward, and decreased sensitivity to non-reward / punishment*? The latter might manifest itself as increased impulsiveness in mania. That is a suggestion that might be considered to be the opposite of what has been described for depression in the previous part of this Section 18.5.

It turns out that there is support for this hypothesis. It indeed appears that the risk for mania is characterized by a hypersensitivity to goal- and reward-relevant cues (Nusslock et al., 2014). This hypersensitivity can lead to an excessive increase in approach-related affect and motivation during life events involving rewards or goal striving and attainment. In the extreme, this excessive increase in reward-related affect is reflected in manic symptoms, such as pursuit of rewarding activities without attention to risks, elevated or irritable mood, decreased need for sleep, increased psychomotor activation, and extreme self-confidence.

Some evidence consistent with the hypothesis is that patients with bipolar I disorder and their relatives showed greater activation of the medial orbitofrontal cortex in response to reward delivery (Wessa et al., 2014). Also, reduced deactivation of the medial orbitofrontal cortex (where rewards are represented) during reward reversal might reflect a reduced error signal in bipolar disorder patients and their relatives in the lateral orbitofrontal cortex. (The activation of the lateral orbitofrontal cortex by non-reward in healthy individuals is illustrated in Fig. 11.16.) This type of responsiveness has been found to be very different in mania, with apparently decreasing activations in the lateral orbitofrontal cortex during expectation of increasing loss, the opposite of what is found in healthy participants (Bermpohl et al., 2010) which we discovered in the orbitofrontal cortex (O'Doherty, Kringelbach, Rolls, Hornak and Andrews, 2001a). In this context, of potentially reduced sensitivity or even abnormal function of the lateral orbitofrontal cortex non-reward system in mania, it is relevant that manic bipolar patients continue to pursue immediate rewards despite negative consequences (Wessa et al., 2014). Further, impulsivity in mania is pervasive, encompassing deficits in attention and behavioral inhibition. In addition, impulsivity is greater if the illness is severe (with for example frequent episodes, substance use disorders, and suicide attempts) (Swann, 2009). The significance of this is that impulsivity may reflect decreased sensitivity to non-reward, which is represented by activations in the lateral orbitofrontal cortex, where non-reward is represented (see above).

Thus mania may reflect a state in which there is decreased sensitivity of non-reward systems and hence increased impulsiveness due to reduced sensitivity of the lateral orbitofrontal cortex, and at the same time, increased sensitivity to reward reflected in activations in the medial orbitofrontal cortex and pregenual cingulate cortex. Although these medial and lateral orbitofrontal cortex systems may show reciprocally related activations within an individual, with for example increasing activations in the medial orbitofrontal cortex to increasing monetary gains and decreasing activations in the lateral orbitofrontal cortex, and vice versa to increasing monetary loss (O'Doherty et al., 2001a), the reward and non-reward systems could be, and indeed are likely to, have their sensitivity set by independent genes, providing a basis for some patients to be depressed, and others to show both mania and depression. Indeed, Rolls' theory of emotion (Rolls, 2014a) (Chapter 11) would go beyond this, and suggest that the sensitivity to many different rewards (e.g. food when hungry, water when thirsty, pleasant touch, sensitivity to reputation), and correspondingly to many different non-rewards, may be set by genes somewhat independently. This provides a relation to personality (Rolls, 2014a), with the implication that people with depression may be particularly sensitive to certain non-rewards or punishers, and people with mania may be particularly sensitive to particular rewards. This has important implications for therapy, which might be well-directed towards particular sensitivities to particular non-rewards and particular rewards in different individuals.

The question then arises of the extent to which attractor network operations contribute to mania. In terms of responses to inputs that increase the expectancy of reward, a short-term attractor system, probably in the orbitofrontal cortex, is likely to be present, to bridge any temporal interval between the expected reward signal and the actual outcome. This could in principle be oversensitive in mania. When the reward, the outcome, is delivered, it might also be useful to have a short-term attractor, to help reset a rule attractor for which stimulus is currently rewarding. However, it would be maladaptive if these reward-expectancy or reward-outcome attractors normally operated for more than perhaps 10 s, for this would tend to break the important contingency between input stimuli and outcomes. In addition to these short-term attractors, there also needs to be a longer term attractor process to reflect mood state, which typically operates on a much longer time scale. This might again be an attractor (with separate competing attractors for different mood states), and this attractor might be re-activated by the longer loop through the language / planning system, which by recalling a recent reward might calculate the long-term benefits, helping to keep the mood state prolonged. This whole 'long-loop' attractor might also be more sensitive in mania. These are interesting concepts for future empirical exploration. There is much left to understand about bipolar disorder (Kato, 2019).

18.6 Attractor stochastic dynamics, aging, and memory

In Section 18.3 I considered how some cognitive symptoms such as poor short-term memory and attention could arise due to reduced depth in the basins of attraction of prefrontal cortical networks, and the effects of noise. The hypothesis is that the reduced depth in the basins of attraction would make short-term memory unstable, so that sometimes the continuing firing of neurons that implement short-term memory would cease, and the system under the influence of noise would fall back out of the short-term memory state into spontaneous firing.

Given that top-down attention requires a short-term memory to hold the object of attention in mind, and that this is the source of the top-down attentional bias that influences competition in other networks that are receiving incoming signals, then disruption of short-term memory is also predicted to impair the stability of attention.

These ideas are elaborated in Section 18.3, where the reduced depth of the basins of attraction in schizophrenia is related to down-regulation of NMDA receptors, or to factors that influence NMDA receptor generated ion channel currents such as dopamine D1 receptors.

Could similar processes, in which the stochasticity of the dynamics is increased because of a reduced depth in the basins of attraction, contribute to the changes in short-term memory and attention that are common in aging? Reduced short-term memory and less good attention are common in aging, as are impairments in episodic memory (Grady, 2008; Dahan et al., 2020). What changes in aging might contribute to a reduced depth in the basins of attraction? Computational approaches to the memory problems in aging are considered next (Rolls and Deco, 2015b; Rolls, 2019a). Some of the changes in the aging brain include impaired synaptic plasticity, and impaired neurogenesis in the dentate gyrus of the hippocampal system (Dahan et al., 2020). The ways in which impaired synaptic plasticity could influence memory are described below in Section 18.6.3. Neurogenesis, considered in Section 9.3.6.6, would if impaired reduce the ability of new items to generate separate patterns of firing in the CA3 neurons of the hippocampal episodic memory system, and thereby impair the formation of new episodic memories.

18.6.1 NMDA receptor hypofunction

One factor is that NMDA receptor functionality tends to decrease with aging (Kelly et al., 2006; Temido-Ferreira et al., 2019; Ploux et al., 2020; Orzylowski et al., 2021). This would act, as investigated in detail in Section 18.3, to reduce the depth of the basins of attraction, both by reducing the firing rate of the neurons in the active attractor, and effectively by decreasing the strength of the potentiated synaptic connections that support each attractor as the currents passing through these potentiated synapses would decrease. These two actions are clarified by considering Equation B.12 on page 835, in which the Energy E reflects the depth of the basin of attraction.

An example of the reductions of firing rate in an attractor network produced by even a small downregulations of the NMDA receptor activated ion channel conductances is shown in Fig. 18.16. The effect of these reductions would be to decrease the depth of the basins of

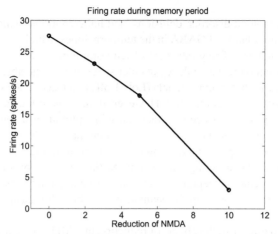

Fig. 18.16 Aging: reductions of NMDA receptor conductances reduce the firing rates (and therefore the stability) of short-term memory networks. Effects of reductions of NMDA receptor conductance on the firing rates of neurons in the short-term memory integrate-and-fire network during the short-term memory period of 4–5 s in the simulations. The firing rates are shown for correct trials only, that is when the spontaneous firing state was stable, and when the firing rate remained high in pool S1 (i.e. greater than 10 spikes/s more than in pool 2) until the end of the trial. (For the reduction of NMDA receptor activated synaptic conductance of 10%, there were no trials on which the memory was correctly maintained during this period, and the rates reflect a value close to the spontaneous firing rate before the memory retrieval cue was applied.) (From Rolls, E.T. and Deco,G. (2015) Stochastic cortical neurodynamics underlying the memory and cognitive changes in aging. Neurobiology of Learning and Memory 118: 150–161. © Elsevier Inc.)

attraction, both by reducing the firing rate, and by producing an effect similar to weakened synaptic strengths, as shown in Equation B.12.

The reduced depth in the basins of attraction could have a number of effects that are relevant to cognitive changes in aging.

First, the stability of short-term memory networks would be impaired, and it might be difficult to hold items in short-term memory for long, as the noise might push the network easily out of its shallow attractor.

Second, top-down attention would be impaired, in two ways. In one, the short-term memory network holding the object of attention in mind would be less stable, so that the source of the top-down bias for the biased competition in other cortical areas might disappear. In a second, and very interestingly, even when the short-term memory for attention is still in its persistent attractor state, it would be less effective as a source of the top-down bias, because the firing rates would be lower, as shown in Fig. 18.16.

Third, the recall of information from episodic memory systems in the temporal lobe (Rolls, 2016b; Dere et al., 2008; Rolls, 2008e) would be impaired. This would arise because the positive feedback from the recurrent collateral synapses that helps the system to fall into a basin of attraction, representing in this case the recalled memory, would be less effective, and so the recall process would be more noisy overall.

Fourth, any reduction of the firing rate of the pyramidal cells caused by NMDA receptor hypofunction (Fig. 18.16) would itself be likely to impair new learning involving LTP.

In addition, if the NMDA receptor hypofunction were expressed not only in the prefrontal cortex where it would affect short-term memory, and in the temporal lobes where it would affect episodic memory, but also in the orbitofrontal cortex, then we would predict some reduction in emotion and motivation with aging, as these functions rely on the orbitofrontal cortex (see Rolls (2019e) and Section 18.3).

Although NMDA hypofunction may contribute to cognitive effects such as poor short-term memory and attention in aging and in schizophrenia, the two states are clearly very different. Part of the difference lies in the positive symptoms of schizophrenia (the psychotic symptoms, such as thought disorder, delusions, and hallucinations) which may be related to the additional downregulation of GABA in the temporal lobes, which would promote too little stability of the spontaneous firing rate state of temporal lobe attractor networks, so that the networks would have too great a tendency to enter states even in the absence of inputs, and to not be controlled normally by input signals (Loh, Rolls and Deco, 2007a,b; Rolls, Loh, Deco and Winterer, 2008d) (see Section 18.3). However, in relation to the cognitive symptoms of schizophrenia, there has always been the fact that schizophrenia is a condition that often has its onset in the late teens or twenties, and I suggest that there could be a link here to changes in NMDA and related receptor functions that are related to aging. In particular, short-term memory is at its peak when young, and it may be the case that by the late teens or early twenties NMDA and related receptor systems (including dopamine) may be less efficacious than when younger, so that the cognitive symptoms of schizophrenia are more likely to occur at this age than earlier.

Possible ways to minimize the effects of reduction in NMDA receptor efficacy with aging may be caffeine (Temido-Ferreira et al., 2019), and d-serine (Ploux et al., 2020).

18.6.2 Dopamine and norepinephrine

D1 receptor blockade in the prefrontal cortex can impair short-term memory (Sawaguchi and Goldman-Rakic, 1991, 1994; Goldman-Rakic, 1999; Castner et al., 2000). Part of the reason for this may be that D1 receptor blockade can decrease NMDA receptor activated ion channel conductances, among other effects (Seamans and Yang, 2004; Durstewitz et al., 1999, 2000a; Brunel and Wang, 2001; Durstewitz and Seamans, 2002) (see further Section 18.3). Thus part of the role of dopamine in the prefrontal cortex in short-term memory can be accounted for by a decreased depth in the basins of attraction of prefrontal attractor networks (Loh, Rolls and Deco, 2007a,b; Rolls, Loh, Deco and Winterer, 2008d). The decreased depth would be due to both the decreased firing rate of the neurons, and the reduced efficacy of the modified synapses as their ion channels would be less conductive (see equation B.12). The reduced depth of the basins of attraction can be thought of as decreasing the signal-to-noise ratio (Loh, Rolls and Deco, 2007b; Rolls, Loh, Deco and Winterer, 2008d). Given that dopaminergic function in the prefrontal cortex may decline with aging (Sikström, 2007), and in conditions in which there are cognitive impairments such as Parkinson's disease, the decrease in dopamine could contribute to the reduced short-term memory and attention in aging.

In attention deficit hyperactivity disorder (ADHD), in which there are attentional deficits including too much distractibility, catecholamine function more generally (dopamine and noradrenaline (i.e. norepinephrine)) may be reduced (Arnsten and Li, 2005), and I suggest that these reductions could produce less stability of short-term memory and thereby attentional states by reducing the depth of the basins of attraction. Indeed, treatment with guanfacine, an adrenoceptor agonist (i.e. working on receptors activated by norepinephrine) can improve cognitive including working memory functions implemented in the dorsolateral prefrontal cortex (Arnsten and Wang, 2016), and this may be helpful in healthy aging.

18.6.3 Impaired synaptic modification

Another factor that may contribute to the cognitive changes in aging is that long-lasting associative synaptic modification as assessed by long-term potentiation (LTP) is more difficult to achieve in older animals and decays more quickly (Barnes, 2003; Burke and Barnes, 2006; Kelly et al., 2006; Dahan et al., 2020; Orzylowski et al., 2021). This would tend to make the synaptic strengths that would support an attractor weaker, and weaken further over the course of time, and thus directly reduce the depth of the attractor basins. This would impact episodic memory, the memory for particular past episodes, such as where one was at breakfast on a particular day, who was present, and what was eaten (Rolls, 2016b, 2008e; Dere et al., 2008). The reduction of synaptic strength over time could also affect short-term memory, which requires that the synapses that support a short-term memory attractor be modified in the first place using LTP, before the attractor is used (Kesner and Rolls, 2001). Part of the mechanism involving the decrease in synaptic plasticity in aging may be a decrease in D-serine, which is a cofactor required for normal operation of the NMDA receptor in synaptic plasticity (Orzylowski et al., 2021).

In view of these changes, boosting glutamatergic transmission is being explored as a means of enhancing cognition and minimizing its decline in aging. Several classes of AMPA receptor potentiators have been described. These molecules bind to allosteric sites on AMPA receptors, slow desensitization, and thereby enhance signalling through the receptors. Some AMPA receptor potentiator agents have been explored in rodent models and are now entering clinical trials (Lynch and Gall, 2006; O'Neill and Dix, 2007). These treatments might increase the depth of the basins of attraction. Agents that activate the glycine or serine modulatory sites on the NMDA receptor (Coyle, 2006; Uno and Coyle, 2019; Ploux et al., 2020) would also be predicted to be useful in healthy aging, and there is some evidence that D-serine administration or agents that influence D-serine can reverse some of the memory problems in aging in humans and in animal models (Orzylowski et al., 2021).

Another factor is that Ca^{2+}-dependent processes affect Ca^{2+} signaling pathways and impair synaptic function in an aging-dependent manner, consistent with the Ca^{2+} hypothesis of brain aging and dementia (Kelly et al., 2006). In particular, an increase in Ca^{2+} conductance can occur in aged neurons, and CA1 pyramidal cells in the aged hippocampus have an increased density of L-type Ca^{2+} channels that might lead to disruptions in Ca^{2+} homeostasis, contributing to the plasticity deficits that occur during aging (Burke and Barnes, 2006; Orzylowski et al., 2021).

18.6.4 Cholinergic function and memory

18.6.4.1 Cholinergic function, memory, and aging

Another factor is acetylcholine. Acetylcholine in the neocortex has its origin largely in the cholinergic neurons in the basal magnocellular forebrain nuclei of Meynert (Mesulam, 1990; Zaborszky et al., 2018, 2008; Galvin et al., 2020). The correlation of clinical dementia ratings with the reductions in a number of cortical cholinergic markers such as choline acetyltransferase, muscarinic and nicotinic acetylcholine receptor binding, as well as levels of acetylcholine, suggested an association of cholinergic hypofunction with cognitive deficits, which led to the formulation of the cholinergic hypothesis of memory dysfunction in senescence and in Alzheimer's disease (Bartus, 2000; Schliebs and Arendt, 2006). Could the cholinergic system alter the function of the cerebral cortex in ways that can be illuminated by stochastic neurodynamics? The dorsolateral prefrontal cortex is a key brain area in working memory (Chapter 13), and acetylcholine working mainly through nicotinic receptors is important in enabling neurons to maintain their firing in attractor states to implement working memory (Galvin et al., 2020). In addition, acetylcholine is important in hippocampal synaptic plasticity and memory (Hasselmo and Giocomo, 2006; Giocomo and Hasselmo, 2007; Hasselmo and Sarter, 2011; Newman et al., 2012; Zaborszky et al., 2018; Rolls, 2021b), as described in Chapter 9.

18.6.4.2 The responses of basal magnocellular forebrain nuclei cholinergic neurons

The cells in the basal magnocellular forebrain nuclei of Meynert lie just lateral to the lateral hypothalamus in the substantia innominata, and extend forward through the preoptic area into the diagonal band of Broca (Mesulam, 1990). These cells, many of which are cholinergic, project directly to the cerebral cortex (Divac, 1975; Kievit and Kuypers, 1975; Mesulam, 1990; Zaborszky et al., 2018; Galvin et al., 2020). These cells provide the major cholinergic input to the cerebral cortex, in that if they are lesioned the cortex is depleted of acetylcholine (Mesulam, 1990). Loss of these cells does occur in Alzheimer's disease, and there is consequently a reduction in cortical acetylcholine in this disease (Mesulam, 1990; Schliebs and Arendt, 2006). This loss of cortical acetylcholine may contribute to the memory loss in Alzheimer's disease, although it may not be the primary factor in the aetiology.

In order to investigate the role of the basal forebrain nuclei in memory, Aigner et al. (1991) made neurotoxic lesions of these nuclei in monkeys. Some impairments on a simple test of recognition memory, delayed non-match-to-sample, were found. Analysis of the effects of similar lesions in rats showed that performance on memory tasks was impaired, perhaps because of failure to attend properly (Muir et al., 1994). Damage to the cholinergic neurons in this region in monkeys with a selective neurotoxin was also shown to impair memory (Easton and Gaffan, 2000; Easton et al., 2002).

There are quite limited numbers of these basal forebrain neurons (in the order of thousands). Given that there are relatively few of these neurons, it is not likely that they carry the information to be stored in cortical memory circuits, for the number of different patterns that could be represented and stored is so small. (The number of different patterns that could be stored is dependent in a leading way on the number of input connections on to each neuron in a pattern associator, see e.g. Rolls (2016b)). With these few neurons distributed throughout the cerebral cortex, the memory capacity of the whole system would be impractically small. This argument alone indicates that these cholinergic neurons are unlikely to carry the information to be stored in cortical memory systems. Instead, they could modulate storage in the cortex of information derived from what provides the numerically major input to cortical neurons, the glutamatergic terminals of other cortical neurons. This modulation may operate by setting thresholds for cortical cells to the appropriate value, or by more directly influencing the cascade of processes involved in long-term potentiation (Rolls, 2016b). There is indeed evidence that acetylcholine is necessary for cortical synaptic modifiability, as shown by studies in which depletion of acetylcholine and noradrenaline impaired cortical LTP/synaptic modifiability (Bear and Singer, 1986). However, non-specific effects of damage to the basal forebrain cholinergic neurons are also likely, with cortical neurons becoming much more sluggish in their responses, and showing much more adaptation, in the absence of cholinergic inputs (Markram and Tsodyks, 1996; Abbott, Varela, Sen and Nelson, 1997) (see later).

The question then arises of whether the basal forebrain cholinergic neurons tonically release acetylcholine, or whether they release it particularly in response to some external influence. To examine this, recordings have been made from basal forebrain neurons, at least some of which project to the cortex (see Rolls (2005a)) and will have been the cholinergic neurons just described.

It has been found that some of these basal forebrain neurons respond to visual stimuli associated with rewards such as food (Rolls, 1975, 1981b,a, 1982, 1986c,a,b, 1990c, 1993, 1999a; Rolls, Burton and Mora, 1976; Burton, Rolls and Mora, 1976; Mora, Rolls and Burton, 1976; Wilson and Rolls, 1990b,a), or with punishment (Rolls, Sanghera and Roper-Hall, 1979b), that others respond to novel visual stimuli (Wilson and Rolls, 1990c), and that others respond to a range of visual stimuli. For example, in one set of recordings, one group of these neurons (1.5%) responded to novel visual stimuli while monkeys performed recognition or visual discrimination tasks (Wilson and Rolls, 1990c).

A complementary group of neurons more anteriorly responded to familiar visual stimuli in the same tasks (Rolls, Perrett, Caan and Wilson, 1982d; Wilson and Rolls, 1990c).

A third group of neurons (5.7%) responded to positively reinforcing visual stimuli in visual discrimination and in recognition memory tasks (Wilson and Rolls, 1990b,a).

In addition, a considerable proportion of these neurons (21.8%) responded to any visual stimuli shown in the tasks, and some (13.1%) responded to the tone cue that preceded the presentation of the visual stimuli in the task, and was provided to enable the monkey to alert to the visual stimuli (Wilson and Rolls, 1990c). None of these neurons responded to touch to the leg which induced arousal, so their responses did not simply reflect arousal.

Neurons in this region receive inputs from the amygdala (Mesulam, 1990; Amaral et al., 1992; Russchen et al., 1985) and orbitofrontal cortex (Rolls et al., 2023c; Rolls, 2022b), and it is probably via the amygdala and orbitofrontal cortex that the information described here reaches the basal forebrain neurons. For example, neurons with similar response properties have been found in the amygdala, and the amygdala appears to be involved in decoding visual stimuli that are associated with reinforcers, or are novel (Rolls, 1990c, 1992b; Davis, 1992; Wilson and Rolls, 1993; Rolls, 2000c; LeDoux, 1995; Wilson and Rolls, 2005; Rolls, 2005a, 2016b). Further, similar neurons responding to rewarding stimuli, aversive stimuli, and to novel stimuli are found in the orbitofrontal cortex (Thorpe, Rolls and Maddison, 1983; Rolls, Browning, Inoue and Hernadi, 2005a; Rolls, 2019f,e) (see Chapter 11).

18.6.4.3 Basal magnocellular forebrain nuclei cholinergic neurons as a cortical strobe to facilitate memory

On the basis of these findings, it is suggested that the normal physiological function of these basal forebrain neurons is to send a general activation signal to the cortex when certain classes of environmental stimulus occur. These stimuli are often stimuli to which behavioral activation is appropriate or required, such as positively or negatively reinforcing visual stimuli, or novel visual stimuli. The effect of the firing of these neurons on the cortex is excitatory, and in this way produces activation. This cortical activation may produce behavioral arousal, and may thus facilitate concentration and attention, which are both impaired in Alzheimer's disease. The reduced arousal and concentration may themselves contribute to the memory disorders. But the acetylcholine released from these basal magnocellular neurons may in addition be more directly necessary for memory formation, for Bear and Singer (1986) showed that long-term potentiation, used as an indicator of the synaptic modification which underlies learning, requires the presence in the cortex of acetylcholine as well as noradrenaline. For comparison, acetylcholine in the hippocampus makes it more likely that LTP will occur, probably through activation of an inositol phosphate second messenger cascade (Markram and Segal, 1992; Seigel and Auerbach, 1996; Hasselmo and Bower, 1993; Hasselmo et al., 1995; Hasselmo, 1999).

The adaptive value of the cortical strobe provided by the basal magnocellular neurons may thus be that it facilitates memory storage especially when significant (e.g. reinforcing) environmental stimuli are detected. This means that memory storage is likely to be conserved (new memories are less likely to be laid down) when significant environmental stimuli are not present. In that the basal forebrain projection spreads widely to many areas of the cerebral cortex, and in that there are relatively few basal forebrain neurons (in the order of thousands), the basal forebrain neurons do not determine the actual memories that are stored. Instead the actual memories stored are determined by the active subset of the thousands of cortical afferents on to a strongly activated cortical neuron (Treves and Rolls, 1994; Rolls and Treves,

1998; Rolls, 2016b). The basal forebrain magnocellular neurons would then according to this analysis when activated increase the probability that a memory would be stored. Impairment of the normal operation of the basal forebrain magnocellular neurons would be expected to interfere with normal memory by interfering with this function, and this interference could contribute in this way to the memory disorder in Alzheimer's disease.

Interesting new evidence is that in humans the cholinergic septal neurons that project to the hippocampus receive inputs in humans from the pregenual anterior cingulate cortex, which in turn receives from the orbitofrontal and ventromedial prefrontal cortex; and the basal forebrain cholinergic neurons that project to the neocortex receive from the medial orbitofrontal cortex (Rolls et al., 2023c). This places the human orbitofrontal cortex in a key position to influence memory consolidation, and indeed to be the origin of the cortical strobe that can increase memory consolidation (Rolls et al., 2023c; Rolls, 2022b). Consistent with this, damage to the ventromedial prefrontal cortex / pregenual anterior cingulate cortex impairs memory consolidation (Rolls, 2022b) (see Section 9.2.8.5). It is accordingly proposed that an additional factor in any decline in memory function in aging could relate to a less strong cortical strobe from the reward / punishment / novelty system in the orbitofrontal cortex, which might itself be less responsive to these emotion-provoking stimuli in some individuals as part of the normal aging process.

Thus one way in which impaired cholinergic neuron function is likely to impair memory is by reducing the depth of the basins of attraction of cortical networks, in that these networks store less strongly the representations that are needed for episodic memory and for short-term memory, thus making the recall of long-term episodic memories less reliable in the face of stochastic noise, and the maintenance of short-term memory less reliable in the face of stochastic noise. Such changes would thereby also impair attention.

18.6.4.4 Basal magnocellular forebrain nuclei cholinergic neurons reduce cortical adaptation

Another property of cortical neurons is that they tend to adapt with repeated input (Abbott, Varela, Sen and Nelson, 1997; Fuhrmann, Markram and Tsodyks, 2002a; Rolls, 2016b). However, this adaptation is most marked in slices, in which there is no acetylcholine. One effect of acetylcholine is to reduce this adaptation (Power and Sah, 2008). The mechanism is understood as follows. The afterpolarization (AHP) that follows the generation of a spike in a neuron is primarily mediated by two calcium-activated potassium currents, I_{AHP} and sI_{AHP} (Sah and Faber, 2002), which are activated by calcium influx during action potentials. The I_{AHP} current is mediated by small conductance calcium-activated potassium (SK) channels, and its time course primarily follows cytosolic calcium, rising rapidly after action potentials and decaying with a time constant of 50 to several hundred milliseconds (Sah and Faber, 2002). In contrast, the kinetics of the sI_{AHP} are slower, exhibiting a distinct rising phase and decaying with a time constant of 1–2 s (Sah, 1996). A variety of neuromodulators, including acetylcholine (ACh), noradrenaline, and glutamate acting via G-protein-coupled receptors, suppress the sI_{AHP} and thus reduce spike-frequency adaptation (Nicoll, 1988).

When recordings are made from single neurons operating in physiological conditions in the awake behaving monkey, peristimulus time histograms of inferior temporal cortex neurons to visual stimuli show only limited adaptation. There is typically an onset of the neuronal response at 80–100 ms after the stimulus, followed within 50 ms by the highest firing rate. There is after that some reduction in the firing rate, but the firing rate is still typically more than half-maximal 500 ms later (see example in Fig. 2.16). Thus under normal physiological conditions, firing rate adaptation can occur, but does not involve a major adaptation, even when cells are responding fast (at e.g. 100 spikes/s) to a visual stimulus. One of the factors that keeps the response relatively maintained may however be the presence of acetylcholine.

The depletion of acetylcholine in aging and some disease states (Schliebs and Arendt, 2011) could lead to less sustained neuronal responses (i.e. more adaptation), and this may contribute to the symptoms found. In particular, the reduced firing rate that may occur as a function of time if acetylcholine is low would gradually over a few seconds reduce the depth of the basin of attraction, and thus destabilize short-term memory when noise is present, by reducing the firing rate component shown in Equation B.12. I suggest that such changes would thereby impair short-term memory, and thus also top-down attention.

This adaptation can be studied by including a time-varying intrinsic (potassium like) conductance in the cell membrane, as described in Section B.6.2. A specific implementation of the spike-frequency adaptation mechanism using Ca^{++}-activated K^+ hyperpolarizing currents (Liu and Wang, 2001) as follows was used, and was also used by Deco and Rolls (2005c) (who also describe two other approaches to adaptation).

We assume that the intrinsic gating of K^+ after-hyper-polarizing current (I_{AHP}) is fast, and therefore its slow activation is due to the kinetics of the cytoplasmic Ca^{2+} concentration. This can be introduced in the model by adding an extra current term in the integrate-and-fire model, i.e. by adding I_{AHP} to the right hand of Equation 18.4, which describes the evolution of the subthreshold membrane potential $V(t)$ of each neuron:

$$C_m \frac{dV(t)}{dt} = -g_m(V(t) - V_L) - I_{syn}(t) \tag{18.4}$$

where $I_{syn}(t)$ is the total synaptic current flow into the cell, V_L is the resting potential, C_m is the membrane capacitance, and g_m is the membrane conductance. The extra current term that is introduced into this equation is as follows:

$$I_{AHP} = -g_{AHP}[Ca^{2+}](V(t) - V_K) \tag{18.5}$$

where V_K is the reversal potential of the potassium channel. Further, each action potential generates a small amount (α) of calcium influx, so that I_{AHP} is incremented accordingly. Between spikes the $[Ca^{2+}]$ dynamics is modelled as a leaky integrator with a decay constant τ_{Ca}. Hence, the calcium dynamics can be described by the following system of equations:

$$\frac{d[Ca^{2+}]}{dt} = -\frac{[Ca^{2+}]}{\tau_{Ca}} \tag{18.6}$$

If $V(t) = \theta$, then $[Ca^{2+}] = [Ca^{2+}] + \alpha$ and $V = V_{reset}$, and these are coupled to the previously-mentioned modified equations. The $[Ca^{2+}]$ is initially set to be 0 μM, τ_{Ca}= 600 ms, $\alpha = 0.005$, V_K=-80 mV and g_{AHP}=7.5 nS.

On the basis of these hypotheses, it is predicted that enhancing cholinergic function will help to reduce the instability of attractor networks involved in short-term memory and attention that may occur in aging.

Part of the interest of this stochastic dynamics approach to aging (Rolls and Deco, 2015b; Rolls, 2019a) is that it provides a way to test combinations of pharmacological treatments, that may together help to minimize the cognitive symptoms of aging. Indeed, the approach facilitates the investigation of drug combinations that may together be effective in doses lower than when only one drug is given. Further, this approach may lead to predictions for effective treatments that need not necessarily restore the particular change in the brain that caused the symptoms, but may find alternative routes to restore the stability of the dynamics.

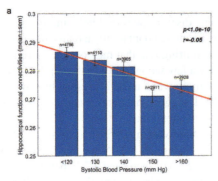 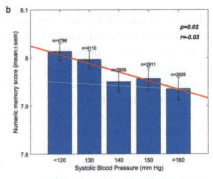

Fig. 18.17 The hippocampus, blood pressure, and memory. a. For 19,507 participants with neuroimaging data from the UK Biobank, there was a graded reduction in the functional connectivity of 88 hippocampal functional connectivity links and systolic blood pressure. The mean functional connectivity ± the sem is shown, together with the number of participants. The line shows the linear regression computed over all 19,507 participants, with age regressed out, and was significant at $p < 10^{-10}$. b. For the same participants there was a graded reduction in the numeric memory score with higher values of blood pressure, with the linear regression coefficient significant at $p < 10^{-10}$ and age regressed out. (From Feng,R., Rolls, E. T., Cheng,W. and Feng,J. (2020) Hypertension is associated with reduced hippocampal connectivity and impaired memory. EBioMedicine 61: 103082.)

18.7 High blood pressure, reduced hippocampal functional connectivity, and impaired memory

In another investigation to help to relate the advances in the computational approaches described in this book to disorders of brain function, we discovered that in the general population (with 19,507 participants in the UK Biobank), there was a linear relation between higher blood pressure, reduced hippocampal functional connectivity with other brain regions, and impaired numeric and prospective memory (all p< 10^{-10}) (see Fig. 18.17) (Feng, Rolls, Cheng and Feng, 2020). Effects of this type are probably related to a number of neurovascular changes that occur in hypertension (Iadecola and Gottesman, 2019), but part of the interest of the new discovery is that effects are found throughout the range of systolic blood pressure on both decreased functional connectivity of the hippocampus and decreased memory performance. These findings have implications for the treatment of hypertension, because the findings show more about the effects of even small increases in blood pressure. It is also of interest and potential clinical relevance that these effects were more evident for systolic blood pressure than for diastolic blood pressure (Feng, Rolls, Cheng and Feng, 2020).

18.8 Brain development, and structural differences in the brain

The differences in functional connectivity described in this Chapter that could produce different dynamics of different brain systems in some mental disorders could be partly related to genetic differences, and partly to the environment. It has recently been shown in several very large-scale studies with thousands of participants that in children or adolescents, there may even be structural differences in the brain that relate to psychiatric and cognitive problems, though again, we do not yet know whether these are related to genetic or environmental effects, or to a combination.

We have discovered that a set of different factors can be associated with reduced area or volume of the orbitofrontal cortex, anterior cingulate and medial prefrontal cortex, the medial temporal lobe, and some related areas; and with behavioral and psychiatric problems including difficult behavior and depression. In one study, this syndrome was associated with prolonged nausea and vomiting during pregnancy of the mothers (Wang, Rolls, Du, Du, Yang, Li, Li, Cheng and Feng, 2020c). In another study, family conflict was associated with a similar reduction of the area and volume of the same brain areas and similar behavioral, psychiatric and cognitive problems; and high parental monitoring (care) of the children with the opposite brain and behavioral differences (Gong, Rolls, Du, Feng and Cheng, 2021). In a third study, reduced area and volume of similar brain areas in the children, and behavioral and psychiatric problems, were associated with a low age of the mother when the child was born (Du, Rolls, Gong, Cao, Vatansever, Zhang, Kang, Cheng and Feng, 2022).

19 Computations by different types of brain, and by artificial neural systems

19.1 Introduction and overview

In this Chapter a comparison is made between computations in the brain and computations performed in computers (Section 19.3). This is intended to be helpful to those engineers, computer scientists, AI specialists and others interested in designing new computers that emulate aspects of brain function. In fact, the whole of this book is intended to be useful for this aim, by setting out what is computed by different brain systems, and what we know about how it is computed. It is essential to know this if an emulation of brain function is to be performed, and this is important to enable this group of scientists to bring their expertise to help understand brain function, and its disorders, better.

The comparison between computation in the brain and computation in computers in Section 19.3 is also intended to be of interest to neuroscientists to emphasize the differences in the implementations of computation in the brain and in computers.

Part of the interest here is that many computer implementations of 'neural networks' implement very different algorithms to those implemented in the brain. This means that there is a lot left not only to learn about the brain, but also to learn from the brain. For example, Section 19.4 specifically compares deep learning in artificial neural networks to the type of self-organising learning implemented in the brain; and Section 19.5 compares reinforcement learning in the brain (and in computers) to other learning systems in the brain.

Section 19.6 raises an important issue for understanding brains (and computers): the relation between explanations at different levels (neurons, networks, the computation that is performed, etc) of how brains and computers work, which is relevant to the mind-brain problem (Rolls, 2020a). Section 19.6.4 considers in particular the levels of investigation that are essential in order to understand how the brain performs it computations.

Section 19.7 considers the pioneering approach taken in this book to biologically plausible computations performed by each of many brain regions.

Section 19.8 is on Brain-Inspired Intelligence: how we can learn from the brain to implement new applications in computers.

Section 19.9 is on Brain-Inspired Medicine: how our developing understanding of how the brain computes has many implications not only for understanding how we as humans operate in health, but also what happens in for example mental disorders (considered in Chapter 18) and in other types of behavior, including behavior driven by our reward systems that can result in overeating and obesity.

Finally, Section 19.10 makes it clear why the focus of this book is on computations in primate (and that very much includes human) brains, rather than on rodent (rat and mice) brains. It is because the systems-level organization of primate including human brains is quite different from that in rodents.

We start in Section 19.2 by making the point that to understand how the brain works, a way forward is to understand how its different systems operate; and how that provides the foundation for how different systems operate together to produce a particular behavior.

That is also an important way forward when aiming to emulate in a computer how the brain performs a particular function.

19.2 Computations that combine different computational systems in the brain to produce behavior

By understanding what is computed in each brain system, how the information is represented, and how each system connects to other systems, we have a foundation for understanding how different brain systems operate together to perform behavioral functions. The ability to understand computationally what each part of the brain computes, and how the results of its computations are represented, is crucial to this aim. Studying each of these systems when the same behavior is being performed is also key to this aim. This approach is feasible, to understand the computations performed by each brain system separately, but while the same behavior is being performed, because there is considerable localisation of function in the brain, as set out by Rolls (2016b).

To model how the brain implements a function such as visual object recognition, or episodic memory, the strategy can next be to combine together the computations performed by several brain systems using information of the type presented in the different Chapters of this book, and in the Appendices. When moving forward to do this, it is suggested that a twofold strategy will be useful. The first part is to utilize the information provided in this book about what is computed in different brain systems, and how it is computed. The second part towards the implementation is to take into account the principles of operation of the cerebral cortex, as set out for example in *Cerebral Cortex: Principles of Operation* (Rolls, 2016b). In that book I did not attempt to produce a theory of how particular different brain systems compute, but instead focussed on the principles of operation and computation of the cortex. Thus what is in these two books complements each other in understanding the computations performed by the brain, and together they provide a foundation for further developments in our understanding, and in applying that understanding. Important applications of these advances are to understanding brain operation in disease, and developing new machines with what might be described as '**Brain-Inspired Intelligence**'.

19.3 Brain computation compared to computation on a digital computer

An important component of the approach taken in this book is to describe what computations are performed, and then how they may be performed. This enables the different levels of analysis in neuroscience to be brought together in a multilevel causal account.

However, the types of computation that are performed by the brain, and the computational style, are very different from the type of computation performed by a digital computer, which performs specified logical / syntactic operations on exact data retrieved from memory, and then stores the exact result back in memory. To highlight some of the principles of brain computation described in this book, and to emphasize how the type of computation is very different from that performed by digital computers, the principles of computation by the brain are compared next with those of a digital computer, with a summary of some of the differences in Table 19.1.

Data addressing. An item of data is retrieved from the memory of a digital computer by providing the address of the data in memory, and then the data can be manipulated (moved,

Table 19.1 Brain computation vs Digital computer computation

Brain Computation	Digital computer computation
1. Dot product similarity followed by a threshold	vs logical functions e.g. AND, NAND, OR
2. 10,000 inputs per neuron	vs several inputs to a logic gate
3. Content-addressable memory	vs data accessed by address
4. Fault tolerant: dot product	vs no inherent fault tolerance
5. Generalization and completion	vs only exact match in the hardware
6. Fast: parallel update of a neuron and of neurons in a network	vs serial processing with fast components
7. Approximate, low precision	vs high precision 64 bit
8. Stochastic spiking noise: probabilistic computation helps originality, creativity	vs noise free implemented by non-linearities
9. Dynamics are parallel e.g. an attractor network retrieves in 1–2 time constants of the synapses	vs inherently serial
10. Heuristics, e.g. Invariant object recognition analyzes only part of a scene.	vs attempt to understand a whole scene
11. Syntax: none inherent	vs syntactical operations on data at an address
12. The architecture adapts by learning to implement the computation.	vs fixed architecture with different software
13. Sparse distributed representation	vs binary encoding in a computer word
14. Mind vs brain	vs software vs hardware

compared, added to the data at another address in the computer etc.) using typically a 32-bit or 64-bit binary word of data. Pointers to memory locations are thus used extensively. In contrast, in the cortex, the data are used as the access key (in for example a pattern associator, autoassociator, and competitive network, see Appendix B), and the neurons with synaptic weights that match the data respond. Memory in the brain is thus **content-addressable**. In one time constant of the synapses / cell membranes, the brain has thus found the correct output. In contrast, in a digital computer a serial search is required, in which the data at every address must be retrieved and compared in turn to the test data to discover if there is a match.

Vector similarity vs logical operations. Cortical computation including that performed by associative memories and competitive networks operates by vector similarity – the dot (inner) product of the input and of the synaptic weight vector of each neuron are produced, and the neurons with the highest dot product will be most activated (Section 1.4 and Appendix B). Even if an exact match is not found, some output is likely to result. In contrast, in a digital computer, logical operations (such as AND, OR, XOR) and exact mathematical operations (such as addition, subtraction, multiplication, and division) are computed. (There is no bitwise similarity between the binary representations of 7 (0111) and 8 (1000).) The similarity computations performed by the brain may be very useful, in enabling similarities to be seen and parallels to be drawn, and this may be an interesting aspect of human creativity, realized for example in *Finnegans's Wake* by James Joyce in which thoughts reached by associative thinking abound. However, the lateral thinking must be controlled, to prevent bizarre similarities being found, and this is argued to be related to the symptoms of schizophrenia in Section 18.3.

Fault tolerance. Because exact computations are performed in a digital computer, there is no in-built fault tolerance or graceful degradation. If one bit of a memory has a fault, the whole memory chip must be discarded. In contrast, the brain is naturally fault tolerant, because it uses vector similarity (by neurons using their input firing rate vectors and synaptic weight vectors) in its calculations, and linked to this, distributed representations. This makes the brain robust developmentally with respect to 'missing synapses', and robust with respect to later losing some synapses or neurons (see Appendix B).

Word length. To enable the vector similarity comparison to have high capacity (for example memory capacity) the 'word length' in the brain is typically long, with between 10,000 and 50,000 synapses onto every neuron being common in cortical areas. (Remember that the leading term in the factor that determines the storage capacity of an associative memory is the number of synapses per neuron – see Sections B.2 and B.3.) In contrast, the word length in typical digital computers at 32 or 64 bits is much shorter, though with the binary and exact encoding used this allows great precision in a digital computer.

Readability of the code. To comment further on the encoding: in the cortex, the code must not be too compact, so that it can be read by neuronally plausible dot product decoding and can use vector similarity to generalize to similar patterns (Rolls, 2016b), as shown in Sections 1.7, B.2.4.3 and C.3.1, and throughout Appendices B and C. In contrast, the binary encoding used in a digital computer is optimally efficient, with one bit stored and retrievable for each binary memory location. However, the computer binary code cannot be read by neuronally plausible dot-product decoding.

Precision. The precision of the components in a digital computer is that every modifiable memory location must store one bit accurately. In contrast, it is of interest that synapses in the brain need not work with exact precision, with for example typically less that one bit per synapse being usable in associative memories (Treves and Rolls, 1991; Rolls and Treves, 1998). The precision of the encoding of information in the firing rate of a neuron is likely to be a few bits – perhaps 3 – as judged by the standard deviation and firing rate range of individual cortical neurons (Appendix C).

The speed of computation. This brings us to the speed of computation. In the brain, considerable information can be read in 20 ms from the firing rate of an individual neuron (e.g. 0.2 bits), leading to estimates of 10–30 bits/s for primate temporal cortex visual neurons (Rolls, Treves and Tovee, 1997b; Rolls and Tovee, 1994), and 2–3 bits/s for rat hippocampal cells (Skaggs, McNaughton, Gothard and Markus, 1993; Rolls, 2016b; Rolls and Treves, 2011) (Appendix C). Though this is very slow compared to a digital computer, the brain does have the advantage that a single neuron receives spikes from thousands of individual neurons, and computes its output from all of these inputs within a period of approximately 10–20 ms (determined largely by the time constant of the synapses) (Rolls, 2016b). Moreover, each neuron, up to at least the order of tens of neurons, conveys independent information, as described in Appendix C.

Parallel vs serial processing. Computation in a conventional digital computer is inherently serial, with a single central processing unit that must fetch the data from a memory address, manipulate the word of data, and store it again at a memory address. In contrast, brain computation is parallel in at least three senses.

First, an individual neuron in performing a dot product between its input firing rate vector and its synaptic weight vector does operate in an analog way to sum all the injected currents through the thousands of synapses to calculate the activation h_i, and fire if a threshold is reached, in a time in the order of the synaptic time constant. To implement this on a digital computer would take $2C$ operations (C multiply operations, and C add operations, where C is the number of synapses per neuron – see Equation 1.1).

Second, each neuron in a single network (e.g. a small region of the cortex with of the order of hundreds of thousands of neurons) does this dot product computation in parallel, followed by interaction through the GABA inhibitory neurons, which again is fast. (It is in the order of the time constant of the synapses involved, operates in continuous time, and does not have to wait at all until the dot product operation of the pyramidal cells has been completed by all neurons given the spontaneous neuronal activity that allows some neurons to reflect their changed inputs rapidly by when the next spike occurs.) This interaction sets the threshold in associative and competitive networks, and helps to set the sparseness of the representation of the population of neurons.

Third, different brain areas operate in parallel. An example is that the ventral visual stream computes object representations, while simultaneously the dorsal visual stream computes (inter alia) the types of global motion described by Rolls and Stringer (2006a) (Section 3.3), including for example a wheel rotating in the same direction as it traverses the visual field. Another example is that within a hierarchical system in the brain, every stage operates simultaneously, as a pipeline processor, with a good example being V1–V2–V4–IT (inferior temporal visual cortex), which can all operate simultaneously as the data are pipelined through (Chapter 2).

We could refer to the computation that takes place in different modules, that is in networks that are relatively separate in terms of the number of connections between modules relative to those within modules, such as those in the dorsal and ventral visual streams, as being parallel computation. Within a single module or network, such as the CA3 region of the hippocampus, or inferior temporal visual cortex, we could refer to the computation as being *parallel distributed computation*, in that the closely connected neurons in the network all contribute to the result of the computation. For example, with distributed representations in an attractor network, all the neurons interact with each other directly and through the inhibitory interneurons to retrieve and then maintain a stable pattern of neuronal firing in short-term memory (Section B.3). In a competitive network involved in pattern categorization, all the neurons interact through the inhibitory interneurons to result in an active population of neurons that represents the best match between the input stimulus and what has been learned previously by the network, with neurons with a poor match being inhibited by neurons with a good match (Section B.4). In a more complicated scenario with closely connected interacting modules, such as the prefrontal cortex and the inferior temporal cortex during top-down attention tasks and more generally forward and backward connections between adjacent cortical areas, we might also use the term parallel distributed computation, as the bottom-up and top-down interactions may be important in how the whole dynamical system of interconnected networks settles (see examples in Sections 13.6.1, 13.4, 2.12, and Appendix B).

Stochastic dynamics and probabilistic computation. Digital computers do not have noise to contend with as part of the computation, as they use binary logic levels, and perform exact computation. In contrast, brain computation is inherently noisy, and this gives it a non-exact, probabilistic, character. One of the sources of noise in the brain is the spiking activity of each neuron. Each neuron must transmit information by spikes, for an all-or-none spike carried along an axon ensures that the signal arrives faithfully, and is not subject to the uncertain cable transmission line losses of analog potentials. But once a neuron needs to spike, then it turns out to be important to have spontaneous activity, so that neurons do not all have to charge up from a hyperpolarized baseline whenever a new input is received. The fact that neurons are kept near threshold, with therefore some spontaneous spiking, is inherent to the rapid operation of for example autoassociative retrieval, as described in Section B.3. But keeping the neurons close to threshold, and the spiking activity received from other neurons, results in spontaneous spike trains that are approximately Poisson, that is with spikes randomly timed for a given mean firing rate. The result of the interaction of all these randomly timed inputs is that in a network of finite size (i.e. with a limited number of neurons) there will be statistical fluctuations, that influence which memory is recalled, which decision is taken, etc. as described in Section 11.5.1 and Chapter 18. Thus brain computation is inherently noisy and probabilistic, and this has many advantages, as described in Section 11.5.1, Chapter 18, and by Rolls and Deco (2010) and Rolls (2016b).

Syntax. Digital computers can perform arbitrary syntactical operations on operands, because they use pointers to address each of the different operands required (corresponding even for example to the subject, the verb, and the object of a sentence). In contrast, as data are not accessed in the brain by pointers that can point anywhere, but instead just having neurons firing to represent a data item, a real problem arises in specifying which neurons firing represent for example the subject, the verb, and the object, and distributed representations potentially make this even more difficult. The brain thus inherently finds syntactical operations difficult (as explained in Section 14.5). We do not know how the brain implements the syntax required for language. But we do know that the firing of neurons conveys 'meaning' based on spatial location in the brain. For example, a neuron firing in V1 indicates that a bar or edge matching the filter characteristic of the neuron is present at a particular location in space. Another neuron in V1 encodes another feature at another position in space. A neuron in the inferior temporal visual cortex indicates (with other neurons helping to form a distributed representation) that a particular object or face is present in the visual scene. Perhaps the implementation of the syntax required for language that is implemented in the brain also utilizes the spatial location of the network in the cortex to help specify what syntactical role the representation should perform. This is a suggestion I make, as it is one way that the brain could deal with the implementation of the syntax required for language (Section 14.5).

Modifiable connectivity. The physical architecture (what is connected to what) of a digital computer is fixed. In contrast, the connectivity of the brain alters as a result of experience and learning, and indeed it is alterations in the strength of the synapses (which implement the connectivity) that underlie learning and memory. Indeed, self-organization in for example competitive networks has a strong influence on how the brain is matched to the statistics of the incoming signals from the world, and of the architecture that develops. In a digital computer, every connection must be specified. In contrast, in the brain there are far too few genes (of order 25,000) for the synaptic connections in the brain (of order 10^{15}, given approximately 10^{11} neurons each with in the order of 10^4 synapses) for the genes to specify every connection[22]. The genes must therefore specify some much more general rules, such as that each CA3 neuron should make approximately 12,000 synapses with other CA3 neurons, and receive approximately 48 synapses from dentate granule cells (see Chapter 9). The actual connections made would then be made randomly within these constraints, and then strengthened or weakened as a result of self-organization based on for example conjunctive pre- and postsynaptic activity. Some of the rules that may be specified genetically have been suggested on the basis of a comparison of the architecture of different brain areas (Rolls and Stringer, 2000; Rolls, 2016b). Moreover, it has been shown that if these rules are selected by a genetic algorithm based on the fitness of the network that self-organizes and learns based on these rules, then architectures are built that solve different computational problems in one-layer networks, including pattern association learning, autoassociation memory, and competitive learning (Rolls and Stringer, 2000; Rolls, 2016b) (see Section B.20). The architecture of the brain is thus interestingly adaptive, but guided in the long term by genetic selection of the

---

[22]For comparison, a computer with 1 Gb of memory has approximately 10^{10} modifiable locations, and if it had a 100 Gb disk that would have approximately 10^{12} modifiable locations.

building rules.

Logic. The learning rules that are implemented in the brain that are most widely accepted are associative, as exemplified by LTP and LTD. This, and the vector similarity operations implemented by neurons, set the stage for processes such as pattern association, autoassociation, and competitive learning to occur naturally, but not for logical operations such as XOR and NAND or arithmetic operations. Of course, the non-linearity inherent in the firing threshold of neurons is important in many of the properties of associative memories and competitive learning, as described in Appendix B, and indeed are how some of the non-linearities that can be seen with attention can arise (Deco and Rolls, 2005b).

Dynamical interaction between modules. Because the brain has populations of neurons that are simultaneously active (operating in parallel), but are interconnected, many properties arise naturally in dynamical neural systems, including the interactions that give rise to top-down attention (Sections 13.4 and 2.12), the effects of mood on memory (Rolls and Stringer, 2001b; Rolls, 2014a) etc. Because simultaneous activity of different computational nodes does not occur in digital computers, these dynamical systems properties that arise from interacting subsystems do not occur naturally in digital computers, though they can be simulated.

The cortex has recurrent excitatory connections within a cortical area, and reciprocal, forward and feedback, connections between adjacent cortical areas in a hierarchy. The excitatory connections enable cortical activity to be maintained over short periods, making short-term memory an inherent property of the cortex. They also provide the autoassociative long-term memory with completion from a partial cue (given associative synaptic modifiability in these connections). However, completion on a digital computer is a difficult and serial process to identify a possible correct partial match. Another comparison is that the short-term memory property of the cortex is part of what makes the cortex a dynamical interacting system, with for example what is in short-term memory in the prefrontal cortex acting to influence memory recall, perception, and even what decision is taken, in other networks, by top-down biased competition (see Sections 13.4 and 2.12). There is a price that the brain pays for this positive feedback inherent in its recurrent cortical circuitry, which is that this circuitry is inherently unstable, and requires strong control by inhibitory interneurons to minimize the risk of epilepsy and other disorders (Chapter 18).

Modular organization. Brain organization is modular, with many relatively independent modules each performing a different function, whereas digital computers typically have a single central processing unit connected to memory. The cortex has many localized modules with dense connectivity within a module, and then connections to a few other modules. The reasons for the modularity of the brain are considered by Rolls (2016b).

Hierarchical organization. As described by Rolls (2016b), many cortical systems are organized hierarchically. A major reason for this is that this enables the connectivity to be kept within the limits of which neurons appear capable (up to 50,000 synapses per neuron), yet also enables global computation (such as the presence of a particular object anywhere in the visual field) to be achieved, as exemplified by VisNet, a model of invariant visual object recognition (see Fig. 2.2 and Chapter 2). Another important reason is that hierarchical organization simplifies the learning that is required at each stage and enables it to be a local operation, in contrast to backpropagation of error networks where similar problems could in principle be solved in a two-layer network (with one hidden layer), but would require training with a non-local learning rule (Appendix C) as well as potentially neurons with very large numbers of connections. Another feature of cortical organization is that the number of areas or levels in any hierarchy in the brain is not more than 4 or 5, because each area requires 20–30 ms of computation and transmission time. (This of course contrasts with the hundreds of successive layers being explored with artificial neural networks, as described in Section B.14, which is completely biologically implausible in terms of response times.)

19.4   A comparison of brain computation with learning in artificial deep learning networks using error backpropagation

Learning in deep networks with error backpropagation (LeCun, Bengio and Hinton, 2015; Lillicrap, Santoro, Marris, Akerman and Hinton, 2020) is described in Section B.12. Attempts to compare the operation of hierarchical convolutional deep neural networks to the operation of the ventral visual cortical stream (Yamins and DiCarlo, 2016; Rajalingham, Issa, Bashivan, Kar, Schmidt and DiCarlo, 2018) are evaluated in Section 2.9.4. Here the biological plausibility and advantages and disadvantages of this deep learning compared with brain computation are considered.

A first problem in terms of biological plausibility of deep networks trained by error backpropagation is that these are typically supervised systems, with a separate teacher for each output neuron informing it how each output neuron should be responding for a given input pattern at the bottom layer of the network (LeCun et al., 2015; Lillicrap et al., 2020). There is no architecture that looks remotely like this in the cerebral cortex, with a separate teacher for each neuron. The only part of the brain where there is what might be a teacher for each neuron is in the cerebellum, where there is a single climbing fibre for each Purkinje cell, and a network with no hidden layers (Chapter 17). Progress is being made in unsupervised training of deep convolutional neural networks (Zhuang, Yan, Nayebi, Schrimpf, Frank, DiCarlo and Yamins, 2021) using for example principles utilised in autoencoders in which higher layers aim to reconstruct the signals in the input layer and update the connections based on the differences (the errors) (Lillicrap et al., 2020), but these still implement convolution and deep learning using non-local learning rules including backpropagation of error to optimize representations, so are still biologically implausible.

But the problem is deeper than that there is no teacher for each output neuron (and the other problems that appear to make deep learning biologically implausible described below). A bigger problem for backpropagation of error networks is that someone has to know what the output should be, for every neuron, that is, backprop is a supervised learning system in that error correction is performed. The great beauty of the brain in contrast is that it is a largely self-organizing system, without a teacher telling each neuron what to do, as is made evident throughout this book, with a simple example of such a system a hierarchically organised set of competitive networks with convergence from stage to stage, as described in Chapter 2. Such self-organizing networks learn what categories to form based on the statistics of the inputs arriving from the world. They often use special adaptations to learn those statistics in a useful way, such as the trace short-term memory learning rule described in Chapter 2 that enables invariant representations to be learned because over short time periods it is likely to be the same object that is being viewed. And they may benefit from guidance (mild supervision) provided by top-down signals from higher layers, as described in Section B.4.5.

In essence, a deep network trained by backpropagation of error tries to achieve an optimal mapping between input patterns and output patterns of neural activity. The number of neurons in each deep layer must be carefully adjusted to ensure that the system does not become just a look-up table, yet has sufficient neurons to enable the mapping and generalization required, and the number of layers is often adjusted to be 100 or more to help to minimize overall errors. But a problem that arises is that what is being represented at each intermediate layer is very difficult to understand, and is likely to yield very little useful information to help understand the brain. There may be a lesson here, as follows:

At each stage of cortical processing, some output is always taken and directed to structures such as the striatum and basal ganglia for use in behavioral output. That is a key aspect of cortical design (Rolls, 2016b). It may reflect an interesting way in which the cortex evolves, by adding new areas each of which can produce useful output. That is not true of deep backprop networks.

An important point is that the brain does not solve a predetermined mapping problem from input to output, as in deep learning. Instead, the general architecture of the brain is specified by a relatively small number of genes that appear to specify what type of neuron connects to what other type to generate the architecture within and between cortical areas (Section B.20 and Chapter 19 of Rolls (2016b)). The brain then builds the details of its synaptic connectivities using self-organizing learning based on the environment in which it finds itself. This view has been developed by comparing the connectivity of different cortical areas, and then allowing genetic algorithms to select different combinations of the connectivity rules to build neural networks in computer simulations that can successfully solve different types of computational problem for which different architectures are needed (Rolls and Stringer, 2000; Rolls, 2016b) (Section B.20).

Another key feature of cortical design is that with its self-organizing principles rather than being taught what to compute, the cortex is able to solve complex problems with just a few layers, e.g. four, as described in Chapter 2 and by Rolls (2016b). The cortex is constrained to a few layers in the hierarchy, because each layer takes about 15 ms to compute including recurrent attractor operations, and the total compute time needs to be kept to less than 100 ms for biological utility. More layers could be tried in artificial self-organizing neural networks.

I hope that those interested in brain-inspired intelligence will look carefully at what the computational problems are that are solved by different parts of the brain, and will not only learn from our current understanding of how the brain performs its computations, but will also suggest new ways in which those computations may be performed. In this context, *Cerebral Cortex: Principles of Operation* (Rolls, 2016b) does set out principles of the organization of the brain many of which underlie its computational abilities and style.

There are other factors that make deep networks trained by backprop biologically implausible. Given that the signed error for a hidden neuron in an error backpropagation network is calculated by propagating backwards information based on the errors of all the output neurons to which a hidden neuron is connected, and all the relevant synaptic weights, and the activations of the output neurons to define the part of the activation function on which they are operating, it is implausible to suppose that the correct information to provide the appropriate signed error for each hidden neuron is propagated backwards between real neurons. A hidden neuron would have to 'know', or receive information about, the errors of all the neurons to which it is connected, and its synaptic weights to them, and their current activations (Section B.12). If there were more than one hidden layer, this would be even more difficult.

To expand on the difficulties: first, there would have to be a mechanism in the brain for providing an appropriate error signal to each output neuron in the network. With the possible exception of the cerebellum, an architecture where a separate error signal could be provided for each output neurons is difficult to identify in the brain. Second, as noted in Chapter 9 and by Rolls (2016b), the backprojection pathways that are present in the cortex seem suited to perform recall (Chapter 9) and to implement top-down attention (Sections 2.12 and B.8.4), and this might make it difficult for them also to have the correct strength to carry the correct error signal.

A problem with the backpropagation of error approach in a biological context is thus that in order to achieve their competence, backpropagation networks use what is almost certainly a learning rule that is much more powerful than those that could be implemented biologically, and achieve their excellent performance by performing the mapping though a minimal number of hidden neurons (Lillicrap, Santoro, Marris, Akerman and Hinton, 2020). In contrast, real neuronal networks in the brain probably use much less powerful learning rules, in which errors are not propagated backwards, and at the same time have very large numbers of hidden neurons, without the bottleneck that helps to provide backpropagation networks with their good performance. A consequence of these differences between backpropagation and biologically plausible networks may be that the way in which biological networks solve difficult problems may be rather different from the way in which backpropagation networks find mappings. Thus the solutions found by connectionist systems may not always be excellent guides to how biologically plausible networks may perform on similar problems. Part of the challenge for future work is to discover how more biologically plausible networks than backpropagation networks can solve comparably hard problems, and then to examine the properties of these networks, as a perhaps more accurate guide to brain computation (Lillicrap, Santoro, Marris, Akerman and Hinton, 2020).

As stated above, it is a major challenge for brain research to discover whether there are algorithms that will solve comparably difficult problems to backpropagation, but with a local learning rule (see also Lillicrap, Santoro, Marris, Akerman and Hinton (2020)). Such algorithms may be expected to require many more hidden neurons than backpropagation networks, in that the brain does not appear to use information bottlenecks to help it solve difficult problems. The issue here is that much of the power of backpropagation algorithms arises because there is a minimal number of hidden neurons to perform the required mapping using typically a final one-layer delta-rule network. Useful generalization arises in such networks because with a minimal number of hidden neurons, the net sets the representation they provide to enable appropriate generalization. The danger with more hidden neurons is that the network becomes a look-up table, with one hidden neuron for every required output, and generalization when the inputs vary becomes poor. The challenge is to find a more biologically plausible type of network that operates with large numbers of neurons, and yet that still provides useful generalization. An example of such an approach is described in Chapter 2 (Rolls, 2021d).

Another key difference between artificial deep learning approaches and real networks in humans and other primates is in the training. For deep learning with supervision, a very large number of exemplars, typically visual images, is presented each with a label to state its category. In contrast primates including humans experience a continuous world in which first one object is encountered for typically many seconds as it is held in the hand and viewed from different angles, or the individual moves round the world for example by crawling and sees the world gradually change as obstacles are moved round or bumped into or grasped. The latter type of real-world training allows temporal and spatial continuities about objects in the world to be learned, and that is the style of training used with VisNet (Chapter 2) in which continuities about visually transforming objects are used to help learn about the properties of objects and how they transform in the real world. With such different styles of training, it is likely to be difficult to use artificial deep learning networks trained by thousands of different labelled exemplars to understand how the real primate including human brain learns about the rules of perception, visual object recognition, etc. It is not clear what would be learned for example if a primate or human brain was trained only on thousands of labelled exemplars, rather than on the continuous input from the world in which the properties of objects and space can be learned as they continuously transform. It is not clear that whatever such an individual learned would be at all like what is learned and is present in a real brain trained in a real natural environment.

What is described here and elsewhere (Rolls, 2016b, 2021d,b) may it is hoped be useful for developing better artificial neural networks and artificial intelligence. For example, convolutional neural networks are typically trained on very large numbers of single training image exemplars (snapshots) of the classes to be learned, and can fail if a few pixels are altered, implying that they learn pixel-level representations. It is proposed that training such networks with different transforms of objects with statistics of how objects transform in short time periods in the real world as in trace rule learning (Chapter 2) would much better enable transform-invariant shape-based representations to be learned, leading to much more powerful performance.

Limitations of current understanding of deep learning networks and how different they are from the computations performed by the brain, and how difficult it would be to implement a backprop equivalent in the brain perhaps with autoencoders without raising many further difficulties, have been highlighted by others (Plebe and Grasso, 2019; Sejnowski, 2020; Lillicrap, Santoro, Marris, Akerman and Hinton, 2020; Bowers, Malhotra, Dujmovic, Montero, Tsvetkov, Biscione, Puebla, Adolfi, Hummel, Heaton, Evans, Mitchell and Blything, 2023). The mild guidance of competitive learning by cortico-cortical backprojections described in Section B.4.5 may provide a brain-feasible and at least biologically plausible approach.

19.5 Reinforcement Learning

Reinforcement learning is another approach to understanding the function of some brain areas that has its origin in the machine learning literature (Sutton and Barto, 1998). Reinforcement learning is described in Section B.17, and evidence that the dopamine neurons encode a reward prediction error signal is described in Section 16.4.3 (Schultz, 2013, 2016c,b, 2017, 2019). Some evaluation about how it fits in with brain design follows.

Reinforcement learning utilizes a single reward or reinforcement signal to train a whole network. This is in contrast with backpropagation of error networks, which typically specify what the output should be of every output neuron for a given input pattern, which is a much more information-rich training signal. Reinforcement learning is thus in a sense simpler in terms of evolutionary design, because the single training signal can be broadcast widely in the neural network, without having to tell individual neurons how to respond, which is biologically implausible.

Reinforcement learning uses a widely broadcast reward prediction error signal to systems in the brain such as the basal ganglia. If there has been very recent neuronal activity at synapses that reflect coactivity of for example stimulus encoding and response encoding neurons, then those synaptic connections are strengthened if the dopamine input is high (see Chapter 16). In this way, stimulus-response habits may be set up in the basal ganglia. A property is that the reward is not part of what is learned, just the stimulus-response connection. So if the reward is devalued, the stimulus-response connection is still there, and the response is elicited when the stimulus occurs, even though the stimulus is no longer a goal for action. A further property is that the dopamine neurons seem to convey just a reward prediction error signal, and do not specify the type of reward, such as food, water, novelty, money etc. So lots of habits may be set up without the goal for which the habit may have been set up specified in the stimulus-response habit.

This is very different from the type of learning implemented in the orbitofrontal cortex to anterior cingulate cortex learning system to perform actions to obtain goals (with the goals the rewards specified by the orbitofrontal cortex) (Rolls, 2019c) (Chapter 12). Here there is a potentially very precise specification of the outcome, and different actions can be learned to obtain different goals, even if the actions are very similar, but the outcomes are different. That is, a precise association is learned between a particular action and a particular outcome. To put it another way: the orbitofrontal cortex provides the anterior cingulate cortex with a high-dimensional reward signal with each type of reward specified as being different to other rewards, and this makes for a much more efficient learning system to enable any of a wide range of actions to be associated rapidly with any of a wide range of reward (see Section 12.2.2). Because the cingulate cortex initiates actions to obtain the goals or rewards specified by the orbitofrontal cortex (Rolls, 2019c), if the reward/goal stimulus is devalued, actions will not be performed. Moreover, the stimulus value can be reset in the orbitofrontal cortex by for example relearning or reversal of a stimulus-reward association, and that learning can be on one trial, again allowing great flexibility of action-outcome learning as implemented in the orbitofrontal cortex / anterior cingulate cortex system (Chapter 12 and Rolls (2019c)).

In comparison, with reinforcement learning and its very general reward prediction error signal, the learning tends to be slow, so that regular associations between a stimulus and a response can be evaluated, and stamped in by the dopamine modulator. If the system is not slow, then the reinforcement learning system risks setting up incorrect stimulus-response associations, because of chance stimulus and response co-occurrence, or because of noise-related effects in the brain.

The orbitofrontal cortex reward evaluation system, followed by an action-outcome system (Rolls, 2019c), thus appears to be a much more powerful learning system than reinforcement learning using a general reward prediction error signal. The reinforcement learning in which the basal ganglia and dopamine system are implicated (Schultz (2016c) and Chapter 16) may have been appropriate at early stages of evolution as it does not require a memory of the response that has just been made apart from a simple eligibility signal for synapses that have recently been active. The striatum and globus pallidus do not implement a short-term memory that could be used for a longer term 'eligibility trace', because the basal ganglia have no recurrent collateral connections to support a short-term memory (Chapter 16). On the other hand, the cingulate cortex as it is neocortex has a highly developed set of recurrent collaterals, and may therefore be much better suited to learning, when the actions may be followed by a delay before the outcome (reward) arrives, and where the results of the previous few choices can be accumulated (Chapter 12 and Rolls (2019c)).

A comparison of the computations involved in reversal learning helps to show why reinforcement learning as implemented in the basal ganglia using dopamine for stimulus–response habit learning is much less efficient than the orbitofrontal cortex – cingulate cortex action–outcome learning system. The learning considered is a visual discrimination task in which a choice of one visual stimulus leads to reward, and of the other to punishment / loss. When this occurs for the dopamine system, the reward prediction errors change, but new stimulus-response connections need to be learned. This may even mean a return to trial and error learning, where many different responses may be tried until a response is found that when following the stimulus leads to a positive reward prediction error. This then takes some time to train the system, for the reasons given above. In contrast, for the orbitofrontal cortex – cingulate cortex action–outcome system, when the reward association of the visual stimuli reverses, on the very next trial after an error, the orbitofrontal cortex expected value representations reverse. Accordingly, the next time a visual stimulus is shown, the correct expected value is sent to the cingulate cortex, which then performs the same action that it has already learned for that expected value input received from the orbitofrontal cortex. (This is described in Chapter 11.) So part of the power of the orbitofrontal cortex – cingulate cortex system is that it is a two stage learning process, and the visual stimulus to reward association process, a stimulus–stimulus learning process implemented in the orbitofrontal cortex, can reverse in one trial, with no new action learning needed.

Additionally, as described above, the cingulate cortex is likely to be able to remember actions for longer times until the outcome becomes known when new actions need to be learned to obtain rewards; and can match actions to particular outcomes (such as food, water, money etc), whereas the reinforcement learning system uses just a single general reward prediction error. It also seems likely that the cingulate cortex has a repertoire of previously learned actions, which can rapidly be associated with new different outcomes by rapid associative learning between actions and outcomes (Rolls, 2019c).

For these reasons, I argue that the orbitofrontal cortex – cingulate cortex action–outcome learning system is a much more powerful way that the brain uses to deal with reward-related learning than the reinforcement learning stimulus-response dopamine reward prediction error habit system. Consistent with this, it is damage to the orbitofrontal cortex that has a great influence on our emotional and reward-related behavior and their disorders including depression, as described in Chapter 11 and elsewhere (Rolls, 2018a, 2019e), whereas the effects of damage to the dopamine system produce major motor problems including Parkinson's disease. In this context, we should remember that stimulus-response learning is a simple type of motor learning.

I have also argued that reward prediction error neurons do not themselves relate to emotion, because emotions can still occur to rewarding or punishing stimuli even when there is no new learning and no reward prediction error (Rolls, 2018a, 2019e) (Chapter 11). That is, emotions are states elicited by rewards or punishers, not by reward prediction errors (Rolls, 2014a, 2018a, 2019e) (Chapter 11).

I thus argue that reinforcement learning in the brain involving dopamine neurons, despite great interest in it (Schultz, 2013, 2016c,b, 2017; O'Doherty et al., 2017), is a rather specialized brain system, and that other processes, described in Chapters 11 and 12 are involved in much reward and goal-related behavior, and in emotion.

The reinforcement learning algorithm can be applied in deep networks (Botvinick et al., 2019), that is, in a network with one or more hidden layers (see Appendix B). Indeed, artificial neural networks of this type have become popular in Artificial Intelligence, and can perform well in Atari video games, Go, and Capture the Flag (Botvinick et al., 2019). However, such systems do require a great deal of training, so produce slow learning. Variations have been tried, such as incorporation of a type of episodic memory about rewards received in previous similar situations, and that can speed up the learning (Botvinick et al., 2019). However, if reinforcement learning in the brain is used mainly in the basal ganglia, then the type of problem to which it is applied is at least usually rather simple, stimulus-response habit learning (see Chapter 16). On the other hand, use of a hippocampal episodic memory system to remember the outcome when a previous situation occurred might be a solution that could be used that would not require reinforcement learning.

19.6 Levels of explanation, and the mind-brain problem

19.6.1 A levels of explanation theory of causality, and the relation between the mind and the brain

We can now understand brain processing from the level of ion channels in neurons, through neuronal biophysics, to neuronal firing, through the computations performed by populations of neurons, and how their activity is reflected by functional neuroimaging, to behavioral and cognitive effects (Rolls, 2016b; Rolls and Deco, 2010; Rolls, 2014a, 2021b). Activity at any one level can be used to understand activity at the next. This raises the philosophical issue of how we should consider causality with these different levels (Rolls, 2020a, 2012e, 2021g,e). Does the brain cause effects in the mind, or do events at the mind level cause brain activity?

What is the relation between the mind and the brain? This is the mind–brain or mind–body problem. Do mental, mind, events cause brain events? Do brain events cause mental effects? What can we learn from the relation between software and hardware in a computer about mind–brain interactions and how causality operates? Neuroscience shows that there is a close relation between mind and matter (captured by the following inverted saying: 'Never matter, no mind').

My view (Rolls, 2016b, 2020a, 2021g,e) is that the relationship between mental events and neurophysiological events is similar to the relationship between the program running in a computer and the hardware of the computer. Does the program (the software loaded onto the computer usually written in a high-level language such as C or Matlab) 'cause' the logic gates (TTL, transistor-transistor logic) of the hardware to move to the next state? And does this hardware state change 'cause' the program to move to its next step or state?

I propose that one way to think about this is that when we are looking at different levels of what is overall the operation of a system, causality can usefully be understood as operating within levels (causing one step of the program to move to the next; or the neurons to move from one state to another), but not between levels (e.g. software to hardware and vice versa). That is, if the events at the different levels of explanation are occurring simultaneously, without a time delay, then my view is that we should not think of causality as operating between levels, but just that what happens at a higher level may be an emergent property of what happens at a lower level. This is the solution I propose to this aspect of the mind-brain problem (Rolls, 2020a, 2021g,e).

Following this thinking, when one step of a process at one level of explanation moves to the next step in time, we can speak of causality that would meet the criteria for Granger causality where one time series, including the time series being considered, can be used to predict the next step in time (Section 13.4) (Granger, 1969; Ge, Feng, Grabenhorst and Rolls, 2012; Bressler and Seth, 2011). In contrast, when we consider the relationship between processes described at different levels of explanation, such as the relation between a step in the hardware in a computer and a step in the software, then these processes may occur simultaneously, and be inextricably linked with each other, and just be different ways of describing the same process, so that temporal (Granger) causality does not apply to this relation between levels, but only within levels. The whole processing can now be specified from the mechanistic level of neuronal firings, etc. up through the computational level to the cognitive and behavioral level.

In the neuroscience-based approach that I propose for the relation between the mind and the brain, the proposal is that events at the sub-neuronal, neuronal, and neuronal network levels take place simultaneously to perform a computation that can be described at a high level as a mental state, with content about the world (Rolls, 2021g). It is argued that as the processes at the different levels of explanation take place at the same time, they are linked by a non-causal relationship: causality can best be described in brains as operating within but not between levels. This mind-brain theory allows mental events to be different in kind from the mechanistic events that underlie them; but does not lead one to argue that mental events cause brain events, or vice versa: they are different levels of explanation of the operation of the computational system (Rolls, 2021g).

The proposal has been developed further (Rolls, 2021e), and it is proposed that causality, at least as it applies to the brain, should satisfy three conditions. First, interventionist tests for causality (Kim, 2011; Woodward, 2015, 2005, 2021b,a, 2020; Craver and Bechtel, 2007) must be satisfied. If one intervenes to remove a potential cause, and the putative effect no longer occurs, then that makes it more likely that the potential cause does cause the putative effect. More formally, where X and Y are variables, X causes Y *iff* there are some possible interventions that would change the value of X and if such intervention were to occur, a regular change in the value of Y would occur (Woodward, 2021b, 2020). Second, the causally related events should be at the same level of explanation. The bases of the argument include the point that the processes that occur at the different levels can occur simultaneously (for example the mental and brain event, or the mathematical or logic operation performed by a computer and the current flow within its arithmetic logic unit), whereas causal processes can be understood to involve sequences of events in time with the operations performed within a level (Rolls, 2021g,e). Third, a temporal order condition must be satisfied, with a suitable time scale in the order of 10 ms for brain processing (to exclude application to quantum physics; and a cause cannot follow an effect) (Rolls, 2021e). Next, although it may be useful for different purposes to describe causality involving the mind and brain at the mental level, or at the brain level, it is argued that the brain level may sometimes be more accurate, for sometimes causal accounts at the mental level may arise from confabulation by the mentalee, whereas understanding exactly what computations have occurred in the brain that result in a choice or action will provide the correct causal account for why a choice or action was made (Rolls, 2021e) (see Section 11.3.9).

19.6.2 Downward or Upward Causality?

In addition, it is argued that possible cases of 'downward causation' (or 'upward causation') can be accounted for by a within-levels-of-explanation account of causality (Rolls, 2021e). One example might be that excessive synaptic pruning or reductions in synaptic transmission produced by lower NMDA receptor efficacy may causally contribute to some of the cognitive and behavioral symptoms of schizophrenia (Rolls, 2021a). As these changes in synaptic transmission relate to the symptoms (which involve the whole person), should this be considered as a case of across-level causation (Woodward, 2021b,a)? (In this case, it would be upward causation, from synapses to cognitive symptoms.) In the present case, my account is that reduced synaptic transmission (caused for example by high synaptic pruning or reduced NMDA receptor conductances) reduces the firing rates of populations of neurons, which destabilizes the attractor neuronal networks in the prefrontal cortex (Rolls, 2021a,b). Now these prefrontal cortex attractor networks are involved in maintaining items in short-term memory, and in holding on-line in short-term memory the top-down bias required to bias processing in some parts of the brain thus providing a mechanism for top-down attention (Rolls, 2021b; Deco and Rolls, 2005b,a; Luo et al., 2013). The computational level of events in the brain thus provides a causal, computational, account of how these synaptic events alter behavior so that attention and short-term memory change. But the causal level is within-level in this approach, at the level of synapses, transmitters, receptors, and neuronal networks; and the behavioral changes occur at the same time, but are descriptions at a higher level of explanation. In such systems we can describe necessary relations between levels, or superveniences between levels of operation of the system, but the mechanistic, causal, computational account is best dealt with in this case at the brain level of explanation.

Another possible case considered as 'downward causation' in physics is when a higher level Law 'causes' an effect at a lower level (Ellis, 2020). Let us take as an example the interaction between neurons in a population that falls into a low energy attractor basin (Hopfield, 1982; Amit, 1989; Amit et al., 1985). This happens to be a system that is highly relevant to understanding the operation of the cerebral cortex, as the most characteristic attribute of cerebral cortex is the highly developed excitatory recurrent collateral local connections between pyramidal cells that enable local attractor networks to be implemented for short-term memory, long-term memory, top-down attention, decision-making, etc. (Rolls, 2016b, 2021b). The interaction between the neurons (equivalent to spins in a physics model) can be analyzed at the population level (but not at the single neuron level) to show how the whole network can fall into an attractor state, and to specify the number of possible attractor states, for example the maximum number of different memory patterns, that can be stored and correctly retrieved.

One concept of causality that has been advanced for systems with different levels is that because a Law can be specified for a system such as the number of stable memory states and hence memory capacity at a high level (the population of neurons level), then that Law or rule of operation formulated at the high level provides 'downward causation' to the lower level (Ellis, 2020), to in this case result in the number of stable attractor basins being limited to what is shown by mathematical analysis using the methods of theoretical physics to be possible (Hopfield, 1982; Amit, 1989; Amit et al., 1985; Treves, 1991b; Treves and Rolls, 1991).

But that is not how I see the system as operating in terms of causality. The individual neurons at the lower level do not wait for a top-down signal from the population level to tell them what to do next. Instead, it just is a property of the whole system that the individual neurons at the lower level operate as neurons each with a certain number of connections to the other neurons, and the result of the lower level interactions between the neurons is that only a certain number of stable states can be stored and correctly retrieved. To elucidate further, when we simulate such an attractor network in a computer, we set up for example neurons with threshold linear activation functions, and modify the synaptic connections between the neurons to store the memory patterns, and then we let the system run (Rolls, 2012b, 2021b). We find that as we increase the number of memory patterns stored in the system, at some point, the critical capacity, the recalled memories become very poor, and the system no longer works as a memory system (Rolls, 2012b). But we do not include in the program that we write that the neuron-level implementation should check up to some higher level to find out if the number of patterns specified by the Law specifying the critical capacity has been exceeded, and if so to fall into a random neuronal firing (or spin) state. Nor is there a high-level part of the program that knows about the equations that specify the capacity and checks if the number of memories to be stored is too high for the critical capacity, and if so causes the lower level to fall into a random spin state (i.e. a random set of neurons firing). So the operation of the system is implemented only at the lower level, and that is where causality acts, by the firing of individual neurons influencing other neurons through the modified synaptic weights. Now of course the operation of the system in terms of its storage capacity can be explained, and analyzed, at the higher level, where the interactions between the whole population of neurons can be understood, and specified as rules or Laws of the operation of the system. But that does not mean that the higher level rules or Laws that describe the operation of the whole system have to act down to the lower level to cause effects there at the low level, whether synchronously, or after a time delay. Thus I reject the concept (Ellis, 2020), at least in relation to the operation of the brain, that Laws that apply at a high level act by 'downward causation' to control the operation of the system at a lower level. The high level Laws just express some properties of the system.

Thus my view of the mind–brain issue is that we are considering the process as a mechanism with different levels of explanation. As described above, we can now understand brain processing from the level of ion channels in neurons, through neuronal biophysics, to neuronal firing, through the computations performed by populations of neurons, to behavioral and cognitive effects, and even perhaps to the phenomenal (feeling) aspects of consciousness (Rolls, 2020a, 2016b). The whole processing is now specified from the mechanistic level of neuronal firings, etc. up through the computational level to the cognitive and behavioral level.

Sometimes the cognitive effects seem remarkable, for example the recall of a whole memory from a part of it, and we describe this as an 'emergent property', but once understood from the mechanistic level upwards, the functions implemented are elegant and wonderful, but understandable and not magical or poorly understood (Rolls, 2016b, 2012e, 2021g,e).

This computational neuroscience levels of explanation approach to causality provides an opportunity to proceed beyond Cartesian dualism (Descartes, 1644) and physical reductionism (Carruthers, 2019) in considering the relations between the mind and the brain. What I propose (Rolls, 2021g,e) is that a necessary relation between the different levels of explanation needs to be established, and that can be done using interventionist tests (Kim, 2011; Woodward, 2015, 2005, 2021b,a, 2020; Craver and Bechtel, 2007) as described above (Section 19.6.1). But because the transitions at the different levels take place simultaneously, we should not think of different levels as causing effects in each other, for the reasons described earlier in this subsection 19.6.2. Instead, we should think of causality as operating within each level, and identifiable by time delays in the causal chain of events within each level of explanation and analysis. In this analysis, time delays (post hoc, ergo propter hoc, 'after that, therefore because of that') are an important property of causality (at the macro not subatomic level). So there is a necessary relation between some brain and mental events, but the relation should be thought of as necessary (when established), but not causal.

The point I make is that however one thinks about causality in such a mechanistic system with interesting 'emergent' computational properties, the system is now well-defined, is no longer mysterious or magical, and we have now from a combination of neuroscience and analyses of the type used in theoretical physics a clear understanding of the properties of neural systems and how cognition emerges from neural mechanisms. There are of course particular problems that remain to be resolved with this approach, such as that of how language is implemented in the brain, but my point is that this mechanistic approach, supported by parsimony, appears to be capable of leading us to a full understanding of brain function, cognition, and behavior. However, the property of phenomenal consciousness is a big step for an 'emergent property', and that hard problem is therefore considered elsewhere (Rolls, 2020a, 2012e, 2021g,e, 2016b, 2004b). A summary follows.

19.6.3 Consciousness - a Higher Order Syntactic Thought theory

The global workspace hypothesis of consciousness holds that many different brain systems need to interact to account for consciousness (Dehaene, 2014; Dehaene et al., 2017; van Vugt et al., 2018; Lau, 2022). However, there are problems with this approach, for example about exactly how global the workspace needs to be for consciousness to suddenly be present (Rolls, 2020a; Lau, 2022). Humans can perform many complex tasks, including apparently driving a car for a short period, without being able to report about the driving if they were thinking about something else, which they can report about. Yet driving a car might be thought to require a rather large workspace. Problems are also raised (Rolls, 2020a) with a version that excludes conceptual (categorical or discrete) representations, and in which phenomenal consciousness can be reduced to physical processes (Carruthers, 2019).

Instead a different levels of explanation approach to the relation between the brain and the mind has been advocated (Rolls, 2020a; Rolls et al., 2022b; Rolls and Deco, 2015a). Further, a different theory of phenomenal consciousness is described, in which there is a particular computational system involved in which Higher Order Syntactic Thoughts (HOSTs) are used to perform credit assignment on first order thoughts of multiple step plans to correct them by manipulating symbols in a syntactic type of working memory (Rolls, 2020a). This provides a good evolutionary reason for the evolution of this kind of computational module, with which, it is proposed, phenomenal consciousness is associated (Rolls, 2020a).

Some advantages of this HOST approach to phenomenal consciousness compared to other Higher Order Thought (HOT) theories (Rosenthal, 2012; Lau and Rosenthal, 2011) have been described (Rolls, 2020a). For example, a multi-step thought or planning system has a potential credit assignment problem (which step in the multistep process caused the process to fail), and the incorrect step needs to be identified, for which a natural method is to think about the plan, and work out which step may have produced the error (Rolls, 2020a). It is hypothesized that the HOST system which requires the ability to manipulate first (or lower) order symbols in working memory might utilize parts of the prefrontal cortex implicated in working memory, and especially the left inferior frontal gyrus, which is involved in language and probably syntactical processing (Rolls, 2020a; Rolls et al., 2022b; Rolls and Deco, 2015a). Overall, the approach advocated is to identify the computations that are linked to consciousness, and to analyze the neural bases of those computations (Rolls, 2020a).

This Higher Order Syntactic Thought theory of consciousness (Rolls, 2020a) differs from that of Lau (2022), who proposes that consciousness involves a higher order monitoring of perceptual reality that could be used to correct problems such an an incorrect threshold for perceptual input. However, that type of problem could include a signal-to-noise ratio problem, which need have nothing to do with consciousness. A simple algorithm can separate neural noise (Lau's source of interference) from a signal. And it is not clear how a Higher Order Thought could correct the engineering issue of a signal to noise ratio problem by adjusting the threshold by just thinking about it. But if the theory (Lau, 2022) is that one needs to reason about the sensory (or any other processing) to see whether it needs to be corrected, then it becomes a theory very much like my HOST theory of consciousness (Rolls, 2020a), except that I argue that the monitoring that is needed and that would be computationally useful is that of thoughts, in which a credit assignment problem could arise, and which could be corrected by a higher order syntactic thought about a lower order syntactic thought, and this would be very useful for any multistep planning (Rolls, 2020a).

I then argue that it is plausible to think that a system that was performing this type of computation, thinking about its own thoughts, with the lower order thoughts grounded in the world, would feel conscious. That is of course a plausibility argument, but a plausible one (Rolls, 2020a, 1997b,a, 2004b, 2007a,b, 2008a, 2010c, 2011b, 2014a). And the HOST theory is testable, for example by intervening by temporary inactivation of this type of computation in the brain, to test whether consciousness is affected by this intervention.

19.6.4 Levels of explanation, and levels of investigation

It will be evident from the approach taken in this book that to understand how the brain works, we need to understand what is computed in each brain area, as well as how it is computed. It should be evident that the level at which information is exchanged between the computing elements of the brain is the firing of single neurons, with the evidence set out by Rolls (2016b) and elsewhere (Rolls, 2021g,e).

It is important to investigate this at the level of single neurons, and populations of single neurons, because neurons often have relatively independent responses as is made clear in Appendix C, so that it is only possible to know what is represented in a brain area by utilising evidence from neuronal firing.

Operating at a higher level, such as the signals measured in functional neuroimaging that reflect the activity of thousands of neurons, does not lend itself well to making computational models of how the brain works, because one does not know exactly what is represented at each successive stage. Thus methods such as fMRI may be useful for obtaining some evidence on the functions of different brain areas, but do need to be complemented where possible by evidence on the firing of neurons (which of course is often not possible in humans).

The architecture of the cerebral cortex is also considerably localised, with among the evolutionary reasons that this design minimises the connection length between neurons, and also the genetic information needed to specify cortical design, as set out in *Cerebral Cortex* (Rolls, 2016b). Those are among the reasons why there are hierarchically organised networks in the brain, with the major connections between adjacent cortical areas in the hierarchy. The level of granularity here corresponds to for example V1, V2, V4, posterior inferior temporal cortex, and anterior inferior temporal cortex, with frequently cytoarchitectural differences between such areas leading to classifications at about the level of Brodmann areas. There is also a finer level of granularity, specified by the radial extents of cortical pyramidal cell dendrites and their axons, which have a high density with a radius of 2–3 mm, and provide a basis for local cortical attractor networks (Rolls, 2016b).

The level of analysis just described, in which the different computational roles of each brain area are addressed using methods such as comparing neuronal activity in different stages of the processing, and double dissociation of the effects of brain lesions or inactivation of neuronal populations, sits uncomfortably with brain networks identified with some neuroimaging approaches in which correlations between the BOLD signals of many brain areas are found, leading to identification of a few brain networks (Ryali, Supekar, Chen, Kochalka, Cai, Nicholas, Padmanabhan and Menon, 2016). If these reflect just descriptions of correlations, that is one thing, but when simple functions are attributed to such networks, then that may be an oversimplification (or indeed misdiagnosis) of exactly what is computed in each brain region, which is the different approach taken here.

For example, these large-scale networks identifiable with neuroimaging correlation-based measures have been described as follows: "The Saliency Network (SN) (Menon and Uddin, 2010) is a limbic-paralimbic network anchored in the anterior insula and dorsal anterior cingulate cortex with prominent subcortical nodes in affective and reward processing regions including the amygdala and ventral striatum. The Saliency Network plays an important role in orienting attention to behaviorally and emotionally salient and rewarding stimuli and facilitating goal-directed behavior. The fronto-parietal Central Executive Network (CEN) is anchored in the dorsolateral prefrontal cortex and supramarginal gyrus and is critical for actively maintaining and manipulating information in working memory. The Default Mode Network (DMN) is anchored in the posterior cingulate cortex, medial prefrontal cortex, medial temporal lobe, and angular gyrus and is involved in self-referential mental activity and autobiographical memory" (Ryali, Supekar, Chen, Kochalka, Cai, Nicholas, Padmanabhan and Menon, 2016).

To take the Saliency Network (Menon and Uddin, 2010) as an example, it is clear that the dorsal anterior insula is the primary taste cortex, and that there is an area ventral to it that is probably visceral/autonomic cortex (Rolls, 2016c; Critchley and Harrison, 2013; Hassanpour et al., 2018), and is shown in the ventral parts of the anterior insula in Fig. 2 of Baylis, Rolls and Baylis (1995). The autonomic cortex during salient and emotional events is likely to produce autonomic output (alterations of heart rate and variability, sweating, and skin conductance), and far from 'altering attention to behaviorally and emotionally salient and reward stimuli' (Menon and Uddin, 2010), it is likely to receive outputs about such stimuli from the orbitofrontal cortex, which has strong connections to it, so that the anterior insular cortex provides a pathway to autonomic output (Rolls, 2016c, 2019e). The taste insula of primates is not involved in taste reward according to the experimental evidence (Rolls, 2016c, 2019e) (Chapter 4). And much of the rest of the insula is involved in somatosensory processing (Chapter 6). And the anterior cingulate cortex receives reward and punishment information from the orbitofrontal cortex, and uses this reward outcome information for action-outcome learning (Rolls, 2019c) (Chapter 12).

So it appears that a lot is lost if simple functions are ascribed to these large-scale human cortical networks such as the saliency network, and such concepts may not have much explanatory value. Instead the goal that I advocate is to identify what computations are performed by each cortical area. Each area will of course transmit information to other specialised cortical areas. And together in their complementary ways they will produce a particular computation of a brain system. The brain regions to which I refer might previously have been defined as for example Brodmann areas based on cytoarchitecture (Section 1.11). But now the Human Connectome Project has moved the enterprise forward, by delineating 360 cortical regions each defined by multiple, multimodal, methods including anatomy, functional connectivity, and task-related activations (Glasser, Coalson, Robinson, Hacker, Harwell, Yacoub, Ugurbil, Andersson, Beckmann, Jenkinson, Smith and Van Essen, 2016a) (Section 1.12), and this now provides a useful current approach to defining cortical regions each of which may have different computational functions. 66 subcortical regions have been added in an extended version of this atlas (Huang, Rolls, Feng and Lin, 2022).

19.7 Biologically plausible computation in the brain: a grand unifying theory?

In an interesting and perceptive review in the journal *Brain* of *Brain Computations: What and How* (Rolls, 2021b), Manohar (2022) raised the question of whether the book provides 'a grand unifying theory' of brain function with the computational neuroscience approach taken in that book. My response to that is that the approach taken in *Brain Computations: What and How* and in the present book *Brain Computations and Connectivity* is indeed aiming to provide exactly that, a comprehensive theory of the operation of the brain, and is pioneering in that it forges and provides the foundation of a biologically plausible computational approach to brain function.

The approach taken is a biologically plausible approach to how the brain computes, rather than invoking the artificial intelligence approach of deep learning to try to account for brain computation. The approach to how the brain computes in this book is biologically plausible in that it utilises only local synaptic modification rules to set up the synaptic connections between neurons, and primarily unsupervised learning, yet considers how far this can take us in understanding how the brain operates. This approach is quite different to the deep learning approach used now in much machine learning and AI, which typically backpropagates an error back down through the network to correct every synaptic weight in all preceding layers of the network (LeCun et al., 2015; Lillicrap et al., 2020), but that is not easily consistent with cortical connectivity and function, as described in Section 19.4. Moreover, the learning in the brain is largely unsupervised, whereas deep learning approaches typically require a supervisor for each output neuron, which in turn requires what must be computed for each output neuron to be specified by the designer of the deep network. The point is developed (in Section 19.4) that machine learning might benefit from understanding some of the unsupervised approaches used by the brain to solve complex problems, including navigation, attention, semantics, and even syntax. The title of this book, *Brain Computations and Connectivity*, refers to the concept that the actual connectivity at the local level of neurons and synapses that is found in the brain, and between brain regions, is important in understanding what and how the brain computes.

In this book, much new evidence has been provided that is important to this biologically plausible computational neuroscience approach in that the connectivity studies of the 360 cortical areas defined in the Human Connectome Project Multimodal Parcellation atlas (HCP-MMP) (Glasser et al., 2016a; Huang et al., 2022) that are described in this book (Huang et al., 2021; Ma et al., 2022a; Rolls et al., 2022a, 2023c,i,d, 2022b, 2023e,h,f,b,a) provide a framework to help understand better what computation is being performed in each of these brain regions, and how the results of that computation are fed primarily to a limited set of further cortical regions to which strong effective connectivity is directed. This book therefore helps to bring the computational neuroscience approach developed in *Cerebral Cortex: Principles of Operation* (Rolls, 2016b) and *Brain Computations: What and How* (Rolls, 2021b) to relate much more closely to the different cortical regions of the human brain, which is a key step in the biologically plausible approach to understanding brain computation developed in this book.

We can then ask whether the biologically plausible networks described in these books (Rolls, 2016b, 2021b, 2023a) are sufficient to account for brain computation.

A pattern association network (Section B.2) is excellent for recalling a stimulus or event with which a stimulus has been associated. A simple example is an association between a previously neutral visual stimulus, such as the sight of an object, with the taste of a food reward, to produce an expected reward value representation, that can be used to guide goal-directed actions to obtain the taste reward outcome. This type of learning is key in emotional learning (Chapter 11). This type of pattern association is also fundamental to how the backprojection pathways from the hippocampus to the neocortex in the brain are used to recall episodic memories to the neocortex (Section 9.3.8), and also to how backprojection pathways are used to implement top-down attention (Section 2.12).

An autoassociation network (Section B.3) performs *the* key type of cortical computation, and is implemented by the highly developed excitatory local recurrent collateral connections between nearby pyramidal cells in the neocortex (Section 1.14.5), or throughout the CA3 neurons of the hippocampus (Chapter 9). One key computational property is that the self-re-excitation of any one of many different sets of neurons with strong connections between them can maintain the firing of that set of neurons to implement short-term memory, and to provide a foundation for working memory and planning (Chapter 13). But this computational ability is useful not only for what we might think of as short-term memory functions, but for many other functions. An important example in sensory cortices is to maintain activity for sufficiently long, in the order of one to several seconds, for the statistics of the world to be able to guide the learning of representations that are useful because they capture the properties of stimuli that all can be produced by the same object or stimulus. A key example is the trace learning rule in VisNet to help learn invariant representations (Section 2.8). A key computational property that is provided here is that this is relatively unsupervised learning: there is no teacher for each output neuron, and no need to prespecify what categories should be formed, which is a limitation of brain computation that is used in typical supervised deep learning artificial neural networks. The point here is that the cortical recurrent collaterals can help to maintain neuronal activity in a population of neurons for sufficiently long to enable invariant representations to be formed based on the statistics of the input from the world. The same principle is useful in coordinate transforms learned by gain modulation (Section 3.5), and in the learning of global motion in the dorsal visual system (Section 3.3).

Another key property of autoassociation networks is that the whole of the representation, for example a whole memory, can be retrieved from any one part. This is key in the mechanisms of episodic memory (Chapter 9). It is emphasised that this is not a property of a pattern association network.

A key feature of pattern association and autoassociation networks in the brain is that they have a high capacity, which is in the order of the number of associatively modifiable synapses on any one neuron in a network with sparse representations (Sections B.2 and B.3). A typical

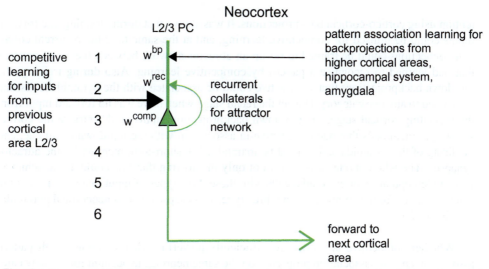

Fig. 19.1 The neocortical model that combines competitive learning using the forward inputs from the preceding cortical region, with associatively modifiable recurrent collateral synapses to form an autoassociation attractor network to maintain neuronal firing for short periods, and with pattern association learning to implement recall or top-down attention using cortico-cortical backprojections. L2/3 PC is a layer 2/3 pyramidal cell. The thick line above the pyramidal cell body is the dendrite, receiving inputs from the previous cortical area and operating by competitive learning using the synapses w^{comp}; from the recurrent collaterals that operate as an attractor network using synapses w^{rec}; and back-projections from higher cortical areas for memory recall and top-down attention that operate by pattern association learning using the synapses w^{bp}. 1-6 : the layers of the neocortex. (Reprinted from Rolls (2021) The connections of neocortical pyramidal cells can implement the learning of new categories, attractor memory, and top-down recall and attention. Brain Structure and Function 226: 2523-2536. © Springer.)

cortical neuron might have approximately 10,000 associatively modifiable synapses, so the storage capacity of a single local neocortical network which might be approximately 1–2 mm in diameter (and containing 100,000 neurons given the diluted connectivity that is a feature of the cortex) could store in the order of 10,000 memories, which is the size of a person's typical working vocabulary. (And that may not be just a co-incidence.)

However a key property of the neocortex is that it learns new representations: it can categorise incoming stimuli for example as one type of object, or another. The key type of biologically plausible network for this type of learning is a competitive network (Section B.4). It can usefully allocate inputs that regularly occur together to form a category defined by their combination or conjunction. Competitive networks with sparse representations can learn to categorise inputs with a fairly high capacity. Moreover, competitive networks implement a type of unsupervised learning.

A very important property of competitive networks is that they can be combined with other synapses on the same neurons that implement short-term memory using attractor dynamics, and with another set of synaptic inputs that learn by pattern association to initiate memory recall later, or to implement top-down attention. This has been tested computationally: all three types of computation can be performed using these three types of computation by populations of such single neurons, and this is proposed to be *the* key feature of the design of the neocortex (Rolls, 2021c).

The architecture that was simulated to prove the operation of this computational combination is shown in Fig. 19.1 (Rolls, 2021c), and is a part of the neocortical architecture illustrated in Fig. 1.17. The computational model combines competitive learning using the forward inputs from the preceding cortical region, with associatively modifiable recurrent collateral synapses to form an autoassociation attractor network to maintain neuronal firing for short periods, and with pattern association learning to implement recall or top-down attention using cortico-cortical backprojections. It was shown that during training, the forward inputs could be utilised for competitive learning, and at the same time the recurrent collateral connections could be trained to set up an attractor network between the set of neurons that had learned to recognise a pattern by competitive learning. Also during training, the top-down backprojections that were active could be associated with the pyramidal cells that responded to any one category. During the recall stage when there was no forward input from the preceding cortical stage, the top-down backprojection inputs could retrieve the correct set of pyramidal cells that had been active in association with the top-down recall cue, and the firing of the pyramidal cells could be maintained in short-term memory by the attractor synapses. The whole model was useful not only in showing that this could all be achieved in a single population of pyramidal cells with these three types of input, but also in showing suitable ranges for the strengths of the three types of synapse on each neocortical pyramidal cell (Rolls, 2021c).

Whether competitive networks are sufficiently powerful, when combined with pattern association and autoassociation properties on the same neurons, to account for the new categories that can be learned, typically in hierarchical networks, remains to be investigated. This is a key frontier for future research: if competitive networks, constructed with the addition of pattern and autoassociators in the neocortex, are not sufficiently powerful to account for the learning of new categories and the formation of semantic networks, then what alternatives are there? Potts attractor networks, which are combinations of attractor networks, may have high storage capacity (Song, Yao and Treves, 2014; Boboeva, Brasselet and Treves, 2018; Ryom, Stendardi, Ciaramelli and Treves, 2023), but it is not clear how useful new representations could be learned by them. So the area of how biologically plausible networks can learn new representations if competitive networks are not sufficiently powerful is of great interest for the future.

Another type of learning that is probably implemented in the brain is reinforcement learning using dopamine as a single reward prediction error signal (Schultz, 2016a,c, 2017). One of its main uses in the brain is for stimulus-response learning of rather fixed habits using the dopamine pathway that projects to the basal ganglia (Schultz, 2016c) (Chapter 16), and that is one of the relatively simple types of learning performed by the brain, and may even predate the neocortex in evolution.

Another type of learning may be some perceptron type of learning with a separate teacher for each neuron (Section B.11) in one part of the brain, the cerebellum, where the teacher may be the climbing fibre which forces a pyramidal cell to learn what is present on its parallel fibre inputs (Chapter 17). However, it is not clear how the teacher knows what to teach in that system.

Novelty detection is relatively easy to set up in neural networks, and is found in for example the orbitofrontal cortex (Rolls, Browning, Inoue and Hernadi, 2005a). The opposite, familiarity detection, which might help to represent one's friends, one's belongings, and one's territory, appears to be represented in the perirhinal cortex (Hölscher, Rolls and Xiang, 2003), and again can be easily learned in neural networks (Rolls, Franco and Stringer, 2005b).

The approach taken in this book and in my previous books (Rolls, 2016b, 2021b) may thus not be a 'a grand unifying theory' (Manohar, 2022) of how the brain works. But it is a pioneering approach to how biologically plausible computation may be performed in very many parts of our brains to implement very many of the wonderful things that our brains can do. It is an open issue at present about whether different principles are needed, and if so, how they are implemented in biologically plausible networks in our brains.

This book is intended to pioneer a foundation for future developments, by setting out what we know about what computations are performed in many different brain regions, how biologically plausible networks could perform the computations in many brain regions, and leaves open the question of whether the computations that are performed might need some more powerful but biologically plausible algorithms than those described here.

This book is also pioneering in that it goes beyond purely theoretical studies of neural networks, and approaches instead what particular networks may be implemented in different brain regions, and how these networks or modules are interconnected to enable processes such as episodic memory, invariant visual object recognition, and emotion to be implemented in the primate including human brain.

A feature of this book is that it highlights many of the fundamental conceptual and empirical discoveries that have been made to help understand cortical function and computation, as seeing what the fundamental discoveries were, and how they were made, is didactically important to help foster future fundamental advances.

19.8 Brain-Inspired Intelligence

One of the aims of this book is to provide for neuroscientists a computational approach to brain function. This is I believe very important, for it takes us beyond metaphors and analogies and word-level descriptions about how the brain works, to well-defined computational hypotheses that allow testing at many levels of explanation, and indeed for the relations between the levels to be understood, as set out in Section 19.6.

Another key aim is to set out for those interested in machine intelligence, what is computed in different brain systems, so that those who wish to learn from or emulate brain function know what each part computes. That is an essential prerequisite for advances to be made, which might not only try to emulate brain function, but to be inspired by it, with possible new ways of solving similar computational problems.

This book also sets out many current hypotheses about how the brain solves these computational problems, and this is likely to be an area in which many advances can be made. Indeed, advances in our understanding of how the brain computes are likely to be facilitated by very large-scale simulations of parts of the brain, to test whether the computational hypotheses scale up appropriately, as well as enabling the machine implementations to be on the same, or a larger, scale than in the real brain. This should thus provide for fruitful advances to be made in both directions, from understanding the brain to machine intelligence; and from large scale simulation on large computers of well formulated computational hypotheses about how the brain computes. But all of this rests on evidence on what is computed in different brain regions, and how it is computed.

Advances in this area are made possible by the way in which the brain is designed compared to a digital computer, as summarized in Section 19.3 and in *Cerebral Cortex: Principles of Operation* (Rolls, 2016b). Key aspects that help us to understand what and how it computes include the following.

Brain functions are considerably localized, due to the importance of minimizing the length of neural connections, and of the simplicity that this offers in the genetic specification of the brain used while it develops, which often relies on proximity rules (Rolls, 2016b). Another key aspect is that the information is transmitted from the basic computing elements, the neurons, by spike trains with one output for each neuron, so that we can listen in to what is being transmitted from one brain area to another, using the methods described in Appendix C.

Further, by making more advances in understanding how genes specify the architecture of the brain (Rolls and Stringer, 2000; Rolls, 2016b), it will be possible in future to use genetic algorithms to design the architecture of brain-like computing devices, which will enable the development of new types of computational solution to problems. Indeed, we were enormously surprised by the solutions found by neural architectures built by genetic algorithms, which frequently found ways to 'cheat', to operate in ways that we had not expected, in order to succeed at the fitness function that we had set (Rolls and Stringer, 2000) (Section B.20). And this was when all that the genetic algorithm had to work with were the building blocks of how genes might specify differences between neural architectures, in contrast to being allowed to explore new specification rules.

It seems as if we have reasonable approaches now, since the start in about 1970, of an understanding of what is computed in many brain systems in the macaque brain, and much of that and the complementary information about the human brain is what has been described in this book. We also have at least the start to approaches about how different brain systems compute. The area of brain function about which we know computationally the least is how language, including syntax and also semantics, are implemented in the brain, and how they operate together. That is an area in which at the computational level our understanding is still very incomplete, and where major advances are needed.

19.9 Brain-Inspired Medicine

There are many applications showing how advances in understanding brain function and computation have led to advances relevant to medicine. Some are highlighted in the following sections. Some others include the use of deep brain stimulation for Parkinson's disease (Little and Brown, 2020), the use of antiphase brain stimulation to cancel for example tremor, and the identification that there are two subtypes of Parkinson's disease, based on an analysis of functional connectivity (Wang, Cheng, Rolls, Dai, Gong, Du, Zhang, Wang, Liu, Wang, Brown and Feng, 2020d).

19.9.1 Computational psychiatry and neurology

As shown in Chapter 18, a number of mental disorders can be understood at least partly in terms of stability of different brain systems. This may be understood in the broader context that stability of a cortical system with positive feedback between its computing elements, the neurons, is a difficult issue to manage. This is compounded by the hypothesis that natural selection may be operating on parameters that influence the stability of different brain systems, in order to search for advantages of different options in different environments or situations.

For example, one strategy might be to make the system very sensitive to non-reward, as this may be adaptive in a number of obvious ways; yet too much sensitivity might lead to depression. Having a smaller degree of sensitivity to non-reward might also be a useful strategy in some circumstances, for it would result in continued trying, even in the face of adversity. This could result in genetic variation in sensitivity to, for example, non-reward, being maintained in the population.

The computational accounts being developed for a number of mental disorders have implications for medical treatment. For example, in depression approaches might be tried of ways to reduce the activity or connectivity of the non-reward lateral orbitofrontal cortex, and to increase the sensitivity or connectivity of the reward-related medial orbitofrontal cortex. In this context, it is interesting that modern antidepressant drugs (e.g SSRIs) do reduce the connectivity of the lateral orbitofrontal cortex back down towards levels in controls; but do not restore the reduced connectivity of the reward-related medial orbitofrontal cortex in depression. That sets a new target for the development of further treatments for depression aimed to facilitate the operation of the reward-related medial orbitofrontal cortex, and the evidence described in Chapter 18 suggests that ketamine may act on the medial orbitofrontal cortex. If the latter turns out to be the case, that opens up possibilities for combined drug treatments that together correct the lateral and the medial orbitofrontal cortex. Similarly, the understanding of brain mechanisms of emotion described in this book suggests that a key brain system in emotion is the orbitofrontal cortex; and that points the way to possible brain stimulation of the orbitofrontal cortex as a new brain area to explore for the possible relief of treatment resistant depression.

However, the computational approach is helpful in another way in understanding and potentially treating some mental disorders, and these treatments might be at the purely behavioral level. For example, the modern computational approach to understanding possible causes of depression indicates that non-reward inputs in which no action is possible might lead to feelings of sadness and depression (Fig. 11.20). In this situation, advice at the behavioral level might be to avoid as much as is reasonable stimuli that are associated with non-reward. In the case of the loss of a loved one, this might lead for example to attempts to divert the mind to other more rewarding thoughts, and divert activities from being constantly focussed on the loss. These types of approach and many others to depression are described further in my book *The Brain, Emotion, and Depression* (Rolls, 2018a, 2022a).

A similar point can be made about attention deficit hyperactivity disorder (ADHD). We have found that the functional connectivity of the visual thalamic nucleus, the lateral geniculate, with early visual cortical areas is higher in ADHD than in controls (Rolls et al., 2021b). An implication is that this may make such individuals more easily distracted and dominated by visual stimuli in the environment, and indeed we have shown that people with ADHD do display very much more screen use (i.e. use of mobile phones, computers, computer games, television, etc) (Yang et al., 2022). There are implications from this neurocomputational approach for treatment at the purely behavioral level, for by understanding this sensitivity of some parts of the brain, advice might include limiting screen use to a reasonable level, and providing a quiet atmosphere for work without environmental distractions. There are opposite differences in schizophrenia, with decreased connectivity of thalamic with visual cortex connectivity (as well as overconnectivity of backprojections from areas concerned with the self and internal thoughts such as the precuneus), as described in Section 18.3 and by Rolls et al. (2021b), and that may also have implications for treatment.

In addition, understanding with computational methods the connectivity of the brain can help to identify subtypes of a disorder. For example, subtypes of depression have been found with and without anxiety as a comorbid condition (Drysdale et al., 2017), and this may be helpful for treatment, as it may be that the subgroups with anxiety are particularly helped by Transcranial Magnetic Stimulation of the lateral orbitofrontal cortex (Feffer, Fettes, Giacobbe, Daskalakis, Blumberger and Downar, 2018).

19.9.2 Reward systems in the brain, and their application to understanding food intake control and obesity

What is computed in reward systems in the brain, and how it is computed, are described in Chapters 4–7, 11, 12, and 16. In this Section, we consider some applications of this understanding.

Different individuals have different sensitivities to rewards, non-reward, etc, and indeed this provides a basis for understanding personality, and motivation (Rolls, 2014a, 2023b). This has application to a number of areas in medicine, of which one is obesity.

Understanding the mechanisms that control appetite is becoming an increasingly important issue, given the increasing incidence of obesity. Obesity affects approximately one third of adults in the United States (with an additional one third falling into the overweight category). In the UK, there has been a three-fold increase since 1980 to a figure of 20% defined by a Body Mass Index > 30, and there is a realization that it is associated with major health risks (with 1000 deaths each week in the UK attributable to obesity). It is important to understand and thereby be able to minimize and treat obesity because many diseases are associated with a body weight that is much above normal. These diseases include hypertension, cardiovascular disease, hypercholesterolaemia, and gall bladder disease; and in addition obesity is associated with some deficits in reproductive function (e.g. ovulatory failure), and with an excess mortality from certain types of cancer (Guyenet and Schwartz, 2012; Myers et al., 2021).

There are many factors that can cause or contribute to obesity in humans (Rolls, 2007g, 2011f, 2012f, 2016g; Myers et al., 2021; Farooqi, 2022). Rapid progress is being made in understanding many of these factors at present with the aim of leading to better ways to minimize and treat obesity. Some of these factors are related to reward systems in the brain (Rolls, 2012f, 2014a, 2016g, 2023f; Rolls et al., 2023g), as described next (see also Section 4.2.10).

The way in which the sensory factors produced by the taste, smell, texture and sight of food interact in the brain with satiety signals (such as gastric distension and satiety-related hormones) to determine the pleasantness and palatability of food, and therefore whether and how much food will be eaten, is described in Chapters 4, 5 and 11. The concept is that convergence of sensory inputs produced by the taste, smell, texture and sight of food occurs in the orbitofrontal cortex to build a representation of food flavor. The orbitofrontal cortex is where the pleasantness and palatability of food are represented, as shown by the discoveries that these representations of food value are only activated if appetite is present and the food is chosen, and correlate with the subjective pleasantness of the food flavor. The orbitofrontal cortex representation of whether food is pleasant (which takes into account any satiety signals present) then drives brain areas such as the striatum and cingulate cortex that then lead to eating behavior.

The fundamental concept this leads to about some of the major causes of obesity is that, over the last 30 years, sensory stimulation produced by the taste, smell, texture and appearance of food, as well as its availability, have increased dramatically, yet the satiety signals produced by stomach distension, satiety hormones etc. summarized in Rolls (2014a) have remained essentially unchanged (see Rolls (2014a) and Rolls (2016g)). The consequence is that the effect on the brain's control system for appetite is to lead to a net average increase in the reward value and palatability of food which over-rides the satiety signals, and contributes to the tendency to be overstimulated by food and to overeat (Rolls, 2014a, 2007g, 2011f, 2012f, 2016g, 2023f; Rolls et al., 2023g).

In this scenario, it is important to understand much better the rules used by the brain to produce the representation of the pleasantness of food and how the system is modulated by eating and satiety. This understanding, and how the sensory factors can be designed and controlled so as not to override satiety signals, are important research areas in the understanding, prevention, and treatment of obesity. Advances in understanding the receptors that encode the taste, olfactory, fat texture (Rolls, 2011e; Rolls et al., 2018b; Rolls, 2020c) and other properties of food, and the processing in the brain of these properties (Rolls, 2014a, 2007g, 2011f, 2012f, 2016g, 2020c, 2023f), are also important in providing the potential to produce highly palatable food that is at the same time nutritious and healthy.

An important aspect of this hypothesis is that different humans may have reward systems that are especially strongly driven by the sensory and cognitive factors that make food highly palatable. In a test of this, we showed that activation to the sight and flavor of chocolate in the orbitofrontal and pregenual cingulate cortex were much higher in chocolate cravers than non-cravers (Rolls and McCabe, 2007). In more detail, the sight of chocolate produced more activation in chocolate cravers than non-cravers in the medial orbitofrontal cortex and ventral striatum. For cravers vs non-cravers, a combination of a picture of chocolate with chocolate in the mouth produced a greater effect than the sum of the components (i.e. supralinearity) in the medial orbitofrontal cortex and pregenual cingulate cortex. Furthermore, the pleasantness ratings of the chocolate and chocolate-related stimuli had higher positive correlations with the fMRI signals in the pregenual cingulate cortex and medial orbitofrontal cortex in the cravers than in the non-cravers. Thus there are differences between cravers and non-cravers in their responses to the reward components of a craved food in the orbitofrontal and pregenual cingulate cortex and a region to which they project the ventral striatum that is implicated in addiction (Rolls, 2019e), and in some of these regions the differences are related to the subjective pleasantness rating value of the craved food (Rolls and McCabe, 2007). It was of interest that there were no differences between the cravers and the non-cravers in the activations in the taste insula to the chocolate, so that the differences found were in the tuning of the reward system and not of the purely sensory system (Rolls and McCabe, 2007). Individual differences in brain responses to images of food have also been described by Beaver et al. (2006).

The concept that individual differences in responsiveness to food reward are reflected in brain activations in regions related to the control food intake (Rolls, 2014a, 2007g, 2011f, 2012f, 2016g) may provide a way for understanding and helping to control food intake. In this context, we should remember that individual differences in the reward systems are to be expected given that variation in these systems is an important part of the process of evolution by natural selection. Research in this area with the aim of understanding the relation between the activation of different brain systems by food, and obesity, is developing (Volkow et al., 2013, 2017).

A factor in obesity is food palatability, which with modern methods of food production can now be greater than would have been the case during the evolution of our feeding control systems. These brain systems evolved so that internal signals from for example gastric distension and glucose utilization could act to decrease the pleasantness of the sensations produced by feeding sufficiently by the end of a meal to stop further eating. However, the greater palatability of modern food may mean that this balance is altered, so that there is a tendency for the greater palatability of food to be insufficiently decreased by a standard amount of food eaten, so that extra food is eaten in a meal (Rolls, 2014a, 2012f, 2016g, 2023f).

Sensory-specific satiety is the decrease in the appetite for a particular food as it is eaten in a meal, without a decrease in the appetite for different foods, as shown above in Section 4.2.5 and Chapters 5 and 11 (Rolls, 2014a, 2016g, 2019e). It is an important factor influencing how much of each food is eaten in a meal, and its evolutionary significance may be to encourage eating of a range of different foods, and thus obtaining a range of nutrients. As a result of sensory-specific satiety, if a wide variety of foods is available, overeating in a meal can occur. Given that it is now possible to make available a very wide range of food flavors, textures, and appearances, and that such foods are readily available, this variety effect may be a factor in promoting excess food intake (Rolls, 2016g).

Another factor that could contribute to obesity is fixed meal times, in that the normal control of food intake by alterations in inter-meal interval is not readily available in humans, and food may be eaten at a meal-time even if hunger is not present (Rolls, 2014a, 2016g). Even more than this, because of the high and easy availability of food (in the home and workplace) and stimulation by advertising, there is a tendency to start eating again when satiety signals after a previous meal have decreased only a little, and the consequence is that the system again becomes overloaded.

Making food salient, for example by placing it on display, may increase food selection particularly in the obese (Schachter, 1971; Rodin, 1976; Cornell et al., 1989), and portion size is a factor, with more being eaten if a large portion of food is presented (Rolls, 2012a), though whether this is a factor that can lead to obesity and not just alter test meal size is not yet clear. The driving effects of visual and other stimuli, including the effects of advertising, on the brain systems that are activated by food reward may be different in different individuals, and may contribute to obesity.

19.9.3 Multiple Routes to Action

Section 11.3.9 describes evidence that there are multiple routes to action, some of which are unconscious (Rolls, 2020a). The gene-specified reward value route to action may perform actions in the interests of the genes. The rational route may perform actions in the interests of the individual. Thus the goals for these routes may be different, and the route that causally accounts of the action performed may be subject to selection by noise-related attractor decision-making networks. This makes human decision-making particularly interesting. Further, although sometimes the reason given by the rational system for an action may be correct, in cases when the rational system initiated the action, on other occasions it may be producing a confabulated account of why an action was performed, if the action was performed by the gene-specified reward-related system. This has broad implications for understanding human behavior (Rolls, 2012e, 2023b), including human economic decision-making (Rolls, 2019d).

19.10 Primates including humans have a different systems-level organisation of many brain systems compared to rodents

Primates including humans have a different systems-level organisation of many brain systems compared to rodents. This is evident for at least the following systems, where rodents refers in particular to neuroscience investigations in rats and mice. This makes rodents in many cases not a good model for systems-level analysis of the computations performed in many primate (including human) brain systems. The focus of this book is therefore on primates including humans, with complementary evidence frequently provided by neurophysiological discoveries in primates, that are important for understanding the computations being performed, and that are closely related to corresponding processing in humans as shown by neuroimaging investigations and the effects of brain damage in humans. The interest here is to understand the human brain in health and disease, including understanding and a foundation that is relevant to treatment in humans.

19.10.1 The visual system

For primate **vision**, the fovea is associated with object recognition for what is at the fovea, and uses a highly developed ventral processing stream to compute transform-invariant representations of objects (Chapter 2). Associated with this foveate vision, primates have a highly developed dorsal visual system to enable fixation of objects, faces, parts of scenes etc (Chapter 3), and computes many coordinate transforms (Chapters 3 and 10). Part of the way that invariant object recognition is solved in the primate and human visual system is by having a high resolution fovea, and performing invariant object recognition for what is at the fovea, and then moving the eyes to fixate on another part of a scene, and perform invariant object recognition for what is then at the fovea. In contrast rodents do not have a fovea but instead have vision with a field of view of 180–270°, do not have highly developed ventral and dorsal visual systems with visual areas in macaques that correspond to areas in humans, and so provide a poor model of primate including human vision. And of course the face identity and face expression systems, important in the primate and human visual system (Chapter 2), are not present in rodents. The very different visual systems of primates and rodents in turn appear to have profound implications on what is represented in the hippocampus, which in primates and humans can be about where an object is seen in a location in a spatial scene (Rolls, 2023c; Rolls and Wirth, 2018), whereas in rodents the emphasis in on the place where the individual is located (O'Keefe and Speakman, 1987; O'Keefe, 1979; O'Keefe and Krupic, 2021).

The differences between the rodent and primate visual system is highlighted by the report that when rodents locomote, the firing of neurons in the primary visual cortex is highly disturbed (Diamanti, Reddy, Schroder, Muzzu, Harris, Saleem and Carandini, 2021), whereas in primates the inferior temporal visual cortex has neuronal responses to visual stimuli that are independent of and not influenced by actions being made to obtain them including reaching to touch a computer screen (Rolls et al., 1977, 2003a). Similarly, visual responses to viewed spatial locations in macaques are not influenced by any locomotion being performed (Rolls et al., 1997a; Georges-François et al., 1999). This provides evidence that the rodent visual system operates far less specifically in terms of its encoding of visual stimuli than in primates, and indicates very poor cortical selectivity in visual cortical regions of rodents.

19.10.2 The taste system

For the **taste** system (Chapter 4), the rodent taste system is organised very differently to the primate taste system in two major ways. First in rodents there are connections from the nucleus of the solitary tract, and then to a taste area not present in primates the pontine taste area, which then sends information subcortically to regions such as the amygdala and hypothalamus (Rolls, 2016c, 2015d; Rolls and Scott, 2003; Scott and Small, 2009; Small and Scott, 2009; Rolls, 2019e). In contrast, in primates the taste system projects from the nucleus of the solitary tract to the thalamus and thence to the insular primary taste cortex. The insular taste cortex then projects into the orbitofrontal cortex (Chapter 4 and Fig. 4.1). Second, in rodents there is evidence that reward value, as assessed by the effects on neuronal responses to taste of feeding to satiety, is present even in the periphery, in for example the nucleus of the solitary tract, with the evidence reviewed by Rolls (2016c) and Rolls (2019e). In contrast, in primates including humans taste and flavor reward are represented in the orbitofrontal cortex (as shown by the effects of devaluation produced by feeding to satiety), but not at earlier stages of processing including the primary taste cortex in the anterior insula (Rolls, 2015d, 2016c, 2019e) (Chapter 4). The implication is that taste, and the closely related olfactory and visual processing that contribute to food reward value and expected value, are much more difficult to understand in rodents than in primates, partly because there is less segregation of 'what' (identity and intensity) from reward / hedonic processing in rodents.

It has been proposed that this great change in the systems-level computational design of the taste system in evolution from rodents to primates is related to the importance of cortical processing for all sensory systems in primates to the object level, so that multimodal representations can be formed about objects independently of whether they are currently rewarding (Rolls, 2019e, 2016b). Part of the value of this reward-independent representation of objects in primates including humans is that the neurons still respond to the object and can learn about the object, for example the location of food, even when the object may not be rewarding. (In rodents, the taste information is broadcast to many subcortical structures from the rodent pontine taste area, so that there is not the more powerful computational design of primates in which multimodal object representations are built before reward-related processing.) Building such multimodal representations in primates, including to the level of semantic descriptions in humans, is much more stable if there are separate representations in each cortical processing system of 'what' object is present, independently of its current reward value.

This evolutionary argument applies also to processing in the olfactory system, and the visual system (Rolls, 2019e, 2016b). Moreover, this evolutionary evidence points to the particular importance of the orbitofrontal cortex and amygdala in primates including humans, as they are the first stages of processing at which reward value, and hence emotion, can be represented (Chapter 11).

19.10.3 The olfactory system

For the **olfactory** system (Chapter 5) there are great differences too in rodents in terms of processing of the reward value of odors. In humans, activity in the pyriform cortex appears to be related to 'what' stimulus is present (its identity), and its intensity, and not to its reward value, in that activations in the human pyriform cortex are linearly related to the intensity rating of odorants, and not to their pleasantness (Grabenhorst, Rolls, Margot, da Silva and Velazco, 2007); in that paying attention to the intensity vs the pleasantness of an odor increases activations in the pyriform cortex (Rolls, Grabenhorst, Margot, da Silva and Velazco, 2008b); and in that activations in the pyriform (primary olfactory) cortex were not decreased by odor devaluation by satiety (Gottfried, 2015). In contrast, in rodents, reducing reward value by feeding to satiety or by administering leptin reduces the neural activity even in the olfactory bulb (Pager, Giachetti, Holley and LeMagnen, 1972; Sun, Tang, Wu, Xu, Zhang, Cao, Zhou, Yu and Li, 2019a). The same points can be made as for taste about the different computations of reward value performed in different parts of the rodent vs primate olfactory system. With the highly developed human orbitofrontal cortex, there is a hedonic map of odor in the medial vs lateral orbitofrontal cortex (see Fig. 5.5 and Rolls et al. (2003c)), and nothing like this is known in rodents. And of course top-down modulation of reward value for olfaction and taste, very evident in humans even from the word level (Chapters 4 and 5), has no correspondent in rodents, yet is probably very important in what makes foods and many other rewards become acceptable in humans (including the effects of advertising). Further, the emphasis on the olfactory system in rodents may bias rodents to spatial representations of the place where they are located, as evident in rodent hippocampal place cells. This is in contrast with the importance of spatial view in primates because of the emphasis in primates on visual processing of representations of viewed spatial locations 'out there', as evident in the responses of primate hippocampal spatial view cells (Chapter 9).

19.10.4 The somatosensory system

For the **somatosensory** system, the representations in the higher cortical parts of the system in the parietal cortex become closely linked to vision, with neurons specialized for reaching towards and then grasping with the correct grip an object being looked at in peripersonal space (Chapters 6 and 10). Nothing similar is present in rodents. An interesting computational feature of this in primates is that the coordinates of where to reach in peripersonal space can be communicated in a sense though the world, for the place to reach is the place currently being visually fixated.

The differences between the primate somatosensory cortex and the rodent somatosensory cortex are enormous. For example, rodents and macaques have for a primary somatosensory cortex area 3b, but macaques have in addition three additional anterior parietal fields including area 1 which processes cutaneous input, area 3a which processes proprioceptive input, and area 2 which integrates cutaneous and proprioceptive inputs (O'Connor, Krubitzer and Bensmaia, 2021). In addition, humans have a great development of the somatosensory hierarchy in the inferior parietal cortex leading to region PF (Fig. 10.1, Chapters 6 and 10) (Rolls et al., 2023f), with little similar in rodents (O'Connor et al., 2021).

19.10.5 The auditory system

For the **auditory** system, the human auditory association cortex in the superior temporal gyrus becomes heavily involved in language processing and especially auditory comprehension of speech, as described in Chapters 7, 8 and 14 (Rolls et al., 2023h). Part of this specialisation involves major connections with the inferior frontal gyrus (Broca's area, involved in speech production).

19.10.6 The hippocampal system, memory, and navigation

The differences for the visual system have major effects on the **hippocampal system**, in which in primates parts of distant visual scenes are represented by spatial view cells that enable objects, rewards, and goals at different locations in a scene to be remembered (Rolls, 2021f), whereas in rodents the emphasis is on place cell representations for where the rodent is located (O'Keefe, 1990; Burgess and O'Keefe, 1996; Hartley, Lever, Burgess and O'Keefe, 2014; O'Keefe and Krupic, 2021) (Chapter 9). This in turn has major effects on navigation, which in primates including humans can be performed relatively easily using visual cells such as spatial view cells that respond to landmarks in scenes (Chapter 10, and Section 9.3.15.5) (Rolls, 2021f, 2023c). Navigation using a topological map of the type believed to be implemented by place cells in rodents is much more complicated, because of the need to constantly make conversions between allocentric spatial 'cognitive' maps, and egocentric, action-based movement systems (Chapter 10). The difference of the primate brain may also lead to differences in the recall of information about episodic events from the hippocampus to the neocortex for use in the neocortex. In primates and humans, with the highly developed temporal lobe, semantic representations can be built using the information recalled from the hippocampus, as described in Chapters 9, 8 and 14. Very little about this is known in rodents, and these temporal lobe neocortical areas are much less developed in rodents.

As described in Section 9.3.15.1, humans normally navigate to a viewed object or reward in a scene such as a building, and non-human primates might locomote to particular locations in the viewed environment with local cues where there are sources of food, water, shelter and a place to sleep etc. In these cases, environmental visual features identify each location, and spatial view cells are ideal for this type of navigation. What is often studied in rodents as a model of navigation without any local cues as in the Morris water maze (Morris, Garrud, Rawlins and O'Keefe, 1982) may not be at all commonly how humans and other primates navigate. Spatial view cells provide the mechanism often used for navigation in humans and other primates which is typically towards visible landmarks such as a building, the top of a hill, etc (Rolls, 2021f, 2023d). Navigation may thus be performed in primates including humans (Rolls, 2021f, 2023a,d) in very different ways to those utilised in rodents, in which local place-associated cues sensed with the vibrissae or olfactory system define places, and idiothetic navigation between such places often in the dark may be important (McNaughton, Barnes, Gerrard, Gothard, Jung, Knierim, Kudrimoti, Qin, Skaggs, Suster and Weaver, 1996; Moser, Rowland and Moser, 2015; Moser, Moser and McNaughton, 2017). Moreover, because of the limited visual acuity of rodents illustrated in Fig. 9.12 in Section 9.2.5, navigation in rodents is unlikely to be towards small objects or rewards located at distant locations in visual scenes, whereas this is typical of navigation in primates including humans implemented using spatial view cells (Rolls, 2023d). Thus navigational strategies, and how they are implemented in the brain, may be very different in primates including humans to those in rodents.

19.10.7 The orbitofrontal cortex and amygdala

The organisation of the **orbitofrontal cortex and amygdala, and reward value systems** is also very different in primates including humans vs rodents (Chapter 11). One difference is that the orbitofrontal cortex is relatively little developed in rodents, yet is one of the major brain areas involved in emotion and motivation in primates including humans (Rolls, 2014a, 2019e). Indeed, it has been argued that the granular prefrontal cortex is a primate innovation (Passingham, 2021), and the implication of the argument is that any areas that might be termed orbitofrontal cortex in rats (Schoenbaum et al., 2009) are homologous only to the agranular parts of the primate orbitofrontal cortex (shaded mid grey in Fig. 11.3), that is to areas 13a, 14c, and the agranular insular areas labelled Ia in Fig. 11.3 (Wise, 2008; Passingham and Wise, 2012). It follows from that argument that for most areas of the orbitofrontal and medial prefrontal cortex in humans and macaques (those shaded light grey in Fig. 11.3), special consideration must be given to research in macaques and humans (Rolls, 2014a, 2017b). As shown in Fig. 11.3, there may be no cortical area in rodents that is homologous to most of the primate including human orbitofrontal cortex (Preuss, 1995; Wise, 2008; Passingham and Wise, 2012; Passingham, 2021).

A second difference is that reward value in primates including humans is represented in the orbitofrontal cortex, and to some extent in the amygdala, but not at earlier cortical areas (Chapter 11 and Fig. 11.1). As shown above, and in more detail in Chapter 8 of Rolls (2019e), reward value is represented early on in sensory processing in rodents, so that any distinction between object identity and object value is much less clear in rodents. An underlying evolutionary advantage for the primate design may be that the great development of the neocortex which enables for example invariant visual object recognition to be performed means that once formed, it is useful to interface this to other modalities to form multimodal object including semantic representations, and this benefits from having 'what' representations in every sensory modality, untrammelled by possible confusion by current reward value. This makes the system not only very different in rodents, but also much more difficult to analyze.

A third key difference is that the primate orbitofrontal cortex has neurons that reverse in one trial in a rule-based system, allowing very rapid updating of reward value representations based on feedback from the environment (Thorpe et al., 1983; Rolls et al., 2020e), and this is likely to have great advantage in social behavior (Chapter 11). I have discussed this with those who work with rodents, and none so far believes that rodents can perform this one-trial rule-based reversal, and indeed evidence that they do not is described in Chapter 11 (e.g. Hervig, Fiddian, Piilgaard, Bozic, Blanco-Pozo, Knudsen, Olesen, Alsio and Robbins (2020)).

A fourth key difference is that in association with the importance of face and voice expression and identity for emotional signals and social behavior in primates including humans, there are highly developed analysis systems for these signals in the temporal cortex (Chapter 2), which in turn projects to the orbitofrontal cortex which is involved in the social and emotional behavior produced by these stimuli (Chapter 11).

A fifth key difference is that the representations in the primate including human orbitofrontal cortex are of the reward value of stimuli, with very little representation of behavioral responses or actions (Chapter 11). In contrast, it has been suggested that in rodents the orbitofrontal cortex provides a cognitive map of state space that could describe its role in value-based decision-making (Wilson, Takahashi, Schoenbaum and Niv, 2014b; Sharpe, Stalnaker,

Schuck, Killcross, Schoenbaum and Niv, 2019). (A state-space representation as described in this context is a mathematical model of a physical system as a set of input, output and state variables related by differential equations or difference equations. State variables are variables whose values evolve through time in a way that depends on the values they have at any given time and also depends on the externally imposed values of input variables. Output variables' values depend on the values of the state variables.) According to this view, the orbitofrontal cortex represents previous stimuli, responses and actions, and other sensory features that occur in association with outcomes in a multidimensional array, and thus supports reinforcement learning implemented elsewhere in the brain. That suggestion is based on findings in rodents (Wilson et al., 2014b). That suggestion does not fit the primate, including human, findings on the orbitofrontal cortex. These findings, described in Chapter 11 and by Rolls (2019e), show that the primate orbitofrontal cortex contains representations of stimulus reward value, and is involved in learning and rapidly updating these reward value representations, but does not have major representations of actions (Thorpe, Rolls and Maddison, 1983; Rolls, 2019f; Padoa-Schioppa and Assad, 2006; Rolls, 2014a; Grattan and Glimcher, 2014; Rolls, 2019e). In another example, although neuronal systems involved in rewarded behavior are present in the mouse orbitofrontal cortex, behavioral responses are also represented (Kuwabara et al., 2020), and not primarily stimulus reward value as in primates. Thus the computations being performed in the rodent orbitofrontal cortex (Izquierdo, 2017; Rolls, 2019e) appear to be different in kind from those in the primate orbitofrontal cortex. Further, the functions of different parts of the rodent orbitofrontal cortex are poorly understood (Izquierdo, 2017; Barreiros et al., 2021).

A sixth key brain difference is that in rodents the amygdala is relatively important in emotion (LeDoux, 2000; LeDoux and Pine, 2016), but the amygdala appears to be overshadowed by the great development of the orbitofrontal cortex in humans, damage to which produces much greater changes in emotional behavior and subjective emotions than does damage to the human amygdala (Chapter 11) (Rolls, 2019e; Rolls et al., 2023b,h). Indeed the rodent and human amygdala appear to share similar functions in producing autonomic and behavioral responses such as freezing, but the human amygdala appears to be little involved in reported, declarative, experienced, emotion, with instead the human orbitofrontal cortex being involved in these major properties of emotion (Rolls et al., 2023h,b; Rolls, 2023b) (Section 11.4).

19.10.8 The cingulate cortex

The **cingulate cortex** in rodents also appears to be different to that in primates. In primates the anterior and mid-cingulate cortex are implicated in action-outcome learning, using information from the orbitofrontal cortex about reward outcomes, and information about actions from the parietal cortex via the posterior cingulate cortex (Rolls (2019c) and Chapter 12). In contrast, in rodents the state space proposals for the rodent 'orbitofrontal cortex' hold that the rodent 'orbitofrontal cortex' is involved in action-outcome learning (Wilson, Takahashi, Schoenbaum and Niv, 2014b; Sharpe, Stalnaker, Schuck, Killcross, Schoenbaum and Niv, 2019). Further, correspondences between the human and macaque anterior cingulate cortex are clear, but what the correspondences are to what is found in 'prelimbic' and related regions in rodents are very unclear, and there may be no clear correspondences (Klein-Flugge, Bongioanni and Rushworth, 2022a).

A further difference is that the rodent is believed not to have an equivalent to the primate posterior cingulate cortex areas 23 and 31 (Vogt, 2009; Rolls, 2019c; Rolls et al., 2023i), yet these regions are important in human episodic memory (Rolls et al., 2023i). Indeed, in humans the posterior cingulate cortex has greater functional connectivity with other cortical regions in females than in males, and this can be related to evidence for better episodic memory in females in humans (Zhang et al., 2023b).

19.10.9 The motor system

The differences in the visual system of primates are also associated with differences in the **motor system**, for there are major specializations in primate parietal, premotor, and motor areas association for grasping and manipulating visually fixated objects and tools, and the precision grip (Chapter 15).

19.10.10 Language

Of course the organisation of brain systems for **language** (Chapters 14 and 8) is very different in humans. However, it is of interest that some parts of the system such as the inferior frontal gyrus and its connections with the anterior temporal cortex that are relevant to language can be identified as systems in non-human primates that will develop into language systems in evolution (Chapter 14).

The focus in this book on brain computations in primates including humans is because a key aim is to understand the human brain and human behavior in health and disease, and most of the systems-level organisation in rodents appears to be very different, and the rodent provides a poor model for the systems-level organisation of the human brain or the non-human primate brain.

Appendix 1 Introduction to linear algebra for neural networks

In this Appendix I review some simple elements of linear algebra relevant to understanding neural networks. This will provide a useful basis for a quantitative understanding of how neural networks operate (see Appendix B).

A.1 Vectors

A vector is an ordered set of numbers. An example of a vector is the set of numbers

$$\begin{bmatrix} 7 \\ 4 \end{bmatrix}$$

If we denote the jth element of this vector as w_j, then $w_1 = 7$, and $w_2 = 4$. We can denote the whole vector by **w**. This notation is very economical. If the vector has 10,000 elements, then we can still refer to it in mathematical operations as **w**. **w** might refer to the vector of 10,000 synaptic weights on the dendrites of a neuron. Another example of a vector is the set of firing rates of the axons that make synapses onto a dendrite, as shown in Fig. 1.2. The firing rate x of each axon forming the input vector can be indexed by j, and is denoted by x_j. The vector would be denoted by **x**.

Certain mathematical operations can be performed with vectors. We start with the operation which is fundamental to simple models of neural networks, the inner product or dot product of two vectors.

A.1.1 The inner or dot product of two vectors

The operation of computing the activation h of a neuron from the firing rate on its input axons multiplied by the corresponding synaptic weight can be expressed as:

$$h = \sum_j x_j w_j \qquad (A.1)$$

where $\sum_j$ indicates that the sum is over the C input axons to each neuron, indexed by j. Denoting the firing rate vector as **x** and the synaptic weight vector as **w**, we can write

$$h = \mathbf{x} \cdot \mathbf{w} \qquad . \qquad (A.2)$$

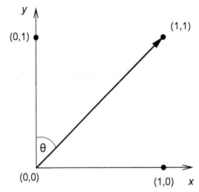

Fig. A.1 Illustration of a vector in a two-dimensional space. The basis for the space is made up of the x axis in the [1,0] direction, and the y axis in the [0,1] direction. (The first element of each vector is then the x value, and the second the y value. The values of x and y for different points, marked by a dot, in the space are shown. The origins of the axes are at point 0,0.) The [1,1] vector projects in the [1,1] (or $45°$) direction to the point 1,1, with length 1.414.

If the weight vector is

$$\mathbf{w} = \begin{bmatrix} 9 \\ 5 \\ 2 \end{bmatrix}$$

and the firing rate input vector is

$$\mathbf{x} = \begin{bmatrix} 3 \\ 6 \\ 7 \end{bmatrix}$$

then we can write

$$\mathbf{x} \cdot \mathbf{w} = (3 \cdot 9) + (6 \cdot 5) + (7 \cdot 2) = 71 \quad . \tag{A.3}$$

Thus in the inner or dot product, we multiply the corresponding terms, and then sum the result. As this is the simple mathematical operation that is used to compute the activation h in the most simplified abstraction of a neuron (see Chapter 1), we see that it is indeed the fundamental operation underlying many types of neural network. We will shortly see that some of the properties of neuronal networks can be understood in terms of the properties of the dot product. We next review a number of basic aspects of vectors and inner products between vectors.

There is a simple geometrical interpretation of vectors, at least in low-dimensional spaces. If we define, for example, x and y axes at right angles to each other in a two-dimensional space, then any two-component vector can be thought of as having a direction and length in that space that can be defined by the values of the two elements of the vector. If the first element is taken to correspond to x and the second to y, then the x axis lies in the direction [1,0] in the space, and the y axis in the direction [0,1], as shown in Fig. A.1. The line to point [1,1] in the space then lies at $45°$ to both axes, as shown in Fig. A.1.

A.1.2 The length of a vector

Consider taking the inner product of a vector

$$\mathbf{w} = \begin{bmatrix} 4 \\ 3 \end{bmatrix}$$

with itself. Then

$$\|\mathbf{w}\| = \sqrt{\mathbf{w} \cdot \mathbf{w}} = \sqrt{4^2 + 3^2} = 5. \tag{A.4}$$

This is the length of the vector. We can represent this operation in the two-dimensional graph shown in Fig. A.1. In this case, the coordinates where vector $\mathbf{w}$ ends in the space are [1,1]. The length of the vector (from [0,0]) to [1,1] is obtained by Pythagoras' theorem. Pythagoras' theorem states that the length of the vector $\mathbf{w}$ is equal to the square root of the sum of the squares of the two sides. Thus we define the length of the vector $\mathbf{w}$ as

$$\|\mathbf{w}\| = \sqrt{\mathbf{w} \cdot \mathbf{w}} \tag{A.5}$$

In the [1,1] case, this value is $\sqrt{2} = 1.414$.

A.1.3 Normalizing the length of a vector

We can scale a vector in such a way that its length is equal to 1 by dividing it by its length. If we form the dot product of two normalized vectors, its maximum value will be 1, and its minimum value -1.

A.1.4 The angle between two vectors: the normalized dot product

The angle between two vectors $\mathbf{x}$ and $\mathbf{w}$ is defined in terms of the inner product as follows:

$$\cos\theta = \frac{\mathbf{x} \cdot \mathbf{w}}{\|\mathbf{x}\| \|\mathbf{w}\|} \tag{A.6}$$

For example, the angle between two vectors

$$\mathbf{x} = \begin{bmatrix} 0 \\ 1 \end{bmatrix} \text{ and } \mathbf{w} = \begin{bmatrix} 1 \\ 1 \end{bmatrix}$$

where the length of vector $\mathbf{x}$ is $\sqrt{0.0 + 1.1} = 1$ and of vector $\mathbf{w}$ is $\sqrt{1.1 + 1.1} = \sqrt{2}$ is

$$\cos\theta = \frac{(0.1) + (1.1)}{1.\sqrt{2}} = 0.707. \tag{A.7}$$

Thus $\theta = \cos^{-1}(0.707) = 45°$.

We can give a simple geometrical interpretation of this as shown in Fig. A.1. However, Equation A.6 is much easier to use in a high-dimensional space!

The dot product reflects the similarity between two vectors. Once the length of the vectors is fixed, the higher their dot product, the more similar are the two vectors. By normalizing the dot product, that is by dividing by the lengths of each vector as shown in Equation A.6, we obtain a value that varies from -1 to $+1$. This normalized dot product is then just the cosine of the angle between the vectors, and is a very useful measure of the similarity between any two vectors, because it always lies in the range -1 to $+1$. It is closely related to the (Pearson product–moment) correlation coefficient between any two vectors, as we see if we write the equation in terms of its components

$$\cos\theta = \frac{\sum_j x_j w_j}{(\sum_j x_j^2)^{1/2}(\sum_j w_j^2)^{1/2}} \quad (A.8)$$

which is just the formula for the correlation coefficient between two sets of numbers with zero mean (or with the mean value removed by subtracting the mean of the components of each vector from each component of that vector).

Now consider two vectors that have a dot product of zero, that is where $\cos\theta = 0$ or the angle between the vectors is 90°. Such vectors are described as orthogonal (literally at right angles) to each other. If our two orthogonal vectors were $\mathbf{x}$ and $\mathbf{w}$, then the activation of the neuron, measured by the dot product of these two vectors, would be zero. If our two orthogonal vectors each had a mean of zero, their correlation would also be zero: the two vectors can then be described as unrelated or independent.

If, instead, the two vectors had zero angle between them, that is if $\cos\theta = 1$, then the dot product would be maximal (given the vectors' lengths), the normalized dot product would be 1, and the two vectors would be described as identical to each other apart from their length. Note that in this case their correlation would also be 1, even if the two vectors did not have zero mean components.

For intermediate similarities of the two vectors, the degree of similarity would be expressed by the relative magnitude of the dot product, or by the normalized dot product of the two vectors, which is just the cosine of the angle between them. These measures are closely related to the correlation between two vectors.

Thus we can think of the simple operation performed by neurons as measuring the similarity between their current input vector and their synaptic weight vector. Their activation, h, is this dot product. It is because of this simple operation that neurons can generalize to similar inputs; can still produce useful outputs if some of their inputs or synaptic weights are damaged or missing, that is they can show graceful degradation or fault tolerance; and can be thought of as learning to point their weight vectors towards input patterns, which is very useful in enabling neurons to categorize their inputs in competitive networks (see Section B.4).

A.1.5 The outer product of two vectors

Let us take a row vector having as components the firing rates of a set of output neurons in a pattern associator or competitive network, which we might denote as $\mathbf{y}$, with components y_i and the index i running from 1 to the number N of output neurons. $\mathbf{y}$ is then a shorthand for writing down each component, e.g. [7,2,5,2,...], to indicate that the firing rate of neuron 1 is 7, etc. To avoid confusion, we continue in the following to denote the firing rate of input neuron j as x_j. Now recall (see Chapter 1 and Section B.2) how the synaptic weights are formed in a pattern associator using a Hebb rule as follows:

$$\delta w_{ij} = \alpha y_i x_j \quad (A.9)$$

where δw_{ij} is the change of the synaptic weight w_{ij} which results from the simultaneous (or conjunctive) presence of presynaptic firing x_j and postsynaptic firing or activation y_i, and α is a learning rate constant which specifies how much the synapses alter on any one pairing. In a more compact vector notation, this expression would be

$$\delta\mathbf{w}_i = \alpha y_i \mathbf{x}' \quad (A.10)$$

where the firing rates on the axons form a column vector with the values, for example, as follows[23]:

$$\mathbf{x}' = \begin{bmatrix} 2 \\ 0 \\ 3 \\ .... \end{bmatrix}$$

The weights are then updated by a change proportional (the α factor) to the following matrix (Table A.1):

Table A.1 Multiplication of a row vector [7 2 5 ....] by a column vector to form the external or tensor product, representing for example the changes to a matrix of synaptic weights $\mathbf{W}$

	[7	2	5	.....]
[2]	14	4	10	......
[0]	0	0	0	......
[3]	21	6	15	......
.....	.....	.....	.....	.....

This multiplication of the two vectors is called the outer, or tensor, product, and forms a matrix, in this case of (alterations to) synaptic weights. Thus we see that the operation of altering synaptic weights in a network can be thought of as forming a matrix of weight changes, which can then be used to alter the existing matrix of synaptic weights.

A.1.6 Linear and non-linear systems

The operations with which we have been concerned in this Appendix so far are linear operations. We should note that if two matrices operate linearly, we can form their product by matrix multiplication, and then replace the two matrices with the single matrix that is their product. We can thus effectively replace two synaptic matrices in a linear multilayer neural network with one synaptic matrix, the product of the two matrices. For this reason, multilayer neural networks if linear cannot achieve more than can be achieved in a single-layer linear network. It is only in non-linear networks that more can be achieved, in terms of mapping input vectors through the synaptic weight matrices, to produce particular mappings to output vectors. Much of the power of many networks in the brain comes from the fact that they are multilayer non-linear networks (in that the computing elements in each network, the neurons, have non-linear properties such as thresholds, and saturation at high levels of output). Because the matrix by matrix multiplication operations of linear algebra cannot be applied directly to the operation of neural networks in the brain, we turn instead back to other aspects of linear algebra, which can help us to understand which classes of pattern can be successfully learned by different types of neural network.

---

[23] The prime after the $\mathbf{x}$ is used here to remind us that this vector is a column vector, which can be thought of as a transformed row vector, and the prime indicates the transformed vector. We do not use the prime for most of this book in order to keep the notation uncluttered.

A.1.7 Linear combinations of vectors, linear independence, and linear separability

We can multiply a vector by a scalar (a single value, e.g. 2) thus:

$$2 \cdot \begin{bmatrix} 4 \\ 1 \\ 3 \end{bmatrix} = \begin{bmatrix} 8 \\ 2 \\ 6 \end{bmatrix}$$

We can add two vectors thus:

$$\begin{bmatrix} 4 \\ 1 \\ 3 \end{bmatrix} + \begin{bmatrix} 2 \\ 7 \\ 2 \end{bmatrix} = \begin{bmatrix} 6 \\ 8 \\ 5 \end{bmatrix}$$

The sum of the two vectors is an example of a linear combination of vectors, which is in general a weighted sum of several vectors, component by component. Thus, the linear combination of vectors $\mathbf{v}_1$, $\mathbf{v}_2$, ... to form a vector $\mathbf{v}_s$ is expressed by the sum

$$\mathbf{v}_s = c_1 \mathbf{v}_1 + c_2 \mathbf{v}_2 + ... \tag{A.11}$$

where c_1 and c_2 are scalars.

By adding vectors in this way, we can produce any vector in the space spanned by a set of vectors as a linear combination of vectors in the set. If in a set of n vectors at least one can be written as a linear combination of the others, then the vectors are described as **linearly dependent**. If in a set of n vectors none can be written as a linear combination of the others, then the vectors are described as **linearly independent**. A linearly independent set of vectors has the properties that any vector in the space spanned by the set can be written in only one way as a linear combination of the set, and the space has dimension $d = n$. In contrast, a vector in a space spanned by a linearly dependent set can be written in an infinite number of equivalent ways, and the dimension d of the space is less than n.

Consider a set of linearly dependent vectors and the d-dimensional space they span. Two subsets of this set are described as **linearly separable** if the vectors of one subset (that is, their endpoints) can be separated from those of the other by a hyperplane, that is a subspace of dimension $d - 1$. Subsets formed from a set of linearly independent vectors are always linearly separable. For example, the four vectors:

$$\begin{bmatrix} 0 \\ 0 \end{bmatrix} \quad \begin{bmatrix} 0 \\ 1 \end{bmatrix} \quad \begin{bmatrix} 1 \\ 0 \end{bmatrix} \quad \begin{bmatrix} 1 \\ 1 \end{bmatrix}$$

are linearly dependent, because the fourth can be formed by a linear combination of the second and third (and also because the first, being the null vector, can be formed by multiplying any other vector by zero, a specific linear combination). In fact, $n = 4$ and $d = 2$. If we split this set into subset A including the first and fourth vector, and subset B including the second and third, the two subsets are not linearly separable, because there is no way to draw a line (which is the subspace of dimension $d - 1 = 1$) to separate the two subsets A and B. We will encounter this set of vectors in Appendix B, and this is the geometrical interpretation of why a one-layer, one-output neuron network cannot separate these patterns. Such a network (a simple perceptron) is equivalent to its (single) weight vector, and in turn the weight vector defines a set of parallel $d - 1$ dimensional hyperplanes. (Here $d = 2$, so a hyperplane is simply a line, any line perpendicular to the weight vector.) No line can be found that separates the first and fourth vector from the second and third, whatever the weight vector the line is perpendicular to, and hence no perceptron exists that performs the required classification (see Section A.2.1). To separate such patterns, a multilayer network with non-linear neurons is needed (see Appendix B).

Any set of linearly independent vectors comprise the basis of the space they span, and they are called basis vectors. All possible vectors in the space spanned by these vectors can be formed as linear combinations of these vectors. If the vectors of the basis are in addition mutually orthogonal, the basis is an orthogonal basis, and it is, further, an orthonormal basis if the vectors are chosen to be of unit length. Given any space of vectors with a preassigned meaning to each of their components (for example the space of patterns of activation, in which each component is the activation of a particular unit), the most natural, canonical choice for a basis is the set of vectors in which each vector has one component, in turn, with value 1, and all the others with value 0. For example, in the $d = 2$ space considered earlier, the natural choice is to take as basis vectors

$$\begin{bmatrix} 1 \\ 0 \end{bmatrix}$$

and

$$\begin{bmatrix} 0 \\ 1 \end{bmatrix}$$

from which all vectors in the space can be created. This can be seen from Fig. A.1. (A vector in the [−1,−1] direction would have the opposite direction of the vector shown in Fig. A.1.)

If we had three vectors that were all in the same plane in a three-dimensional (x, y, z) space, then the space they spanned would be less than three-dimensional. For example, the three vectors

$$\begin{bmatrix} 1 \\ 0 \\ 0 \end{bmatrix} \quad \begin{bmatrix} 0 \\ 1 \\ 0 \end{bmatrix} \quad \begin{bmatrix} -1 \\ -1 \\ 0 \end{bmatrix}$$

all lie in the same z plane, and span only a two-dimensional space. (All points in the space could be shown in the plane of the paper in Fig. A.1.)

A.2 Application to understanding simple neural networks

The operation of simple one-layer networks can be understood in terms of these concepts.

A.2.1 Capability and limitations of single-layer networks: linear separability and capacity

Single-layer perceptrons perform pattern classification, and can be trained by an associative (Hebb) learning rule or by an error-correction (delta) rule (see Appendix B). That is, each neuron classifies the input patterns it receives into classes determined by the teacher. Single-layer perceptrons are thus supervised networks, with a separate teacher for each output neuron. The classification is most clearly understood if the output neurons are binary, or are strongly non-linear, but the network will still try to obtain an optimal mapping with linear or near-linear output neurons.

When each neuron operates as a binary classifier, we can consider how many input patterns p can be classified by each neuron, and the classes of pattern that can be correctly classified. The result is that the maximum number of patterns that can be correctly classified by a neuron with C inputs is

$$p_{\max} = 2C \tag{A.12}$$

when the inputs have random continuous-valued inputs, but the patterns must be linearly separable (see Hertz et al. (1991)). More generally, a network with a single binary unit can implement a classification between two subspaces of a space of possible input patterns provided that the p actual patterns given as examples of the correct classification are linearly separable.

The linear separability requirement can be made clear by considering a geometric interpretation of the logical AND problem, which is linearly separable, and the XOR (exclusive OR) problem, which is not linearly separable. The truth tables for the AND and XOR functions are shown in Table A.2 (there are two inputs, x_1 and x_2, and one output neuron):

Table A.2 Truth table for AND and XOR functions performed by a single output neuron with two inputs. 1 = active or firing; 0 = inactive.

Inputs		Output	
x_1	x_2	AND	XOR
0	0	0	0
1	0	0	1
0	1	0	1
1	1	1	0

For the AND function, we can plot the mapping required in a 2D graph as shown in Fig. A.2. A line can be drawn to separate the input coordinates for which 0 is required as the output from those for which 1 is required as the output. The problem is thus linearly separable. A neuron with two inputs can set its weights to values which draw this line through this space, and such a one-layer network can thus solve the AND function.

For the XOR function, we can plot the mapping required in a 2D graph as shown in Fig. A.3. No straight line can be drawn to separate the input coordinates for which 0 is required as the output from those for which 1 is required as the output. The problem is thus not linearly separable. For a one-layer network, no set of weights can be found that will perform the XOR, or any other non-linearly separable function.

Although the inability of one-layer networks with binary neurons to solve non-linearly separable problems is a limitation, it is not in practice a major limitation on the processing that can be performed in a neural network for a number of reasons. First, if the inputs can take continuous values, then if the patterns are drawn from a random distribution, the one-layer

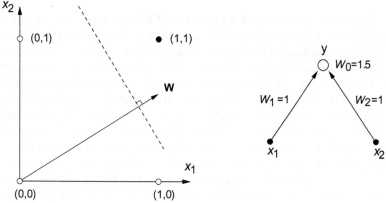

Fig. A.2 Left: the AND function shown in a 2D space. Input values for the two neurons are shown along the two axes of the space. The outputs required are plotted at the coordinates where the inputs intersect, and the values of the output required are shown as an open circle for 0, and a filled circle for 1. The AND function is linearly separable, in that a line can be drawn in the space which separates the coordinates for which 0 output is required from those from which a 1 output is required. **W** shows the direction of the weight vector. Right: a one-layer neural network can set its two weights w_1 and w_2 to values which allow the output neuron to be activated only if both inputs are present. In this diagram, w_0 is used to set a threshold for the neuron, and is connected to an input with value 1. The neuron thus fires only if the threshold of 1.5 is exceeded, which happens only if both inputs to the neuron are 1.

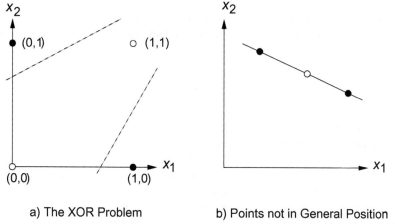

a) The XOR Problem   b) Points not in General Position

Fig. A.3 The XOR function shown in a 2D space. Input values for the two neurons are shown along the two axes of the space. The outputs required are plotted at the coordinates where the inputs intersect, and the values of the output required are shown as an open circle for 0, and a filled circle for 1. The XOR function is not linearly separable, in that a line cannot be drawn in the space to separate the coordinates for those from which a 0 output is required from those from which a 1 output is required. A one-layer neural network cannot set its two weights to values which allow the output neuron to be activated appropriately for the XOR function.

network can map up to $2C$ of them. Second, as described for pattern associators, and for one-layer error-correcting perceptrons (see Appendix B), these networks could be preceded by an expansion recoding network such as a competitive network with more output than input neurons. This effectively provides a two-layer network for solving the problem, and multilayer networks are in general capable of solving arbitrary mapping problems. Ways in which such multilayer networks might be trained are discussed in Chapter 2 and Appendix B.

More generally, a binary output unit provides by its operation a hyperplane (the hyperplane orthogonal to its synaptic weight vector as shown in Fig. A.2) that divides the input space in two. The input space is of dimension C, if C is the number of input axons or connections. A one-layer network with a number n of binary output units is equivalent to n hyperplanes, that could potentially divide the input space into as many as 2^n regions, each corresponding to input patterns leading to a different output. However the number p of *arbitrary* examples of the correct classification (each example consisting of an input pattern and its required correct output) that the network may be able to implement is well below 2^n, and in fact depends on C not on n. This is because for p too large it will be impossible to position the n weight vectors such that all examples of input vectors for which the first output unit is required to be 'on' fall on one side of the hyperplane associated with the first weight vector, all those for which it is required to be 'off' fall on the other side, and simultaneously the same holds with respect to the second output unit (a different dichotomy), the third, and so on. The limit on p, which can be thought of also as the number of independent associations implemented by the network, when this is viewed as a heteroassociator (i.e. pattern associator) with binary outputs, can be calculated with the Gardner method (Gardner, 1987, 1988) and depends on the statistics of the patterns. For input patterns that are also binary, random and with equal probability for each of the two states on every unit, the limit is $p_c = 2C$ (see further Appendix B, and Rolls and Treves (1998) Appendix A3).

A.2.2 Non-linear networks: neurons with non-linear activation functions

These concepts also help one to understand further the limitation of linear systems, and the power of non-linear systems. Consider the dot product operation by which the neuronal activation h is computed:

$$h = \sum_j x_j w_j. \tag{A.13}$$

If the output firing is just a linear function of the activation, any input pattern will produce a non-zero output unless it happens to be exactly orthogonal to the weight vector. For positive-only firing rates and synaptic weights, being orthogonal means taking non-zero values only on non-corresponding components. Since with distributed representations the non-zero components of different input firing vectors will in general be overlapping (i.e. some corresponding components in both firing rate vectors will be on, that is the vectors will overlap), this will result effectively in interference between any two different patterns that for example have to be associated to different outputs. Thus a basic limitation of linear networks is that they can perform pattern association perfectly only if the input patterns $\mathbf{x}$ are orthogonal; and for positive-only patterns that represent actual firing rates only if the different firing rate vectors are non-overlapping. Further, linear networks cannot of course perform any classification, just because they act linearly. (Classification implies producing output states that are clearly defined as being in one class, and not in other classes.) For example, in a linear network, if a pattern is presented that is intermediate between two patterns $\mathbf{v}_1$ and $\mathbf{v}_2$, such as $c_1\mathbf{v}_1 + c_2\mathbf{v}_2$, then the output pattern will be a linear combination of the outputs produced by $\mathbf{v}_1$ and $\mathbf{v}_2$ (e.g. $c_1\mathbf{o}_1 + c_2\mathbf{o}_2$), rather than being classified into $\mathbf{o}_1$ or $\mathbf{o}_2$. In contrast, with non-linear neurons, the patterns need not be orthogonal, only linearly separable, for a one-layer network to be able to correctly classify the patterns (provided that a sufficiently powerful learning rule is used – see Appendix B).

The networks just described, and most of those described in this book, are trained with a local learning rule, in which the pre- and post-synaptic terms needed to alter the synaptic weights are available locally in the synapses, in terms for example of the release of transmitter from the presynaptic terminal, and the depolarization of the postsynaptic neuron. This type of network is considered because this is a biologically plausible constraint (see Section 19.4). It is much less biologically plausible to use an algorithm such as multilayer error backpropagation which calculates the correction to the value of a synapse that is needed taking into account the values of the errors of the neurons at later stages of the system and the strengths of all the synapses to these neurons (see Section B.12). This use of a local learning rule is a major difference of the networks described in this book, which is directed at neurally plausible computation, from connectionist and artificial neural networks, which typically assume non-local learning rules and which therefore operate very differently from real neural networks in the brain (see Section B.12, McLeod, Plunkett and Rolls (1998), and Lillicrap et al. (2020)).

A.2.3 Non-linear networks: neurons with non-linear activations

Most of the networks described in this book calculate the activation h of each neuron as the linear product of the input firing weighted by the synaptic weight vector (see Equation A.13). This corresponds in a real neuron to receiving currents from each of its synapses which sum to produce depolarization of the neuronal cell body and the spike initiation region which is located very close to the cell body. This is a reasonable reflection of what does happen in many neurons, especially those with large dendrites such as pyramidal cells (Koch, 1999). This calculation of the activation h by a linear summation not only approximates to what happens in many real neurons, but is also a useful simplification which makes tractable the analysis of many classes of network that utilize such neurons. These analyses provide insight into the operation of networks of neurons, even if the linear summation assumption is not perfectly realized. Having computed the activation linearly, the neurons do of course for essentially all the networks described in this book, then utilize a non-linear activation function, which, as described above, provides the networks with much of their interesting computational power. Given that the activation functions of the neurons are non-linear, some non-linearity in the summation expressed in Equation A.13 may in practice be lumped into the non-linearity in the activation function.

However, another class of neuron that is implemented in some networks in the brain utilizes non-linearity in the calculation of the activation h of the neuron, which reflects a local product of two inputs to a neuron. This could arise for example if one synapse makes a presynaptic contact with another synapse which in turn connects to the dendrite, or if two synapses are close together on a thin dendrite. In such situations, the current injected into the neuron could reflect the conjoint firing of the two classes of input (Koch, 1999). The dendrite as a whole could then sum all such products into the cell body, leading to the description **Sigma-Pi**. This could be expressed by equation A.14

$$h = \sum_j \sum_k w_{jk} x_j x^c{}_k \qquad (A.14)$$

where x_j is the firing rate of input cell j, $x^c{}_k$ is the firing rate of input cell k of class c, and w_{jk} is the connection strength. Such Sigma-Pi neurons were utilized in the model described in Section B.5.5 of how idiothetic inputs could update a continuous attractor network. Another possible application is to learning invariant representations in neural networks. For example, the x^c input in equation A.14 could be a signal that varies with the shift required to compute translation invariance, effectively mapping the appropriate set of x_j inputs through to the output neurons depending on the shift required (Mel, Ruderman and Archie, 1998; Mel and Fiser, 2000; Olshausen, Anderson and Van Essen, 1993, 1995).

To train such a Sigma-Pi network requires that combinations of the two presynaptic inputs to a neuron be learned onto a neuron, using for example associativity with the post-synaptic term y, as exemplified in Equation A.15

$$\delta w_{jk} = \alpha y x_j x^c{}_k. \tag{A.15}$$

This learning principle is exemplified in the model described in Section B.5.5 of how idiothetic inputs could update a continuous attractor network to perform path integration.

Sigma-Pi networks are clearly very powerful, but require rather specialized anatomical and biophysical arrangements (see Koch (1999) and Mel et al. (2017)), and hence we do not use them unless they become very necessary in models of neural network operations in the brain. We have shown that in at least some applications such as path integration, it is possible to replace a Sigma-Pi network with a competitive network followed by a pattern association network (Stringer and Rolls, 2006).

Appendix 2 Neuronal network models

B.1 Introduction

Formal models of neural networks are needed in order to provide a basis for understanding the processing and memory functions performed by real neuronal networks in the brain. The formal models included in this Appendix all describe fundamental types of network found in different brain regions, and the computations they perform. Each of the types of network described can be thought of as providing one of the fundamental building blocks that the brain uses. Often these building blocks are combined within a brain area to perform a particular computation.

The aim of this Appendix is to describe a set of fundamental networks used by the brain, including the parts of the brain involved in memory, attention, decision-making, and the building of perceptual representations. As each type of network is introduced, we will point briefly to parts of the brain in which each network is found. Understanding these models provides a basis for understanding the theories of how different types of brain computations are performed. The descriptions of these networks are kept relatively concise in this Appendix. More detailed descriptions of some of the quantitative aspects of storage in pattern associators and autoassociators are provided in the Appendices of Rolls and Treves (1998) *Neural Networks and Brain Function*. Another book that provides a clear and quantitative introduction to some of these networks is Hertz, Krogh and Palmer (1991) *Introduction to the Theory of Neural Computation*, and other useful sources include Dayan and Abbott (2001), Gerstner et al. (2014) (who focus on neuronal dynamics), Amit (1989) (for attractor networks), Koch (1999) (for a biophysical approach), Wilson (1999) (on spiking networks), and Rolls (2016b).

Some of the background to the operation of the types of neuronal network described here, including a brief review of the evidence on neuronal structure and function, and on synaptic plasticity and the rules by which synaptic strength is modified, much based on studies with long-term potentiation, is provided in Chapter 1.

The network models on which we focus in this Appendix utilize a local learning rule, that is a rule for synaptic modification, in which the signals needed to alter the synaptic strength are present in the pre- and post-synaptic neurons. We focus on these networks because use of a local learning rule is biologically plausible. We discuss the issue of biological plausibility of the networks described, and show how they differ from less biologically plausible networks such as multilayer backpropagation of error networks, in Section 19.4.

B.2 Pattern association memory

A fundamental operation of most nervous systems is to learn to associate a first stimulus with a second that occurs at about the same time, and to retrieve the second stimulus when the first is presented. The first stimulus might be the sight of food, and the second stimulus the taste of food. After the association has been learned, the sight of food would enable its taste to be retrieved. In classical conditioning, the taste of food might elicit an unconditioned response of salivation, and if the sight of the food is paired with its taste, then the sight of that food would

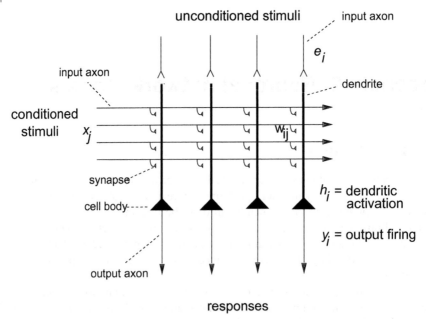

Fig. B.1 A pattern association memory. An unconditioned stimulus has activity or firing rate e_i for the ith neuron, and produces firing y_i of the ith neuron. An unconditioned stimulus may be treated as a vector, across the set of neurons indexed by i, of activity **e**. The firing rate response can also be thought of as a vector of firing **y**. The conditioned stimuli have activity or firing rate x_j for the jth axon, which can also be treated as a vector **x**.

by learning come to produce salivation. Pattern associators are thus used where the outputs of the visual system interface to learning systems in the orbitofrontal cortex and amygdala that learn associations between the sight of objects and their taste or touch in stimulus–reinforcer association learning (see Chapter 11). Pattern association is also used throughout the cerebral (neo)cortical areas, as it is the architecture that describes the backprojection connections from one cortical area to the preceding cortical area (see Chapters 1, 9 and 13). Pattern association thus contributes to implementing top-down influences in attention, including the effects of attention from higher to lower cortical areas, and thus between the visual object and spatial processing streams (Rolls and Deco, 2002) (see Chapter 13); the effects of mood on memory and visual information processing (Rolls and Stringer, 2001b); the recall of visual memories; and the operation of short-term memory systems (see Section 13.6.1).

B.2.1 Architecture and operation

The essential elements necessary for pattern association, forming what could be called a prototypical pattern associator network, are shown in Fig. B.1. What we have called the second or unconditioned stimulus pattern is applied through unmodifiable synapses generating an input to each neuron, which, being external with respect to the synaptic matrix we focus on, we can call the external input e_i for the ith neuron. [We can also treat this as a vector, **e**, as indicated in the legend to Fig. B.1. Vectors and simple operations performed with them are summarized in Appendix A. This unconditioned stimulus is dominant in producing or forcing the firing of the output neurons (y_i for the ith neuron, or the vector **y**)]. At the same time, the first or conditioned stimulus pattern consisting of the set of firings on the horizontally running input axons in Fig. B.1 (x_j for the jth axon) (or equivalently the vector **x**) is applied through modifiable synapses w_{ij} to the dendrites of the output neurons. The synapses are modifiable in such a way that if there is presynaptic firing on an input axon x_j paired during learning with postsynaptic activity on neuron i, then the strength or weight w_{ij} between that axon and the dendrite increases. This simple learning rule is often called the Hebb rule, after Donald Hebb who in 1949 formulated the hypothesis that if the firing of one neuron was regularly associated with another, then the strength of the synapse or synapses between the neurons should increase[24]. After learning, presenting the pattern x on the input axons will activate the dendrite through the strengthened synapses. If the cue or conditioned stimulus pattern is the same as that learned, the postsynaptic neurons will be activated, even in the absence of the external or unconditioned input, as each of the firing axons produces through a strengthened synapse some activation of the postsynaptic element, the dendrite. The total activation h_i of each postsynaptic neuron i is then the sum of such individual activations. In this way, the 'correct' output neurons, that is those activated during learning, can end up being the ones most strongly activated, and the second or unconditioned stimulus can be effectively recalled. The recall is best when only strong activation of the postsynaptic neuron produces firing, that is if there is a threshold for firing, just like real neurons. The advantages of this are evident when many associations are stored in the memory, as will soon be shown.

Next we introduce a more precise description of the above by writing down explicit mathematical rules for the operation of the simple network model of Fig. B.1, which will help us to understand how pattern association memories in general operate. (In this description we introduce simple vector operations, and, for those who are not familiar with these, refer the reader to Appendix A.) We have denoted above a conditioned stimulus input pattern as x. Each of the axons has a firing rate, and if we count or index through the axons using the subscript j, the firing rate of the first axon is x_1, of the second x_2, of the jth x_j, etc. The whole set of axons forms a vector, which is just an ordered (1, 2, 3, etc.) set of elements. The firing rate of each axon x_j is one element of the firing rate vector x. Similarly, using i as the index, we can denote the firing rate of any output neuron as y_i, and the firing rate output vector as y. With this terminology, we can then identify any synapse onto neuron i from neuron j as w_{ij} (see Fig. B.1). In this book, the first index, i, always refers to the receiving neuron (and thus signifies a dendrite), while the second index, j, refers to the sending neuron (and thus signifies a conditioned stimulus input axon in Fig. B.1). We can now specify the learning and retrieval operations as follows:

B.2.1.1 Learning

The firing rate of every output neuron is forced to a value determined by the unconditioned (or external or forcing stimulus) input e_i. In our simple model this means that for any one neuron i,

$$y_i = \mathrm{f}(e_i) \tag{B.1}$$

which indicates that the firing rate is a function of the dendritic activation, taken in this case to reduce essentially to that resulting from the external forcing input (see Fig. B.1). The function f is called the activation function (see Fig. 1.3), and its precise form is irrelevant, at least during this learning phase. For example, the function at its simplest could be taken to be linear, so that the firing rate would be just proportional to the activation.

The Hebb rule can then be written as follows:

$$\delta w_{ij} = \alpha y_i x_j \tag{B.2}$$

---

[24] In fact, the terms in which Hebb put the hypothesis were a little different from an association memory, in that he stated that if one neuron regularly comes to elicit firing in another, then the strength of the synapses should increase. He had in mind the building of what he called cell assemblies. In a pattern associator, the conditioned stimulus need not produce before learning any significant activation of the output neurons. The connection strengths must simply increase if there is associated pre- and postsynaptic firing when, in pattern association, most of the postsynaptic firing is being produced by a different input.

where δw_{ij} is the change of the synaptic weight w_{ij} that results from the simultaneous (or conjunctive) presence of presynaptic firing x_j and postsynaptic firing or activation y_i, and α is a learning rate constant that specifies how much the synapses alter on any one pairing.

The Hebb rule is expressed in this multiplicative form to reflect the idea that both presynaptic and postsynaptic activity must be present for the synapses to increase in strength. The multiplicative form also reflects the idea that strong pre- and postsynaptic firing will produce a larger change of synaptic weight than smaller firing rates. It is also assumed for now that before any learning takes place, the synaptic strengths are small in relation to the changes that can be produced during Hebbian learning. We will see that this assumption can be relaxed later when a modified Hebb rule is introduced that can lead to a reduction in synaptic strength under some conditions.

B.2.1.2 Recall

When the conditioned stimulus is present on the input axons, the total activation h_i of a neuron i is the sum of all the activations produced through each strengthened synapse w_{ij} by each active neuron x_j. We can express this as

$$h_i = \sum_{j=1}^{C} x_j w_{ij} \tag{B.3}$$

where $\sum_{j=1}^{C}$ indicates that the sum is over the C input axons (or connections) indexed by j to each neuron.

The multiplicative form here indicates that activation should be produced by an axon only if it is firing, and only if it is connected to the dendrite by a strengthened synapse. It also indicates that the strength of the activation reflects how fast the axon x_j is firing, and how strong the synapse w_{ij} is. The sum of all such activations expresses the idea that summation (of synaptic currents in real neurons) occurs along the length of the dendrite, to produce activation at the cell body, where the activation h_i is converted into firing y_i. This conversion can be expressed as

$$y_i = \text{f}(h_i) \tag{B.4}$$

where the function f is again the activation function. The form of the function now becomes more important. Real neurons have thresholds, with firing occurring only if the activation is above the threshold. A threshold linear activation function is shown in Fig. 1.3b on page 8. This has been useful in formal analysis of the properties of neural networks. Neurons also have firing rates that become saturated at a maximum rate, and we could express this as the sigmoid activation function shown in Fig. 1.3c. Yet another simple activation function, used in some models of neural networks, is the binary threshold function (Fig. 1.3d), which indicates that if the activation is below threshold, there is no firing, and that if the activation is above threshold, the neuron fires maximally. Whatever the exact shape of the activation function, some non-linearity is an advantage, for it enables small activations produced by interfering memories to be minimized, and it can enable neurons to perform logical operations, such as to fire or respond only if two or more sets of inputs are present simultaneously.

B.2.2 A simple model

An example of these learning and recall operations is provided in a simple form as follows. The neurons will have simple firing rates, which can be 0 to represent no activity, and 1 to indicate high firing. They are thus binary neurons, which can assume one of two firing rates. If we have a pattern associator with six input axons and four output neurons, we could represent the network before learning, with the same layout as in Fig. B.1, as shown in Fig. B.2:

```
           U C S
           1 1 0 0
           ↓ ↓ ↓ ↓
    CS
    1 →   0 0 0 0
    0 →   0 0 0 0
    1 →   0 0 0 0
    0 →   0 0 0 0
    1 →   0 0 0 0
    0 →   0 0 0 0
```

Fig. B.2 Pattern association: before synaptic modification. The unconditioned stimulus (UCS) firing rates are shown as 1 if high and 0 if low as a row vector being applied to force firing of the four output neurons. The six conditioned stimulus (CS) firing rates are shown as a column vector being applied to the vertical dendrites of the output neurons which have initial synaptic weights of 0.

where $\mathbf{x}$ or the conditioned stimulus (CS) is 101010, and $\mathbf{y}$ or the firing produced by the unconditioned stimulus (UCS) is 1100. (The arrows indicate the flow of signals.) The synaptic weights are initially all 0.

After pairing the CS with the UCS during one learning trial, some of the synaptic weights will be incremented according to Equation B.2, so that after learning this pair the synaptic weights will become as shown in Fig. B.3:

```
           U C S
           1 1 0 0
           ↓ ↓ ↓ ↓
    CS
    1 →   1 1 0 0
    0 →   0 0 0 0
    1 →   1 1 0 0
    0 →   0 0 0 0
    1 →   1 1 0 0
    0 →   0 0 0 0
```

Fig. B.3 Pattern association: after synaptic modification. The synapses where there is conjunctive pre- and post-synaptic activity have been strengthened to value 1.

We can represent what happens during recall, when, for example, we present the CS that has been learned, as shown in Fig. B.4:

```
              CS
     1 →     1  1  0  0
     0 →     0  0  0  0
     1 →     1  1  0  0
     0 →     0  0  0  0
     1 →     1  1  0  0
     0 →     0  0  0  0
             ↓  ↓  ↓  ↓

             3  3  0  0  Activation h_i
             1  1  0  0  Firing y_i
```

Fig. B.4 Pattern association: recall. The activation h_i of each neuron i is converted with a threshold of 2 to the binary firing rate y_i (1 for high, and 0 for low).

The activation of the four output neurons is 3300, and if we set the threshold of each output neuron to 2, then the output firing is 1100 (where the binary firing rate is 0 if below threshold, and 1 if above). The pattern associator has thus achieved recall of the pattern 1100, which is correct.

We can now illustrate how a number of different associations can be stored in such a pattern associator, and retrieved correctly. Let us associate a new CS pattern 110001 with the UCS 0101 in the same pattern associator. The weights will become as shown next in Fig. B.5 after learning:

```
                      U  C  S
                      0  1  0  1
                      ↓  ↓  ↓  ↓
              CS
              1 →     1  2  0  1
              1 →     0  1  0  1
              0 →     1  1  0  0
              0 →     0  0  0  0
              0 →     1  1  0  0
              1 →     0  1  0  1
```

Fig. B.5 Pattern association: synaptic weights after learning a second pattern association.

If we now present the second CS, the retrieval is as shown in Fig. B.6:

```
              CS
      1 →    1  2  0  1
      1 →    0  1  0  1
      0 →    1  1  0  0
      0 →    0  0  0  0
      0 →    1  1  0  0
      1 →    0  1  0  1
              ↓  ↓  ↓  ↓

             1  4  0  3   Activation hᵢ
             0  1  0  1   Firing yᵢ
```

Fig. B.6 Pattern association: recall with the second CS.

The binary output firings were again produced with the threshold set to 2. Recall is perfect.

This illustration shows the value of some threshold non-linearity in the activation function of the neurons. In this case, the activations did reflect some small cross-talk or interference from the previous pattern association of CS1 with UCS1, but this was removed by the threshold operation, to clean up the recall firing. The example also shows that when further associations are learned by a pattern associator trained with the Hebb rule, Equation B.2, some synapses will reflect increments above a synaptic strength of 1. It is left as an exercise to the reader to verify that recall is still perfect to CS1, the vector 101010. (The activation vector **h** is 3401, and the output firing vector **y** with the same threshold of 2 is 1100, which is perfect recall.)

B.2.3 The vector interpretation

The way in which recall is produced, Equation B.3, consists for each output neuron i of multiplying each input firing rate x_j by the corresponding synaptic weight w_{ij} and summing the products to obtain the activation h_i. Now we can consider the firing rates x_j where j varies from 1 to N', the number of axons, to be a vector. (A vector is simply an ordered set of numbers – see Appendix A.) Let us call this vector **x**. Similarly, on a neuron i, the synaptic weights can be treated as a vector, $\mathbf{w}_i$. (The subscript i here indicates that this is the weight vector on the ith neuron.) The operation we have just described to obtain the activation of an output neuron can now be seen to be a simple multiplication operation of two vectors to produce a single output value (called a scalar output). This is the inner product or dot product of two vectors, and can be written

$$h_i = \mathbf{x} \cdot \mathbf{w}_i. \tag{B.5}$$

The inner product of two vectors indicates how similar they are. If two vectors have corresponding elements the same, then the dot product will be maximal. If the two vectors are similar but not identical, then the dot product will be high. If the two vectors are completely different, the dot product will be 0, and the vectors are described as orthogonal. (The term orthogonal means at right angles, and arises from the geometric interpretation of vectors, which is summarized in Appendix A.) Thus the dot product provides a direct measure of how similar two vectors are.

It can now be seen that a fundamental operation many neurons perform is effectively to compute how similar an input pattern vector **x** is to their stored weight vector $\mathbf{w}_i$. The similarity measure they compute, the dot product, is a very good measure of similarity, and indeed, the standard (Pearson product–moment) correlation coefficient used in statistics is the same as a normalized dot product with the mean subtracted from each vector, as shown in Appendix A. (The normalization used in the correlation coefficient results in the coefficient varying always between $+1$ and -1, whereas the actual scalar value of a dot product clearly depends on the length of the vectors from which it is calculated.)

With these concepts, we can now see that during learning, a pattern associator adds to its weight vector a vector $\delta\mathbf{w}_i$ that has the same pattern as the input pattern **x**, if the postsynaptic neuron i is strongly activated. Indeed, we can express Equation B.2 in vector form as

$$\delta\mathbf{w}_i = \alpha y_i \mathbf{x}. \tag{B.6}$$

We can now see that what is recalled by the neuron depends on the similarity of the recall cue vector $\mathbf{x}_r$ to the originally learned vector **x**. The fact that during recall the output of each neuron reflects the similarity (as measured by the dot product) of the input pattern $\mathbf{x}_r$ to each of the patterns used originally as **x** inputs (conditioned stimuli in Fig. B.1) provides a simple way to appreciate many of the interesting and biologically useful properties of pattern associators, as described next.

B.2.4 Properties

B.2.4.1 Generalization

During recall, pattern associators generalize, and produce appropriate outputs if a recall cue vector $\mathbf{x}_r$ is similar to a vector that has been learned already. This occurs because the recall operation involves computing the dot (inner) product of the input pattern vector $\mathbf{x}_r$ with the synaptic weight vector $\mathbf{w}_i$, so that the firing produced, y_i, reflects the similarity of the current input to the previously learned input pattern **x**. (Generalization will occur to input cue or conditioned stimulus patterns $\mathbf{x}_r$ that are incomplete versions of an original conditioned stimulus **x**, although the term completion is usually applied to the autoassociation networks described in Section B.3.)

This is an extremely important property of pattern associators, for input stimuli during recall will rarely be absolutely identical to what has been learned previously, and automatic generalization to similar stimuli is extremely useful, and has great adaptive value in biological systems.

Generalization can be illustrated with the simple binary pattern associator considered above. (Those who have appreciated the vector description just given might wish to skip this illustration.) Instead of the second CS, pattern vector 110001, we will use the similar recall cue 110100, as shown in Fig. B.7:

```
                    CS
            1 →     1   2   0   1
            1 →     0   1   0   1
            0 →     1   1   0   0
            1 →     0   0   0   0
            0 →     1   1   0   0
            0 →     0   1   0   1
                    ↓   ↓   ↓   ↓

                    1   3   0   2   Activation $h_i$
                    0   1   0   1   Firing $y_i$
```

Fig. B.7 Pattern association: generalization using an input vector similar to the second CS.

It is seen that the output firing rate vector, 0101, is exactly what should be recalled to CS2 (and not to CS1), so correct generalization has occurred. Although this is a small network trained with few examples, the same properties hold for large networks with large numbers of stored patterns, as described more quantitatively in Section B.2.7.1 on capacity below and in Appendix A3 of Rolls and Treves (1998).

B.2.4.2 Graceful degradation or fault tolerance

If the synaptic weight vector w_i (or the weight matrix, which we can call W) has synapses missing (e.g. during development), or loses synapses, then the activation h_i or h is still reasonable, because h_i is the dot product (correlation) of x with w_i. The result, especially after passing through the activation function, can frequently be perfect recall. The same property arises if for example one or some of the conditioned stimulus (CS) input axons are lost or damaged. This is a very important property of associative memories, and is not a property of conventional computer memories, which produce incorrect data if even only 1 storage location (for 1 bit or binary digit of data) of their memory is damaged or cannot be accessed. This property of graceful degradation is of great adaptive value for biological systems.

We can illustrate this with a simple example. If we damage two of the synapses in Fig. B.6 to produce the synaptic matrix shown in Fig. B.8 (where x indicates a damaged synapse which has no effect, but was previously 1), and now present the second CS, the retrieval is as follows:

```
                    CS
            1 →     1   2   0   1
            1 →     0   1   0   x
            0 →     1   1   0   0
            0 →     0   0   0   0
            0 →     1   x   0   0
            1 →     0   1   0   1
                    ↓   ↓   ↓   ↓

                    1   4   0   2   Activation $h_i$
                    0   1   0   1   Firing $y_i$
```

Fig. B.8 Pattern association: graceful degradation when some synapses are damaged (x).

The binary output firings were again produced with the threshold set to 2. The recalled vector, 0101, is perfect. This illustration again shows the value of some threshold non-linearity in the activation function of the neurons. It is left as an exercise to the reader to verify that recall is still perfect to CS1, the vector 101010. (The output activation vector **h** is 3301, and the output firing vector **y** with the same threshold of 2 is 1100, which is perfect recall.)

B.2.4.3 The importance of distributed representations for pattern associators

A distributed representation is one in which the firing or activity of all the elements in the vector is used to encode a particular stimulus. For example, in a conditioned stimulus vector CS1 that has the value 101010, we need to know the state of all the elements to know which stimulus is being represented. Another stimulus, CS2, is represented by the vector 110001. We can represent many different events or stimuli with such overlapping sets of elements, and because in general any one element cannot be used to identify the stimulus, but instead the information about which stimulus is present is distributed over the population of elements or neurons, this is called a distributed representation (see Section 1.7). If, for binary neurons, half the neurons are in one state (e.g. 0), and the other half are in the other state (e.g. 1), then the representation is described as fully distributed. The CS representations above are thus fully distributed. If only a smaller proportion of the neurons is active to represent a stimulus, as in the vector 100001, then this is a sparse representation. For binary representations, we can quantify the sparseness by the proportion of neurons in the active (1) state.

In contrast, a local representation is one in which all the information that a particular stimulus or event has occurred is provided by the activity of one of the neurons, or elements in the vector. One stimulus might be represented by the vector 100000, another stimulus by the vector 010000, and a third stimulus by the vector 001000. The activity of neuron or element 1 would indicate that stimulus 1 was present, and of neuron 2, that stimulus 2 was present. The representation is local in that if a particular neuron is active, we know that the stimulus represented by that neuron is present. In neurophysiology, if such cells were present, they might be called 'grandmother cells' (cf. Barlow (1972), (1995); see Chapter 1 and Appendix C), in that one neuron might represent a stimulus in the environment as complex and specific as one's grandmother. Where the activity of a number of cells must be taken into account in order to represent a stimulus (such as an individual taste), then the representation is sometimes described as using ensemble encoding.

The properties just described for associative memories, generalization, and graceful degradation are only implemented if the representation of the CS or **x** vector is distributed. This occurs because the recall operation involves computing the dot (inner) product of the input pattern vector $\mathbf{x}_r$ with the synaptic weight vector $\mathbf{w}_i$. This allows the activation h_i to reflect the similarity of the current input pattern to a previously learned input pattern **x** only if several or many elements of the **x** and $\mathbf{x}_r$ vectors are in the active state to represent a pattern. If local encoding were used, e.g. 100000, then if the first element of the vector (which might be the firing of axon 1, i.e. x_1, or the strength of synapse $i1$, w_{i1}) is lost, the resulting vector is not similar to any other CS vector, and the activation is 0. In the case of local encoding, the important properties of associative memories, generalization and graceful degradation do not thus emerge. Graceful degradation and generalization are dependent on distributed representations, for then the dot product can reflect similarity even when some elements of the vectors involved are altered. If we think of the correlation between Y and X in a graph, then this correlation is affected only a little if a few X, Y pairs of data are lost (see Appendix A).

B.2.5 Prototype extraction, extraction of central tendency, and noise reduction

If a set of similar conditioned stimulus vectors **x** are paired with the same unconditioned stimulus e_i, the weight vector $\mathbf{w}_i$ becomes (or points towards) the sum (or with scaling, the average) of the set of similar vectors **x**. This follows from the operation of the Hebb rule in Equation B.2. When tested at recall, the output of the memory is then best to the average input pattern vector denoted $<\mathbf{x}>$. If the average is thought of as a prototype, then even though the prototype vector $<\mathbf{x}>$ itself may never have been seen, the best output of the neuron or network is to the prototype. This produces 'extraction of the prototype' or 'central tendency'. The same phenomenon is a feature of human memory performance (see McClelland and Rumelhart (1986) Chapter 17), and this simple process with distributed representations in a neural network accounts for the psychological phenomenon.

If the different exemplars of the vector **x** are thought of as noisy versions of the true input pattern vector $<\mathbf{x}>$ (with incorrect values for some of the elements), then the pattern associator has performed 'noise reduction', in that the output produced by any one of these vectors will represent the output produced by the true, noiseless, average vector $<\mathbf{x}>$.

B.2.6 Speed

Recall is very fast in a real neuronal network, because the conditioned stimulus input firings x_j ($j = 1, C$ axons) can be applied simultaneously to the synapses w_{ij}, and the activation h_i can be accumulated in one or two time constants of the dendrite (e.g. 10–20 ms). Whenever the threshold of the cell is exceeded, it fires. Thus, in effectively one step, which takes the brain no more than 10–20 ms, all the output neurons of the pattern associator can be firing with rates that reflect the input firing of every axon. This is very different from a conventional digital computer, in which computing h_i in Equation B.3 would involve C multiplication and addition operations occurring one after another, or $2C$ time steps.

The brain performs parallel computation in at least two senses in even a pattern associator. One is that for a single neuron, the separate contributions of the firing rate x_j of each axon j multiplied by the synaptic weight w_{ij} are computed in parallel and added in the same timestep. The second is that this can be performed in parallel for all neurons $i = 1, N$ in the network, where there are N output neurons in the network. It is these types of parallel and time-continuous (see Section B.6) processing that enable these classes of neuronal network in the brain to operate so fast, in effectively so few steps.

Learning is also fast ('one-shot') in pattern associators, in that a single pairing of the conditioned stimulus **x** and the unconditioned stimulus (UCS) **e** which produces the unconditioned output firing **y** enables the association to be learned. There is no need to repeat the pairing in order to discover over many trials the appropriate mapping. This is extremely important for biological systems, in which a single co-occurrence of two events may lead to learning that could have life-saving consequences. (For example, the pairing of a visual stimulus with a potentially life-threatening aversive event may enable that event to be avoided in future.) Although repeated pairing with small variations of the vectors is used to obtain the useful properties of prototype extraction, extraction of central tendency, and noise reduction, the essential properties of generalization and graceful degradation are obtained with just one pairing. The actual time scales of the learning in the brain are indicated by studies of associative synaptic modification using long-term potentiation paradigms (LTP, see Section 1.6). Co-occurrence or near simultaneity of the CS and UCS is required for periods of as little as 100 ms, with expression of the synaptic modification being present within typically a few seconds.

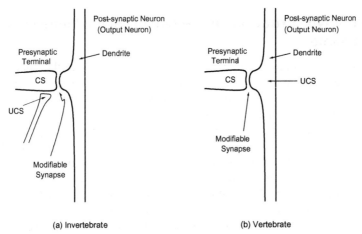

(a) Invertebrate (b) Vertebrate

Fig. B.9 (b) In vertebrate pattern association learning, the unconditioned stimulus (UCS) may be made available at all the conditioned stimulus (CS) terminals onto the output neuron because the dendrite of the postsynaptic neuron is electrically short, so that the effect of the UCS spreads for long distances along the dendrite. (a) In contrast, in at least some invertebrate association learning systems, the unconditioned stimulus or teaching input makes a synapse onto the presynaptic terminal carrying the conditioned stimulus.

B.2.7 Local learning rule

The simplest learning rule used in pattern association neural networks, a version of the Hebb rule, is, as shown in Equation B.2 above,

$$\delta w_{ij} = \alpha y_i x_j.$$

This is a local learning rule in that the information required to specify the change in synaptic weight is available locally at the synapse, as it is dependent only on the presynaptic firing rate x_j available at the synaptic terminal, and the postsynaptic activation or firing y_i available on the dendrite of the neuron receiving the synapse (see Fig. B.9b). This makes the learning rule biologically plausible, in that the information about how to change the synaptic weight does not have to be carried from a distant source, where it is computed, to every synapse. Such a non-local learning rule would not be biologically plausible, in that there are no appropriate connections known in most parts of the brain to bring in the synaptic training or teacher signal to every synapse.

Evidence that a learning rule with the general form of Equation B.2 is implemented in at least some parts of the brain comes from studies of long-term potentiation, described in Section 1.6. Long-term potentiation (LTP) has the synaptic specificity defined by Equation B.2, in that only synapses from active afferents, not those from inactive afferents, become strengthened. Synaptic specificity is important for a pattern associator, and most other types of neuronal network, to operate correctly. The number of independently modifiable synapses on each neuron is a primary factor in determining how many different memory patterns can be stored in associative memories (see Sections B.2.7.1 and B.3.3.7).

Another useful property of real neurons in relation to Equation B.2 is that the postsynaptic term, y_i, is available on much of the dendrite of a cell, because the electrotonic length of the dendrite is short. In addition, active propagation of spiking activity from the cell body along the dendrite may help to provide a uniform postsynaptic term for the learning. Thus if a neuron is strongly activated with a high value for y_i, then any active synapse onto the cell will be capable of being modified. This enables the cell to learn an association between the pattern of activity on all its axons and its postsynaptic activation, which is stored as an addition to its weight vector $\mathbf{w}_i$. Then later on, at recall, the output can be produced as a vector dot product operation between the input pattern vector $\mathbf{x}$ and the weight vector $\mathbf{w}_i$, so that the output of the cell can reflect the correlation between the current input vector and what has previously been learned by the cell.

It is interesting that at least many invertebrate neuronal systems may operate very differently from those described here, as described by Rolls and Treves (1998) (see Fig. B.9a). If there were 5,000 conditioned stimulus inputs to a neuron, the implication is that every one would need to have a presynaptic terminal conveying the same UCS to each presynaptic terminal, which is hardly plausible. The implication is that at least some invertebrate neural systems operate very differently to those in vertebrates and, in such systems, the useful properties that arise from using distributed CS representations such as generalization would not arise in the same simple way as a property of the network.

B.2.7.1 Capacity

The question of the storage capacity of a pattern associator is considered in detail in Appendix A3 of Rolls and Treves (1998). It is pointed out there that, for this type of associative network, the number of memories that it can hold simultaneously in storage has to be analyzed together with the retrieval quality of each output representation, and then only for a given quality of the representation provided in the input. This is in contrast to autoassociative nets (Section B.3), in which a critical number of stored memories exists (as a function of various parameters of the network), beyond which attempting to store additional memories results in it becoming impossible to retrieve essentially anything. With a pattern associator, instead, one will always retrieve something, but this something will be very small (in information or correlation terms) if too many associations are simultaneously in storage and/or if too little is provided as input.

The conjoint quality–capacity input analysis can be carried out, for any specific instance of a pattern associator, by using formal mathematical models and established analytical procedures (see e.g. Treves (1995), Rolls and Treves (1998), Treves (1990) and Rolls and Treves (1990)). This, however, has to be done case by case. It is anyway useful to develop some intuition for how a pattern associator operates, by considering what its capacity would be in certain well-defined simplified cases.

Linear associative neuronal networks These networks are made up of units with a linear activation function, which appears to make them unsuitable to represent real neurons with their positive-only firing rates. However, even purely linear units have been considered as provisionally relevant models of real neurons, by assuming that the latter operate sometimes in the linear regime of their transfer function. (This implies a high level of spontaneous activity, and may be closer to conditions observed early on in sensory systems rather than in areas more specifically involved in memory.) As usual, the connections are trained by a Hebb (or similar) associative learning rule. The capacity of these networks can be defined as the total number of associations that can be learned independently of each other, given that the linear nature of these systems prevents anything more than a linear transform of the inputs. This implies that if input pattern C can be written as the weighted sum of input patterns A and B, the output to C will be just the same weighted sum of the outputs to A and B. If there are N' input axons, then there can be only at most N' mutually independent input patterns (i.e. none able to be written as a weighted sum of the others), and therefore the capacity of linear networks, defined above, is just N', or equal to the number of inputs to each neuron. In general, a random set of less than N' vectors (the CS input pattern vectors) will tend to be mutually independent but not mutually orthogonal (at 90 deg to each other) (see Appendix A). If they are not orthogonal (the normal situation), then the dot product of them is not 0, and the output pattern activated by one of the input vectors will be partially activated by other input pattern vectors, in accordance with how similar they are (see Equations B.5 and B.6).

This amounts to interference, which is therefore the more serious the less orthogonal, on the whole, is the set of input vectors.

Since input patterns are made of elements with positive values, if a simple Hebbian learning rule like the one of Equation B.2 is used (in which the input pattern enters directly with no subtraction term), the output resulting from the application of a stored input vector will be the sum of contributions from all other input vectors that have a non-zero dot product with it (see Appendix A), and interference will be disastrous. The only situation in which this would not occur is when different input patterns activate completely different input lines, but this is clearly an uninteresting circumstance for networks operating with distributed representations. A solution to this issue is to use a modified learning rule of the following form:

$$\delta w_{ij} = \alpha y_i (x_j - x) \tag{B.7}$$

where x is a constant, approximately equal to the average value of x_j. This learning rule includes (in proportion to y_i) increasing the synaptic weight if $(x_j - x) > 0$ (long-term potentiation), and decreasing the synaptic weight if $(x_j - x) < 0$ (heterosynaptic long-term depression). It is useful for x to be roughly the average activity of an input axon x_j across patterns, because then the dot product between the various patterns stored on the weights and the input vector will tend to cancel out with the subtractive term, except for the pattern equal to (or correlated with) the input vector itself. Then up to N' input vectors can still be learned by the network, with only minor interference (provided of course that they are mutually independent, as they will in general tend to be).

Table B.1 Effects of pre- and post-synaptic activity on synaptic modification

		Post-synaptic activation	
		0	high
Presynaptic firing	0	No change	Heterosynaptic LTD
	high	Homosynaptic LTD	LTP

This modified learning rule can also be described in terms of a contingency table (Table B.1) showing the synaptic strength modifications produced by different types of learning rule, where LTP indicates an increase in synaptic strength (called long-term potentiation in neurophysiology), and LTD indicates a decrease in synaptic strength (called long-term depression in neurophysiology). Heterosynaptic long-term depression is so-called because it is the decrease in synaptic strength that occurs to a synapse that is other than that through which the postsynaptic cell is being activated. This heterosynaptic long-term depression is the type of change of synaptic strength that is required (in addition to LTP) for effective subtraction of the average presynaptic firing rate, in order, as it were, to make the CS vectors appear more orthogonal to the pattern associator. The rule is sometimes called the Singer–Stent rule, after work by Singer (1987) and Stent (1973), and was discovered in the brain by Levy (Levy, 1985; Levy and Desmond, 1985) (see also Brown, Kairiss and Keenan (1990b)). Homosynaptic long-term depression is so-called because it is the decrease in synaptic strength that occurs to a synapse which is (the same as that which is) active. For it to occur, the postsynaptic neuron must simultaneously be inactive, or have only low activity. (This rule is sometimes called the BCM rule after the paper of Bienenstock, Cooper and Munro (1982); see Rolls and

Deco (2002), Chapter 7).

Associative neuronal networks with non-linear neurons With non-linear neurons, that is with at least a threshold in the activation function so that the output firing y_i is 0 when the activation h_i is below the threshold, the capacity can be measured in terms of the number of different clusters of output pattern vectors that the network produces. This is because the non-linearities now present (one per output neuron) result in some clustering of the outputs produced by all possible (conditioned stimulus) input patterns **x**. Input patterns that are similar to a stored input vector can produce, due to the non-linearities, output patterns even closer to the stored output; and vice versa, sufficiently dissimilar inputs can be assigned to different output clusters thereby increasing their mutual dissimilarity. As with the linear counterpart, in order to remove the correlation that would otherwise occur between the patterns because the elements can take only positive values, it is useful to use a modified Hebb rule of the form shown in Equation B.7.

With fully distributed output patterns, the number p of associations that leads to different clusters is of order C, the number of input lines (axons) per output neuron (that is, of order N' for a fully connected network), as shown in Appendix A3 of Rolls and Treves (1998). If sparse patterns are used in the output, or alternatively if the learning rule includes a non-linear postsynaptic factor that is effectively equivalent to using sparse output patterns, the coefficient of proportionality between p and C can be much higher than one, that is, many more patterns can be stored than inputs onto each output neuron (see Appendix A3 of Rolls and Treves (1998)). Indeed, the number of different patterns or prototypes p that can be stored can be derived for example in the case of binary units (Gardner, 1988) to be

$$p \approx C/[a_o log(1/a_o)] \tag{B.8}$$

where a_o is the sparseness of the output firing pattern **y** produced by the unconditioned stimulus. p can in this situation be much larger than C (see Appendix A3 of Rolls and Treves (1998), Rolls and Treves (1990) and Treves (1990)). This is an important result for encoding in pattern associators, for it means that provided that the activation functions are non-linear (which is the case with real neurons), there is a very great advantage to using sparse encoding, for then many more than C pattern associations can be stored. Sparse representations may well be present in brain regions involved in associative memory for this reason (see Appendix C).

The non-linearity inherent in the NMDA receptor-based Hebbian plasticity present in the brain may help to make the stored patterns more sparse than the input patterns, and this may be especially beneficial in increasing the storage capacity of associative networks in the brain by allowing participation in the storage of especially those relatively few neurons with high firing rates in the exponential firing rate distributions typical of neurons in sensory systems (see Appendix C).

Dilution of the connectivity in pattern association networks can help to maximize capacity by reducing the probability of more than one synapse between an input and output neuron (Rolls, 2015a).

B.2.7.2 Interference

Interference occurs in linear pattern associators if two vectors are not orthogonal, and is simply dependent on the angle between the originally learned vector and the recall cue or CS vector (see Appendix A), for the activation of the output neuron depends simply on the dot product of the recall vector and the synaptic weight vector (equation B.5). Also in non-linear pattern associators (the interesting case for all practical purposes), interference may occur if two CS patterns are not orthogonal, though the effect can be controlled with sparse encoding

Input A	1	0	1
Input B	0	1	1
Required Output	1	1	0

Fig. B.10 A non-linearly separable mapping.

of the UCS patterns, effectively by setting high thresholds for the firing of output units. In other words, the CS vectors need not be strictly orthogonal, but if they are too similar, some interference will still be likely to occur.

The fact that interference is a property of neural network pattern associator memories is of interest, for interference is a major property of human memory. Indeed, the fact that interference is a property of human memory and of neural network association memories is entirely consistent with the hypothesis that human memory is stored in associative memories of the type described here, or at least that network associative memories of the type described represent a useful exemplar of the class of parallel distributed storage network used in human memory.

It may also be suggested that one reason that interference is tolerated in biological memory is that it is associated with the ability to generalize between stimuli, which is an invaluable feature of biological network associative memories, in that it allows the memory to cope with stimuli that will almost never be identical on different occasions, and in that it allows useful analogies that have survival value to be made.

B.2.7.3 Expansion recoding

If patterns are too similar to be stored in associative memories, then one solution that the brain seems to use repeatedly is to expand the encoding to a form in which the different stimulus patterns are less correlated, that is, more orthogonal, before they are presented as CS stimuli to a pattern associator. The problem can be highlighted by a non-linearly separable mapping (which captures part of the eXclusive OR (XOR) problem), in which the mapping that is desired is as shown in Fig. B.10. The neuron has two inputs, A and B.

This is a mapping of patterns that is impossible for a one-layer network, because the patterns are not linearly separable[25]. A solution is to remap the two input lines A and B to three input lines 1–3, that is to use expansion recoding, as shown in Fig. B.11. This can be performed by a competitive network (see Section B.4). The synaptic weights on the dendrite of the output neuron could then learn the following values using a simple Hebb rule, Equation B.2, and the problem could be solved as in Fig. B.12. The whole network would look like that shown in Fig. B.11.

Competitive networks could help with this type of recoding, and could provide very useful preprocessing for a pattern associator in the brain (Rolls and Treves, 1998; Rolls, 2016b). It is possible that the lateral nucleus of the amygdala performs this function, for it receives inputs from the temporal cortical visual areas, and may preprocess them before they become the inputs to associative networks at the next stage of amygdala processing (Rolls, 2016b, 2014a). The granule cells of the cerebellum may operate similarly (Chapter 17).

---

[25] See Appendix A. There is no set of synaptic weights in a one-layer net that could solve the problem shown in Fig. B.10. Two classes of patterns are not linearly separable if no hyperplane can be positioned in their N-dimensional space so as to separate them (see Appendix A). The XOR problem has the additional constraint that $A = 0, B = 0$ must be mapped to Output = 0.

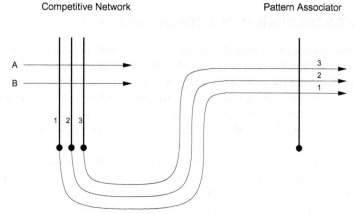

Fig. B.11 Expansion recoding. A competitive network followed by a pattern associator that can enable patterns that are not linearly separable to be learned correctly.

	Synaptic weight
Input 1 (A=1, B=0)	1
Input 2 (A=0, B=1)	1
Input 3 (A=1, B=1)	0

Fig. B.12 Synaptic weights on the dendrite of the output neuron in Fig. B.11.

B.2.8 Implications of different types of coding for storage in pattern associators

Throughout this section, we have made statements about how the properties of pattern associators – such as the number of patterns that can be stored, and whether generalization and graceful degradation occur – depend on the type of encoding of the patterns to be associated. (The types of encoding considered, local, sparse distributed, and fully distributed, are described above.) We draw together these points in Table B.2.

Table B.2 Coding in associative memories*

	Local	Sparse distributed	Fully distributed
Generalization, completion, graceful degradation	No	Yes	Yes
Number of patterns that can be stored	N (large)	of order $C/[a_o \log(1/a_o)]$ (can be larger)	of order C (usually smaller than N)
Amount of information in each pattern (values if binary)	Minimal ($\log(N)$ bits)	Intermediate ($Na_o \log(1/a_o)$ bits)	Large (N bits)

* N refers here to the number of output units, and C to the average number of inputs to each output unit. a_o is the sparseness of output patterns, or roughly the proportion of output units activated by a UCS pattern. Note: logs are to the base 2.

The amount of information that can be stored in each pattern in a pattern associator is considered in Appendix A3 of Rolls and Treves (1998). That Appendix has been made available at https://www.oxcns.org, and contains a quantitative approach to the capacity of pattern association networks that has not been published elsewhere.

In conclusion, the architecture and properties of pattern association networks make them very appropriate for stimulus–reinforcer association learning. Their high capacity enables them to learn the reinforcement associations for very large numbers of different stimuli.

B.3 Autoassociation or attractor memory

Autoassociative memories, or attractor neural networks, store memories, each one of which is represented by a pattern of neural activity. The memories are stored in the recurrent synaptic connections between the neurons of the network, for example in the recurrent collateral connections between cortical pyramidal cells. Autoassociative networks can then recall the appropriate memory from the network when provided with a fragment of one of the memories. This is called completion. Many different memories can be stored in the network and retrieved correctly. A feature of this type of memory is that it is content addressable; that is, the information in the memory can be accessed if just the contents of the memory (or a part of the contents of the memory) are used. This is in contrast to a conventional computer, in which the address of what is to be accessed must be supplied, and used to access the contents of the memory. Content addressability is an important simplifying feature of this type of memory, which makes it suitable for use in biological systems. The issue of content addressability will be amplified below.

An autoassociation memory can be used as a short-term memory, in which iterative processing round the recurrent collateral connection loop keeps a representation active by continuing neuronal firing. The short-term memory reflected in continuing neuronal firing for several hundred milliseconds after a visual stimulus is removed which is present in visual cortical areas such as the inferior temporal visual cortex (see Chapter 2) is probably implemented in this way. This short-term memory is one possible mechanism that contributes to the implementation of the trace memory learning rule which can help to implement invariant object recognition as described in Chapter 2. Autoassociation memories also appear to be used in a short-term memory role in the prefrontal cortex. In particular, the temporal visual cortical areas have connections to the ventrolateral prefrontal cortex which help to implement the short-term memory for visual stimuli (in for example delayed match to sample tasks, and visual search tasks, as described in Section 13.6.1). In an analogous way the parietal cortex has connections to the dorsolateral prefrontal cortex for the short-term memory of spatial responses (see Section 13.6.1). These short-term memories provide a mechanism that enables attention to be maintained through backprojections from prefrontal cortex areas to the temporal and parietal areas that send connections to the prefrontal cortex, as described in Chapter 13. Autoassociation networks implemented by the recurrent collateral synapses between cortical pyramidal cells also provide a mechanism for constraint satisfaction and also noise reduction whereby the firing of neighbouring neurons can be taken into account in enabling the network to settle into a state that reflects all the details of the inputs activating the population of connected neurons, as well as the effects of what has been set up during developmental plasticity as well as later experience. Attractor networks are also effectively implemented by virtue of the forward and backward connections between cortical areas (see Sections 9.3.8 and 13.6.1). An autoassociation network with rapid synaptic plasticity can learn each memory in one trial. Because of its 'one-shot' rapid learning, and ability to complete, this type of network is well suited for episodic memory storage, in which each past episode must be stored and recalled later from a fragment, and kept separate from other episodic memories (see Chapter 9).

B.3.1 Architecture and operation

The prototypical architecture of an autoassociation memory is shown in Fig. B.13. The external input e_i is applied to each neuron i by unmodifiable synapses. This produces firing y_i of each neuron, or a vector of firing on the output neurons **y**. Each output neuron i is connected by a recurrent collateral connection to the other neurons in the network, via mod-

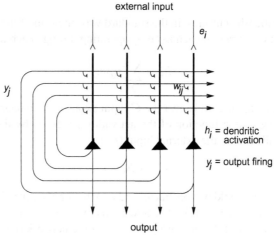

Fig. B.13 The architecture of an autoassociative neural network.

ifiable connection weights w_{ij}. This architecture effectively enables the output firing vector **y** to be associated during learning with itself. Later on, during recall, presentation of part of the external input will force some of the output neurons to fire, but through the recurrent collateral axons and the modified synapses, other neurons in **y** can be brought into activity. This process can be repeated a number of times, and recall of a complete pattern may be perfect. Effectively, a pattern can be recalled or recognized because of associations formed between its parts. This of course requires distributed representations.

Next we introduce a more precise and detailed description of the above, and describe the properties of these networks. Ways to analyze formally the operation of these networks are introduced in Appendix A4 of Rolls and Treves (1998) and by Amit (1989).

B.3.1.1 Learning

The firing of every output neuron i is forced to a value y_i determined by the external input e_i. Then a Hebb-like associative local learning rule is applied to the recurrent synapses in the network:

$$\delta w_{ij} = \alpha y_i y_j. \tag{B.9}$$

It is notable that in a fully connected network, this will result in a symmetric matrix of synaptic weights, that is the strength of the connection from neuron 1 to neuron 2 will be the same as the strength of the connection from neuron 2 to neuron 1 (both implemented via recurrent collateral synapses).

It is a factor that is sometimes overlooked that there must be a mechanism for ensuring that during learning y_i does approximate e_i, and must not be influenced much by activity in the recurrent collateral connections, otherwise the new external pattern **e** will not be stored in the network, but instead something will be stored that is influenced by the previously stored memories. It is thought that in some parts of the brain, such as the hippocampus, there are processes that help the external connections to dominate the firing during learning (see Chapter 9, Treves and Rolls (1992) and Rolls and Treves (1998)).

B.3.1.2 Recall

During recall, the external input e_i is applied, and produces output firing, operating through the non-linear activation function described below. The firing is fed back by the recurrent collateral axons shown in Fig. B.13 to produce activation of each output neuron through the modified synapses on each output neuron. The activation h_i produced by the recurrent collateral effect on the ith neuron is, in the standard way, the sum of the activations produced in proportion to the firing rate of each axon y_j operating through each modified synapse w_{ij}, that is,

$$h_i = \sum_j y_j w_{ij} \tag{B.10}$$

where $\sum_j$ indicates that the sum is over the C input axons to each neuron, indexed by j.

The output firing y_i is a function of the activation produced by the recurrent collateral effect (internal recall) and by the external input (e_i):

$$y_i = \text{f}(h_i + e_i) \tag{B.11}$$

The activation function should be non-linear, and may be for example binary threshold, linear threshold, sigmoid, etc. (see Fig. 1.3). The threshold at which the activation function operates is set in part by the effect of the inhibitory neurons in the network (not shown in Fig. B.13). The connectivity is that the pyramidal cells have collateral axons that excite the inhibitory interneurons, which in turn connect back to the population of pyramidal cells to inhibit them by a mixture of shunting (divisive) and subtractive inhibition using GABA (gamma-aminobutyric acid) terminals, as described in Section B.6. There are many fewer inhibitory neurons than excitatory neurons (in the order of 5–10%, see Table 1.8) and of connections to and from inhibitory neurons (see Table 1.8), and partly for this reason the inhibitory neurons are considered to perform generic functions such as threshold setting, rather than to store patterns by modifying their synapses. Similar inhibitory processes are assumed for the other networks described in this Appendix. The non-linear activation function can minimize interference between the pattern being recalled and other patterns stored in the network, and can also be used to ensure that what is a positive feedback system remains stable. The network can be allowed to repeat this recurrent collateral loop a number of times. Each time the loop operates, the output firing becomes more like the originally stored pattern, and this progressive recall is usually complete within 5–15 iterations.

B.3.2 Introduction to the analysis of the operation of autoassociation networks

With complete connectivity in the synaptic matrix, and the use of a Hebb rule, the matrix of synaptic weights formed during learning is symmetric. The learning algorithm is fast, 'one-shot', in that a single presentation of an input pattern is all that is needed to store that pattern.

During recall, a part of one of the originally learned stimuli can be presented as an external input. The resulting firing is allowed to iterate repeatedly round the recurrent collateral system, gradually on each iteration recalling more and more of the originally learned pattern. Completion thus occurs. If a pattern is presented during recall that is similar but not identical to any of the previously learned patterns, then the network settles into a stable recall state in which the firing corresponds to that of the previously learned pattern. The network can thus generalize in its recall to the most similar previously learned pattern. The activation function of the neurons should be non-linear, since a purely linear system would not produce any categorization of the input patterns it receives, and therefore would not be able to effect anything more than a trivial (i.e. linear) form of completion and generalization.

Recall can be thought of in the following way, relating it to what occurs in pattern associators. The external input $\mathbf{e}$ is applied, produces firing $\mathbf{y}$, which is applied as a recall cue on the recurrent collaterals as $\mathbf{y}^{\text{T}}$. (The notation $\mathbf{y}^{\text{T}}$ signifies the transpose of $\mathbf{y}$, which is implemented by the application of the firing of the neurons $\mathbf{y}$ back via the recurrent collateral axons as the next set of inputs to the neurons.) The activity on the recurrent collaterals is then multiplied by the synaptic weight vector stored during learning on each neuron to produce the new activation h_i which reflects the similarity between $\mathbf{y}^T$ and one of the stored patterns. Partial recall has thus occurred as a result of the recurrent collateral effect. The activations h_i after thresholding (which helps to remove interference from other memories stored in the network, or noise in the recall cue) result in firing y_i, or a vector of all neurons $\mathbf{y}$, which is already more like one of the stored patterns than, at the first iteration, the firing resulting from the recall cue alone, $\mathbf{y} = \mathbf{f}(\mathbf{e})$. This process is repeated a number of times to produce progressive recall of one of the stored patterns.

Autoassociation networks operate by effectively storing associations between the elements of a pattern. Each element of the pattern vector to be stored is simply the firing of a neuron. What is stored in an autoassociation memory is a set of pattern vectors. The network operates to recall one of the patterns from a fragment of it. Thus, although this network implements recall or recognition of a pattern, it does so by an association learning mechanism, in which associations between the different parts of each pattern are learned. These memories have sometimes been called autocorrelation memories (Kohonen, 1977), because they learn correlations between the activity of neurons in the network, in the sense that each pattern learned is defined by a set of simultaneously active neurons. Effectively each pattern is associated by learning with itself. This learning is implemented by an associative (Hebb-like) learning rule.

The system formally resembles spin glass systems of magnets analyzed quantitatively in statistical mechanics. This has led to the analysis of (recurrent) autoassociative networks as dynamical systems made up of many interacting elements, in which the interactions are such as to produce a large variety of basins of attraction of the dynamics. Each basin of attraction corresponds to one of the originally learned patterns, and once the network is within a basin it keeps iterating until a recall state is reached that is the learned pattern itself or a pattern closely similar to it. (Interference effects may prevent an exact identity between the recall state and a learned pattern.) This type of system is contrasted with other, simpler, systems of magnets (e.g. ferromagnets), in which the interactions are such as to produce only a limited number of related basins, since the magnets tend to be, for example, all aligned with each other. The states reached within each basin of attraction are called attractor states, and the analogy between autoassociator neural networks and physical systems with multiple attractors was drawn by Hopfield (1982) in a very influential paper. He was able to show that the recall state can be thought of as the local minimum in an energy landscape, where the energy would be defined as

$$E = -\frac{1}{2} \sum_{i,j} w_{ij}(y_i - <y>)(y_j - <y>). \tag{B.12}$$

This Equation can be understood in the following way. If two neurons are both firing above their mean rate (denoted by $<y>$), and are connected by a weight with a positive value, then the firing of these two neurons is consistent with each other, and they mutually support each other, so that they contribute to the system's tendency to remain stable. If across the whole network such mutual support is generally provided, then no further change will take place, and the system will indeed remain stable. If, on the other hand, either of our pair of neurons was not firing, or if the connecting weight had a negative value, the neurons would not support each other, and indeed the tendency would be for the neurons to try to alter ('flip' in the case of binary units) the state of the other. This would be repeated across the whole network until a situation in which most mutual support, and least 'frustration', was reached. What makes it possible to define an energy function and for these points to hold is that the matrix is symmetric (see Hopfield (1982), Hertz, Krogh and Palmer (1991), Amit (1989)).

Physicists have generally analyzed a system in which the input pattern is presented and then immediately removed, so that the network then 'falls' without further assistance (in what is referred to as the unclamped condition) towards the minimum of its basin of attraction. A more biologically realistic system is one in which the external input is left on contributing to the recall during the fall into the recall state. In this clamped condition, recall is usually faster, and more reliable, so that more memories may be usefully recalled from the network. The approach using methods developed in theoretical physics has led to rapid advances in the understanding of autoassociative networks, and its basic elements are described in Appendix A4 of Rolls and Treves (1998), and by Hertz, Krogh and Palmer (1991) and Amit (1989).

B.3.3 Properties

The internal recall in autoassociation networks involves multiplication of the firing vector of neuronal activity by the vector of synaptic weights on each neuron. This inner product vector multiplication allows the similarity of the firing vector to previously stored firing vectors to be provided by the output (as effectively a correlation), if the patterns learned are distributed. As a result of this type of 'correlation computation' performed if the patterns are distributed, many important properties of these networks arise, including pattern completion (because part of a pattern is correlated with the whole pattern), and graceful degradation (because a damaged synaptic weight vector is still correlated with the original synaptic weight vector). Some of these properties are described next.

B.3.3.1 Completion

Perhaps the most important and useful property of these memories is that they complete an incomplete input vector, allowing recall of a whole memory from a small fraction of it. The memory recalled in response to a fragment is that stored in the memory that is closest in pattern similarity (as measured by the dot product, or correlation). Because the recall is iterative and progressive, the recall can be perfect.

This property and the associative property of pattern associator neural networks are very similar to the properties of human memory. This property may be used when we recall a part of a recent memory of a past episode from a part of that episode. The way in which this could be implemented in the hippocampus is described in Chapter 9.

B.3.3.2 Generalization

The network generalizes in that an input vector similar to one of the stored vectors will lead to recall of the originally stored vector, provided that distributed encoding is used. The principle by which this occurs is similar to that described for a pattern associator.

B.3.3.3 Graceful degradation or fault tolerance

If the synaptic weight vector $\mathbf{w}_i$ on each neuron (or the weight matrix) has synapses missing (e.g. during development), or loses synapses (e.g. with brain damage or ageing), then the activation h_i (or vector of activations $\mathbf{h}$) is still reasonable, because h_i is the dot product (correlation) of $\mathbf{y}^T$ with $\mathbf{w}_i$. The same argument applies if whole input axons are lost. If an output neuron is lost, then the network cannot itself compensate for this, but the next network in the brain is likely to be able to generalize or complete if its input vector has some elements missing, as would be the case if some output neurons of the autoassociation network were damaged.

B.3.3.4 Prototype extraction, extraction of central tendency, and noise reduction

These arise when a set of similar input pattern vectors $\{\mathbf{e}\}$ (which induce firing of the output neurons $\{\mathbf{y}\}$) are learned by the network. The weight vectors $\mathbf{w}_i$ (or strictly $\mathbf{w}_i^T$) become (or point towards) the average $\{<\mathbf{y}>\}$ of that set of similar vectors. This produces 'extraction of the prototype' or 'extraction of the central tendency', and 'noise reduction'. This process can result in better recognition or recall of the prototype than of any of the exemplars, even though the prototype may never itself have been presented. The general principle by which the effect occurs is similar to that by which it occurs in pattern associators. It of course only occurs if each pattern uses a distributed representation.

Related to outputs of the visual system to long-term memory systems (see Chapter 9), there has been intense debate about whether when human memories are stored, a prototype of what is to be remembered is stored, or whether all the instances or the exemplars are each stored separately so that they can be individually recalled (McClelland and Rumelhart (1986), Chapter 17, p. 172). Evidence favouring the prototype view is that if a number of different examples of an object are shown, then humans may report more confidently that they have seen the prototype before than any of the different exemplars, even though the prototype has never been shown (Posner and Keele, 1968; Rosch, 1975). Evidence favouring the view that exemplars are stored is that in categorization and perceptual identification tasks the responses made are often sensitive to the congruity between particular training stimuli and particular test stimuli (Brooks, 1978; Medin and Schaffer, 1978; Jacoby, 1983a,b; Whittlesea, 1983). It is of great interest that both types of phenomena can arise naturally out of distributed information storage in a neuronal network such as an autoassociator. This can be illustrated by the storage in an autoassociation memory of sets of stimuli that are all somewhat different examples of the same pattern. These can be generated, for example, by randomly altering each of the input vectors from the input stimulus. After many such randomly altered exemplars have been learned by the network, recall can be tested, and it is found that the network responds best to the original (prototype) input vector, with which it has never been presented. The reason for this is that the autocorrelation components that build up in the synaptic matrix with repeated presentations of the exemplars represent the average correlation between the different elements of the vector, and this is highest for the prototype. This effect also gives the storage some noise immunity, in that variations in the input that are random noise average out, while the signal that is constant builds up with repeated learning.

B.3.3.5 Speed

The recall operation is fast on each neuron on a single iteration, because the pattern $\mathbf{y}^T$ on the axons can be applied simultaneously to the synapses $\mathbf{w}_i$, and the activation h_i can be accumulated in one or two time constants of the dendrite (e.g. 10–20 ms). If a simple implementation of an autoassociation net such as that described by Hopfield (1982) is simulated on a computer, then 5–15 iterations are typically necessary for completion of an incomplete input cue $\mathbf{e}$. This might be taken to correspond to 50–200 ms in the brain, rather too slow for any one local network in the brain to function. However, it has been shown that if the neurons are treated not as McCulloch–Pitts neurons which are simply 'updated' at each iteration, or cycle of timesteps (and assume the active state if the threshold is exceeded), but instead are analyzed and modelled as 'integrate-and-fire' neurons in real continuous time, then the network can effectively 'relax' into its recall state very rapidly, in one or two time constants of the synapses (see Section B.6 and Treves (1993), Battaglia and Treves (1998a) and Appendix A5 of Rolls and Treves (1998)). This corresponds to perhaps 20 ms in the brain.

One factor in this rapid dynamics of autoassociative networks with brain-like 'integrate-and-fire' membrane and synaptic properties is that with some spontaneous activity, some of the neurons in the network are close to threshold already before the recall cue is applied, and hence some of the neurons are very quickly pushed by the recall cue into firing, so that information starts to be exchanged very rapidly (within 1–2 ms of brain time) through the modified synapses by the neurons in the network. The progressive exchange of information starting early on within what would otherwise be thought of as an iteration period (of perhaps 20 ms, corresponding to a neuronal firing rate of 50 spikes/s) is the mechanism accounting for rapid recall in an autoassociative neuronal network made biologically realistic in this way. Further analysis of the fast dynamics of these networks if they are implemented in a biologically plausible way with 'integrate-and-fire' neurons is provided in Section B.6, in Appendix A5 of Rolls and Treves (1998), and by Treves (1993). *The general approach applies to other networks with recurrent connections, not just autoassociators, and the fact that such networks can operate much faster than it would seem from simple models that follow discrete time dynamics is probably a major factor in enabling these networks to provide some of the building blocks of brain function.*

Learning is fast, 'one-shot', in that a single presentation of an input pattern **e** (producing **y**) enables the association between the activation of the dendrites (the post-synaptic term h_i) and the firing of the recurrent collateral axons $\mathbf{y}^T$, to be learned. Repeated presentation with small variations of a pattern vector is used to obtain the properties of prototype extraction, extraction of central tendency, and noise reduction, because these arise from the averaging process produced by storing very similar patterns in the network.

B.3.3.6 Local learning rule

The simplest learning used in autoassociation neural networks, a version of the Hebb rule, is (as in equation B.9)

$$\delta w_{ij} = \alpha y_i y_j.$$

The rule is a local learning rule in that the information required to specify the change in synaptic weight is available locally at the synapse, as it is dependent only on the presynaptic firing rate y_j available at the synaptic terminal, and the postsynaptic activation or firing y_i available on the dendrite of the neuron receiving the synapse. This makes the learning rule biologically plausible, in that the information about how to change the synaptic weight does not have to be carried to every synapse from a distant source where it is computed. As with pattern associators, since firing rates are positive quantities, a potentially interfering correlation is induced between different pattern vectors. This can be removed by subtracting the mean of the presynaptic activity from each presynaptic term, using a type of long-term depression. This can be specified as

$$\delta w_{ij} = \alpha y_i (y_j - z) \tag{B.13}$$

where α is a learning rate constant. This learning rule includes (in proportion to y_i) increasing the synaptic weight if $(y_j - z) > 0$ (long-term potentiation), and decreasing the synaptic weight if $(y_j - z) < 0$ (heterosynaptic long-term depression). This procedure works optimally if z is the average activity $<y_j>$ of an axon across patterns.

Evidence that a learning rule with the general form of Equation B.9 is implemented in at least some parts of the brain comes from studies of long-term potentiation, described in Section 1.6. One of the important potential functions of heterosynaptic long-term depression is its ability to allow in effect the average of the presynaptic activity to be subtracted from the presynaptic firing rate (see Appendix A3 of Rolls and Treves (1998), and Rolls and Treves (1990)).

Autoassociation networks can be trained with the error-correction or delta learning rule described in Section B.11. Although a delta rule is less biologically plausible than a Hebb-like rule, a delta rule can help to store separately patterns that are very similar (see McClelland and Rumelhart (1989) and Hertz, Krogh and Palmer (1991)).

B.3.3.7 Capacity

One measure of storage capacity is to consider how many orthogonal patterns could be stored, as with pattern associators. If the patterns are orthogonal, there will be no interference between them, and the maximum number p of patterns that can be stored will be the same as the number N of output neurons in a fully connected network. Although in practice the patterns that have to be stored will hardly be orthogonal, this is not a purely academic speculation, since it was shown how one can construct a synaptic matrix that effectively orthogonalizes any set of (linearly independent) patterns (Kohonen, 1977, 1989; Personnaz, Guyon and Dreyfus, 1985; Kanter and Sompolinsky, 1987). However, this matrix cannot be learned with a local, one-shot learning rule, and therefore its interest for autoassociators in the brain is limited. The more general case of random non-orthogonal patterns, and of Hebbian learning rules, is considered next. However, it is important to reduce the correlations between patterns to be stored in an autoassociation network to not limit the capacity (Marr, 1971; Kohonen, 1977, 1989; Kohonen et al., 1981; Sompolinsky, 1987; Rolls and Treves, 1998; Boboeva et al., 2018; Rolls, 2023d; Ryom et al., 2023), and in the brain mechanisms to perform pattern separation are frequently present (Rolls, 2016f), including granule cells, as shown in many places in this book.

With non-linear neurons used in the network, the capacity can be measured in terms of the number of input patterns **y** (produced by the external input **e**, see Fig. B.13) that can be stored in the network and recalled later whenever the network settles within each stored pattern's basin of attraction. The first quantitative analysis of storage capacity (Amit, Gutfreund and Sompolinsky, 1987) considered a fully connected Hopfield (1982) autoassociator model, in which units are binary elements with an equal probability of being 'on' or 'off' in each pattern, and the number C of inputs per unit is the same as the number N of output units. (Actually it is equal to $N-1$, since a unit is taken not to connect to itself.) Learning is taken to occur by clamping the desired patterns on the network and using a modified Hebb rule, in which the mean of the presynaptic and postsynaptic firings is subtracted from the firing on any one learning trial (this amounts to a covariance learning rule, and is described more fully in Appendix A4 of Rolls and Treves (1998)). With such fully distributed random patterns, the number of patterns that can be learned is (for C large) $p \approx 0.14C = 0.14N$, hence well below what could be achieved with orthogonal patterns or with an 'orthogonalizing' synaptic matrix. Many variations of this 'standard' autoassociator model have been analyzed subsequently.

Treves and Rolls (1991) have extended this analysis to autoassociation networks that are much more biologically relevant in the following ways. First, some or many connections between the recurrent collaterals and the dendrites are missing (this is referred to as diluted connectivity, and results in a non-symmetric synaptic connection matrix in which w_{ij} does not equal w_{ji}, one of the original assumptions made in order to introduce the energy formalism in the Hopfield model). Second, the neurons need not be restricted to binary threshold neurons, but can have a threshold linear activation function (see Fig. 1.3). This enables the neurons to assume real continuously variable firing rates, which are what is found in the brain (Rolls and Tovee, 1995b; Treves, Panzeri, Rolls, Booth and Wakeman, 1999). Third, the representation need not be fully distributed (with half the neurons 'on', and half 'off'), but instead can have a small proportion of the neurons firing above the spontaneous rate, which is what is found in parts of the brain such as the hippocampus that are involved in memory (see Treves and Rolls

(1994), and Chapter 6 of Rolls and Treves (1998)). Such a representation is defined as being sparse, and the sparseness a of the representation can be measured, by extending the binary notion of the proportion of neurons that are firing, as

$$a = \frac{(\sum_{i=1}^{N} y_i/N)^2}{\sum_{i=1}^{N} y_i^2/N} \qquad (B.14)$$

where y_i is the firing rate of the ith neuron in the set of N neurons. Treves and Rolls (1991) have shown that such a network does operate efficiently as an autoassociative network, and can store (and recall correctly) a number of different patterns p as follows

$$p \approx \frac{C^{RC}}{a \ln(\frac{1}{a})} k \qquad (B.15)$$

where C^{RC} is the number of synapses on the dendrites of each neuron devoted to the recurrent collaterals from other neurons in the network, and k is a factor that depends weakly on the detailed structure of the rate distribution, on the connectivity pattern, etc., but is roughly in the order of 0.2–0.3.

The main factors that determine the maximum number of memories that can be stored in an autoassociative network are thus the number of connections on each neuron devoted to the recurrent collaterals, and the sparseness of the representation. For example, for $C^{RC} = 12,000$ and $a = 0.02$, p is calculated to be approximately 36,000. This storage capacity can be realized, with little interference between patterns, if the learning rule includes some form of heterosynaptic long-term depression that counterbalances the effects of associative long-term potentiation (Treves and Rolls (1991); see Appendix A4 of Rolls and Treves (1998)). It should be noted that the number of neurons N (which is greater than C^{RC}, the number of recurrent collateral inputs received by any neuron in the network from the other neurons in the network) is not a parameter that influences the number of different memories that can be stored in the network. The implication of this is that increasing the number of neurons (without increasing the number of connections per neuron) does not increase the number of different patterns that can be stored (see Rolls and Treves (1998) Appendix A4), although it may enable simpler encoding of the firing patterns, for example more orthogonal encoding, to be used. This latter point may account in part for why there are generally in the brain more neurons in a recurrent network than there are connections per neuron (see e.g. Chapter 9).

The non-linearity inherent in the NMDA receptor-based Hebbian plasticity present in the brain may help to make the stored patterns more sparse than the input patterns, and this may be especially beneficial in increasing the storage capacity of associative networks in the brain by allowing participation in the storage of especially those relatively few neurons with high firing rates in the exponential firing rate distributions typical of neurons in sensory systems (see Sections B.4.9.3 and C.3.1).

B.3.3.8 Context

The environmental context in which learning occurs can be a very important factor that affects retrieval in humans and other animals. Placing the subject back into the same context in which the original learning occurred can greatly facilitate retrieval.

Context effects arise naturally in association networks if some of the activity in the network reflects the context in which the learning occurs. Retrieval is then better when that context is present, for the activity contributed by the context becomes part of the retrieval cue for the memory, increasing the correlation of the current state with what was stored. (A strategy for retrieval arises simply from this property. The strategy is to keep trying to recall as many fragments of the original memory situation, including the context, as possible, as this will provide a better cue for complete retrieval of the memory than just a single fragment.)

The effects that mood has on memory including visual memory retrieval may be accounted for by backprojections from brain regions such as the amygdala and orbitofrontal cortex in which the current mood, providing a context, is represented, to brain regions involved in memory such as the perirhinal cortex, and in visual representations such as the inferior temporal visual cortex (see Rolls and Stringer (2001b)). The very well-known effects of context in the human memory literature could arise in the simple way just described. An implication of the explanation is that context effects will be especially important at late stages of memory or information processing systems in the brain, for there information from a wide range of modalities will be mixed, and some of that information could reflect the context in which the learning takes place. One part of the brain where such effects may be strong is the hippocampus, which is implicated in the memory of recent episodes, and which receives inputs derived from most of the cortical information processing streams, including those involved in space (see Chapter 9).

B.3.3.9 Mixture states

If an autoassociation memory is trained on pattern vectors $\mathbf{A}$, $\mathbf{B}$, and $\mathbf{A} + \mathbf{B}$ (i.e. $\mathbf{A}$ and $\mathbf{B}$ are both included in the joint vector $\mathbf{A} + \mathbf{B}$; that is if the vectors are not linearly independent), then the autoassociation memory will have difficulty in learning and recalling these three memories as separate, because completion from either $\mathbf{A}$ or $\mathbf{B}$ to $\mathbf{A} + \mathbf{B}$ tends to occur during recall. (The ability to separate such patterns is referred to as configurational learning in the animal learning literature, see e.g. Sutherland and Rudy (1991).) This problem can be minimized by re-representing $\mathbf{A}$, $\mathbf{B}$, and $\mathbf{A} + \mathbf{B}$ in such a way that they are different vectors before they are presented to the autoassociation memory. This can be performed by recoding the input vectors to minimize overlap using, for example, a competitive network, and possibly involving expansion recoding, as described for pattern associators (see Section B.2, Fig. B.11). It is suggested that this is a function of the dentate granule cells in the hippocampus, which precede the CA3 recurrent collateral network (Treves and Rolls, 1992, 1994; Rolls, 2018b) (see Chapter 9).

B.3.3.10 Memory for sequences

One of the first extensions of the standard autoassociator paradigm that has been explored in the literature is the capability to store and retrieve not just individual patterns, but whole sequences of patterns. Hopfield (1982), suggested that this could be achieved by adding to the standard connection weights, which associate a pattern with itself, a new, asymmetric component, which associates a pattern with the next one in the sequence. In practice this scheme does not work very well, unless the new component is made to operate on a slower time scale than the purely autoassociative component (Kleinfeld, 1986; Sompolinsky and Kanter, 1986). With two different time scales, the autoassociative component can stabilize a pattern for a while, before the heteroassociative component moves the network, as it were, into the next pattern. The heteroassociative retrieval cue for the next pattern in the sequence is just the previous pattern in the sequence. A particular type of 'slower' operation occurs if the asymmetric component acts after a delay τ. In this case, the network sweeps through the sequence, staying for a time of order τ in each pattern.

One can see how the necessary ingredient for the storage of sequences is only a minor departure from purely Hebbian learning: in fact, the (symmetric) autoassociative component of the weights can be taken to reflect the Hebbian learning of strictly simultaneous conjunctions of pre- and post-synaptic activity, whereas the (asymmetric) heteroassociative component can be implemented by Hebbian learning of each conjunction of postsynaptic activity with presynaptic activity shifted a time τ in the past. Both components can then be seen as resulting from a generalized Hebbian rule, which increases the weight whenever postsynaptic activity is paired with presynaptic activity occurring within a given time range, which may extend from a few hundred milliseconds in the past up to include strictly simultaneous activity. This is similar to a trace rule (see Chapter 2), which itself matches very well the observed conditions for induction of long-term potentiation, and appears entirely plausible. The learning rule necessary for learning sequences, though, is more complex than a simple trace rule in that the time-shifted conjunctions of activity that are encoded in the weights must in retrieval produce activations that are time-shifted as well (otherwise one falls back into the Hopfield (1982) proposal, which does not quite work). The synaptic weights should therefore keep separate 'traces' of what was simultaneous and what was time-shifted during the original experience, and this is not very plausible.

Levy and colleagues (Levy, Wu and Baxter, 1995; Wu, Baxter and Levy, 1996) have investigated these issues further, and the temporal asymmetry that may be present in LTP (see Section 1.6) has been suggested as a mechanism that might provide some of the temporal properties that are necessary for the brain to store and recall sequences (Minai and Levy, 1993; Abbott and Blum, 1996; Markram, Pikus, Gupta and Tsodyks, 1998; Abbott and Nelson, 2000). A problem with this suggestion is that, given that the temporal dynamics of attractor networks are inherently very fast when the networks have continuous dynamics (see Section B.6), and that the temporal asymmetry in LTP may be in the order of only milliseconds to a few tens of milliseconds (see Section 1.6), the recall of the sequences would be very fast, perhaps 10–20 ms per step of the sequence, with every step of a 10-step sequence effectively retrieved and gone in a quick-fire session of 100–200 ms.

Rolls and Stringer (see Rolls and Kesner (2006b)) have suggested that the over-rapid replay of a sequence of memories stored in an autoassociation network such as CA3 if it included asymmetric synaptic weights to encode a sequence could be controlled by the physical inputs from the environment. If a sequence of places 1, 2, and 3 had been learned by the use of an asymmetric trace learning rule implemented in the CA3 network, then the firing initiated by place 1 would reflect (by the learned association) a small component of place 2 (which might be used to guide navigation to place 2, and which might be separated out from place 1 better by the competitive network action in CA1), but would not move fully away from representing place 1 until the animal moved away from place 1, because of the clamping effect on the CA3 firing of the external input representing place 1 to the recurrent network. In this way, the physical constraints of movements between the different places in the environment would control the speed of readout from the sequence memory. In the network of Rolls and Stringer (see Rolls and Kesner (2006b)), CA3 might, by the continuing firing implemented by autoassociation, allow one item to be held in short-term memory until the next item arrives for heteroassociation. This would enable long time gaps within the sequence during training to be bridged.

Another way in which a delay could be inserted in a recurrent collateral path in the brain is by inserting another cortical area in the recurrent path. This could fit in with the cortico-cortical backprojection connections described in Fig. 9.2 with return projections to the entorhinal cortex, which might then send information back into the hippocampus, which would introduce some conduction delay (Panzeri, Rolls, Battaglia and Lavis, 2001). Another possibility is that the connections between the deep and the superficial layers of the entorhinal cortex help to close a loop from entorhinal cortex through hippocampal circuitry and back to the entorhinal cortex (van Haeften et al., 2003). Another suggestion is that the CA3 system holds by continuing firing a memory for event 1, which can then be associated with event 2 at the CA3 to CA1 synapses if event 2 activates CA1 neurons by the direct entorhinal input (Levy, 1989).

Another proposal is that sequence memory can be implemented by using synaptic adaptation to effectively encode the order of the items in a sequence (Deco and Rolls, 2005c) (see Section B.10). Whenever the attractor system is quenched into inactivity, the next member of the sequence emerges out of the spontaneous activity, because the least recently activated member of the sequence has the least synaptic or neuronal adaptation. This could be implemented in recurrent networks such as the CA3 or the prefrontal cortex.

For the recall of which item occurred most recently in short-term memory, the sequence type of memory would be possible, but difficult because once a sequence has been recalled, a system has to "manipulate" the items, picking out which is later (or earlier) in the sequence. A simpler possibility is to use a short term form of long term potentiation (LTP) which decays, and, then the latest of two items can be picked out because when it is seen again, the neuronal response is larger than to the earlier items (Rolls and Deco, 2002; Renart et al., 2001). This type of memory does not explicitly encode sequences, but instead reflects just how recently an item occurred. This could be implemented at any synapses in the system (e.g. in CA3 or CA1), and does not require recurrent collateral connectivity.

Using a single attractor network to store sequences does thus not turn out to be very efficient. One solution that the brain uses instead to implement sequence memory are associations made to hippocampal time cells, as described in Section 9.3.4 (Rolls and Mills, 2019) together with the neural network computations that may produce time cells.

B.3.4 Diluted connectivity and the storage capacity of attractor networks

Rolls (2012b) investigated how diluted connectivity can increase the storage capacity of attractor networks, by reducing the probability that there will be more than one synaptic connection between any pair of neurons, which would distort the landscape of the basins of attraction.

B.3.4.1 The autoassociative or attractor network architecture being studied

The architecture and functional properties of autoassociative or attractor networks are described in detail by Hertz et al. (1991), by Amit (1989), and earlier in Section B.3. Here it is assumed that the memory patterns are stored in the autoassociative network by an associative (or Hebbian) learning process in an architecture of the type shown in Fig. B.13 as follows. The firing of every output neuron i is forced to a value y_i determined by the external input e_i. Then a Hebb-like associative local learning rule is applied to the recurrent synapses in the network:

$$\delta w_{ij} = \alpha y_i y_j. \tag{B.16}$$

where α is a learning rate constant, and y_j is the presynaptic firing rate.

During recall, the external input e_i is applied, and produces output firing, operating through the non-linear activation function described below. The firing is fed back by the recurrent collateral axons shown in Fig. B.13 to produce activation of each output neuron through the modified synapses on each output neuron. The activation h_i produced by the recurrent collateral effect on the ith neuron is the sum of the activations produced in proportion to the firing rate of each axon y_j operating through each modified synapse w_{ij}, that is,

$$h_i = \sum_j^C y_j w_{ij} \tag{B.17}$$

where $\sum_{j}^{C}$ indicates that the sum is over the C input axons to each neuron, indexed by j.

The output firing y_i is a function of the activation produced by the recurrent collateral effect (internal recall) and by the external input (e_i):

$$y_i = \mathrm{f}(h_i + e_i). \tag{B.18}$$

The activation function should be non-linear, and may be for example binary threshold, linear threshold, sigmoid, etc. (Hopfield, 1982; Hertz et al., 1991; Rolls, 2016b) (Fig. 1.3 and Section B.3).

B.3.4.2 The storage capacity of attractor networks with diluted connectivity

With non-linear neurons used in the network, the capacity can be measured in terms of the number of input memory patterns **y** (each a firing rate vector comprised by the firing rate of each neuron forming a vector of firing rates across the population of neurons) produced by the external input **e**, see Fig. B.13), that can be stored in the network and recalled later, even from a fragment of the stored memory pattern, whenever the network settles within each stored pattern's basin of attraction. The accuracy of the recall of each memory pattern can be measured by the correlation between the recalled firing rate vector and the stored firing rate vector. The first quantitative analysis of storage capacity, measured by the number of memory patterns that can be stored and later recalled correctly, considered a fully connected Hopfield (1982) autoassociator model, in which neurons are binary elements with an equal probability of being 'on' or 'off' in each pattern, and the number C of inputs per neuron is the same as the number N of output units (Amit, Gutfreund and Sompolinsky, 1987). (Actually it is equal to $N - 1$, since a neuron is taken not to connect to itself.) Learning is taken to occur by clamping the desired patterns on the network and using a modified Hebb rule, in which the mean of the presynaptic and postsynaptic firings is subtracted from the firing on any one learning trial (this amounts to a covariance learning rule, and is described more fully in Appendix A4 of Rolls and Treves (1998), and is shown in Equation B.21). With such fully distributed binary random patterns, the number of patterns that can be learned is (for C large) $p \approx 0.14C = 0.14N$, hence well below what could be achieved with orthogonal patterns or with an 'orthogonalizing' synaptic matrix (Hopfield, 1982; Amit et al., 1987). Many variations of this 'standard' autoassociator model have been analyzed subsequently (Amit, 1989; Hertz et al., 1991; Rolls and Treves, 1998).

This analysis has been extended to autoassociation networks that are much more biologically relevant in the following ways (Treves, 1990, 1991b; Treves and Rolls, 1991; Rolls, Treves, Foster and Perez-Vicente, 1997c; Rolls and Treves, 1998; Rolls, 2016b). First, some or many connections between the recurrent collaterals and the dendrites are missing (this is referred to as diluted connectivity, and results in a non-symmetric synaptic connection matrix in which w_{ij} does not equal w_{ji}, one of the original assumptions made in order to introduce the energy formalism in the Hopfield (1982) model). Second, the neurons need not be restricted to binary threshold neurons, but can have a threshold linear activation function (see Fig. 1.3). This enables the neurons to assume real continuously graded firing rates to different stimuli (Treves, 1990; Treves and Rolls, 1991), which are what is found in the brain (Rolls and Tovee, 1995b; Treves, Panzeri, Rolls, Booth and Wakeman, 1999; Rolls, 2016b; Rolls and Treves, 2011). Third, the representation need not be fully distributed (with half the neurons 'on', and half 'off'), but instead can have a small proportion of the neurons firing above the spontaneous rate (Treves and Rolls, 1991), which is what is found in parts of the brain such as the hippocampus that are involved in memory (Rolls, 2016b) (Appendix C). Such a representation is defined as being sparse, and the sparseness a of the representation can be measured, by extending the binary notion of the proportion of neurons that are firing, as

$$a = (\sum_{i=1}^{N} y_i/N)^2 / \sum_{i=1}^{N} y_i^2/N \tag{B.19}$$

where y_i is the firing rate of the ith neuron in the set of N neurons. Treves and Rolls (1991) have shown that such a network does operate efficiently as an autoassociative network, and can store (and recall correctly) a number of different patterns p as follows

$$p \approx \frac{C^{\mathrm{RC}}}{a \ln(\frac{1}{a})} k \tag{B.20}$$

where C^{RC} is the number of synapses on the dendrites of each neuron devoted to the recurrent collaterals from other neurons in the network, and k is a factor that depends weakly on the detailed structure of the rate distribution, on the connectivity pattern, etc., but is roughly in the order of 0.2–0.3.

The main factors that determine the maximum number of memories that can be stored in an autoassociative network are thus the number of connections on each neuron devoted to the recurrent collaterals, and the sparseness of the representation (Treves, 1991b; Treves and Rolls, 1991; Rolls and Treves, 1998; Rolls, 2016b) (Section B.3). For example, for $C^{\mathrm{RC}} = 12,000$ and $a = 0.02$, p is calculated to be approximately 36,000. This storage capacity can be realized, with little interference between patterns, if the learning rule includes some form of heterosynaptic long-term depression that counterbalances the effects of associative long-term potentiation (Treves and Rolls (1991); see Appendix A4 of Rolls and Treves (1998)). It should be noted that the number of neurons N (which is greater than C^{RC}, the number of recurrent collateral inputs received by any neuron in the network from the other neurons in the network) is not a parameter that influences the number of different memories that can be stored in the network. The implication of this is that increasing the number of neurons (without increasing the number of connections per neuron) does not increase the number of different patterns that can be stored (see Rolls and Treves (1998) Appendix A4), although it may enable simpler encoding of the firing patterns, for example more orthogonal encoding, to be used. *This latter point may account in part for why there are generally in the cerebral cortex more neurons in a recurrent network than there are connections per neuron (Rolls, 2016b), which is an important principle of cortical function.* In addition, the random stochastic fluctuations (or 'noise' (Rolls and Deco, 2010)) related to the finite number of spiking neurons is smaller with diluted compared to fully connected networks when the number of connections C per neuron and hence the storage capacity is equated (Rolls and Webb, 2012).

B.3.4.3 The network simulated

The network can be described under four headings which correspond to the four stages in which the simulation of the network operates. The formal specification of the operation of the network is the same as that of the network analyzed by Treves (1990) (see also Treves (1991b)) and simulated by Rolls, Treves, Foster and Perez-Vicente (1997c), except where indicated. First, the patterns that the net is to be trained on are binary, that is, a fraction of the neurons, which defines the sparseness a, are 1, and the remainder are 0. Second, the weights are set according to a Hebbian covariance rule. Third, the weight matrix is ablated, that is a proportion of its elements are probabilistically set to zero, to achieve an effective dilution of recurrent connectivity. In other tests, in addition, some of the synaptic weights are multiplied by 2, 3 etc as defined by a Poisson distribution to investigate the effects of multiple synaptic connections between some of the neurons. Fourth, the net undergoes testing with incomplete persistent external cues until the state has settled into retrieval or otherwise.

Pattern generation

Random binary patterns with a sparseness a of 0.1 were used.

The sparseness of the retrieved patterns was measured, to ensure that the network was operating in such a way that the sparseness of the retrieved patterns was close to that of the stored patterns. In these simulations, in contrast to earlier simulations (Rolls, Treves, Foster and Perez-Vicente, 1997c), the sparseness was set by altering the threshold T_{thr} for the activation of a neuron to produce firing in such a way that the sparseness reached a value of $a=0.1$. This has the advantage that it can be implemented by an automatic algorithm, and ensures that the sparseness of the retrieved pattern is close to the value desired of a.

Learning

The learning mechanism is a form of Hebbian covariance synaptic modification, a one-step application of a simple rule which takes account of simple pairwise covariance relationships within each pattern. The exact rule is as follows. Note that the form of the covariance rule is commutative with respect to units i and j, therefore forcing a fully connected net with such a rule to have symmetric weights.

$$w_{ij} = \frac{1}{Na^2} \sum_{\mu=1}^{p} (y_i^\mu - a)(y_j^\mu - a) \tag{B.21}$$

where w_{ij} is the weight between units i and j. y_i^μ represents the firing rate of unit i within pattern μ. This is a simple covariance rule, and a represents the mean activity in the neuronal network.

Connectivity

Networks with asymmetrical dilution of the connectivity were investigated. The dilution applied is described below where the effects of different types of dilution, and of some probability of multiple synapses between pairs of neurons, are analyzed. The total number of neurons is N, each neuron receives exactly C inputs, the dilution is C/N, and $p = \alpha C$ is the number of patterns stored in the net. The critical loading of the net, when it fails to operate as a memory, is denoted as α_c.

Testing recall by the net

During recall, the activity of each neuron in the network was asynchronously updated according to a rule which, by analogy with the theoretical analysis, considered a local field h_i at each unit i consisting of an internal field and external field, as follows:

$$h_i = \sum_{j(\neq i)} w_{ij} y_j + \sum_\mu s^\mu \frac{e_i^\mu}{a} \tag{B.22}$$

where y_j represents the output of neuron j, and s^μ represents the relative strength of pattern μ, see below.

The external field (the last term in the above Equation with e_i^μ the firing rate of the external input to neuron i produced by the pattern μ) is equivalent to the clamping, persistent external cue, which is believed to be provided by for example the direct perforant path afferents into CA3 from entorhinal cortex (Treves and Rolls, 1992). The ratio between the average number of perforant path synapses per CA3 cell and that of the recurrent collaterals is in this model allowed to determine their relative influence on the firing of CA3 cells. Anatomical evidence available from the rat suggests that the ratio of the external input (the retrieval cue) to the internal recall provided by the recurrent collaterals should be in the order of 0.25 (see Treves and Rolls (1992)), and s^μ was set to produce this ratio (for example when the retrieval cue had a correlation of 0.5 with the originally learned pattern).

The internal field (the first term in the above Equation) is equivalent to the recurrent activation provided by the recurrent collaterals in CA3. This is implemented through a standard autoassociation update rule involving weighted inputs from each of the other units. As explained above, this is qualified by the connectivity enforced through zero weights.

The activation function of the neurons is a threshold linear function of the local field h_i, with a gain factor g described by Treves (1990) set to 0.5, and with the threshold T_{thr} adjusted after each iteration in the recall to produce a retrieval sparseness that was close to 0.1 (which was the sparseness of the stored patterns), as described above.

$$y = \begin{cases} g(h - T_{\text{thr}}), & h > T_{\text{thr}} \\ 0, & h < T_{\text{thr}} \end{cases}$$

The recall of the net was measured by the correlation of the retrieved pattern with that stored, when incomplete retrieval cues were used. The performance of the network was also measured by the information retrievable from the network in bits per synapse about the set of stored patterns, as follows

$$I = \frac{\alpha}{\log 2} \sum_{k=0}^{m} \sum_{l=0}^{n} c_k^l \log \frac{c_k^l}{c_k c^l} \tag{B.23}$$

with Treves (1990) and Rolls (2016b) providing further details. Briefly, for each element of the retrieved network state and the corresponding stored pattern, the firing was first discretized into bins, and then the expression above was evaluated. In the above, c_k is the probability that the pattern element is in the kth bin of m bins, c^l is the probability that the retrieved element is in the lth bin of n bins, and c_k^l is the probability that the retrieved element is in the lth bin, and the pattern element is in the kth bin. In the implementation of this calculation, due to practical limitations, both the patterns and network states were binned into 15 bins. Note that the factor α means that the result is in bits per synapse, which is proportional to the total information stored in, and retrievable from, the whole network.

Parameters

The network functioned with a set of parameters chosen to be biologically relevant. Where the parameters are not in correspondence with measurable quantities, they were optimized to the values required for the theory to apply (Treves, 1990). This subsection details some of these parameters, and the reason for their choice.

The total number of neurons in the net was set to 1000 for the results reported.

The gain parameter, equivalent to the gradient of the linear threshold function producing the output of each unit from its incoming local field, was tested at a number of different values, and found to be optimal in the region of $g = 0.5$ for binary neurons. The actual value of g used was 0.5 for the binary patterns.

The loading α was expressed as the ratio p/C, where p is the number of patterns stored, and C is the number of connections per neuron. The loading was varied between 0.1 and 1.2 to investigate the maximum value of the storage capacity α_c, in terms of patterns, as well as to investigate the effect of over-loading. The number of patterns was varied from 40 to 480. The net was allowed to iterate for a maximum of 30 epochs.

B.3.4.4 The effects of diluted connectivity on the storage capacity of attractor networks

First a model of how the connections may be set up between neurons is formulated. The initial value of the synaptic weights is 0. This is only the prescription for whether a neuron i will receive a synaptic connection from neuron j. Let us assume that some genetic factors set the number of connections to be received by a neuron of class A from class B to be a constant C (Rolls and Stringer, 2000), the number of neurons in the network to be N, and the average connection probability to be p, so that $C = pN$. Previous analyses (Treves and Rolls, 1991; Treves, 1991b; Rolls and Treves, 1998) have assumed that when diluted connectivity is present there are exactly C connections onto each neuron i, that $C < N$, that the connections between pairs of neurons need not be reciprocal and symmetrical, and that there is at most 1 connection from neuron i to neuron j and vice versa. It is this last condition that is relaxed in this investigation (Rolls, 2012b), to examine the consequence of different scenarios that might arise according to different prescriptions for determining whether there is a synaptic connection between any two neurons in the network. Three prescriptions are considered.

Full connectivity

With full connectivity, there is one and only one synapse in a given direction between neurons i and j, and all neurons are reciprocally connected with equal weights in the two directions. This situation arises in a fully connected autoassociation network trained with an associative (Hebbian) synaptic modification rule, which produces a symmetric synaptic weight matrix (Section B.3).

Although this is the system favoured for formal analysis (Hopfield, 1982; Amit, 1989), I suggest that this would be extremely difficult for real biological systems to set up. There would have to be a biological system that would have to detect whether among something in the order of say 10,000 synapses being received by neuron i, there was more than one from neuron j. This is rejected as being implausible. There would also have to be a mechanism for ensuring that every neuron in the set of N neurons had at least 1 connection to every other neuron in the set of N neurons. This is rejected as being implausible. There would also need to be a way for genes to specify that a particular set of N neurons specified a particular network. This is rejected as being implausible. Thus it is argued that fully connected networks are unlikely to be found in the brain if they are set up by a simple mechanism such as a neuron making synapses at random with nearby neurons, which is consistent with the evidence (Hill, Wang, Riachi, Schürmann and Markram, 2012). Thus this genetically simple mechanism to prescribe connections for neurons to make would not lead to a fully connected network.

Connectivity with on average one synapse in a given direction between neurons j and i

Let us assume that among a population of N neurons, a biological process forms connections at random to any one neuron i from the other neurons j until the average number of connections to any neuron i from any one neuron j is 1. In this situation, some neurons i will receive more than one connection from neuron j, and some will receive 0 connections from neuron j. In fact, the number of connections received by neuron i from neuron j will follow approximately a Poisson distribution with mean (λ) = 1. Given that all neurons are trained using an associative synaptic modification rule of the form shown in Equation B.16, this will mean that some neuron pairs will have a synaptic strength that is twice, three times, etc. the strength of the connections between the neurons with one synapse between them. It is suggested, and tested next, that the consequences of this are that the energy landscape is considerably distorted. Hopfield (1982) was able to show that in a fully connected network trained associatively the recall state can be thought of as the local minimum in an energy

Table B.3 The probability of different numbers of connections X between neurons for different values of λ, the average number of connections between neurons in the network, based on a Poisson distribution. The column labelled $C(N = 1000)$ shows the numbers of synaptic connections to a neuron i multiplied by X in prescribing a network with N=1000 neurons with λ=1.

X	λ=1	$C(N=1000)$	λ=0.1	λ=0.04
0	0.3679	368	0.9048	0.9608
1	0.3679	368	0.0905	0.0384
2	0.1839	184	0.0045	0.0008
3	0.0613	61	0.0002	0.0000
4	0.0153	15	0.0000	0.0000
5	0.0031	3	0.0000	0.0000
6	0.0005	0.5	0.0000	0.0000

landscape, where the energy would be defined as

$$E = -\frac{1}{2} \sum_{i,j} w_{ij} (y_i - <y>)(y_j - <y>). \tag{B.24}$$

This Equation can be understood in the following way. If two neurons are both firing above their mean rate (denoted by $<y>$), and are connected by a weight with a positive value, then the firing of these two neurons is consistent with each other, and they mutually support each other, so that they contribute to the system's tendency to remain stable. If across the whole network such mutual support is generally provided, then no further change will take place, and the system will indeed remain stable. If, on the other hand, either of our pair of neurons was not firing, or if the connecting weight had a negative value, the neurons would not support each other, and indeed the tendency would be for the neurons to try to alter ('flip' in the case of binary units) the state of the other. This would be repeated across the whole network until a situation in which most mutual support, and least 'frustration', was reached. What makes it possible to define an energy function and for these points to hold is that the matrix is symmetric (see Hopfield (1982), Hertz, Krogh and Palmer (1991), Amit (1989)).

It is shown next by simulations that if connectivity of the type defined in this section is present, with some pairs of neurons having several connections between them, then the energy landscape is distorted in such a way that there are deep energy minima in some parts of the energy landscape, and this reduces the capacity of the network, that is, its ability to store 0.14 N binary patterns with sparseness a=0.5 (Hopfield, 1982), or a larger number of patterns with more sparse representations as shown in Equations B.20 and B.15 (Treves and Rolls, 1991).

Simulations were run with the attractor network described in Section B.3.4.3 and by Rolls, Treves, Foster and Perez-Vicente (1997c) with 1000 neurons (Rolls, 2012b). The sparseness of the randomly chosen binary patterns was 0.1. The connectivity was set to have a mean number of connections between any pair of neurons, λ, equal to 1.0 with a Poisson distribution, resulting in the number of connections between pairs of neurons shown in Table B.3. The algorithm for setting the number of connections was to select an output neuron i, and then set it to have exactly the number of inputs from each of the other neurons in the network (chosen in a random sequence to prevent connections from a neuron already chosen) shown in Table B.3. This resulted in an asymmetric connection matrix with each neuron i having exactly the number of 0, single, double, etc synaptic connections to other neurons in the network shown in Table B.3. In practice, the algorithm was applied after training by multiplying the synaptic weights by the values shown in Table B.3. The resulting synaptic connectivity matrix thus reflected what would be produced by any one neuron having a mean number of connections with other neurons set according to a Poisson distribution with the mean number

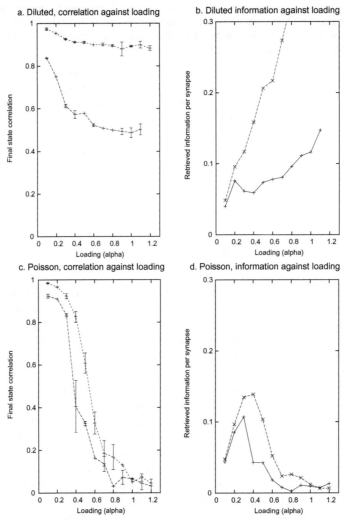

Fig. B.14 (a, b). The performance of the attractor network with diluted connectivity only with λ=1 for the average number of connections received by each output neuron. In this case, there were 368 weights of zero, and the remainder were multiplied by 1. (c, d). The performance of the attractor network with the numbers of connections between neurons specified by the full Poisson distribution shown in Table B.3 diluted connectivity only with λ=1 for the average number of connections received by each output neuron. In this case, there were 368 weights of zero, and 368 were multiplied by 1, 184 by 2, 61 by 3, etc. (a,c). The correlation of the final state of the network after recall with the stored pattern, as a function of loading $\alpha = p/C$. The two lines in each graph correspond to two retrieval cue levels: the lower line is for a cue correlated 0.5–0.55 with the original stored pattern, and the upper line is for a cue correlation of 0.9–0.95. The error bars represent the standard deviations. (b,d). The information retrieved in bits per synapse after recall with the stored pattern, as a function of loading $\alpha = p/C$. (From Edmund T. Rolls (2012) Advantages of dilution in the connectivity of attractor networks in the brain. Biologically Inspired Cognitive Architectures 1: 44–54. Copyright © Elsevier B.V.)

of connections between any pair of neurons, λ, equal to 1. In some cases a pair of neurons would have no synaptic connections, and in other cases 1, 2, 3 etc synaptic connections as shown by the probabilities and numbers for a network of 1000 neurons shown in Table B.3.

Fig. B.14a,b shows the results of applying just the degree of dilution of the synaptic weights indicated in Table B.3 as the baseline control condition, without any double, triple etc synapses. In this case, there were 368 weights of zero out of the starting number of C=1000, and the remainder were multiplied by 1. The correlation of the final state of the network after recall with the stored pattern, as a function of loading $\alpha = p/C$, is shown in Fig. B.14a. The two lines in each graph correspond to two retrieval cue levels: the lower line is for a retrieval cue correlated 0.5–0.55 with the original stored pattern, and the upper line is for a retrieval cue correlation of 0.9–0.95. The information retrieved in bits per synapse after recall with the stored pattern, as a function of loading $\alpha = p/C$ is shown in Fig. B.14b. (In this Figure, the loading value α shown on the abscissa refers to the fully connected case with C=1000 connections per neuron, and should be multiplied by 1.58 given that with the dilution there are in fact C=638 connections per neuron, as shown in Table B.3.) The results in Fig. B.14a,b show good performance up to high loading levels when only dilution of the connectivity is present, and there are no multiple synapses between neuron pairs present.

These results emphasize that with diluted connectivity, and asymmetric connections between pairs of neurons, the attractor network still displays its predicted memory capacity, and ability to complete memories from incomplete patterns (Treves and Rolls, 1991; Treves, 1991b; Bovier and Gayrard, 1992; Perez Castillo and Skantzos, 2004; Rolls et al., 1997c; Rolls and Treves, 1998).

Fig. B.14c,d shows the results of applying the identical degree of dilution of the synaptic weights to that used in Fig. B.14a,b, but now with the number of double, triple etc weight synapses indicated in Table B.3 column 3. At low levels of loading $\alpha \leq 0.4$ the performance is as good as or better than the control baseline dilution-only simulation shown in Fig. B.14a,b, but at higher loading levels the performance drops off very greatly (Fig. B.14c,d). Fig. B.14a,b shows that α_c, the critical loading capacity of the network beyond which the memory fails and little information can be retrieved from it, is approximately 0.4. With just diluted connectivity, without multiple synaptic connections, the critical capacity α_c was higher than 1.2, as shown in Fig. B.14a,b.

It is therefore concluded (Rolls, 2012b) that prescription 2 (section B.3.4.4) for setting the connectivity is seriously flawed, as it reduces the capacity of the attractor network, i.e. the number of patterns that it can store per synapse onto each neuron (Treves and Rolls, 1991; Rolls, 2016b), because of the multiple synapses found between a proportion of the neurons. The interpretation of the loss of capacity with some multiple synapses present is that this distorts the energy landscape by producing irregular deep and broad areas which attract patterns that are some distance away, so that it is not possible to have a large number of approximately equal-size basins of attraction in the energy landscape. The interpretation of the somewhat better performance at low loading with some multiple synapses present is that if there are few basins present, but they are deep and large due to the multiple synapses, then patterns some distance away can be drawn into a nearby attractor, which, given large spacing between the attractor basins, is likely to be the correct attractor basin.

I further hypothesize that double synapses would distort the patterns being stored if they are graded (for example having an exponential distribution of firing rates across the population of neurons for any one stimulus), which is typical of neural representations (Treves, 1990; Rolls, 2016b; Rolls and Treves, 2011; Rolls et al., 1997c; Franco et al., 2007; Rolls and Treves, 2011) (Appendix C). It is possible that the graded firing rate representation could no longer be accurately stored: the graded representation would be distorted by the extra firing of neurons with double connections. Simulations of the type described by Rolls, Treves, Foster and Perez-Vicente (1997c) could be performed to check whether this becomes an issue, depending on the number of double, triple etc synapses between some neuron pairs.

Diluted connectivity with $C < N$

Let us assume that among a population of N neurons, a biological process forms connections at random between any pair of neurons, so that in the resulting network there are C incoming connections to any of N neurons, with $C < N$. Assuming symmetry, this implies that the number L_{ij} of the connections from any neuron j to any neuron i follows a Binomial distribution Bin $\left(C, \frac{1}{N-1}\right)$:

$$\text{Prob}\{L_{ij} = k\} = \frac{C!}{k!(C-k)!}\left(\frac{1}{N-1}\right)^k\left(1 - \frac{1}{N-1}\right)^{C-k} \quad \text{(B.25)}$$
$$= \frac{C(C-1)\ldots(C-k+1)}{1\cdot 2\cdot\ldots k}(N-1)^{C-k}$$

where k is between 0 and C. When $C = \lambda N$ and $N \to \infty$, this distribution is well approximated by the Poisson distribution with mean λ.

For example, let us assume a diluted connectivity with the average number of connections per neuron λ=0.1. We set up connections with the same general prescription as in prescription 2 (Section B.3.4.4). However, if $\lambda = 0.1$, the probability that any two neurons will have two connections between them is 0.0045, as shown in Table B.3. (In a network with N=1000 neurons, there would be 91 single connections onto each neuron, and only 5 double connections onto each neuron, with no triple connections.) This is a much smaller probability. Additional simulations of the type illustrated in Fig. B.14 were performed with $\lambda = 0.1$. The results showed that having this small proportion of double strength synapses in the network produced very little reduction in the correlation of the retrieved patterns with those stored, or in the capacity of the attractor network to store many patterns using the type of analysis shown in Fig. B.14c,d. The number of patterns that can be stored is still of order C (Treves and Rolls, 1991), with the constant k in Equation B.20 little affected by this small number of multiple connections between pairs of neurons.

This scenario applies in the real brain. For example, an estimate for the dilution C/N in the neocortex might be 0.1. (For the neocortex, assuming 10,000 recurrent collaterals per pyramidal cell, that the density of pyramidal cells is 30,000 / mm^3 (Rolls, 2016b), that the radius of the recurrent collaterals is 1 mm, and that we are dealing with the superficial (or deep) layers of the cortex with a depth of approximately 1 mm, the dilution between the superficial (or deep) pyramidal cells would be approximately 0.1.)

A similar but somewhat more diluted scenario applies in the hippocampus. In the rat hippocampus, there are $N = 300,000$ CA3 neurons, and each neuron receives $C = 12,000$ synapses (see Fig. 9.23) (Rolls, 1990b; Treves and Rolls, 1992). (It is assumed that each CA3 neuron correspondingly makes 12,000 recurrent collateral synapses.) The dilution of this network C/N thus equals 0.04. In a network with N=1000 neurons and λ=0.04, there would be 38 single synapses onto each neuron, and only 1 double synapse, as is evident from Table B.3. This low number of double synapses, with no triple etc synapses, has little effect on the operation of the network, as shown by further simulations of the type illustrated in Fig. B.14 (Rolls, 2012b). It is proposed that this network operates as an autoassociation or attractor network, and is key to how the hippocampus operates to store episodic memories (Rolls, 1996d, 2016b, 2010b) (see Chapter 2 of Rolls (2016b)), and here the number of different memories that can be stored in the network is at a premium, and is provided for by this level of dilution of the connectivity which ensures few multiple synapses between any pair of neurons.

B.3.4.5 Synthesis of the effects of diluted connectivity in attractor networks

The results of the simulations (Rolls, 2012b) therefore support the proposal made by Rolls (2012b) that the reason why networks in the neocortex and hippocampal cortex have diluted connectivity is that the diluted connectivity ensures that the energy landscape and thereby the memory capacity is not disturbed by multiple connections between pairs of neurons, with the network still operating correctly in the diluted regime where C/N is in the range 0.1–0.01 (Treves, 1991b; Rolls et al., 1997c; Rolls and Treves, 1998; Rolls, 2016b). The somewhat greater dilution of connectivity (with fewer multiple synapses) in the hippocampal CA3 network (0.04) than the estimate of its value in the neocortex (0.1) may be related to the great importance of achieving a high memory capacity with good retrieval of all stored patterns in the hippocampus where this may be useful for episodic memory, for which memory capacity in a single network is important (Rolls, 2016b, 2010b) (Chapter 9).

In both these types of cortex, there is evidence that the excitatory interconnections between neurons are associatively modifiable, and that the system supports attractor dynamics that enable memories to be stored (Section B.3). One of the points made here is that with a local associative rule, the presynaptic and the postsynaptic activity at a given synapse to determine the strength of that connection between a pair of neurons, which is a widely held assumption (Rolls and Treves, 1998; Rolls, 2016b), then consequences of the type described here on memory capacity would ensue. A difference between these cortical structures is that the CA3 network is a single network allowing any representation to be associated with any other representation, providing an implementation of episodic memory (Rolls, 2016b, 2010b; Kesner and Rolls, 2015). In contrast, the neocortex has local connectivity with a radius of approximately 2 mm, and this enables the whole of the cerebral cortex to have many separate attractor networks, each storing a large number of memories (O'Kane and Treves, 1992; Rolls, 2016b).

Another potential advantage of diluted connectivity in which the number of neurons N is greater than C^{RC}, the number of recurrent collateral inputs received by any neuron in the network from the other neurons in the network, is that this may enable simpler encoding of the firing patterns, for example more orthogonal encoding, to be used. For example, much of the information available from the firing rates of a population of neurons about which stimulus was presented can be read by a decoding procedure as simple as a dot product, which is what neurons compute using their synaptic weight vector, and which is very biologically plausible (Rolls, 2016b; Rolls and Treves, 2011) (Appendix C).

Another advantage of diluted recurrent collateral connectivity is that it can increase the storage capacity α_c of autoassociation (attractor) networks, that is the number of patterns that can be stored per recurrent collateral synapse (Treves and Rolls, 1991). (This useful effect applies provided that representations are not too sparse, because when the sparseness is very low, $a << 0.01$, the performance becomes similar to that of a fully connected network (see Treves and Rolls (1991) Fig. 5a; and Rolls and Treves (1998) Fig. A4.2.)

Another advantage of diluted connectivity (for the same number of connections per neuron) is that this increases the stability and accuracy of the network as there is less spiking-related noise producing stochastic fluctuations in the diluted network (which has more neurons in it), with little cost in increased decision times (Rolls and Webb, 2012).

Very diluted connectivity in feedforward networks (for example, competitive networks) can also play a role in pattern separation, by encouraging different output neurons to respond to different, random, combinations of the inputs because each neuron is connected to a different combination of inputs (Rolls, 2016b,f). This finds application in the brain in for example the dentate granule cell mossy fibre to CA3 connections which are very dilute but strong. The architecture helps grid cell representations to be transformed into place or spatial view representations (Treves and Rolls, 1992; Rolls, Stringer and Elliot, 2006c; Rolls and Kesner, 2006b; Rolls, 2016b, 2010b).

In summary, Rolls (2012b) proposed that the reason why networks in the neocortex and hippocampal cortex have diluted connectivity in the recurrent collateral connections is that the diluted connectivity ensures that the energy landscape and thereby the memory capacity is not disturbed by multiple connections between pairs of neurons, with the network still operating correctly in the diluted regime where C/N is in the range 0.1–0.01 (Treves, 1991b; Rolls et al., 1997c; Rolls and Treves, 1998; Rolls, 2016b). It was shown that having a proportion of multiple connections between neurons in an attractor network trained by an associative rule produces a major reduction in $\alpha_c = p/C$, the memory capacity of the network beyond which adding further memories drastically impairs the ability of the network to retrieve any memories. That important reason for dilution in the connectivity of cortical networks, which helps them to be specified by relatively few and simple genetic rules consistent with a limited number of genes in the whole genome in the order of 25,000 compared to the number of synapses which is in the order of 10^{15} (Rolls and Stringer, 2000; Rolls, 2016b), is accompanied by other advantages of the dilution of cortical connectivity elucidated by Rolls (2012b).

B.3.5 Use of autoassociation networks in the brain

Because of its 'one-shot' rapid learning, and ability to complete, this type of network is well suited for episodic memory storage, in which each episode must be stored and recalled later from a fragment, and kept separate from other episodic memories. It does not take a long time (the 'many epochs' of backpropagation networks) to train this network, because it does not have to 'discover the structure' of a problem. Instead, it stores information in the form in which it is presented to the memory, without altering the representation. An autoassociation network may be used for this function in the CA3 region of the hippocampus (see Chapter 9, and Rolls and Treves (1998) Chapter 6).

An autoassociation memory can also be used as a short-term memory, in which iterative processing round the recurrent collateral loop keeps a representation active until another input cue is received. This may be used to implement many types of short-term memory in the brain (see Section 13.6.1). For example, it may be used in the perirhinal cortex and adjacent temporal lobe cortex to implement short-term visual object memory (Miyashita and Chang, 1988; Amit, 1995; Hirabayashi, Takeuchi, Tamura and Miyashita, 2013); in the dorsolateral prefrontal cortex to implement a short-term memory for spatial responses (Goldman-Rakic, 1996); and in the prefrontal cortex to implement a short-term memory for where eye movements should be made in space (see Section 13.6.1 and Rolls (2016b)). Such an autoassociation memory in the temporal lobe visual cortical areas may be used to implement the firing that continues for often 300 ms after a very brief (16 ms) presentation of a visual stimulus (Rolls and Tovee, 1994) (see e.g. Fig. C.19), and may be one way in which a short memory trace is implemented to facilitate invariant learning about visual stimuli (see Chapter 2). In all these cases, the short-term memory may be implemented by the recurrent excitatory collaterals that connect nearby pyramidal cells in the cerebral cortex. The connectivity in this system, that is the probability that a neuron synapses on a nearby neuron, may be in the region of 10% (Braitenberg and Schüz, 1991; Abeles, 1991; Rolls, 2016b).

The recurrent connections between nearby neocortical pyramidal cells may also be important in defining the response properties of cortical cells, which may be triggered by external inputs (from for example the thalamus or a preceding cortical area), but may be considerably dependent on the synaptic connections received from nearby cortical pyramidal cells.

The cortico-cortical backprojection connectivity described in Chapters 1, and 9 can be interpreted as a system that allows the forward-projecting neurons in one cortical area to be linked autoassociatively with the backprojecting neurons in the next cortical area (see Chapter 9). This would be implemented by associative synaptic modification in for example the backprojections. This particular architecture may be especially important in constraint satisfaction (as well as recall), that is it may allow the networks in the two cortical areas to settle into a mutually consistent state. This would effectively enable information in higher cortical areas, which would include information from more divergent sources, to influence the response properties of neurons in earlier cortical processing stages. This is an important function in cortical information processing of interacting associative networks.

For semantic memory, different cortical regions may specialize in different attributes of a semantic memory, e.g. an individual with attributes such as the sight of the face, the sound of the voice, the location where they work, etc. Semantic memories could be formed by coupling many such attractor networks together, in what are described as Potts attractor networks (Treves, 2005; Kropff and Treves, 2005; Boboeva, Brasselet and Treves, 2018; Ryom, Stendardi, Ciaramelli and Treves, 2023). An interesting issue arises though that if similar features (e.g. the sounds of the voices of several of the individuals are similar) are present in such compositional memories in the semantic representations of different individual items, this effectively increases the correlations between the items in the whole memory, and this can reduce somewhat the total memory capacity that might be expected (Ryom, Stendardi, Ciaramelli and Treves, 2023). Given that the formation of semantic memories is facilitated by the recall of episodic memory from the hippocampus (Section 9.2.8.5), it is proposed that an important contribution of the hippocampus to semantic memories is that pattern separation performed by the hippocampal system including the dentate granule cells (Rolls, 2016f), helps to reduce the correlations between the different semantic memories formed by hippocampus to neocortical recall. How semantic representations are stored using coupled attractor networks is a topic of current interest.

B.4 Competitive networks, including self-organizing maps

B.4.1 Function

Competitive neural networks learn to categorize input pattern vectors. Each category of inputs activates a different output neuron (or set of output neurons – see below). The categories formed are based on similarities between the input vectors. Similar, that is correlated, input vectors activate the same output neuron. In that the learning is based on similarities in the input space, and there is no external teacher that forces classification, this is an unsupervised network. The term categorization is used to refer to the process of placing vectors into categories based on their similarity. The term classification is used to refer to the process of placing outputs in particular classes as instructed or taught by a teacher. Examples of classifiers are pattern associators, one-layer delta-rule perceptrons, and multilayer perceptrons taught by error backpropagation (see Sections B.2, B.3, B.11 and B.12). In supervised networks there is usually a teacher for each output neuron.

The categorization produced by competitive nets is of great potential importance in perceptual systems including the whole of the visual cortical processing hierarchies, as described in Chapter 2. Each category formed reflects a set or cluster of active inputs x_j that occur together. This cluster of coactive inputs can be thought of as a feature, and the competitive network can be described as building feature analyzers, where a feature can now be defined as a correlated set of inputs. During learning, a competitive network gradually discovers these features in the input space, and the process of finding these features without a teacher is referred to as self-organization.

Another important use of competitive networks is to remove redundancy from the input space, by allocating output neurons to reflect a set of inputs that co-occur.

Another important aspect of competitive networks is that they separate patterns that are somewhat correlated in the input space, to produce outputs for the different patterns that are less correlated with each other, and may indeed easily be made orthogonal to each other. This has been referred to as orthogonalization.

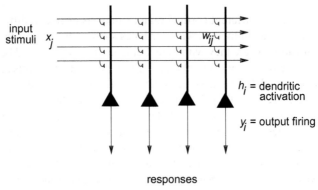

Fig. B.15 The architecture of a competitive network.

Another important function of competitive networks is that partly by removing redundancy from the input information space, they can produce sparse output vectors, without losing information. We may refer to this as sparsification.

B.4.2 Architecture and algorithm

B.4.2.1 Architecture

The basic architecture of a competitive network is shown in Fig. B.15. It is a one-layer network with a set of inputs that make modifiable excitatory synapses w_{ij} with the output neurons. The output cells compete with each other (for example by mutual inhibition) in such a way that the most strongly activated neuron or neurons win the competition, and are left firing strongly. The synaptic weights, w_{ij}, are initialized to random values before learning starts. If some of the synapses are missing, that is if there is randomly diluted connectivity, that is not a problem for such networks, and can even help them (see below).

In the brain, the inputs arrive through axons, which make synapses with the dendrites of the output or principal cells of the network. The principal cells are typically pyramidal cells in the cerebral cortex. In the brain, the principal cells are typically excitatory, and mutual inhibition between them is implemented by inhibitory interneurons, which receive excitatory inputs from the principal cells. The inhibitory interneurons then send their axons to make synapses with the pyramidal cells, typically using GABA (gamma-aminobutyric acid) as the inhibitory transmitter.

B.4.2.2 Algorithm

1. Apply an input vector **x** and calculate the activation h_i of each neuron

$$h_i = \sum_j x_j w_{ij} \qquad (B.26)$$

where the sum is over the C input axons, indexed by j. (It is useful to normalize the length of each input vector **x**. In the brain, a scaling effect is likely to be achieved both by feedforward inhibition, and by feedback inhibition among the set of input cells (in a preceding network) that give rise to the axons conveying **x**.)

The output firing y_i^1 is a function of the activation of the neuron

$$y_i^1 = f(h_i). \qquad (B.27)$$

The function f can be linear, sigmoid, monotonically increasing, etc. (see Fig. 1.3).

2. Allow competitive interaction between the output neurons by a mechanism such as lateral or mutual inhibition (possibly with self-excitation), to produce a contrast-enhanced version of the firing rate vector

$$y_i = g(y_i^1). \tag{B.28}$$

Function g is typically a non-linear operation, and in its most extreme form may be a winner-take-all function, in which after the competition one neuron may be 'on', and the others 'off'. Algorithms that produce softer competition without a single winner to produce a distributed representation are described in Section B.4.9.4 below. Grossberg (2021) has described suitable mathematical formulations.

3. Apply an associative Hebb-like learning rule

$$\delta w_{ij} = \alpha y_i x_j. \tag{B.29}$$

4. Normalize the length of the synaptic weight vector on each dendrite to prevent the same few neurons always winning the competition:

$$\sum_j (w_{ij})^2 = 1. \tag{B.30}$$

(A less efficient alternative is to scale the sum of the weights to a constant, e.g. 1.0.)

5. Repeat steps 1–4 for each different input stimulus **x**, in random sequence, a number of times.

B.4.3 Properties

B.4.3.1 Feature discovery by self-organization

Each neuron in a competitive network becomes activated by a set of consistently coactive, that is correlated, input axons, and gradually learns to respond to that cluster of coactive inputs. We can think of competitive networks as discovering features in the input space, where features can now be defined by a set of consistently coactive inputs. Competitive networks thus show how feature analyzers can be built, with no external teacher. The feature analyzers respond to correlations in the input space, and the learning occurs by self-organization in the competitive network. Competitive networks are therefore well suited to the analysis of sensory inputs. Ways in which they may form fundamental building blocks of sensory systems are described in Chapter 2.

The operation of competitive networks can be visualized with the help of Fig. B.16. The input patterns are represented as dots on the surface of a sphere. (The patterns are on the surface of a sphere because the patterns are normalized to the same length.) The directions of the weight vectors of the three neurons are represented by '×'s. The effect of learning is to move the weight vector of each of the neurons to point towards the centre of one of the clusters of inputs. If the neurons are winner-take-all, the result of the learning is that although there are correlations between the input stimuli, the outputs of the three neurons are orthogonal. In this sense, orthogonalization is performed. At the same time, given that each of the patterns within a cluster produces the same output, the correlations between the patterns within a cluster become higher. In a winner-take-all network, the within-pattern correlation becomes 1, and the patterns within a cluster have been placed within the same category.

B.4.3.2 Removal of redundancy

In that competitive networks recode sets of correlated inputs to one or a few output neurons, then redundancy in the input representation is removed. Identifying and removing redundancy

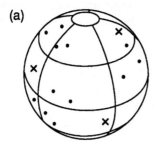 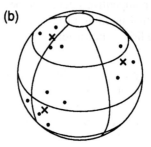

Fig. B.16 Competitive learning. The dots represent the directions of the input vectors, and the '×'s the weights for each of three output neurons. (a) Before learning. (b) After learning. (After Rumelhart,D.E. and Zipser,D. (1985) Feature discovery by competitive learning. Cognitive Science 9: 75–112.)

in sensory inputs is an important part of processing in sensory systems (cf. Barlow (1989)), in part because a compressed representation is more manageable as an output of sensory systems. The reason for this is that neurons in the receiving systems, for example pattern associators in the orbitofrontal cortex or autoassociation networks in the hippocampus, can then operate with the limited numbers of inputs that each neuron can receive. For example, although the information that a particular face is being viewed is present in the 10^6 fibres in the optic nerve, the information is unusable by associative networks in this form, and is compressed through the visual system until the information about which of many hundreds of faces is present can be represented by less than 100 neurons in the temporal cortical visual areas (Rolls, Treves and Tovee, 1997b; Abbott, Rolls and Tovee, 1996). (Redundancy can be defined as the difference between the maximum information content of the input data stream (or channel capacity) and its actual content; see Appendix C.)

The recoding of input pattern vectors into a more compressed representation that can be conveyed by a much reduced number of output neurons of a competitive network is referred to in engineering as vector quantization. With a winner-take-all competitive network, each output neuron points to or stands for one of or a cluster of the input vectors, and it is more efficient to transmit the states of the few output neurons than the states of all the input elements. (It is more efficient in the sense that the information transmission rate required, that is the capacity of the channel, can be much smaller.) Vector quantization is of course possible when the input representation contains redundancy.

B.4.3.3 Orthogonalization and categorization

Figure B.16 shows visually how competitive networks reduce the correlation between different clusters of patterns, by allocating them to different output neurons. This is described as orthogonalization. It is a process that is very usefully applied to signals before they are used as inputs to associative networks (pattern associators and autoassociators) trained with Hebbian rules (see Sections B.2 and B.3), because it reduces the interference between patterns stored in these memories. The opposite effect in competitive networks, of bringing closer together very similar input patterns, is referred to as categorization.

These two processes are also illustrated in Fig. B.17, which shows that in a competitive network, very similar input patterns (with correlations higher in this case than approximately 0.8) produce more similar outputs (close to 1.0), whereas the correlations between pairs of input patterns that are smaller than approximately 0.7 become much smaller in the output representation. (This simulation used soft competition between neurons with graded firing rates.)

Further analyses of the operation of competitive networks, and how diluted connectivity

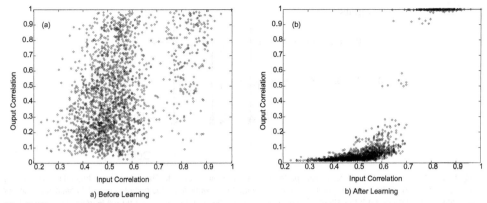

Fig. B.17 Orthogonalization and categorization in a competitive network: (a) before learning; (b) after learning. The correlations between pairs of output vectors (abscissa) are plotted against the correlations of the corresponding pairs of input vectors that generated the output pair, for all possible pairs in the input set. The competitive net learned for 16 cycles. One cycle consisted of presenting the complete input set of stimuli in a renewing random sequence. The correlation measure shown is the cosine of the angle between two vectors (i.e. the normalized dot product). The network used had 64 input axons to each of 8 output neurons. The net was trained with 64 stimuli, made from 8 initial random binary vectors with each bit having a probability of 0.5 of being 1, from each of which 8 noisy exemplars were made by randomly altering 10 % of the 64 elements. Soft competition was used between the output neurons. (A normalized exponential activation function described in Section B.4.9.4 was used to implement the soft competition.) The sparseness a of the input patterns thus averaged 0.5; and the sparseness a of the output firing vector after learning was close to 0.17 (i.e. after learning, primarily one neuron was active for each input pattern; before learning, the average sparseness of the output patterns produced by each of the inputs was 0.39).

can help the operation of competitive networks, are provided elsewhere (Rolls, 2016f) (see also Section 7.4 of Rolls (2016b)). Dilution in the connectivity of competitive networks can help to break the symmetry, so that some neurons are likely to be allocated to some patterns, and other neurons to other patterns (because of the particular set of input connections of each neuron), and this can help to stabilize a competitive network, by making it difficult for neurons to drift during further learning if the input patterns drift (Rolls, 2016f,b). In such a system, multiple connections from some input neurons to an output neuron might even be advantageous, for the reasons just given. This emphasizes the point that multiple connections between neurons are found in some parts of the cortex, including for example thalamo-cortical inputs and cortico-cortical forward projections, where a strong selective drive to some neurons may be important (Rolls, 2016b).

B.4.3.4 Sparsification

Competitive networks can produce more sparse representations than those that they receive, depending on the degree of competition. With the greatest competition, winner-take-all, only one output neuron remains active, and the representation is at its most sparse. This effect can be understood further using Figs. B.16 and B.17. This sparsification is useful to apply to representations before input patterns are applied to associative networks, because sparse representations allow many different pattern associations or memories to be stored in these networks (see Sections B.2 and B.3).

B.4.3.5 Capacity

In a competitive net with N output neurons and a simple winner-take-all rule for the competition, it is possible to learn up to N output categories, in that each output neuron may be allocated a category. When the competition acts in a less rudimentary way, the number of categories that can be learned becomes a complex function of various factors, including the number of modifiable connections per cell and the degree of dilution, or incompleteness, of the connections. Such a function has not yet been described analytically in general, but an

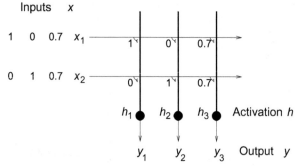

Fig. B.18 Separation of linearly dependent patterns by a competitive network. The network was trained on patterns 10, 01, and 11, applied on the inputs x_1 and x_2. After learning, the network allocated output neuron 1 to pattern 10, neuron 2 to pattern 01, and neuron 3 to pattern 11. The weights in the network produced during the learning are shown. Each input pattern was normalized to unit length, and thus for pattern 11, x_1=0.7 and x_2=0.7, as shown. Because the weight vectors were also normalized to unit length, w_{31}=0.7 and w_{32}=0.7.

upper bound on it can be deduced for the particular case in which the learning is fast, and can be achieved effectively in one shot, or one presentation of each pattern. In that case, the number of categories that can be learned (by the self-organizing process) will at most be equal to the number of associations that can be formed by the corresponding pattern associators, a process that occurs with the additional help of the driving inputs, which effectively determine the categorization in the pattern associator.

Separate constraints on the capacity result if the output vectors are required to be strictly orthogonal. Then, if the output firing rates can assume only positive values, the maximum number p of categories arises, obviously, in the case when only one output neuron is firing for any stimulus, so that up to N categories are formed. If ensemble encoding of output neurons is used (soft competition), again under the orthogonality requirement, then the number of output categories that can be learned will be reduced according to the degree of ensemble encoding. The p categories in the ensemble-encoded case reflect the fact that the between-cluster correlations in the output space are lower than those in the input space. The advantages of ensemble encoding are that dendrites are more evenly allocated to patterns (see Section B.4.9.5), and that correlations between different input stimuli can be reflected in correlations between the corresponding output vectors, so that later networks in the system can generalize usefully. This latter property is of crucial importance, and is utilized for example when an input pattern is presented that has not been learned by the network. The relative similarity of the input pattern to previously learned patterns is indicated by the relative activation of the members of an ensemble of output neurons. This makes the number of different representations that can be reflected in the output of competitive networks with ensemble encoding much higher than with winner-take-all representations, even though with soft competition all these representations cannot strictly be learned.

B.4.3.6 Separation of non-linearly separable patterns

A competitive network can not only separate (e.g. by activating different output neurons) pattern vectors that overlap in almost all elements, but can also help with the separation of vectors that are not linearly separable. An example is that three patterns **A**, **B**, and **A+B** will lead to three different output neurons being activated (see Fig. B.18). For this to occur, the length of the synaptic weight vectors must be normalized (to for example unit length), so that they lie on the surface of a sphere or hypersphere (see Fig. B.16). (If the weight vectors of each neuron are scaled to the same sum, then the weight vectors do not lie on the surface of a hypersphere, and the ability of the network to separate patterns is reduced.)

The property of pattern separation makes a competitive network placed before an autoassociation (or pattern association) network very valuable, for it enables the autoassociator to store the three patterns separately, and to recall **A+B** separately from **A** and **B**. This is referred to as the configuration learning problem in animal learning theory (Sutherland and Rudy, 1991). Placing a competitive network before a pattern associator will enable a linearly inseparable problem to be solved. For example, three different output neurons of a two-input competitive network could respond to the patterns 01, 10, and 11, and a pattern associator can learn different outputs for neurons 1–3, which are orthogonal to each other (see Fig. B.11). This is an example of expansion recoding (cf. Marr (1969), who used a different algorithm to obtain the expansion). The sparsification that can be produced by the competitive network can also be advantageous in preparing patterns for presentation to a pattern associator or autoassociator, because the sparsification can increase the number of memories that can be associated or stored.

B.4.3.7 Stability

These networks are generally stable if the input statistics are stable. If the input statistics keep varying, then the competitive network will keep following the input statistics. If this is a problem, then a critical period in which the input statistics are learned, followed by stabilization, may be useful. This appears to be a solution used in developing sensory systems, which have critical periods beyond which further changes become more difficult. An alternative approach taken by Carpenter and Grossberg in their 'Adaptive Resonance Theory' (Carpenter, 1997; Grossberg, 2021) is to allow the network to learn only if it does not already have categorizers for a pattern (see Hertz, Krogh and Palmer (1991), p. 228).

Diluted connectivity can help stability, by making neurons tend to find inputs to categorize in only certain parts of the input space, and then making it difficult for the neuron to wander randomly throughout the space later (Rolls, 2016f,b).

B.4.3.8 Frequency of presentation

If some stimuli are presented more frequently than others, then there will be a tendency for the weight vectors to move more rapidly towards frequently presented stimuli, and more neurons may become allocated to the frequently presented stimuli. If winner-take-all competition is used, the result is that the neurons will tend to become allocated during the learning process to the more frequently presented patterns. If soft competition is used, the tendency of neurons to move from patterns that are infrequently or never presented can be reduced by making the competition fairly strong, so that only a few neurons show any learning when each pattern is presented. Provided that the competition is moderately strong (see Section B.4.9.4), the result is that more neurons are allocated to frequently presented patterns, but one or some neurons are allocated to infrequently presented patterns. These points can all be easily demonstrated in simulations.

In an interesting development, it has been shown that if objects consisting of groups of features are presented during training always with another object present, then separate representations of each object can be formed provided that each object is presented many times, but on each occasion is paired with a different object (Stringer and Rolls, 2008; Stringer, Rolls and Tromans, 2007b). This is related to the fact that in this scenario the frequency of co-occurrence of features within the same object is greater than that of features between different objects (see Section 2.8.6.2).

B.4.3.9 Comparison to principal component analysis (PCA) and cluster analysis

Although competitive networks find clusters of features in the input space, they do not perform hierarchical cluster analysis as typically performed in statistics. In hierarchical cluster analysis, input vectors are joined starting with the most correlated pair, and the level of the joining of vectors is indicated. Competitive nets produce different outputs (i.e. activate different output neurons) for each cluster of vectors (i.e. perform vector quantization), but do not compute the level in the hierarchy, unless the network is redesigned (see Hertz, Krogh and Palmer (1991)).

The feature discovery can also be compared to principal component analysis (PCA). (In PCA, the first principal component of a multidimensional space points in the direction of the vector that accounts for most of the variance, and subsequent principal components account for successively less of the variance, and are mutually orthogonal.) In competitive learning with a winner-take-all algorithm, the outputs are mutually orthogonal, but are not in an ordered series according to the amount of variance accounted for, unless the training algorithm is modified. The modification amounts to allowing each of the neurons in a winner-take-all network to learn one at a time, in sequence. The first neuron learns the first principal component. (Neurons trained with a modified Hebb rule learn to maximize the variance of their outputs – see Hertz, Krogh and Palmer (1991).) The second neuron is then allowed to learn, and because its output is orthogonal to the first, it learns the second principal component. This process is repeated. Details are given by Hertz, Krogh and Palmer (1991), but as this is not a biologically plausible process, it is not considered in detail here.

I note that simple competitive learning is very helpful biologically, because it can separate patterns, but that a full ordered set of principal components as computed by PCA would probably not be very useful in biologically plausible networks. The point here is that biological neuronal networks may operate well if the variance in the input representation is distributed across many input neurons, whereas principal component analysis would tend to result in most of the variance being allocated to a few neurons, and the variance being unevenly distributed across the neurons.

B.4.4 Utility of competitive networks in information processing by the brain

B.4.4.1 Feature analysis and preprocessing

Neurons that respond to correlated combinations of their inputs can be described as feature analyzers. Neurons that act as feature analyzers perform useful preprocessing in many sensory systems (see e.g. Chapter 8 of Rolls and Treves (1998) and Rolls (2021b)). The power of competitive networks in multistage hierarchical processing to build combinations of what is found at earlier stages, and thus effectively to build higher-order representations, is also described in Chapter 2 of this book. An interesting development is that competitive networks can learn about individual objects even when multiple objects are presented simultaneously, provided that each object is presented several times more frequently than it is paired with any other individual object (Stringer and Rolls, 2008) (see Section 2.8.6.2). This property arises because learning in competitive networks is primarily about forming representations of objects defined by a high correlation of coactive features in the input space (Stringer and Rolls, 2008; Rolls, 2021d).

B.4.4.2 Removal of redundancy

The removal of redundancy by competition is thought to be a key aspect of how sensory systems, including the ventral cortical visual system, operate. Competitive networks can also be thought of as performing dimension reduction, in that a set of correlated inputs may be responded to as one category or dimension by a competitive network. The concept of redundancy removal can be linked to the point that individual neurons trained with a modified Hebb rule point their weight vector in the direction of the vector that accounts for most of the variance in the input, that is (acting individually) they find the first principal component of the input space (see Section B.4.3.9 and Hertz, Krogh and Palmer (1991)). Although networks with anti-Hebbian synapses between the principal cells (in which the anti-Hebbian learning forces neurons with initially correlated activity to effectively inhibit each other) (Földiák, 1991), and networks that perform Independent Component Analysis (Bell and Sejnowski, 1995), could in principle remove redundancy more effectively, it is not clear that they are implemented biologically. In contrast, competitive networks are more biologically plausible, and illustrate redundancy reduction. The more general use of an unsupervised competitive preprocessor is discussed below (see Fig. B.25).

B.4.4.3 Orthogonalization

The orthogonalization performed by competitive networks is very useful for preparing signals for presentation to pattern associators and autoassociators, for this re-representation decreases interference between the patterns stored in such networks. Indeed, this can be essential if patterns are overlapping and not linearly independent, e.g. 01, 10, and 11. If three such binary patterns were presented to an autoassociative network, it would not form separate representations of them, because either of the patterns 01 or 10 would result by completion in recall of the 11 pattern. A competitive network allows a separate neuron to be allocated to each of the three patterns, and this set of orthogonal representations can be learned by associative networks (see Fig. B.18).

B.4.4.4 Sparsification

The sparsification performed by competitive networks is very useful for preparing signals for presentation to pattern associators and autoassociators, for this re-representation increases the number of patterns that can be associated or stored in such networks (see Sections B.2 and B.3).

B.4.4.5 Brain systems in which competitive networks may be used for orthogonalization and sparsification

One system is the hippocampus, in which the dentate granule cells are believed to operate as a competitive network in order to prepare signals for presentation to the CA3 autoassociative network (see Chapter 9). In this case, the operation is enhanced by expansion recoding, in that (in the rat) there are approximately three times as many dentate granule cells as there are cells in the preceding stage, the entorhinal cortex. This expansion recoding will itself tend to reduce correlations between patterns (cf. Marr (1970), and Marr (1969)).

Also in the hippocampus, the CA1 neurons are thought to act as a competitive network that recodes the separate representations of each of the parts of an episode that must be separately represented in CA3, into a form more suitable for the recall using pattern association performed by the backprojections from the hippocampus to the cerebral cortex (see Chapter 9 and Rolls and Treves (1998) Chapter 6).

The granule cells of the cerebellum may perform a similar function, but in this case the principle may be that each of the very large number of granule cells receives a very small

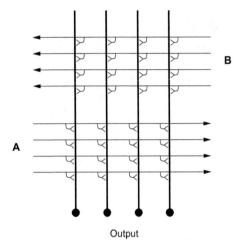

Fig. B.19 Competitive net receiving a normal forward set of inputs **A**, but also another set of inputs **B** that can be used to influence the categories formed in response to **A** inputs. The inputs **B** might be backprojection inputs.

random subset of inputs, so that the outputs of the granule cells are decorrelated with respect to the inputs (Marr (1969); see Chapter 17).

B.4.5 Guidance of competitive learning

Although competitive networks are primarily unsupervised networks, it is possible to influence the categories found by supplying a second input, as follows (Rolls, 1989a). Consider a competitive network as shown in Fig. B.19 with the normal set of inputs **A** to be categorized, and with an additional set of inputs **B** from a different source. Both sets of inputs work in the normal way for a competitive network, with random initial weights, competition between the output neurons, and a Hebb-like synaptic modification rule that normalizes the lengths of the synaptic weight vectors onto each neuron. The idea then is to use the **B** inputs to influence the categories formed by the **A** input vectors. The influence of the **B** vectors works best if they are orthogonal to each other. Consider any two **A** vectors. If they occur together with the same **B** vector, then the categories produced by the **A** vectors will be more similar than they would be without the influence of the **B** vectors. The categories will be pulled closer together if soft competition is used, or will be more likely to activate the same neuron if winner-take-all competition is used. Conversely, if any two **A** vectors are paired with two different, preferably orthogonal, **B** vectors, then the categories formed by the **A** vectors will be drawn further apart than they would be without the **B** vectors. The differences in categorization remain present after the learning when just the **A** inputs are used.

This guiding function of one of the inputs is one way in which the consequences of sensory stimuli could be fed back to a sensory system to influence the categories formed when the **A** inputs are presented. This could be one function of backprojections in the cerebral cortex (Rolls, 1989c,a) (Chapter 9). In this case, the **A** inputs of Fig. B.19 would be the forward inputs from a preceding cortical area, and the **B** inputs backprojecting axons from the next cortical area, or from a structure such as the amygdala or hippocampus. If two **A** vectors were both associated with positive reinforcement that was fed back as the same **B** vector from another part of the brain, then the two **A** vectors would be brought closer together in the representational space provided by the output of the neurons. If one of the **A** vectors was associated with positive reinforcement, and the other with negative reinforcement, then the output representations of the two **A** vectors would be further apart. This is one way in which external signals could influence in a mild way the categories formed in sensory systems.

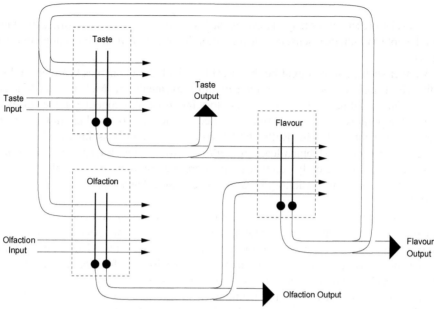

Fig. B.20 A two-layer set of competitive nets in which feedback from layer 2 can influence the categories formed in layer 1. Layer 2 could be a higher cortical visual area with convergence from earlier cortical visual areas (see Chapter 2). In the example, taste and olfactory inputs are received by separate competitive nets in layer 1, and converge into a single competitive net in layer 2. The categories formed in layer 2 (which may be described as representing 'flavor') may be dominated by the relatively orthogonal set of a few tastes that are received by the net. When these layer 2 categories are fed back to layer 1, they may produce in layer 1 categories in, for example, the olfactory network that reflect to some extent the flavor categories of layer 2, and are different from the categories that would otherwise be formed to a large set of rather correlated olfactory inputs. A similar principle may operate in any multilayer hierarchical cortical processing system, such as the ventral visual system, in that the categories that can be formed only at later stages of processing may help earlier stages to form categories relevant to what can be identified at later stages.

Another is that if any **B** vector only occurred for important sensory **A** inputs (as shown by the immediate consequences of receiving those sensory inputs), then the **A** inputs would simply be more likely to have any representation formed than otherwise, due to strong activation of neurons only when combined **A** and **B** inputs are present.

A similar architecture could be used to provide mild guidance for one sensory system (e.g. olfaction) by another (e.g. taste), as shown in Fig. B.20. (Another example of where this architecture could be used is convergence in the visual system at the next cortical stage of processing, with guiding feedback to influence the categories formed in the different regions of the preceding cortical area, as illustrated in Chapter 9.) The idea is that the taste inputs would be more orthogonal to each other than the olfactory inputs, and that the taste inputs would influence the categories formed in the olfactory input categorizer in layer 1, by feedback from a convergent net in layer 2. The difference from the previous architecture is that we now have a two-layer net, with unimodal or separate networks in layer 1, each feeding forward to a single competitive network in layer 2. The categories formed in layer 2 reflect the co-occurrence of a particular taste with particular odors (which together form flavor in layer 2). Layer 2 then provides feedback connections to both the networks in layer 1. It can be shown in such a network that the categories formed in, for example, the olfactory net in layer 1 are influenced by the tastes with which the odors are paired. The feedback signal is built only in layer 2, after there has been convergence between the different modalities. This architecture captures some of the properties of sensory systems, in which there are unimodal processing cortical areas followed by multimodal cortical areas. The multimodal cortical areas can build representations that represent the unimodal inputs that tend to co-occur, and the higher level representations may in turn, by the highly developed cortico-cortical backprojections, be able to influence sensory categorization in earlier cortical processing areas (Rolls, 1989a).

Another such example might be the effect by which the phonemes heard are influenced by the visual inputs produced by seeing mouth movements (cf. McGurk and MacDonald (1976)). This could be implemented by auditory inputs coming together in the cortex in the superior temporal sulcus onto neurons activated by the sight of the lips moving (recorded during experiments of Baylis, Rolls and Leonard (1987), and Hasselmo, Rolls, Baylis and Nalwa (1989b)), using Hebbian learning with co-active inputs. Backprojections from such multimodal areas to the early auditory cortical areas could then influence the responses of auditory cortex neurons to auditory inputs (see Section B.9 and Fig. B.41, and cf. Calvert et al. (1997)).

A similar principle may operate in any multilayer hierarchical cortical processing system, such as the ventral visual system, in that the categories that can be formed only at later stages of processing may help earlier stages to form categories relevant to what can be identified at the later stages as a result of the operation of backprojections (Rolls, 1989a). The idea that the statistical correlation between the inputs received by neighbouring processing streams can be used to guide unsupervised learning within each stream has also been developed by Becker and Hinton (1992) and others (see Phillips, Kay and Smyth (1995)). The networks considered by these authors self-organize under the influence of collateral connections, such as may be implemented by cortico-cortical connections between parallel processing systems in the brain. They use learning rules that, although somewhat complex, are still local in nature, and tend to optimize specific objective functions. The locality of the learning rule, and the simulations performed so far, raise some hope that, once the operation of these types of networks is better understood, they might achieve similar computational capabilities to backpropagation networks (see Section B.12) while retaining biological plausibility.

B.4.6 Topographic map formation

A simple modification to the competitive networks described so far enables them to develop topological maps. In such maps, the closeness in the map reflects the similarity (correlation) between the features in the inputs. The modification that allows such maps to self-organize is to add short-range excitation and long-range inhibition between the neurons. The function to be implemented has a spatial profile that is described as having a Mexican hat shape (see Fig. B.21). The effect of this connectivity between neurons, which need not be modifiable, is to encourage neurons that are close together to respond to similar features in the input space, and to encourage neurons that are far apart to respond to different features in the input space. When these response tendencies are present during learning, the feature analyzers that are built by modifying the synapses from the input onto the activated neurons tend to be similar if they are close together, and different if far apart. This is illustrated in Figs. B.22 and B.23. Feature maps built in this way were described by von der Malsburg (1973) and Willshaw and von der Malsburg (1976). It should be noted that the learning rule needed is simply the modified Hebb rule described above for competitive networks, and is thus local and biologically plausible. (For computational convenience, the algorithm that Kohonen (Kohonen, 1982, 1989, 1995) has mainly used does not use Mexican hat connectivity between the neurons, but instead arranges that when the weights to a winning neuron are updated, so to a smaller extent are those of its neighbours – see further Hertz, Krogh and Palmer (1991).)

A very common characteristic of connectivity in the brain, found for example throughout the neocortex, consists of short-range excitatory connections between neurons, with inhibition mediated via inhibitory interneurons. The density of the excitatory connectivity even

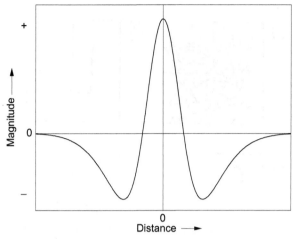

Fig. B.21 Mexican hat lateral spatial interaction profile.

falls gradually as a function of distance from a neuron, extending typically a distance in the order of 1 mm from the neuron (Braitenberg and Schüz, 1991), contributing to a spatial function quite like that of a Mexican hat. (Longer-range inhibitory influences would form the negative part of the spatial response profile.) This supports the idea that topological maps, though in some cases probably seeded by chemoaffinity, could develop in the brain with the assistance of the processes just described. It is noted that some cortico-cortical connections even within an area may be longer, skipping past some intermediate neurons, and then making connections after some distance with a further group of neurons. Such longer-range connections are found for example between different columns with similar orientation selectivity in the primary visual cortex. The longer range connections may play a part in stabilizing maps, and again in the exchange of information between neurons performing related computations, in this case about features with the same orientations.

If a low-dimensional space, for example the orientation sensitivity of cortical neurons in the primary visual cortex (which is essentially one-dimensional, the dimension being angle), is mapped to a two-dimensional space such as the surface of the cortex, then the resulting map can have long spatial runs where the value along the dimension (in this case orientation tuning) alters gradually, and continuously. Such self-organization can account for many aspects of the mapping of orientation tuning, and of ocular dominance columns, in V1 (Miller, 1994; Harris, Ermentrout and Small, 1997). If a high-dimensional information space is mapped to the two-dimensional cortex, then there will be only short runs of groups of neurons with similar feature responsiveness, and then the map must fracture, with a different type of feature mapped for a short distance after the discontinuity. This is exactly what Rolls suggests is the type of topology found in the anterior inferior temporal visual cortex, with the individual groupings representing what can be self-organized by competitive networks combined with a trace rule as described in Section 2.8. Here, visual stimuli are not represented with reference to their position on the retina, because here the neurons are relatively translation invariant. Instead, when recording here, small clumps of neurons with similar responses may be encountered close together, and then one moves into a group of neurons with quite different feature selectivity (personal observations). This topology will arise naturally, given the anatomical connectivity of the cortex with its short-range excitatory connections, because there are very many different objects in the world and different types of features that describe objects, with no special continuity between the different combinations of features possible.

Rolls' hypothesis contrasts with the view of Tanaka (1996), who has claimed that the

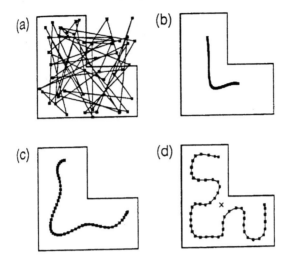

Fig. B.22 Kohonen feature mapping from a two-dimensional L-shaped region to a linear array of 50 units. Each unit has 2 inputs. The input patterns are the X,Y coordinates of points within the L-shape shown. In the diagrams, each point shows the position of a weight vector. Lines connect adjacent units in the 1 D (linear) array of 50 neurons. The weights were initialized to random values within the unit square (a). During feature mapping training, the weights evolved through stages (b) and (c) to (d). By stage (d) the weights have formed so that the positions in the original input space are mapped to a 1 D vector in which adjacent points in the input space activate neighbouring units in the linear array of output units. (Reproduced from Hertz,J.A., Krogh,A. and Palmer,R.G. (1991) Introduction to the Theory of Neural Computation. Addison-Wesley: Wokingham, UK. Fig. 9.13.)

inferior temporal cortex provides an alphabet of visual features arranged in discrete modules. The type of mapping found in higher cortical visual areas as proposed by Rolls implies that topological self-organization is an important way in which maps in the brain are formed, for it seems most unlikely that the locations in the map of different types of object seen in an environment could be specified genetically (Rolls and Stringer, 2000). Consistent with this, Tsao, Freiwald, Tootell and Livingstone (2006) described with macaque fMRI 'anterior face patches' at A15 to A22. A15 might correspond to where we have analyzed face-selective neurons (it might translate to 3 mm posterior to our sphenoid reference, see Section 2.4), and at this level there are separate regions specialized for face identity in areas TEa and TEm on the ventral lip of the superior temporal sulcus and the adjacent gyrus, and for face expression and movement in the cortex deep in the superior temporal sulcus (Hasselmo, Rolls and Baylis, 1989a; Baylis, Rolls and Leonard, 1987; Rolls, 2007e). The 'middle face patch' of Tsao, Freiwald, Tootell and Livingstone (2006) was at A6, which is probably part of the posterior inferior temporal cortex, and, again consistent with self-organizing map principles, has a high concentration of face-selective neurons within the patch.

The biological utility of developing such topology-preserving feature maps may be that if the computation requires neurons with similar types of response to exchange information more than neurons involved in different computations (which is more than reasonable), then the total length of the connections between the neurons is minimized if the neurons that need to exchange information are close together (cf. Cowey (1979), Durbin and Mitchison (1990)). Examples of this include the separation of color constancy processing in V4 from global motion processing in MT as follows (see Chapter 3 of Rolls and Deco (2002)). In V4, to compute color constancy, an estimate of the illuminating wavelengths can be obtained by summing the outputs of the pyramidal cells in the inhibitory interneurons over several degrees of visual space, and subtracting this from the excitatory central ON color-tuned region of the receptive field by (subtractive) feedback inhibition. This enables the cells to discount the illuminating

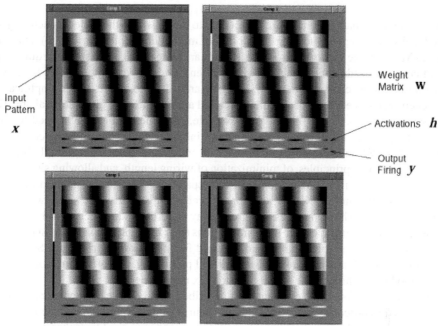

Fig. B.23 Example of a one-dimensional topological map that self-organized from inputs in a low-dimensional space. The network has 64 neurons (vertical elements in the diagram) and 64 inputs per neuron (horizontal elements in the diagram). The four different diagrams represent the net tested with different input patterns. The input patterns x are displayed at the left of each diagram, with white representing firing and black not firing for each of the 64 inputs. The central square of each diagram represents the synaptic weights of the neurons, with white representing a strong weight. The row vector below each weight matrix represents the activations of the 64 output neurons, and the bottom row vector the output firing y. The network was trained with a set of 8 binary input patterns, each of which overlapped in 8 of its 16 'on' elements with the next pattern. The diagram shows that as one moves through correlations in the input space (top left to top right to bottom left to bottom right), so the output neurons activated move steadily across the output array of neurons. Closely correlated inputs are represented close together in the output array of neurons. The way in which this occurs can be seen by inspection of the weight matrix. The network architecture was the same as for a competitive net, except that the activations were converted linearly into output firings, and then each neuron excited its neighbours and inhibited neurons further away. This lateral inhibition was implemented for the simulation by a spatial filter operating on the output firings with the following filter weights (cf. Fig. B.21): 5, 5, 5, 5, 5, 5, 5, 5, 5, 10, 10, 10, 10, 10, 10, 10, 10, 10, 5, 5, 5, 5, 5, 5, 5, 5 which operated on the 64-element firing rate vector.

wavelength, and thus compute color constancy. For this computation, no inputs from motion-selective cells (which in the dorsal stream are color insensitive) are needed. In MT, to compute global motion (e.g. the motion produced by the average flow of local motion elements, exemplified for example by falling snow), the computation can be performed by averaging in the larger (several degrees) receptive fields of MT the local motion inputs received by neurons in earlier cortical areas (V1 and V2) with small receptive fields (see Chapter 3 of Rolls and Deco (2002) and Rolls and Stringer (2006a)). For this computation, no input from color cells is useful. Having separate areas (V4 and MT) for these different computations minimizes the wiring lengths, for having intermingled color and motion cells in a single cortical area would increase the average connection length between the neurons that need to be connected for the computations being performed. Minimizing the total connection length between neurons in the brain is very important in order to keep the size of the brain relatively small.

Placing close to each other neurons that need to exchange information, or that need to receive information from the same source, or that need to project towards the same destination, may also help to minimize the complexity of the rules required to specify cortical (and indeed brain) connectivity (Rolls and Stringer, 2000). For example, in the case of V4 and MT, the connectivity rules can be simpler (e.g. connect to neurons in the vicinity, rather than look for color-, or motion-marked cells, and connect only to the cells with the correct genetically specified label specifying that the cell is either part of motion or of color processing). Further, the V4 and MT example shows that how the neurons are connected can be specified quite simply, but of course it needs to be specified to be different for different computations. Specifying a general rule for the classes of neurons in a given area also provides a useful simplification to the genetic rules needed to specify the functional architecture of a given cortical area (Rolls and Stringer, 2000). In our V4 and MT example, the genetic rules would need to specify the rules separately for different populations of inhibitory interneurons if the computations performed by V4 and MT were performed with intermixed neurons in a single brain area. Together, these two principles, of minimization of wiring length, and allowing simple genetic specification of wiring rules, may underlie the separation of cortical visual information processing into different (e.g. ventral and dorsal) processing streams. The same two principles operating within each brain processing stream may underlie (taken together with the need for hierarchical processing to enable the computations to be biologically plausible in terms of the number of connections per neuron, and the need for local learning rules, see Section 19.4) much of the overall architecture of visual cortical processing, and of information processing and its modular architecture throughout the cortex more generally.

The rules of information exchange just described could also tend to produce more gross topography in cortical regions. For example, neurons that respond to animate objects may have certain visual feature requirements in common, and may need to exchange information about these features. Other neurons that respond to inanimate objects might have somewhat different visual feature requirements for their inputs, and might need to exchange information strongly. (For example, selection of whether an object is a chisel or a screwdriver may require competition by mutual (lateral) inhibition to produce the contrast enhancement necessary to result in unambiguous neuronal responses.) The rules just described would account for neurons with responsiveness to inanimate and animate objects tending to be grouped in separate parts of a cortical map or representation, and thus separately susceptible to brain damage (see e.g. Farah (1990), Farah (2000)).

B.4.7 Invariance learning by competitive networks

In conventional competitive learning, the weight vector of a neuron can be thought of as moving towards the centre of a cluster of similar overlapping input stimuli (Rumelhart and Zipser, 1985; Hertz, Krogh and Palmer, 1991; Rolls and Treves, 1998; Rolls and Deco, 2002; Perry, Rolls and Stringer, 2006; Rolls, 2016b). The weight vector points towards the centre of the set of stimuli in the category. The different training stimuli that are placed into the same category (i.e. activate the same neuron) are typically overlapping in that the pattern vectors are correlated with each other. Figure B.24a illustrates this.

For the formation of invariant representations, there are multiple occurrences of the object at different positions in the space. The object at each position represents a different transform (whether in position, size, view etc.) of the object. The different transforms may be uncorrelated with each other, as would be the case for example with an object translated so far in the space that there would be no active afferents in common between the two transforms. Yet we need these two orthogonal patterns to be mapped to the same output. It may be a very elongated part of the input space that has to be mapped to the same output in invariance learning. These concepts are illustrated in Fig. B.24b.

Objects in the world have temporal and spatial continuity. That is, the statistics of the world are such that we tend to look at one object for some time, during which it may be transforming continuously from one view to another. The temporal continuity property is used in trace rule invariance training, in which a short-term memory in the associative learning rule

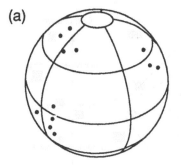 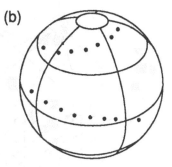

Fig. B.24 (a) Conventional competitive learning. A cluster of overlapping input patterns is categorized as being similar, and this is implemented by a weight vector of an output neuron pointing towards the centre of the cluster. Three clusters are shown, and each cluster might after training have a weight vector pointing towards it. (b) Invariant representation learning. The different transforms of an object may span an elongated region of the space, and the transforms at the far ends of the space may have no overlap (correlation), yet the network must learn to categorize them as similar. The different transforms of two different objects are represented.

normally used to train competitive networks is used to help build representations that reflect the continuity in time that characterizes the different transforms of each object, as described in Chapter 2. The transforms of an object also show spatial continuity, and this can also be used in invariance training in what is termed continuous spatial transform learning, described in Section 2.8.11.

In conventional competitive learning the overall weight vector points to the prototypical representation of the object. The only sense in which after normal competitive training (without translations etc) the network generalizes is with respect to the dot product similarity of any input vector compared to the central vector from the training set that the network learns. Continuous spatial transformation learning works by providing a set of training vectors that overlap, and between them cover the whole space over which an invariant transform of the object must be learned. Indeed, it is important for continuous spatial transformation learning that the different exemplars of an object are sufficiently close that the similarity of adjacent training exemplars is sufficient to ensure that the same postsynaptic neuron learns to bridge the continuous space spanned by the whole set of training exemplars of a given object (Stringer, Perry, Rolls and Proske, 2006; Perry, Rolls and Stringer, 2006; Rolls, 2021d). This will enable the postsynaptic neuron to span a very elongated space of the different transforms of an object, as described in Section 2.8.11.

B.4.8 Radial Basis Function networks

As noted above, a competitive network can act as a useful preprocessor for other networks. In the neural examples above, competitive networks were useful preprocessors for associative networks. Competitive networks are also used as preprocessors in artificial neural networks, for example in hybrid two-layer networks such as that illustrated in Fig. B.25. The competitive network is advantageous in this hybrid scheme, because as an unsupervised network, it can relatively quickly (with a few presentations of each stimulus) discover the main features in the input space, and code for them. This leaves the second layer of the network to act as a supervised network (taught for example by the delta rule, see Section B.11), which learns to map the features found by the first layer into the output required. This learning scheme is very much faster than that of a (two-layer) backpropagation network, which learns very

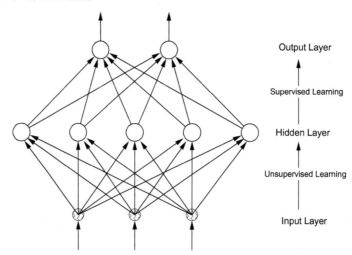

Fig. B.25 A hybrid network, in which for example unsupervised learning rapidly builds relatively orthogonal representations based on input differences, and this is followed by a one-layer supervised network (taught for example by the delta rule) that learns to classify the inputs based on the categorizations formed in the hidden/intermediate layer.

slowly because it takes it a long time to perform the credit assignment to build useful feature analyzers in layer one (the hidden layer) (see Section B.12).

The general scheme shown in Fig. B.25 is used in radial basis function (RBF) neural networks. The main difference from what has been described is that in an RBF network, the hidden neurons do not use a winner-take-all function (as in some competitive networks), but instead use a normalized activation function in which the measure of distance from a weight vector of the neural input is (instead of the dot product $\mathbf{x} \cdot \mathbf{w}_i$ used for most of the networks described in this book), a Gaussian measure of distance:

$$y_i = \frac{\exp[-(\mathbf{x} - \mathbf{w}_i)^2 / 2\sigma_i^2]}{\sum_k \exp[-(\mathbf{x} - \mathbf{w}_k)^2 / 2\sigma_k^2]}. \tag{B.31}$$

The effect is that the response y_i of neuron i is a maximum if the input stimulus vector $\mathbf{x}$ is centred at $\mathbf{w}_i$, the weight vector of neuron i (this is the upper term in Equation B.31). The magnitude is normalized by dividing by the sum of the activations of all the k neurons in the network. If the input vector $\mathbf{x}$ is not at the centre of the receptive field of the neuron, then the response is decreased according to how far the input vector is from the weight vector $\mathbf{w}_i$ of the neuron, with the weighting decreasing as a Gaussian function with a standard deviation of σ. The idea is like that implemented with soft competition, in that the relative response of different neurons provides an indication of where the input pattern is in relation to the weight vectors of the different neurons. The rapidity with which the response falls off in a Gaussian radial basis function neuron is set by σ_i, which is adjusted so that for any given input pattern vector, a number of RBF neurons are activated. The positions in which the RBF neurons are located (i.e. the directions of their weight vectors, $\mathbf{w}$) are determined usually by unsupervised learning, e.g. the vector quantization that is produced by the normal competitive learning algorithm. The first layer of an RBF network is not different in principle from a network with soft competition, and it is not clear how biologically a Gaussian activation function would be implemented, so the treatment is not developed further here (see Hertz, Krogh and Palmer (1991), Poggio and Girosi (1990a), and Poggio and Girosi (1990b) for further details).

B.4.9 Further details of the algorithms used in competitive networks

B.4.9.1 Normalization of the inputs

Normalization is useful because in step 1 of the training algorithm described in Section B.4.2.2, the neuronal activations, formed by the inner product of the pattern and the normalized weight vector on each neuron, are scaled in such a way that they have a maximum value of 1.0. This helps different input patterns to be equally effective in the learning process. A way in which this normalization could be achieved by a layer of input neurons is given by Grossberg (1976a, 2021). In the brain, a number of factors may contribute to normalization of the inputs. One factor is that a set of input axons to a neuron will come from another network in which the firing is controlled by inhibitory feedback, and if the numbers of axons involved is large (hundreds or thousands), then the inputs will be in a reasonable range. Second, there is increasing evidence that the different classes of input to a neuron may activate different types of inhibitory interneuron (e.g. Buhl, Halasy and Somogyi (1994)), which terminate on separate parts of the dendrite, usually close to the site of termination of the corresponding excitatory afferents. This may allow separate feedforward inhibition for the different classes of input. In addition, the feedback inhibitory interneurons also have characteristic termination sites, often on or close to the cell body, where they may be particularly effective in controlling firing of the neuron by shunting (divisive) inhibition, rather than by scaling a class of input (see Section B.6).

B.4.9.2 Normalization of the length of the synaptic weight vector on each dendrite

This is necessary to ensure that one or a few neurons do not always win the competition. (If the weights on one neuron were increased by simple Hebbian learning, and there was no normalization of the weights on the neuron, then it would tend to respond strongly in the future to patterns with some overlap with patterns to which that neuron has previously learned, and gradually that neuron would capture a large number of patterns.) A biologically plausible way to achieve this weight adjustment is to use a modified Hebb rule:

$$\delta w_{ij} = \alpha y_i (x_j - w_{ij}) \tag{B.32}$$

where α is a constant, and x_j and w_{ij} are in appropriate units. In vector notation,

$$\delta \mathbf{w}_i = \alpha y_i (\mathbf{x} - \mathbf{w}_i) \tag{B.33}$$

where $\mathbf{w}_i$ is the synaptic weight vector on neuron i. This implements a Hebb rule that increases synaptic strength according to conjunctive pre- and post-synaptic activity, and also allows the strength of each synapse to decrease in proportion to the firing rate of the postsynaptic neuron (as well as in proportion to the existing synaptic strength). This results in a decrease in synaptic strength for synapses from weakly active presynaptic neurons onto strongly active postsynaptic neurons. Such a modification in synaptic strength is termed heterosynaptic long-term depression in the neurophysiological literature, referring to the fact that the synapses that weaken are other than those that activate the neuron.

This is an important computational use of heterosynaptic long-term depression (LTD). In that the amount of decrease of the synaptic strength depends on how strong the synapse is already, the rule is compatible with what is frequently reported in studies of LTD (see Section 1.6). This rule can maintain the sums of the synaptic weights on each dendrite to be very similar without any need for explicit normalization of the synaptic strengths, and is useful in competitive nets. This rule was used by Willshaw and von der Malsburg (1976). As is made clear with the vector notation above, the modified Hebb rule moves the direction of the weight vector $\mathbf{w}_i$ towards the current input pattern vector $\mathbf{x}$ in proportion to the difference between these two vectors and the firing rate y_i of neuron i.

If explicit weight (vector length) normalization is needed, the appropriate form of the modified Hebb rule is:

$$\delta w_{ij} = \alpha y_i(x_j - y_i w_{ij}). \tag{B.34}$$

This rule, formulated by Oja (1982), makes weight decay proportional to y_i^2, normalizes the synaptic weight vector (see Hertz, Krogh and Palmer (1991)), is still a local learning rule, and is known as the Oja rule.

B.4.9.3 Non-linearity in the learning rule

Non-linearity in the learning rule can assist competition (Rolls, 1990b, 1996d). For example, in the brain, long-term potentiation typically occurs only when strong activation of a neuron has produced sufficient depolarization for the voltage-dependent NMDA receptors to become unblocked, allowing Ca^{2+} to enter the cell (see Section 1.6). This means that synaptic modification occurs only on neurons that are strongly activated, effectively assisting competition to select few winners. The learning rule can be written:

$$\delta w_{ij} = \alpha m_i x_j \tag{B.35}$$

where m_i is a (e.g. threshold) non-linear function of the post-synaptic firing y_i which mimics the operation of the NMDA receptors in learning. (It is noted that in associative networks the same process may result in the stored pattern being more sparse than the input pattern, and that this may be beneficial, especially given the exponential firing rate distribution of neurons, in helping to maximize the number of patterns stored in associative networks (see Sections B.2, B.3, and C.3.1).

B.4.9.4 Competition

In a simulation of a competitive network, a single winner can be selected by searching for the neuron with the maximum activation. If graded competition is required, this can be achieved by an activation function that increases greater than linearly. In some of the networks we have simulated (Rolls, 1990b, 1989a; Wallis and Rolls, 1997), raising the activation to a fixed power, typically in the range 2–5, and then rescaling the outputs to a fixed maximum (e.g. 1) is simple to implement. In a real neuronal network, winner-take-all competition can be implemented using mutual (lateral) inhibition between the neurons with non-linear activation functions, and self-excitation of each neuron (see e.g. Grossberg (1976a), Grossberg (1988), Hertz, Krogh and Palmer (1991), and Grossberg (2021)).

Another method to implement soft competition in simulations is to use the normalized exponential or 'softmax' activation function for the neurons (Bridle (1990); see Bishop (1995)):

$$y = \exp(h) / \sum_i \exp(h_i) . \tag{B.36}$$

This function specifies that the firing rate of each neuron is an exponential function of the activation, scaled by the whole vector of activations h_i, $i = 1, N$. The exponential function (in increasing supralinearly) implements soft competition, in that after the competition the faster firing neurons are firing relatively much faster than the slower firing neurons. In fact, the strength of the competition can be adjusted by using a 'temperature' T greater than 0 as follows:

$$y = \exp(h/T) / \sum_i \exp(h_i/T). \tag{B.37}$$

Very low temperatures increase the competition, until with $T \to 0$, the competition becomes 'winner-take-all'. At high temperatures, the competition becomes very soft. (When using the function in simulations, it may be advisable to prescale the firing rates to for example the range 0–1, both to prevent machine overflow, and to set the temperature to operate on a constant range of firing rates, as increasing the range of the inputs has an effect similar to decreasing T.)

The softmax function has the property that activations in the range $-\infty$ to $+\infty$ are mapped into the range 0 to 1.0, and the sum of the firing rates is 1.0. This facilitates interpretation of the firing rates under certain conditions as probabilities, for example that the competitive network firing rate of each neuron reflects the probability that the input vector is within the category or cluster signified by that output neuron (see Bishop (1995)).

B.4.9.5 Soft competition

The use of graded (continuous valued) output neurons in a competitive network, and soft competition rather than winner-take-all competition, has the value that the competitive net generalizes more continuously to an input vector that lies between input vectors that it has learned. Also, with soft competition, neurons with only a small amount of activation by any of the patterns being used will nevertheless learn a little, and move gradually towards the patterns that are being presented. The result is that with soft competition, the output neurons all tend to become allocated to one of the input patterns or one of the clusters of input patterns.

B.4.9.6 Untrained neurons

In competitive networks, especially with winner-take-all or finely tuned neurons, it is possible that some neurons remain unallocated to patterns. This may be useful, in case patterns in the unused part of the space occur in future. Alternatively, unallocated neurons can be made to move towards the parts of the space where patterns are occurring by allowing such losers in the competition to learn a little. Another mechanism is to subtract a bias term μ_i from y_i, and to use a 'conscience' mechanism that raises μ_i if a neuron wins frequently, and lowers μ_i if it wins infrequently (Grossberg, 1976b; Bienenstock, Cooper and Munro, 1982; De Sieno, 1988).

B.4.9.7 Large competitive nets: further aspects

If a large neuronal network is considered, with the number of synapses on each neuron in the region of 10,000, as occurs on large pyramidal cells in some parts of the brain, then there is a potential disadvantage in using neurons with synaptic weights that can take on only positive values. This difficulty arises in the following way. Consider a set of positive normalized input firing rates and synaptic weight vectors (in which each element of the vector can take on any value between 0.0 and 1.0). Such vectors of random values will on average be more highly aligned with the direction of the central vector (1,1,1,...,1) than with any other vector. An example can be given for the particular case of vectors evenly distributed on the positive 'quadrant' of a high-dimensional hypersphere: the average overlap (i.e. normalized dot product) between two binary random vectors with half the elements on and thus a sparseness of 0.5 (e.g. a random pattern vector and a random dendritic weight vector) will be approximately 0.5, while the average overlap between a random vector and the central vector will be approximately 0.707. A consequence of this will be that if a neuron begins to learn towards several input pattern vectors it will get drawn towards the average of these input patterns which will be closer to the 1,1,1,...,1 direction than to any one of the patterns. As a dendritic weight vector moves towards the central vector, it will become more closely aligned with more and more input patterns so that it is more rapidly drawn towards the central vector. The end result is that in large nets of this type, many of the dendritic weight vectors will point towards the central vector. This effect is not seen so much in small systems, since the fluctuations in the magnitude of the overlaps are sufficiently large that in most cases a dendritic weight vector will have an input pattern very close to it and thus will not learn towards the centre. In large systems, the fluctuations in the overlaps between random vectors become smaller by a factor of $\frac{1}{\sqrt{N}}$ so that the dendrites will not be particularly close to any of the input patterns.

One solution to this problem is to allow the elements of the synaptic weight vectors to take negative as well as positive values. This could be implemented in the brain by feedforward inhibition. A set of vectors taken with random values will then have a reduced mean correlation between any pair, and the competitive net will be able to categorize them effectively. A system with synaptic weights that can be negative as well as positive is not physiologically plausible, but we can instead imagine a system with weights lying on a hypersphere in the positive quadrant of space but with additional inhibition that results in the cumulative effects of some input lines being effectively negative. This can be achieved in a network by using positive input vectors, positive synaptic weight vectors, and thresholding the output neurons at their mean activation. A large competitive network of this general nature does categorize well, and has been described more fully elsewhere (Bennett, 1990). In a large network with inhibitory feedback neurons, and principal cells with thresholds, the network could achieve at least in part an approximation to this type of thresholding useful in large competitive networks.

A second way in which nets with positive-only values of the elements could operate is by making the input vectors sparse and initializing the weight vectors to be sparse, or to have a reduced contact probability. (A measure a of neuronal population sparseness is defined (as before) in Equation B.38:

$$a = \frac{(\sum_{i=1}^{N} y_i/N)^2}{\sum_{i=1}^{N} y_i^2/N} \tag{B.38}$$

where y_i is the firing rate of the ith neuron in the set of N neurons.) For relatively small net sizes simulated ($N = 100$) with patterns with a sparseness a of, for example, 0.1 or 0.2, learning onto the average vector can be avoided. However, as the net size increases, the sparseness required does become very low. In large nets, a greatly reduced contact probability between neurons (many synapses kept identically zero, i.e. diluted connectivity) would prevent learning of the average vector, thus allowing categorization to occur (Rolls, 2016f,b). Reduced contact probability will, however, prevent complete alignment of synapses with patterns, so that the performance of the network will be affected.

B.5 Continuous attractor networks

B.5.1 Introduction

Single-cell recording studies have shown that some neurons represent the current position along a continuous physical dimension or space even when no inputs are available, for example in darkness (see Chapter 9). Examples include neurons that represent the positions of the eyes (i.e. eye direction with respect to the head), the place where the animal is looking in space, head direction, and the place where the animal is located. In particular, examples of such classes of cells include head direction cells in rats (Ranck, 1985; Taube, Muller and Ranck, 1990a; Taube, Goodridge, Golob, Dudchenko and Stackman, 1996; Muller, Ranck and Taube, 1996) and primates (Robertson, Rolls, Georges-François and Panzeri, 1999), which respond maximally when the animal's head is facing in a particular preferred direction; place cells in rats (O'Keefe and Dostrovsky, 1971; McNaughton, Barnes and O'Keefe, 1983;

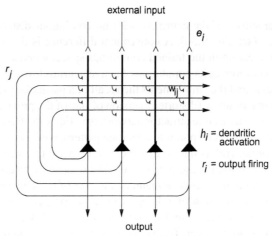

Fig. B.26 The architecture of a continuous attractor neural network (CANN).

O'Keefe, 1984; Muller, Kubie, Bostock, Taube and Quirk, 1991; Markus, Qin, Leonard, Skaggs, McNaughton and Barnes, 1995) that fire maximally when the animal is in a particular location; and spatial view cells in primates that respond when the monkey is looking towards a particular location in space (Rolls, Robertson and Georges-François, 1997a; Georges-François, Rolls and Robertson, 1999; Robertson, Rolls and Georges-François, 1998; Rolls, 2023c). In the parietal cortex there are many spatial representations, in several different coordinate frames (see Chapters 3 and 10, and Andersen, Batista, Snyder, Buneo and Cohen (2000)), and they have some capability to remain active during memory periods when the stimulus is no longer present. Even more than this, the dorsolateral prefrontal cortex networks to which the parietal networks project have the capability to maintain spatial representations active for many seconds or minutes during short-term memory tasks, when the stimulus is no longer present (see Section 13.6.1). In this section, we describe how such networks representing continuous physical space could operate. The locations of such spatial networks in the brain are the parietal areas, the prefrontal areas that implement short-term spatial memory and receive from the parietal cortex (see Section 13.6.1), and the hippocampal system which combines information about objects from the inferior temporal visual cortex with spatial information (see Chapter 9).

A class of network that can maintain the firing of its neurons to represent any location along a continuous physical dimension such as spatial position, head direction, etc. is a 'Continuous Attractor' neural network (CANN). It uses excitatory recurrent collateral connections between the neurons to reflect the distance between the neurons in the state space of the animal (e.g. head direction space). These networks can maintain the bubble of neural activity constant for long periods wherever it is started to represent the current state (head direction, position, etc) of the animal, and are likely to be involved in many aspects of spatial processing and memory, including spatial vision. Global inhibition is used to keep the number of neurons in a bubble or packet of actively firing neurons relatively constant, and to help to ensure that there is only one activity packet. Continuous attractor networks can be thought of as very similar to autoassociation or discrete attractor networks (described in Section B.3), and have the same architecture, as illustrated in Fig. B.26. The main difference is that the patterns stored in a CANN are continuous patterns, with each neuron having broadly tuned firing which decreases with for example a Gaussian function as the distance from the optimal firing location of the cell is varied, and with different neurons having tuning that overlaps throughout the space. Such tuning is illustrated in Fig. 9.30. For comparison, the autoassociation networks described in Section B.3 have discrete (separate) patterns (each pattern implemented by the firing of a particular subset of the neurons), with no continuous distribution of the patterns throughout the space (see Fig. 9.30). A consequent difference is that the CANN can maintain its firing at any location in the trained continuous space, whereas a discrete attractor or autoassociation network moves its population of active neurons towards one of the previously learned attractor states, and thus implements the recall of a particular previously learned pattern from an incomplete or noisy (distorted) version of one of the previously learned patterns. The energy landscape of a discrete attractor network (see Equation B.12) has separate energy minima, each one of which corresponds to a learned pattern, whereas the energy landscape of a continuous attractor network is flat, so that the activity packet remains stable with continuous firing wherever it is started in the state space. (The state space refers to the set of possible spatial states of the animal in its environment, e.g. the set of possible head directions.)

In Section B.5.2, we first describe the operation and properties of continuous attractor networks, which have been studied by for example Amari (1977), Zhang (1996), and Taylor (1999), and then, following Stringer, Trappenberg, Rolls and De Araujo (2002b), address four key issues about the biological application of continuous attractor network models.

One key issue in such continuous attractor neural networks is how the synaptic strengths between the neurons in the continuous attractor network could be learned in biological systems (Section B.5.3).

A second key issue in such continuous attractor neural networks is how the bubble of neuronal firing representing one location in the continuous state space should be updated based on non-visual cues to represent a new location in state space (Section B.5.5). This is essentially the problem of path integration: how a system that represents a memory of where the agent is in physical space could be updated based on idiothetic (self-motion) cues such as vestibular cues (which might represent a head velocity signal), or proprioceptive cues (which might update a representation of place based on movements being made in the space, during for example walking in the dark).

A third key issue is how stability in the bubble of activity representing the current location can be maintained without much drift in darkness, when it is operating as a memory system (Section B.5.6).

A fourth key issue is considered in Section B.5.8 in which we describe networks that store both continuous patterns and discrete patterns (see Fig. 9.30), which can be used to store for example the location in (continuous, physical) space where an object (a discrete item) is present.

B.5.2 The generic model of a continuous attractor network

The generic model of a continuous attractor is as follows. (The model is described in the context of head direction cells, which represent the head direction of rats (Taube et al., 1996; Muller et al., 1996) and macaques (Robertson, Rolls, Georges-François and Panzeri, 1999), and can be reset by visual inputs after gradual drift in darkness.) The model is a recurrent attractor network with global inhibition. It is different from a Hopfield attractor network primarily in that there are no discrete attractors formed by associative learning of discrete patterns. Instead there is a set of neurons that are connected to each other by synaptic weights w_{ij} that are a simple function, for example Gaussian, of the distance between the states of the agent in the physical world (e.g. head directions) represented by the neurons. Neurons that represent similar states (locations in the state space) of the agent in the physical world have strong synaptic connections, which can be set up by an associative learning rule, as described in Section B.5.3. The network updates its firing rates by the following 'leaky-integrator' dynamical Equations. The continuously changing activation h_i^{HD} of each head direction cell i is governed by the Equation

$$\tau \frac{dh_i^{\text{HD}}(t)}{dt} = -h_i^{\text{HD}}(t) + \frac{\phi_0}{C^{\text{HD}}} \sum_j (w_{ij} - w^{\text{inh}}) r_j^{\text{HD}}(t) + I_i^V, \qquad (B.39)$$

where r_j^{HD} is the firing rate of head direction cell j, w_{ij} is the excitatory (positive) synaptic weight from head direction cell j to cell i, w^{inh} is a global constant describing the effect of inhibitory interneurons, and τ is the time constant of the system[26]. The term $-h_i^{\text{HD}}(t)$ indicates the amount by which the activation decays (in the leaky integrator neuron) at time t. (The network is updated in a typical simulation at much smaller timesteps than the time constant of the system, τ.) The next term in Equation B.39 is the input from other neurons in the network r_j^{HD} weighted by the recurrent collateral synaptic connections w_{ij} (scaled by a constant ϕ_0 and C^{HD} which is the number of synaptic connections received by each head direction cell from other head direction cells in the continuous attractor). The term I_i^V represents a visual input to head direction cell i. Each term I_i^V is set to have a Gaussian response profile in most continuous attractor networks, and this sets the firing of the cells in the continuous attractor to have Gaussian response profiles as a function of where the agent is located in the state space (see e.g. Fig. 9.30 on page 385), but the Gaussian assumption is not crucial. (It is known that the firing rates of head direction cells in both rats (Taube, Goodridge, Golob, Dudchenko and Stackman, 1996; Muller, Ranck and Taube, 1996) and macaques (Robertson, Rolls, Georges-François and Panzeri, 1999) are approximately Gaussian.) When the agent is operating without visual input, in memory mode, then the term I_i^V is set to zero. The firing rate r_i^{HD} of cell i is determined from the activation h_i^{HD} and the sigmoid function

$$r_i^{\text{HD}}(t) = \frac{1}{1 + e^{-2\beta(h_i^{\text{HD}}(t) - \alpha)}}, \qquad (B.40)$$

where α and β are the sigmoid threshold and slope, respectively.

B.5.3 Learning the synaptic strengths between the neurons that implement a continuous attractor network

So far we have said that the neurons in the continuous attractor network are connected to each other by synaptic weights w_{ij} that are a simple function, for example Gaussian, of the distance between the states of the agent in the physical world (e.g. head directions, spatial views etc) represented by the neurons. In many simulations, the weights are set by formula to have weights with these appropriate Gaussian values. However, Stringer, Trappenberg, Rolls and De Araujo (2002b) showed how the appropriate weights could be set up by learning. They started with the fact that since the neurons have broad tuning that may be Gaussian in shape, nearby neurons in the state space will have overlapping spatial fields, and will thus be co-active to a degree that depends on the distance between them. They postulated that therefore the synaptic weights could be set up by associative learning based on the co-activity of the neurons produced by external stimuli as the animal moved in the state space. For example, head direction cells are forced to fire during learning by visual cues in the environment that produce Gaussian firing as a function of head direction from an optimal head direction for each cell. The learning rule is simply that the weights w_{ij} from head direction cell j with firing rate r_j^{HD} to head direction cell i with firing rate r_i^{HD} are updated according to an associative (Hebb) rule

$$\delta w_{ij} = k r_i^{\text{HD}} r_j^{\text{HD}} \qquad (B.41)$$

---

[26] Note that for this section, we use r rather than y to refer to the firing rates of the neurons in the network, remembering that, because this is a recurrently connected network (see Fig. B.13), the output from a neuron y_i might be the input x_j to another neuron.

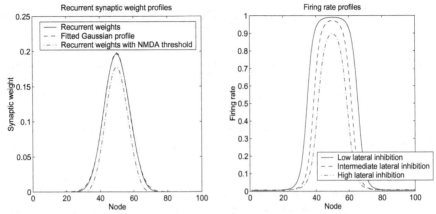

Fig. B.27 Training the weights in a continuous attractor network with an associative rule (equation B.41). Left: the trained recurrent synaptic weights from head direction cell 50 to the other head direction cells in the network arranged in head direction space (solid curve). The dashed line shows a Gaussian curve fitted to the weights shown in the solid curve. The dash-dot curve shows the recurrent synaptic weights trained with rule Equation (B.41), but with a non-linearity introduced that mimics the properties of NMDA receptors by allowing the synapses to modify only after strong postsynaptic firing is present. Right: the stable firing rate profiles forming an activity packet in the continuous attractor network during the testing phase when the training (visual) inputs are no longer present. The firing rates are shown after the network has been initially stimulated by visual input to initialize an activity packet, and then allowed to settle to a stable activity profile without visual input. The three graphs show the firing rates for low, intermediate and high values of the lateral inhibition parameter w^{inh}. For both left and right plots, the 100 head direction cells are arranged according to where they fire maximally in the head direction space of the agent when visual cues are available. (After Stringer,S.M., Trappenberg,T.P., Rolls,E.T. and De Araujo,I.E.T. (2002) Self-organizing continuous attractor networks and path integration: One-dimensional models of head direction cells. Network: Computation in Neural Systems 13: 217–242. © Informa Ltd.)

where δw_{ij} is the change of synaptic weight and k is the learning rate constant. During the learning phase, the firing rate r_i^{HD} of each head direction cell i might be the following Gaussian function of the displacement of the head from the optimal firing direction of the cell

$$r_i^{\text{HD}} = e^{-s_{\text{HD}}^2/2\sigma_{\text{HD}}^2}, \quad (\text{B.42})$$

where s_{HD} is the difference between the actual head direction x (in degrees) of the agent and the optimal head direction x_i for head direction cell i, and σ_{HD} is the standard deviation.

Stringer, Trappenberg, Rolls and De Araujo (2002b) showed that after training at all head directions, the synaptic connections develop strengths that are an almost Gaussian function of the distance between the cells in head direction space, as shown in Fig. B.27 (left). Interestingly if a non-linearity is introduced into the learning rule that mimics the properties of NMDA receptors by allowing the synapses to modify only after strong postsynaptic firing is present, then the synaptic strengths are still close to a Gaussian function of the distance between the connected cells in head direction space (see Fig. B.27, left). They showed that after training, the continuous attractor network can support stable activity packets in the absence of visual inputs (see Fig. B.27, right) provided that global inhibition is used to prevent all the neurons becoming activated. (The exact stability conditions for such networks have been analyzed by Amari (1977)). Thus Stringer, Trappenberg, Rolls and De Araujo (2002b) demonstrated biologically plausible mechanisms for training the synaptic weights in a continuous attractor using a biologically plausible local learning rule.

Stringer, Trappenberg, Rolls and De Araujo (2002b) went on to show that if there was a short term memory trace built into the operation of the learning rule, then this could help to produce smooth weights in the continuous attractor if only incomplete training was available, that is if the weights were trained at only a few locations. The same rule can take advantage in training the synaptic weights of the temporal probability distributions of firing when they happen to reflect spatial proximity. For example, for head direction cells the agent will necessarily move through similar head directions before reaching quite different head directions, and so the temporal proximity with which the cells fire can be used to set up the appropriate synaptic weights. This new proposal for training continuous attractor networks can also help to produce broadly tuned spatial cells even if the driving (e.g. visual) input (I_i^V in Equation B.39) during training produces rather narrowly tuned neuronal responses. The learning rule with such temporal properties is a memory trace learning rule that strengthens synaptic connections between neurons, based on the temporal probability distribution of the firing. There are many versions of such rules (Rolls and Milward, 2000; Rolls and Stringer, 2001a), which are described more fully in Chapter 2, but a simple one that works adequately is

$$\delta w_{ij} = k \bar{r}_i^{HD} \bar{r}_j^{HD} \tag{B.43}$$

where δw_{ij} is the change of synaptic weight, and $\bar{r}^{HD}$ is a local temporal average or trace value of the firing rate of a head direction cell given by

$$\bar{r}^{HD}(t + \delta t) = (1 - \eta) r^{HD}(t + \delta t) + \eta \bar{r}^{HD}(t) \tag{B.44}$$

where η is a parameter set in the interval [0,1] which determines the contribution of the current firing and the previous trace. For $\eta = 0$ the trace rule (B.43) becomes the standard Hebb rule (B.41), while for $\eta > 0$ learning rule (B.43) operates to associate together patterns of activity that occur close together in time. The rule might allow temporal associations to influence the synaptic weights that are learned over times in the order of 1 s. The memory trace required for operation of this rule might be no more complicated than the continuing firing that is an inherent property of attractor networks, but it could also be implemented by a number of biophysical mechanisms, discussed in Chapter 2. Finally, we note that some long-term depression (LTD) in the learning rule could help to maintain the weights of different neurons equally potent (see Section B.4.9.2 and Equation B.32), and could compensate for irregularity during training in which the agent might be trained much more in some than other locations in the space (see Stringer, Trappenberg, Rolls and De Araujo (2002b)).

B.5.4 The capacity of a continuous attractor network: multiple charts and packets

The capacity of a continuous attractor network can be approached on the following bases. First, as there are no discrete attractor states, but instead a continuous physical space is being represented, some concept of spatial resolution must be brought to bear, that is the number of different positions in the space that can be represented. Second, the number of connections per neuron in the continuous attractor will directly influence the number of different spatial positions (locations in the state space) that can be represented. Third, the sparseness of the representation can be thought of as influencing the number of different spatial locations (in the continuous state space) that can be represented, in a way analogous to that described for discrete attractor networks in Equation B.14 (Battaglia and Treves, 1998b). That is, if the tuning of the neurons is very broad, then fewer locations in the state space may be represented. Fourth, and very interestingly, if representations of different continuous state spaces, for example maps or charts of different environments, are stored in the same network, there may be little cost of adding extra maps or charts. The reason for this is that the large part of the interference between the different memories stored in such a network arises from the correlations between the different positions in any one map, which are typically relatively high because quite broad tuning of individual cells is common. In contrast, there are in general low correlations between the representations of places in different maps or charts, and therefore many different maps can be simultaneously stored in a continuous attractor network (Battaglia and Treves, 1998b).

For a similar reason, it is even possible to have the activity packets that operate in different spaces simultaneously active in a single continuous attractor network of neurons, and to move independently of each other in their respective spaces or charts (Stringer, Rolls and Trappenberg, 2004).

B.5.5 Continuous attractor models: path integration

So far, we have considered how spatial representations could be stored in continuous attractor networks, and how the activity can be maintained at any location in the state space in a form of short-term memory when the external (e.g. visual) input is removed. However, many networks with spatial representations in the brain can be updated by internal, self-motion (i.e. idiothetic), cues even when there is no external (e.g. visual) input. Examples are head direction cells in the presubiculum of rats and macaques, place cells in the rat hippocampus, and spatial view cells in the primate hippocampus (see Chapter 9). The major question arises about how such idiothetic inputs could drive the activity packet in a continuous attractor network and, in particular, how such a system could be set up biologically by self-organizing learning.

One approach to simulating the movement of an activity packet produced by idiothetic cues (which is a form of path integration whereby the current location is calculated from recent movements) is to employ a look-up table that stores (taking head direction cells as an example), for every possible head direction and head rotational velocity input generated by the vestibular system, the corresponding new head direction (Samsonovich and McNaughton, 1997). Another approach involves modulating the strengths of the recurrent synaptic weights in the continuous attractor on one but not the other side of a currently represented position, so that the stable position of the packet of activity, which requires symmetric connections in different directions from each node, is lost, and the packet moves in the direction of the temporarily increased weights, although no possible biological implementation was proposed of how the appropriate dynamic synaptic weight changes might be achieved (Zhang, 1996). Another mechanism (for head direction cells) (Skaggs, Knierim, Kudrimoti and McNaughton, 1995) relies on a set of cells, termed (head) rotation cells, which are co-activated by head direction cells and vestibular cells and drive the activity of the attractor network by anatomically distinct connections for clockwise and counter-clockwise rotation cells, in what is effectively a look-up table. However, no proposal had been made about how this could be achieved by a biologically plausible learning process for most approaches to path integration in continuous attractor networks, which relied heavily on rather artificial pre-set synaptic connectivities.

In that context Stringer, Trappenberg, Rolls and De Araujo (2002b) introduced a proposal with more biological plausibility about how the synaptic connections from idiothetic inputs to a continuous attractor network can be learned by a self-organizing learning process. The essence of the hypothesis is described with Fig. B.28. The continuous attractor synaptic weights w^{RC} are set up under the influence of the external visual inputs I^V as described in Section B.5.3. At the same time, the idiothetic synaptic weights w^{ID} (in which the ID refers to the fact that they are in this case produced by idiothetic inputs, produced by cells that fire to represent the velocity of clockwise and anticlockwise head rotation), are set up by associating the change of head direction cell firing that has just occurred (detected by a trace memory mechanism described below) with the current firing of the head rotation cells r^{ID}. For example, when the trace memory mechanism incorporated into the idiothetic synapses w^{ID} detects that the head direction cell firing is at a given location (indicated by the firing r^{HD}) and is moving clockwise (produced by the altering visual inputs I^V), and there is

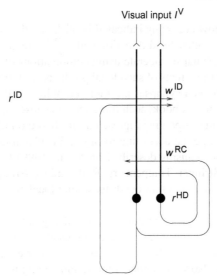

Fig. B.28 General network architecture for a one-dimensional continuous attractor model of head direction cells which can be updated by idiothetic inputs produced by head rotation cell firing r^{ID}. The head direction cell firing is r^{HD}, the continuous attractor synaptic weights are w^{RC}, the idiothetic synaptic weights are w^{ID}, and the external visual input is I^{V}. (After Stringer,S.M., Trappenberg,T.P., Rolls,E.T. and De Araujo,I.E.T. (2002) Self-organizing continuous attractor networks and path integration: One-dimensional models of head direction cells. Network: Computation in Neural Systems 13: 217–242. © Informa Ltd.)

simultaneous clockwise head rotation cell firing, the synapses w^{ID} learn the association, so that when that rotation cell firing occurs later without visual input, it takes the current head direction firing in the continuous attractor into account, and moves the location of the head direction attractor in the appropriate direction.

For the learning to operate, the idiothetic synapses onto head direction cell i with firing r_i^{HD} need two inputs: the memory traced term from other head direction cells $\bar{r}_j^{\mathrm{HD}}$ (given by Equation B.44), and the head rotation cell input with firing r_k^{ID}; and the learning rule can be written

$$\delta w_{ijk}^{\mathrm{ID}} = \tilde{k}\, r_i^{\mathrm{HD}}\, \bar{r}_j^{\mathrm{HD}}\, r_k^{\mathrm{ID}}, \tag{B.45}$$

where $\tilde{k}$ is the learning rate associated with this type of synaptic connection. The head rotation cell firing (r_k^{ID}) could be as simple as one set of cells that fire for clockwise head rotation (for which k might be 1), and a second set of cells that fire for anticlockwise head rotation (for which k might be 2).

After learning, the firing of the head direction cells would be updated in the dark (when $I_i^V = 0$) by idiothetic head rotation cell firing r_k^{ID} as follows

$$\tau \frac{dh_i^{\mathrm{HD}}(t)}{dt} = -h_i^{\mathrm{HD}}(t) + \frac{\phi_0}{C^{\mathrm{HD}}} \sum_j (w_{ij} - w^{inh}) r_j^{\mathrm{HD}}(t) + I_i^V$$

$$+ \phi_1 \left(\frac{1}{C^{\mathrm{HD}} \times \mathrm{ID}} \sum_{j,k} w_{ijk}^{\mathrm{ID}} r_j^{\mathrm{HD}} r_k^{\mathrm{ID}} \right). \tag{B.46}$$

Equation B.46 is similar to Equation B.39, except for the last term, which introduces the effects of the idiothetic synaptic weights w_{ijk}^{ID}, which effectively specify that the current firing of head direction cell i, r_i^{HD}, must be updated by the previously learned combination of the particular head rotation now occurring indicated by r_k^{ID}, and the current head direction indicated by the firings of the other head direction cells r_j^{HD} indexed through j[27]. This makes it clear that the idiothetic synapses operate using combinations of inputs, in this case of two inputs. Neurons that sum the effects of such local products are termed Sigma-Pi neurons (see Section A.2.3). Although such synapses are more complicated than the two-term synapses used throughout the rest of this book, such three-term synapses appear to be useful to solve the computational problem of updating representations based on idiothetic inputs in the way described. Synapses that operate according to Sigma-Pi rules might be implemented in the brain by a number of mechanisms described by Koch (1999) (Section 21.1.1), Jonas and Kaczmarek (1999), and Stringer, Trappenberg, Rolls and De Araujo (2002b), including having two inputs close together on a thin dendrite, so that local synaptic interactions would be emphasized.

Simulations demonstrating the operation of this self-organizing learning to produce movement of the location being represented in a continuous attractor network were described by Stringer, Trappenberg, Rolls and De Araujo (2002b), and one example of the operation is shown in Fig. B.29. They also showed that, after training with just one value of the head rotation cell firing, the network showed the desirable property of moving the head direction being represented in the continuous attractor by an amount that was proportional to the value of the head rotation cell firing. Stringer, Trappenberg, Rolls and De Araujo (2002b) also describe a related model of the idiothetic cell update of the location represented in a continuous attractor, in which the rotation cell firing directly modulates in a multiplicative way the strength of the recurrent connections in the continuous attractor in such a way that clockwise rotation cells modulate the strength of the synaptic connections in the clockwise direction in the continuous attractor, and vice versa.

It should be emphasized that although the cells are organized in Fig. B.29 according to the spatial position being represented, there is no need for cells in continuous attractors that represent nearby locations in the state space to be close together, as the distance in the state space between any two neurons is represented by the strength of the connection between them, not by where the neurons are physically located. This enables continuous attractor networks to represent spaces with arbitrary topologies, as the topology is represented in the connection strengths (Stringer, Trappenberg, Rolls and De Araujo, 2002b; Stringer, Rolls, Trappenberg and De Araujo, 2002a; Stringer, Rolls and Trappenberg, 2005; Stringer and Rolls, 2002). Indeed, it is this that enables many different charts each with its own topology to be represented in a single continuous attractor network (Battaglia and Treves, 1998b).

In the network described so far, self-organization occurs, but one set of synapses is Sigma-Pi. We have gone on to show that the Sigma-Pi synapses are not necessary, and can be replaced by a competitive network that learns to respond to combinations of the spatial position and the idiothetic velocity, as illustrated in Fig. B.30 (Stringer and Rolls, 2006).

B.5.6 Stabilization of the activity packet within the continuous attractor network when the agent is stationary

With irregular learning conditions (in which identical training with high precision of every node cannot be guaranteed), the recurrent synaptic weights between nodes in the continuous attractor will not be of the perfectly regular and symmetric form normally required in a continuous attractor neural network. This can lead to drift of the activity packet within the

---

[27]The term $\phi_1/C^{\text{HD}\times\text{ID}}$ is a scaling factor that reflects the number $C^{\text{HD}\times\text{ID}}$ of inputs to these synapses, and enables the overall magnitude of the idiothetic input to each head direction cell to remain approximately the same as the number of idiothetic connections received by each head direction cell is varied.

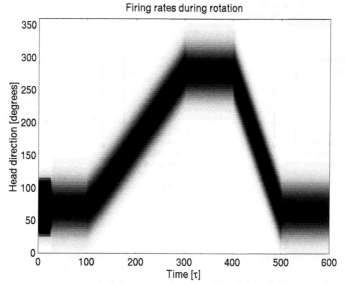

Fig. B.29 Idiothetic update of the location represented in a continuous attractor network. The firing rate of the cells with optima at different head directions (organized according to head direction on the ordinate) is shown by the blackness of the plot, as a function of time. The activity packet was initialized to a head direction of 75 degrees, and the packet was allowed to settle without visual input. For timestep=0 to 100 there was no rotation cell input, and the activity packet in the continuous attractor remained stable at 75 degrees. For timestep=100 to 300 the clockwise rotation cells were active with a firing rate of 0.15 to represent a moderate angular velocity, and the activity packet moved clockwise. For timeste=300 to 400 there was no rotation cell firing, and the activity packet immediately stopped, and remained still. For timestep=400 to 500 the anti-clockwise rotation cells had a high firing rate of 0.3 to represent a high velocity, and the activity packet moved anticlockwise with a greater velocity. For timestep=500 to 600 there was no rotation cell firing, and the activity packet immediately stopped. (After Stringer,S.M., Trappenberg,T.P., Rolls,E.T. and De Araujo,I.E.T. (2002) Self-organizing continuous attractor networks and path integration: One-dimensional models of head direction cells. Network: Computation in Neural Systems 13: 217–242. © Informa Ltd.)

continuous attractor network of e.g. head direction cells when no visual cues are present, even when the agent is not moving. This drift is a common property of the short-term memories of spatial position implemented in the brain, which emphasizes the computational problems that can arise in continuous attractor networks if the weights between nodes are not balanced in different directions in the space being represented. An approach to stabilizing the activity packet when it should not be drifting in real nervous systems, which does help to minimize the drift that can occur, is now described.

The activity packet may be stabilized within a continuous attractor network, when the agent is stationary and the network is operating in memory mode without an external stabilizing input, by enhancing the firing of those cells that are already firing. In biological systems this might be achieved through mechanisms for short-term synaptic enhancement (Koch, 1999). Another way is to take advantage of the non-linearity of the activation function of neurons with NMDA receptors, which only contribute to neuronal firing once the neuron is sufficiently depolarized (Wang, 1999). The effect is to enhance the firing of neurons that are already reasonably well activated. The effect has been utilized in a model of a network with recurrent excitatory synapses that can maintain active an arbitrary set of neurons that are initially sufficiently strongly activated by an external stimulus (see Lisman, Fellous and Wang (1998), and, for a discussion on whether these networks could be used to implement short-term memories, see Kesner and Rolls (2001)).

We have incorporated this non-linearity into a model of a head direction continuous attractor network by adjusting the sigmoid threshold α_i (see Equation B.40) for each head direction cell i as follows (Stringer, Trappenberg, Rolls and De Araujo, 2002b). If the head

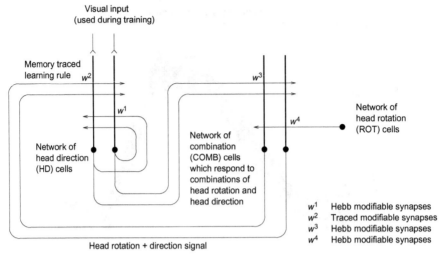

Fig. B.30 Network architecture for a two-layer self-organizing neural network model of the head direction system. The network architecture contains a layer of head direction (HD) cells representing the head direction of the agent, a layer of combination (COMB) cells representing a combination of head direction and rotational velocity, and a layer of rotation (ROT) cells which become active when the agent rotates. There are four types of synaptic connection in the network, which operate as follows. The w^1_{ij} synapses are Hebb-modifiable recurrent connections between head direction cells. These connections help to support stable packets of activity within this continuous attractor layer of head direction cells in the absence of visual input. The combination cells receive inputs from the head direction cells through the Hebb-modifiable w^3_{ij} synapses, and inputs from the rotation cells through the Hebb-modifiable w^4_{ij} synapses. These synaptic inputs encourage combination cells by competitive learning to respond to particular combinations of head direction and rotational velocity. In particular, the combination cells only become significantly active when the agent is rotating. The head direction cells receive inputs from the combination cells through the w^2_{ij} synapses. The $w^2_{i,j}$ synapses are trained using a 'trace' learning rule, which incorporates a temporal trace of recent combination cell activity. This rule introduces an asymmetry into the w^2_{ij} weights, which plays an important role in shifting the activity packet through the layer of head direction cells during path integration in the dark. (After Stringer,S.M. and Rolls, E. T. (2006) Self-organizing path integration using a linked continuous attractor and competitive network: path integration of head direction. Network: Computation in Neural Systems 17: 419–445. © Informa Ltd.)

direction cell firing rate r_i^{HD} is lower than a threshold value, γ, then the sigmoid threshold α_i is set to a relatively high value α^{high}. Otherwise, if the head direction cell firing rate r_i^{HD} is greater than or equal to the threshold value, γ, then the sigmoid threshold α_i is set to a relatively low value α^{low}. It was shown that this procedure has the effect of enhancing the current position of the activity packet within the continuous attractor network, and so prevents the activity packet drifting erratically due to the noise in the recurrent synaptic weights produced for example by irregular learning. An advantage of using the non-linearity in the activation function of a neuron (produced for example by the operation of NMDA receptors) is that this tends to enable packets of activity to be kept active without drift even when the packet is not in one of the energy minima that can result from irregular learning (or from diluted connectivity in the continuous attractor as described below). Thus use of this non-linearity increases the number of locations in the continuous physical state space at which a stable activity packet can be maintained (Stringer, Trappenberg, Rolls and De Araujo, 2002b).

The same process might help to stabilize the activity packet against drift caused by the probabilistic spiking of neurons in the network (cf. Section 11.5.1).

B.5.7 Continuous attractor networks in two or more dimensions

Some types of spatial representation used by the brain are of spaces that exist in two or more dimensions. Examples are the two- (or three-) dimensional space representing where one is looking at in a spatial scene. Another is the two- (or three-) dimensional space representing where one is located. It is possible to extend continuous attractor networks to operate in higher dimensional spaces than the one-dimensional spaces considered so far (Taylor, 1999; Stringer, Rolls, Trappenberg and De Araujo, 2002a). Indeed, it is also possible to extend the analyses of how idiothetic inputs could be used to update two-dimensional state spaces, such as the locations represented by place cells in rats (Stringer, Rolls, Trappenberg and De Araujo, 2002a) and the location at which one is looking represented by primate spatial view cells (Stringer, Rolls and Trappenberg, 2005; Stringer and Rolls, 2002). Interestingly, the number of terms in the synapses implementing idiothetic update do not need to increase beyond three (as in Sigma-Pi synapses) even when higher dimensional state spaces are being considered (Stringer, Rolls, Trappenberg and De Araujo, 2002a). Also interestingly, a continuous attractor network can in fact represent the properties of very high dimensional spaces, because the properties of the spaces are captured by the connections between the neurons of the continuous attractor, and these connections are of course, as in the world of discrete attractor networks, capable of representing high dimensional spaces (Stringer, Rolls, Trappenberg and De Araujo, 2002a). With these approaches, continuous attractor networks have been developed of the two-dimensional representation of rat hippocampal place cells with idiothetic update by movements in the environment (Stringer, Rolls, Trappenberg and De Araujo, 2002a), and of primate hippocampal spatial view cells with idiothetic update by eye and head movements (Stringer, Rolls and Trappenberg, 2005; Rolls and Stringer, 2005; Stringer and Rolls, 2002). Continuous attractor models with some similar properties have also been applied to understanding motor control, for example the generation of a continuous movement in space (Stringer and Rolls, 2007; Stringer, Rolls and Taylor, 2007a).

B.5.8 Mixed continuous and discrete attractor networks

It has now been shown that attractor networks can store both continuous patterns and discrete patterns, and can thus be used to store for example the location in (continuous, physical) space where an object (a discrete item) is present (see Fig. 9.30 and Rolls, Stringer and Trappenberg (2002)). In this network, when events are stored that have both discrete (object) and continuous (spatial) aspects, then the whole place can be retrieved later by the object, and the object can be retrieved by using the place as a retrieval cue. Such networks are likely to be present in parts of the brain that receive and combine inputs both from systems that contain representations of continuous (physical) space, and from brain systems that contain representations of discrete objects, such as the inferior temporal visual cortex. One such brain system is the hippocampus, which appears to combine and store such representations in a mixed attractor network in the CA3 region, which thus is able to implement episodic memories which typically have a spatial component, for example where an item such as a key is located (see Chapter 9). This network thus shows that in brain regions where the spatial and object processing streams are brought together, then a single network can represent and learn associations between both types of input. Indeed, in brain regions such as the hippocampal system, it is essential that the spatial and object processing streams are brought together in a single network, for it is only when both types of information are in the same network that spatial information can be retrieved from object information, and vice versa, which is a fundamental property of episodic memory (see Chapter 9). It may also be the case that in the prefrontal cortex, attractor networks can store both spatial and discrete (e.g. object-based) types of information in short-term memory (see Section 13.6.1).

B.6 Network dynamics: the integrate-and-fire approach

The concept that attractor (autoassociation) networks can operate very rapidly if implemented with neurons that operate dynamically in continuous time was introduced in Section B.3.3.5. The result described was that the principal factor affecting the speed of retrieval is the time constant of the synapses between the neurons that form the attractor ((Treves, 1993; Rolls and Treves, 1998; Battaglia and Treves, 1998a; Panzeri, Rolls, Battaglia and Lavis, 2001). This was shown analytically by Treves (1993), and described by Rolls and Treves (1998) Appendix 5. We now describe in more detail the approaches that produce these results, and the actual results found on the speed of processing.

The networks described so far in this chapter, and analyzed in Appendices 3 and 4 of Rolls and Treves (1998), were described in terms of the steady-state activation of networks of neuron-like units. Those may be referred to as 'static' properties, in the sense that they do not involve the time dimension. In order to address 'dynamical' questions, the time dimension has to be reintroduced into the formal models used, and the adequacy of the models themselves has to be reconsidered in view of the specific properties to be discussed.

Consider for example a real network whose operation has been described by an autoassociative formal model that acquires, with learning, a given attractor structure. How does the state of the network approach, in real time during a retrieval operation, one of those attractors? How long does it take? How does the amount of information that can be read off the network's activity evolve with time? Also, which of the potential steady states is indeed a stable state that can be reached asymptotically by the net? How is the stability of different states modulated by external agents? These are examples of dynamical properties, which to be studied require the use of models endowed with some dynamics.

B.6.1 From discrete to continuous time

Already at the level of simple models in which each unit is described by an input–output relation, one may introduce equally simple 'dynamical' rules, in order both to fully specify the model, and to simulate it on computers. These rules are generally formulated in terms of 'updatings': time is considered to be discrete, a succession of time steps, and at each time step the output of one or more of the units is set, or updated, to the value corresponding to its input variable. The input variable may reflect the outputs of other units in the net as updated at the previous time step or, if delays are considered, the outputs as they were at a prescribed number of time steps in the past. If all units in the net are updated together, the dynamics is referred to as parallel; if instead only one unit is updated at each time step, the dynamics is sequential. (One main difference between the Hopfield (1982) model of an autoassociator and a similar model considered earlier by Little (1974) is that the latter was based on parallel rather than sequential dynamics.) Many intermediate possibilities obviously exist, involving the updating of groups of units at a time. The order in which sequential updatings are performed may for instance be chosen at random at the beginning and then left the same in successive cycles across all units in the net; or it may be chosen anew at each cycle; yet a third alternative is to select at each time step a unit, at random, with the possibility that a particular unit may be selected several times before some of the other ones are ever updated. The updating may also be made probabilistic, with the output being set to its new value only with a certain probability, and otherwise remaining at the current value.

Variants of these dynamical rules have been used for decades in the analysis and computer simulation of physical systems in statistical mechanics (and field theory). They can reproduce in simple but effective ways the stochastic nature of transitions among discrete quantum states, and they have been subsequently considered appropriate also in the simulation of neural network models in which units have outputs that take discrete values, implying that a change from one value to another can only occur in a sudden jump. To some extent, different rules are equivalent, in that they lead, in the evolution of the activity of the net along successive steps and cycles, to the same set of possible steady states. For example, it is easy to realize that when no delays are introduced, states that are stable under parallel updating are also stable under sequential updating. The reverse is not necessarily true, but on the other hand states that are stable when updating one unit at a time are stable irrespective of the updating order. Therefore, static properties, which can be deduced from an analysis of stable states, are to some extent robust against differences in the details of the dynamics assigned to the model. (This is a reason for using these dynamical rules in the study of the thermodynamics of physical systems.) Such rules, however, bear no relation to the actual dynamical processes by which the activity of real neurons evolves in time, and are therefore inadequate for the discussion of dynamical issues in neural networks.

A first step towards realism in the dynamics is the substitution of discrete time with continuous time. This somewhat parallels the substitution of the discrete output variables of the most rudimentary models with continuous variables representing firing rates. Although continuous output variables may evolve also in discrete time, and as far as static properties are concerned differences are minimal, with the move from discrete to continuous outputs the main raison d'etre for a dynamics in terms of sudden updatings ceases to exist, since continuous variables can change continuously in continuous time. A paradox arises immediately, however, if a continuous time dynamics is assigned to firing rates. The paradox is that firing rates, although in principle continuous if computed with a generic time-kernel, tend to vary in jumps as new spikes – essentially discrete events – come to be included in the kernel. To avoid this paradox, a continuous time dynamics can be assigned, instead, to instantaneous continuous variables such as membrane potentials. Hopfield (1984), among others, has introduced a model of an autoassociator in which the output variables represent membrane potentials and evolve continuously in time, and has suggested that under certain conditions the stable states attainable by such a network are essentially the same as for a network of binary units evolving in discrete time. If neurons in the central nervous system communicated with each other via the transmission of graded membrane potentials, as they do in some peripheral and invertebrate neural systems, this model could be an excellent starting point. The fact that, centrally, transmission is primarily via the emission of discrete spikes makes a model based on membrane potentials as output variables inadequate to correctly represent spiking dynamics.

B.6.2 Continuous dynamics with discontinuities

In principle, a solution would be to keep the membrane potential as the basic dynamical variable, evolving in continuous time, and to use as the output variable the spike emission times, as determined by the rapid variation in membrane potential corresponding to each spike. A point-like neuron can generate spikes by altering the membrane potential V according to continuous equations of the Hodgkin–Huxley type:

$$C\frac{dV}{dt} = g_0(V_{\text{rest}} - V) + g_{\text{Na}}mh^3(V_{\text{Na}} - V) + g_{\text{K}}n^4(V_{\text{K}} - V) + I \tag{B.47}$$

$$\tau_m \frac{dm}{dt} = m_\infty(V) - m \tag{B.48}$$

$$\tau_h \frac{dh}{dt} = h_\infty(V) - h \tag{B.49}$$

$$\tau_n \frac{dn}{dt} = n_\infty(V) - n. \tag{B.50}$$

The changes in the membrane potential, driven by the input current I, interact with the opening and closing of intrinsic conductances (here a sodium conductance, whose channels are gated by the 'particles' m and h, and a potassium conductance, whose channels are gated by n; Hodgkin and Huxley (1952)). These equations provide an effective description, phenomenological but broadly based on physical principles, of the conductance changes underlying action potentials, and they are treated in any standard neurobiology text.

From the point of view of formal models of neural networks, this level of description is too complicated to be the basis for an analytic understanding of the operation of networks, and it must be simplified. The most widely used simplification is the so-called integrate-and-fire model (see for example MacGregor (1987) and Brunel and Wang (2001)), which is legitimized by the observation that (sodium) action potentials are typically brief and self-similar events. If, in particular, the only relevant variable associated with the spike is its time of emission (at the soma, or axon hillock), which essentially coincides with the time the potential V reaches a certain threshold level V_{thr}, then the conductance changes underlying the rest of the spike can be omitted from the description, and substituted with the ad hoc prescription that (i) a spike is emitted, with its effect on receiving units and on the unit itself; and (ii) after a brief time corresponding to the duration of the spike plus a refractory period, the membrane potential is reset and resumes its integration of the input current I. After a spike the membrane potential is taken to be reset to a value V_{reset}. This type of simplified dynamics of the membrane potentials is thus in continuous time with added discontinuities: continuous in between spikes, with discontinuities occurring at different times for each neuron in a population, every time a neuron emits a spike.

A leaky integrate-and-fire neuron can be modelled as follows (see also Section 11.5.1.2 and Fig. 11.34). The model describes the depolarization of the membrane potential V (which typically is dynamically changing as a result of the synaptic effects described below between approximately –70 and –50 mV) until threshold V_{thr} (typically –50 mV) is reached when a spike is emitted and the potential is reset to V_{reset} (typically –55 mV). The membrane time constant τ_m is set by the membrane capacitance C_m and the membrane leakage conductance g_m where $\tau_m = C_m/g_m$. V_L denotes the resting potential of the cell, typically –70 mV. Changes in the membrane potential are defined by the following equation

$$C_m \frac{dV(t)}{dt} = g_m(V_L - V(t)) + \sum_j g_j(V_{\text{AMPA}} - V(t)) + \sum_j g_j(V_{\text{GABA}} - V(t)). \quad \text{(B.51)}$$

The first term on the right of the equation describes how the membrane potential decays back towards the resting potential of the cell depending on how far the cell potential V is from the resting potential V_L, and the membrane leak conductance g_m. The second term on the right represents the excitatory synaptic current that could be injected through AMPA receptors. This is a sum over all AMPA synapses indexed by j on the cell. At each synapse, the current is driven into the cell by the difference between the membrane potential V and the reversal potential V_{AMPA} of the channels opened by AMPA receptors, weighted by the synaptic conductance g_j. This synaptic conductance changes dynamically as a function of the time since a spike reached the synapse, as shown below. Due to their reversal potential V_{AMPA} of typically 0 mV, these currents will tend to depolarize the cell, that is to move the membrane potential towards the firing threshold. The third term on the right represents the inhibitory synaptic current that could be injected through GABA receptors. Due to their reversal potential V_{GABA} of typically –70 mV, these currents will tend to hyperpolarize the cell, that is to move the membrane potential away from the firing threshold. There may be other types of receptor on a cell, for example NMDA receptors, and these operate analogously though with interesting differences, as described in Section B.6.3.

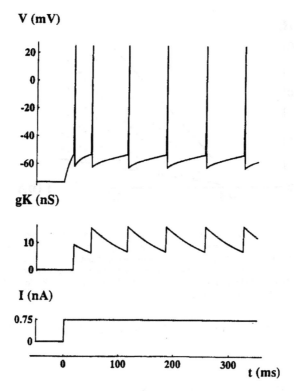

Fig. B.31 Model behavior of an integrate-and-fire neuron: the membrane potential and adaptation-producing potassium conductance in response to a step of injected current. The spikes were added to the graph by hand, as they do not emerge from the simplified voltage equation. (From Treves, A. (1993) Mean-field analysis of neuronal spike dynamics. Network: Computation in Neural Systems 4: 259–284. Copyright © Taylor and Francis Ltd.)

The opening of each synaptic conductance g_j is driven by the arrival of spikes at the presynaptic terminal j, and its closing can often be described as a simple exponential process. A simplified equation for the dynamics of $g_j(t)$ is then

$$\frac{dg_j(t)}{dt} = -\frac{g_j(t)}{\tau} + \Delta g_j \sum_l \delta(t - \Delta t - t_l). \tag{B.52}$$

According to the above equation, each synaptic conductance opens instantaneously by a fixed amount Δg_j a time Δt after the emission of the presynaptic spike at t_l. Δt summarizes delays (axonal, synaptic, and dendritic), and each opening superimposes linearly, without saturating, on previous openings. The value of τ in this equation will be different for AMPA receptors (typically 2–10 ms), NMDA receptors (typically 100 ms), and GABA receptors (typically 10 ms).

In order to model the phenomenon of adaptation in the firing rate, prominent especially with pyramidal cells, it is possible to include a time-varying intrinsic (potassium-like) conductance in the cell membrane (Brown, Gähwiler, Griffith and Halliwell, 1990a) (shown as g_K in equations B.53 and B.54). This can be done by specifying that this conductance, which if open tends to shunt the membrane and thus to prevent firing, opens by a fixed amount with the potential excursion associated with each spike, and then relaxes exponentially to its closed state. In this manner sustained firing driven by a constant input current occurs at lower rates after the first few spikes, in a way similar, if the relevant parameters are set appropriately, to the behavior observed in vitro of many pyramidal cells (for example, Lanthorn, Storm and Andersen (1984), Mason and Larkman (1990)).

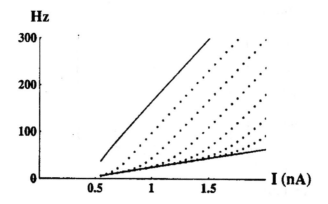

Fig. B.32 Current-to-frequency transduction in a pyramidal cell modelled as an integrate-and-fire neuron. The top solid curve is the firing frequency in the absence of adaptation, $\Delta g_K = 0$. The dotted curves are the instantaneous frequencies computed as the inverse of the ith interspike interval (top to bottom, $i = 1, ..., 6$). The bottom solid curve is the adapted firing curve ($i \to \infty$). With or without adaptation, the input–output transform is close to threshold–linear. (From Treves, A. (1993) Mean-field analysis of neuronal spike dynamics. Network: Computation in Neural Systems 4: 259–284. Copyright © Taylor and Francis Ltd.)

The equations for the dynamics of each neuron with adaptation are then

$$C_m \frac{dV(t)}{dt} = g_m(V_L - V(t)) + \sum_j g_j(V_{AMPA} - V(t)) + \sum_j g_j(V_{GABA} - V(t)) + g_K(t)(V_K - V(t))$$

(B.53)

and

$$\frac{dg_K(t)}{dt} = -\frac{g_K(t)}{\tau_K} + \sum_k \Delta g_K \delta(t - t_k)$$

(B.54)

supplemented by the prescription that when at time $t = t_{k+1}$ the potential reaches the level V_{thr}, a spike is emitted, and hence included also in the sum of Equation B.54, and the potential resumes its evolution according to Equation B.53 from the reset level V_{reset}. The resulting behavior is exemplified in Fig. B.31, while Fig. B.32 shows the input–output transform (current to frequency transduction) operated by an integrate-and-fire unit of this type with firing rate adaptation. One should compare this with the transduction operated by real cells, as exemplified for example in Fig. 1.4.

It should be noted that synaptic conductance dynamics is not always included in integrate-and-fire models: sometimes it is substituted with current dynamics, which essentially amounts to neglecting non-linearities due to the appearance of the membrane potential in the driving force for synaptic action (see for example, Amit and Tsodyks (1991), Gerstner (1995)); and sometimes it is simplified altogether by assuming that the membrane potential undergoes small sudden jumps when it receives instantaneous pulses of synaptic current (see the review in Gerstner (1995)). The latter simplification is quite drastic and changes the character of the dynamics markedly; whereas the former can be a reasonable simplification in some circumstances, but it produces serious distortions in the description of inhibitory $GABA_A$ currents, which, having an equilibrium (Cl^-) synaptic potential close to the operating range of the membrane potential, are quite sensitive to the instantaneous value of the membrane potential itself.

B.6.3 An integrate-and-fire implementation

In this subsection the mathematical equations that describe the spiking activity and synapse dynamics in some of the integrate-and-fire simulations performed by Rolls and Deco (Deco and Rolls, 2003; Deco, Rolls and Horwitz, 2004; Deco and Rolls, 2005d,c,b, 2006; Loh, Rolls and Deco, 2007a; Rolls, Loh and Deco, 2008c; Rolls, Grabenhorst and Deco, 2010b,c; Insabato, Pannunzi, Rolls and Deco, 2010; Deco, Rolls and Romo, 2010; Rolls and Deco, 2011b; Webb, Rolls, Deco and Feng, 2011; Rolls and Webb, 2012; Rolls, Webb and Deco, 2012; Martinez-Garcia, Rolls, Deco and Romo, 2011; Rolls, Dempere-Marco and Deco, 2013; Rolls and Deco, 2015a,b, 2016) are set out, in order to show in more detail how an integrate-and-fire simulation is implemented. The equations follow in general the formulation described by Brunel and Wang (2001), though each simulation describes its own architecture to be simulated and neurocomputational questions to be addressed, with additional dynamics introduced where described to implement synaptic facilitation and/or synaptic adaptation (Rolls, 2016b).

Each neuron is described by an integrate-and-fire model. The subthreshold membrane potential $V(t)$ of each neuron evolves according to the following equation:

$$C_m \frac{dV(t)}{dt} = -g_m(V(t) - V_L) - I_{\text{syn}}(t) \tag{B.55}$$

where $I_{\text{syn}}(t)$ is the total synaptic current flow into the cell, V_L is the resting potential, C_m is the membrane capacitance, and g_m is the membrane conductance. When the membrane potential $V(t)$ reaches the threshold V_{thr} a spike is generated, and the membrane potential is reset to V_{reset}. The neuron is unable to spike during the first τ_{ref} which is the absolute refractory period.

The total synaptic current is given by the sum of glutamatergic excitatory components (NMDA and AMPA) and inhibitory components (GABA). The external excitatory contributions (ext) from outside the network are produced through AMPA receptors ($I_{\text{AMPA,ext}}$), while the excitatory recurrent synapses (rec) within the network act through AMPA and NMDA receptors ($I_{\text{AMPA,rec}}$ and $I_{\text{NMDA,rec}}$). The total synaptic current is therefore given by:

$$I_{\text{syn}}(t) = I_{\text{AMPA,ext}}(t) + I_{\text{AMPA,rec}}(t) + I_{\text{NMDA,rec}}(t) + I_{\text{GABA}}(t) \tag{B.56}$$

where

$$I_{\text{AMPA,ext}}(t) = g_{\text{AMPA,ext}}(V(t) - V_E) \sum_{j=1}^{N_{\text{ext}}} s_j^{\text{AMPA,ext}}(t) \tag{B.57}$$

$$I_{\text{AMPA,rec}}(t) = g_{\text{AMPA,rec}}(V(t) - V_E) \sum_{j=1}^{N_E} w_j s_j^{\text{AMPA,rec}}(t) \tag{B.58}$$

$$I_{\text{NMDA,rec}}(t) = \frac{g_{\text{NMDA,rec}}(V(t) - V_E)}{(1 + [\text{Mg}^{++}] \exp(-0.062V(t))/3.57)} \sum_{j=1}^{N_E} w_j s_j^{\text{NMDA,rec}}(t) \tag{B.59}$$

$$I_{\text{GABA}}(t) = g_{\text{GABA}}(V(t) - V_I) \sum_{j=1}^{N_I} s_j^{\text{GABA}}(t) \tag{B.60}$$

In the preceding equations the reversal potential of the excitatory synaptic currents $V_E = 0$ mV and of the inhibitory synaptic currents $V_I = -70$ mV. The different form for the NMDA receptor-activated channels implements the voltage-dependence of NMDA receptors. This voltage-dependency, and the long time constant of the NMDA receptors, are important in the effects produced through NMDA receptors (Brunel and Wang, 2001; Wang, 1999). The synaptic strengths w_j are specified in the papers by Rolls and Deco cited above, and depend on the architecture being simulated. The fractions of open channels s are given by:

$$\frac{ds_j^{\text{AMPA,ext}}(t)}{dt} = -\frac{s_j^{\text{AMPA,ext}}(t)}{\tau_{\text{AMPA}}} + \sum_k \delta(t - t_j^k) \tag{B.61}$$

$$\frac{ds_j^{\text{AMPA,rec}}(t)}{dt} = -\frac{s_j^{\text{AMPA,rec}}(t)}{\tau_{\text{AMPA}}} + \sum_k \delta(t - t_j^k) \tag{B.62}$$

$$\frac{ds_j^{\text{NMDA,rec}}(t)}{dt} = -\frac{s_j^{\text{NMDA,rec}}(t)}{\tau_{\text{NMDA,decay}}} + \alpha x_j(t)(1 - s_j^{\text{NMDA,rec}}(t)) \tag{B.63}$$

$$\frac{dx_j(t)}{dt} = -\frac{x_j(t)}{\tau_{\text{NMDA,rise}}} + \sum_k \delta(t - t_j^k) \tag{B.64}$$

$$\frac{ds_j^{\text{GABA}}(t)}{dt} = -\frac{s_j^{\text{GABA}}(t)}{\tau_{\text{GABA}}} + \sum_k \delta(t - t_j^k) \tag{B.65}$$

where the sums over k represent a sum over spikes emitted by presynaptic neuron j at time t_j^k. The value of $\alpha = 0.5$ ms^{-1}.

Typical values of the conductances for pyramidal neurons are: $g_{\text{AMPA,ext}}$=2.08, $g_{\text{AMPA,rec}}$=0.052, $g_{\text{NMDA,rec}}$=0.164, and g_{GABA}=0.67 nS; and for interneurons: $g_{\text{AMPA,ext}}$=1.62, $g_{\text{AMPA,rec}}$=0.0405, $g_{\text{NMDA,rec}}$=0.129 and g_{GABA}=0.49 nS.

A full list of the values of the parameters used is given in Section B.8.3 and in each of the papers cited above in this Section B.6.3.

B.6.4 The speed of processing of one-layer attractor networks with integrate-and-fire neurons

Given that the analytic approach to the rapidity of the dynamics of attractor networks with integrate-and-fire dynamics (Treves, 1993; Rolls and Treves, 1998) applies mainly when the state is close to the attractor basin, it is of interest to check the performance of such networks by simulation when the completion of partial patterns that may be towards the edge of the attractor basin can be tested. Simmen, Rolls and Treves (1996a) and Treves, Rolls and Simmen (1997) made a start with this, and showed that retrieval could indeed be fast, within 1–2 time constants of the synapses. However, they found that they could not load the systems they simulated with many patterns, and the firing rates during the retrieval process tended to be unstable. The cause of this turned out to be that the inhibition they used to maintain the activity level during retrieval was subtractive, and it turns out that divisive (shunting) inhibition is much more effective in such networks, as described by Rolls and Treves (1998) in Appendix 5. Divisive inhibition is likely to be organized by inhibitory inputs that synapse close to the cell body (where the reversal potential is close to that of the channels opened by GABA receptors), in contrast to synapses on dendrites, where the different potentials result in opening of the same channels producing hyperpolarization (that is an effectively subtractive influence with respect to the depolarizing currents induced by excitatory (glutamate-releasing) terminals). Battaglia and Treves (1998a) therefore went on to study networks with neurons where the inhibitory neurons could be made to be divisive by having them synapse close to the cell body in neurons modelled with multiple (ten) dendritic compartments. The excitatory inputs terminated on the compartments more distant from the cell body in the model. They found that with this divisive inhibition, the neuronal firing during retrieval was kept under much better control, and the number of patterns that could be successfully stored and retrieved was much higher. Some details of their simulation follow.

Battaglia and Treves (1998a) simulated a network of 800 excitatory and 200 inhibitory cells in its retrieval of one of a number of memory patterns stored in the synaptic weights representing the excitatory-to-excitatory recurrent connections. The memory patterns were assigned at random, drawing the value of each unit in each of the patterns from a binary distribution with sparseness 0.1, that is a probability of 1 in 10 for the unit to be active in the pattern. No baseline excitatory weight was included, but the modifiable weights were instead constrained to remain positive (by clipping at zero synaptic modifications that would make a synaptic weight negative), and a simple exponential decay of the weight with successive modifications was also applied, to prevent runaway synaptic modifications within a rudimentary model of forgetting. Both excitation on inhibitory units and inhibition were mediated by non-modifiable uniform synaptic weights, with values chosen so as to satisfy stability conditions of the type shown in Equations A5.13 of Rolls and Treves (1998). Both inhibitory and excitatory neurons were of the general integrate-and-fire type, but excitatory units had in addition an extended dendritic cable, and they received excitatory inputs only at the more distal end of the cable, and inhibitory inputs spread along the cable. In this way, inhibitory inputs reached the soma of excitatory cells with variable delays, and in any case earlier than synchronous excitatory inputs, and at the same time they could shunt the excitatory inputs, resulting in a largely multiplicative form of inhibition (Abbott, 1991). The uniform connectivity was not complete, but rather each type of unit could contact units of the other type with a probability of 0.5, and the same was true for inhibitory-to-inhibitory connections.

After 100 (simulated) ms of activity evoked by external inputs uncorrelated with any of the stored patterns, a cue was provided that consisted of the external input becoming correlated with one of the patterns, at various levels of correlation, for 300 ms. After that, external inputs were removed, but when retrieval operated successfully the activity of the units remained strongly correlated with the memory pattern, or even reached a higher level of correlation if a rather corrupted cue had been used, so that, if during the 300 ms the network had stabilized into a state rather distant from the memory pattern, it got much closer to it once the cue was removed. All correlations were quantified using information measures (see Appendix C)), in terms of mutual information between the firing rate pattern across units and the particular memory pattern being retrieved, or in terms of mutual information between the firing rate of one unit and the set of patterns, or, finally, in terms of mutual information between the decoded firing rates of a subpopulation of 10 excitatory cells and the set of memory patterns. The same algorithms were used to extract information measures as were used for example by Rolls, Treves, Tovee and Panzeri (1997d) with real neuronal data from inferior temporal cortex neurons (see further (Rolls and Treves, 2011)). The firing rates were measured over sliding windows of 30 ms, after checking that shorter windows produced noisier measures. The effect of using a relatively long window, 30 ms, for measuring rates is an apparent linear early rise in information values with time. Nevertheless, in the real system the activity of these cells is 'read' by other cells receiving inputs from them, and that in turn have their own membrane capacitance-determined characteristic time for integrating input activity, a time broadly in the order of 30 ms. Using such a time window for integrating firing rates did not therefore artificially slow down the read-out process.

It was shown that the time course of different information measures did not depend significantly on the firing rates prevailing during the retrieval state, nor on the resistance–capacitance-determined membrane time constants of the units. Figure B.33 shows that the rise in information after providing the cue at time = 100 ms followed a roughly exponential approach to its steady-state value, which continued until the steady state switched to a new

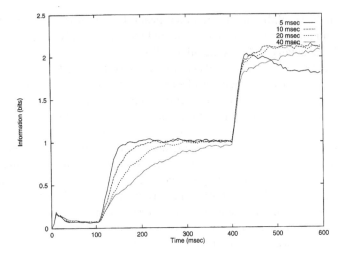

Fig. B.33 The speed of memory retrieval in an integrate-and-fire attractor network is very fast: in the order of 1.5 times the time constants of the recurrent collateral synapses. Time course of the transinformation about which memory pattern had been selected, as decoded from the firing rates of 10 randomly selected excitatory units. Excitatory conductances closed exponentially with time constants of 5, 10, 20 and 40 ms (curves from top to bottom). A cue of correlation 0.2 with the memory pattern was presented from 100 to 400 ms, uncorrelated external inputs with the same mean strength and sparseness as the cue were applied at earlier times, and no external inputs were applied at later times. (From Battaglia,F. and Treves,A. (1998) Stable and rapid recurrent processing in realistic autoassociative memories. Neural Computation 10: 431–450. © Massachusetts Institute of Technology.)

value when the retrieval cue was removed at time = 400 ms. The time constant of the approach to the first steady state was a linear function, as shown in Fig. B.33, of the time constant for excitatory conductances, as predicted by the analysis. (The proportionality factor in the Figure is 2.5, or a collective time constant 2.5 times longer than the synaptic time constant.) The approach to the second steady-state value was more rapid, and the early apparent linear rise prevented the detection of a consistent exponential mode. Therefore, it appears that the cue leads to the basin of attraction of the correct retrieval state by activating transient modes, whose time constant is set by that of excitatory conductances; once the network is in the correct basin, its subsequent reaching the 'very bottom' of the basin after the removal of the cue is not accompanied by any prominent transient mode (see further Battaglia and Treves (1998a)).

Overall, these simulations confirm that recurrent networks, in which excitation is mediated mainly by fast (AMPA, see Section 1.6) channels, can reach asynchronous steady firing states very rapidly, over a few tens of milliseconds, and the rapid approach to steady state is reflected in the relatively rapid rise of information quantities that measure the speed of the operation in functional terms. If the AMPA receptor time constant is 10 ms in the brain, the implication is that the attractor network would fall into its attractor basin in 15 ms.

An analysis based on integrate-and-fire model units thus indicates that recurrent dynamics can be so fast as to be practically indistinguishable from purely feedforward dynamics, in contradiction to what simple intuitive arguments would suggest. This makes it hazardous to draw conclusions on the underlying circuitry on the basis of the experimentally observed speed with which selective neuronal responses arise, as attempted by Thorpe and Imbert (1989). The results also show that networks that implement feedback processing can settle into a global retrieval state very rapidly, and that rapid processing is not just a feature of feedforward networks.

We return to the intuitive understanding of this rapid processing. The way in which networks with continuous dynamics (such as networks made of real neurons in the brain, and networks modelled with integrate-and-fire neurons) can be conceptualized as settling so fast into their attractor states is that spontaneous activity in the network ensures that some neurons are close to their firing threshold when the retrieval cue is presented, so that the firing of these neurons is influenced within 1–2 ms by the retrieval cue. These neurons then influence other neurons within milliseconds (given the point that some other neurons will be close to threshold) through the modified recurrent collateral synapses that store the information. In this way, the neurons in networks with continuous dynamics can influence each other within a fraction of the synaptic time constant, and retrieval can be very rapid.

B.6.5 The speed of processing of a four-layer hierarchical network with integrate-and-fire attractor dynamics in each layer

Given that the visual system has a whole series of cortical areas organized predominantly hierarchically (e.g. V1 to V2 to V4 to inferior temporal cortex), the issue arises of whether the rapid information processing that can be performed for object recognition is predominantly feedforward, or whether there is sufficient time for feedback processing within each cortical area implemented by the local recurrent collaterals to contribute to the visual information processing being performed. Some of the constraints are as follows.

An analysis of response latencies indicates that there is sufficient time for only 10–20 ms per processing stage in the visual system. In the primate cortical ventral visual system the response latency difference between neurons in layer $4C\beta$ of V1 and inferior temporal cortical cells is approximately 60 ms (Bullier and Nowak, 1995; Nowak and Bullier, 1997; Schmolesky, Wang, Hanes, Thompson, Leutgeb, Schall and Leventhal, 1998). For example, the latency of the responses of neurons in V1 is approximately 30–40 ms (Celebrini, Thorpe, Trotter and Imbert, 1993), and in the temporal cortex visual areas approximately 80–110 ms (Baylis, Rolls and Leonard, 1987; Sugase, Yamane, Ueno and Kawano, 1999). Given that there are 4–6 stages of processing in the ventral visual system from V1 to the anterior inferior temporal cortex, the difference in latencies between each ventral cortical stage is on this basis approximately 10 ms (Rolls, 1992a; Oram and Perrett, 1994). Information theoretic analyses of the responses of single visual cortical cells in primates reveal that much of the information that can be extracted from neuronal spike trains is often found to be present in periods as short as 20–30 ms (Tovee, Rolls, Treves and Bellis, 1993; Tovee and Rolls, 1995; Heller, Hertz, Kjaer and Richmond, 1995; Rolls, Tovee and Panzeri, 1999b). Backward masking experiments indicate that each cortical area needs to fire for only 20–30 ms to pass information to the next stage (Rolls and Tovee, 1994; Rolls, Tovee, Purcell, Stewart and Azzopardi, 1994b; Kovacs, Vogels and Orban, 1995; Rolls, Tovee and Panzeri, 1999b; Rolls, 2003) (see Section C.3.4). Rapid serial visual presentation of image sequences shows that cells in the temporal visual cortex are still face selective when faces are presented at the rate of 14 ms/image (Keysers, Xiao, Foldiak and Perrett, 2001). Finally, event-related potential studies in humans provide strong evidence that the visual system is able to complete some analyses of complex scenes in less than 150 ms (Thorpe, Fize and Marlot, 1996).

To investigate whether feedback processing within each layer could contribute to information processing in such a multilayer system in times as short as 10–20 ms per layer, Panzeri, Rolls, Battaglia and Lavis (2001) simulated a four-layer network with attractor networks in each layer. The network architecture is shown schematically in Fig. B.34. All the neurons realized integrate-and-fire dynamics, and indeed the individual layers and neurons were implemented very similarly to the implementation used by Battaglia and Treves (1998a). In particular, the current flowing from each compartment of the multicompartment neurons to the external medium was expressed as:

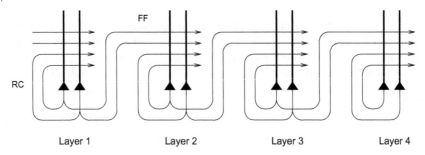

Fig. B.34 Model for the speed of operation of a cortical hierarchical network with attractor dynamics at each stage. The structure of the excitatory connections in the network. There are feedforward (FF) connections between each layer and the next, and excitatory recurrent collaterals (RC) in each layer. Inhibitory connections are also present within each layer, but they are not shown in this Figure. (After Panzeri,S., Rolls, E. T., Battaglia,F. and Lavis,R. (2001) Speed of feedforward and recurrent processing in multilayer networks of integrate-and-fire neurons. Network: Computation in Neural Systems 12: 423–440. © Informa Ltd.)

$$I(t) = g_{\text{leak}}(V(t) - V^0) + \sum_j g_j(t)(V(t) - V_j), \quad \text{(B.66)}$$

where g_{leak} is a constant passive leakage conductance, V^0 the membrane resting potential, $g_j(t)$ the value of the jth synapse conductance at time t, and V_j the reversal potential of the jth synapse. $V(t)$ is the potential in the compartment at time t. The most important parameter in the simulation, the AMPA inactivation time constant, was set to 10 ms. The recurrent collateral (RC) integration time constant of the membrane of excitatory cells was 20 ms long for the simulations presented. The synaptic conductances decayed exponentially in time, obeying the Equation

$$\frac{dg_j}{dt} = -\frac{g_j}{\tau_j} + \Delta g_j \sum_k \delta(t - \Delta t - t_k^j), \quad \text{(B.67)}$$

where τ_j is the synaptic decay time constant, Δt is a delay term summarizing axonal and synaptic delays, and Δg_j is the amount that the conductance is increased when the pre-synaptic unit fires a spike. Δg_j thus represents the (unidirectional) coupling strength between the pre-synaptic and the post-synaptic cell. t_k^j is the time at which the pre-synaptic unit fires its kth spike.

An example of the rapid information processing of the system is shown in Fig. B.35, obtained under conditions in which the local recurrent collaterals can contribute to correct performance because the feedforward (FF) inputs from the previous stage are noisy. (The noise implemented in these simulations was some imperfection in the FF signals produced by some alterations to the FF synaptic weights.) Figure B.35 shows that, when the FF carry an incomplete signal, some information is still transmitted successfully in the 'No RC' condition (in which the recurrent collateral connections in each layer are switched off), and with a relatively short latency. However, the noise term in the FF synaptic strengths makes the retrieval fail more and more layer by layer. When in contrast the recurrent collaterals (RC) are present and operating after Hebbian training, the amount of information retrieved is now much higher, because the RC are able to correct a good part of the erroneous information injected into the neurons by the noisy FF synapses. In Layer 4, 66 ms after cue injection in Layer 1, the information in the Hebbian RC case is 0.2 bits higher than that provided by the FF connections in the 'No RC' condition. This shows that the RC are able to retrieve information in Layer 4 that is not available by any other purely FF mechanism after only roughly 50–55 ms from the time when Layer 1 responds. (This corresponds to 17–18 ms per layer.)

A direct comparison of the latency differences in layers 1–4 of the integrate-and-fire network simulated by Panzeri, Rolls, Battaglia and Lavis (2001) is shown in Fig. B.36. The

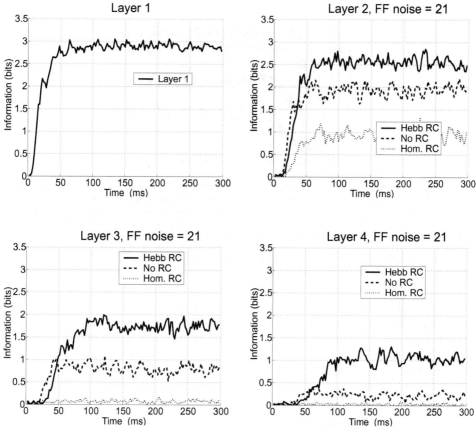

Fig. B.35 The speed of information processing in a 4-layer network with integrate-and-fire attractor dynamics at each stage requires only about 1.5 times the synaptic time constant for each stage or layer. The information time course of the average information carried by the responses of a population of 30 excitatory neurons in each layer. In the simulations considered here, there is noise in the feedforward (FF) synapses. Layer 1 was tested in just one condition. Layers 2–4 are tested in three different conditions: No RC (in which the recurrent collateral synaptic effects do not operate), Hebbian RC (in which the recurrent collaterals have been trained by as associative rule and can help pattern retrieval in each layer), and a control condition named Homogeneous RC (in which the recurrent collaterals could inject current into the neurons, but no useful information was provided by them because they were all set to the same strength). (After Panzeri,S., Rolls, E. T., Battaglia,F. and Lavis,R. (2001) Speed of feedforward and recurrent processing in multilayer networks of integrate-and-fire neurons. Network: Computation in Neural Systems 12: 423–440. © Informa Ltd.)

results are shown for the Hebbian condition illustrated in Fig. B.35, and separate curves are shown for each of the layers 1–4. The Figure shows that, with the time constant of the synapses set to 10 ms, the network can operate with full utilization of and benefit from recurrent processing within each layer in a time which enables the signal to propagate through the 4-layer system with a time course of approximately 17 ms per layer.

The overall results of Panzeri, Rolls, Battaglia and Lavis (2001) were as follows. Through the implementation of continuous dynamics, latency differences were found in information retrieval of only 5 ms per layer when local excitation was absent and processing was purely feedforward. However, information latency differences increased significantly when non-associative local excitation (simulating spontaneous firing or unrelated inputs present in the brain) was included. It was also found that local recurrent excitation through associatively modified synapses can contribute significantly to processing in as little as 15 ms per layer, including the feedforward and local feedback processing. Moreover, and in contrast to purely feed-forward processing, the contribution of local recurrent feedback was useful and approximately this rapid even when retrieval was made difficult by noise. These findings provide ev-

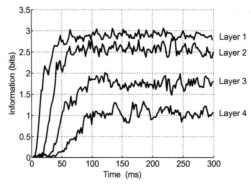

Fig. B.36 The speed of information processing in a 4-layer network with integrate-and-fire attractor dynamics at each stage requires only about 1.5 times the synaptic time constant for each stage or layer. The information time course of the average information carried by the responses of a population of 30 excitatory neurons in each layer. The results are shown for the Hebbian condition illustrated in Fig. B.35, and separate curves are shown for each of the layers 1–4. The Figure shows that, with the time constant of the synapses set to 10 ms, the network can operate with full utilization of and benefit from recurrent processing within each layer in a time in the order of 17 ms per layer. (After Panzeri,S., Rolls, E. T., Battaglia,F. and Lavis,R. (2001) Speed of feedforward and recurrent processing in multilayer networks of integrate-and-fire neurons. Network: Computation in Neural Systems 12: 423–440. © Informa Ltd.)

idence that cortical information processing can be very fast even when local recurrent circuits are critically involved. The time cost of this recurrent processing is minimal when compared with a feedforward system with spontaneous firing or unrelated inputs already present, and the performance is better than that of a purely feedforward system when noise is present.

It is concluded that local feedback loops within each cortical area can contribute to fast visual processing and cognition.

B.6.6 Spike response model

In this section, I describe another mathematical approach that models the activity of single spiking neurons. This model captures the principal effects of real neurons in a realistic way and is simple enough to permit analytical calculations (Gerstner, Ritz and Van Hemmen, 1993; Gerstner and Kistler, 2002; Gerstner, Kistler, Naud and Paninski, 2014). In contrast to some integrate-and-fire models (Tuckwell, 1988), which are essentially given by differential equations, the spike-response model is based on response kernels that describe the integrated effect of spike reception or emission on the membrane potential. In this model, spikes are generated by a threshold process (i.e. the firing time t' is given by the condition that the membrane potential reaches the firing threshold θ; that is, $h(t') = \theta$). Figure B.37 (bottom) shows schematically the spike-generating mechanism.

The membrane potential is given by the integration of the input signal weighted by a kernel defined by the Equations

$$h(t') = h^{\mathrm{refr}}(t') + h^{\mathrm{syn}}(t') \tag{B.68}$$

$$h^{\mathrm{refr}}(t') = \int_0^\infty \eta^{\mathrm{refr}}(z)\delta(t' - z - t'_{\mathrm{last}})dz \tag{B.69}$$

$$h^{\mathrm{syn}}(t') = \sum_j J_j \int_0^\infty \Lambda(z', t' - t'_{\mathrm{last}})s(t' - z')dz' . \tag{B.70}$$

The kernel $\eta^{\mathrm{refr}}(z)$ is the refractory function. If we consider only absolute refractoriness, $\eta^{\mathrm{refr}}(z)$ is given by:

$$\eta^{\mathrm{refr}}(z) = \begin{cases} -\infty & \text{for } 0 < z \leq \tau^{\mathrm{refr}} \\ 0 & \text{for } z \geq \tau^{\mathrm{refr}} \end{cases} \tag{B.71}$$

where τ^{refr} is the absolute refractory time. The time t'_{last} corresponds to the last postsynaptic spike (i.e. the most recent firing of the particular neuron). The second response function is the synaptic kernel $\Lambda(z', t' - t'_{\text{last}})$. It describes the effect of an incoming spike on the membrane potential at the soma of the postsynaptic neuron, and it eventually includes also the dependence on the state of the receiving neuron through the difference $t' - t'_{\text{last}}$ (i.e. through the time that has passed since the last postsynaptic spike). The input spike train yields $s(t' - z') = \sum_i \delta(t' - z' - t_{ij})$, t_{ij} being the ith spike at presynaptic input j. In order to simplify the discussion and without losing generality, let us consider only a single synaptic input, and therefore we can remove the subindex j. In addition, we assume that the synaptic strength J is positive (i.e. excitatory). Integrating Equations B.69 and B.70, we obtain

$$h(t') = \eta^{\text{refr}}(t' - t'_{\text{last}}) + J \sum_i \Lambda(t' - t_i, t' - t'_{\text{last}}) \qquad (B.72)$$

Synaptic kernels are of the form

$$\Lambda(t' - t_i, t' - t'_{\text{last}}) = \mathrm{H}(t' - t_i)\mathrm{H}(t_i - t'_{\text{last}})\Psi(t' - t_i) \qquad (B.73)$$

where $\mathrm{H}(s)$ is the step (or Heaviside) function which vanishes for $s \leq 0$ and takes a value of 1 for $s > 0$. After firing, the membrane potential is reset according to the renewal hypothesis.

This spike-response model is not used in the models described in this book, but is presented to show alternative approaches to modelling the dynamics of network activity.

B.7 Network dynamics: introduction to the mean-field approach

Model neurons whose potential and conductances follow the integrate-and-fire equations in Section B.6 can be assembled together in a model network of any composition and architecture. It is convenient to imagine that units (neurons) are grouped into classes, such that the parameters quantifying the electrophysiological properties of the units are uniform, or nearly uniform, within each class, while the parameters assigned to synaptic connections are uniform or nearly uniform for all connections from a given presynaptic class to another given postsynaptic class. The parameters that have to be set in a model at this level of description are quite numerous, as listed in Tables B.4 and B.5.

In the limit in which the parameters are constant within each class or pair of classes, a mean-field treatment can be applied to analyze a model network, by summing equations that describe the dynamics of individual units to obtain a more limited number of equations that describe the dynamical behavior of groups of units (Frolov and Medvedev, 1986). The treatment is exact in the further limit in which very many units belong to each class, and is an approximation if each class includes just a few units. Suppose that N_C is the number of classes defined. Summing equations B.53 and B.54 across units of the same class results in N_C functional equations describing the evolution in time of the fraction of cells of a particular class that at a given instant have a given membrane potential. In other words, from a treatment in which the evolution of the variables associated with each unit is followed separately, one moves to a treatment based on density functions, in which the common behavior of units of the same class is followed together, keeping track solely of the portion of units at any given value of the membrane potential. Summing equation B.52 across connections with the same class of origin and destination results in $N_C \times N_C$ equations describing the dynamics of the overall summed conductance opened on the membrane of a cell of a particular class by all

Table B.4 Cellular parameters (chosen according to the class of each unit)

V_{rest} Resting potential
V_{thr} Threshold potential
V_{ahp} Reset potential
V_{K} Potassium conductance equilibrium potential
C Membrane capacitance
τ_{K} Potassium conductance time constant
g_0 Leak conductance
Δg_{K} Extra potassium conductance following a spike
Δt Overall transmission delay

Table B.5 Synaptic parameters (chosen according to the classes of presynaptic and postsynaptic units)

V_α Synapse equilibrium potential
τ_α Synaptic conductance time constant
Δg_α Conductance opened by one presynaptic spike
Δt_α Delay of the connection

the cells of another given class. A more explicit derivation of mean-field equations is given by Treves (1993) and in Section B.8.

The system of mean-field equations can have many types of asymptotic solutions for long times, including chaotic, periodic, and stationary ones. The stationary solutions are stationary in the sense of the mean fields, but in fact correspond to the units of each class firing tonically at a certain rate. They are of particular interest as the dynamical equivalent of the steady states analyzed by using non-dynamical model networks. In fact, since the neuronal current-to-frequency transfer function resulting from the dynamical equations is rather similar to a threshold linear function (see Fig. B.32), and since each synaptic conductance is constant in time, the stationary solutions are essentially the same as the states described using model networks made up of threshold linear, non-dynamical units. Thus the dynamical formulation reduces to the simpler formulation in terms of steady-state rates when applied to asymptotic stationary solutions; but, among simple rate models, it is equivalent only to those that allow description of the continuous nature of neuronal output, and not to those, for example based on binary units, that do not reproduce this fundamental aspect. The advantages of the dynamical formulation are that (i) it enables one to describe the character and prevalence of other types of asymptotic solutions, and (ii) it enables one to understand how the network reaches, in time, the asymptotic behavior.

The development of this mean-field approach, and the foundations for its application to models of cortical visual processing and attention, are described in Section B.8.

B.8 Mean-field based neurodynamics

A model of brain functions requires the choice of an appropriate theoretical framework, which permits the investigation and simulation of large-scale biologically realistic neural networks. Starting from the mathematical models of biologically realistic single neurons (i.e. spiking neurons), one can derive models that describe the joint activity of pools (i.e. populations) of equivalent neurons. This kind of neurodynamical model at the neuronal assembly level is motivated by the experimental observation that cortical neurons of the same type that are near to each other tend to receive similar inputs. As described in the previous section, it is convenient in this simplified approach to neural dynamics to consider all neurons of the same type in a small cortical volume as a computational unit of a neural network. This computational unit is called a neuronal pool or assembly. The mathematical description of the dynamical evolution of neuronal pool activity in multimodular networks, associated with different cortical areas, establishes the roots of the dynamical approach that are used in Chapter 13 and Section 11.5.1, and in Rolls and Deco (2002) Chapters 9–11. In this Section (B.8), we introduce the mathematical fundamentals utilized for a neurodynamical description of pool activity (see also Section B.8.2). Beginning at the microscopic level and using single spiking neurons to form the pools of a network, we derive the mathematical formulation of the neurodynamics of cell assemblies. Further, we introduce the basic architecture of neuronal pool networks that fulfil the basic mechanisms consistent with the biased competition hypothesis. Each of these networks corresponds to cortical areas that also communicate with each other. We describe therefore the dynamical interaction between different modules or networks, which will be the basis for the implementation of attentional top-down bias.

B.8.1 Population activity

We now introduce thoroughly the concept of a neuronal pool and the differential equations representing the neurodynamics of pool activity.

Starting from individual spiking neurons one can derive a differential equation that describes the dynamical evolution of the averaged activity of a pool of extensively many equivalent neurons. Several areas of the brain contain groups of neurons that are organized in populations of units with (somewhat) similar properties (though in practice the neurons convey independent information, as described in Appendix C). These groups for mean-field modelling purposes are usually called pools of neurons and are constituted by a large and similar population of identical spiking neurons that receive similar external inputs and are mutually coupled by synapses of similar strength. Assemblies of motor neurons (Kandel, Koester, Mack and Siegelbaum, 2021) and the columnar organization in the visual and somatosensory cortex (Hubel and Wiesel, 1962; Mountcastle, 1957) are examples of these pools. Each single cell in a pool can be described by a spiking model, e.g. the spike response model presented in Section B.6.6. Due to the fact that for large-scale cortical modelling, neuronal pools form a relevant computational unit, we adopt a population code. We take the activity level of each pool of neurons as the relevant dependent variable rather than the spiking activity of individual neurons. We therefore derive a dynamical model for the mean activity of a neural population. In a population of M neurons, the mean activity $A(t)$ is determined by the proportion of active neurons by counting the number of spikes $n_{\text{spikes}}(t, t + \Delta t)$ in a small time interval Δt and dividing by M and by Δt (Gerstner, 2000), i.e. formally

$$A(t) = \lim_{\Delta t \to 0} \frac{n_{\text{spikes}}(t, t + \Delta t)}{M \Delta t}. \tag{B.74}$$

As indicated by Gerstner (2000), and as depicted in Fig. B.37, the concept of pool activity is quite different from the definition of the average firing rate of a single neuron. Contrary to the concept of temporal averaging over many spikes of a single cell, which requires that the input is slowly varying compared with the size of the temporal averaging window, a coding scheme based on pool activity allows rapid adaptation to real-world situations with quickly changing inputs. It is possible to derive dynamical equations for pool activity levels by utilizing the mean-field approximation (Wilson and Cowan, 1972; Abbott, 1991; Amit and Tsodyks, 1991). The mean-field approximation consists of replacing the temporally averaged

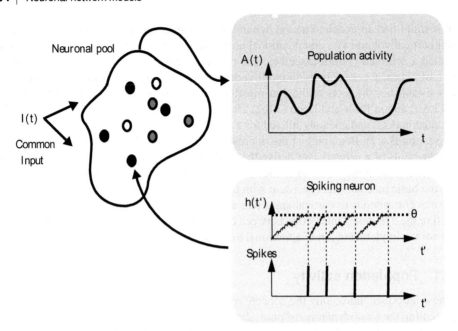

Fig. B.37 Population averaged rate of a neuronal pool of spiking neurons (top) and the action potential generating mechanism of single neurons (bottom). In a neuronal pool, the mean activity $A(t)$ is determined by the proportion of active neurons by counting the number of spikes in a small time interval Δt and dividing by the number of neurons in the pool and by Δt. Spikes are generated by a threshold process. The firing time t' is given by the condition that the membrane potential $h(t')$ reaches the firing threshold θ. The membrane potential $h(t')$ is given by the integration of the input signal weighted by a given kernel (see text for details). (From Rolls, E. T. and Deco,G. (2002) Computational Neuroscience of Vision. Oxford University Press: Oxford.)

discharge rate of a cell with an equivalent momentary activity of a neural population (ensemble average) that corresponds to the assumption of ergodicity. According to this approximation, we categorize each cell assembly by means of its activity $A(t)$. A pool of excitatory neurons without external input can be described by the dynamics of the pool activity given by

$$\tau \frac{\partial A(t)}{\partial t} = -A(t) + q\mathrm{F}(A(t)) \tag{B.75}$$

where the first term on the right hand side is a decay term and the second term takes into account the excitatory stimulation between the neurons in the pool. In the previous equation, the non-linearity

$$\mathrm{F}(x) = \frac{1}{T_r - \tau \log(1 - \frac{1}{\tau x})} \tag{B.76}$$

is the response function (transforming current into discharge rate) for a spiking neuron with deterministic input, membrane time constant τ, and absolute refractory time T_r. Equation B.75 was derived by Gerstner (2000) assuming adiabatic conditions. Gerstner (2000) has shown that the population activity in a homogeneous population of neurons can be described by an integral equation. A systematic reduction of the integral equation to a single differential equation of the form B.75 always supposes that the activity changes only slowly compared with the typical interval length. In other words, the mean-field approach described in the above equations and utilized in parts of Chapters 2 and 13, and Section 11.5.1 generates a dynamics that neglects fast, transient behavior. This means that we are assuming that rapid oscillations (and synchronization) do not play a computational role at least for the brain functions that we will consider. Rapid oscillations of neural activity could have a relevant functional role, namely of dynamical cooperation between pools in the same or different brain areas. It is well known in the theory of dynamical systems that the synchronization of oscillators is a cooperative phenomenon. Cooperative mechanisms might complement the competitive mechanisms on which this computational cortical model is based.

An example of the application of the mean field approach, used in a model of decision-making (Deco and Rolls, 2006), is provided in Section B.8.2, with the parameters used provided in Section B.8.3. The mean-field analysis described is consistent with the integrate-and-fire spiking simulation described in Section B.6.3, that is, the same parameters used in the mean-field analysis can then be used in the integrate-and-fire simulations. Part of the value of the mean-field analysis is that it provides a way of determining the parameters that will lead to the specified steady state behavior (in the absence of noise), and these parameters can then be used in a well-defined system for the integrate-and-fire simulations to investigate the full dynamics of the system in the presence of the noise generated by the random spike timings of the neurons.

Ways in which noise can be introduced into the mean-field approach are described by Rolls and Deco (2010).

B.8.2 The mean-field approach used in a model of decision-making

The mean-field approximation used by Deco and Rolls (2006) was derived by Brunel and Wang (2001), assuming that the network of integrate-and-fire neurons is in a stationary state. This mean-field formulation includes synaptic dynamics for AMPA, NMDA and GABA activated ion channels (Brunel and Wang, 2001). In this formulation the potential of a neuron is calculated as:

$$\tau_x \frac{dV(t)}{dt} = -V(t) + \mu_x + \sigma_x \sqrt{\tau_x} \eta(t) \tag{B.77}$$

where $V(t)$ is the membrane potential, x labels the populations, τ_x is the effective membrane time constant, μ_x is the mean value the membrane potential would have in the absence of spiking and fluctuations, σ_x measures the magnitude of the fluctuations, and η is a Gaussian process with absolute exponentially decaying correlation function with time constant τ_{AMPA}. The quantities μ_x and σ_x^2 are given by:

$$\mu_x = \frac{(T_{ext}\nu_{ext} + T_{AMPA}n_x^{AMPA} + \rho_1 n_x^{NMDA})V_E + \rho_2 n_x^{NMDA}\langle V \rangle + T_I n_x^{GABA}V_I + V_L}{S_x} \tag{B.78}$$

$$\sigma_x^2 = \frac{g_{AMPA,ext}^2(\langle V \rangle - V_E)^2 N_{ext}\nu_{ext}\tau_{AMPA}^2 \tau_x}{g_m^2 \tau_m^2}. \tag{B.79}$$

where ν_{ext} Hz is the external incoming spiking rate, $\tau_m = C_m/g_m$ with the values for the excitatory or inhibitory neurons depending on the population considered, and the other quantities are given by:

$$S_x = 1 + T_{\text{ext}}\nu_{\text{ext}} + T_{\text{AMPA}}n_x^{\text{AMPA}} + (\rho_1 + \rho_2)n_x^{\text{NMDA}} + T_{\text{I}}n_x^{\text{GABA}} \tag{B.80}$$

$$\tau_x = \frac{C_{\text{m}}}{g_{\text{m}}S_x} \tag{B.81}$$

$$n_x^{\text{AMPA}} = \sum_{j=1}^{p} r_j w_{jx}^{\text{AMPA}} \nu_j \tag{B.82}$$

$$n_x^{\text{NMDA}} = \sum_{j=1}^{p} r_j w_{jx}^{\text{NMDA}} \psi(\nu_j) \tag{B.83}$$

$$n_x^{\text{GABA}} = \sum_{j=1}^{p} r_j w_{jx}^{\text{GABA}} \nu_j \tag{B.84}$$

$$\psi(\nu) = \frac{\nu \tau_{\text{NMDA}}}{1 + \nu \tau_{\text{NMDA}}}\left(1 + \frac{1}{1 + \nu \tau_{\text{NMDA}}} \sum_{n=1}^{\infty} \frac{(-\alpha \tau_{\text{NMDA,rise}})^n T_n(\nu)}{(n+1)!}\right) \tag{B.85}$$

$$T_n(\nu) = \sum_{k=0}^{n} (-1)^k \binom{n}{k} \frac{\tau_{\text{NMDA,rise}}(1 + \nu \tau_{\text{NMDA}})}{\tau_{\text{NMDA,rise}}(1 + \nu \tau_{\text{NMDA}}) + k\tau_{\text{NMDA,decay}}} \tag{B.86}$$

$$\tau_{\text{NMDA}} = \alpha \tau_{\text{NMDA,rise}} \tau_{\text{NMDA,decay}} \tag{B.87}$$

$$T_{\text{ext}} = \frac{g_{\text{AMPA,ext}}\tau_{\text{AMPA}}}{g_{\text{m}}} \tag{B.88}$$

$$T_{\text{AMPA}} = \frac{g_{\text{AMPA,rec}}N_{\text{E}}\tau_{\text{AMPA}}}{g_{\text{m}}} \tag{B.89}$$

$$\rho_1 = \frac{g_{\text{NMDA}}N_{\text{E}}}{g_{\text{m}}J} \tag{B.90}$$

$$\rho_2 = \beta \frac{g_{\text{NMDA}}N_{\text{E}}(\langle V_x \rangle - V_{\text{E}})(J-1)}{g_{\text{m}}J^2} \tag{B.91}$$

$$J = 1 + \gamma \exp(-\beta \langle V_x \rangle) \tag{B.92}$$

$$T_{\text{I}} = \frac{g_{\text{GABA}}N_{\text{I}}\tau_{\text{GABA}}}{g_{\text{m}}} \tag{B.93}$$

$$\langle V_x \rangle = \mu_x - (V_{\text{thr}} - V_{\text{reset}})\nu_x \tau_x, \tag{B.94}$$

where p is the number of excitatory populations, r_x is the fraction of neurons in the excitatory population x, w_{jx} the weight of the connections from population x to population j, ν_x is the spiking rate of the population x, $\gamma = [\text{Mg}^{++}]/3.57$, $\beta = 0.062$ and the average membrane potential $\langle V_x \rangle$ has a value between -55 mV and -50 mV.

The spiking rate of a population as a function of the defined quantities is then given by:

$$\nu_x = \phi(\mu_x, \sigma_x), \tag{B.95}$$

where

$$\phi(\mu_x, \sigma_x) = \left(\tau_{\text{rp}} + \tau_x \int_{\beta(\mu_x,\sigma_x)}^{\alpha(\mu_x,\sigma_x)} du\sqrt{\pi}\exp(u^2)[1+\text{erf}(u)]\right)^{-1} \tag{B.96}$$

$$\alpha(\mu_x, \sigma_x) = \frac{(V_{\text{thr}} - \mu_x)}{\sigma_x}\left(1 + 0.5\frac{\tau_{\text{AMPA}}}{\tau_x}\right) + 1.03\sqrt{\frac{\tau_{\text{AMPA}}}{\tau_x}} - 0.5\frac{\tau_{\text{AMPA}}}{\tau_x} \tag{B.97}$$

$$\beta(\mu_x, \sigma_x) = \frac{(V_{\text{reset}} - \mu_x)}{\sigma_x} \tag{B.98}$$

with erf(u) the error function and τ_{rp} the refractory period which is considered to be 2 ms for excitatory neurons and 1 ms for inhibitory neurons. To solve the equations defined by (B.95) for all xs we integrate numerically (B.94) and the differential Equation B.99, which has fixed point solutions corresponding to Equation B.95:

$$\tau_x \frac{d\nu_x}{dt} = -\nu_x + \phi(\mu_x, \sigma_x). \tag{B.99}$$

The values of the parameters used in a mean-field analysis of decision-making are provided in Section B.8.3, with further details of the parameters in Chapter 11.5.1.

B.8.3 The model parameters used in the mean-field analyses of decision-making

The fixed parameters of the model are shown in Table B.6, and not only provide information about the values of the parameters used in the simulations, but also enable them to be compared to experimentally measured values.

Table B.6 Parameters used in the integrate-and-fire simulations

N_E	800
N_I	200
r	0.1
w_+	2.2
w_I	1.015
N_{ext}	800
ν_{ext}	2.4 kHz
C_m (excitatory)	0.5 nF
C_m (inhibitory)	0.2 nF
g_m (excitatory)	25 nS
g_m (inhibitory)	20 nS
V_L	−70 mV
V_{thr}	−50 mV
V_{reset}	−55 mV
V_E	0 mV
V_I	−70 mV
$g_{\text{AMPA,ext}}$ (excitatory)	2.08 nS
$g_{\text{AMPA,rec}}$ (excitatory)	0.104 nS
g_{NMDA} (excitatory)	0.327 nS
g_{GABA} (excitatory)	1.25 nS
$g_{\text{AMPA,ext}}$ (inhibitory)	1.62 nS
$g_{\text{AMPA,rec}}$ (inhibitory)	0.081 nS
g_{NMDA} (inhibitory)	0.258 nS
g_{GABA} (inhibitory)	0.973 nS
$\tau_{\text{NMDA,decay}}$	100 ms
$\tau_{\text{NMDA,rise}}$	2 ms
τ_{AMPA}	2 ms
τ_{GABA}	10 ms
α	0.5 ms^{-1}

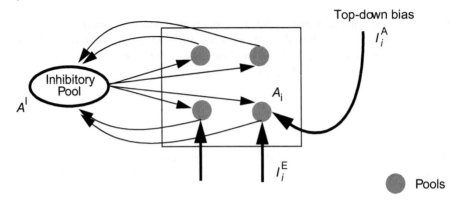

Fig. B.38 Basic computational module for biased competition: a competitive network with external top-down bias. Excitatory pools with activity A_i for the ith pool are connected with a common inhibitory pool with activity A^I in order to implement a competition mechanism. I_i^E is the external sensory input to the cells in pool i, and I_i^A attentional top-down bias, an external input coming from higher modules. The external top-down bias can shift the competition in favour of a specific pool or group of pools. This architecture is similar to that shown in Fig. B.19, but with competition between pools of similar neurons. (After Rolls, E. T. and Deco,G. (2002) Computational Neuroscience of Vision. Oxford University Press: Oxford.)

B.8.4 A basic computational module based on biased competition

We are interested in the neurodynamics of modules composed of several pools that implement a competitive mechanism[28]. This can be achieved by connecting the pools of a given module with a common inhibitory pool, as is schematically shown in Fig. B.38.

In this way, the more pools of the module that are active, the more active the common inhibitory pool will be, and consequently, the more feedback inhibition will affect the pools in the module, such that only the most excited group of pools will survive the competition. On the other hand, external top-down bias could shift the competition in favour of a specific group of pools. This basic computational module implements therefore the biased competition hypothesis described in Chapter 13. Let us assume that there are m pools in a given module. The system of differential equations describing the dynamics of such a module is given by two differential equations, both of the type of equation B.75. The first differential equation describes the dynamics of the activity level of the excitatory pools (pyramidal neurons) and is mathematically expressed by

$$\tau \frac{\partial A_i(t)}{\partial t} = -A_i(t) + a\mathrm{F}(A_i(t)) - b\mathrm{F}(A^I(t)) + \\ I_0 + I_i^E(t) + I_i^A(t) + \nu \quad ; \qquad \text{for } i = 1, ..., m \qquad (\text{B}.100)$$

and the second one describes the dynamics of the activity level of the common inhibitory pool for each feature dimension (stellate neurons)

$$\tau_p \frac{\partial A^I(t)}{\partial t} = -A^I(t) + c \sum_{i=1}^{m} \mathrm{F}(A_i(t)) - d\mathrm{F}(A^I(t)) \qquad (\text{B}.101)$$

where $A_i(t)$ is the activity for pool i, $A^I(t)$ is the activity in the inhibitory pool, I_0 is a diffuse spontaneous background input, $I^E(t)$ is the external sensory input to the cells in pool i, and ν is additive Gaussian noise. The attentional top-down bias $I_i^A(t)$ is defined as an external input coming from higher modules that is not explicitly modelled.

A qualitative description of the main fixed point attractors of the system of differential Equations B.100 and B.101 was provided by Usher and Niebur (1996). Basically, we will

---

[28] These neurodynamics are used in Chapter 13.

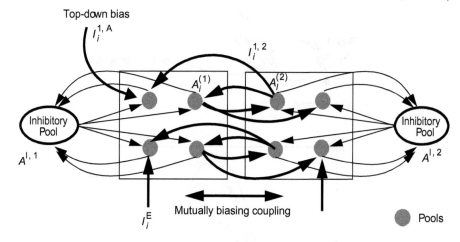

Fig. B.39 Two competitive networks mutually biased through intermodular connections. The activity $A_i^{(1)}$ of the ith excitatory pool in module 1 (on the left) and of the lth excitatory pool in module 2 (on the right) are connected by the mutually biasing coupling $I_i^{1,2}$. The architecture could implement top-down feedback originating from the interaction between brain areas that are explicitly modelled in the system. (Module 2 might be the higher module.) The external top-down bias $I_i^{1,A}$ corresponds to the coupling to pool i of module 1 from brain area A that is not explicitly modelled in the system. (After Rolls, E. T. and Deco,G. (2002) Computational Neuroscience of Vision. Oxford University Press: Oxford.)

be interested in the fixed points corresponding to zero activity and larger activation. The parameters will therefore be fixed such that the dynamics evolves to these attractors.

B.8.5 Multimodular neurodynamical architectures

In order to model complex psychophysically and neuropsychologically relevant brain functions such as visual search or object recognition (see e.g. Chapter 13 and Rolls and Deco (2002)), we must take into account the computational role of individual brain areas and their mutual interaction. The macroscopic phenomenological behavior will therefore be the result of the mutual interaction of several computational modules.

The dynamical coupling of different basic modules in a multimodular architecture can be described, in our neurodynamical framework, by allowing mutual interaction between pools belonging to different modules. Figure B.39 shows this idea schematically. The system of differential equations describing the global dynamics of such a multimodular system is given by a set of equations of the type of Equation B.75.

The excitatory pools belonging to a module obey the following equations:

$$\tau \frac{\partial A_i^{(j)}(t)}{\partial t} = -A_i^{(j)}(t) + a\mathrm{F}(A_i^{(j)}(t)) - b\mathrm{F}(A^{I,j}(t)) +$$
$$I_i^{j,k} + I_0 + I_i^E(t) + I_i^A(t) + \nu \qquad \text{for } i = 1, ..., m \quad \text{(B.102)}$$

and the corresponding inhibitory pools evolve according to

$$\tau_p \frac{\partial A^{I,j}(t)}{\partial t} = -A^{I,j}(t) + c \sum_{i=1}^{m} \mathrm{F}(A_i^{(j)}(t)) - d\mathrm{F}(A^{I,j}(t)). \quad \text{(B.103)}$$

The mutual coupling $I_i^{j,k}$ between module (j) and (k) is given by

$$I_i^{j,k} = \sum_l W_{il} \mathrm{F}(I_l^{(k)}(t)) \quad \text{(B.104)}$$

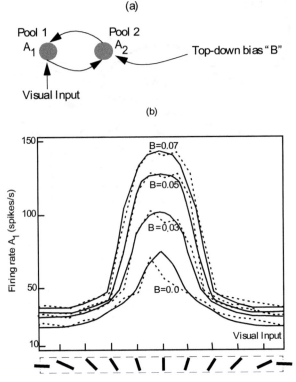

Fig. B.40 (a) The basic building block of the top-down attentional system utilizes non-specific competition between pools within the same module and specific mutual facilitation between pools in different modules. Excitatory neuronal pools within the same module compete with each other through one or more inhibitory neuronal pool(s) I_I with activity A^{I_I}. Excitatory pool 1 (with activity A_1) receives a bottom-up (visual) input I_1^V, and excitatory pool 2 receives a top-down ('attentional') bias input I_2^A. Excitatory neuronal pools in the two different modules can excite each other via mutually biased coupling. (b) The effect of altering the bias input B to pool 2 on the responses or activity of pool 1 to its orientation-tuned visual input (see text). (After Rolls, E. T. and Deco,G. (2002) Computational Neuroscience of Vision. Oxford University Press: Oxford.)

where W_{il} is the synaptic coupling strength between the pool i of module (j) and pool l of module (k). This mutual coupling term can be interpreted as a top-down bias originating from the interaction between brain areas that is explicitly modelled in our system. On the other hand, the external top-down bias I_i^A corresponds to the coupling with brain areas A that are not explicitly modelled in our system.

Additionally, it is interesting to note that the top-down bias in this kind of architecture modulates the response of the pool activity in a multiplicative manner. Responses of neurons in parietal area 7a are modulated by combined eye and head movement, exhibiting a multiplicative gain modulation that modifies the amplitude of the neural responses to retinal input but does not change the preferred retinal location of a cell, nor in general the width of the receptive field (Brotchie, Andersen, Snyder and Goodman, 1995). It has also been suggested that multiplicative gain modulation might play a role in translation invariant object representation (Salinas and Abbott, 1997). We use this multiplicative effect for formulating an architecture for attentional gain modulation, which can contribute to correct translation invariant object recognition in ways described in Chapter 13.

We show now that multiplicative-like responses can arise from the top-down biased mutual interaction between pools. Another alternative architecture that can also perform product operations on additive synaptic inputs was proposed by Salinas and Abbott (1996). Our basic architecture for showing this multiplicative effect is presented schematically in Fig. B.40a.

Two pools are mutually connected via fixed weights. The first pool or unit receives a bottom-up visual input I_1^V, modelled by the response of a vertically oriented complex cell. The second pool receives a top-down attentional bias $I_2^A = B$. The two pools are mutually coupled with unity weight. The equations describing the activities of the two pools are given by:

$$\tau \frac{\partial A_1(t)}{\partial t} = -A_1(t) + \alpha F(A_1(t)) + I_o + I_1^V + \nu \quad \text{(B.105)}$$

$$\tau \frac{\partial A_2(t)}{\partial t} = -A_2(t) + \alpha F(A_2(t)) + I_o + I_2^A + \nu \quad \text{(B.106)}$$

where A_1 and A_2 are the activities of pool 1 and pool 2 respectively, $\alpha = 0.95$ is the coefficient of recurrent self-excitation of the pool, ν is the noise input to the pool drawn from a normal distribution $N(\mu = 0, \sigma = 0.02)$, and $I_o = 0.025$ is a direct current biasing input to the pool.

Simulation of the above dynamical equations produces the results shown in Fig. B.40b. The orientation tuning curve of unit (or pool) 1 was modulated by a top-down bias B introduced to unit (pool) 2. The gain modulation was transmitted through the coupling from pool 2 to pool 1 after a few steps of evolution of the dynamical equations. Without the feedback from unit 2, unit 1 exhibits the orientation tuning curve shown as $(B = 0)$. As B increased, the increase in pool 1's response to the vertical bar was significantly greater than the increase in its response to the horizontal bar. Therefore, the attentional gain modulation produced in pool 1 through the mutual coupling was not a simple additive effect, but had a strong multiplicative component. The net effect was that the width of the orientation tuning curve of the cell was roughly preserved under attentional modulation. This was due to the non-linearity in the activation function.

This finding is basically consistent with the effect of attention on the orientation tuning curves of neurons in V4 (McAdams and Maunsell, 1999).

Summarizing, the neurodynamics of the competitive mechanisms between neuronal pools, and their mutual gain modulation, are the two main ingredients used for a cortical architecture that models attention and different kinds of object search in a visual scene (see Chapter 13, and Rolls and Deco (2002) Chapters 9–11 which are available at https://www.oxcns.org).

B.9 Interacting attractor networks

It is prototypical of the cerebral neocortical areas that there are recurrent collateral connections between the neurons within an area or module, and forward connections to the next cortical area in the hierarchy, which in turn sends backprojections (see Section 9.3.8). This architecture, made explicit in Fig. 13.10, immediately suggests, given that the recurrent connections within a module, and the forward and backward connections, are likely to be associatively modifiable, that the operation incorporates at least to some extent, interactions between coupled attractor (autoassociation) networks. For these reasons, it is important to analyze the rules that govern the interactions between coupled attractor networks. This has been done using the formal type of model described in Section 13.6.2.2.

One boundary condition is when the coupling between the networks is so weak that there is effectively no interaction. This holds when the coupling parameter g between the networks is less than approximately 0.002, where the coupling parameter indicates the relative strength of the inter-modular to the intra-modular connections, and measures effectively the relative strengths of the currents injected into the neurons by the inter-modular relative to the intra-modular (recurrent collateral) connections (Renart, Parga and Rolls, 1999b). At the other

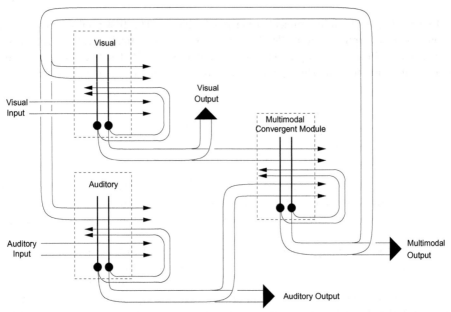

Fig. B.41 A two-layer set of attractor nets in which feedback from layer 2 can influence the states reached in layer 1. Layer 2 could be a higher cortical visual area with convergence from earlier cortical visual areas (see Chapter 2). Layer 2 could also be a multimodal area receiving inputs from unimodal visual and auditory cortical areas, as labelled. Each of the 3 modules has recurrent collateral synapses that are trained by an associative synaptic learning rule, and also inter-modular synaptic connections in the forward and backward direction that are also associatively trained. Attractors are formed within modules, the different modules interact, and attractors are also formed by the forward and backward inter-modular connections. The higher area may not only affect the states reached during attractor settling in the input layers, but may also, as a result of this, influence the representations that are learned in earlier cortical areas. A similar principle may operate in any multilayer hierarchical cortical processing system, such as the ventral visual system, in that the categories that can be formed only at later stages of processing may help earlier stages to form categories relevant to what can be diagnosed at later stages.

extreme, if the coupling parameter is strong, all the networks will operate as a single attractor network, together able to represent only one state (Renart, Parga and Rolls, 1999b). This critical value of the coupling parameter (at least for reciprocally connected networks with symmetric synaptic strengths) is relatively low, in the region of 0.024 (Renart, Parga and Rolls, 1999b). This is one reason why cortico-cortical backprojections are predicted to be quantitatively relatively weak, and for this reason it is suggested end on the apical parts of the dendrites of cortical pyramidal cells (see Section 9.3.8). In the strongly coupled regime when the system of networks operates as a single attractor, the total storage capacity (the number of patterns that can be stored and correctly retrieved) of all the networks will be set just by the number of synaptic connections onto any single neuron received from other neurons in the network, a number in the order of a few thousand (see Section B.3). This is one reason why connected cortical networks are thought not to act in the strongly coupled regime, because the total number of memories that could be represented in the whole of the cerebral cortex would be so small, in the order of a few thousand, depending on the sparseness of the patterns (see Equation B.15) (O'Kane and Treves, 1992).

Between these boundary conditions, that is in the region where the inter-modular coupling parameter g is in the range 0.002–0.024, it has been shown that interesting interactions can occur (Renart, Parga and Rolls, 1999b,a). In a bimodular architecture, with forward and backward connections between the modules, the capacity of one module can be increased, and an attractor is more likely to be found under noisy conditions, if there is a consistent pattern in the coupled attractor. By consistent we mean a pattern that during training was linked associatively by the forward and backward connections, with the pattern being retrieved in the first module. This provides a quantitative model for understanding some of the effects that backprojections can produce by supporting particular states in earlier cortical areas (Renart, Parga and Rolls, 1999b). The total storage capacity of the two networks is however, in line with O'Kane and Treves (1992), not a great deal greater than the storage capacity of one of the modules alone. Thus the help provided by the attractors in falling into a mutually compatible global retrieval state (in e.g. the scenario of a hierarchical system) is where the utility of such coupled attractor networks must lie. Another interesting application of such weakly coupled attractor networks is in coupled perceptual and short-term memory systems in the brain, described in Section 13.6.1 and Chapter 13.

In a trimodular attractor architecture shown in Fig. B.41 (which is similar to the architecture of the multilayer competitive net illustrated in Fig. B.20 but has recurrent collateral connections within each module), further interesting interactions occur that account for effects such as the McGurk effect, in which what is seen affects what is heard (Renart, Parga and Rolls, 1999a). The effect was originally demonstrated with the perception of auditory syllables, which were influenced by what is seen (McGurk and MacDonald, 1976). The trimodular architecture (studied using similar methods to those used by Renart, Parga and Rolls (1999b) and frequently utilizing scenarios in which first a stimulus was presented to a module, then removed during a memory delay period in which stimuli were applied to other modules) showed a phase with $g < 0.005$ in which the modules operated in an isolated way.

With g in the range 0.005–0.012, an 'independent' regime existed in which each module could be in a separate state to the others, but in which interactions between the modules occurred, which could assist or hinder retrieval in a module depending on whether the states in the other modules were consistent or inconsistent. It is in this 'independent' regime that a module can be in a continuing attractor that can provide other modules with a persistent external modulatory input that is helpful for tasks such as making comparisons between stimuli processed sequentially (as in delayed match-to-sample tasks and visual search tasks) (see Section 13.6.1). In this regime, if the modules are initially quiescent, then application of a stimulus to one input module propagates to the central module, and from it to the non-stimulated input module as well (see Fig. B.41).

When g grows beyond 0.012, the picture changes and the independence between the modules is lost. The delay activity states found in this region (of the phase space) *always* involve the three modules in attractors correlated with consistent features associated in the synaptic connections. Also, since g is now larger, changes in the properties of the external stimuli have more impact on the delay activity states. The general trend seen in this phase under the change of stimulus after a previous consistent attractor has been reached is that, first, if the second stimulus is not effective enough (it is weak or brief), it is unable to move any of the modules from their current delay activity states. If the stimulus is made more effective, then as soon as it is able to change the state of the stimulated input module, the internal and non-stimulated input modules follow, and the whole network moves into the new consistent attractor selected by the second stimulus. In this case, the interaction between the modules is so large that it does not allow contradictory local delay activity states to coexist, and the network is described as being in a 'locked' state.

The conclusion is that the most interesting scenario for coupled attractor networks is when they are weakly coupled (in the trimodular architecture $0.005 < g < 0.012$), for then interactions occur whereby how well one module responds to its own inputs can be influenced by the states of the other modules, but it can retain partly independent representations. This emphasizes the importance of weak interactions between coupled modules in the brain (Renart, Parga and Rolls, 1999b,a, 2000).

These generally useful interactions between coupled attractor networks can be useful in implementing top-down constraint satisfaction (see Section 9.3.8) and short-term memory (see Section 13.6.1). One type of constraint satisfaction in which they are also probably important is cross-modal constraint satisfaction, which occurs for example when the sight of the lips moving assists the hearing of syllables. If the experimenter mismatches the visual and auditory inputs, then auditory misperception can occur, as in the McGurk effect. In such experiments (McGurk and MacDonald, 1976) the subject receives one stimulus through the auditory pathway (e.g. the syllables *ga-ga*) and a *different* stimulus through the visual pathway (e.g. the lips of a person performing the movements corresponding to the syllables *ba-ba* on a video monitor). These stimuli are such that their acoustic waveforms as well as the lip motions needed to pronounce them are rather different. One can then assume that although they share the same vowel 'a', the internal representation of the syllables is dominated by the consonant, so that the representations of the syllables *ga-ga* and *ba-ba* are not correlated either in the primary visual cortical areas or in the primary auditory ones. At the end of the experiment, the subject is asked to repeat what he heard. When this procedure is repeated with many subjects, it is found that roughly 50% of them claim to have heard either the auditory stimulus (*ga-ga*), or the visual one (*ba-ba*). The rest of the subjects report to have heard neither the auditory nor the visual stimuli, but actually a combination of the two (e.g. *gabga*) or even something else including phonemes not presented auditorially or visually (e.g. *gagla*).

Renart, Parga and Rolls (1999a) were able to show that the McGurk effect can be accounted for by the operation of coupled attractor networks of the form shown in Fig. B.41. One input module is for the auditory input, the second is for the visual input, and both converge into a higher area which represents the syllable formed on the evidence of combination of the two inputs. There are backprojections from the convergent module back to the input modules. Persistent (continuing) inputs were applied to both the inputs, and during associative training of all the weights the visual and auditory inputs corresponded to the same syllable. When tested with inconsistent visual and auditory inputs, it was found for g between ~ 0.10 and ~ 0.11, the convergent module can either remain in a symmetric state in which it represents a mixture of the two inputs, or choose between one of the inputs, with either situation being stable. For lower g the convergent module always settles into a state corresponding to the input in one of the input modules. It is the random fluctuations produced during the convergence to the attractor that determine the pattern selected by the convergent module. When the convergent module becomes correlated with *one* of its stored patterns, the signal back-projected to the input module stimulated with the feature associated with that pattern becomes stronger and the overlap in this module is increased. Thus, with low values of the inter-module coupling parameter g, situations are found in which sometimes the input to one module dominates, and sometimes the input to the other module dominates what is represented in the convergent module, and sometimes mixture states are stable in the convergent module. This model can thus account for the influences that visual inputs can have on what is heard, in for example the McGurk effect.

The interactions between coupled attractor networks can lead to the following effects. Facilitation can occur in a module if its external input is matched by an input from another module, whereas suppression in a module of its response to an external input can occur if the two inputs mismatch. This type of interaction can be used in imaging studies to identify brain regions where different signals interact with each other. One example is to locate brain regions where multimodal inputs converge. If the inputs in two sensory modalities are consistent based on previous experience, then facilitation will occur, whereas if they are inconsistent, suppression of the activity in a module can occur. This is one of the effects described in the bimodular and trimodular architectures investigated by Renart, Parga and Rolls (1999b), Renart, Parga and Rolls (1999a) and Rolls and Stringer (2001b), and found in architectures such as that illustrated in Fig. B.41.

If a multimodular architecture is trained with each of many patterns (which might be visual stimuli) in one module associated with one of a few patterns (which might be mood states) in a connected module, then interesting effects due to this asymmetry are found, as described by Rolls and Stringer (2001b).

An interesting issue that arises is how rapidly a system of interacting attractor networks such as that illustrated in Fig. B.41 settles into a stable state. Is it sufficiently rapid for the interacting attractor effects described to contribute to cortical information processing? It is likely that the settling of the whole system is quite rapid, if it is implemented (as it is in the brain) with synapses and neurons that operate with continuous dynamics, where the time constant of the synapses dominates the retrieval speed, and is in the order of 15 ms for each module, as described in Section B.6 and by Panzeri, Rolls, Battaglia and Lavis (2001). In that Section, it is shown that a multimodular attractor network architecture can process information in approximately 15 ms per module (assuming an inactivation time constant for the synapses of 10 ms), and similarly fast settling may be expected of a system of the type shown in Fig. B.41.

B.10 Sequence memory implemented by adaptation in an attractor network

Sequence memory can be implemented by using synaptic adaptation (Rolls, 2016b) to effectively encode the order of the items in a sequence, as described by Deco and Rolls (2005c) and used in the model of syntax (Rolls and Deco, 2015a) (Section 14.5). Whenever the attractor system is quenched into inactivity, the next member of the sequence emerges out of the spontaneous activity, because the least recently activated member of the sequence has the least synaptic or neuronal adaptation. This mechanism could be implemented in recurrent networks such as the hippocampal CA3, prefrontal cortex, language areas of cortex, etc.

B.11 Perceptrons and one-layer error correction networks

The networks described in the next two Sections (B.11 and B.12) are capable of mapping a set of inputs to a set of required outputs using correction when errors are made. Although some of the networks are very powerful in the types of mapping they can perform, the power is obtained at the cost of learning algorithms that do not use local learning rules. A local learning rule specifies that synaptic strengths should be altered on the basis of information available locally at the synapse, for example the activity of the presynaptic and the post-synaptic neurons. Because the networks described here do not use local learning rules, their biological plausibility remains at present uncertain. One of the aims of future research must be to determine whether comparably difficult problems to those solved by the networks described in Sections B.11 and B.12 can be solved by biologically plausible neuronal networks.

We now describe one-layer networks taught by an error correction algorithm. The term *perceptron* refers strictly to networks with binary threshold activation functions. The outputs might take the values only 1 or 0 for example. The term perceptron arose from networks designed originally to solve perceptual problems (Rosenblatt, 1961; Minsky and Papert, 1969), and these networks are referred to briefly below. If the output neurons have continuous-valued firing rates, then a more general error-correcting rule called the delta rule is used, and is introduced in this Section (B.11). For such networks, the activation function may be linear, or it may be non-linear but monotonically increasing, without a sharp threshold, as in the sigmoid activation function (see Fig. 1.3).

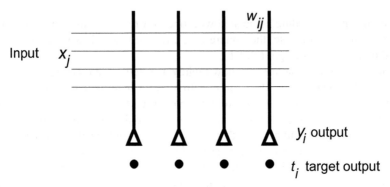

Fig. B.42 One-layer perceptron.

B.11.1 Architecture and general description

The one-layer error-correcting network has a set of inputs that it is desired to map or classify into a set of outputs (see Fig. B.42). During learning, an input pattern is selected, and produces output firing by activating the output neurons through modifiable synapses, which then fire as a function of their typically non-linear activation function. The output of each neuron is then compared with a target output for that neuron given that input pattern, an error between the actual output and the desired output is determined, and the synaptic weights on that neuron are then adjusted to minimize the error. This process is then repeated for all patterns until the average error across patterns has reached a minimum. A one-layer error-correcting network can thus produce output firing for each pattern in a way that has similarities to a pattern associator. It can perform more powerful mappings than a pattern associator, but requires an error to be computed for each neuron, and for that error to affect the synaptic strength in a way that is not altogether local. A more detailed description follows.

These one-layer networks have a target for each output neuron (for each input pattern). They are thus an example of a supervised network. With the one-layer networks taught with the delta rule or perceptron learning rule described next, there is a separate teacher for each output neuron, as shown in Fig. B.42.

B.11.2 Generic algorithm for a one-layer error correction network

For each input pattern and desired target output:

1. Apply an input pattern to produce input firing **x**, and obtain the activation of each neuron in the standard way by computing the dot product of the input pattern and the synaptic weight vector. The synaptic weight vector can be initially zero, or have random values.

$$h_i = \sum_j x_j w_{ij} \qquad (B.107)$$

where $\sum_j$ indicates that the sum is over the C input axons (or connections) indexed by j to each neuron.

2. Apply an activation function to produce the output firing y_i:

$$y_i = f(h_i) . \qquad (B.108)$$

This activation function f may be sigmoid, linear, binary threshold, linear threshold, etc. If the activation function is non-linear, this helps to classify the inputs into distinct output patterns, but a linear activation function may be used if an optimal linear mapping is desired (see

Adaline and Madaline, below).

3. Calculate the difference for each cell i between the target output t_i and the actual output y_i produced by the input, which is the error Δ_i

$$\Delta_i = t_i - y_i. \tag{B.109}$$

4. Apply the following learning rule, which corrects the (continuously variable) weights according to the error and the input firing x_j

$$\delta w_{ij} = k(t_i - y_i)x_j \tag{B.110}$$

where k is a constant that determines the learning rate. This is often called the delta rule, the Widrow–Hoff rule, or the LMS (least mean squares) rule (see below).

5. Repeat steps 1–4 for all input pattern – output target pairs until the root mean square error becomes zero or reaches a minimum.

In general, networks taught by the delta rule may have linear, binary threshold, or non-linear but monotonically increasing (e.g. sigmoid) activation functions, and may be taught with binary or continuous input patterns (see Rolls and Treves (1998), Chapter 5). The properties of these variations are made clear next.

B.11.3 Capability and limitations of single-layer error-correcting networks

Perceptrons perform pattern classification. That is, each neuron classifies the input patterns it receives into classes determined by the teacher. This is thus an example of a supervised network, with a separate teacher for each output neuron. The classification is most clearly understood if the output neurons are binary, or are strongly non-linear, but the network will still try to obtain an optimal mapping with linear or near-linear output neurons.

When each neuron operates as a binary classifier, we can consider how many input patterns p can be classified by each neuron, and the classes of pattern that can be correctly classified. The result is that the maximum number of patterns that can be correctly classified by a neuron with C inputs is

$$p_{\max} = 2C \tag{B.111}$$

when the inputs have random continuous-valued inputs, but the patterns must be linearly separable (see Section A.2.1, and Hertz, Krogh and Palmer (1991)). For a one-layer network, no set of weights can be found that will perform the XOR (exclusive OR), or any other non-linearly separable function (see Appendix A).

Although the inability of one-layer networks with binary neurons to solve non-linearly separable problems is a limitation, it is not in practice a major limitation on the processing that can be performed in a neural network for a number of reasons. First, if the inputs can take continuous values, then if the patterns are drawn from a random distribution, the one-layer network can map up to $2C$ of them. Second, as described for pattern associators, the perceptron could be preceded by an expansion recoding network such as a competitive network with more output than input neurons. This effectively provides a two-layer network for solving the problem, and multilayer networks are in general capable of solving arbitrary mapping problems. Ways in which such multilayer networks might be trained are discussed later in this Appendix.

We now return to the issue of the capacity of one-layer perceptrons, that is, how many patterns p can be correctly mapped to correct binary outputs if the input patterns are linearly separable.

B.11.3.1 Output neurons with continuous values, and random patterns

Before treating this case, I note that if the inputs are orthogonal, then just as in the pattern associator, C patterns can be correctly classified, where there are C inputs, x_j, $(j = 1, C)$, per neuron. The argument is the same as for a pattern associator.

We consider next the capacity of a one-layer error-correcting network that learns patterns drawn from a random distribution. For neurons with continuous output values, whether the activation function is linear or not, the capacity (for fully distributed inputs) is set by the criterion that the set of input patterns must be linearly independent (see Hertz, Krogh and Palmer (1991)). (Three patterns are linearly independent if any one cannot be formed by addition (with scaling allowed) of the other two patterns – see Appendix A.) Given that there can be a maximum of C linearly independent patterns in a C-dimensional space (see Appendix A), the capacity of the perceptron with such patterns is C patterns. If we choose p random patterns with continuous values, then they will be linearly independent for $p \leq C$ (except for cases with very low probability when the randomly chosen values may not produce linearly independent patterns). (With random continuous values for the input patterns, it is very unlikely that the addition of any two, with scaling allowed, will produce a third pattern in the set.) Thus with continuous valued input patterns,

$$p_{\max} = C. \qquad (B.112)$$

If the inputs are not linearly independent, networks trained with the delta rule produce a least mean squares (LMS) error (optimal) solution (see below).

B.11.3.2 Output neurons with binary threshold activation functions

Let us consider here strictly defined perceptrons, that is, networks with (binary) threshold output neurons, and taught by the perceptron learning procedure.

Capacity with fully distributed output patterns

The condition here for correct classification is that described in Appendix A for the AND and XOR functions, that the patterns must be linearly separable. If we consider random continuous-valued inputs, then the capacity is

$$p_{\max} = 2C \qquad (B.113)$$

(see Cover (1965), Hertz, Krogh and Palmer (1991); this capacity is the case with C large, and the number of output neurons small). The interesting point to note here is that, even with fully distributed inputs, a perceptron is capable of learning more (fully distributed) patterns than there are inputs per neuron. This formula is in general valid for large C, but happens to hold also for the AND function illustrated in Appendix A.2.1.

Sparse encoding of the patterns

If the output patterns $\mathbf{y}$ are sparse (but still distributed), then just as with the pattern associator, it is possible to map many more than C patterns to correct outputs. Indeed, the number of different patterns or prototypes p that can be stored is

$$p \approx C/a \qquad (B.114)$$

where a is the sparseness of the target pattern t. p can in this situation be much larger than C (cf. Rolls and Treves (1990), and Rolls and Treves (1998) Appendix A3).

Perceptron convergence theorem

It can be proved that such networks will learn the desired mapping in a finite number of steps (Block, 1962; Minsky and Papert, 1969; Hertz, Krogh and Palmer, 1991). (This of course depends on there being such a mapping, the condition for this being that the input patterns are linearly separable.) This is important, for it shows that single-layer networks can be proved to be capable of solving certain classes of problem.

As a matter of history, Minsky and Papert (1969) went on to emphasize the point that no one-layer network can correctly classify non-linearly separable patterns. Although it was clear that multilayer networks can solve such mapping problems, Minsky and Papert were pessimistic that an algorithm for training such a multilayer network would be found. Their emphasis that neural networks might not be able to solve general problems in computation, such as computing the XOR, which is a non-linearly separable mapping, resulted in a decline in research activity in neural networks. In retrospect, this was unfortunate, for humans are rather poor at solving parity problems such as the XOR (Thorpe, O'Regan and Pouget, 1989), yet can perform many other useful neural network operations very quickly. Algorithms for training multilayer perceptrons were gradually discovered by a number of different investigators, and became widely known after the publication of the algorithm described by Rumelhart, Hinton and Williams (1986b), and Rumelhart, Hinton and Williams (1986a). Even before this, interest in neural network pattern associators, autoassociators and competitive networks was developing (see Hinton and Anderson (1981), Kohonen (1977), Kohonen (1988)), but the acceptance of the backpropagation or error algorithm for training multilayer perceptrons led to a great rise in interest in neural networks, partly for use in connectionist models of cognitive function (McClelland and Rumelhart, 1986; McLeod, Plunkett and Rolls, 1998), and partly for use in applications (Bishop, 1995; LeCun, Bengio and Hinton, 2015; Lillicrap, Santoro, Marris, Akerman and Hinton, 2020).

In that perceptrons can correctly classify patterns provided only that they are linearly separable, but pattern associators are more restricted, perceptrons are more powerful learning devices than Hebbian pattern associators.

B.11.3.3 Gradient descent for neurons with continuous-valued outputs

We now consider networks trained by the delta (error correction) rule B.110, and having continuous-valued outputs. The activation function may be linear or non-linear, but provided that it is differentiable (in practice, does not include a sharp threshold), the network can be thought of as gradually decreasing the error on every learning trial, that is as performing some type of gradient descent down a continuous error function. The concept of gradient descent arises from defining an error ϵ for a neuron as

$$\epsilon = \sum_{\mu}(t^{\mu} - y^{\mu})^2 \qquad \text{(B.115)}$$

where μ indexes the patterns learned by the neuron. The error function for a neuron in the direction of a particular weight would have the form shown in Fig. B.43. The delta rule can be conceptualized as performing gradient descent of this error function, in that for the jth synaptic weight on the neuron

$$\delta w_j = -k\partial\epsilon/\partial w_j \qquad \text{(B.116)}$$

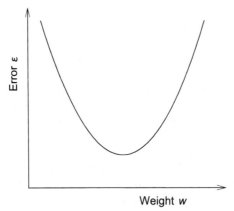

Fig. B.43 The error function ϵ for a neuron in the direction of a particular weight w.

where $\partial \epsilon / \partial w_j$ is just the slope of the error curve in the direction of w_j in Fig. B.43. This will decrease the weight if the slope is positive and increase the weight if the slope is negative. Given Equation B.109, and recalling that $h = \sum_j x_j w_j$, Equation B.43 becomes

$$\delta w_j = -k \partial / \partial w_j \sum_\mu [(t^\mu - f(h^\mu))^2] \tag{B.117}$$

$$= 2k \sum_\mu [(t^\mu - y^\mu)] f'(h) x_j \tag{B.118}$$

where $f'(h)$ is the derivative of the activation function. Provided that the activation function is monotonically increasing, its derivative will be positive, and the sign of the weight change will only depend on the mean sign of the error. Equation B.118 thus shows one way in which, from a gradient descent conceptualization, Equation B.110 can be derived.

With linear output neurons, this gradient descent is proved to reach the correct mapping (see Hertz, Krogh and Palmer (1991)). (As with all single-layer networks with continuous-valued output neurons, a perfect solution is only found if the input patterns are linearly independent. If they are not, an optimal mapping is achieved, in which the sum of the squares of the errors is a minimum.) With non-linear output neurons (for example with a sigmoid activation function), the error surface may have local minima, and is not guaranteed to reach the optimal solution, although typically a near-optimal solution is achieved. Part of the power of this gradient descent conceptualization is that it can be applied to multilayer networks with neurons with non-linear but differentiable activation functions, for example with sigmoid activation functions (see Hertz, Krogh and Palmer (1991)).

B.11.4 Properties

The properties of single-layer networks trained with a delta rule (and of perceptrons) are similar to those of pattern associators trained with a Hebbian rule in many respects (see Section B.2). In particular, the properties of generalization and graceful degradation are similar, provided that (for both types of network) distributed representations are used. The main differences are in the types of pattern that can be separated correctly, the learning speed (in that delta-rule networks can take advantage of many training trials to learn to separate patterns that could not be learned by Hebbian pattern associators), and in that the delta-rule network needs an error term to be supplied for each neuron, whereas an error term does not have to be supplied for a pattern associator, just an unconditioned or forcing stimulus. Given these overall similarities and differences, the properties of one-layer delta-rule networks are considered here briefly.

B.11.4.1 Generalization

During recall, delta-rule one-layer networks with non-linear output neurons produce appropriate outputs if a recall cue vector $\mathbf{x}_r$ is similar to a vector that has been learned already. This occurs because the recall operation involves computing the dot (inner) product of the input pattern vector $\mathbf{x}_r$ with the synaptic weight vector $\mathbf{w}_i$, so that the firing produced, y_i, reflects the similarity of the current input to the previously learned input pattern $\mathbf{x}$. Distributed representations are needed for this property. If two patterns that a delta-rule network has learned to separate are very similar, then the weights of the network will have been adjusted to force the different outputs to occur correctly. At the same time, this will mean that the way in which the network generalizes in the space between these two vectors will be very sharply defined. (Small changes in the input vector will force it to be classified one way or the other.)

B.11.4.2 Graceful degradation or fault tolerance

One-layer delta-rule networks show graceful degradation provided that the input patterns $\mathbf{x}$ are distributed.

B.11.4.3 Prototype extraction, extraction of central tendency, and noise reduction

These occur as for pattern autoassociators.

B.11.4.4 Speed

Recall is very fast in a one-layer pattern associator or perceptron, because it is a feedforward network (with no recurrent or lateral connections). Recall is also fast if the neuron has cell-like properties, because the stimulus input firings x_j ($j = 1, C$ axons) can be applied simultaneously to the synapses w_{ij}, and the activation h_i can be accumulated in one or two time constants of the synapses and dendrite (e.g. 10–20 ms) (see Section B.6.5). Whenever the threshold of the cell is exceeded, it fires. Thus, in effectively one time step, which takes the brain no more than 10–20 ms, all the output neurons of the delta-rule network can be firing with rates that reflect the input firing of every axon.

Learning is as fast ('one-shot') in perceptrons as in pattern associators if the input patterns are orthogonal. If the patterns are not orthogonal, so that the error correction rule has to work in order to separate patterns, then the network may take many trials to achieve the best solution (which will be perfect under the conditions described above).

B.11.4.5 Non-local learning rule

The learning rule is not truly local, as it is in pattern associators, autoassociators, and competitive networks, in that with one-layer delta-rule networks, the information required to change each synaptic weight is not available in the presynaptic terminal (reflecting the presynaptic rate) and the postsynaptic activation. Instead, an error for the neuron must be computed, possibly by another neuron, and then this error must be conveyed back to the postsynaptic neuron to provide the postsynaptic error term, which together with the presynaptic rate determines how much the synapse should change, as in equation B.110,

$$\delta w_{ij} = k(t_i - y_i)x_j$$

where $(t_i - y_i)$ is the error.

A rather special architecture would be required if the brain were to utilize delta-rule error-correcting learning. One such architecture might require each output neuron to be supplied with its own error signal by another neuron. The possibility (Albus, 1971) that this is implemented in one part of the brain, the cerebellum, is described in Chapter 17. Another functional architecture would require each neuron to compute its own error by subtracting its current activation by its x inputs from another set of afferents providing the target activation for that neuron. A neurophysiological architecture and mechanism for this is not currently known.

B.11.4.6 Interference

Interference is less of a property of single-layer delta rule networks than of pattern autoassociators and autoassociators, in that delta rule networks can learn to separate patterns even when they are highly correlated. However, if patterns are not linearly independent, then the delta rule will learn a least mean squares solution, and interference can be said to occur.

B.11.4.7 Expansion recoding

As with pattern associators and autoassociators, expansion recoding can separate input patterns into a form that makes them learnable, or that makes learning more rapid with only a few trials needed, by delta rule networks. It has been suggested that this is the role of the granule cells in the cerebellum, which provide for expansion recoding by 1,000:1 of the mossy fibre inputs before they are presented by the parallel fibres to the cerebellar Purkinje cells (Marr, 1969; Albus, 1971; Rolls and Treves, 1998) (Chapter 17).

B.11.4.8 Utility of single-layer error-correcting networks in information processing by the brain

In the cerebellum, each output cell, a Purkinje cell, has its own climbing fibre, that distributes from its inferior olive cell its terminals throughout the dendritic tree of the Purkinje cell. It is this climbing fibre that controls whether learning of the x inputs supplied by the parallel fibres onto the Purkinje cell occurs, and it has been suggested that the function of this architecture is for the climbing fibre to bring the error term to every part of the postsynaptic neuron (Chapter 17). This rather special arrangement with each output cell apparently having its own teacher is probably unique in the brain, and shows the lengths to which the brain might need to go to implement a teacher for each output neuron. The requirement for error-correction learning is to have the neuron forced during a learning phase into a state that reflects its error while presynaptic afferents are still active, and rather special arrangements are needed for this.

B.12 Multilayer perceptrons: backpropagation of error networks

B.12.1 Introduction

So far, we have considered how error can be used to train a one-layer network using a delta rule. Minsky and Papert (1969) emphasized the fact that one-layer networks cannot solve certain classes of input–output mapping problems (as described above). It was clear then that these restrictions would not apply to the problems that can be solved by feedforward multi-layer networks, if they could be trained. A multilayer feedforward network has two or more connected layers, in which connections allow activity to be projected forward from one layer to the next, and in which there are no lateral connections within a layer. Such a multilayer network has an output layer (which can be trained with a standard delta rule using an error provided for each output neuron), and one or more hidden layers, in which the neurons do not receive separate error signals from an external teacher. (Because they do not provide the

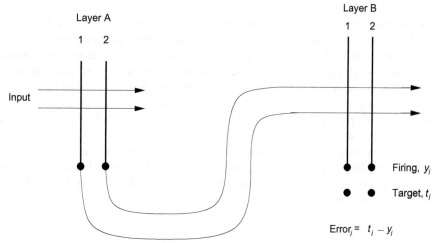

Fig. B.44 A two-layer perceptron. Inputs are applied to layer A through modifiable synapses. The outputs from layer A are applied through modifiable synapses to layer B. Layer B can be trained using a delta rule to produce firing y_i which will approach the target t_i. It is more difficult to modify the weights in layer A, because appropriate error signals must be backpropagated from layer B.

outputs of the network directly, and do not directly receive their own teaching error signal, these layers are described as hidden.) To solve an arbitrary mapping problem (in which the inputs are not linearly separable), a multilayer network could have a set of hidden neurons that would remap the inputs in such a way that the output layer can be provided with a linearly separable problem to solve using training of its weights with the delta rule. The problem was: how could the synaptic weights into the hidden neurons be trained in such a way that they would provide an appropriate representation? Minsky and Papert (1969) were pessimistic that such a solution would be found and, partly because of this, interest in computations in neural networks declined for many years. Although some work in neural networks continued in the following years (e.g. (Marr, 1969, 1970, 1971; Willshaw and Longuet-Higgins, 1969; Willshaw, 1981; Malsburg, 1973; Grossberg, 1976a,b; Arbib, 1964; Amari, 1982; Amari, Yoshida and Kanatani, 1977)), widespread interest in neural networks was revived by the type of approach to associative memory and its relation to human memory taken by the work described in the volume edited by Hinton and Anderson (1981), and by Kohonen (Kohonen, 1977, 1989). Soon after this, a solution to training a multilayer perceptron using backpropagation of error became widely known (Rumelhart, Hinton and Williams, 1986b,a) (although earlier solutions had been found), and very great interest in neural networks and also in neural network approaches to cognitive processing (connectionism) developed (Rumelhart and McClelland, 1986; McClelland and Rumelhart, 1986; McLeod, Plunkett and Rolls, 1998).

B.12.2 Architecture and algorithm

An introduction to the way in which a multilayer network can be trained by backpropagation of error is described next, with further details provided elsewhere (LeCun, Bengio and Hinton, 2015; Lillicrap, Santoro, Marris, Akerman and Hinton, 2020). Then we consider whether such a training algorithm is biologically plausible. More formal accounts of the training algorithm for multilayer perceptrons (sometimes abbreviated MLP) are given by Rumelhart, Hinton and Williams (1986b), Rumelhart, Hinton and Williams (1986a), Hertz, Krogh and Palmer (1991), LeCun, Bengio and Hinton (2015), and Lillicrap, Santoro, Marris, Akerman and Hinton (2020), and below.

Consider the two-layer network shown in Fig. B.44. Inputs to the hidden neurons in layer

A feed forward activity to the output neurons in layer B. The neurons in the network have a sigmoid activation function. One reason for such an activation function is that it is non-linear, and non-linearity is needed to enable multilayer networks to solve difficult (non-linearly separable) problems. (If the neurons were linear, the multilayer network would be equivalent to a one-layer network, which cannot solve such problems.) Neurons B1 and B2 of the output layer, B, are each trained using a delta rule and an error computed for each output neuron from the target output for that neuron when a given input pattern is being applied to the network. Consider now the error that needs to be used to train neuron A1 by a delta rule. This error clearly influences the error of neuron B1 in a way that depends on the magnitude of the synaptic weight from neuron A1 to B1; and on the error of neuron B2 in a way that depends on the magnitude of the synaptic weight from neuron A1 to B2. In other words, the error for neuron A1 depends on:

the weight from A1 to B1 $(w_{11}) \cdot$ error of neuron B1
+ the weight from A1 to B2 $(w_{21}) \cdot$ error of neuron B2.

In this way, the error calculation can be propagated backwards through the network to any neuron in any hidden layer, so that each neuron in the hidden layer can be trained, once its error is computed, by a delta rule (which uses the computed error for the neuron and the presynaptic firing at the synapse to correct each synaptic weight). For this to work, the way in which each neuron is activated and sends a signal forward must be continuous (not binary), so that the extent to which there is an error in, for example, neuron B1 can be related back in a graded way to provide a continuously variable correction signal to previous stages. This is one of the requirements for enabling the network to descend a continuous error surface. The activation function must be non-linear (e.g. sigmoid) for the network to learn more than could be learned by a single-layer network. (Remember that a multilayer linear network can always be made equivalent to a single-layer linear network, and that there are some problems that cannot be solved by single-layer networks.) For the way in which the error of each output neuron should be taken into account to be specified in the error correction rule, the position at which the output neuron is operating on its activation function must also be taken into account. For this, the slope of the activation function is needed, and because the slope is needed, the activation function must be differentiable. Although we indicated use of a sigmoid activation function, other activation functions that are non-linear and monotonically increasing (and differentiable) can be used. (For further details, see Rumelhart, Hinton and Williams (1986b), Rumelhart, Hinton and Williams (1986a), and Hertz, Krogh and Palmer (1991)).

More formally, the operation of a backpropagation of error network can be described as follows (Fig. B.45) (LeCun, Bengio and Hinton, 2015; Lillicrap, Santoro, Marris, Akerman and Hinton, 2020). Fig. B.45a shows how a multilayer neural network (shown by the connected dots) can distort the input space to make the classes of data (examples of which are on the red and blue lines) linearly separable. Note how a regular grid (shown on the left) in the input space is also transformed (shown in the middle panel) by hidden units. This is an illustrative example with only two input units, two hidden units and one output unit, but the networks may contain hundreds of thousands of units.

Fig. B.45b shows how the chain rule of derivatives tells us how two small effects (that of a small change of x on y, and that of y on z) are composed. A small change Δx in x gets transformed first into a small change Δx in y by getting multiplied by $\partial y / \partial x$ (that is, the definition of partial derivative). Similarly, the change Δy creates a change Δz in z. Substituting one equation into the other gives the chain rule of derivatives – how Δx gets turned into Δz through multiplication by the product of $\partial y / \partial x$ and $\partial z / \partial x$. It also works when x, y and z are vectors (and the derivatives are Jacobian matrices).

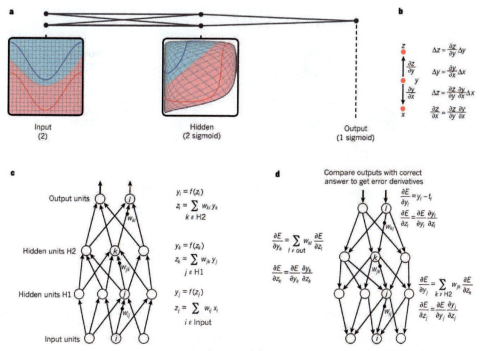

Fig. B.45 Multilayer neural networks and backpropagation (see text). a. How a multilayer neural network (shown by the connected dots) can distort the input space to make the classes of data (examples of which are on the red and blue lines) linearly separable. b. A chain rule of derivatives. c. Equations used for computing the forward pass in a neural net with two hidden layers and one output layer. d. The equations used for computing the backward pass (see text). Note that the indices use different conventions to those used in the remainder of this book. (Reproduced from Yann LeCun, Yoshua Bengio and Geoffrey Hinton (2015) Deep learning. Nature 521: 436–444. Copyright © Springer Nature.)

Fig. B.45c shows the equations used for computing the forward pass in a neural net with two hidden layers and one output layer, each constituting a module through which one can backpropagate gradients. At each layer, we first compute the total input z to each unit, which is a weighted sum of the outputs of the units in the layer below. Then a non-linear function $f(.)$ is applied to z to get the output of the unit. For simplicity, bias terms are omitted. The non-linear function used is now typically the rectified linear unit (ReLU) $f(z) = \max(0, z)$ (known in neuroscience as a threshold linear activation function), although sigmoid activation functions have been used.

Fig. B.45d shows the equations used for computing the backward pass. At each hidden layer we compute the error derivative with respect to the output of each unit, which is a weighted sum of the error derivatives with respect to the total inputs to the units in the layer above. We then convert the error derivative with respect to the output into the error derivative with respect to the input by multiplying it by the gradient of $f(z)$. At the output layer, the error derivative with respect to the output of a unit is computed by differentiating the cost function. This gives $y_l - t_l$ if the cost function for unit l is $0.5(y_l - t_l)^2$, where t_l is the target value. Once the $\partial E/\partial z_k$ is known, the error-derivative for the weight w_{jk} on the connection from unit j in the layer below is $y_j \partial E/\partial z_k$.

Once we have this error derivative for a single neuron, we can update the weights into that neuron by performing a gradient descent step in the direction specified by the derivative to minimize the cost function (see LeCun, Bengio and Hinton (2015) and Lillicrap, Santoro, Marris, Akerman and Hinton (2020)).

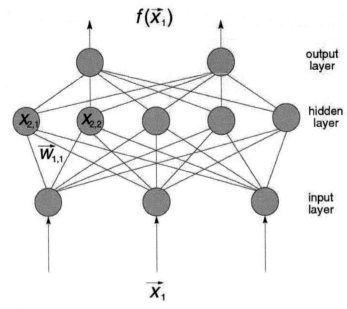

Fig. B.46 Artificial neural feedforward network used for backpropagation of error learning. This network has three layers, but a deep network might have 100 layers. The mathematical symbols correspond to those used in Equation B.119. (Reproduced from Plebe,A. and Grasso,G. (2019) The unbearable shallow understanding of deep learning. Minds and Machines 29: 515–553. Copyright © Springer Nature.)

Another way of describing backpropagation of error learning is as follows (Plebe and Grasso, 2019). They start with a deep network with several layers that is in essence a feedforward network, shown in Fig. B.46. The values of the units are computed with the following equations:

$$\mathbf{x}_1 = \mathbf{A}^{(I)} \mathbf{x} + \mathbf{b}^{(I)},$$
$$\hat{f}(\mathbf{x}) = \mathbf{A}^{(O)} \mathbf{x}_N + \mathbf{b}^{(O)}, \quad \text{(B.119)}$$
$$x_{i,k} = h\left(\mathbf{w}_{i,k} \mathbf{x}_{i-1} - \theta_{i,k}\right) \quad 1 < i < N.$$

The first (bottom) layer, ruled by Equations B.119, provides input values to the network, normalized with the linear operators $\mathbf{A}^{(I)}$ and $\mathbf{b}^{(I)}$. The top layer is where the output data appear. The entire feedforward network can be expressed as a function $\hat{f}(\mathbf{x})$ of the input vector $\mathbf{x}$, and, as described by Equations B.119, it is normalized again to meet the desired data range. The real work is done by the layers in between, according to Equation B.119. In a layer i, each unit $x_{i,k}$ sums up all the values from the previous level, weighted by parameters $\mathbf{w}_{i,k}$, and the result is modified by a non-linear activation function $h(.)$, such as the sigmoid or the hyperbolic tangent.

The backpropagation learning rule specifies how to train the connections between the units, from examples of the desired function between known inputs and outputs. With $\mathbf{w}$ the vector of all learnable parameters in a network, such as $\mathbf{w}_{i,k}$ in Equation B.119, and $\mathscr{L}\mathbf{x},\mathbf{w}$ a measure of the error of the network with parameters $\mathbf{w}$ when applied to the sample $\mathbf{x}$, the backpropagation of error learning rule updates the parameters iteratively, according to the following formula:

$$\mathbf{w}_{t+1} = \mathbf{w}_{t+1} - \eta \nabla_w \mathscr{L}(\mathbf{x}_t, \mathbf{w}_t) \quad \text{(B.120)}$$

where t spans over all available samples x_t, and η is the learning rate (Plebe and Grasso, 2019). By iterating this procedure many times, the network gradually converges to approximate the unknown function sampled at $\mathbf{x}_t$.

B.12.3 Properties of multilayer networks trained by error backpropagation

B.12.3.1 Arbitrary mappings

Arbitrary mappings of non-linearly separable patterns can be achieved. For example, such networks can solve the XOR problem, and parity problems in general of which XOR is a special case. (The parity problem is to determine whether the sum of the (binary) bits in a vector is odd or even.) Multilayer feedforward backpropagation of error networks are not guaranteed to converge to the best solution, and may become stuck in local minima in the error surface. However, they generally perform very well.

B.12.3.2 Fast operation

The network operates as a feedforward network, without any recurrent or feedback processing. Thus (once it has learned) the network operates very quickly, with a time proportional to the number of layers.

B.12.3.3 Learning speed

The learning speed can be very slow, taking many thousands of trials. The network learns to gradually approximate the correct input–output mapping required, but the learning is slow because of the credit assignment problem for neurons in the hidden layers. The credit assignment problem refers to the issue of how much to correct the weights of each neuron in the hidden layer. As the example above shows, the error for a hidden neuron could influence the errors of many neurons in the output layers, and the error of each output neuron reflects the error from many hidden neurons. It is thus difficult to assign credit (or blame) on any single trial to any particular hidden neuron, so an error must be estimated, and the net run until the weights of the crucial hidden neurons have become altered sufficiently to allow good performance of the network. Another factor that can slow learning is that if a neuron operates close to a horizontal part of its activation function, then the output of the neuron will depend rather little on its activation, and correspondingly the error computed to backpropagate will depend rather little on the activation of that neuron, so learning will be slow.

More general approaches to this issue suggest that the number of training trials for such a network will (with a suitable training set) be of the same order of magnitude as the number of synapses in the network (see Cortes, Jaeckel, Solla, Vapnik and Denker (1996)).

B.12.3.4 Number of hidden neurons and generalization

Backpropagation networks are generally intended to discover regular mappings between the input and output, that is mappings in which generalization will occur usefully. If there were one hidden neuron for every combination of inputs that had to be mapped to an output, then this would constitute a look-up table, and no generalization between similar inputs (or inputs not yet received) would occur. The best way to ensure that a backpropagation network learns the structure of the problem space is to set the number of neurons in the hidden layers close to the minimum that will allow the mapping to be implemented. This forces the network not to operate as a look-up table. A problem is that there is no general rule about how many hidden neurons are appropriate, given that this depends on the types of mappings required. In practice, these networks are sometimes trained with different numbers of hidden neurons, until the minimum number required to perform the required mapping has been approximated.

The lack of biological plausibility of backpropagation of error deep networks in considered in Section 19.4, and limitations of current understanding have been highlighted (Plebe and Grasso, 2019; Sejnowski, 2020). One limitation of deep networks trained by backpropagation is that anything that requires reasoning (like programming or applying the scientific method), long-term planning, and algorithmic data manipulation is out of reach for deep-learning models, no matter how much data you throw at them (Plebe and Grasso, 2019). Deep networks trained by error backpropagation are not a solution to general artificial intelligence (Plebe and Grasso, 2019).

B.13 Deep learning using stochastic gradient descent

The most popular approach in deep learning is a slight modification of backpropagation, in Equation B.121 used for stochastic gradient descent (Plebe and Grasso, 2019), where $\mathbf{w}$ is the vector of all learnable parameters in a network, such as $\mathbf{w}_{i,k}$ in Equation B.119, and $\mathscr{L}\mathbf{x},\mathbf{w}$ a measure of the error of the network with parameters $\mathbf{w}$ when applied to the sample $\mathbf{x}$:

$$\mathbf{w}_{t+1} = \mathbf{w}_t - \eta \nabla_w \frac{1}{M} \sum_i^M \mathscr{L}\left(\mathbf{x}_i, \mathbf{w}_t\right) \tag{B.121}$$

where instead of computing the gradients over a single sample t as in backpropagation (Equation B.120), a stochastic estimation is made over a random subset of size M of the entire dataset, and at each iteration step t a different subset, with the same size, is sampled. This way, the parameters at the next iteration step are determined by the parameters at the previous iteration step adjusted by the mean sampled gradient over M samples. The term 'backpropagation' is now out of fashion, and techniques related to Equation B.121 are referred to as stochastic gradient descent (Plebe and Grasso, 2019).

B.14 Deep convolutional networks

Although not biologically plausible, a class of artificial network that was inspired by neuroscience (Fukushima, 1980, 1988) is the convolution network (LeCun, Kavukcuoglu and Farabet, 2010; LeCun, Bengio and Hinton, 2015; Bengio, Goodfellow and Courville, 2017). This type of network is described here, to compare to biologically plausible networks. A deep convolutional network is a multilayer network that is trained by backpropagation of error and that has convergence from stage to stage.

In more detail, the architecture of a typical convolution network (ConvNet) is structured as a series of stages (LeCun, Bengio and Hinton, 2015). The first few stages are composed of two types of layers: convolutional layers and pooling layers.

Units in a convolutional layer are organized in feature maps, within which each unit is connected to local patches in the feature maps of the previous layer through a set of weights called a filter bank. The result of this local weighted sum is then passed through a non-linearity such as a ReLU (a threshold-linear activation function). All units in a feature map share the same filter bank. To be more specific: the local patch of one layer that connects to a neuron in the next layer may be 3x3 units. Whatever weights are learned by backpropagation are the same for all the units across the layer, and this is achieved artificially, effectively by copying the weights laterally. There may be different feature maps in a layer (e.g. for different colors), and each uses a different filter bank. The reason for this architecture is twofold. First, in array data such as images, local groups of values are often highly correlated, forming distinctive local motifs that are easily detected. Second, the local statistics of images and other signals are invariant to location. In other words, if a motif can appear in one part of the image, it could appear anywhere, hence the idea of units at different locations sharing the same weights and detecting the same pattern in different parts of the array. Mathematically, the filtering operation performed by a feature map is a discrete convolution, hence the name.

Although the role of the convolutional layer is to detect local conjunctions of features from the previous layer, the role of the pooling layer is to merge semantically similar features into one. Because the relative positions of the features forming a motif can vary somewhat, reliably detecting the motif can be done by coarse-graining the position of each feature. A typical pooling unit computes the maximum of a local patch of units in one feature map (or in a few feature maps). To be more specific: a pooling neuron may take the maximum input from a 2 unit x 2 unit patch of units in its input convolution layer. Neighbouring pooling units take input from patches that are shifted by more than one row or column, thereby reducing the dimension of the representation and creating an invariance to small shifts and distortions. The 'stride' may be 2. A convolution net architecture might have these tiny local convolution then pooling of 'max' operator pairs of layers stacked 140 or more on top of one another. Or the architecture might be varied, with several convolution layers before the next pooling layer. At the top of the system, there may be more convolutional and fully-connected pooling layers. To train a ConvNet, stochastic gradient descent is used in conjunction with the gradients computed by backpropagation of error to update the weights to minimize the errors of the output units. The targets for the individual units in the output layer are decided by the experimenter, and might include for one neuron cars, for another neuron bicycles, etc. The whole net is trained with in the order of one million exemplars.

Thus in a convolution network, layers typically alternate, with one layer performing the convolution and filtering followed by a non-linear function such as a threshold linear function (an 'S' layer), and the next layer performing 'pooling' over the neurons in the previous layer (a 'C' layer), to help with transform invariance. The alternation of 'S' and 'C' layers follows the suggestion of Hubel and Wiesel (1962) that complex cells might compute their responses by summing over a set of simple cells. However, there is no evidence for any alternation of S and C layers in most of the primate ventral visual system. The general idea though is that some neurons in the net need to learn to respond to feature combinations, and this is the function of the convolution layer; and the system also needs to do something to cope with transform invariance, and this is done by the max function layers.

The concept of copying weights laterally was used in the Neocognitron (Fukushima, 1980) (Section 2.6.6.2), and has the machine advantages that only one small region is learned, and that the 'filters' or neurons are uniformly good (or bad) throughout a layer. The convolution operator in a convolution network has this effect. This lateral copying is of course biologically implausible, and is not used in VisNet (Chapter 2).

With its powerful backpropagation training algorithm, and very large numbers of training trials, a convolution net can learn to activate the correct output neuron in the output layer for a category of object with good accuracy which may be commercially useful (LeCun, Bengio and Hinton, 2015). However, unlike VisNet, there is no attempt in general to teach the network transform invariance by presenting images with spatial continuity, and no attempt to take advantage of the statistics of the world to help it learn which transforms are probably of the same object by capitalising on temporal continuity. The network is very biologically implausible, in that each unit (or 'neuron') receives from only typically a 3 x 3 or 2 x 2 unit patch of the preceding area (i.e. the receptive fields are small); by using lateral weight copying within a layer; by having up to 140 or more layers stacked on top of each other in the hierarchy; by using the non biologically plausible backpropagation of error training algorithm; and by using a teacher for every neuron in the output layer (Rolls, 2021d; Bowers et al., 2023).

An attempt to compare the operation of such networks to the operation of the ventral visual cortical stream (Yamins and DiCarlo, 2016; Rajalingham, Issa, Bashivan, Kar, Schmidt and DiCarlo, 2018) is evaluated in Section 2.9.4 (Rolls, 2021d).

B.15 Contrastive Hebbian learning: the Boltzmann machine

In a move towards a learning rule that is more local than in backpropagation networks, yet that can solve similar mapping problems in a multilayer architecture, we describe briefly contrastive Hebbian learning. The multilayer architecture has forward connections through the network to the output layer, and a set of matching backprojections from the output layer through each of the hidden layers to the input layer. The forward connection strength between any pair of neurons has the same value as the backward connection strength between the same two neurons, resulting in a symmetric set of forward and backward connection strengths. An input pattern is applied to the multilayer network, and an output is computed using normal feedforward activation processing with neurons with a sigmoid (non-linear and monotonically increasing) activation function. The output firing then via the backprojections is used to create firing of the input neurons. This process is repeated until the firing rates settle down, in an iterative way (which is similar to the settling of the autoassociative nets described in Section B.3). After settling, the correlations between any two neurons are remembered, for this type of unclamped operation, in which the output neurons fire at the rates that the process just described produces. The correlations reflect the normal presynaptic and postsynaptic terms used in the Hebb rule, e.g. $(x_j y_i)^{uc}$, where 'uc' refers to the unclamped condition, and as usual x_j is the firing rate of the input neuron, and y_i is the activity of the receiving neuron. The output neurons are then clamped to their target values, and the iterative process just described is repeated, to produce for every pair of synapses in the network $(x_j y_i)^c$, where the c refers now to the clamped condition. An error correction term for each synapse is then computed from the difference between the remembered correlation of the unclamped and the clamped conditions, to produce a synaptic weight correction term as follows:

$$\delta w_{ij} = k[(x_j y_i)^c - (x_j y_i)^{uc}], \tag{B.122}$$

where k is a learning rate constant. This process is then repeated for each input pattern to output pattern to be learned. The whole process is then repeated many times with all patterns until the output neurons fire similarly in the clamped and unclamped conditions, that is until the errors have become small. Further details are provided by Hinton and Sejnowski (1986). The version described above is the mean field (or deterministic) Boltzmann machine (Peterson and Anderson, 1987; Hinton, 1989). It is sometimes called the '**wake - sleep**' algorithm (Hinton et al., 1995), because when the system is unclamped, with no input, it might be likened to a sleeping or dreaming state. More traditionally, a Boltzmann machine updates one randomly chosen neuron at a time, and each neuron fires with a probability that depends on its activation (Ackley, Hinton and Sejnowski, 1985; Hinton and Sejnowski, 1986). The latter version makes fewer theoretical assumptions, while the former may operate an order of magnitude faster (Hertz, Krogh and Palmer, 1991).

In terms of biological plausibility, it certainly is the case that there are backprojections between adjacent cortical areas (see Chapters 1 and 9). Indeed, there are as many backprojections between adjacent cortical areas as there are forward projections. The backward projections seem to be more diffuse than the forward projections, in that they connect to a wider region of the preceding cortical area than the region that sends the forward projections. If the backward and the forward synapses in such an architecture were Hebb-modifiable, then there is a possibility that the backward connections would be symmetric with the forward connections. Indeed, such a connection scheme would be useful to implement top-down recall, as summarized in Chapter 9 and described by Rolls and Treves (1998) in their Chapter 6. What seems less biologically plausible is that after an unclamped phase of operation, the correlations between all pairs of neurons would be remembered, there would then be a clamped phase of operation with each output neuron clamped to the required rate for that particular input pattern, and then the synapses would be corrected by an error correction rule that would require a comparison of the correlations between the neuronal firing of every pair of neurons in the unclamped and clamped conditions.

Although this algorithm has the disadvantages that it is not very biologically plausible, and does not operate as well as standard backpropagation, it has been made use of by O'Reilly and Munakata (2000) in approaches to connectionist modelling in cognitive neuroscience.

B.16 Deep Belief Networks

Another artificial network is a Deep Belief Network which is a probabilistic model composed of many Restricted Boltzmann Machines (RBMs) stacked on top of each other with each layer trained on the output of the previous one (Hinton et al., 2006). A restricted Boltzmann Machine (in contrast to a traditional Boltzmann Machine) has no lateral connections within layers, and the connectivity is relaxed to be undirected. This results in the units in a particular layer being conditionally independent given a set of observed activations in the other. This is a key difference that allows for the efficient learning and inference within these models. Each subsequent layer acts like constraints on the activities of the one below. This is a greedy training process and will probably not yield an optimum representation for the entire hierarchy, primarily because the individual layers are trained in isolation. (Once a layer is trained the weights are frozen.) This inefficiency however can be remedied by a relatively small amount of fine tuning (generative or discriminative) after the stack is complete (Hinton and Salakhutdinov, 2006). It should be noted that a Deep Belief Network itself is not a deep Restricted Boltzmann Machine. The lower layers do not themselves define an undirected model, and only the top-most two layers keep their undirected nature. However there has been work on modifications that restore the undirected nature of the lower layers allowing inference within the lower layers to make use of top-down connectivity as well as the usual bottom-up connectivity (Salakhutdinov and Larochelle, 2010).

The operation of deep belief networks can be summarized as follows (Plebe and Grasso, 2019). The procedure is to take two adjacent layers in a feedforward network, and train them as Boltzmann Machines. The procedure starts with the input and the first hidden layer, so that it is possible to use the inputs of the dataset to train the unsupervised Boltzmann Machine model. Then, this model is used to generate a new dataset, just by processing all the inputs. This new set is used to train the next couple of layers. This procedure is a sort of pre-training that gives a first shape to all the connections in the network, to be further refined by ordinary backpropagation using both the inputs and the known outputs of the dataset (Plebe and Grasso, 2019).

Deep belief networks do have the advantage, like VisNet, that they are unsupervised, and do not need a teacher for every output neuron to help teach the system how to respond. However, scaling such models to full-sized, high-dimensional images remains a difficult problem. To address this a pooling operation has been tested within a deep belief network, and this can help to form transform-invariant representations (Lee et al., 2011). However, their training algorithm remains very biologically implausible.

B.17 Reinforcement learning

In supervised networks, an error signal is provided for each output neuron in the network, and whenever an input to the network is provided, the error signals specify the magnitude and direction of the error in the output produced by each neuron. These error signals are then used to correct the synaptic weights in the network in such a way that the output errors for each input pattern to be learned gradually diminish over trials (see Sections B.11 and B.12). These networks have an architecture that might be similar to that of the pattern associator shown in Fig. B.1, except that instead of an unconditioned stimulus, there is an error correction signal provided for each output neuron. Such a network trained by an error correcting (or delta) rule is known as a one-layer perceptron. The architecture is not very plausible for most brain regions, in that it is not clear how an individual error signal could be computed for each of thousands of neurons in a network, and fed into each neuron as its error signal and then used in a delta rule synaptic correction (see Section B.11).

The architecture can be generalized to a multilayer feedforward architecture with many layers between the input and output (Rumelhart, Hinton and Williams, 1986a), but the learning is very non-local and rather biologically implausible (see Section B.12), in that an error term (magnitude and direction) for each neuron in the network must be computed from the errors and synaptic weights of all subsequent neurons in the network that any neuron influences, usually on a trial-by-trial basis, by a process known as error backpropagation. Thus although computationally powerful, an issue with perceptrons and multilayer perceptrons that makes them generally biologically implausible for many brain regions is that a separate error signal must be supplied for each output neuron, and that with multilayer perceptrons, computed error backpropagation must occur.

When operating in an environment, usually a simple binary or scalar signal representing success or failure of the whole network or organism is received. This is usually action-dependent feedback that provides a single evaluative measure of the success or failure. Evaluative feedback tells the learner whether or not, and possibly by how much, its behavior has improved; or it provides a measure of the 'goodness' of the behavior. Evaluative feedback does not directly tell the learner what it should have done, and although it may provide an index of the degree (i.e. magnitude) of success, it does not include directional information telling the learner how to change its behavior towards a target, as does error-correction learning (see Barto (1995)). Partly for this reason, there has been some interest in networks that can be taught with such a single reinforcement signal. In this Section (B.17), approaches to such networks are described. It is noted that such networks are classified as reinforcement networks in which there is a single teacher, and that these networks attempt to perform an optimal mapping between an input vector and an output neuron or set of neurons. They thus solve the same class of problems as single layer and multilayer perceptrons. They should be distinguished from pattern-association networks in the brain, which might learn associations between previously neutral stimuli and primary reinforcers such as taste (signals which might be interpreted appropriately by a subsequent part of the brain), but do not attempt to produce arbitrary mappings between an input and an output, using a single reinforcement signal.

A class of problems to which such reinforcement networks might be applied are motor-control problems. It was to such a problem that Barto and Sutton (Barto, 1985; Sutton and Barto, 1981, 2018) applied a reinforcement learning algorithm, the associative reward–penalty algorithm described next. The algorithm can in principle be applied to multilayer networks, and the learning is relatively slow. The algorithm is summarized in Section B.17.1 and by Hertz, Krogh and Palmer (1991). More recent developments in reinforcement learning (see Sections B.17.2 and B.17.3) have been described (Dayan and Abbott, 2001; Sutton and Barto,

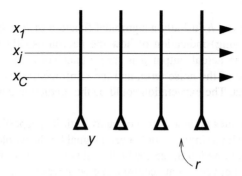

Fig. B.47 A network trained by a single reinforcement input r. The inputs to each neuron are $x_j, j = 1, C$; and y is the output of one of the output neurons.

2018; Collins and Cockburn, 2020; Botvinick, Wang, Dabney, Miller and Kurth-Nelson, 2020).

B.17.1 Associative reward–penalty algorithm of Barto and Sutton

The terminology of Barto and Sutton is followed here (see Barto (1985)).

B.17.1.1 Architecture

The architecture, shown in Fig. B.47, uses a single reinforcement signal, r, = +1 for reward, and –1 for penalty. The inputs x_j take real (continuous) values. The output of a neuron, y, is binary, +1 or –1. The weights on the output neuron are designated w_j.

B.17.1.2 Operation

1. An input vector is applied to the network, and produces activation, h, in the normal way as follows:

$$h = \sum_{j=1}^{C} x_j w_j \tag{B.123}$$

where $\sum_{j=1}^{C}$ indicates that the sum is over the C input axons (or connections) indexed by j to each neuron.

2. The output y is calculated from the activation with a noise term η included. The principle of the network is that if the added noise on a particular trial helps performance, then whatever change it leads to should be incorporated into the synaptic weights, in such a way that the next time that input occurs, the performance is improved.

$$y = \begin{cases} +1 & \text{if } h + \eta \geq 0, \\ -1 & \text{else.} \end{cases} \tag{B.124}$$

where η = the noise added on each trial.

3. Learning rule. The weights are changed as follows:

$$\delta w_j = \begin{cases} \rho(y - \mathrm{E}[y|h])x_j & \text{if } r = +1, \\ \rho\lambda(-y - \mathrm{E}[y|h])x_j & \text{if } r = -1. \end{cases} \tag{B.125}$$

ρ and λ are learning-rate constants. (They are set so that the learning rate is higher when positive reinforcement is received than when negative reinforcement is received.) $\mathrm{E}[y|h]$ is the expectation of y given h (usually a sigmoidal function of h with the range ± 1). $\mathrm{E}[y|h]$ is a (continuously varying) indication of how the neuron usually responds to the current input pattern, i.e. if the actual output y is larger than normally expected, by computing $h = \sum w_j x_j$, because of the noise term, and the reinforcement is +1, increase the weight from x_j; and vice versa. The expectation could be the prediction generated before the noise term is incorporated.

This network combines an associative capacity with its properties of generalization and graceful degradation, with a single 'critic' or error signal for the whole network (Barto, 1985). [The term $y - \mathrm{E}[y|h]$ in Equation B.125 can be thought of as an error for the output of the neuron: it is the difference between what occurred, and what was expected to occur. The synaptic weight is adjusted according to the sign and magnitude of the error of the postsynaptic firing, multiplied by the presynaptic firing, and depending on the reinforcement r received. The rule is similar to a Hebb synaptic modification rule (equation B.2), except that the postsynaptic term is an error instead of the postsynaptic firing rate, and the learning is modulated by the reinforcement.] The network can solve difficult problems (such as balancing a pole by moving a trolley that supports the pole from side to side, as the pole starts to topple). Although described for single-layer networks, the algorithm can be applied to multilayer networks. The learning rate is very slow, for there is a single reinforcement signal on each trial for the whole network, not a separate error signal for each neuron in the network as is the case in a perceptron trained with an error rule (see Section B.11).

This associative reward–penalty reinforcement-learning algorithm is certainly a move towards biological relevance, in that learning with a single reinforcer can be achieved. That single reinforcer might be broadcast throughout the system by a general projection system. It is not clear yet how a biological system might store the expected output $\mathrm{E}[y|h]$ for comparison with the actual output when noise has been added, and might take into account the sign and magnitude of this difference. Nevertheless, this is an interesting algorithm, which is related to the temporal difference reinforcement learning algorithm described in Section B.17.3.

B.17.2 Reward prediction error or delta rule learning, and classical conditioning

In classical or Pavlovian associative learning, a number of different types of association may be learned (Rolls, 2014a; Cardinal, Parkinson, Hall and Everitt, 2002). This type of associative learning may be performed by networks with the general architecture and properties of pattern associators (see Section B.2 and Fig. B.1). However, the time course of the acquisition and extinction of these associations can be expressed concisely by a modified type of learning rule in which an error correction term is used (introduced in Section B.17.1), rather than the postsynaptic firing y itself as in Equation B.2. Use of this modified, error correction, type of learning also enables some of the properties of classical conditioning to be explained (see Dayan and Abbott (2001) for review), and this type of learning is therefore described briefly here. The rule is known in learning theory as the Rescorla–Wagner rule, after Rescorla and Wagner (1972).

The Rescorla–Wagner rule is a version of error correction or delta-rule learning (see Section B.11), and is based on a simple linear prediction of the expected reward value, denoted by v, associated with a stimulus representation x ($x = 1$ if the stimulus is present, and $x = 0$ if the stimulus is absent). The **expected reward value** v is expressed as the input stimulus variable x multiplied by a weight w

$$v = wx. \tag{B.126}$$

The **reward prediction error** is the difference between the expected reward value v and the actual **reward outcome** r obtained, i.e.

$$\Delta = r - v \qquad (B.127)$$

where Δ is the reward prediction error. The value of the weight w is learned by a rule designed to minimize the expected squared error $<(r-v)^2>$ between the actual reward outcome r and the predicted reward value v. The angle brackets indicate an average over the presentations of the stimulus and reward. The delta rule will perform the required type of learning:

$$\delta w = k(r - v)x \qquad (B.128)$$

where δw is the change of synaptic weight, k is a constant that determines the learning rate, and the term $(r-v)$ is the reward prediction error Δ (equivalent to the error in the postsynaptic firing, rather than the postsynaptic firing y itself as in Equation B.2). Application of this rule during conditioning with the stimulus x presented on every trial results in the weight w approaching the asymptotic limit $w = r$ exponentially over trials as the error Δ becomes zero. In extinction, when $r = 0$, the weight (and thus the output of the system) exponentially decays to $w = 0$. This rule thus helps to capture the time course over trials of the acquisition and extinction of conditioning. The rule also helps to account for a number of properties of classical conditioning, including blocking, inhibitory conditioning, and overshadowing (see Dayan and Abbott (2001)).

How this functionality is implemented in the brain is not yet clear. We consider one suggestion (Schultz et al., 1995b; Schultz, 2004, 2006, 2013) after we introduce a further sophistication of reinforcement learning which allows the time course of events within a trial to be taken into account.

B.17.3 Temporal Difference (TD) learning

An important advance in the area of reinforcement learning was the introduction of algorithms that allow for learning to occur when the reinforcement is delayed or received over a number of time steps, and which allow effects within a trial to be taken into account (Sutton and Barto, 1998, 1990, 2018). A solution to these problems is the addition of an adaptive critic that learns through a time difference (TD) algorithm how to predict the future value of the reinforcer. The time difference algorithm takes into account not only the current reinforcement just received, but also a temporally weighted average of errors in predicting future reinforcements. The temporal difference error is the error by which any two temporally adjacent error predictions are inconsistent (see Barto (1995)). The output of the critic is used as an effective reinforcer instead of the instantaneous reinforcement being received (see Sutton and Barto (1998), Sutton and Barto (1990), and Barto (1995)). This is a solution to the temporal credit assignment problem, and enables future rewards to be predicted. Summaries are provided by Doya (1999), Schultz, Dayan and Montague (1997), Dayan and Abbott (2001) and Sutton and Barto (2018). The application of temporal difference learning to invariant object and face recognition is described in Section 2.8.4.3.

In reinforcement learning, a learning agent takes an *action* $\mathbf{u}(t)$ in response to the *state* $\mathbf{x}(t)$ of the environment, which results in the change of the state

$$\mathbf{x}(t+1) = \mathbf{F}(\mathbf{x}(t), \mathbf{u}(t)), \qquad (B.129)$$

and the delivery of the reinforcement signal, or *reward*

$$r(t+1) = \mathbf{R}(\mathbf{x}(t), \mathbf{u}(t)). \qquad (B.130)$$

In the above equations, **x** is a vector representation of inputs x_j, and Equation B.129 indicates that the next state $\mathbf{x}(t+1)$ at time $(t+1)$ is a function F of the state at the previous time step of the inputs and actions at that time step in a closed system. In equation B.130 the reward at the next time step is determined by a reward function R which uses the current sensory inputs and action taken. The time t may refer to time within a trial.

The goal is to find a *policy* function G which maps sensory inputs **x** to actions

$$\mathbf{u}(t) = G(\mathbf{x}(t)) \tag{B.131}$$

which maximizes the cumulative sum of the rewards based on the sensory inputs.

The current action $\mathbf{u}(t)$ affects all future states and accordingly all future rewards. The maximization is realized by the use of the *value function* V of the states to predict, given the sensory inputs **x**, the cumulative sum (possibly discounted as a function of time) of all future rewards $V(\mathbf{x})$ (possibly within a learning trial) as follows:

$$V(\mathbf{x}) = E[r(t+1) + \gamma r(t+2) + \gamma^2 r(t+3) + ...] \tag{B.132}$$

where $r(t)$ is the reward at time t, and $E[\cdot]$ denotes the expected value of the sum of future rewards up to the end of the trial. $0 \leq \gamma \leq 1$ is a discount factor that makes rewards that arrive sooner more important than rewards that arrive later, according to an exponential decay function. (If $\gamma = 1$ there is no discounting.) It is assumed that the presentation of future cues and rewards depends only on the current sensory cues and not the past sensory cues. The right-hand side of Equation B.132 is evaluated for the dynamics in equations B.129–B.131 with the initial condition $\mathbf{x}(t) = \mathbf{x}$. The two basic ingredients in reinforcement learning are the estimation (which we term $\hat{V}$) of the value function V, and then the improvement of the policy or action **u** using the value function (Sutton and Barto, 2018).

The basic algorithm for learning the value function is to minimize the *temporal difference* (TD) *error* $\Delta(t)$ for time t within a trial, and this is computed by a 'critic' for the estimated value predictions $\hat{V}(\mathbf{x}(t))$ at successive time steps as

$$\Delta(t) = [r(t) + \gamma \hat{V}(\mathbf{x}(t))] - \hat{V}(\mathbf{x}(t-1)) \tag{B.133}$$

where $\hat{V}(\mathbf{x}(t)) - \hat{V}(\mathbf{x}(t-1))$ is the difference in the reward value prediction at two successive time steps, giving rise to the terminology temporal difference learning. If we introduce the term $\hat{v}$ as the estimate of the cumulated reward by the end of the trial, we can define it as a function $\hat{V}$ of the current sensory input $\mathbf{x}(t)$, i.e. $\hat{v} = \hat{V}(\mathbf{x})$, and we can also write equation B.133 as

$$\Delta(t) = r(t) + \gamma \hat{v}(t) - \hat{v}(t-1) \tag{B.134}$$

which draws out the fact that it is differences at successive timesteps in the reward value predictions $\hat{v}$ that are used to calculate Δ.

$\Delta(t)$ is used to improve the estimates $\hat{v}(t)$ by the 'critic', and can also be used (by an 'actor') to learn appropriate actions.

For example, when the value function is represented (in the critic) as

$$\hat{V}(\mathbf{x}(t)) = \sum_{j=1}^{n} w_j^C x_j(t) \tag{B.135}$$

the learning algorithm for the (value) weight w_j^C in the critic is given by

$$\delta w_j^C = k_c \Delta(t) x_j(t-1) \tag{B.136}$$

where δw_j^C is the change of synaptic weight, k_c is a constant that determines the learning rate for the sensory input x_j, and $\Delta(t)$ is the Temporal Difference error at time t. Under certain conditions this learning rule will cause the estimate $\hat{v}$ to converge to the true value (Dayan and Sejnowski, 1994).

A simple way of improving the policy of the actor is to take a stochastic action

$$u_i(t) = g(\sum_{j=1}^{n} w_{ij}^A x_j(t) + \mu_i(t)), \tag{B.137}$$

where g() is a scalar version of the policy function G, w_{ij}^A is a weight in the actor, and $\mu_i(t)$ is a noise term. The TD error $\Delta(t)$ as defined in Equation B.133 then signals the unexpected delivery of the reward $r(t)$ or the increase in the state value $\hat{V}(\mathbf{x}(t))$ above expectation, possibly due to the previous choice of action $u_i(t-1)$. The learning algorithm for the action weight w_{ij}^A in the actor is given by

$$\delta w_{ij}^A = k_a \Delta(t)(u_i(t-1) - <u_i>)x_j(t-1), \tag{B.138}$$

where $<u_i>$ is the average level of the action output, and k_a is a learning rate constant in the actor.

Thus, the TD error $\Delta(t)$, which signals the error in the reward prediction at time t, works as the main teaching signal in both learning the value function (implemented in the critic), and the selection of actions (implemented in the actor). The usefulness of a separate critic is that it enables the TD error to be calculated based on the difference in reward value predictions at two successive time steps as shown in Equation B.133.

The algorithm has been applied to modelling the time course of classical conditioning (Sutton and Barto, 1990). The algorithm effectively allows the future reinforcement predicted from past history to influence the responses made, and in this sense allows behavior to be guided not just by immediate reinforcement, but also by 'anticipated' reinforcements. Different types of temporal difference learning are described by Sutton and Barto (2018). An application is to the analysis of decisions when future rewards are discounted with respect to immediate rewards (Dayan and Abbott, 2001; Tanaka et al., 2004). Another application is to the learning of sequences of actions to take within a trial (Suri and Schultz, 1998).

The possibility that dopamine neuron firing may provide an error signal useful in training neuronal systems to predict reward has been discussed in Section 16.4.3. It has been proposed that the firing of the dopamine neurons can be thought of as an error signal about reward prediction, in that the firing occurs in a task when a reward is given, but then moves forward in time within a trial to the time when a stimulus is presented that can be used to predict when the taste reward will be obtained (Schultz et al., 1995b; Schultz, 2013, 2017, 2019) (see Fig. 16.12). The argument is that there is no prediction error when the taste reward is obtained if it has been signalled by a preceding conditioned stimulus, and that is why the dopamine midbrain neurons do not respond at the time of taste reward delivery, but instead, at least during training, to the onset of the conditioned stimulus (Waelti, Dickinson and Schultz, 2001). If a different conditioned stimulus is shown that normally predicts that no taste reward will be given, there is no firing of the dopamine neurons to the onset of that conditioned stimulus.

This hypothesis has been built into models of learning in which the error signal is used to train synaptic connections in dopamine pathway recipient regions (such as presumably the striatum and orbitofrontal cortex) (Houk, Adams and Barto, 1995; Schultz, 2004; Schultz, Dayan and Montague, 1997; Waelti, Dickinson and Schultz, 2001; Dayan and Abbott, 2001; Schultz, 2013, 2016c). Some difficulties with the hypothesis are discussed in Section 16.4.3 on page 688. The difficulties include the fact that dopamine is released in large quantities by aversive stimuli (see Section 16.4.3); that error computations for differences between the expected reward and the actual reward received on a trial are computed in the primate orbitofrontal cortex, where expected reward, actual reward, and error neurons are all found, and lesions of which impair the ability to use changes in reward contingencies to reverse behavior (see Section 11.3.4); that the tonic, sustained, firing of the dopamine neurons in the delay period of a task with probabilistic rewards may reflect reward uncertainty, and not the expected reward, nor the magnitude of the prediction error (see Section 16.4.3 and Shizgal and Arvanitogiannis (2003)); and that reinforcement learning is suited to setting up connections that might be required in fixed tasks such as motor habit or sequence learning, for reinforcement learning algorithms seek to set weights correctly in an 'actor', but are not suited to tasks where rules must be altered flexibly, as in rapid one-trial reversal, for which a very different type of mechanism is described in Section 11.5.3 (Deco and Rolls, 2005d; Rolls and Deco, 2016).

The temporal difference approach to reinforcement learning using an actor-critic approach has a weakness that although it can be used to predict internal signals during reinforcement learning in some tasks, it does not directly address learning with respect to actions that are not taken. Q-learning can be considered as an extension of TD learning which adds additional terms to take into account signals from actions that are not taken, for example information gained by observation of others (Montague, King-Casas and Cohen, 2006). In more detail, action-value-learning models do not learn about the values of states, and instead learn directly about the values of specific actions available within each given state. Thus, the corresponding TD prediction error is computed in accordance with differences in successive predictions about the values of actions as opposed to states. An action-value-learning model such as the Q-learning model may learn more quickly than the actor/critic model (Colas et al., 2017; O'Doherty et al., 2017).

Reinforcement learning models have been used to model in fMRI studies where reward prediction error may be represented in the brain, with one area in which reward prediction error is represented the ventral striatum (Hare et al., 2008; Colas et al., 2017; O'Doherty et al., 2017). A useful toolkit for estimating reward prediction error has been described (Piray et al., 2019) and is available at https://payampiray.github.io/cbm.

Overall, reinforcement learning algorithms are certainly a move towards biological relevance, in that learning with a single reinforcer can be achieved in systems that might learn motor habits or fixed sequences. Whether a single prediction error is broadcast throughout a neural system by a general projection system, such as the dopamine pathways in the brain, which distribute to large parts of the striatum and the prefrontal cortex, remains to be clearly established (see further Chapter 11, Section 16.4.3), though using a modulator of synaptic learning may be computationally useful (Fremaux and Gerstner, 2015).

B.18 Learning in the neocortex

The neocortex builds new representations. This happens in every sensory system, as described in Chapters 2 – 7. The representations might be of new objects, new faces, new voices, new flavors, etc. The representations formed are different from each other; are sparse but distributed; and need to be readable by simple neuronal networks such as pattern association and autoassociation networks. In this section I bring together some of the principles that appear to be involved, building on the principles described in earlier Chapters and models in this book, and in *Cerebral Cortex: Principles of Operation* (Rolls, 2016b).

A canonical circuit for neocortex is shown in Fig. 1.17, with the architectural anatomy and it computational implications discussed in Chapters 1 and 18 of *Cerebral Cortex* (Rolls, 2016b).

A first computational component is competitive learning, as described in Section B.4. This is the key feature, and involves primarily inputs from a preceding cortical area that synapse into pyramidal neurons, as shown in Fig. 1.17. If it is a primary sensory cortical area, the input is likely to come from the thalamus, and may be relayed through stellate cells in the granular layer 4. It is proposed that these inputs to the neocortex reach the thousands of synapses on the superficial pyramidal cells in layers 2 and 3 (L2/3 PC in Fig. 1.17), and form a competitive network (Rolls, 2021c). The synapses are associatively modifiable, and involve some type of long-term synaptic depression which tends to normalize the total synaptic strength from these inputs, as is required for a competitive network. The inhibition needed for the competitive learning is from the local inhibitory neurons, which provide feedback inhibition from the pyramidal cells. The inhibition is over a short range in the order of 2 mm, so that the neurons compete to learn different categories of input within that radius. The degree of inhibition sets the sparseness of the representation.

The competitive learning operates in conjunction with feedforward connectivity from stage to stage of the type illustrated in Fig. 2.2. This, in combination with the feature hierarchy approach described in Section 2.6.6, enables neurons at successive stage of a hierarchy to represent information that involves a convergence of information from preceding cortical areas that may itself involve feature combinations from the preceding cortical area. The multiple layer feature hierarchy approach is an elegant way of combining different types of information to form feature combination neurons that represent quite selective combinations that happen to be present in the environment, without requiring enormous numbers of synaptic connections onto the final categorising neurons. The information combined in this way need not be from a single processing stream. This would result in feature combination neurons, which then represent a category in the world. The information from a cortical area is passed up the hierarchy from the layer 2 and 3 pyramidal cells, as shown in Fig. 1.17 in which they are labelled 'forward to next cortical area L4', although they also synapse heavily onto the superficial pyramidal cells in the next layer. The operation of this hierarchy can be fast, because each cortical area receives inputs from the preceding cortical area on its superficial pyramidal cells, and those pyramidal cell pass their firing directly to the layer 2 and 3 pyramidal cells in the next cortical area in the hierarchy.

The categories learned in a cortical area could be influenced by top-down effects of backprojections from a higher part of the system that when it categorises better has backprojection information that may support the formation of useful categories at the earlier stage, as described in Section B.4.5. These backprojection synapses are shown in Fig. 1.17. These backprojection synapses need to be associatively modifiable in order to implement memory recall, as described in Chapter 9.

If invariant representations are needed, as in transform invariant object recognition, then learning from the statistics in the world over short time periods using trace rule (i.e. slow) learning appears to be a very useful way to assist the formation of the correct feature combination neurons that will respond to different transforms of the same object, as described in Section 2.8. The recurrent collateral connections rc between the superficial pyramidal cells may play an important role in such invariance learning, by operating as an attractor network that keeps the superficial pyramidal cells firing for short period in the order of 100 ms – 1 s to help with the short term memory trace rule learning described in Chapters 2 and 3. To implement such an attractor network, the recurrent collateral connections need to be associatively modifiable (Rolls, 2021c).

Once these category-forming processes involving especially competitive learning and a feedforward hierarchical convergence have resulted in neurons representing new categories, another key feature of neocortical architecture, the recurrent collateral connections between pyramidal cells within a short radius in the order or 2 mm, are likely to become involved.

These do not help in the formation of new categories, but operating as an autoassociation network, as described in Section B.3, will form associations between the features encoded by nearby neurons (Rolls, 2021c) (Fig. 19.1). This means that later on, if some of the usual features are missing, for example the eyes are not visible due to dark glasses, the same object or person representation will become active, because of the completion properties of auto-association networks described in Section B.3. Key evidence that this does occur is that if a stimulus is shown that is ambiguous for a category, perhaps because it is a morph between categories, then the neocortical network will fall into a state where it will represent one of the categories, or another (Akrami, Liu, Treves and Jagadeesh, 2009). This is likely to be useful, not only for taking advantage of the best set of inputs that best represent the category over a population of neurons, but also for the extremely important computation of allowing a short term memory of that category, and keeping it active, for example until another stimulus arrives in the environment to which associations can be learned; or in trace rule slow learning of invariant representations (Rolls, 2021d,c).

The recurrent collaterals between nearby neocortical pyramidal cells may also be useful in building semantic representations in the anterior temporal lobe, as described in Chapter 8.

The layer 5 pyramidal cells (L5 PC in Fig. 1.17) receive inputs from the pyramidal cells in the superficial cortical layers, and are an important source, if not the only source (Markov et al., 2013, 2014a), of the backprojections to layer 1 of the preceding cortical area referred to above. The neurons have their own highly developed recurrent collateral connections, which make operation as some form of attractor network likely (Rolls and Mills, 2017).

The layer 5 pyramidal cells also project to the striatum, which provides an important output of every cortical area, and that may help in the initiation of a single stream of movement and action, as described in Chapter 16. The layer 6 pyramidal cells receive from the layer 5 pyramidal cells, and project to the thalamus, where they may serve a feedback function to control the level of afferent input to each cortical area.

These principles of operation are elucidated and extended throughout this book, and what is in this section (B.18) is just a summary. Further evidence on the operation of cortical circuitry is provided in Rolls (2016b), Singer, Sejnowski and Rakic (2019), Rolls (2021c), and Rolls and Mills (2017).

B.19 Forgetting in cortical associative neural networks, and memory reconsolidation

Forgetting is an important feature of associative neural networks and the brain, and is important in their successful operation. There are a number of different mechanisms for forgetting, and a number of different reasons why forgetting is important in particular classes of network.

Consider attractor, that is autoassociation, networks, which are used for short-term memory, episodic memory, etc. These networks have a critical storage capacity, as described in Section B.3, and if this is exceeded, most of the memories in the network become unretrievable. It is therefore crucial to have a mechanism for forgetting in these networks.

One mechanism is decay of synaptic strength. The simple forgetting mechanism is just an exponential decay of the synaptic value back to its baseline, which may be exponential in time or in the number of learning changes incurred (Nadal, Toulouse, Changeux and Dehaene, 1986). This form of forgetting does not require keeping track of each individual change and preserves linear superposition, that is each memory is added linearly to previous memories, as provided for by Equation B.9 on page 833. In calculating the storage capacity of pattern associators and of autoassociators, the inclusion or exclusion of simple exponential decay does not change significantly the calculation of capacity, and only results in a different prefactor (one 2.7 times the other) for the maximum number of associations that can be stored. Therefore a forgetting mechanism as simple as exponential decay is normally omitted, and one has just to remember that its inclusion would reduce the critical capacity obtained to roughly 0.37 of that without the decay. This type of memory has been called a palimpsest.

Another form of forgetting, which is potentially interesting in terms of biological plausibility, is implemented by setting limits to the range allowed for each synaptic strength or weight (Parisi, 1986). As a particular synapse hits the upper or lower limit on its range, it is taken to be unable to further modify in the direction that would take it beyond the limit. Only after modifications in the opposite direction have taken it away from the limit does the synapse regain its full plasticity. A forgetting scenario of this sort requires a slightly more complicated formal analysis (since it violates linear superposition of different memories), but it effectively results in a progressive, exponential degradation of older memories similar to that produced by straight exponential decay of synaptic weights.

A combined forgetting rule that may be particularly attractive in the context of modelling synapses between pyramidal cells is implemented by setting a lower limit, that is, zero, on the excitatory weight (just requiring that the associated conductance be a non-negative quantity!), and allowing exponential decay of the value of the weight with time. Again, this type of combined forgetting rule places demands on the analytical techniques that have to be used to calculate the storage capacity, but leads to functionally similar effects (Rolls and Treves, 1998).

Two conditions under which synaptic strengths may decrease are described in Fig. 1.6. Heterosynaptic long-term depression, which can occur for inactive presynaptic terminals on active postsynaptic neurons, can be useful computationally in the following ways. First, it is a useful way to subtract the effect of the mean presynaptic firing rate of each neuron in a pattern associator, which removes the effect of the mean firing rate in increasing the correlation between different input patterns used in the network, as is made evident in Equation B.7. This orthogonalizing effect helps to maximize the storage capacity of pattern associators. The same situation applies to autoassociation (attractor) networks (see Equation B.13). This decrease of firing rate for inactive inputs may of course result in some loss of memories previously stored in these association networks, if a particular synapse had been strengthened as part of a previous memory. Homosynaptic long-term depression might contribute to a similar function.

Heterosynaptic long-term depression (LTD) is also useful in competitive networks, for it provides a way for the synaptic weight vectors of different neurons to be kept of approximately equal length, and this is important to ensure that the different categories of input patterns find different output neurons to activate. In the case of competitive networks, the appropriate effect is achieved if the subtractive term in the presynaptic component depends on the existing strength of the synapse, as shown in Equation B.32. The fact that in studies of LTD it is sometimes remarked that LTD is easier to demonstrate after LTP has been induced lends support to the likelihood that LTD of the form indicated in Equation B.32 that depends on the existing synaptic strength is implemented in the brain. Because of the computational significance of LTD that depends on the existing strength of synapses for competitive networks, it would be useful to see further experimental exploration of this.

Forgetting in attractor networks takes two forms that can be clearly distinguished. One is that the current attractor state implemented by the continuing firing of one set of neurons in the network is labile, and may be interrupted by a strong new input which forces the network into a new attractor state, or may be interrupted by quenching effects through non-specific effects implemented through for example inhibitory neurons (Section 11.5.3). Both these effects could be facilitated by synaptic or neuronal adaptation, as described in Section 11.5.3.

The second form of forgetting in attractor networks is of the strengthened synaptic connections that specify each of the different attractor memories in the network. If the network is to be used for large numbers of different short-term memories, then these synaptic weights must decay or be overwritten by LTD as described above. This is likely to be required for short-term memory networks in the prefrontal cortex which must adapt themselves to be capable of storing the particular stimuli and actions that may be required in particular tasks (Rolls, 2016b), in short-term memory networks that implement the visuo-spatial scratchpad, etc. We may note that because short-term memory networks have these two different aspects, once an attractor set of synaptic connections has been imprinted in a network by synaptic modification, then no further synaptic modification is necessary to use that network repeatedly for holding the neurons in one of the stored attractors active to implement the short-term memory in a delay period (Kesner and Rolls, 2001).

Forgetting may be less important in semantic networks. (Semantic networks store structured information with appropriate associative links and hierarchical structure, for example a family tree, or one's geographical knowledge (McClelland and Rumelhart, 1986).) We may note that because any one associative memory network has a memory capacity that is related to the number of associative synapses onto each neuron from other neurons in the network, semantic memory is likely to involve connections between modules in the cortex, where each module might be defined by a 1–3 mm region of cortex with high local connectivity between the neurons. For this type of memory, forgetting is not so much the requirement as incorporating new semantic knowledge, that is making new appropriate links, and perhaps weakening existing links. In this scenario, the fact that when a memory is retrieved, as would occur when a sematic memory is being updated or extended, then it may need to be reconsolidated, suggests a possible useful function for memory reconsolidation (see below), as it could facilitate the restructuring of a semantic memory. In contrast, such restructuring would not be a very useful property of an episodic memory, in which each episode must be clearly distinguished from others.

Reconsolidation refers to a process in which after a memory has been stored, it may be weakened or lost if recall is performed during the presence of a protein synthesis inhibitor (Debiec, LeDoux and Nader, 2002; Debiec, Doyere, Nader and LeDoux, 2006; Haubrich and Nader, 2018). The implication that has been drawn is that whenever a memory is recalled, some reconsolidation process requiring protein synthesis may be needed.

One possible function of reconsolidation is that it may allow some restructuring of a memory, as described above, though this might be useful more in semantic than episodic memory systems.

A second possible computational function is that reconsolidation might be useful as a mechanism to ensure that whenever a memory is retrieved, additional LTP (long-term potentiation of synaptic strength) is not added to the existing LTP. This could be achieved if during the recall process the memory strength is reset to a low value from which it is then strengthened. Indeed, a potential problem with memory systems is what separates storage from recall, in that whenever recall occurs, pre- and post-synaptic activity is present at the relevant synapses for the memory, and thus one might expect another round of synaptic strengthening to occur. Reconsolidation, by effectively resetting the baseline of synaptic strength during recall, might then provide for the restrengthened synapses not to be stronger than they were before the memory recall. A relevant point here is that in associative memories, the amount of information stored and retrieved from any one synapse is quite low, in the order of 0.2–0.3 bits for autoassociators (Rolls and Treves, 1998; Treves and Rolls, 1991) and a little higher for pattern associators (Rolls and Treves, 1998), so that in any case having synaptic strengths that could be repeatedly strengthened by superposition of different memories with distributed representations and with precision maintained at each strengthening would not appear to be a necessary property of the synapses in such memory systems. Under these circumstances, allowing during recall a weakening of a memory, and then its reconsolidation from a relatively fixed baseline might not lead to loss of useful information, and might be a possible solution to continually strengthening synapses every time a memory is recalled.

A third possible computational function of reconsolidation is that it could enable the selective retention of 'useful' memories (or in fact memories being used), and the forgetting of memories not being used, as follows. Consider a memory system in which there is slow exponential decay of synaptic strength with time, a not altogether unlikely scenario given the properties of a biological system. In this situation memories will gradually be lost, perhaps with a different time course in different memory systems, which might be in the order of days, weeks, months or years. In this scenario, if a piece of information was actually recalled because an environmental situation occurred in which for example there was a retrieval cue for a memory, then that memory (i.e. the synaptic strengths) would by reconsolidation be strengthened back to near its initial value. That memory would then be strong and available for future use, compared to other memories not recalled that would be passively decaying. The passive decay of memories not being recalled and reset by reconsolidation would be useful in cleaning out the memory stores so that any critical capacity was not reached, and at the same time in minimizing interference (due to generalization to similar patterns) between memories in store. An example might be the number of one's hotel room, which while it is being repeatedly recalled for use while in that hotel and thus restored, would then decay passively and gradually be lost when it was not longer being actively recalled and hence reconsolidated. One could propose that in some memory systems the passive decay might be relatively rapid, occurring within hours or days. An example might be the dorsolateral prefrontal cortex, where depending on the requirements of the short-term memory or planning tasks being performed, synapses might by reconsolidation keep representations used in attractor networks available while a given task was being performed. However, when that task was no longer being performed, passive synaptic decay would mean that neurons allocated to that task would gradually decline, and instead new attractor landscapes (i.e. memories) could be set up for new tasks or planning, without interference from representations that were previously being used. There is some evidence at the phenomenological level that neuronal representations are made and kept relevant to whatever task is being performed (Miller et al., 2003; Everling et al., 2006), and I have just proposed a possible mechanism for this implemented by reconsolidation.

Memories stored early in life may be stored better, and later recalled better, than those stored later in life. There are a number of possible reasons for this. One is that the transmitters that generally facilitate synaptic modification, such as acetylcholine and noradrenaline (see Section 18.6.4), may become depleted with ageing.

Another mechanism, not necessarily independent, is that new synaptic modification, as assessed by long-term potentiation (LTP), appears to be less long-lasting with ageing (Burke and Barnes, 2006; Barnes, 2011). Another mechanism may be that storing memories in a flat energy landscape (i.e. without much prior synaptic modification) may help these memories to stand out from those added later. While this would not be a natural property of the type of autoassociation palimpsest memory described above, it could be a property of the way in which an episodic memory stored in the hippocampus may be retrieved into the neocortex where it can be incorporated into a semantic memory (see Chapter 9), the relevant example of which in this case would be an autobiographical memory.

In semantic memories, it could be that the first stored links tend to provide the framework around which other information is structured.

Another factor in the apparent strength of early memories may be that some may be stored with an affective component, and this may not only make the memory strong by activation of the cholinergic and related systems described in Section 18.6.4, but may also mean that part at least of the memory is stored in different brain structures such as the amygdala which may have relatively more persistent and less flexible or reversible memories than other memory systems.

Another factor in the importance and stability of synaptic modification early in life arises in perceptual systems, in which it is important to allow neurons to become tuned to the statistics of for example the visual environment, but once feature analyzers have been formed, stability of the feature analyzers in early cortical processing layers may be important so that later stages in the hierarchy can perform reliable object recognition which achieves stability only if the input filters to the system do not keep changing (see Chapter 2). This could be the importance of a critical period for learning early on in perceptual development.

Sleep has been proposed as a state in which useful forgetting or consolidation of memories could occur. One suggestion was that if deep basins of attraction formed in a memory network, then this could impair performance, as the memories in the basins would tend to be recalled whatever the retrieval cue. If noise, present in the disorganized patterns of neural firing during sleep, caused these memories to be recalled, this would indicate that they were 'parasitic', and the suggestion was that associative synaptic weakening (LTD) of synapses of neurons with high firing during sleep would tend to decrease the depth of those basins of attraction, and improve the performance of the memory (Crick and Mitchison, 1995). At least at the formal level of neural networks, the suggestion does have some merit as a possible way to 'clean up' associative networks, even if it is not a process implemented in the brain. Although the idea of some role of sleep in memory remains active, this remains to be fully established (Walker and Stickgold, 2006), and indeed there is evidence that quiet waking may be relevant rather than sleep per se (Dastgheib et al., 2022). That would fit much better with my theory of memory consolidation which proposes that recall from the hippocampus to the neocortex and active reorganization of the information during waking to organize it in relation to existing semantic information may be much more relevant (Rolls, 2022b) (Section 9.2.8.5).

The idea that sleep could be a time when memories are unloaded from the hippocampus to be consolidated in long term, possibly semantic, memories during sleep (Marr, 1971) (allowing hippocampal episodic memories to then be overwritten by new episodic memories) continues to be explored. (David Marr heard this considered in a lecture at Cambridge by Larry Weiskrantz in 1967.) It has been shown for example that after hippocampal spatial representations have been altered by experience during the day, these changes are reflected in 'replay' neuronal activity in the neocortex during sleep (Wilson and McNaughton, 1993; Wilson, 2002; Chen and Wilson, 2017; Foster, 2017). The type of experience might involve repeated locomotion between two places, and the place fields of rat hippocampal neurons for those places may become associated with each other because of coactivity of the neurons representing the frequently visited places. The altered co-firing of the hippocampal neurons for those places may then be reflected in neocortical representations of those places. This could then result in altered representations in the neocortex, if LTP occurs during sleep in the neocortex. Of course, any change in neocortical neuronal activity might just reflect the altered representations in the hippocampus, which would be expected to influence the neocortical representations via hippocampo-neocortical backprojections, even without any neocortical learning (see Chapter 9). However, the evidence that sleep is critically involved in memory consolidation, and even that replay is involved in memory consolidation, is now receiving critical re-evaluation, for replay can occur in waking, and may represent trajectories never taken by the animal (Findlay, Tononi and Cirelli, 2020).

In conclusion, we have seen in this Section that forgetting has important functions in the cortex, and is a necessary property of many different types of memory system if they are to continue to function efficiently and to allow new learning in the same networks in the brain. This is especially likely to apply to the episodic memory system implemented in the hippocampus, because there is a single network in CA3 (Chapter 9). In semantic memories in the anterior temporal lobe, the challenge is more to incorporate new information to update previous representations, rather than to over-write them (see Chapter 8).

B.20 Genes and self-organization build neural networks in the cortex

B.20.1 Introduction

Analysis of the structure and function of different cortical areas is starting to reveal how the operation of networks of neurons may implement the functions of each cortical area. The question then arises as part of understanding cortical and indeed brain function of how the networks found in different cortical and brain areas actually have evolved, and how their basic architecture may be specified by genes and then built using self-organisation and environmental input during development.

To address these fundamental issues, I compared the architecture and networks found in different brain areas, and in particular how they differ from each other, to formulate hypotheses about a set of parameters that may be specified by genes that could lead to the building during development of the neuronal network functional architectures found in different cortical regions (Rolls and Stringer, 2000). The choice of parameters was guided not only by comparison of the functional architecture of different brain regions, but also by what parameters, if specified by genes, could with a reasonably small set of genes actually build the networks found in different brain regions. The concept is that if these parameters are specified by different genes, then genetic reproduction and natural selection using these parameters could lead to the evolution of neuronal networks in our brains well adapted for different functions.

A second aim is to show how the sufficiency of the general approach, and the appropriateness of the particular parameters selected, can be tested and investigated using genetic algorithms which actually use the hypothesised genes to specify networks. We showed this by implementing a genetic algorithm, and testing whether it can search the high dimensional space provided by the suggested parameters to specify and build neuronal networks that will solve particular computational problems (Rolls and Stringer, 2000).

A third aim could be, if we start to understand how genes and self-organisation build networks in the brain using a set of biologically plausible components, to provide a foundation for building artificial neural networks with again relatively few 'genes', but with genes now able to specify much more powerful computer architectures than those found in the brain.

The computational problems we choose to test are simple and well defined problems that can be solved by one-layer networks, and that as shown in this book capture some of the architectural properties of different cortical areas, and are some of the building blocks of cortical function (Rolls and Stringer, 2000). These problems are pattern association, autoassociation, and unsupervised categorization as can be performed by a competitive network, which require quite different architectures for them to be solved (see Chapter 1 including Fig. 1.7 and earlier parts if this Appendix B).

Because the problems to be solved are well specified, we can define a good fitness measure for the operation of each class of network, which will be used to guide the evolution by reproduction involving genetic variation and selection in each generation. Although we do not suppose that the actual parameters chosen for illustration are necessarily those specified by mammalian genes, they have been chosen because they seem reasonable given the differences in the functional architecture of different brain areas, and allow illustration of the overall concept about how different network architectures found in different brain regions evolve.

Although these computational problems to be solved were chosen to have well understood one-layer neural network solutions, now that this general approach has been established (Rolls and Stringer, 2000), it will be of great interest in future to examine problems that are solved by multilayer networks in the brain (e.g. invariant object recognition (Chapter 2) and episodic memory (Chapter 9), in order to understand how brain mechanisms to solve complex problems may evolve and how they may operate.

The first example of the networks to be investigated was pattern association networks in which one input (e.g. an unconditioned stimulus) drives the output neurons through unmodifiable synapses, and a second input (e.g. a conditioned stimulus) has associatively modifiable synapses onto the output neurons, so that by associative learning it can come to produce the same output as the unconditioned stimulus (Section B.2). Pattern association memory may be implemented in structures such as the amygdala and orbitofrontal cortex to implement stimulus-reward. Pattern association learning may also be used in the connections of back-projecting neurons in the cerebral cortex onto the apical dendrites of neurons in the preceding cortical area to implement memory recall.

A second example is autoassociation networks characterized by recurrent collateral axons with associatively modifiable synapses (Section B.3), which may implement functions such as short term memory in the cerebral cortex, and episodic memory in the hippocampus.

A third example is competitive learning (Section B.4), where there is one major set of inputs to a network connected with associatively modifiable synapses, and mutual (e.g. lateral) inhibition between the output neurons (through e.g. inhibitory feedback neurons). Competitive networks can be used to build feature analyzers by learning to respond to clusters of inputs which tend to co-occur, and may be fundamental building blocks of perceptual systems. Allowing short range excitatory connections between neurons (as in the cerebral cortex) and longer range inhibitory connections can lead to the formation of topographic maps where the closeness in the map reflects the similarity between the inputs being mapped.

B.20.2 Hypotheses about the genes that could build different types of neuronal network in different brain areas

The hypotheses for the genes that might specify the different types of neuronal network in different brain areas are now introduced. The hypotheses are based on knowledge of the architectures of different brain regions, which are described in Chapter 1 and in sources such as the following (Shepherd, 2004; Shepherd and Grillner, 2010; Braitenberg and Schüz, 1991, 1998; Peters and Jones, 1984; Somogyi et al., 1998; Harris and Mrsic-Flogel, 2013; Kubota, 2014; Harris and Shepherd, 2015; Shepherd and Rowe, 2017), and on a knowledge of some of the parameters that influence the operation of neuronal networks. These genes were used in the simulations in which evolution of the architectures was explored using genetic algorithms. The emphasis in this section is on the rationale for suggesting different genes. A more formal specification of the genes, together with additional information on how they were implemented in the simulations, is provided in Section B.20.4.2. It may also be noted that large numbers of genes will be needed to specify for example the operation of a neuron. This Section focusses on those genes that, given the basic building blocks of neurons, may specify the differences in the functional architecture of different regions of the cerebral cortex.

The overall concept is as follows. There are far too few genes (in humans 20,000–25,000 protein coding genes (Human Genome Sequencing, 2004)) to specify each synapse (i.e. which neuron is connected to which other neuron, and with what connection strength) in the brain. (The number of synapses in the human brain, with 10^{10} - 10^{11} neurons in the brain, and perhaps an average of 10,000 synapses each, is in the order of 10^{14} - 10^{15}). In any case, brain design is likely to be more flexible if the actual strength of each synapse is set up by self-organisation and experience. On the other hand, brain connectivity is far from random.

In more detail, a key constraint for building the cortex is that this has to be performed with relatively few genes for each cortical or brain region. Given that humans have fewer than 25,000 genes (with perhaps a further 5000 non-protein-coding regulators (Espinos et al., 2022) that are likely to be important in humans (Zwir et al., 2022)), it is unlikely that more than 20% of the 25,000 (say 5000) are used to specify brain connectivity. If there are 180 cortical regions that can be identified in one hemisphere (in the HCP-MMP atlas (Glasser et al., 2016a; Huang et al., 2022)), then taking that number of 180, assuming that the other hemisphere uses many of the same genes, and the rest of the brain, might require say 250 brain regions to be specified. That might mean only 20 genes for specifying the specific connectivity of a brain region that makes it different from other brain regions. That type of argument leads to the hypothesis that the genes may specify to define one brain region as being different from another a few classes of neuron for each brain region that would have as specifiers what classes of other neurons they should connect to in the input and outputs regions of each brain region (Rolls and Stringer, 2000). This type of argument guided the hypotheses about what was being specified by genes to provide a basis on which self-organisation could build useful connectivity of individual networks in the brain, and also the whole brain. This is a key aspect of what is implied by the title of this book: *Brain Computations and Connectivity*: it is a fundamental part of understanding the brain to understand how its connectivity is built. Of course many more genes may be needed to specify each brain region, but those genes could be common among many brain regions. What is sought here are the specifiers that may define what is different about the connectivity of each brain region. Even though the actual hypotheses described so far for what these genes specify may develop over time, the overall approach taken here to how brains may be built by genes and self-organisation is what is important.

Some indications about what is specified can be gathered by considering the connectivity of the hippocampus (Chapter 9). The CA3 pyramidal cells each receive approximately 50 mossy fibre synapses from dentate granule cells, 12,000 synapses from other CA3 cells formed from recurrent collaterals, and 3,600 perforant path synapses originating from entorhinal cortex neurons (see Fig. 9.23). In the preceding stage, the 1,000,000 dentate granule cells (the numbers given are for the rat) receive one main source of input, from the entorhinal cortex, and each makes approximately 14 synapses with CA3 cells.

Specification of neuron classes, and of connection rules between classes

On the basis of considerations of this type for many different brain areas, it is postulated that for each class of cell the genome specifies the approximate numbers of synapses the class will receive from a specified other class (including itself, for recurrent collaterals), and the approximate number of synapses its axons will make onto specified classes of target cells (including itself). The individual neurons with which synapses are made are not specified, but are chosen randomly, though sometimes under a constraint (specified by another gene) about how far away the axon should travel in order to make connections with other neurons. One parameter value of the latter gene might specify the widespread recurrent collateral system of the CA3 neurons (Chapter 9). Another value for the latter might specify much more limited spread of recurrent collaterals with the overall density decreasing rapidly from the cell of origin, which, as in the neocortex and if accompanied by longer range inhibitory processes implemented by feedback inhibitory neurons, would produce center-surround organisation, and tend to lead to the formation of topological maps (see Section B.4.6) and to local attractor networks.

The actual mechanism by which this specification of connection rules between classes of neuron is implemented would presumably involve some (genetically specified) chemical recognition process, together with the production of a limited quantity of a trophic substance that would limit the number of synapses from, and made to, each other class of cell. Consistent with this fundamental hypothesis, gene knockout investigations show that for example different genes specify the NMDA receptors in the cell classes: dentate gyrus, CA3, and CA1 (Nakazawa et al., 2002, 2003, 2004; Huerta et al., 2000). Genetic specifiers for connectivity in the neocortex are being considered (Schmidt and Polleux, 2021).

Some of these processes would of course be occurring primarily during development (ontogenesis), when simple rules such as making local connections as a function of distance away would be adequate to specify the connectivity, without the need for long pathway connection routes (such as between the substantia nigra and the striatum) to be genetically encoded. It is presumably because of the complex genetic specification that would be required to specify in the adult brain the route to reach all target neurons that epigenetic factors are so important in embryological development, and that as a general rule the formation of new neurons is not allowed in adult mammalian brains apart from in the hippocampal dentate gyrus (Section 9.3.6.6) (Rolls, 2016b).

It is a feature of brain neuronal network design that not only is which class of neuron to connect to apparently specified, but also approximately where on the dendrite the connections from each other class of neuron should be received. For example, in the CA3 system, the mossy fibres synapse closest to the cell body (where they can have a strong influence on the cell), the CA3 recurrent collaterals synapse on the next part of the dendrite, and the entorhinal inputs synapse on the more distal ends of the dendrites. The effect of the proximal relative to the more distal synapses will depend on a number of factors, including for distal inputs whether proximal inputs are active and thereby operating as current shunts producing division, and on the diameter of the dendrite, which will set its cable properties (Koch, 1999). If the dendritic cable diameter is specified as large, all inputs (including distal inputs) will sum reasonably linearly to inject current into the cell body.

Although inhibitory neurons have not been included in the examples already given, similar specifications would be applicable, including for example a simple specification of the different parts of the dendrite on which different classes of inhibitory neuron synapse (Kubota, 2014), and hence whether the effect is subtractive or shunting (Koch, 1999). In cortical areas, both feedforward and feedback inhibition (the latter from pyramidal cells via inhibitory neurons back to the same population of pyramidal cells) could be produced by a simple genetic specification of this type.

Specification of synaptic learning rules

Next, the nature of the synaptic connections, and the learning rule for synaptic modifiability, must be specified. One gene specifies in the simulation described later whether a given neuron class is excitatory or inhibitory. In the brain, this gene (or genes) would specify the transmitter (or transmitters in some cases) that are released, with the actual effects of for example glutamate being excitatory, and gamma-amino-butyric acid (GABA) inhibitory. The learning rule implemented at each synapse is determined by another gene (or genes). One possible effect specified is no synaptic modification. Another is a Hebb rule of associative synaptic plasticity (increase the synaptic strength if both presynaptic and postsynaptic activity are high, the simple rule implemented by associative long-term potentiation (LTP)). For this, the genes might specify NMDA (n-methyl-d-aspartate) receptors on the post-synaptic neurons together with the linked intracellular processes that implement LTP (Bliss and Collingridge, 2013; Takeuchi et al., 2014; Bliss and Collingridge, 2019; Moser et al., 2021) (Section 1.6). Another possible effect is long-term depression (LTD). This may be heterosynaptic, that is the synaptic weight may be decreased if there is high post-synaptic activity but low presynaptic activity. Part of the utility of this in the brain is that when combined with LTP in pattern associators and autoassociators the effect is to remove the otherwise positive correlation that would be produced between different input patterns if all patterns are specified by positive-only firing rates, as they are in the brain. The effect of removing this correlation is to reduce interference between patterns, and to maximize the storage capacity (see earlier in this Appendix B). A further useful property of heterosynaptic LTD is that it can help to maintain the total synaptic strength onto a neuron constant, by decreasing synaptic strengths from inputs to a neuron which are inactive when the neuron is currently firing. This can be very useful in competitive networks to prevent some winning neurons from continually increasing their synaptic strength so that they win to all patterns, and can in addition be seen as part of the process by which the synaptic weight vector is moved to point in the direction of a current input pattern of neuronal activity (see Section B.4). Another type of LTD is homosynaptic, in which the synaptic strength decreases if there is high presynaptic activity but low or moderate postsynaptic activity. This might be useful in autoassociative synaptic networks, as combined with LTP and heterosynaptic LTD it can produce a covariance-like learning rule.

Another learning rule of potential biological importance is a trace learning rule, in which for example the post-synaptic term is a short term average in an associative Hebb-like learning rule. This encourages neurons to respond to the current stimulus in the same way as they did to previous stimuli. This is useful if the previous stimuli are different views etc of the same object (which they tend statistically to be in our visual world), because this promotes invariant responses to different versions of the same object. Use of such a rule has been proposed to be one way in which networks can learn invariant responses (Rolls, 2012d, 2021d) (Chapter 2). Such a trace could be implemented in real neurons by a number of different mechanisms, including slow unbinding of glutamate from the NMDA receptor (which may take 100 ms or more), and maintaining a trace of previous neuronal activity by using short term autoassociative attractor memories implemented by recurrent collaterals in the cerebral neocortex (Rolls and Treves, 1998) (Section 1.14.5 and Chapter 13).

Other types of synaptic modification that may be genetically specified include non-associative LTP (as may be implemented by the hippocampal mossy fibre synapses), and non-associative LTD. Other genes working with these may set parameters such as the rapidity with which synapses learn (which in a structure such as the hippocampus may be very fast, in one trial, to implement memory of a particular episode, and in structures such as the basal ganglia may be slow to enable the learning of motor habits based on very many trials of experience); and the initial and maximal values of synapses (e.g. the mossy fibre synapses onto hippocampal CA3 cells can achieve high values).

Specification of the operation of neurons

Another set of genes specifies some of the biophysical parameters that control the operation of individual neurons (see Koch (1999) for background). One gene (in a simulation, or biologically perhaps several) specifies how the activation h_i of a neuron i is calculated. A linear sum of the inputs r'_j weighted by the synaptic weights w_{ij} is the standard one used in most models of biologically plausible neuronal networks (Section 19.4), and those simulated here, as follows:

$$h_i = \sum_j r'_j w_{ij} \qquad (B.139)$$

where $\sum_j$ indicates that the sum is over the C input axons (or connections) indexed by j. An alternative is that there is non-linearity in this process, produced for example by local interactions in dendrites, including local shunting, affected most notably by the cable diameter of the dendrite, which is what such genes may control. For most pyramidal cells, the dendrite diameter is sufficiently large that linear summation to produce the net current injected into the cell bodies is a reasonable approximation (Koch, 1999).

Several further genes set the activation function of the neuron. (The activation function is the relation between the activation of the neuron and its firing. Examples are shown in Fig. 1.3). One possibility is linear. A second, and the most biologically plausible, is to have a threshold, followed by a part of the curve where the firing rate increases approximately linearly with the activation, followed by a part of the curve where the firing rate gradually saturates to a maximum. This function can be captured by for example a sigmoid activation function as follows:

$$r_i = \frac{1}{1+e^{-2\beta(h_i-\alpha)}} \qquad (B.140)$$

where α and β are the sigmoid threshold and slope, respectively. The output of this function, also sometimes known as the logistic function, is 0 for an input of $-\infty$, 0.5 for h_i equal to α, and 1 for $+\infty$. For this type of activation function, at least two genes would be needed (and biologically there would probably be several to specify the biophysical parameters), one to control the threshold, and a second to control the slope. A third possibility is to have a binary threshold, producing a neuron which moves from zero activity below threshold to maximal firing above threshold. This activation function is sometimes used in mathematical modelling because of its analytic tractability.

One variable that is controlled by the threshold (and to some extent the slope) of the activation function is the proportion of neurons in a population that are likely to be firing for any one input. This is the population sparseness of the representation. If the neurons have a binary activation function, the population sparseness may be measured just by the proportion of active neurons, and takes the value 0.5 for a fully distributed representation, in which half of the neurons are active. For neurons with continuous activation functions, the population sparseness a may be defined as

$$a = \frac{(\sum_i r_i/N)^2}{\sum_i r_i^2/N} \qquad (B.141)$$

where N is the number of neurons in the population and r_i is the rate of the ith neuron in the population (Appendix B). This works also for binary neurons. To provide precise control of the sparseness in some of the simulations described below we made provision for this to be controlled as an option directly by one gene, rather than being determined indirectly by the threshold and slope gene-specified parameters of the sigmoid activation function shown in Eq. B.140.

B.20.3 Genetic selection of neuronal network parameters to produce different network architectures with different functions

Given the proposals just described for the types of parameter that are determined by different genes, we describe next how gene selection is postulated to lead to the evolution of neuronal networks adapted for particular (computational) functions. The description is phrased in terms of simulations of the processes using genetic algorithms, as investigations of this type enable the processes to be studied precisely. The processes involve reproduction, ontogenesis

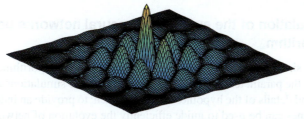

Fig. B.48 A landscape with a broadly unimodal space but with many local optima that is susceptible to genetic search to find the top of the highest peak.

followed by tests of how well the offspring can learn to solve particular problems, and natural selection.

First, a selection of genes is made for a set of G genotypes in a population, which should be of a certain minimum size for evolution to work correctly. The genes are set out on a chromosome (or chromosomes). (Effects of gene linkage on a chromosome are not considered here.) Each set of genes is a genotype. The selection of individual genotypes from which to breed is made a probabilistic function which increases with the fitness of the genotype, measured by a fitness function that is quantified by how well that genotype builds an individual that can solve the computational problem that is set.

Having chosen two genotypes in this way, two genotypes to specify two new (haploid) offspring for the next generation are made by the genetic processes of sexual reproduction involving both gene recombination and mutation, which occur with specified probabilities. This process is repeated until G genotypes have been produced. Then G individuals are built with the network architectures specified by the G genotypes. The fitness of these individuals is then measured by how well they perform at the computational problem set.

In order to solve the computational problem, the networks are trained by presenting the set of input patterns, and adjusting the synaptic weights in the network according to the learning rules specified by the genotype of that individual. The individuals then breed again with a probability of being selected for reproduction that is proportional to their fitness relative to that of the whole population.

This process is allowed to proceed for many generations, during which the fitness of the best individual in the population, and the average fitness, both increase if evolution is working.

This type of genetic process is an efficient method of searching through a high dimensional space (the space specified by the genes), particularly where the space has many local optima so that simple hill climbing is inefficient, and where there is a single measure of fitness (Holland, 1975; Ackley, 1987; Goldberg, 1989). An example of such a landscape is shown in two dimensions in Fig. B.48. The sexual reproduction by allowing recombination of genes facilitates local hill-climbing in such a landscape. However, once the top of the local hill is reached, the process may become stuck at the top of the hill. Mutations have the effect of allowing a random jump to another part of the space, where the local hill-climbing can begin all over again. The combination of sexual reproduction and occasional mutations is an efficient way to find the top of the highest hill in the landscape, and this is part of the mathematical basis for how evolution works by using natural selection operating on changes made using both sexual reproduction and occasional mutations.

An additional useful feature of genetic search is that past gene combinations, useful possibly in other contexts, can remain in the population for a number of generations, and can then be reused later on, without the need to search for those gene combinations again. This re-use of past combinations is one of the features of genetic search that can make it powerful, rapid, and show sudden jumps forward.

B.20.4 Simulation of the evolution of neural networks using a genetic algorithm

Next I describe simulations of these processes using a genetic algorithm, in order to make explicit some of the parameters hypothesized. The aims of the simulations are to demonstrate the feasibility and details of the hypotheses and approach; to provide an indication of whether the proposed genes can be used to guide efficiently the evolution of networks that can solve computational problems of the type solved by the brain; and to provide a tool for investigating in more detail both the parameters that can best and biologically plausibly be genetically specified to define neural networks in the brain, and more complicated multilayer networks that operate to solve computationally difficult problems such as episodic memory or invariant visual object recognition. The proposals were tested to determine whether three different types of one-layer network with different architectures appropriate for solving different computational problems evolve depending on the computational problem set (Rolls and Stringer, 2000). The problems were those appropriate for the pattern associator, autoassociator, and competitive networks shown schematically in Fig. 1.7.

B.20.4.1 The neural networks

The neural networks considered have a number of classes of neuron. Within a class, a gene allows the number of neurons to vary from 1 up to N. For the simulations described here, N was set to 100. Within a class, the genetic specification of a neuron is homogeneous, with the neurons for that class having, for example, identical activation functions and connectivity probabilities. The number of classes will depend on the individual task, e.g. pattern association, autoassociation, competitive nets, etc, which can be described as one-layer networks, with one layer of computing elements between the input and output (see Fig. 1.7). However, in our simulations there is typically an input layer where patterns are presented, and an output layer where the performance of the network is tested. For the simulations described, the number of classes was set to allow one-layer networks such as these to be built, but the number of layers that could be formed is in principle under genetic control, and indeed multilayer networks can be formed if there is a sufficient number of classes of neuron. Regarding the implementation of inter-layer connection topologies, the neurons in individual layers exist in a circular arrangement, and connections to a cell in one layer are derived from a topologically related region of the preceding layer. Connections to individual neurons may then be established according to either a uniform or Gaussian probability distribution centered on the topologically corresponding location in the sending layer.

On discrete time steps each neuron i calculates a weighted sum of its inputs as shown in Equation B.139. This is in principle the subject of genetic modification (see below), but the gene specifying this was set for the simulations described here to this type of calculation of the neuronal activation. Next the neuronal firing r_i is calculated, using for example the standard sigmoid function shown in Equation B.140 and allowing α and β the sigmoid threshold and slope to evolve genetically. Next, there is an optional procedure that can be specified by the experimenter to be called to set the sparseness of the firing rates r_i of a class of neuron according to Equation B.141, with a being allowed to evolve. This specification is used in the simulations, but in the cortex in this and other similar cases a number of genes would specify factors that influence this, such as in this case the strength of the feedback inhibition implemented by inhibitory neurons. After the neuronal outputs r_i have been calculated, the synaptic weights w_{ij} are updated according to one of a number of different learning rules, which are capable of implementing for example both long term potentiation (LTP) and long term depression (LTD), as described below, and which are genetically selected. For example, the standard Hebb rule takes the form

$$\Delta w_{ij} = k r_i r'_j, \tag{B.142}$$

where r'_j is the presynaptic firing rate and k is the learning rate.

B.20.4.2 The specification of the genes

The genes that specify the architecture and operation of the network are described next. In principle, each gene evolves genetically, but for particular runs, particular genes can be set to specified values to allow investigation of how other genes are selected when there are particular constraints.

Each neural network architecture is described by a genotype consisting of a single chromosome of the following form

$$\text{chromosome} = \begin{bmatrix} \mathbf{c}_1 \\ \mathbf{c}_2 \\ \vdots \\ \mathbf{c}_n \end{bmatrix} \tag{B.143}$$

where $\mathbf{c}_l$ is a vector containing the genes specifying the properties of neurons in class l, and n is the total number of classes that is set manually at the beginning of a run of the simulation. The vectors $\mathbf{c}_l$ take the form

$$\mathbf{c}_l = \begin{bmatrix} \mathbf{g}_l \\ \mathbf{h}_{l1} \\ \mathbf{h}_{l2} \\ \vdots \\ \mathbf{h}_{ln} \end{bmatrix} \tag{B.144}$$

where the vector $\mathbf{g}_l$ contains the *intra*-class properties for class l, and the vectors $\mathbf{h}_{lm}$ contain the *inter*-class connection properties to class l from class m where m is in the range 1 to n.

The vector of intra-class properties takes the form

$$\mathbf{g}_l = \begin{bmatrix} b_l \\ \alpha_l \\ \beta_l \\ a_l \end{bmatrix} \tag{B.145}$$

where we have the following definitions for intra-class genes.

(1) b_l is the number of neurons in class l. b_l is an integer bounded between 2 and N, which was set to 100 for the simulations described here. Individual classes are restricted to contain more than one neuron since a key strategy we have adopted for enhancing the biological plausibility is to evolve classes composed of a number of neurons with homogeneous genetic specifications rather than to specify genetically the properties of individual single neurons.

(2) α_l is the threshold of the sigmoid transfer function in Equation B.140 for class l. α_l is a real number bounded within the interval [0.0,200.0].

(3) β_l is the slope of the sigmoid transfer function in Equation B.140 for class l. β_l is a real number bounded within the interval [0.0,200.0]. We note that low values of the slope will effectively specify a nearly linear activation function, whereas high values of the slope specify a nearly binary activation function (see Fig. 1.3).

(4) a_l is the sparseness of firing rates within class l as defined by Equation B.141. By definition a_l is a real number bounded within the interval [0.0,1.0]. However, in practice we ensure a minimum firing sparseness by setting a_l to lie within the interval [$1.0/b_l$,1.0], where b_l is the number of neurons in class l. With binary neurons with output r equal to either 0 or 1, setting $a_l \geq 1.0/b_l$ ensures that at least one neuron is firing. For the simulations described in this Chapter, when this gene was being used, a was set to 0.5 and produced a binary firing rate distribution with a sparseness of 0.5 unless otherwise specified. The alternative way of calculating the firing rates was to allow genes α and β specifying the sigmoid activation function to evolve.

The vectors of inter-class connection genes specify the connections to class l from class m, and take the form

$$\mathbf{h}_{lm} = \begin{bmatrix} r_{lm} \\ s_{lm} \\ c_{lm} \\ e_{lm} \\ z_{lm} \\ t_{lm} \\ p_{lm} \\ \sigma_{lm} \\ q_{lm} \\ f_{lm} \\ k_{lm} \\ d_{lm} \\ u_{lm} \\ v_{lm} \end{bmatrix} \quad (B.146)$$

where we have the following definitions for inter-class genes.

(1) r_{lm} controls the inter-layer connection topology in that it helps to govern which neurons in class m make connections with individual neurons in class l. The exact definition of r_{lm} depends on the type of probability distribution used to make the connections, which is governed by the gene s_{lm} described below. For $s_{lm} = 0$, connections are established according to a uniform distribution, and r_{lm} specifies the number of neurons within the spatial region from which connections may be made. For $s_{lm} = 1$, connections are established according to a Gaussian distribution, where r_{lm} specifies the standard deviation of the distribution. For the Gaussian distribution, individual connections originate with 68% probability from within a region of 1 standard deviation away. These real valued variates are then rounded to their nearest integer values. As noted in section B.20.2, connection topologies are characteristically different for different connection types such as CA3 recurrent collateral connections, which are widespread, and intra-module connections in the cerebral cortex. This parameter may also be set by genetic search to enable the region of effect of inhibitory feedback neurons to be just greater than the region within which excitatory neurons receive their input; and to enable topographic maps to be built by arranging for the lateral excitatory connections to operate within a smaller range than inhibitory connections. This parameter may also be set to enable multilayer networks to be built with feedforward connectivity which is from a small region of the preceding layer, but which over many layers allows an output neuron to receive from any part of the input space, as happens in many sensory systems in which topology is gradually lost and as is implemented in a model of the operation of the visual cortical areas (Chapter 2). For the simulations described here, this gene was set to 100 to allow global con-

nectivity, and thus to not specify local connectivity.

(2) s_{lm} specifies for the region gene r_{lm} the connection probability distribution to class l from class m. s_{lm} takes the following values.

- $s_{lm} = 0$: Connections are established according to a uniform probability distribution within the region r_{lm}.
- $s_{lm} = 1$: Connections are established according to a Gaussian probability distribution. r_{lm} specifies the size of the region from which there is a 68% probability of individual connections originating.

In the experiments described here, the values of s were set to 0.

(3) c_{lm} is the number of connections each neuron in class l receives from neurons in class m. c_{lm} takes integer values from 0 to b_m (the number of neurons within class m). These connections are made probabilistically, selecting for each class l of neuron c_{lm} connections from class m. The probabilistic connections are selected either from a uniform probability distribution (as used here), or according to a Gaussian probability distribution. In both cases the local spatial connectivity within the two classes l and m is specified by the region parameter gene r_{lm}.

(4) e_{lm} specifies whether synapses to class l from class m are excitatory or inhibitory. e_{lm} takes the following values.

- $e_{lm} = 0$: Connections are inhibitory
- $e_{lm} = 1$: Connections are excitatory

For inhibitory connections with $e=0$, the weights in Equation (B.139) are scaled by -1, and no learning is allowed to take place.

(5) z_{lm} specifies whether connections from class m to class l are additive or divisive. z_{lm} takes the following values.

- $z_{lm} = 0$: Connections are divisive
- $z_{lm} = 1$: Connections are additive

  This gene selects whether the neuronal activation h_i is calculated according to linear summation of the input firing rates r'_j weighted by the synaptic strengths w_{ij}, as specified by Eq. B.139, and as used throughout by setting $z_{lm} = 1$; or whether with $z_{lm} = 0$ there is local computation on a dendrite including perhaps local summation of excitatory inputs and shunting effects produced by inhibitory inputs or inputs close to the cell body. The most important physical property of a neuron that would implement the effects of this gene would be the diameter of the dendrite (see Section B.20.2 and (Koch, 1999)). If set so that $z_{lm} = 0$ for local multiplicative and divisive effects to operate, it would be reasonable and in principle straightforward to extend the genome to include genes which specify where on the dendrite with respect to the cell body synapses are made from class m to class l neurons, the cable properties of the dendrite, etc.

(6) t_{lm} specifies how the synaptic weights to class l from class m are initialised at the start of a simulation. t_{lm} takes the following values.

- $t_{lm} = 0$: Synaptic weights are set to zero. This might be optimal for the conditioned stimulus inputs for a pattern associator, or the recurrent collateral connections in an autoassociator, for then existing connections would not produce interference in the synaptic

connections being generated during the associative learning. This would produce a non-operating network if used in a competitive network, for an input could not produce any output.
- $t_{lm} = 1$: Synaptic weights are set to a uniform deviate in the interval [0,1] scaled by the constant value encoded on the genome as q_{lm} (described below).
- $t_{lm} = 2$: Synaptic weights are set to the constant value encoded on the genome as q_{lm} (described below). This could be useful in an associative network if a learning rule that allowed synaptic weights to decrease as well as increase was specified genetically, because this would potentially allow correlations between the input patterns due to positive-only firing rates to be removed, yet prevent the synapses from hitting the floor of zero, which could lose information (Rolls and Treves, 1998).
- $t_{lm} = 3$: Synaptic weights are set to a Gaussian function of distance x away from the afferent neuron in class l. This function takes the form

$$f(x) = \frac{1}{\sigma\sqrt{2\Pi}} e^{-x^2/2\sigma^2}$$

where σ is the standard deviation. This would be an alternative way to implement local spatial connectivity effects to those implemented by r_{lm}.

(7) p_{lm} is the scale factor used for synaptic weight initialisation with a Gaussian distribution (i.e. for $t_{lm} = 3$). p_{lm} is a real number bounded within the interval [0.0,100.0].

(8) σ_{lm} is the standard deviation used for synaptic weight initialisation with a Gaussian distribution (i.e. for $t_{lm} = 3$). σ_{lm} is a real number bounded within the interval [0.001,10.0]. σ_{lm} is restricted to be greater than 0.001 to avoid a singularity that would occur in the Gaussian function for $\sigma_{lm} = 0.0$.

(9) q_{lm} is the scale factor used for synaptic weight initialisation for $t_{lm} = 1$ and $t_{lm} = 2$ (see above). q_{lm} is a real number bounded within the interval [0.0,100.0]. If t_{lm} is 1 or 2, q_{lm} would be expected to be small for pattern associators and autoassociators (as described above).

(10) f_{lm} specifies which learning rule is used to update weights at synapses to class l from class m. f_{lm} takes the following values.
- $f_{lm} = 0$: Learning rule 0 (no learning) $\Delta w_{ij} = 0$.
- $f_{lm} = 1$: Learning rule 1 (Hebb rule) $\Delta w_{ij} = kr_i r'_j$.
- $f_{lm} = 2$: Learning rule 2 (modified Hebb rule) $\Delta w_{ij} = kr_i(r'_j - <r'_j>)$ where $<.>$ indicates an average value. In this rule LTP is incorporated with heterosynaptic LTD set to keep the average weight unchanged. Use of this rule can help to remove the correlations between the input patterns produced by positive-only firing rates (Rolls and Treves, 1998). If this rule is selected, it will work best if the synaptic weight initialisation selected genetically is not zero (to allow the weights to decrease without hitting a floor), and is optimally a constant (so that noise is not added to the synaptic weights which implement the association).
- $f_{lm} = 3$: Learning rule 3 (modified Hebb rule) $\Delta w_{ij} = kr_i(r'_j - w_{ij})$. This rule has the effect of helping to maintain the sum of the synaptic weights on a neuron approximately constant, and is therefore helpful in competitive networks (Rolls and Treves, 1998). This rule accords with the neurophysiological observation that it is easier to demonstrate LTD after LTP has been produced.
- $f_{lm} = 4$: Learning rule 4 (covariance rule) $\Delta w_{ij} = k(r_i - <r_i>)(r'_j - <r'_j>)$.

- $f_{lm} = 5$: Learning rule 5 (homosynaptic LTD with LTP) $\Delta w_{ij} = k(r_i - <r_i>)r'_j$.
- $f_{lm} = 6$: Learning rule 6 (non-associative LTP) $\Delta w_{ij} = kr'_j$. This rule may be implemented in the hippocampal mossy fibre synapses.
- $f_{lm} = 7$: Learning rule 7 (non-associative LTD) $\Delta w_{ij} = -kr'_j$.
- $f_{lm} = 8$: Learning rule 8 (trace learning rule) $\Delta w_{ij} = k\bar{r}_i^\tau r'^\tau_j$ where the trace $\bar{r}_i^\tau$ is updated according to

$$\bar{r}_i^\tau = (1-\eta)r_i^\tau + \eta\bar{r}_i^{\tau-1} \tag{B.147}$$

and we have the following definitions: $\bar{r}_i^\tau$ is the trace value of the output of the neuron at time step τ, and η is a trace parameter which determines the time or number of presentations of exemplars of stimuli over which the trace decays exponentially. The optimal value of η varies with the presentation sequence length. Further details, and a hypothesis about how this type of learning rule could contribute to the learning of invariant representations, are provided in Chapter 2. For the simulations described by Rolls and Stringer (2000), this learning rule was disabled.

(11) k_{lm} is the learning rate k for synaptic weights to class l from class m. k_{lm} is a real number bounded within the interval $[0.0, 10.0]$.

(12) d_{lm} is the maximum size allowed for the absolute value of synaptic weight updates from class m to class l. d_{lm} is a real number bounded within the interval $[0.0, 10.0]$.

(13) u_{lm} is the maximum size allowed for synaptic weights to class l from class m. u_{lm} is a real number bounded within the interval $[-100.0, 100.0]$.

(14) v_{lm} is the minimum size allowed for synaptic weights to class l from class m. v_{lm} is a real number bounded within the interval $[-100.0, 100.0]$.

Implementation details are that v is bounded to be less than u; and that during initialisation of the synaptic weights, v and u are applied after the other initialisation parameters have operated.

B.20.4.3 The genetic algorithm, and general procedure

The genetic algorithm used was a conventional one described by Goldberg (1989). Each individual genotype was a haploid chromosome of the type just defined. The values for the genes in the initial chromosome were chosen at random from the possible values. (In this simulation, if a value in the genotype was one of a large number of possible values, then a single integer or real-valued gene was used, whereas in the brain we would expect several genes to be used, with perhaps each of the several genes coding for different parts of the range with different precision. For example, c_{lm}, the number of synaptic connections to a neuron in class l from a neuron in class m, is to be chosen from 2 to 100 in the simulation, and uses a single integer. In the brain, where we might expect the number of connections per neuron to vary in the range 5 to 50,000, one possible scenario is that 5 different genes would be used, coding for the values 5, 50, 500, 5,000 and 50,000. We would thus expect that the number of genes required to specify the part of the genotype described here would increase by a factor in the order of 5 in the brain.)

There was a set number of genotypes (and hence individuals) per generation, which was 100 for the simulations described. (Too small a number reduces the amount of diversity in the population sufficiently to lead to poor performance of the genetic evolution.) From each genotype an individual network was constructed, with all connections being chosen probabilistically within the values specified by the genotype, and with a uniform probability distribution (i.e. s_{lm} was set to 0 for the simulations described), and the initial values for the synapses were also chosen as proscribed by the genotype. That individual was then tested on the computation being studied, e.g. pattern association, and the fitness (performance) of the network was measured. The actual testing involved presenting the set of patterns to be learned (as specified below for each network) to the network while allowing learning to occur, and then testing the performance of the network by presenting the same, similar, or incomplete test patterns and measuring the output of the network. The fitness measure used for each class of network is defined below. This process was repeated until a fitness measure had been obtained for each of the genotypes.

The next generation of genotypes was then bred by reproduction from the previous genotypes. Two genotypes were selected for reproduction with a probability that was proportional to their fitness relative to the sum of the fitnesses of all individuals in that generation. That is, the probability P_i of an individual i being selected is given by

$$P_i = \frac{F_i}{\sum_j F_j} \qquad (B.148)$$

where F_j is the fitness of an individual genotype j, and the sum $\sum_j F_j$ is over all individuals in the population. The genotypes were then bred to produce two offspring genotypes using the processes of recombination and mutation. The probability of recombination was set to 0.4 (so that it occurred with a 40% chance for every breeding pair in every generation), and the probability of mutation of each gene was set to 0.05. The computational background to this is that recombination allows a non-linear search of a high dimensional space in which gene complexes or combinations may be important, allowing local performance hills in the space to be detected, and performance once in a local hill to improve. Mutation on the other hand enables occasional moves to be tried to other parts of the space, usually with poorer performance, but occasionally moving a genotype away from a well explored location to a new area to explore. Both processes enable the search to be much more efficient in a high dimensional space with multiple performance hills or mountains than with simple gradient ascent, which will climb the first hill found, and become stuck there (Ackley, 1987; Goldberg, 1989). The recombination took place with respect to a random point on the chromosome each time it occurred. The mutation also took place at a random place on the chromosome each time it occurred, and the single gene being mutated was altered to a new random value within the range specified for that gene.

This reproduction process was repeated until sufficient individual genotypes for the next generation (100 unless otherwise stated) had been produced. The fitness of those genotypes was then measured by building and testing the networks they specified as previously outlined. Then the whole reproduction, ontogenesis, and testing to measure fitness, processes were repeated for many generations, to determine whether the fitness would increase, and if so, what solutions were found for the successful networks.

B.20.4.4 Pattern association networks

The operation of the system simulated is described briefly for the three networks, emphasizing the generic points. Details of the simulations and the explorations with them are described by Rolls and Stringer (2000).

The computational problem set was to associate pairs of random binary patterns of 1s and 0s with sparseness of 0.5 (i.e. with half the elements 0 and the other half 1s), an appropriate problem for a pattern association net (Appendix B). There were 10 pattern pairs, which places

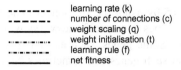
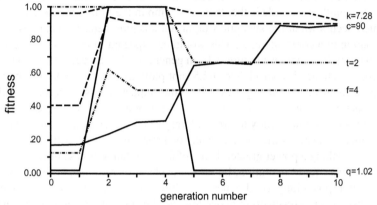

Fig. B.49 Fitness of the best genotype in the pattern association task as a function of the number of generations, together with the values of selected genes. The simulation is performed with the firing rates assigned binary values of 0 or 1 according to the neuronal activations, with the proportion of neurons firing set by the firing rate sparsity gene a. The parameters shown all refer to connections from class 1 (the input neurons) to class 2 (the output neurons). The final values of the parameters are shown at the end of each plot. For example, the genetic algorithm set the number of connections onto each output neuron as 90, a relatively high number (the maximum was 100), which results in a high memory capacity, which was what the fitness function was set to optimize. (After Rolls, E. T. and Stringer, S. M. 2000. On the design of neural networks in the brain by genetic evolution. Prog Neurobiol 61: 557-579.)

a reasonable load on the network (Rolls and Treves, 1998) (Section B.2). There were two classes of neuron. One of the patterns of the pair, the unconditioned stimulus, was set during learning to activate the 100 output neurons (class 2) during learning, while the other pattern of the pair, the conditioned stimulus, was provided by the firing of 100 input neurons (class 1). The fitness measure was obtained by providing each conditioned stimulus (or a fraction of it), and measuring the correlation of the output vector of firing rates, r_i where $i = 1$ to 100, with that which was presented as the unconditioned stimulus during learning. This correlation measure ranges from 1.0 for perfect recall to 0.0 (obtained for example if the output of the pattern associator is 0). The fitness measure that was used in most runs was the square of this correlation (used to increase the selectivity of the fitness function). (In practice, a pattern associator with associatively modifiable synapses, random patterns, and the sizes and loading of the networks used here can achieve a maximum correlation of approximately 1.000.) It may be noted that the genetics could form connections onto individual neurons of any number (up to $N = 100$, the number of input and output neurons in the network) and type between classes 1 to 2 (feedforward connections), and 2 to 2 (recurrent collaterals), 2 to 1, and 1 to 1. For the simulations performed, the operation of inhibitory feedback neurons was not explicitly studied, although when using the sigmoid activation function the neurons had to select a threshold (by altering α_l).

The values of the fitness measures for a typical run of the simulations are shown in Fig. B.49, along with the values of specific genes. The genes shown are key connection properties from class 1 to class 2, and are: learning rate k_{21}, number of connections c_{21}, weight scaling q_{21}, weight initialisation option t_{21}, and the learning rule f_{21}. The fitness measure is the fitness of the best genotype in the population, and for this run the sparseness of the output representation was set to the value of 0.5 by using the sparseness gene set to this value. It is shown that evolution to produce genotypes that specify networks with high performance occurred over a number of generations. Some genes, such as that specifying the learning rule, settled down early, and changes in such genes can sometimes be seen to be reflected in jumps in the fitness measure. An example in Fig. B.49 is the learning rule, which settled down (for the best genotype) by generation 3 to a value of 4 which selects the covariance learning rule. Another example is that there is a jump in the fitness measure from generation 4 to 5 which occurs when the synaptic weight initialisation gene t_{21} changes from a Gaussian distribution to a constant value. This would be expected to increase the performance in these simulations. The increase in fitness from generation 7 to 8 occurred when the minimum weight gene v_{21} changed from 11.6 to -62.5 (not plotted), which would also be expected to increase performance. For other genes, where the impact is less or zero, the values of the genes can fluctuate throughout evolution, because they are not under selection pressure, in that they do not contribute greatly to fitness. Every run of the simulation eventually produced networks with perfect performance. The selection pressure (relative to other genotypes) could be increased by taking a power greater than 1 of the correlation fitness measure. A high value could produce very rapid evolution, but at the expense of minimising diversity early on in evolution so that potentially good genes were lost from the population, with then a longer time being taken later to reach optimal performance because of the need to rely on mutations. Low values resulted in slow evolution. In practice, raising the correlation fitness measure to a power of 1 (no change) or 2 produced the best evolution.

The best networks all had close to 100 excitatory feedforward connections (gene c_{21}) to each class 2 (output) neuron from the class 1 (input) neurons, which is the minimal number necessary for optimal performance of a fully loaded pattern associator and the maximum number allowed. Moreover, the excitatory feed forward connections for all the successful networks were specified as associative, and in particular f_{21} was selected for these networks as 2 or 4. distributions to achieve optimal results in a pattern associator.

To help understand in full detail the actual gene selections found by the genetic algorithm in the simulations, we were able to simulate the pattern associator with manually selected gene combinations for the feedforward connections from class 1 to class 2. In particular, we calculated the network fitnesses for particular combinations of learning rule f_{21}, weight initialisation option t_{21}, and weight scaling q_{21}. This optional facility of the simulator allowed systematic investigation of the effects of one gene, which could be held fixed at a particular value, on the values of the other genes selected during evolution. Examples of the usefulness of this approach are described by Rolls and Stringer (2000).

B.20.4.5 Autoassociative networks

The computational problem set was to learn random binary pattern vectors (of 1s and 0s with sparseness of 0.5, i.e. with half the elements 0 and the other half 1s), and then to recall the whole pattern when only half of it was presented. This is called completion, and is an appropriate test for an autoassociator (Section B.3). An additional criterion, inherent in the way the simulation was run, was to perform retrieval by using iterated processing in an attractor-like state of steady memory retrieval like that of continuing neuronal firing in a short-term memory (Section B.3).

Most runs of the simulation produced networks with optimal performance. The best networks all had close to 100 excitatory recurrent collateral feedback connections from the output neurons (class 1) to themselves, which is the minimal number necessary for optimal performance of a fully loaded autoassociator given that there are 100 output neurons and that this is the maximum number allowed. The successful networks also had all evolved to use either the covariance or the heterosynaptic LTD learning rule (Rolls and Stringer, 2000), which are necessary for good performance of the autoassociation network (Section B.3).

B.20.4.6 Competitive networks

The computational problem set was to learn to place into separate categories 20 binary pattern vectors each 100 elements long. First, 5 exemplar patterns were randomly generated with 50 1s and 50 0s. Then, for each exemplar, 3 further patterns were created by mutating 20 of the bits from 0 to 1 or 1 to 0. This gave a total of 20 patterns that could be placed in 5 similarity categories. There were two classes of neuron. Class 1 was the input class, consisted of 100 neurons, and was set to fire according to which input pattern was being presented. Class 2 was the output class. Connections were possible from class 1 to 2, from class 1 to 1, from class 2 to 1, and from class 2 to 2. The network shown in Fig. B.15, if trained with learning rule 3 and given a powerful and widespread lateral inhibition scheme can solve this problem (Section B.4). The fitness measure used assessed how well the competitive net was able to classify the 20 patterns into their respective 5 categories.

The simulation runs typically converged to use learning rules 2 or 3, although learning rule 3 appeared to offer the best performance. Learning rule 3 involves LTP, plus LTD proportional to the existing value of the synaptic weight. This is the only rule which actually encourages the synaptic weight vectors of the different output (class 2) neurons to have a similar and limited total value. Use of a learning rule such as this (or explicit normalization of the length of the synaptic weight vector of each neuron), is advantageous in competitive networks, because it prevents any one neuron from learning to respond to all the input patterns (Section B.4). The fact that this learning rule was never chosen by the successful genotypes in the associative nets, but was generally chosen for the competitive nets, is evidence that the genetic evolution was leading to appropriate architectures for different computational problems. Learning rule 0 (no learning) was never chosen by the successful genotypes, and in addition we verified that good solutions to the problem set could not be produced without learning.

Another characteristic of the successful genotypes was that there appeared to be less selection pressure on c_{21} the number of connections to a class 2 from a class 1 neuron, with some highly fit nets having relatively low values for c_{21}. Such diluted connectivity can be useful in competitive networks, because it helps to ensure that different input patterns activate different output neurons (Section B.4) (Rolls, 2016f,b). Low values were never chosen for the best genotypes in the associative networks, where full connectivity is advantageous for full capacity.

B.20.5 Evaluation of the gene-based evolution of single-layer networks

The simulations described by Rolls and Stringer (2000) showed that the overall conception of using genes which control processes of the type described can, when combinations are searched through using genetic evolution utilising a single performance measure, lead to the specification of neural networks that can solve different computational problems, each of which requires a different functional architecture.

The actual genes hypothesized were based on a comparison of the functional neuronal network architectures of many mammalian brain regions, and were well able to specify the architectures described here. However, the research described is intended as a foundation for further exploration of exactly which genes are used biologically to specify real architectures in the mammalian brain which perform particular computations. We note in this context that it may be the case that exhaustive analysis of the genetic specification of an invertebrate with a small number of neurons does not reveal the principles involved in building complex nervous systems and networks of the type addressed here. The genetic specification for simple nervous systems could be considerably different, with much more genetic specification of the properties of particular synapses to produce a particular more fixed network in terms both of which identified neuron is connected to which, and what the value of the synaptic connection strength between each neuron is. In contrast, in the approach taken here, there are not identifiable particular neurons with particular connections to other identifiable neurons, but instead a specification of the general statistics of the connectivity, with large numbers of neurons connecting according to general rules, and the performance of the network being greatly influenced by learning of the appropriate values of the connection strengths between neurons based on the co-activity of neurons, and the nature of the modifiable synaptic connection between them.

The particular hypotheses about the genes that could specify the functional architecture of simple networks in the brain were shown by the work described here to be sufficient to specify some different neuronal network architectures for use in a system that builds computationally useful architectures using a gene selection process based on fitness. The genes hypothesized may be taken as a guide to the types of genes that could be used to specify the functional architecture of real biological nervous systems, but the gene specification postulated and simulated can be simply revised based on empirical discoveries about the real genes. One choice made here was to specify the genes with respect to the receiving neuron. The reason for this, rather than specification with respect to the sending neuron, was that many of the controlling properties of the network architecture and performance are in the post-synaptic neuron. Examples of these properties include the type of post-synaptic receptor (e.g. NMDA receptors to specify associatively modifiable connections), and the cable properties of the postsynaptic neuron. The specification of the receiving neuron does include the appropriate information about the sending neuron, in that for example gene c_{lm} does specify (by identifier m) the identity of the sending population. This implies that when a neuron makes an output connection (through its synapses), the neuron class of the sending neuron is available (as a chemical recognition identifier) at the synaptic terminal. However, in principle, in terms of actually building a network, it would be possible to have the genetic specifiers listed as being properties of the sending neuron.

Another aspect of the gene specifiers hypothesized here is that there was no gene for how many output connections a class of neurons should make to another class. One reason for this is that the networks can be built numerically without such a specifier, as it is unnecessary if the total numbers of neurons of two classes is specified, and the number of connections received by one class of neuron from the other is specified. However, the number of output connections made to another class of neuron might be specified in real biological systems, and neuron numbers might adjust to reflect this type of constraint, which is a possible way to think about cell death during development. If there is local output connectivity within a certain spatial range, this will also act as a factor that determines the number of output connections made by neurons, and indeed this does seem a possible gene in real biological systems. Indeed, in real systems the single gene specifying the region of connectivity (r_{lm}) here might be replaced by different spatial genes specifying the extent of the dendrites of the receiving neuron, and extent of the axonal arborization for the outputs.

It is emphasized that a number of the genes specified here for the simulations might be replaced in real biological systems with several genes operating at a lower level, or in more detail, to implement the function proposed for each gene specified here. The reason for selecting the particular genes hypothesized here is that they serve as a guide to how in principle neuronal networks could be specified genetically in complex neural systems where the functional architecture is being selected for by genetic evolution. Specification of genes as operating at the level described here provides a useful heuristic for investigation by simulation of how evolution may operate to produce neuronal networks with particular computational properties. Once the processes have been investigated and understood with genes operating at the level described here, subsequent investigations that use genes that are more and more biologically accurate and detailed would be facilitated and are envisaged. The approach allows continual updating of the genotype used in the simulations to help understand the implications of new discoveries in neurobiology.

The number of genes used in simulations of the type described here is now considered, remembering that biologically several genes might be required to specify at least some of the genes used in the simulations. The number of genes for each class of neuron in the simulations was 4 + (the number of classes of neuron from which the class receives connections × 14). In the brain, if there were on average five classes of neuron from which each class of neuron received connections, this would result in 4 + 5 × 14 = 74 genes per class of neuron. If there were on average five classes of neuron per network, this would yield 370 genes per network. 100 such networks would require 37,000 genes, though in practice fewer might be needed, as some parameters might be assigned to be the same for many classes of neuron in different networks. For example, the overall functional architecture of the cerebral neocortex appears to follow the same general design for different architectonic areas (Braitenberg and Schüz, 1991; Peters and Jones, 1984; Somogyi et al., 1998; Douglas et al., 2004; Pandya et al., 2015), so much of the neocortex may use one generic network specification, with a few genes used to tweak the parameters for each different architectonic area. (An extension of the idea presented here would allow such a generic specification of the architecture of an area of the cerebral neocortex, and then allow genes to connect different areas with the same generic though locally tweaked architecture.) A factor working in the opposite direction is the fact that a single gene taking an integer or real value was used to specify some of the parameters in the simulation, whereas biologically several genes might be needed to represent such a wide range of parameter values with low, though sufficient, precision as described in Section B.20.4.3.

Although with 100 individuals per generation, and approximately 64 genes for each genotype (for networks with 2 classes of genes, each connected to each other as well as to themselves) each with several at least possible values, the search might be predicted to be long, in practice the genetic search was often quite short. Part of the reason for this is that some genes made a crucial difference, for example the gene specifying the learning rule, and were selected early on in evolution, usually being present in at least some of the genotypes in the initial population. Because these genes had such a dramatic effect on fitness, they were almost always selected for the next generation, and successive generations then had to search the smaller space of the remaining genes only some of which had a substantial impact on performance. Some genes, such at that specifying the learning rule, do indeed often settle down early, and changes in these genes can sometimes be seen to be reflected in jumps in the fitness measure. For other genes, where the impact is less or zero, the values of the genes can fluctuate throughout evolution, because they are not under selection pressure, in that they do not contribute greatly to fitness.

Although therefore in some senses the actual evolution investigated here takes place rapidly and apparently quite easily, this is part of the point of this research, that is to demonstrate that the particular genes identified as those which might allow the networks to be found in different brain areas to be built, and implemented in the simulations, can actually build these networks, and moreover can do so efficiently when using genetic search. However, the networks tested by Rolls and Stringer (2000) are single layer networks, and multilayer networks, with correspondingly more parameter combinations to be explored, will doubtless take longer to evolve in future simulations. Genetic search of the parameter space should then become even more evident as a good procedure, because of its power in searching high dimensional spaces with many local optima and in which the parameters combine non-linearly; because of its use of a single measure of performance; and because of its ability to reuse genetic codes still present in a diverse population but originally developed for a different purpose. The intention however here is to specify the principles involved. Of course, there are many more details of the networks that could be explored by the existing gene specification, including inhibitory interneurons. Simulations of this type will not only enable the evolution and development of more complex multilayer networks to be explored, but will also enable the utility of the specification of different parameters by different genes to be explored, including details of where inputs end on dendrites, dendritic biophysical properties, and thus eventually networks that operate to simulate also the dynamics of the operation of real neural networks in the brain (Treves, 1993; Battaglia and Treves, 1998a; Panzeri et al., 2001; Rolls and Deco, 2010) (Section B.6).

B.20.6 The gene-based evolution of multi-layer cortical systems

We followed up these advances by simulating a two-layer network which was intended to show next how a two-layer network might evolve by the mathematical processes implemented by genetics. The system we chose was the dentate granule cells followed by the CA3 network. We used a cost function that was intended to capture the theoretical utility of the dentate granule cells acting as an orthogonalizing process to perform pattern separation to increase the storage capacity of the CA3 when correlated patterns were presented to the system (Chapter 9).

The results were disappointing. It seemed difficult for the fitness function to optimize the architecture of both the layers simultaneously. Perhaps the minima in this landscape were so dependent on what was happening in each of the layers that a solution was very difficult.

This leads me to the following new hypotheses. One hypothesis is that because of the complexity of the solution landscape being optimized by the fitness function and genetic variation and selection, a mechanism that may be used in evolution (with full generality to the whole process of evolution by neo-Darwinian mechanisms) is to allow one subsystem to evolve, fix its parameters, and then allow the next subsystem in the hierarchy to evolve, then fix this, and so on. In the context of cortical processing, the proposal is that the first cortical area (sometimes referred to here as layer in the network of cortical areas) in the system would evolve, and then become fixed, allowing little further variation, and providing stable inputs for the next layer to evolve to do what it can with the outputs of the preceding layer. This would be repeated for layer after layer in the hierarchy. The process would be efficient, in the sense that genetic evolution would need to search only one layer of the system at a time for a useful advance, measured by an increase in fitness. This would greatly simplify the exploration of high dimensional spaces being performed by genetic evolution. In this evolutionary process, each new added layer (i.e. cortical area) would have a useful function, implemented by the outputs taken from layers 5 and 6 of every cortical area to the basal ganglia, cerebellum, thalamus etc., thus providing a potential advantage for each new added cortical area.

This hypothesis raises the important question of how gene-based evolution would be switched on for an early layer of the system, but then switched off so that the next layer in the hierarchy could evolve later in evolutionary history. One possibility is that genes that have already built early layers of the system or hierarchy show less variation in terms of mutation and recombination, perhaps because of where they are located on a chromosome.

In the context of the brain, a related process may be that after an early layer in a cortical hierarchy has self-organized during development, learning in that cortical layer may be switched off, by switching off its synaptic plasticity, to leave a stable base for the next layer to learn. Consistent with this, there is plasticity in the primary visual cortex, V1, in an early stage of cortical development, so that binocular neurons can be formed to implement stereopsis (Blakemore et al., 1978; LeVay et al., 1980). After a 'critical period', the plasticity in V1 is switched off, and later stages of the hierarchy can learn, and be subject to evolution by genetic variation and natural selection. Indeed, our evidence is that plasticity in the primate inferior temporal visual cortex remains present in adulthood (Rolls et al., 1989a).

There may thus be interesting computational advantages of ontogeny recapitulating phylogeny in this case. For both development, and for evolution, the process of finding useful solutions by selection may be simplified by allowing primarily one stage or layer in the system to be developing or evolving at any one time, to reduce the dimensionality of the space being searched at any one time.

An implication is that the inferior temporal visual cortex is not a fixed structure, and that any changes that genes make in its architecture can influence its function throughout life, and may this have a strong impact on fitness. In any case, it is suggested that genetic variation and natural selection are largely switched off for early layers in the cortical hierarchy, so that genetic variation and natural selection operate mainly on the top layers of the hierarchy, enabling new processing layers to be added to an existing hierarchy and shaped by evolution to perform useful functions, without interference cause by simultaneous evolution of the early layers of the hierarchy. Consistent with this hypothesis, many genes are involved in timing when other genes are expressed.

B.20.7 Summary

1. Gene-based variation operated on by natural selection to promote fitness provides a basis for the design of the cortex during evolution.
2. It is proposed that genes specify a relatively small number of parameters for each class of neuron in a given cortical area, including the classes of neurons to which each class should make synapses. This provides a basis for one cortical area to make the appropriate connections to other cortical areas.
3. Specifying a few parameters for each class of cortical neuron enables relatively few genes, in the order of thousands, to specify the architecture and connectivity of the cerebral cortex.
4. Simulations are described which show that specification of relatively few parameters by genes can enable neural networks to evolve to optimise fitness functions that specify particular results of cortical computations. The genes specify relatively few rules of connectivity of the neural architecture, and learning in the phenotype sets the synaptic weights.

B.21 Highlights

1. The operation and properties of biologically plausible pattern association networks, auto-association networks, and competitive networks are described.
2. The operation of perceptrons, backpropagation networks, and deep learning networks is described.
3. Biological plausibility is a key issue when considering how computations are performed in the brain.
4. Some of the relatively unsupervised ways in which the brain learns are likely to be of interest for machine learning.

5. An interesting feature of brain connectivity and computation is how it evolves using genetic specification by a relatively few connection parameters for each brain region in combination with self-organisation.

Appendix 3 Neuronal encoding, and information theory

In order to understand what is computed in the brain, and how it is computed, it is essential to understand how information is represented in the brain. Is it by the firing rates of neurons, by the latency of neuronal responses, by the order in which action potentials arrive in different neurons, by any stimulus-dependent cross-correlations between the firing of different neurons, etc? It is essential to understand how information is encoded by single neurons, and by populations of neurons. Neuronal encoding, and the use of information theory to analyze it, are described in this Appendix, and by Rolls and Treves (2011).

We have seen that one parameter that influences the number of memories that can be stored in an associative memory is the sparseness of the representation, and it is therefore important to be able to quantify the sparseness of the representations.

We have also seen that the properties of an associative memory system depend on whether the representation is distributed or local (grandmother cell like), and it is important to be able to assess this quantitatively for neuronal representations.

It is also necessary to know how the information is encoded in order to understand how memory systems operate. Is the information that must be stored and retrieved present in the firing rates (the number of spikes in a fixed time), or is it present in synchronized firing of subsets of neurons? This has implications for how each stage of processing would need to operate. If the information is present in the firing rates, how much information is available from the spiking activity in a short period, of for example 20 or 50 ms? For each stage of cortical processing to operate quickly (in for example 20 ms), it is necessary for each stage to be able to read the code being provided by the previous cortical area within this order of time. Thus understanding the neural code is fundamental to understanding how each stage of processing works in the brain, and for understanding the speed of processing at each stage.

To treat all these questions quantitatively, we need quantitative ways of measuring sparseness, and also ways of measuring the information available from the spiking activity of single neurons and populations of neurons, and these are the topics addressed in this Appendix, together with some of the main results obtained, which provide answers to these questions.

Because single neurons are the computing elements of the brain and send the results of their processing by spiking activity to other neurons, we can understand brain processing by understanding what is encoded by the neuronal firing at each stage of the brain (e.g. each cortical area), and determining how what is encoded changes from stage to stage. Each neuron responds differently to a set of stimuli (with each neuron tuned differently to the members of the set of stimuli), and it is this that allows different stimuli to be represented. We can only address the richness of the representation therefore by understanding the differences in the responses of different neurons, and the impact that this has on the amount of information that is encoded. These issues can only be adequately and directly addressed at the level of the activity of single neurons and of populations of single neurons, and understanding at this neuronal level (rather than at the level of thousands or millions of neurons as revealed by functional neuroimaging) is essential for understanding brain computation.

Information theory provides the means for quantifying how much neurons communicate to other neurons, and thus provides a quantitative approach to fundamental questions about information processing in the brain. To investigate what in neuronal activity carries information, one must compare the amounts of information carried by different codes, that is different descriptions of the same activity, to provide the answer. To investigate the speed of information transmission, one must define and measure information rates from neuronal responses. To investigate to what extent the information provided by different cells is redundant or instead independent, again one must measure amounts of information in order to provide quantitative evidence. To compare the information carried by the number of spikes, by the timing of the spikes within the response of a single neuron, and by the relative time of firing of different neurons reflecting for example stimulus-dependent neuronal synchronization, information theory again provides a quantitative and well-founded basis for the necessary comparisons. To compare the information carried by a single neuron or a group of neurons with that reflected in the behavior of the human or animal, one must again use information theory, as it provides a single measure which can be applied to the measurement of the performance of all these different cases. In all these situations, there is no quantitative and well-founded alternative to information theory.

This Appendix briefly introduces the fundamental elements of information theory in Section C.1. A more complete treatment can be found in many books on the subject (e.g. Abramson (1963), Hamming (1990), and Cover and Thomas (1991)), including also Rieke, Warland, de Ruyter van Stevenick and Bialek (1997) which is specifically about information transmitted by neuronal firing. Section C.2 discusses the extraction of information measures from neuronal activity, in particular in experiments with mammals, in which the central issue is how to obtain accurate measures in conditions of limited sampling, that is where the numbers of trials of neuronal data that can be obtained are usually limited by the available recording time. Section C.3 summarizes some of the main results obtained so far on neuronal encoding. The essential terminology is summarized in a Glossary at the end of this Appendix in Section C.4. The approach taken in this Appendix is based on and updated from that provided by Rolls and Treves (1998), Rolls (2016b), and Rolls and Treves (2011).

Readers who wish to see the main findings on neuronal encoding and how information is represented by neuronal firing in the primate brain may wish to skip to Section C.3.

C.1 Information theory and its use in the analysis of formal models

Although information theory was a surprisingly late starter as a mathematical discipline, having being developed and formalized by C. Shannon (1948), the intuitive notion of information is immediate to us. It is also very easy to understand why we use logarithms in order to quantify this intuitive notion, of how much we know about something, and why the resulting quantity is always defined in relative rather than absolute terms. An introduction to information theory is provided next, with a more formal summary given in Section C.1.3.

C.1.1 The information conveyed by definite statements

Suppose somebody, who did not know, is told that Reading is a town west of London. How much information is he given? Well, that depends. He may have known it was a town in England, but not whether it was east or west of London; in which case the new information amounts to the fact that of two *a priori* (i.e. initial) possibilities (E or W), one holds (W). It is also possible to interpret the statement in the more precise sense, that Reading is west of

London, rather than east, north or south, i.e. one out of four possibilities; or else, west rather that north-west, north, etc. Clearly, the larger the number k of *a priori* possibilities, the more one is actually told, and a measure of information must take this into account. Moreover, we would like independent pieces of information to just add together. For example, our person may also be told that Cambridge is, out of l possible directions, north of London. Provided nothing was known on the mutual location of Reading and Cambridge, there are now overall $k \times l$ *a priori* (initial) possibilities, only one of which remains *a posteriori* (after receiving the information). Given that the number of possibilities for independent events are multiplicative, but that we would like the measure of information to be additive, we use logarithms when we measure information, as logarithms have this property. We thus define the amount I of information gained when we are informed in which of k possible locations Reading is located as

$$I(k) = \log_2 k. \tag{C.1}$$

Then when we combine independent information, for example producing $k \times l$ possibilities from independent events with k and l possibilities respectively, we obtain

$$I(k \times l) = \log_2(k \times l) = \log_2 k + \log_2 l = I(k) + I(l). \tag{C.2}$$

Thus in our example, the information about Cambridge adds up to that about Reading. We choose to take logarithms in base 2 as a mere convention, so that the answer to a yes/no question provides one unit, or bit, of information. Here it is just for the sake of clarity that we used different symbols for the number of possible directions with respect to which Reading and Cambridge are localized; if both locations are specified for example in terms of E, SE, S, SW, W, NW, N, NE, then obviously $k = l = 8, I(k) = I(l) = 3$ bits, and $I(k \times l) = 6$ bits. An important point to note is that the *resolution* with which the direction is specified determines the amount of information provided, and that in this example, as in many situations arising when analysing neuronal codings, the resolution could be made progressively finer, with a corresponding increase in information proportional to the log of the number of possibilities.

C.1.2 The information conveyed by probabilistic statements

The situation becomes slightly less trivial, and closer to what happens among neurons, if information is conveyed in less certain terms. Suppose for example that our friend is told, instead, that Reading has odds of 9 to 1 to be west, rather than east, of London (considering now just two *a priori* possibilities). He is certainly given some information, albeit less than in the previous case. We might put it this way: out of 18 equiprobable *a priori* possibilities (9 west + 9 east), 8 (east) are eliminated, and 10 remain, yielding

$$I = \log_2(18/10) = \log_2(9/5) \tag{C.3}$$

as the amount of information given. It is simpler to write this in terms of probabilities

$$I = \log_2 P^{\text{posterior}}(W)/P^{\text{prior}}(W) = \log_2(9/10)/(1/2) = \log_2(9/5). \tag{C.4}$$

This is of course equivalent to saying that the amount of information given by an uncertain statement is equal to the amount given by the absolute statement

$$I = -\log_2 P^{\text{prior}}(W) \tag{C.5}$$

minus the amount of uncertainty remaining after the statement, $I = -\log_2 P^{\text{posterior}}(W)$. A successive clarification that Reading is indeed west of London carries

$$I' = \log_2((1)/(9/10)) \tag{C.6}$$

bits of information, because 9 out of 10 are now the *a priori* odds, while *a posteriori* there is certainty, $P^{\text{posterior}}(W) = 1$. In total we would seem to have

$$I^{\text{TOTAL}} = I + I' = \log_2(9/5) + \log_2(10/9) = 1 \text{ bit} \tag{C.7}$$

as if the whole information had been provided at one time. This is strange, given that the two pieces of information are clearly not independent, and only independent information should be additive. In fact, we have cheated a little. Before the clarification, there was still one residual possibility (out of 10) that the answer was 'east', and this must be taken into account by writing

$$I = P^{\text{posterior}}(W) \log_2 \frac{P^{\text{posterior}}(W)}{P^{\text{prior}}(W)} + \tag{C.8}$$

$$P^{\text{posterior}}(E) \log_2 \frac{P^{\text{posterior}}(E)}{P^{\text{prior}}(E)}$$

as the information contained in the first message. This little detour should serve to emphasize two aspects that are easy to forget when reasoning intuitively about information, and that in this example cancel each other. In general, when uncertainty remains, that is there is more than one possible *a posteriori* state, one has to average information values for each state with the corresponding *a posteriori* probability measure. In the specific example, the sum $I + I'$ totals slightly *more* than 1 bit, and the amount in excess is precisely the information 'wasted' by providing *correlated* messages.

C.1.3 Information sources, information channels, and information measures

In summary, the expression quantifying the information provided by a definite statement that event s, which had an *a priori* probability $P(s)$, has occurred is

$$I(s) = \log_2(1/P(s)) = -\log_2 P(s), \tag{C.9}$$

whereas if the statement is probabilistic, that is several *a posteriori* probabilities remain non-zero, the correct expression involves summing over all possibilities with the corresponding probabilities:

$$I = \sum_s \left[P^{\text{posterior}}(s) \log_2 \frac{P^{\text{posterior}}(s)}{P^{\text{prior}}(s)} \right]. \tag{C.10}$$

When considering a discrete set of mutually exclusive events, it is convenient to use the metaphor of a set of *symbols* comprising an *alphabet* S. The occurrence of each event is then referred to as the emission of the corresponding symbol by an information *source*. The *entropy* of the source, H, is the average amount of information per source symbol, where the average is taken across the alphabet, with the corresponding probabilities

$$H(S) = -\sum_{s \in S} P(s) \log_2 P(s). \tag{C.11}$$

An information *channel* receives symbols s from an alphabet S and emits symbols s' from alphabet S'. If the *joint* probability of the channel receiving s and emitting s' is given by the product

$$P(s, s') = P(s)P(s') \tag{C.12}$$

for any pair s, s', then the input and output symbols are *independent* of each other, and the channel transmits zero information. Instead of joint probabilities, this can be expressed with conditional probabilities: the conditional probability of s' given s is written $P(s'|s)$, and if the two variables are independent, it is just equal to the unconditional probability $P(s')$. In general, and in particular if the channel does transmit information, the variables are not independent, and one can express their joint probability in two ways in terms of conditional probabilities

$$P(s,s') = P(s'|s)P(s) = P(s|s')P(s'), \qquad (C.13)$$

from which it is clear that

$$P(s'|s) = P(s|s')\frac{P(s')}{P(s)}, \qquad (C.14)$$

which is called Bayes' theorem (although when expressed as here in terms of probabilities it is strictly speaking an identity rather than a theorem). The information transmitted by the channel conditional to its having emitted symbol s' (or specific transinformation, $I(s')$) is given by Equation C.10, once the unconditional probability $P(s)$ is inserted as the prior, and the conditional probability $P(s|s')$ as the posterior:

$$I(s') = \sum_s P(s|s') \log_2 \frac{P(s|s')}{P(s)}. \qquad (C.15)$$

Symmetrically, one can define the transinformation conditional to the channel having received symbol s

$$I(s) = \sum_{s'} P(s'|s) \log_2 \frac{P(s'|s)}{P(s')}. \qquad (C.16)$$

Finally, the average transinformation, or **mutual information**, can be expressed in fully symmetrical form

$$I = \sum_s P(s) \sum_{s'} P(s'|s) \log_2 \frac{P(s'|s)}{P(s')} \qquad (C.17)$$

$$= \sum_{s,s'} P(s,s') \log_2 \frac{P(s,s')}{P(s)P(s')}.$$

The **mutual information** can also be expressed as the entropy of the source using alphabet S minus the *equivocation* of S with respect to the new alphabet S' used by the channel, written

$$I = H(S) - H(S|S') \equiv H(S) - \sum_{s'} P(s')H(S|s'). \qquad (C.18)$$

A channel is characterized, once the alphabets are given, by the set of conditional probabilities for the output symbols, $P(s'|s)$, whereas the unconditional probabilities of the input symbols $P(s)$ depend of course on the source from which the channel receives. Then, the *capacity* of the channel can be defined as the maximal mutual information across all possible sets of input probabilities $P(s)$. Thus, the information transmitted by a channel can range from zero to the lower of two independent upper bounds: the entropy of the source, and the capacity of the channel.

C.1.4 The information carried by a neuronal response and its averages

Considering the processing of information in the brain, we are often interested in the amount of information the response r of a neuron, or of a population of neurons, carries about an event happening in the outside world, for example a stimulus s shown to the animal. Once the inputs and outputs are conceived of as sets of symbols from two alphabets, the neuron(s) may be regarded as an information channel. We may denote with P(s) the *a priori* probability that the particular stimulus s out of a given set was shown, while the conditional probability P($s|r$) is the *a posteriori* probability, that is updated by the knowledge of the response r. The response-specific transinformation

$$I(r) = \sum_s P(s|r) \log_2 \frac{P(s|r)}{P(s)} \tag{C.19}$$

takes the extreme values of $I(r) = -\log_2 P(s(r))$ if r unequivocally determines $s(r)$ (that is, P($s|r$) equals 1 for that one stimulus and 0 for all others); and $I(r) = \sum_s P(s) \log_2(P(s)/P(s)) = 0$ if there is no relation between s and r, that is they are independent, so that the response tells us nothing new about the stimulus and thus P($s|r$) = P(s).

This is the information conveyed by each particular response. One is usually interested in further averaging this quantity over all possible responses r,

$$<I> = \sum_r P(r) \left[\sum_s P(s|r) \log_2 \frac{P(s|r)}{P(s)} \right]. \tag{C.20}$$

The angular brackets <> are used here to emphasize the averaging operation, in this case over responses. Denoting with P(s, r) the *joint probability* of the pair of events s and r, and using Bayes' theorem, this reduces to the symmetric form (equation C.18) for the **mutual information** $I(S, R)$

$$<I> = \sum_{s,r} P(s, r) \log_2 \frac{P(s, r)}{P(s)P(r)} \tag{C.21}$$

which emphasizes that responses tell us about stimuli just as much as stimuli tell us about responses. This is, of course, a general feature, independent of the two variables being in this instance stimuli and neuronal responses. In fact, what is of interest, besides the mutual information of Equations C.20 and C.21, is often the information specifically conveyed about each stimulus,

$$I(s) = \sum_r P(r|s) \log_2 \frac{P(r|s)}{P(r)} \tag{C.22}$$

which is a direct quantification of the variability in the responses elicited by that stimulus, compared to the overall variability. Since P(r) is the probability distribution of responses averaged across stimuli, it is again evident that the stimulus-specific information measure of Equation C.22 depends not only on the stimulus s, but also on all other stimuli used. Likewise, the mutual information measure, despite being of an average nature, is dependent on what set of stimuli has been used in the average. This emphasizes again the relative nature of all information measures. More specifically, it underscores the relevance of using, while measuring the information conveyed by a given neuronal population, stimuli that are either representative of real-life stimulus statistics, or of particular interest for the properties of the population being examined[29].

---

[29]The quantity $I(s, R)$, which is what is shown in Equation C.22 and where R draws attention to the fact that this quantity is calculated across the full set of responses R, has also been called the stimulus-specific surprise, see DeWeese and Meister (1999). Its average across stimuli is the mutual information $I(S, R)$.

C.1.4.1 A numerical example

To make these notions clearer, we can consider a specific example in which the response of a neuron to the presentation of, say, one of four visual stimuli (A, B, C, D) is recorded for 10 ms, during which the neuron emits either 0, 1, or 2 spikes, but no more. Imagine that the neuron tends to respond more vigorously to visual stimulus B, less to C, even less to A, and never to D, as described by the table of conditional probabilities P($r|s$) shown in Table C.1. Then, if different visual stimuli are presented with equal probability, the table of joint

Table C.1 The conditional probabilities P($r|s$) that different neuronal responses (r=0, 1, or 2 spikes) will be produced by each of four stimuli (A–D).

	r=0	r=1	r=2
s=A	0.6	0.4	0.0
s=B	0.0	0.2	0.8
s=C	0.4	0.5	0.1
s=D	1.0	0.0	0.0

probabilities P(s, r) will be as shown in Table C.2. From these two tables one can compute

Table C.2 Joint probabilities P(s, r) that different neuronal responses (r=0, 1, or 2 spikes) will be produced by each of four equiprobable stimuli (A–D).

	r=0	r=1	r=2
s=A	0.15	0.1	0.0
s=B	0.0	0.05	0.2
s=C	0.1	0.125	0.025
s=D	0.25	0.0	0.0

various information measures by directly applying the definitions above. Since visual stimuli are presented with equal probability, P(s) = $1/4$, the entropy of the stimulus set, which corresponds to the maximum amount of information any transmission channel, no matter how efficient, could convey on the identity of the stimuli, is $H_s = -\sum_s [P(s) \log_2 P(s)] =$ $-4[(1/4) \log_2(1/4)] = \log_2 4 = 2$ bits. There is a more stringent upper bound on the mutual information that this cell's responses convey on the stimuli, however, and this second bound is the channel capacity T of the cell. Calculating this quantity involves maximizing the mutual information across prior visual stimulus probabilities, and it is a bit complicated to do, in general. In our particular case the maximum information is obtained when only stimuli B and D are presented, each with probability 0.5. The resulting capacity is $T = 1$ bit. We can easily calculate, in general, the entropy of the responses. This is not an upper bound characterizing the source, like the entropy of the stimuli, nor an upper bound characterizing the channel, like the capacity, but simply a bound on the mutual information for this specific combination of source (with its related visual stimulus probabilities) and channel (with its conditional probabilities). Since only three response levels are possible within the short recording window, and they occur with uneven probability, their entropy is considerably lower than H_s, at $H_r = -\sum_r P(r) \log_2 P(r) = -P(0) \log_2 P(0) - P(1) \log_2 P(1) - P(2) \log_2 P(2) =$ $-0.5 \log_2 0.5 - 0.275 \log_2 0.275 - 0.225 \log_2 0.225 = 1.496$ bits. The actual average information I that the responses transmit about the stimuli, which is a measure of the correlation in the variability of stimuli and responses, does not exceed the absolute variability of either stimuli (as quantified by the first bound) or responses (as quantified by the last bound), nor the capacity of the channel. An explicit calculation using the joint probabilities of the second table in expression C.21 yields $I = 0.733$ bits. This is of course only the average value, averaged both across stimuli and across responses.

The information conveyed by a particular response can be larger. For example, when the cell emits two spikes it indicates with a relatively large probability stimulus B, and this is reflected in the fact that it then transmits, according to expression C.19, $I(r = 2) = 1.497$ bits, more than double the average value.

Similarly, the amount of information conveyed about each individual visual stimulus varies with the stimulus, depending on the extent to which it tends to elicit a differential response. Thus, expression C.22 yields that only $I(s = C) = 0.185$ bits are conveyed on average about stimulus C, which tends to elicit responses with similar statistics to the average statistics across stimuli, and are therefore not easily interpretable. On the other hand, exactly 1 bit of information is conveyed about stimulus D, since this stimulus never elicits any response, and when the neuron emits no spike there is a probability of $1/2$ that the stimulus was stimulus D.

C.1.5 The information conveyed by continuous variables

A general feature, relevant also to the case of neuronal information, is that if, among a *continuum* of *a priori* possibilities, only one, or a discrete number, remains *a posteriori*, the information is strictly infinite. This would be the case if one were told, for example, that Reading is exactly 10' west, 1' north of London. The *a priori* probability of precisely this set of coordinates among the continuum of possible ones is zero, and then the information diverges to infinity. The problem is only theoretical, because in fact, with continuous distributions, there are always one or several factors that limit the resolution in the *a posteriori* knowledge, rendering the information finite. Moreover, when considering the mutual information in the conjoint probability of occurrence of two sets, e.g. stimuli and responses, it suffices that at least one of the sets is discrete to make matters easy, that is, finite. Nevertheless, the identification and appropriate consideration of these resolution-limiting factors in practical cases may require careful analysis.

C.1.5.1 Example: the information retrieved from an autoassociative memory

One example is the evaluation of the information that can be retrieved from an autoassociative memory. Such a memory stores a number of firing patterns, each one of which can be considered, as in Appendix B, as a vector $\mathbf{r}^\mu$ with components the firing rates $\{r_i^\mu\}$, where the subscript i indexes the neuron (and the superscript μ indexes the pattern). In retrieving pattern μ, the network in fact produces a distinct firing pattern, denoted for example simply as $\mathbf{r}$. The quality of retrieval, or the similarity between $\mathbf{r}^\mu$ and $\mathbf{r}$, can be measured by the average mutual information

$$<I(\mathbf{r}^\mu, \mathbf{r})> = \sum_{\mathbf{r}^\mu,\mathbf{r}} P(\mathbf{r}^\mu, \mathbf{r}) \log_2 \frac{P(\mathbf{r}^\mu,\mathbf{r})}{P(\mathbf{r}^\mu)P(\mathbf{r})} \quad \text{(C.23)}$$

$$\approx \sum_i \sum_{r_i^\mu, r_i} P(r_i^\mu, r_i) \log_2 \frac{P(r_i^\mu,r_i)}{P(r_i^\mu)P(r_i)}.$$

In this formula the 'approximately equal' sign $\approx$ marks a simplification that is not necessarily a reasonable approximation. If the simplification is valid, it means that in order to extract an information measure, one need not compare whole vectors (the entire firing patterns) with each other, and may instead compare the firing rates of individual cells at storage and retrieval, and sum the resulting single-cell information values. The validity of the simplification is a matter that will be discussed later and that has to be verified, in the end, experimentally, but for the purposes of the present discussion we can focus on the single-cell terms. If either r_i or r_i^μ has a continuous distribution of values, as it will if it represents not the number of spikes emitted in a fixed window, but more generally the firing rate of neuron i computed by convolving the firing train with a smoothing kernel, then one has to deal with probability densities, which we denote as $p(r)\mathrm{d}r$, rather than the usual probabilities $\mathrm{P}(r)$. Substituting $p(r)\mathrm{d}r$ for $\mathrm{P}(r)$ and $p(r^\mu, r)\mathrm{d}r\mathrm{d}r^\mu$ for $\mathrm{P}(r^\mu, r)$, one can write for each single-cell contribution (omitting the cell index i)

$$< I(r^\mu, r) >_i = \int \mathrm{d}r^\mu \mathrm{d}r \; p(r^\mu, r) \log_2 \frac{p(r^\mu, r)}{p(r^\mu)p(r)} \qquad (C.24)$$

and we see that the differentials $\mathrm{d}r^\mu \mathrm{d}r$ cancel out between numerator and denominator inside the logarithm, rendering the quantity well defined and finite. If, however, r^μ were to *exactly* determine r, one would have

$$p(r^\mu, r)\mathrm{d}r^\mu \mathrm{d}r = p(r^\mu)\delta(r - r(r^\mu))\mathrm{d}r^\mu \mathrm{d}r = p(r^\mu)\mathrm{d}r^\mu \qquad (C.25)$$

and, by losing one differential on the way, the mutual information would become infinite. It is therefore important to consider what prevents r^μ from fully determining r in the case at hand – in other words, to consider the sources of noise in the system. In an autoassociative memory storing an extensive number of patterns (see Appendix A4 of Rolls and Treves (1998)), one source of noise always present is the interference effect due to the concurrent storage of all other patterns. Even neglecting other sources of noise, this produces a finite resolution width ρ, which allows one to write an expression of the type $p(r|r^\mu)\mathrm{d}r = \exp -(r-r(r^\mu))^2/2\rho^2 \mathrm{d}r$ which ensures that the information is finite as long as the resolution ρ is larger than zero.

One further point that should be noted, in connection with estimating the information retrievable from an autoassociative memory, is that the mutual information between the current distribution of firing rates and that of the stored pattern does not coincide with the information *gain* provided by the memory device. Even when firing rates, or spike counts, are all that matter in terms of information carriers, as in the networks considered in this book, one more term should be taken into account in evaluating the information gain. This term, to be subtracted, is the information contained in the external input that elicits the retrieval. This may vary a lot from the retrieval of one particular memory to the next, but of course an efficient memory device is one that is able, when needed, to retrieve much more information than it requires to be present in the inputs, that is, a device that produces a large information gain.

Finally, one should appreciate the conceptual difference between the information a firing pattern carries about another one (that is, about the pattern stored), as considered above, and two different notions: (a) the information produced by the network in selecting the correct memory pattern and (b) the information a firing pattern carries about something in the outside world. Quantity (a), the information intrinsic to selecting the memory pattern, is ill defined when analysing a real system, but is a well-defined and particularly simple notion when considering a formal model. If p patterns are stored with equal strength, and the selection is errorless, this amounts to $\log_2 p$ bits of information, a quantity often, but not always, small compared with the information in the pattern itself. Quantity (b), the information conveyed about some outside correlate, is not defined when considering a formal model that does not include an explicit account of what the firing of each cell represents, but is well defined and measurable from the recorded activity of real cells. It is the quantity considered in the numerical example with the four visual stimuli, and it can be generalized to the information carried by the activity of several cells in a network, and specialized to the case that the network operates as an associative memory. One may note, in this case, that the capacity to retrieve memories with high fidelity, or high information content, is only useful to the extent that the representation to be retrieved carries that amount of information about something relevant – or, in other words, that it is pointless to store and retrieve with great care largely meaningless messages. This type of argument has been used to discuss the role of the mossy fibres in the operation of the CA3 network in the hippocampus (Treves and Rolls, 1992; Rolls and Treves, 1998).

C.2 Estimating the information carried by neuronal responses

C.2.1 The limited sampling problem

We now discuss in more detail the application of these general notions to the information transmitted by neurons. Suppose, to be concrete, that an animal has been presented with stimuli drawn from a discrete set, and that the responses of a set of C cells have been recorded following the presentation of each stimulus. We may choose any quantity or set of quantities to characterize the responses; for example let us assume that we consider the firing rate of each cell, r_i, calculated by convolving the spike response with an appropriate smoothing kernel. The response space is then C times the continuous set of all positive real numbers, $(\mathbf{R}/2)^C$. We want to evaluate the average information carried by such responses about which stimulus was shown. In principle, it is straightforward to apply the above formulas, e.g. in the form

$$< I(s, \mathbf{r}) > = \sum_s P(s) \int \Pi_i \mathrm{d}r_i \; p(\mathbf{r}|s) \log_2 \frac{p(\mathbf{r}|s)}{p(\mathbf{r})} \tag{C.26}$$

where it is important to note that $p(\mathbf{r})$ and $p(\mathbf{r}|s)$ are now probability densities defined over the high-dimensional vector space of multi-cell responses. The product sign Π signifies that this whole vector space has to be integrated over, along all its dimensions. $p(\mathbf{r})$ can be calculated as $\sum_s p(\mathbf{r}|s) P(s)$, and therefore, in principle, all one has to do is to estimate, from the data, the conditional probability densities $p(\mathbf{r}|s)$ – the distributions of responses following each stimulus. In practice, however, in contrast to what happens with formal models, in which there is usually no problem in calculating the exact probability densities, real data come in limited amounts, and thus sample only sparsely the vast response space. This limits the accuracy with which, from the experimental *frequency* of each possible response, we can estimate its *probability*, in turn seriously impairing our ability to estimate $< I >$ correctly. We refer to this as the limited sampling problem. This is a purely technical problem that arises, typically when recording from mammals, because of external constraints on the duration or number of repetitions of a given set of stimulus conditions. With computer simulation experiments, and also with recordings from, for example, insects, sufficient data can usually be obtained that straightforward estimates of information are accurate enough (Strong, Koberle, de Ruyter van Stevenick and Bialek, 1998; Golomb, Kleinfeld, Reid, Shapley and Shraiman, 1994). The problem is, however, so serious in connection with recordings from monkeys and rats in which limited numbers of trials are usually available for neuronal data, that it is worthwhile to discuss it, in order to appreciate the scope and limits of applying information theory to neuronal processing.

In particular, if the responses are continuous quantities, the probability of observing exactly the same response twice is infinitesimal. In the absence of further manipulation, this would imply that each stimulus generates its own set of unique responses, therefore any response that has actually occurred could be associated unequivocally with one stimulus, and the mutual information would always equal the entropy of the stimulus set. This absurdity shows that in order to estimate probability densities from experimental frequencies, one has to resort to some *regularizing* manipulation, such as smoothing the point-like response values by convolution with suitable kernels, or binning them into a finite number of discrete bins.

C.2.1.1 Smoothing or binning neuronal response data

The issue is how to estimate the underlying probability distributions of neuronal responses to a set of stimuli from only a limited number of trials of data (e.g. 10–30) for each stimulus. Several strategies are possible. One is to discretize the response space into bins, and estimate the probability density as the histogram of the fraction of trials falling into each bin. If the bins are too narrow, almost every response is in a different bin, and the estimated information will be overestimated. Even if the bin width is increased to match the standard deviation of each underlying distribution, the information may still be overestimated. Alternatively, one may try to 'smooth' the data by convolving each response with a Gaussian with a width set to the standard deviation measured for each stimulus. Setting the standard deviation to this value may actually lead to an underestimation of the amount of information available, due to oversmoothing. Another possibility is to make a bold assumption as to what the general shape of the underlying densities should be, for example a Gaussian. This may produce closer estimates. Methods for regularizing the data are discussed further by Rolls and Treves (1998) in their Appendix A2, where a numerical example is given.

C.2.1.2 The effects of limited sampling

The crux of the problem is that, whatever procedure one adopts, limited sampling tends to produce distortions in the estimated probability densities. The resulting mutual information estimates are intrinsically biased. The bias, or average error of the estimate, is upward if the raw data have not been regularized much, and is downward if the regularization procedure chosen has been heavier. The bias can be, if the available trials are few, much larger than the true information values themselves. This is intuitive, as fluctuations due to the finite number of trials available would tend, on average, to either produce or emphasize differences among the distributions corresponding to different stimuli, differences that are preserved if the regularization is 'light', and that are interpreted in the calculation as carrying genuine information. This is illustrated with a quantitative example by Rolls and Treves (1998) in their Appendix A2.

Choosing the right amount of regularization, or the best regularizing procedure, is not possible *a priori*. Hertz, Kjaer, Eskander and Richmond (1992) have proposed the interesting procedure of using an artificial neural network to regularize the raw responses. The network can be trained on part of the data using backpropagation, and then used on the remaining part to produce what is in effect a clever data-driven regularization of the responses. This procedure is, however, rather computer intensive and not very safe, as shown by some self-evident inconsistency in the results (Heller, Hertz, Kjaer and Richmond, 1995). Obviously, the best way to deal with the limited sampling problem is to try and use as many trials as possible. The improvement is slow, however, and generating as many trials as would be required for a reasonably unbiased estimate is often, in practice, impossible.

C.2.2 Correction procedures for limited sampling

The above point, that data drawn from a single distribution, when artificially paired, at random, to different stimulus labels, results in 'spurious' amounts of apparent information, suggests a simple way of checking the reliability of estimates produced from real data (Optican, Gawne, Richmond and Joseph, 1991). One can disregard the true stimulus associated with each response, and generate a randomly reshuffled pairing of stimuli and responses, which should therefore, being not linked by any underlying relationship, carry no mutual information about each other. Calculating, with some procedure of choice, the spurious information obtained in this way, and comparing with the information value estimated with the same procedure for the real pairing, one can get a feeling for how far the procedure goes into eliminating the apparent information due to limited sampling. Although this spurious information, I_s, is only indicative of the amount of bias affecting the original estimate, a simple heuristic trick (called 'bootstrap'[30]) is to subtract the spurious from the original value, to obtain a somewhat 'corrected' estimate. This procedure can result in quite accurate estimates (see Rolls and Treves (1998), Tovee, Rolls, Treves and Bellis (1993))[31].

A different correction procedure (called 'jack-knife') is based on the assumption that the bias is proportional to $1/N$, where N is the number of responses (data points) used in the estimation. One computes, beside the original estimate $< I_N >$, N auxiliary estimates $< I_{N-1} >_k$, by taking out from the data set response k, where k runs across the data set from 1 to N. The corrected estimate

$$< I > = N < I_N > -(1/N) \sum_k (N-1) < I_{N-1} >_k \qquad (C.27)$$

is free from bias (to leading order in $1/N$), if the proportionality factor is more or less the same in the original and auxiliary estimates. This procedure is very time-consuming, and it suffers from the same imprecision of any algorithm that tries to determine a quantity as the result of the subtraction of two large and nearly equal terms; in this case the terms have been made large on purpose, by multiplying them by N and $N - 1$.

A more fundamental approach (Miller, 1955) is to derive an analytical expression for the bias (or, more precisely, for its leading terms in an expansion in $1/N$, the inverse of the sample size). This allows the estimation of the bias from the data itself, and its subsequent subtraction, as discussed in Treves and Panzeri (1995) and Panzeri and Treves (1996). Such a procedure produces satisfactory results, thereby lowering the size of the sample required for a given accuracy in the estimate by about an order of magnitude (Golomb, Hertz, Panzeri, Treves and Richmond, 1997). However, it does not, in itself, make possible measures of the information contained in very complex responses with few trials. As a rule of thumb, the number of trials per stimulus required for a reasonable estimate of information, once the subtractive correction is applied, is of the order of the effectively independent (and utilized) bins in which the response space can be partitioned (Panzeri and Treves, 1996). This correction procedure is the one that we use standardly (Rolls, Treves, Tovee and Panzeri, 1997d; Rolls, Critchley and Treves, 1996a; Rolls, Treves, Robertson, Georges-François and Panzeri, 1998b; Booth and Rolls, 1998; Rolls, Tovee and Panzeri, 1999b; Rolls, Franco, Aggelopoulos and Jerez, 2006b).

C.2.3 The information from multiple cells: decoding procedures

The bias of information measures grows with the dimensionality of the response space, and for all practical purposes the limit on the number of dimensions that can lead to reasonably accurate direct measures, even when applying a correction procedure, is quite low, two to three. This implies, in particular, that it is not possible to apply Equation C.26 to extract

---

[30] In technical usage bootstrap procedures utilize random pairings of responses with stimuli with replacement, while shuffling procedures utilize random pairings of responses with stimuli without replacement.

[31] Subtracting the 'square' of the spurious fraction of information estimated by this bootstrap procedure as used by Optican, Gawne, Richmond and Joseph (1991) is unfounded and does not work correctly (see Rolls and Treves (1998) and Tovee, Rolls, Treves and Bellis (1993)).

the information content in the responses of several cells (more than two to three) recorded simultaneously. One way to address the problem is then to apply some strong form of regularization to the multiple cell responses. Smoothing has already been mentioned as a form of regularization that can be tuned from very soft to very strong, and that preserves the structure of the response space. Binning is another form, which changes the nature of the responses from continuous to discrete, but otherwise preserves their general structure, and which can also be tuned from soft to strong. Other forms of regularization involve much more radical transformations, or changes of variables.

Of particular interest for information estimates is a change of variables that transforms the response space into the stimulus set, by applying an algorithm that derives a predicted stimulus from the response vector, i.e. the firing rates of all the cells, on each trial. Applying such an algorithm is called decoding. Of course, the predicted stimulus is not necessarily the same as the actual one. Therefore the term decoding should not be taken to imply that the algorithm works successfully, each time identifying the actual stimulus. The predicted stimulus is simply a function of the response, as determined by the algorithm considered. Just as with any regularizing transform, it is possible to compute the mutual information between actual stimuli s and predicted stimuli s', instead of the original one between stimuli s and responses r. Since information about (real) stimuli can only be lost and not be created by the transform, the information measured in this way is bound to be lower in value than the real information in the responses. If the decoding algorithm is efficient, it manages to preserve nearly all the information contained in the raw responses, while if it is poor, it loses a large portion of it. If the responses themselves provided all the information about stimuli, and the decoding is optimal, then predicted stimuli coincide with the actual stimuli, and the information extracted equals the entropy of the stimulus set.

The procedure for extracting information values after applying a decoding algorithm is indicated in Fig. C.1 (in which s? is s'). The underlying idea indicated in Fig. C.1 is that if we know the average firing rate of each cell in a population to each stimulus, then on any single trial we can guess (or decode) the stimulus that was present by taking into account the responses of all the cells. The decoded stimulus is s', and the actual stimulus that was shown is s. What we wish to know is how the percentage correct, or better still the information, based on the evidence from any single trial about which stimulus was shown, increases as the number of cells in the population sampled increases. We can expect that the more cells there are in the sample, the more accurate the estimate of the stimulus is likely to be. If the encoding was local, the number of stimuli encoded by a population of neurons would be expected to rise approximately linearly with the number of neurons in the population. In contrast, with distributed encoding, provided that the neuronal responses are sufficiently independent, and are sufficiently reliable (not too noisy), information from the ensemble would be expected to rise linearly with the number of cells in the ensemble, and (as information is a log measure) the number of stimuli encodable by the population of neurons might be expected to rise exponentially as the number of neurons in the sample of the population was increased.

Table C.3 Decoding. s' is the decoded stimulus, i.e. that predicted from the neuronal responses r.

$$s \quad \Rightarrow \quad r \quad \rightarrow \quad s'$$
$$I(s,r)$$
$$I(s,s')$$

The procedure is schematized in Table C.3 where the double arrow indicates the transformation from stimuli to responses operated by the nervous system, while the single arrow indicates the further transformation operated by the decoding procedure. $I(s, s')$ is the mut-

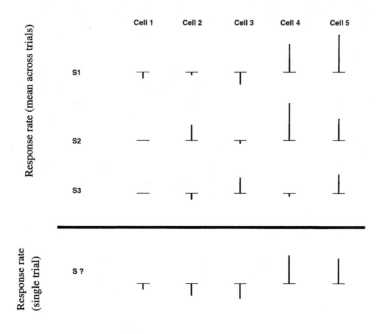

Fig. C.1 Decoding which stimulus (S1–S3) was present with a set of neuronal responses on a single trial to stimulus 'S ?'. The information available from multiple cells can then be calculated by comparing the decoded stimuli to the real stimuli that were presented. The figure shows the average response for each of several cells (Cell 1, etc.) to each of several stimuli (S1, etc.). The change of firing rate from the spontaneous rate is indicated by the vertical line above or below the horizontal line, which represents the spontaneous rate. We can imagine guessing or predicting from such a table the predicted stimulus S? (i.e. s') that was present on any one trial. (After Rolls, E. T., Treves, A. and Tovee, M.J. (1997) The representational capacity of the distributed encoding of information provided by populations of neurons in the primate temporal visual cortex. Experimental Brain Research 114: 149–162. © Springer Nature.)

ual information between the actual stimuli s and the stimuli s' that are predicted to have been shown based on the decoded responses.

A slightly more complex variant of this procedure is a decoding step that extracts from the response on each trial not a single predicted stimulus, but rather probabilities that each of the possible stimuli was the actual one. The joint probabilities of actual and posited stimuli can be averaged across trials, and information computed from the resulting probability matrix $(S \times S)$. Computing information in this way takes into account the relative uncertainty in assigning a predicted stimulus to each trial, an uncertainty that is instead not considered by the previous procedure based solely on the identification of the maximally likely stimulus (Treves, 1997). *Maximum likelihood* information values I_{ml} based on a single stimulus tend therefore to be higher than *probability* information values I_p based on the whole set of stimuli, although in very specific situations the reverse could also be true.

The same correction procedures for limited sampling can be applied to information values computed after a decoding step. Values obtained from maximum likelihood decoding, I_{ml}, suffer from limited sampling more than those obtained from probability decoding, I_p, since each trial contributes a whole 'brick' of weight $1/N$ (N being the total number of trials), whereas with probabilities each brick is shared among several slots of the $(S \times S)$ probability matrix. The neural network procedure devised by Hertz, Kjaer, Eskander and Richmond (1992) can in fact be thought of as a decoding procedure based on probabilities, which deals with limited sampling not by applying a correction but rather by strongly regularizing the original responses.

When decoding is used, the rule of thumb becomes that the minimal number of trials per stimulus required for accurate information measures is roughly equal to the size of the stimulus set, if the subtractive correction is applied (Panzeri and Treves, 1996). This correction procedure is applied as standard in our multiple cell information analyses that use decoding (Rolls, Treves and Tovee, 1997b; Booth and Rolls, 1998; Rolls, Treves, Robertson, Georges-François and Panzeri, 1998b; Franco, Rolls, Aggelopoulos and Treves, 2004; Aggelopoulos, Franco and Rolls, 2005; Rolls, Franco, Aggelopoulos and Jerez, 2006b).

C.2.3.1 Decoding algorithms

Any transformation from the response space to the stimulus set could be used in decoding, but of particular interest are the transformations that either approach optimality, so as to minimize information loss and hence the effect of decoding, or else are implementable by mechanisms that *could* conceivably be operating in the real system, so as to extract information values that could be extracted by the system itself.

The optimal transformation is in theory well-defined: one should estimate from the data the conditional probabilities $P(r|s)$, and use Bayes' rule to convert them into the conditional probabilities $P(s'|r)$. Having these for any value of r, one could use them to estimate I_p, and, after selecting for each particular real response the stimulus with the highest conditional probability, to estimate I_{ml}. To avoid biasing the estimation of conditional probabilities, the responses used in estimating $P(r|s)$ should not include the particular response for which $P(s'|r)$ is going to be derived (jack-knife cross-validation). In practice, however, the estimation of $P(r|s)$ in usable form involves the fitting of some simple function to the responses. This need for fitting, together with the approximations implied in the estimation of the various quantities, prevents us from defining the really optimal decoding, and leaves us with various algorithms, depending essentially on the fitting function used, which are hopefully close to optimal in some conditions. We have experimented extensively with two such algorithms, that both approximate Bayesian decoding (Rolls, Treves and Tovee, 1997b). Both these algorithms fit the response vectors produced over several trials by the cells being recorded to a product of conditional probabilities for the response of each cell given the stimulus. In one case, the single cell conditional probability is assumed to be Gaussian (truncated at zero); in the other it is assumed to be Poisson (with an additional weight at zero). Details of these algorithms are given by Rolls, Treves and Tovee (1997b).

Biologically plausible decoding algorithms are those that limit the algebraic operations used to types that could be easily implemented by neurons, e.g. dot product summations, thresholding and other single-cell non-linearities, and competition and contrast enhancement among the outputs of nearby cells. There is then no need for ever fitting functions or other sophisticated approximations, but of course the degree of arbitrariness in selecting a particular algorithm remains substantial, and a comparison among different choices based on which yields the higher information values may favour one choice in a given situation and another choice with a different data set.

To summarize, the key idea in decoding, in our context of estimating information values, is that it allows substitution of a possibly very high-dimensional response space (which is difficult to sample and regularize) with a reduced object much easier to handle, that is with a discrete set equivalent to the stimulus set. The mutual information between the new set and the stimulus set is then easier to estimate even with limited data, and if the assumptions about population coding, underlying the particular decoding algorithm used, are justified, the value obtained approximates the original target, the mutual information between stimuli and responses. For each response recorded, one can use all the responses except for that one to generate estimates of the average response vectors (the average response for each neuron in the population) to each stimulus. Then one considers how well the selected response vector matches the average response vectors, and uses the degree of matching to estimate, for all stimuli, the probability that they were the actual stimuli. The form of the matching embodies the general notions about population encoding, for example the 'degree of matching' might be simply the dot product between the current vector and the average vector ($\mathbf{r}^{av}$), suitably normalized over all average vectors to generate probabilities

$$P(s'|\mathbf{r}(s)) = \frac{\mathbf{r}(s) \cdot \mathbf{r}^{av}(s')}{\sum_{s''} \mathbf{r}(s) \cdot \mathbf{r}^{av}(s'')} \tag{C.28}$$

where s'' is a dummy variable. (This is called dot product decoding in Fig. 2.18.) One ends up, then, with a table of conjoint probabilities $P(s, s')$, and another table obtained by selecting for each trial the most likely (or predicted) single stimulus s^p, $P(s, s^p)$. Both s' and s^p stand for all possible stimuli, and hence belong to the same set S. These can be used to estimate mutual information values based on probability decoding (I_p) and on maximum likelihood decoding (I_{ml}):

$$<I_p> = \sum_{s \in S} \sum_{s' \in S} P(s, s') \log_2 \frac{P(s, s')}{P(s)P(s')} \tag{C.29}$$

and

$$<I_{ml}> = \sum_{s \in S} \sum_{s^p \in S} P(s, s^p) \log_2 \frac{P(s, s^p)}{P(s)P(s^p)} . \tag{C.30}$$

Examples of the use of these procedures are available (Rolls, Treves and Tovee, 1997b; Booth and Rolls, 1998; Rolls, Treves, Robertson, Georges-François and Panzeri, 1998b; Rolls, Aggelopoulos, Franco and Treves, 2004; Franco, Rolls, Aggelopoulos and Treves, 2004; Rolls, Franco, Aggelopoulos and Jerez, 2006b), and some of the results obtained are described in Section C.3.

C.2.4 Information in the correlations between the spikes of different cells: a decoding approach

Simultaneously recorded neurons sometimes shows cross-correlations in their firing, that is the firing of one is systematically related to the firing of the other cell. One example of this is neuronal response synchronization. The cross-correlation, to be defined below, shows the time difference between the cells at which the systematic relation appears. A significant peak or trough in the cross-correlation function could reveal a synaptic connection from one cell to the other, or a common input to each of the cells, or any of a considerable number of other possibilities. If the synchronization occurred for only some of the stimuli, then the presence of the significant cross-correlation for only those stimuli could provide additional evidence separate from any information in the firing rate of the neurons about which stimulus had been shown. Information theory in principle provides a way of quantitatively assessing the relative contributions from these two types of encoding, by expressing what can be learned from each type of encoding in the same units, bits of information.

Figure C.2 illustrates how synchronization occurring only for some of the stimuli could be used to encode information about which stimulus was presented. In the Figure the spike

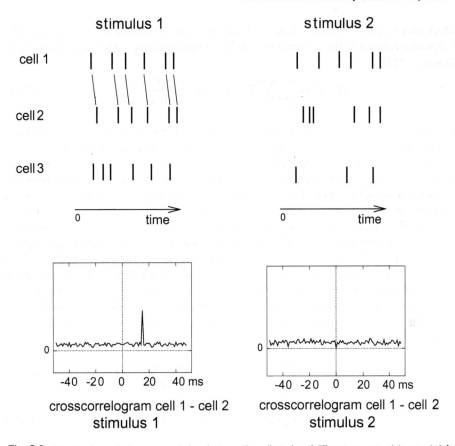

Fig. C.2 Stimulus-dependent cross-correlations between the spike trains of different neurons might encode information. The responses of three cells to two different stimuli are shown on one trial. Cell 3 reflects which stimulus was shown in the number of spikes produced, and this can be measured as spike count or rate information. Cells 1 and 2 have no spike count or rate information, because the number of spikes is not different for the two stimuli. Cells 1 and 2 do show some synchronization, reflected in the cross-correlogram, that is stimulus dependent, as the synchronization is present only when stimulus 1 is shown. The contribution of this effect is measured as the stimulus-dependent synchronization information. (From Rolls, E. T. and Treves.A. (2011) The neuronal encoding of information in the brain. Progress in Neurobiology 95: 448–490. © Elsevier Ltd.)

trains of three neurons are shown after the presentation of two different stimuli on one trial. As shown by the cross-correlogram in the lower part of the figure, the responses of cell 1 and cell 2 are synchronized when stimulus 1 is presented, as whenever a spike from cell 1 is emitted, another spike from cell 2 is emitted after a short time lag. In contrast, when stimulus 2 is presented, synchronization effects do not appear. Thus, based on a measure of the synchrony between the responses of cells 1 and 2, it is possible to obtain some information about what stimulus has been presented. The contribution of this effect is measured as the stimulus-dependent synchronization information. Cells 1 and 2 have no information about what stimulus was presented from the number of spikes, as the same number is found for both stimuli. Cell 3 carries information in the spike count in the time window (which is also called the firing rate) about what stimulus was presented. (Cell 3 emits 6 spikes for stimulus 1 and 3 spikes for stimulus 2.)

The example shown in Fig. C.2 is for the neuronal responses on a single trial. Given that the neuronal responses are variable from trial to trial, we need a method to quantify the information that is gained from a single trial of spike data in the context of the measured variability in the responses of all of the cells, including how the cells' responses covary in a way which may be partly stimulus-dependent, and may include synchronization effects. The direct approach is to apply the Shannon mutual information measure (Shannon, 1948; Cover and Thomas, 1991)

$$I(s, \mathbf{r}) = \sum_{s \in S} \sum_{\mathbf{r}} P(s, \mathbf{r}) \log_2 \frac{P(s, \mathbf{r})}{P(s)P(\mathbf{r})}, \quad (C.31)$$

where $P(s, \mathbf{r})$ is a probability table embodying a relationship between the variable s (here, the stimulus) and $\mathbf{r}$ (a vector where each element is the firing rate of one neuron).

However, because the probability table of the relation between the neuronal responses and the stimuli, $P(s, \mathbf{r})$, is so large (given that there may be many stimuli, and that the response space which has to include spike timing is very large), in practice it is difficult to obtain a sufficient number of trials for every stimulus to generate the probability table accurately, at least with data from mammals in which the experiment cannot usually be continued for many hours of recording from a whole population of cells. To circumvent this undersampling problem, Rolls, Treves and Tovee (1997b) developed a decoding procedure (described in Section C.2.3), in which an estimate (or guess) of which stimulus (called s') was shown on a given trial is made from a comparison of the neuronal responses on that trial with the responses made to the whole set of stimuli on other trials. One then obtains a conjoint probability table $P(s, s')$, and then the mutual information based on probability estimation (PE) decoding (I_p) between the estimated stimuli s' and the actual stimuli s that were shown can be measured:

$$< I_p > = \sum_{s \in S} \sum_{s' \in S} P(s, s') \log_2 \frac{P(s, s')}{P(s)P(s')} \quad (C.32)$$

$$= \sum_{s \in S} P(s) \sum_{s' \in S} P(s'|s) \log_2 \frac{P(s'|s)}{P(s')}. \quad (C.33)$$

These measurements are in the low dimensional space of the number of stimuli, and therefore the number of trials of data needed for each stimulus is of the order of the number of stimuli, which is feasible in experiments. In practice, it is found that for accurate information estimates with the decoding approach, the number of trials for each stimulus should be at least twice the number of stimuli (Franco, Rolls, Aggelopoulos and Treves, 2004).

The nature of the decoding procedure is illustrated in Fig. C.3. The left part of the diagram shows the average firing rate (or equivalently spike count) responses of each of 3 cells (labelled as Rate Cell 1,2,3) to a set of 3 stimuli. The last row (labelled Response single trial) shows the data that might be obtained from a single trial and from which the stimulus that was shown (St. ?) must be estimated or decoded, using the average values across trials shown in the top part of the table, and the probability distribution of these values. The decoding step essentially compares the vector of responses on trial St.? with the average response vectors obtained previously to each stimulus. This decoding can be as simple as measuring the correlation, or dot (inner) product, between the test trial vector of responses and the response vectors to each of the stimuli. This procedure is very neuronally plausible, in that the dot product between an input vector of neuronal activity and the synaptic response vector on a single neuron (which might represent the average incoming activity previously to that stimulus) is the simplest operation that it is conceived that neurons might perform (Rolls and Treves, 1998; Rolls and Deco, 2002; Rolls, 2016b). Other decoding procedures include a Bayesian procedure based on a Gaussian or Poisson assumption of the spike count distributions as described in detail by Rolls, Treves and Tovee (1997b). The Gaussian one is what we have used (Franco, Rolls, Aggelopoulos and Treves, 2004; Aggelopoulos, Franco and Rolls, 2005), and it is described below.

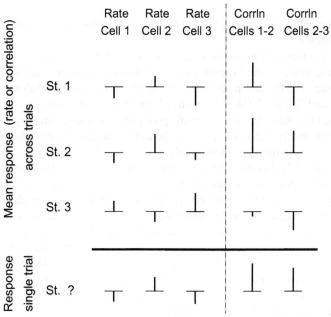

Fig. C.3 Decoding stimulus-dependent cross-correlations between the spike trains of different neurons that might encode information. The left part of the diagram shows the average firing rate (or equivalently spike count) responses of each of 3 cells (labelled as Rate Cell 1,2,3) to a set of 3 stimuli. The right two columns show a measure of the cross-correlation (averaged across trials) for some pairs of cells (labelled as Corrln Cells 1–2 and 2–3). The last row (labelled Response single trial) shows the data that might be obtained from a single trial and from which the stimulus that was shown (St. ? or s') must be estimated or decoded, using the average values across trials shown in the top part of the table. From the responses on the single trial, the most probable decoded stimulus is stimulus 2, based on the values of both the rates and the cross-correlations. (After Franco,L., Rolls, E. T., Aggelopoulos,N.C. and Treves,A. (2004) The use of decoding to analyze the contribution to the information of the correlations between the firing of simultaneously recorded neurons. Experimental Brain Research 155: 370–384. © Springer Nature.)

The new step taken by Franco, Rolls, Aggelopoulos and Treves (2004) is to introduce into the Table Data(s, r) shown in the upper part of Fig. C.3 new columns, shown on the right of the diagram, containing a measure of the cross-correlation (averaged across trials in the upper part of the table) for some pairs of cells (labelled as Corrln Cells 1–2 and 2–3). The decoding procedure can then take account of any cross-correlations between pairs of cells, and thus measure any contributions to the information from the population of cells that arise from cross-correlations between the neuronal responses. If these cross-correlations are stimulus-dependent, then their positive contribution to the information encoded can be measured. This is the new concept for information measurement from neuronal populations introduced by Franco, Rolls, Aggelopoulos and Treves (2004). We describe next how the cross-correlation information can be introduced into the Table, and then how the information analysis algorithm can be used to measure the contribution of different factors in the neuronal responses to the information that the population encodes.

To test different hypotheses, the decoding can be based on all the columns of the Table (to provide the total information available from both the firing rates and the stimulus-dependent synchronization), on only the columns with the firing rates (to provide the information available from the firing rates), and only on the columns with the cross-correlation values (to provide the information available from the stimulus-dependent cross-correlations). Any information from stimulus-dependent cross-correlations will not necessarily be orthogonal to the rate information, and the procedures allow this to be checked by comparing the total information to that from the sum of the two components. If cross-correlations are present but are not stimulus-dependent, these will not contribute to the information available about which stimulus was shown.

The measure of the synchronization introduced into the Table Data(s, r) on each trial is, for example, the value of the Pearson cross-correlation coefficient calculated for that trial at the appropriate lag for cell pairs that have significant cross-correlations (Franco, Rolls, Aggelopoulos and Treves, 2004). This value of this Pearson cross-correlation coefficient for a single trial can be calculated from pairs of spike trains on a single trial by forming for each cell a vector of 0s and 1s, the 1s representing the time of occurrence of spikes with a temporal resolution of 1 ms. Resulting values within the range -1 to 1 are shifted to obtain positive values. An advantage of basing the measure of synchronization on the Pearson cross-correlation coefficient is that it measures the amount of synchronization between a pair of neurons independently of the firing rate of the neurons. The lag at which the cross-correlation measure was computed for every single trial, and whether there was a significant cross-correlation between neuron pairs, can be identified from the location of the peak in the cross-correlogram taken across all trials. The cross-correlogram is calculated by, for every spike that occurred in one neuron, incrementing the bins of a histogram that correspond to the lag times of each of the spikes that occur for the other neuron. The raw cross-correlogram is corrected by subtracting the "shift predictor" cross-correlogram (which is produced by random re-pairings of the trials), to produce the corrected cross-correlogram.

Further details of the decoding procedures are as follows (see Rolls, Treves and Tovee (1997b) and Franco, Rolls, Aggelopoulos and Treves (2004)). The full probability table estimator (PE) algorithm uses a Bayesian approach to extract $P(s'|\mathbf{r})$ for every single trial from an estimate of the probability $P(\mathbf{r}|s')$ of a stimulus–response pair made from all the other trials (as shown in Bayes' rule shown in Equation C.34) in a cross-validation procedure described by Rolls et al. (1997b).

$$P(s'|\mathbf{r}) = \frac{P(\mathbf{r}|s')P(s')}{P(\mathbf{r})}. \tag{C.34}$$

where $P(\mathbf{r})$ (the probability of the vector containing the firing rate of each neuron, where each element of the vector is the firing rate of one neuron) is obtained as:

$$P(\mathbf{r}) = \sum_{s'} P(\mathbf{r}|s')P(s'). \tag{C.35}$$

This requires knowledge of the response probabilities $P(\mathbf{r}|s')$ which can be estimated for this purpose from $P(\mathbf{r}, s')$, which is equal to $P(s') \prod_c P(r_c|s')$, where r_c is the firing rate of cell c. I note that $P(r_c|s')$ is derived from the responses of cell c from all of the trials except for the current trial for which the probability estimate is being made. The probabilities $P(r_c|s')$ are fitted with a Gaussian (or Poisson) distribution whose amplitude at r_c gives $P(r_c|s')$. By summing over different test trial responses to the same stimulus s, we can extract the probability that by presenting stimulus s the neuronal response is interpreted as having been elicited by stimulus s',

$$P(s'|s) = \sum_{\mathbf{r} \in \text{test}} P(s'|\mathbf{r})P(\mathbf{r}|s). \tag{C.36}$$

After the decoding procedure, the estimated relative probabilities (normalized to 1) were averaged over all 'test' trials for all stimuli, to generate a (Regularized) table $P^R{}_N(s, s')$ describing the relative probability of each pair of actual stimulus s and posited stimulus s' (computed with N trials). From this probability table the mutual information measure (I_p) was calculated as described above in Equation C.33.

We also generate a second (Frequency) table $P^F_N(s, s^p)$ from the fraction of times an actual stimulus s elicited a response that led to a predicted (single most likely) stimulus s^p. From this probability Table the mutual information measure based on maximum likelihood decoding (I_{ml}) was calculated with Equation C.37:

$$< I_{ml} > = \sum_{s \in S} \sum_{s^p \in S} P(s, s^p) \log_2 \frac{P(s, s^p)}{P(s) P(s^p)} \ . \tag{C.37}$$

A detailed comparison of maximum likelihood and probability decoding is provided by Rolls, Treves and Tovee (1997b), but I note here that probability estimate decoding is more regularized (see below) and therefore may be safer to use when investigating the effect on the information of the number of cells. For this reason, the results described by Franco, Rolls, Aggelopoulos and Treves (2004) were obtained with probability estimation (PE) decoding. The maximum likelihood decoding does give an immediate measure of the percentage correct.

Another approach to decoding is the dot product (DP) algorithm which computes the normalized dot products between the current firing vector **r** on a "test" (i.e. the current) trial and each of the mean firing rate response vectors in the "training" trials for each stimulus s' in the cross-validation procedure. (The normalized dot product is the dot or inner product of two vectors divided by the product of the length of each vector. The length of each vector is the square root of the sum of the squares.) Thus, what is computed are the cosines of the angles of the test vector of cell rates with, in turn for each stimulus, the mean response vector to that stimulus. The highest dot product indicates the most likely stimulus that was presented, and this is taken as the predicted stimulus s^p for the probability table $P(s, s^p)$. (It can also be used to provide percentage correct measures.)

I note that any decoding procedure can be used in conjunction with information estimates both from the full probability table (to produce I_p), and from the most likely estimated stimulus for each trial (to produce I_{ml}).

Because the probability tables from which the information is calculated may be unregularized with a small number of trials, a bias correction procedure to correct for the undersampling is applied, as described in detail by Rolls, Treves and Tovee (1997b) and Panzeri and Treves (1996). In practice, the bias correction that is needed with information estimates using the decoding procedures described by Franco, Rolls, Aggelopoulos and Treves (2004) and by Rolls et al. (1997b) is small, typically less than 10% of the uncorrected estimate of the information, provided that the number of trials for each stimulus is in the order of twice the number of stimuli. We also note that the distortion in the information estimate from the full probability table needs less bias correction than that from the predicted stimulus table (i.e. maximum likelihood) method, as the former is more regularized because every trial makes some contribution through much of the probability table (see Rolls et al. (1997b)). We further note that the bias correction term becomes very small when more than 10 cells are included in the analysis (Rolls et al., 1997b).

Examples of the use of these procedures are available (Franco, Rolls, Aggelopoulos and Treves, 2004; Aggelopoulos, Franco and Rolls, 2005), and some of the results obtained are described in Section C.3.

C.2.5 Information in the correlations between the spikes of different cells: a second derivative approach

Another information theory-based approach to stimulus-dependent cross-correlation information has been developed as follows by Panzeri, Schultz, Treves and Rolls (1999a) and Rolls,

Franco, Aggelopoulos and Reece (2003b). A problem that must be overcome is the fact that with many simultaneously recorded neurons, each emitting perhaps many spikes at different times, the dimensionality of the response space becomes very large, the information tends to be overestimated, and even bias corrections cannot save the situation. The approach described in this Section (C.2.5) limits the problem by taking short time epochs for the information analysis, in which low numbers of spikes, in practice typically 0, 1, or 2, spikes are likely to occur from each neuron.

In a sufficiently short time window, at most two spikes are emitted from a population of neurons. Taking advantage of this, the response probabilities can be calculated in terms of pairwise correlations. These response probabilities are inserted into the Shannon information formula C.38 to obtain expressions quantifying the impact of the pairwise correlations on the information $I(t)$ transmitted in a short time t by groups of spiking neurons:

$$I(t) = \sum_{s \in S} \sum_{\mathbf{r}} P(s, \mathbf{r}) \log_2 \frac{P(s, \mathbf{r})}{P(s)P(\mathbf{r})} \qquad (C.38)$$

where $\mathbf{r}$ is the firing rate response vector comprised by the number of spikes emitted by each of the cells in the population in the short time t, and $P(s, \mathbf{r})$ refers to the joint probability distribution of stimuli with their respective neuronal response vectors.

The information depends upon the following two types of correlation:

C.2.5.1 The correlations in the neuronal response variability from the average to each stimulus (sometimes called "noise" correlations) γ:

$\gamma_{ij}(s)$ (for $i \neq j$) is the fraction of coincidences above (or below) that expected from uncorrelated responses, relative to the number of coincidences in the uncorrelated case (which is $\overline{n}_i(s)\overline{n}_j(s)$, the bar denoting the average across trials belonging to stimulus s, where $n_i(s)$ is the number of spikes emitted by cell i to stimulus s on a given trial)

$$\gamma_{ij}(s) = \frac{\overline{n_i(s)n_j(s)}}{(\overline{n}_i(s)\overline{n}_j(s))} - 1, \qquad (C.39)$$

and is named the 'scaled cross-correlation density'. It can vary from -1 to ∞; negative $\gamma_{ij}(s)$'s indicate anticorrelation, whereas positive $\gamma_{ij}(s)$'s indicate correlation[32]. $\gamma_{ij}(s)$ can be thought of as the amount of trial by trial concurrent firing of the cells i and j, compared to that expected in the uncorrelated case. $\gamma_{ij}(s)$ (for $i \neq j$) is the 'scaled cross-correlation density' (Aertsen, Gerstein, Habib and Palm, 1989; Panzeri, Schultz, Treves and Rolls, 1999a), and is sometimes called the "noise" correlation (Gawne and Richmond, 1993; Shadlen and Newsome, 1995, 1998; Panzeri, Moroni, Safaai and Harvey, 2022).

---

[32]$\gamma_{ij}(s)$ is an alternative, which produces a more compact information analysis, to the neuronal cross-correlation based on the Pearson correlation coefficient $\rho_{ij}(s)$ (equation C.40), which normalizes the number of coincidences above independence to the standard deviation of the number of coincidences expected if the cells were independent. The normalization used by the Pearson correlation coefficient has the advantage that it quantifies the strength of correlations between neurons in a rate-independent way. For the information analysis, it is more convenient to use the scaled correlation density $\gamma_{ij}(s)$ than the Pearson correlation coefficient, because of the compactness of the resulting formulation, and because of its scaling properties for small t. $\gamma_{ij}(s)$ remains finite as $t \to 0$, thus by using this measure we can keep the t expansion of the information explicit. Keeping the time-dependence of the resulting information components explicit greatly increases the amount of insight obtained from the series expansion. In contrast, the Pearson noise-correlation measure applied to short timescales approaches zero at short time windows:

$$\rho_{ij}(s) \equiv \frac{\overline{n_i(s)n_j(s)} - \overline{n}_i(s)\overline{n}_j(s)}{\sigma_{n_i(s)}\sigma_{n_j(s)}} \simeq t \qquad \gamma_{ij}(s) = \sqrt{\overline{r}_i(s)\overline{r}_j(s)}, \qquad (C.40)$$

where $\sigma_{n_i(s)}$ is the standard deviation of the count of spikes emitted by cell i in response to stimulus s.

C.2.5.2 The correlations in the mean responses of the neurons across the set of stimuli (sometimes called "signal" correlations) ν:

$$\nu_{ij} = \frac{<\overline{n}_i(s)\overline{n}_j(s)>_s}{<\overline{n}_i(s)>_s<\overline{n}_j(s)>_s} - 1 = \frac{<\overline{r}_i(s)\overline{r}_j(s)>_s}{<\overline{r}_i(s)>_s<\overline{r}_j(s)>_s} - 1 \qquad (C.41)$$

where $\overline{r}_i(s)$ is the mean rate of response of cell i (among C cells in total) to stimulus s over all the trials in which that stimulus was present. ν_{ij} can be thought of as the degree of similarity in the mean response profiles (averaged across trials) of the cells i and j to different stimuli. ν_{ij} is sometimes called the "signal" correlation (Gawne and Richmond, 1993; Shadlen and Newsome, 1995, 1998; Panzeri, Moroni, Safaai and Harvey, 2022).

Stimulus-independent 'noise' correlations can decrease the amount of encoded information about a stimulus if they increase the overlap between the distributions of the neuronal rates from the population. This is probably the typical case, though the opposite might occur (Panzeri et al., 2022). Stimulus-dependent 'noise' correlations, that vary in sign and/or strength across stimuli, might provide a separate channel for stimulus information encoding and might increase the amount of information that could be decoded. An example might be temporal synchronisation of the responses of different neurons only on trials on which a particular stimulus was shown (Panzeri et al., 2022). One way to measure how the effects of the correlations in the activity of populations of simultaneously recorded neurons influence the total information that can be encoded is to shuffle the data across trials for each neuron in the population (Panzeri et al., 2022). In practice, 'noise' correlations tend to decrease the information that can be decoded from populations of neurons (Panzeri et al., 2022). However, many of these analyses (Panzeri et al., 2022) assume that for example temporal synchrony between the firing of particular pairs of neurons is actually being measured in the brain and taken into account in decoding the information, and that is not at all clear. Overall, 'noise' correlations are not likely to increase the information that is used in the brain, and if anything may decrease the information that is being used by the brain. Further evidence is provided in Section C.3.7.

C.2.5.3 Information in the cross-correlations in short time periods

In the short timescale limit, the first (I_t) and second (I_{tt}) information derivatives describe the information $I(t)$ available in the short time t

$$I(t) = t\, I_t + \frac{t^2}{2} I_{tt} \, . \qquad (C.42)$$

(The zeroth order, time-independent term is zero, as no information can be transmitted by the neurons in a time window of zero length. Higher order terms are also excluded as they become negligible.)

The instantaneous information rate I_t is[33]

$$I_t = \sum_{i=1}^{C} \left\langle \overline{r}_i(s) \log_2 \frac{\overline{r}_i(s)}{\langle \overline{r}_i(s') \rangle_{s'}} \right\rangle_s . \qquad (C.43)$$

This formula shows that this information rate (the first time derivative) should not be linked to a high signal to noise ratio, but only reflects the extent to which the mean responses of each

---

[33] Note that s' is used in Equations C.43 and C.44 just as a dummy variable to stand for s, as there are two summations performed over s.

cell are distributed across stimuli. It does not reflect anything of the variability of those responses, that is of their noisiness, nor anything of the correlations among the mean responses of different cells.

The effect of (pairwise) correlations between the cells begins to be expressed in the second time derivative of the information. The expression for the instantaneous information 'acceleration' I_{tt} (the second time derivative of the information) breaks up into three terms:

$$I_{tt} = \frac{1}{\ln 2} \sum_{i=1}^{C} \sum_{j=1}^{C} \langle \bar{r}_i(s) \rangle_s \langle \bar{r}_j(s) \rangle_s \left[\nu_{ij} + (1+\nu_{ij}) \ln(\frac{1}{1+\nu_{ij}}) \right]$$
$$+ \sum_{i=1}^{C} \sum_{j=1}^{C} \left[\langle \bar{r}_i(s) \bar{r}_j(s) \gamma_{ij}(s) \rangle_s \right] \log_2(\frac{1}{1+\nu_{ij}})$$
$$+ \sum_{i=1}^{C} \sum_{j=1}^{C} \left\langle \bar{r}_i(s) \bar{r}_j(s)(1+\gamma_{ij}(s)) \log_2 \left[\frac{(1+\gamma_{ij}(s)) \langle \bar{r}_i(s') \bar{r}_j(s') \rangle_{s'}}{\langle \bar{r}_i(s') \bar{r}_j(s')(1+\gamma_{ij}(s')) \rangle_{s'}} \right] \right\rangle_s . \quad \text{(C.44)}$$

The first of these terms is all that survives if there is no noise correlation at all. Thus the *rate component* of the information is given by the sum of I_t (which is always greater than or equal to zero) and of the first term of I_{tt} (which is instead always less than or equal to zero).

The second term is non-zero if there is some correlation in the variance to a given stimulus, even if it is independent of which stimulus is present; this term thus represents the contribution of *stimulus-independent noise correlation* to the information.

The third component of I_{tt} represents the contribution of *stimulus-modulated noise correlation*, as it becomes non-zero only for stimulus-dependent noise correlations. These last two terms of I_{tt} together are referred to as the correlational components of the information.

The application of this approach to measuring the information in the relative time of firing of simultaneously recorded cells, together with further details of the method, are described by Panzeri, Treves, Schultz and Rolls (1999b), Rolls, Franco, Aggelopoulos and Reece (2003b), and Rolls, Aggelopoulos, Franco and Treves (2004), and in Section C.3.7.

Further approaches to measuring how the correlations in the activity of populations of simultaneously recorded neurons influences the total information that can be encoded include shuffling the data across trials for each neuron in the population (Panzeri et al., 2022).

C.3 Neuronal encoding: results obtained from applying information-theoretic analyses

How is information encoded in cortical areas such as the inferior temporal visual cortex? Can we read the code being used by the cortex? What are the advantages of the encoding scheme used for the neuronal network computations being performed in different areas of the cortex? These are some of the key issues considered in this Section (C.3). Because information is exchanged between the computing elements of the cortex (the neurons) by their spiking activity, which is conveyed by their axon to synapses onto other neurons, the appropriate level of analysis is how single neurons, and populations of single neurons, encode information in their firing. More global measures that reflect the averaged activity of large numbers of neurons (for example, PET (positron emission tomography) and fMRI (functional magnetic resonance imaging), EEG (electroencephalographic recording), and ERPs (event-related potentials)) cannot reveal how the information is represented, or how the computation is being performed.

Although information theory provides the natural mathematical framework for analysing the performance of neuronal systems, its applications in neuroscience have been for many years rather sparse and episodic (e.g. MacKay and McCulloch (1952); Eckhorn and Popel (1974); Eckhorn and Popel (1975); Eckhorn, Grusser, Kroller, Pellnitz and Popel (1976); Rolls and Treves (2011); Meshulam, Gauthier, Brody, Tank and Bialek (2017); and Panzeri et al. (2022)). One reason for this limited application of information theory has been the great effort that was apparently required, due essentially to the limited sampling problem, in order to obtain accurate results. Another reason has been the hesitation in analysing as a single complex 'black-box' large neuronal systems all the way from some external, easily controllable inputs, up to neuronal activity in some central cortical area of interest, for example including all visual stations from the periphery to the end of the ventral visual stream in the temporal lobe. In fact, two important bodies of work, that have greatly helped revive interest in applications of the theory in recent years, both sidestep these two problems. The problem with analyzing a huge black-box is avoided by considering systems at the sensory periphery; the limited sampling problem is avoided either by working with insects, in which sampling can be extensive (Bialek, Rieke, de Ruyter van Steveninck and Warland, 1991; de Ruyter van Steveninck and Laughlin, 1996; Rieke, Warland, de Ruyter van Steveninck and Bialek, 1997), or by utilizing a formal model instead of real data (Atick and Redlich, 1990; Atick, 1992). Both approaches have provided insightful quantitative analyses that have been extended to more central mammalian systems (see e.g. Atick, Griffin and Relich (1996)).

In the treatment provided here, we focus on applications to the mammalian brain, using examples from a whole series of investigations on information representation in visual cortical areas, the original papers on which refer to related publications.

C.3.1 The sparseness of the distributed encoding used by the brain

Some of the types of representation that might be found at the neuronal level are summarized next (cf. Section 1.7). A **local representation** is one in which all the information that a particular stimulus or event occurred is provided by the activity of one of the neurons. This is sometimes called a grandmother cell representation, because in a famous example, a single neuron might be active only if one's grandmother was being seen (see Barlow (1995)). A **fully distributed representation** is one in which all the information that a particular stimulus or event occurred is provided by the activity of the full set of neurons. If the neurons are binary (for example, either active or not), the most distributed encoding is when half the neurons are active for any one stimulus or event. A **sparse distributed representation** is a distributed representation in which a small proportion of the neurons is active at any one time.

C.3.1.1 Single neuron sparseness a^s

Equation C.45 defines a measure of the single neuron sparseness, a^s:

$$a^s = \frac{(\sum_{s=1}^{S} y_s/S)^2}{(\sum_{s=1}^{S} y_s^2)/S} \tag{C.45}$$

where y_s is the mean firing rate of the neuron to stimulus s in the set of S stimuli (Rolls and Treves, 1998). For a binary representation, a^s is 0.5 for a fully distributed representation, and $1/S$ if a neuron responds to one of a set of S stimuli. Another measure of sparseness is the kurtosis of the distribution, which is the fourth moment of the distribution. It reflects the length of the tail of the distribution. (An actual distribution of the firing rates of a neuron to a set of 65 stimuli is shown in Fig. C.4. The sparseness a^s for this neuron was 0.69 (see Rolls, Treves, Tovee and Panzeri (1997d).)

It is important to understand and quantify the sparseness of representations in the brain, because many of the useful properties of neuronal networks such as generalization and completion only occur if the representations are not local (see Appendix B), and because the value of the sparseness is an important factor in how many memories can be stored in such neural networks. Relatively sparse representations (low values of a^s) might be expected in memory systems as this will increase the number of different memories that can be stored and retrieved. Less sparse representations might be expected in sensory systems, as this could allow more information to be represented (see Table B.2).

Barlow (1972) proposed a single neuron doctrine for perceptual psychology. He proposed that sensory systems are organized to achieve as complete a representation as possible with the minimum number of active neurons. He suggested that at progressively higher levels of sensory processing, fewer and fewer cells are active, and that each represents a more and more specific happening in the sensory environment. He suggested that 1,000 active neurons (which he called cardinal cells) might represent the whole of a visual scene. An important principle involved in forming such a representation was the reduction of redundancy. The implication of Barlow's (1972) approach was that when an object is being recognized, there are, towards the end of the visual system, a small number of neurons (the cardinal cells) that are so specifically tuned that the activity of these neurons encodes the information that one particular object is being seen. (He thought that an active neuron conveys something of the order of complexity of a word.) The encoding of information in such a system is described as local, in that knowing the activity of just one neuron provides evidence that a particular stimulus (or, more exactly, a given 'trigger feature') is present. Barlow (1972) eschewed 'combinatorial rules of usage of nerve cells', and believed that the subtlety and sensitivity of perception results from the mechanisms determining when a single cell becomes active. In contrast, with distributed or ensemble encoding, the activity of several or many neurons must be known in order to identify which stimulus is present, that is, to read the code. It is the relative firing of the different neurons in the ensemble that provides the information about which object is present.

At the time Barlow (1972) wrote, there was little actual evidence on the activity of neurons in the higher parts of the visual and other sensory systems. There is now considerable evidence, which is now described.

First, it has been shown that the representation of which particular object (face) is present is actually rather distributed. Baylis, Rolls and Leonard (1985) showed this with the responses of temporal cortical neurons that typically responded to several members of a set of five faces, with each neuron having a different profile of responses to each face (see examples in Fig. 2.17 on page 76). It would be difficult for most of these single cells to tell which of even five faces, let alone which of hundreds of faces, had been seen. (At the same time, the neurons discriminated between the faces reliably, as shown by the values of d', taken, in the case of the neurons, to be the number of standard deviations of the neuronal responses that separated the response to the best face in the set from that to the least effective face in the set. The values of d' were typically in the range 1–3.)

Second, the distributed nature of the representation can be further understood by the finding that the firing rate probability distribution of single neurons, when a wide range of natural visual stimuli are being viewed, is approximately exponential, with rather few stimuli producing high firing rates, and increasingly large numbers of stimuli producing lower and lower firing rates, as illustrated in Fig. C.5a (Rolls and Tovee, 1995b; Baddeley, Abbott, Booth, Sengpiel, Freeman, Wakeman and Rolls, 1997; Treves, Panzeri, Rolls, Booth and Wakeman, 1999; Franco, Rolls, Aggelopoulos and Jerez, 2007).

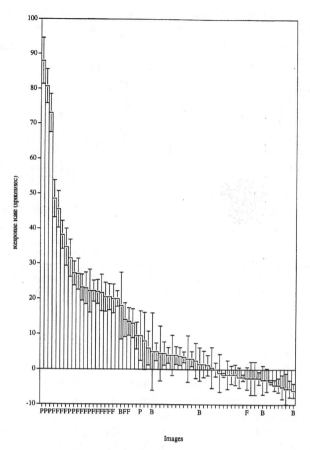

Fig. C.4 Single neuron sparseness. Firing rate distribution of a single neuron in the temporal visual cortex to a set of 23 face (F) and 45 non-face images of natural scenes. The firing rate to each of the 68 stimuli is shown. The neuron does not respond to just one of the 68 stimuli. Instead, it responds to a small proportion of stimuli with high rates, to more stimuli with intermediate rates, and to many stimuli with almost no change of firing. This is typical of the distributed representations found in temporal cortical visual areas. (After Rolls, E. T. and Tovee, M.J. (1995) Sparseness of the neuronal representation of stimuli in the primate temporal visual cortex. Journal of Neurophysiology 73: 713–726.)

For example, the responses of a set of temporal cortical neurons to 23 faces and 42 non-face natural images were measured, and a distributed representation was found (Rolls and Tovee, 1995b). The tuning was typically graded, with a range of different firing rates to the set of faces, and very little response to the non-face stimuli (see example in Fig. C.4). The spontaneous firing rate of the neuron in Fig. C.4 was 20 spikes/s, and the histogram bars indicate the change of firing rate from the spontaneous value produced by each stimulus. Stimuli that are faces are marked F, or P if they are in profile. B refers to images of scenes that included either a small face within the scene, sometimes as part of an image that included a whole person, or other body parts, such as hands (H) or legs. The non-face stimuli are unlabelled. The neuron responded best to three of the faces (profile views), had some response to some of the other faces, and had little or no response, and sometimes had a small decrease of firing rate below the spontaneous firing rate, to the non-face stimuli. The sparseness value a^s for this cell across all 68 stimuli was 0.69, and the response sparseness a_r^s (based on the evoked responses minus the spontaneous firing of the neuron) was 0.19. It was found that the sparseness of the representation of the 68 stimuli by each neuron had an average across all neurons of 0.65 (Rolls and Tovee, 1995b). This indicates a rather distributed representation. (If neurons had a continuum of firing rates equally distributed between zero and maximum

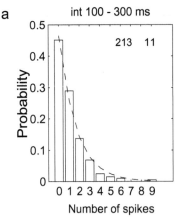 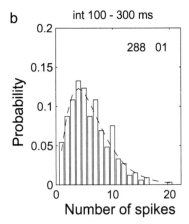

Fig. C.5 Firing rate probability distributions. These are shown for two neurons in the inferior temporal visual cortex tested with a set of 20 face and non-face stimuli. (a) A neuron with a good fit to an exponential probability distribution (dashed line). (b) A neuron that did not fit an exponential firing rate distribution (but which could be fitted by a gamma distribution, dashed line). The firing rates were measured in an interval 100–300 ms after the onset of the visual stimuli, and similar distributions are obtained in other intervals. (After Franco,L., Rolls, E. T., Aggelopoulos,N.C. and Jerez,J.M. (2007) Neuronal selectivity, population sparseness, and ergodicity in the inferior temporal visual cortex. Biological Cybernetics 96: 547-560. © Springer Nature.)

rate, a^s would be 0.75, while if the probability of each response decreased linearly, to reach zero at the maximum rate, a^s would be 0.67).

I comment that these values for a do not seem very sparse. But these values are calculated using the raw firing rates of the neurons, on the basis that these would be what a receiving neuron would receive as its input representation. However, neocortical neurons have a spontaneous firing rate of several spikes/s (with a lower value of 0.75 spikes/s for hippocampal pyramidal cells), and if this spontaneous value is subtracted from the firing rates to yield a 'response sparseness' a_r, this value is considerably lower. For example, the sparseness a of inferior temporal cortex responses to a set of 68 stimuli had an average across all neurons that we analyzed in this study of 0.65 (Rolls and Tovee, 1995b). If the spontaneous firing rate was subtracted from the firing rate of the neuron to each stimulus, so that the changes of firing rate, i.e., the responses of the neurons, were used in the sparseness calculation, then the 'response sparseness' had a lower value, with a mean of $a_r=0.33$ for the population of neurons, or 0.60 if calculated over the set of faces rather than over all the face and non-face stimuli. Further, the true sparseness of the representation is probably much less than this, for this is calculated only over the neurons that had responses to some of these stimuli. There were many more neurons that had no response to the stimuli. At least 10 times the number of inferior temporal cortex neurons had no responses to this set of 68 stimuli. So the true sparseness would be much lower that this value of 0.33. Further, it is important to remember the relative nature of sparseness measures, which (like the information measures to be discussed below) depend strongly on the stimulus set used. Thus we can reject a cardinal cell representation. As shown below, the readout of information from these cells is actually much better in any case than would be obtained from a local representation, and this makes it unlikely that there is a further population of neurons with very specific tuning that use local encoding.

These data provide a clear answer to whether these neurons are grandmother cells: they are not, in the sense that each neuron has a graded set of responses to the different members of a set of stimuli, with the prototypical distribution similar to that of the neuron illustrated in Fig. C.4. On the other hand, each neuron does respond very much more to some stimuli than to many others, and in this sense is tuned to some stimuli.

Figure C.5 shows data of the type shown in Fig. C.4 as firing rate probability density

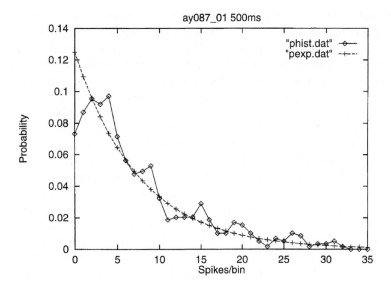

Fig. C.6 Firing rate probability distribution for a single neuron, using natural world image statistics. The probability of different firing rates measured in short (e.g. 100 ms or 500 ms) time windows of a temporal cortex neuron calculated over a 5 min period in which the macaque watched a video showing natural scenes, including faces. An exponential fit (+) to the data (diamonds) is shown. (After Baddeley,R.J., Abbott,L.F., Booth,M.J.A., Sengpiel,F., Freeman,T., Wakeman,E.A., and Rolls, E. T. (1997) Responses of neurons in primary and inferior temporal visual cortices to natural scenes. Proceedings of the Royal Society B 264: 1775-1783.)

functions, that is as the probability that the neuron will be firing with particular rates. These data were from inferior temporal cortex neurons, and show when tested with a set of 20 face and non-face stimuli how fast the neuron will be firing in a period 100–300 ms after the visual stimulus appears (Franco, Rolls, Aggelopoulos and Jerez, 2007). Figure C.5a shows an example of a neuron where the data fit an exponential firing rate probability distribution, with many occasions on which the neuron was firing with a very low firing rate, and decreasingly few occasions on which it fired at higher rates. This shows that the neuron can have high firing rates, but only to a few stimuli. Figure C.5b shows an example of a neuron where the data do not fit an exponential firing rate probability distribution, with insufficiently few very low rates. Of the 41 responsive neurons in this data set, 15 had a good fit to an exponential firing rate probability distribution; the other 26 neurons did not fit an exponential but did fit a gamma distribution in the way illustrated in Fig. C.5b. For the neurons with an exponential distribution, the mean firing rate across the stimulus set was 5.7 spikes/s, and for the neurons with a gamma distribution was 21.1 spikes/s (t=4.5, df=25, $p < 0.001$). It may be that neurons with high mean rates to a stimulus set tend to have few low rates ever, and this accounts for their poor fit to an exponential firing rate probability distribution, which fits when there are many low firing rate values in the distribution as in Fig. C.5a.

The large set of 68 stimuli used by Rolls and Tovee (1995b) was chosen to produce an approximation to a set of stimuli that might be found to natural stimuli in a natural environment, and thus to provide evidence about the firing rate distribution of neurons to natural stimuli. Another approach to the same fundamental question was taken by Baddeley, Abbott, Booth, Sengpiel, Freeman, Wakeman, and Rolls (1997) who measured the firing rates over short periods of individual inferior temporal cortex neurons while monkeys watched continuous videos of natural scenes. They found that the firing rates of the neurons were again approximately exponentially distributed (see Fig. C.6), providing further evidence that this type of representation is characteristic of inferior temporal cortex (and indeed also V1) neurons.

The actual distribution of the firing rates to a wide set of natural stimuli is of interest, because it has a rather stereotypical shape, typically following a graded unimodal distribution with a long tail extending to high rates (see for example Figs. C.5a and C.6). The mode of the distribution is close to the spontaneous firing rate, and sometimes it is at zero firing. If the number of spikes recorded in a fixed time window is taken to be constrained by a fixed maximum rate, one can try to interpret the distribution observed in terms of optimal information transmission (Shannon, 1948), by making the additional assumption that the coding is noiseless. An exponential distribution, which maximizes entropy (and hence information transmission for noiseless codes) is the most efficient in terms of energy consumption if its mean takes an optimal value that is a decreasing function of the relative metabolic cost of emitting a spike (Levy and Baxter, 1996). This argument would favour sparser coding schemes the more energy expensive neuronal firing is (relative to rest). Although the tail of actual firing rate distributions is often approximately exponential (see for example Figs. C.5a and C.6; Baddeley, Abbott, Booth, Sengpiel, Freeman, Wakeman and Rolls (1997); Rolls, Treves, Tovee and Panzeri (1997d); and Franco, Rolls, Aggelopoulos and Jerez (2007)), the maximum entropy argument cannot apply as such, because noise is present and the noise level varies as a function of the rate, which makes entropy maximization different from information maximization. Moreover, a mode at low but non-zero rate, which is often observed (see e.g. Fig. C.5b), is inconsistent with the energy efficiency hypothesis.

A simpler explanation for the characteristic firing rate distribution arises by appreciating that the value of the activation of a neuron across stimuli, reflecting a multitude of contributing factors, will typically have a Gaussian distribution; and by considering a physiological input–output transform (i.e. activation function), and realistic noise levels. In fact, an input–output transform that is supralinear in a range above threshold results from a fundamentally linear transform and fluctuations in the activation, and produces a variance in the output rate, across repeated trials, that increases with the rate itself, consistent with common observations. At the same time, such a supralinear transform tends to convert the Gaussian tail of the activation distribution into an approximately exponential tail, without implying a fully exponential distribution with the mode at zero. Such basic assumptions yield excellent fits with observed distributions (Treves, Panzeri, Rolls, Booth and Wakeman, 1999), which often differ from exponential in that there are too few very low rates observed, and too many low rates (Rolls, Treves, Tovee and Panzeri, 1997d; Franco, Rolls, Aggelopoulos and Jerez, 2007).

This peak at low but non-zero rates may be related to the low firing rate spontaneous activity that is typical of many cortical neurons. Keeping the neurons close to threshold in this way may maximize the speed with which a network can respond to new inputs (because time is not required to bring the neurons from a strongly hyperpolarized state up to threshold). The advantage of having low spontaneous firing rates may be a further reason why a curve such as an exponential cannot sometimes be exactly fitted to the experimental data.

A conclusion of this analysis was that the firing rate distribution may arise from the threshold non-linearity of neurons combined with short-term variability in the responses of neurons (Treves, Panzeri, Rolls, Booth and Wakeman, 1999).

However, given that the firing rate distribution for some neurons is approximately exponential, some properties of this type of representation are worth elucidation. The sparseness of such an exponential distribution of firing rates is 0.5. This has interesting implications, for to the extent that the firing rates are exponentially distributed, this fixes an important parameter of cortical neuronal encoding to be close to 0.5. Indeed, only one parameter specifies the shape of the exponential distribution, and the fact that the exponential distribution is at least a close approximation to the firing rate distribution of some real cortical neurons implies that the sparseness of the cortical representation of stimuli is kept under precise control. The utility of this may be to ensure that any neuron receiving from this representation can

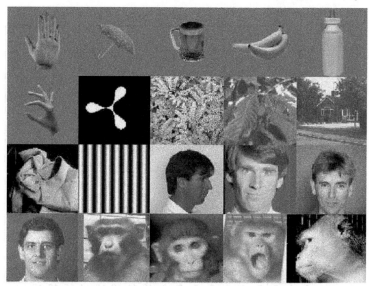

Fig. C.7 The set of 20 stimuli used to investigate the tuning of inferior temporal cortex neurons by Franco, Rolls, Aggelopoulos and Jerez 2007. These objects and faces are typical of those encoded in the ways described here by inferior temporal cortex neurons. The code can be read off simply from the firing rates of the neurons about which object or face was shown, and many of the neurons have invariant responses. (After Franco,L., Rolls, E. T., Aggelopoulos,N.C. and Jerez,J.M. (2007) Neuronal selectivity, population sparseness, and ergodicity in the inferior temporal visual cortex. Biological Cybernetics 96: 547-560. © Springer Nature.)

perform a dot product operation between its inputs and its synaptic weights that produces similarly distributed outputs; and that the information being represented by a population of cortical neurons is kept high. It is interesting to realize that the representation that is stored in an associative network (see Appendix B) may be more sparse than the 0.5 value for an exponential firing rate distribution, because the non-linearity of learning introduced by the voltage dependence of the NMDA receptors (see Appendix B) effectively means that synaptic modification in, for example, an autoassociative network will occur only for the neurons with relatively high firing rates, i.e. for those that are strongly depolarized.

The single neuron selectivity reflects response distributions of individual neurons across time to different stimuli. As we have seen, part of the interest of measuring the firing rate probability distributions of individual neurons is that one form of the probability distribution, the exponential, maximizes the entropy of the neuronal responses for a given mean firing rate, which could be used to maximize information transmission consistent with keeping the firing rate on average low, in order to minimize metabolic expenditure (Levy and Baxter, 1996; Baddeley, Abbott, Booth, Sengpiel, Freeman, Wakeman and Rolls, 1997). Franco, Rolls, Aggelopoulos and Jerez (2007) showed that while the firing rates of some single inferior temporal cortex neurons (tested in a visual fixation task to a set of 20 face and non-face stimuli illustrated in Fig. C.7) do fit an exponential distribution, and others with higher spontaneous firing rates do not, as described above, it turns out that there is a very close fit to an exponential distribution of firing rates if all spikes from all the neurons are considered together. This interesting result is shown in Fig. C.8.

One implication of the result shown in Fig. C.8 is that a neuron with inputs from the inferior temporal visual cortex will receive an exponential distribution of firing rates on its afferents, and this is therefore the type of input that needs to be considered in theoretical models of neuronal network function in the brain (see Appendix B). The second implication is that at the level of single neurons, an exponential probability density function is consistent with minimizing energy utilization, and maximizing information transmission, for a given mean

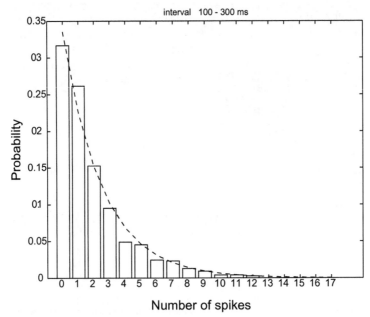

Fig. C.8 The firing rate probability distribution of single neurons is approximately exponential. An exponential firing rate probability distribution obtained by pooling the firing rates of a population of 41 inferior temporal cortex neurons tested to a set of 20 face and non-face stimuli. The firing rate probability distribution for the 100–300 ms interval following stimulus onset was formed by adding the spike counts from all 41 neurons, and across all stimuli. The fit to the exponential distribution (dashed line) was high. (After Franco,L., Rolls, E. T., Aggelopoulos,N.C. and Jerez,J.M. (2007) Neuronal selectivity, population sparseness, and ergodicity in the inferior temporal visual cortex. Biological Cybernetics 96: 547–560. © Springer Nature.)

firing rate (Levy and Baxter, 1996; Baddeley, Abbott, Booth, Sengpiel, Freeman, Wakeman and Rolls, 1997).

C.3.1.2 Population sparseness a^p

If instead we consider the responses of a population of neurons taken at any one time (to one stimulus), we might also expect a sparse graded distribution, with few neurons firing fast to a particular stimulus. It is important to measure the population sparseness, for this is a key parameter that influences the number of different stimuli that can be stored and retrieved in networks such as those found in the cortex with recurrent collateral connections between the excitatory neurons, which can form autoassociation or attractor networks if the synapses are associatively modifiable (Hopfield, 1982; Treves and Rolls, 1991; Rolls and Treves, 1998; Rolls and Deco, 2002; Rolls, 2016b) (see Appendix B). Further, in physics, if one can predict the distribution of the responses of the system at any one time (the population level) from the distribution of the responses of a component of the system across time, the system is described as ergodic, and a necessary condition for this is that the components are uncorrelated (Lehky, Sejnowski and Desimone, 2005). Considering this in neuronal terms, the average sparseness of a population of neurons over multiple stimulus inputs must equal the average selectivity to the stimuli of the single neurons within the population provided that the responses of the neurons are uncorrelated (Földiák, 2003).

The sparseness a^p of the population code may be quantified (for any one stimulus) as

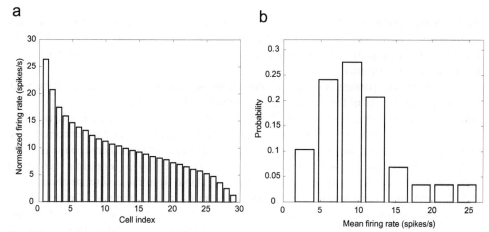

Fig. C.9 Population sparseness. (a) The firing rates of a population of inferior temporal cortex neurons to any one stimulus from a set of 20 face and non-face stimuli. The rates of each neuron were normalized to the same average value of 10 spikes/s, then for each stimulus, the cell firing rates were placed in rank order, and then the mean firing rates of the first ranked cell, second ranked cell, etc. were taken. The graph thus shows how, for any one stimulus picked at random, the expected normalized firing rates of the population of neurons. (b) The population normalized firing rate probability distributions for any one stimulus. This was computed effectively by taking the probability density function of the data shown in (a). (After Franco,L., Rolls, E. T., Aggelopoulos,N.C. and Jerez,J.M. (2007) Neuronal selectivity, population sparseness, and ergodicity in the inferior temporal visual cortex. Biological Cybernetics 96: 547–560. © Springer Nature.)

$$a^p = \frac{(\sum_{n=1}^{N} y_n/N)^2}{(\sum_{n=1}^{N} y_n^2)/N} \tag{C.46}$$

where y_n is the mean firing rate of neuron n in the set of N neurons.

This measure, a^p, of the sparseness of the representation of a stimulus by a population of neurons has a number of advantages. One is that it is the same measure of sparseness that has proved to be useful and tractable in formal analyses of the capacity of associative neural networks and the interference between stimuli that use an approach derived from theoretical physics (Rolls and Treves, 1990; Treves, 1990; Treves and Rolls, 1991; Rolls and Treves, 1998) (see Appendix B). I note that high values of a^p indicate broad tuning of the population, and that low values of a^p indicate sparse population encoding.

Franco, Rolls, Aggelopoulos and Jerez (2007) measured the population sparseness of a set of 29 inferior temporal cortex neurons to a set of 20 stimuli that included faces and objects (see Fig. C.7). Figure C.9a shows, for any one stimulus picked at random, the normalized firing rates of the population of neurons. The rates are ranked with the neuron with the highest rate on the left. For different stimuli, the shape of this distribution is on average the same, though with the neurons in a different order. (The rates of each neuron were normalized to a mean of 10 spikes/s before this graph was made, so that the neurons can be combined in the same graph, and so that the population sparseness has a defined value, as described by Franco, Rolls, Aggelopoulos and Jerez (2007).) The population sparseness a^p of this normalized (i.e. scaled) set of firing rates is 0.77.

Figure C.9b shows the probability distribution of the normalized firing rates of the population of (29) neurons to any stimulus from the set. This was calculated by taking the probability distribution of the data shown in Fig. C.9a. This distribution is not exponential because of the normalization of the firing rates of each neuron, but becomes exponential as shown in Fig. C.8 without the normalization step.

A very interesting finding of Franco, Rolls, Aggelopoulos and Jerez (2007) was that when the single cell sparseness a^s and the population sparseness a^p were measured from the same set of neurons in the same experiment, the values were very close, in this case 0.77. (This was found for a range of measurement intervals after stimulus onset, and also for a larger population of 41 neurons.)

The single cell sparseness a^s and the population sparseness a^p can take the same value if the response profiles of the neurons are uncorrelated, that is each neuron is independently tuned to the set of stimuli (Lehky et al., 2005). Franco, Rolls, Aggelopoulos and Jerez (2007) tested whether the response profiles of the neurons to the set of stimuli were uncorrelated in two ways. In a first test, they found that the mean (Pearson) correlation between the response profiles computed over the 406 neuron pairs was low, 0.049 ± 0.013 (sem). In a second test, they computed how the multiple cell information available from these neurons about which stimulus was shown increased as the number of neurons in the sample was increased, and showed that the information increased approximately linearly with the number of neurons in the ensemble. The implication is that the neurons convey independent (non-redundant) information, and this would be expected to occur if the response profiles of the neurons to the stimuli are uncorrelated.

We now consider the concept of ergodicity. The single neuron selectivity, a^s, reflects response distributions of individual neurons across time and therefore stimuli in the world (and has sometimes been termed "lifetime sparseness"). The population sparseness a^p reflects response distributions across all neurons in a population measured simultaneously (to for example one stimulus). The similarity of the average values of a^s and a^p (both 0.77 for inferior temporal cortex neurons (Franco, Rolls, Aggelopoulos and Jerez, 2007)) indicates, we believe for the first time experimentally, that the representation (at least in the inferior temporal cortex) is ergodic. The representation is ergodic in the sense of statistical physics, where the average of a single component (in this context a single neuron) across time is compared with the average of an ensemble of components at one time (cf. Masuda and Aihara (2003) and Lehky et al. (2005)). This is described further next.

In comparing the neuronal selectivities a^s and population sparsenesses a^p, we formed a table in which the columns represent different neurons, and the stimuli different rows (Földiák, 2003). We are interested in the probability distribution functions (and not just their summary values a^s, and a^p), of the columns (which represent the individual neuron selectivities) and the rows (which represent the population tuning to any one stimulus). We could call the system strongly ergodic (cf. Lehky et al. (2005)) if the selectivity (probability density or distribution function) of each individual neuron is the same as the average population sparseness (probability density function). (Each neuron would be tuned to different stimuli, but have the same shape of the probability density function.) We have seen that this is not the case, in that the firing rate probability distribution functions of different neurons are different, with some fitting an exponential function, and some a gamma function (see Fig. C.5). We can call the system weakly ergodic if individual neurons have different selectivities (i.e. different response probability density functions), but the average selectivity (measured in our case by $< a^s >$) is the same as the average population sparseness (measured by $< a^p >$), where $< ... >$ indicates the ensemble average. We have seen that for inferior temporal cortex neurons the neuron selectivity probability density functions are different (see Fig. C.5), but that their average $< a^s >$ is the same as the average (across stimuli) $< a^p >$ of the population sparseness, 0.77, and thus conclude that the representation in the inferior temporal visual cortex of objects and faces is weakly ergodic (Franco, Rolls, Aggelopoulos and Jerez, 2007).

I note that weak ergodicity necessarily occurs if $< a^s >$ and $< a^p >$ are the same and the neurons are uncorrelated, that is each neuron is independently tuned to the set of stimuli (Lehky et al., 2005). The fact that both hold for the inferior temporal cortex neurons studied by Franco, Rolls, Aggelopoulos and Jerez (2007) thus indicates that their responses are uncorrelated, and this is potentially an important conclusion about the encoding of stimuli by these neurons. This conclusion is confirmed by the linear increase in the information with the number of neurons which is the case not only for this set of neurons (Franco, Rolls, Aggelopoulos and Jerez, 2007), but also in other data sets for the inferior temporal visual cortex (Rolls, Treves and Tovee, 1997b; Booth and Rolls, 1998). Both types of evidence thus indicate that the encoding provided by at least small subsets (up to e.g. 20 neurons) of inferior temporal cortex neurons is approximately independent (non-redundant), which is an important principle of cortical encoding.

C.3.1.3 Comparisons of sparseness between areas: the hippocampus, insula, orbitofrontal cortex, and amygdala

In the study of Franco, Rolls, Aggelopoulos and Jerez (2007) on inferior temporal visual cortex neurons, the selectivity of individual cells for the set of stimuli, or single cell sparseness a^s, had a mean value of 0.77. This is close to a previously measured estimate, 0.65, which was obtained with a larger stimulus set of 68 stimuli (Rolls and Tovee, 1995b). Thus the single neuron probability density functions in these areas do not produce very sparse representations. Therefore the goal of the computations in the inferior temporal visual cortex may not be to produce sparse representations (as has been proposed for V1 (Field, 1994; Olshausen and Field, 1997; Vinje and Gallant, 2000; Olshausen and Field, 2004)). Instead one of the goals of the computations in the inferior temporal visual cortex may be to compute invariant representations of objects and faces (Rolls, 2000a; Rolls and Deco, 2002; Rolls, 2007e; Rolls and Stringer, 2006b) (see Chapter 2), and to produce not very sparse distributed representations in order to maximize the information represented (see Table B.2 on page 831). In this context, it is very interesting that the representations of different stimuli provided by a population of inferior temporal cortex neurons are decorrelated, as shown by the finding that the mean (Pearson) correlation between the response profiles to a set of 20 stimuli computed over 406 neuron pairs was low, 0.049 ± 0.013 (sem) (Franco, Rolls, Aggelopoulos and Jerez, 2007). The implication is that decorrelation is being achieved in the inferior temporal visual cortex, but not by forming a sparse code. It will be interesting to investigate the mechanisms for this.

In contrast, the representation in some memory systems may be more sparse (Rolls and Treves, 2011; Rolls, 2023d). For example, in the hippocampus in which spatial view cells are found in macaques, further analysis (Rolls and Treves, 2011) of data described by Rolls, Treves, Robertson, Georges-François and Panzeri (1998b) shows that for the representation of 64 locations around the walls of the room, the mean single cell sparseness a^s was 0.34 ± 0.13 (sd), and the mean population sparseness a^p was 0.33 ± 0.11. The more sparse representation is consistent with the view that the hippocampus is involved in storing memories, and that for this, more sparse representations than in perceptual areas are relevant. These sparseness values are for spatial view neurons, but it is possible that when neurons respond to combinations of spatial view and object (Rolls, Xiang and Franco, 2005c), or of spatial view and reward (Rolls and Xiang, 2005), the representations are more sparse. It is of interest that the mean firing rate of these spatial view neurons across all spatial views was 1.77 spikes/s (Rolls, Treves, Robertson, Georges-François and Panzeri, 1998b). (The mean spontaneous firing rate of the neurons was 0.1 spikes/s, and the average across neurons of the firing rate for the most effective spatial view was 13.2 spikes/s.) It is also notable that weak ergodicity is implied for this brain region too (given the similar values of a^s and a^p), and the underlying basis for this is that the response profiles of the different hippocampal neurons to the spatial views are uncorrelated. Further support for these conclusions is that the information about spatial view increases linearly with the number of hippocampal spatial view neurons (Rolls, Treves, Robertson, Georges-François and Panzeri, 1998b), again providing evidence that the response profiles of the different neurons are uncorrelated. The representations in the hippocampus may be more sparse than this, in line with the observation that in rodents, hippocampal neurons may have place fields in only one of several environments.

Further evidence is now available on ergodicity in three further brain areas, the macaque insular primary taste cortex, the orbitofrontal cortex, and the amygdala (Rolls, Critchley, Verhagen and Kadohisa, 2010a). In all these brain areas sets of neurons were tested with an identical set of 24 oral taste, temperature, and texture stimuli. (The stimuli were: Taste - 0.1 M NaCl (salt), 1 M glucose (sweet), 0.01 M HCl (sour), 0.001 M quinine HCl (bitter), 0.1 M monosodium glutamate (umami), and water; Temperature - 10°C, 37°C and 42°C; flavor - blackcurrant juice; viscosity - carboxymethyl-cellulose 10 cPoise, 100 cPoise, 1000 cPoise and 10000 cPoise; fatty / oily - single cream, vegetable oil, mineral oil, silicone oil (100 cPoise), coconut oil, and safflower oil; fatty acids - linoleic acid and lauric acid; capsaicin; and gritty texture.) Further analysis of data described by Verhagen, Kadohisa and Rolls (2004) showed that in the primary taste cortex the mean value of a^s across 58 neurons was 0.745 and of a^p (normalized) was 0.708. Further analysis of data described by Rolls, Verhagen and Kadohisa (2003e), Verhagen, Rolls and Kadohisa (2003), Kadohisa, Rolls and Verhagen (2004) and Kadohisa, Rolls and Verhagen (2005a) showed that in the orbitofrontal cortex the mean value of a^s across 30 neurons was 0.625 and of a^p was 0.611. Further analysis of data described by Kadohisa, Rolls and Verhagen (2005b) showed that in the amygdala the mean value of a^s across 38 neurons was 0.811 and of a^p was 0.813. Thus in all these cases, the mean value of a^s is close to that of a^p, and weak ergodicity is implied (Rolls and Treves, 2011). The values of a^s and a^p are also relatively high, implying the importance of representing large amounts of information in these brain areas about this set of stimuli by using a very distributed code, and also perhaps about the stimulus set, some members of which may be rather similar to each other.

C.3.2 The information from single neurons

Examples of the responses of single neurons (in this case in the inferior temporal visual cortex) to sets of objects and/or faces (of the type illustrated in Fig. C.7) are shown in Figs. 2.16, 2.17 and C.4. We now consider how much information these types of neuronal response convey about the set of stimuli S, and about each stimulus s in the set. The mutual information $I(S, R)$ that the set of responses R encode about the set of stimuli S is calculated with Equation C.21 and corrected for the limited sampling using the analytic bias correction procedure described by Panzeri and Treves (1996) as described in detail by Rolls, Treves, Tovee and Panzeri (1997d). The information $I(s, R)$ about each single stimulus s in the set S, termed the stimulus-specific information (Rolls, Treves, Tovee and Panzeri, 1997d) or stimulus-specific surprise (DeWeese and Meister, 1999), obtained from the set of the responses R of the single neuron is calculated with Equation C.22 and corrected for the limited sampling using the analytic bias correction procedure described by Panzeri and Treves (1996) as described in detail by Rolls, Treves, Tovee and Panzeri (1997d). (The average of $I(s, R)$ across stimuli is the mutual information $I(S, R)$.)

Figure C.10 shows the stimulus-specific information $I(s, R)$ available in the neuronal response about each of 20 face stimuli calculated for the neuron (am242) whose firing rate response profile to the set of 65 stimuli is shown in Fig. C.4. Unless otherwise stated, the information measures given are for the information available on a single trial from the firing rate of the neuron in a 500 ms period starting 100 ms after the onset of the stimuli. It is shown in Fig. C.10 that 2.2, 2.0, and 1.5 bits of information were present about the three face stimuli to which the neuron had the highest firing rate responses. The neuron conveyed some but smaller amounts of information about the remaining face stimuli. The average information

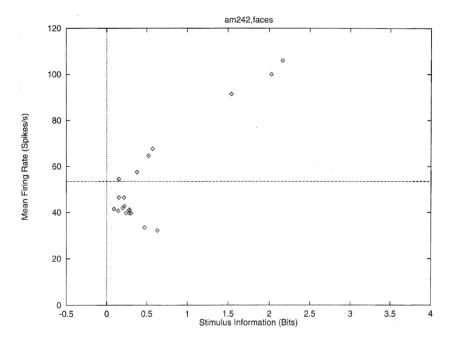

Fig. C.10 The stimulus-specific information $I(s, R)$ available in the response of the same single neuron as in Fig. C.4 about each of the stimuli in the set of 20 face stimuli (abscissa), with the firing rate of the neuron to the corresponding stimulus plotted as a function of this on the ordinate. The horizontal line shows the mean firing rate across all stimuli. (Reproduced from Rolls, E. T., Treves, A., Tovee, M. and Panzeri, S. (1997) Information in the neuronal representation of individual stimuli in the primate temporal visual cortex. Journal of Computational Neuroscience 4: 309–333. © Springer Nature.)

$I(S, R)$ about this set (S) of 20 faces for this neuron was 0.55 bits. The average firing rate of this neuron to these 20 face stimuli was 54 spikes/s. It is clear from Fig. C.10 that little information was available from the responses of the neuron to a particular face stimulus if that response was close to the average response of the neuron across all stimuli. At the same time, it is clear from Fig. C.10 that information was present depending on how far the firing rate to a particular stimulus was from the average response of the neuron to the stimuli. Of particular interest, it is evident that information is present from the neuronal response about which face was shown if that neuronal response was below the average response, as well as when the response was greater than the average response.

One intuitive way to understand the data shown in Fig. C.10 is to appreciate that low probability firing rate responses, whether they are greater than or less than the mean response rate, convey much information about which stimulus was seen. This is of course close to the definition of information. Given that the firing rates of neurons are always positive, and follow an asymmetric distribution about their mean, it is clear that deviations above the mean have a different probability to occur than deviations by the same amount below the mean. One may attempt to capture the relative likelihood of different firing rates above and below the mean by computing a z score obtained by dividing the difference between the mean response to each stimulus and the overall mean response by the standard deviation of the response to that stimulus. The greater the number of standard deviations (i.e. the greater the z score) from the mean response value, the greater the information might be expected to be. We therefore show in Fig. C.11 the relation between the z score and $I(s, R)$. (The z score was calculated by obtaining the mean and standard deviation of the response of a neuron to a particular stimulus s, and dividing the difference of this response from the mean response to all stimuli by the

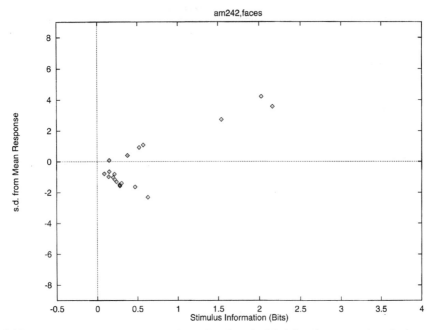

Fig. C.11 The relation for a single cell between the number of standard deviations the response to a stimulus was from the average response to all stimuli (see text, z score) plotted as a function of $I(s, R)$, the information available about the corresponding stimulus, s. (Reproduced from Rolls, E. T., Treves, A., Tovee, M. and Panzeri, S. (1997) Information in the neuronal representation of individual stimuli in the primate temporal visual cortex. Journal of Computational Neuroscience 4: 309–333. © Springer Nature.)

calculated standard deviation for that stimulus.) This results in a C-shaped curve in Figs. C.10 and C.11, with more information being provided by the cell the further its response to a stimulus is in spikes per second or in z scores either above or below the mean response to all stimuli (which was 54 spikes/s). The specific C-shape is discussed further in Section C.3.4.

The information $I(s, R)$ about each stimulus in the set of 65 stimuli is shown in Fig. C.12 for the same neuron, am242. The 23 face stimuli in the set are indicated by a diamond, and the 42 non-face stimuli by a cross. Using this much larger and more varied stimulus set, which is more representative of stimuli in the real world, a C-shaped function again describes the relation between the information conveyed by the cell about a stimulus and its firing rate to that stimulus. In particular, this neuron reflected information about most, but not all, of the faces in the set, that is those faces that produced a higher firing rate than the overall mean firing rate to all the 65 stimuli, which was 31 spikes/s. In addition, it conveyed information about the majority of the 42 non-face stimuli by responding at a rate below the overall mean response of the neuron to the 65 stimuli. This analysis usefully makes the point that the information available in the neuronal responses about which stimulus was shown is relative to (dependent upon) the nature and range of stimuli in the test set of stimuli.

This evidence makes it clear that a single cortical visual neuron tuned to faces conveys information not just about one face, but about a whole set of faces, with the information conveyed on a single trial related to the difference in the firing rate response to a particular stimulus compared to the average response to all stimuli.

The analyses just described for neurons with visual responses are general, in that they apply in a very similar way to olfactory neurons recorded in the macaque orbitofrontal cortex (Rolls, Critchley and Treves, 1996a; Rolls, Critchley, Verhagen and Kadohisa, 2010a).

The neurons in this sample reflected in their firing rates for the post-stimulus period 100 to 600 ms on average 0.36 bits of mutual information about which of 20 face stimuli was

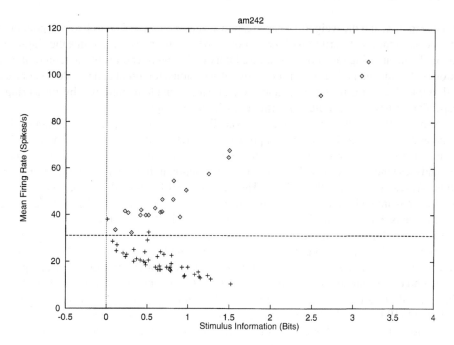

Fig. C.12 The information $I(s, R)$ available in the response of the same neuron about each of the stimuli in the set of 23 face and 42 non-face stimuli (abscissa), with the firing rate of the neuron to the corresponding stimulus plotted as a function of this on the ordinate. The 23 face stimuli in the set are indicated by a diamond, and the 42 non-face stimuli by a cross. The horizontal line shows the mean firing rate across all stimuli. (Reproduced from Rolls, E. T., Treves, A., Tovee, M. and Panzeri, S. (1997) Information in the neuronal representation of individual stimuli in the primate temporal visual cortex. Journal of Computational Neuroscience 4: 309–333. © Springer Nature.)

presented (Rolls, Treves, Tovee and Panzeri, 1997d). Similar values have been found in other experiments (Tovee, Rolls, Treves and Bellis, 1993; Tovee and Rolls, 1995; Rolls, Tovee and Panzeri, 1999b; Rolls, Franco, Aggelopoulos and Jerez, 2006b). The information in short temporal epochs of the neuronal responses is described in Section C.3.4.

C.3.3 The information from single neurons: temporal codes versus rate codes within the spike train of a single neuron

In the third of a series of papers that analyze the response of single neurons in the primate inferior temporal cortex to a set of static visual stimuli, Optican and Richmond (1987) applied information theory in a particularly direct and useful way. To ascertain the relevance of stimulus-locked temporal modulations in the firing of those neurons, they compared the amount of information about the stimuli that could be extracted from just the firing rate, computed over a relatively long interval of 384 ms, with the amount of information that could be extracted from a more complete description of the firing, that included temporal modulation. To derive this latter description (the temporal code within the spike train of a single neuron) they applied principal component analysis (PCA) to the temporal response vectors recorded for each neuron on each trial. The PCA helped to reduce the dimensionality of the neuronal response measurements. A temporal response vector was defined as a vector with as components the firing rates in each of 64 successive 6 ms time bins. The (64×64) covariance matrix was calculated across all trials of a particular neuron, and diagonalized. The first few eigenvectors of the matrix, those with the largest eigenvalues, are the principal components of the response, and the weights of each response vector on these four to five components can be used as a reduced description of the response, which still preserves, unlike the single value giving the mean firing rate along the entire interval, the main features of the temporal modulation within the interval. Thus a four- to five-dimensional temporal code could be contrasted with a one-dimensional rate code, and the comparison made quantitative by measuring the respective values for the mutual information with the stimuli.

Although the initial claim (Optican, Gawne, Richmond and Joseph, 1991; Eskandar, Richmond and Optican, 1992), that the temporal code carried nearly three times as much information as the rate code, was later found to be an artefact of limited sampling, and more recent analyses tend to minimize the additional information in the temporal description (Tovee, Rolls, Treves and Bellis, 1993; Heller, Hertz, Kjaer and Richmond, 1995), this type of application has immediately appeared straightforward and important, and it has led to many developments. By concentrating on the code expressed in the output rather than on the characterization of the neuronal channel itself, this approach is not affected much by the potential complexities of the preceding black box. Limited sampling, on the other hand, is a problem, particularly because it affects much more codes with a larger number of components, for example the four to five components of the PCA temporal description, than the one-dimensional firing rate code. This is made evident in the paper by Heller, Hertz, Kjaer and Richmond (1995), in which the comparison is extended to several more detailed temporal descriptions, including a binary vector description in which the presence or not of a spike in each 1 ms bin of the response constitutes a component of a 320-dimensional vector. Obviously, this binary vector must contain at least all the information present in the reduced descriptions, whereas in the results of Heller, Hertz, Kjaer and Richmond (1995), despite the use of a sophisticated neural network procedure to control limited sampling biases, the binary vector appears to be the code that carries the least information of all. In practice, with the data samples available in the experiments that have been done, and even when using analytic procedures to control limited sampling (Panzeri and Treves, 1996), reliable comparison can be made only with up to two- to three-dimensional codes.

Tovee, Rolls, Treves and Bellis (1993) and Tovee and Rolls (1995) obtained further evidence that little information was encoded in the temporal aspects of firing within the spike train of a single neuron in the inferior temporal cortex by taking short epochs of the firing of neurons, lasting 20 ms or 50 ms, in which the opportunity for temporal encoding would be limited (because there were few spikes in these short time intervals). They found that a considerable proportion (30%) of the information available in a long time period of 400 ms utilizing temporal encoding within the spike train was available in time periods as short as 20 ms when only the number of spikes was taken into account.

Overall, the main result of these analyses applied to the responses to static stimuli in the temporal visual cortex of primates is that not much more information (perhaps only up to 10% more) can be extracted from temporal codes than from the firing rate measured over a judiciously chosen interval (Tovee, Rolls, Treves and Bellis, 1993; Heller, Hertz, Kjaer and Richmond, 1995). Indeed, it turns out that even this small amount of 'temporal information' is related primarily to the onset latency of the neuronal responses to different stimuli, rather than to anything more subtle (Tovee, Rolls, Treves and Bellis, 1993). Consistent with this point, in earlier visual areas the additional 'temporally encoded' fraction of information can be larger, due especially to the increased relevance, earlier on, of precisely locked transient responses (Kjaer, Hertz and Richmond, 1994; Golomb, Kleinfeld, Reid, Shapley and Shraiman, 1994; Heller, Hertz, Kjaer and Richmond, 1995). This is because if the responses to some stimuli are more transient and to others more sustained, this will result in more information if the temporal modulation of the response of the neuron is taken into account. However, the relevance of more substantial temporal codes for static visual stimuli remains to be demonstrated.

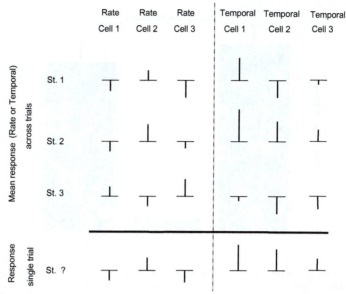

Fig. C.13 Decoding rate and temporal measures of neural responses that might encode information about which stimulus had been presented on a single trial. The upper left part of the diagram shows the average firing rate (or equivalently spike count) responses of each of 3 cells (labelled as Rate Cell 1,2,3) to a set of 3 stimuli. The upper right three columns show the average across trials of a measure of temporal aspects of the neural response, for example latency for each cell. The bottom row (labelled Response single trial) shows the data that might be obtained from a single trial and from which the stimulus that was shown (St. ? or s') must be estimated or decoded, using the average values across trials shown in the top part of the table. From the responses on the single trial, the most probable decoded stimulus is stimulus 2, based on the values of both the rates and the temporal measures. With this decoding procedure, the information can then be measured with the multiple cell information algorithm described by Rolls, Treves and Tovee (1997b) Rolls, Treves and Tovee (1997b). (From Verhagen,J.V., Baker,K.L., Vasan,G., Pieribone,V.A. and Rolls, E. T. (2023) Odor encoding by signals in the olfactory bulb. Journal of Neurophysiology 129:431-444. doi: 10.1152/jn.00449.2022.)

For non-static visual stimuli and for other cortical systems, similar analyses have largely yet to be carried out, although clearly one expects to find much more prominent temporal effects e.g. in the auditory system (Nelken, Prut, Vaadia and Abeles, 1994; deCharms and Merzenich, 1996), for reasons similar to those just annunciated.

Evidence that is consistent with what has just been described for the visual system has been found in another brain system, the olfactory system. We measured the information available about which of six odors had been presented by measuring the presynaptic signals from populations of 28–57 glomeruli in the olfactory bulb of the mouse using optical imaging (Verhagen, Baker, Vasan, Pieribone and Rolls, 2023) (see Section 5.2.1). The information was measured with the multiple cell information analysis method described in Section C.2.4 with the code available as described in Section D.7 and the decoding procedure for temporal aspects of neuronal responses illustrated in Fig. C.13.

We found that although there was a little information in the time course of the response (effectively the latency), there was much more information in the activity (reflecting the neuronal firing rates) of the glomeruli about which odor had been presented (Fig. C.14). Importantly, the total information from both the rates and the latencies was not greater than that from the rates alone, showing that the latency information is redundant with respect to the rate information. (The total information from the rates and latencies was a little lower than from the rates alone, because the latency values added noise to what could be decoded from the rates.) Thus in this olfactory system too, the information is encoded in the rates, and useful extra information is not provided by the latency / time course of the neural response.

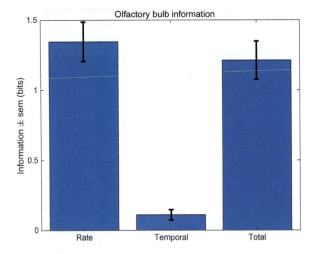

Fig. C.14 The information about which of 6 odors was presented from signals in the mouse olfactory bulb glomeruli from the 'Rate', latency ('Temporal'), and from both the rates and time courses ('Total'). The mean and standard error of the information was measured in 10 experiments in each of which the information from a population of 28–57 glomeruli was measured with the multiple cell information algorithm described by Rolls, Treves and Tovee (1997b). (Data from Verhagen,J.V., Baker,K.L., Vasan,G., Pieribone,V.A. and Rolls, E. T. (2023) Odor encoding by signals in the olfactory bulb. Journal of Neurophysiology 129: 431-444. doi: 10.1152/jn.00449.2022.)

C.3.4 The information from single neurons: the speed of information transfer

It is intuitive that if short periods of firing of single cells are considered, there is less time for temporal modulation effects. The information conveyed about stimuli by the firing rate and that conveyed by more detailed temporal codes become similar in value. When the firing periods analyzed become shorter than roughly the mean interspike interval, even the statistics of firing rate values on individual trials cease to be relevant, and the information content of the firing depends solely on the mean firing rates across all trials with each stimulus. This is expressed mathematically by considering the amount of information provided as a function of the length t of the time window over which firing is analyzed, and taking the limit for $t \to 0$ (Skaggs, McNaughton, Gothard and Markus, 1993; Panzeri, Biella, Rolls, Skaggs and Treves, 1996). To first order in t, only two responses can occur in a short window of length t: either the emission of an action potential, with probability tr_s, where r_s is the mean firing rate calculated over many trials using the same window and stimulus; or no action potential, with probability $1 - tr_s$. Inserting these conditional probabilities into Equation C.22, taking the limit and dividing by t, one obtains for the derivative of the stimulus-specific transinformation

$$dI(s)/dt = r_s \log_2(r_s/<r>) + (<r> - r_s)/\ln 2, \tag{C.47}$$

where $<r>$ is the grand mean rate across stimuli. This formula thus gives the rate, in bits/s, at which information about a stimulus begins to accumulate when the firing of a cell is recorded. Such an information rate depends only on the mean firing rate to that stimulus and on the grand mean rate across stimuli. As a function of r_s, it follows the U-shaped curve in Fig. C.15. The curve is universal, in the sense that it applies irrespective of the detailed firing statistics of the cell, and it expresses the fact that the emission or not of a spike in a short window conveys information in as much as the mean response to a given stimulus is above or below the overall mean rate. No information is conveyed about those stimuli the mean response to which is the same as the overall mean. In practice, although the curve describes

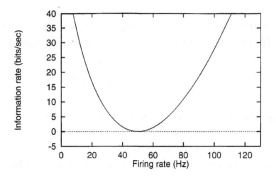

Fig. C.15 Time derivative of the stimulus-specific information as a function of firing rate, for a cell firing at a grand mean rate of 50 Hz. For different grand mean rates, the graph would simply be rescaled.

only the universal behavior of the initial slope of the specific information as a function of time, it approximates well the full stimulus-specific information $I(s, R)$ computed even over rather long periods (Rolls, Critchley and Treves, 1996a; Rolls, Treves, Tovee and Panzeri, 1997d).

Averaging Equation C.47 across stimuli one obtains the time derivative of the mutual information. Further dividing by the overall mean rate yields the adimensional quantity

$$\chi = \sum_s P(s)(r_s/<r>) \log_2(r_s/<r>) \tag{C.48}$$

which measures, in bits, the mutual information per spike provided by the cell (Bialek, Rieke, de Ruyter van Steveninck and Warland, 1991; Skaggs, McNaughton, Gothard and Markus, 1993). One can prove that this quantity can range from 0 to $\log_2(1/a)$

$$0 < \chi < \log_2(1/a), \tag{C.49}$$

where a is the single neuron sparseness a^s defined in Section C.3.1.1. For mean rates r_s distributed in a nearly binary fashion, χ is close to its upper limit $\log_2(1/a)$, whereas for mean rates that are nearly uniform, or at least unimodally distributed, χ is relatively close to zero (Panzeri, Biella, Rolls, Skaggs and Treves, 1996). In practice, whenever a large number of more or less 'ecological' stimuli are considered, mean rates are not distributed in arbitrary ways, but rather tend to follow stereotyped distributions (which for some neurons approximate an exponential distribution of firing rates – see Section C.3.1 (Treves, Panzeri, Rolls, Booth and Wakeman, 1999; Baddeley, Abbott, Booth, Sengpiel, Freeman, Wakeman and Rolls, 1997; Rolls and Treves, 1998; Rolls and Deco, 2002; Franco, Rolls, Aggelopoulos and Jerez, 2007; Rolls, 2016b; Rolls and Treves, 2011)), and as a consequence χ and a (or, equivalently, its logarithm) tend to covary (rather than to be independent variables (Skaggs and McNaughton, 1992)). Therefore, measuring sparseness is in practice nearly equivalent to measuring information per spike, and the rate of rise in mutual information, $\chi <r>$, is largely determined by the sparseness a and the overall mean firing rate $<r>$.

An important point to note from the above is that the 'bits per spike' information measure (Skaggs et al., 1993) is in practice closely equivalent to measuring the sparseness a of the representation, and is not a true measure of information that takes into account the variability of the relation between the stimulus and the neuronal firing. An intuitive understanding is that if a representation is sparse, then when a neuron does fire, the 'bits per spike' will be high, because a spike is a low probability event with sparse representations, and therefore when a spike does occur, it can be thought of as a high information event. The 'bits per spike' measure I_b is calculated as follows for firing rates accumulated in different bins each with a different duration, where the bins might correspond to stimuli, spatial locations, etc.

$$I_b = \sum_i \frac{\lambda_i}{\bar{\lambda}} \log_2 \left(\frac{\lambda_i}{\bar{\lambda}}\right) p_i \qquad (C.50)$$

where λ_i is the firing rate in bin i, $\bar{\lambda}$ is the mean firing rate, and p_i is the fraction of the time spent in bin i.

The important point to note about the single-cell information rate $\chi <r>$ is that, to the extent that different cells express non-redundant codes, as discussed below, the instantaneous *information flow* across a population of C cells can be taken to be simply $C\chi <r>$, and this quantity can easily be measured directly without major limited sampling biases, or else inferred indirectly through measurements of the sparseness a. Values for the information rate $\chi <r>$ that have been published range from 2–3 bits/s for rat hippocampal cells (Skaggs, McNaughton, Gothard and Markus, 1993), to 10–30 bits/s for primate temporal cortex visual cells (Rolls, Treves and Tovee, 1997b), and could be compared with analogous measurements in the sensory systems of frogs and crickets, in the 100–300 bits/s range (Rieke, Warland and Bialek, 1993).

If the first time-derivative of the mutual information measures information flow, successive derivatives characterize, at the single-cell level, different firing modes. This is because whereas the first derivative is universal and depends only on the mean firing rates to each stimulus, the next derivatives depend also on the variability of the firing rate around its mean value, across trials, and take different forms in different firing regimes. Thus they can serve as a measure of discrimination among firing regimes with limited variability, for which, for example, the second derivative is large and positive, and firing regimes with large variability, for which the second derivative is large and negative. Poisson firing, in which in every short period of time there is a fixed probability of emitting a spike irrespective of previous firing, is an example of large variability, and the second derivative of the mutual information can be calculated to be

$$d^2 I/dt^2 = [\ln a + (1-a)] <r>^2 /(a \ln 2), \qquad (C.51)$$

where a is the single neuron sparseness a^s defined in Section C.3.1.1. This quantity is always negative. Strictly periodic firing is an example of zero variability, and in fact the second time-derivative of the mutual information becomes infinitely large in this case (although actual information values measured in a short time interval remain of course finite even for exactly periodic firing, because there is still some variability, ± 1, in the number of spikes recorded in the interval). Measures of mutual information from short intervals of firing of temporal cortex visual cells have revealed a degree of variability intermediate between that of periodic and of Poisson regimes (Rolls, Treves, Tovee and Panzeri, 1997d). Similar measures can also be used to contrast the effect of the graded nature of neuronal responses, once they are analyzed over a finite period of time, with the information content that would characterize neuronal activity if it reduced to a binary variable (Panzeri, Biella, Rolls, Skaggs and Treves, 1996). A binary variable with the same degree of variability would convey information at the same instantaneous rate (the first derivative being universal), but in for example 20–30% reduced amounts when analyzed over times of the order of the interspike interval or longer.

Utilizing these approaches, Tovee, Rolls, Treves and Bellis (1993) and Tovee and Rolls (1995) measured the information available in short epochs of the firing of single neurons, and found that a considerable proportion of the information available in a long time period of 400 ms was available in time periods as short as 20 ms and 50 ms. For example, in periods of 20 ms, 30% of the information present in 400 ms using temporal encoding with the first three

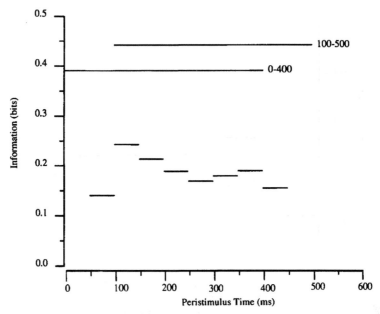

Fig. C.16 The average information I(S,R) available in short temporal epochs (50 ms as compared to 400 ms) of the spike trains of single inferior temporal cortex neurons about which face had been shown. (From Tovee,M.J. and Rolls, E.T.(1995) Information encoding in short firing rate epochs by single neurons in the primate temporal visual cortex. Visual Cognition 2: 35–58. © Informa Ltd.)

principal components was available. Moreover, the exact time when the epoch was taken was not crucial, with the main effect being that rather more information was available if information was measured near the start of the spike train, when the firing rate of the neuron tended to be highest (see Figs. C.16 and C.17). The conclusion was that much information was available when temporal encoding could not be used easily, that is in very short time epochs of 20 or 50 ms.

It is also useful to note from Figs. C.16, C.17 and 2.16 the typical time course of the responses of many temporal cortex visual neurons in the awake behaving primate. Although the firing rate and availability of information is highest in the first 50–100 ms of the neuronal response, the firing is overall well sustained in the 500 ms stimulus presentation period. Cortical neurons in the primate temporal lobe visual system, in the taste cortex (Rolls, Yaxley and Sienkiewicz, 1990), and in the olfactory cortex (Rolls, Critchley and Treves, 1996a), do not in general have rapidly adapting neuronal responses to sensory stimuli. This may be important for associative learning: the outputs of these sensory systems can be maintained for sufficiently long while the stimuli are present for synaptic modification to occur. Although rapid synaptic adaptation within a spike train is seen in some experiments in brain slices (Markram and Tsodyks, 1996; Abbott, Varela, Sen and Nelson, 1997), it is not a very marked effect in at least some brain systems in vivo, when they operate in normal physiological conditions with normal levels of acetylcholine, etc.

To pursue this issue of the speed of processing and information availability even further, Rolls, Tovee, Purcell, Stewart and Azzopardi (1994b) and Rolls and Tovee (1994) limited the period for which visual cortical neurons could respond by using backward masking. In this paradigm, a short (16 ms) presentation of the test stimulus (a face) was followed after a delay of 0, 20, 40, 60, etc. ms by a masking stimulus (which was a high contrast set of letters) (see Fig. C.18). They showed that the mask did actually interrupt the neuronal response, and that at the shortest interval between the stimulus and the mask (a delay of 0 ms, or a 'Stimulus Onset

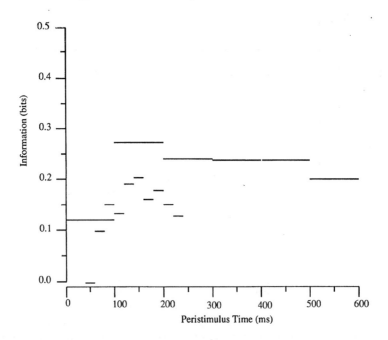

Fig. C.17 The average information I(S,R) available in short temporal epochs (20 ms and 100 ms) of the spike trains of single inferior temporal cortex neurons about which face had been shown. (From Tovee,M.J. and Rolls, E.T.(1995) Information encoding in short firing rate epochs by single neurons in the primate temporal visual cortex. Visual Cognition 2: 35–58. © Informa Ltd.)

Asynchrony' of 20 ms), the neurons in the temporal cortical areas fired for approximately 30 ms (see Fig. C.19). Under these conditions, the subjects could identify which of five faces had been shown much better than chance. Interestingly, under these conditions, when the inferior temporal cortex neurons were firing for 30 ms, the subjects felt that they were guessing, and conscious perception was minimal (Rolls, Tovee, Purcell, Stewart and Azzopardi, 1994b), the neurons conveyed on average 0.10 bits of information (Rolls, Tovee and Panzeri, 1999b). With a stimulus onset asynchrony of 40 ms, when the inferior temporal cortex neurons were firing for 50 ms, not only did the subjects' performance improve, but the stimuli were now perceived clearly, consciously, and the neurons conveyed on average 0.16 bits of information. This has contributed to the view that consciousness has a higher threshold of activity *in a given pathway*, in this case a pathway for face analysis, than does unconscious processing and performance using the same pathway (Rolls, 2003, 2006a).

The issue of how rapidly information can be read from neurons is crucial and fundamental to understanding how rapidly memory systems in the brain could operate in terms of reading the code from the input neurons to initiate retrieval, whether in a pattern associator or auto-association network (see Appendix B). This is also a crucial issue for understanding how any stage of cortical processing operates, given that each stage includes associative or competitive network processes that require the code to be read before it can pass useful output to the next stage of processing (see Chapter 2; Rolls and Deco (2002); Rolls (2016b); and Panzeri, Rolls, Battaglia and Lavis (2001)). For this reason, we have performed further analyses of the speed of availability of information from neuronal firing, and the neuronal code. A rapid readout of information from any one stage of for example visual processing is important, for the ventral visual system is organized as a hierarchy of cortical areas, and the neuronal response latencies are approximately 100 ms in the inferior temporal visual cortex, and 40–50

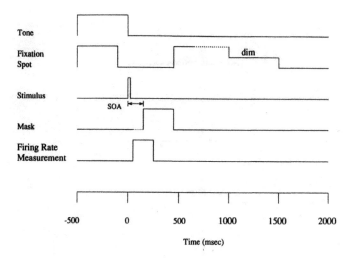

Fig. C.18 Backward masking paradigm. The visual stimulus appeared at time 0 for 16 ms. The time between the start of the visual stimulus and the masking image is the Stimulus Onset Asynchrony (SOA). A visual fixation task was being performed to ensure correct fixation of the stimulus. In the fixation task, the fixation spot appeared in the middle of the screen at time −500 ms, was switched off 100 ms before the test stimulus was shown, and was switched on again at the end of the mask stimulus. Then when the fixation spot dimmed after a random time, fruit juice could be obtained by licking. No eye movements could be performed after the onset of the fixation spot. (After Rolls, E. T. and Tovee,M.J. (1994) Processing speed in the cerebral cortex and the neurophysiology of visual masking. Proceedings of the Royal Society, B, 257: 9–15. © Royal Society.)

ms in the primary visual cortex, allowing only approximately 50–60 ms of processing time for V1–V2–V4–inferior temporal cortex (Baylis, Rolls and Leonard, 1987; Nowak and Bullier, 1997; Rolls and Deco, 2002). There is much evidence that the time required for each stage of processing is relatively short. For example, in addition to the evidence already presented, visual stimuli presented in succession approximately 15 ms apart can be separately identified (Keysers and Perrett, 2002); and the reaction time for identifying visual stimuli is relatively short and requires a relatively short cortical processing time (Rolls, 2003; Bacon-Mace et al., 2005).

In this context, Delorme and Thorpe (2001) have suggested that just one spike from each neuron is sufficient, and indeed it has been suggested that the order of the first spike in different neurons may be part of the code (Delorme and Thorpe, 2001; Thorpe, Delorme and Van Rullen, 2001; VanRullen, Guyonneau and Thorpe, 2005). (Implicit in the spike order hypothesis is that the first spike is particularly important, for it would be difficult to measure the order for anything other than the first spike.) An alternative view is that the number of spikes in a fixed time window over which a postsynaptic neuron could integrate information is more realistic, and this time might be in the order of 20 ms for a single receiving neuron, or much longer if the receiving neurons are connected by recurrent collateral associative synapses and so can integrate information over time (Deco and Rolls, 2006; Rolls and Deco, 2002; Panzeri, Rolls, Battaglia and Lavis, 2001; Rolls, 2016b). Although the number of spikes in a short time window of e.g. 20 ms is likely to be 0, 1, or 2, the information available may be more than that from the first spike alone, and Rolls, Franco, Aggelopoulos and Jerez (2006b) examined this by measuring neuronal activity in the inferior temporal visual cortex, and then applying quantitative information theoretic methods to measure the information transmitted by single spikes, and within short time windows.

The cumulative single cell information about which of the twenty stimuli (Fig. C.7) was shown from all spikes and from the first spike starting at 100 ms after stimulus onset is shown in Fig. C.20. A period of 100 ms is just longer than the shortest response latency of the

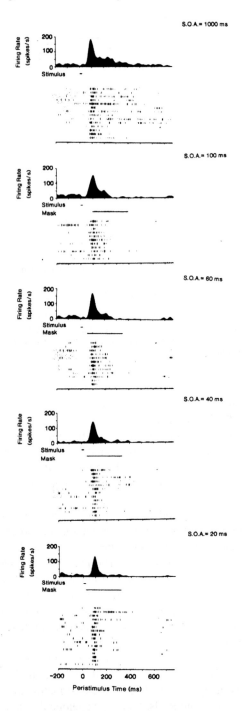

Fig. C.19 Firing of a temporal cortex cell to a 20 ms presentation of a face stimulus when the face was followed with different stimulus onset asynchronies (SOAs) by a masking visual stimulus. At an SOA of 20 ms, when the mask immediately followed the face, the neuron fired for only approximately 30 ms, yet identification above change (by 'guessing') of the face at this SOA by human observers was possible. (After Rolls, E. T. and Tovee,M.J. (1994) Processing speed in the cerebral cortex and the neurophysiology of visual masking. Proceedings of the Royal Society, B, 257: 9–15; and Rolls, E. T., Tovee,M.J., Purcell,D.G., Stewart,A.L. and Azzopardi,P. (1994) The responses of neurons in the temporal cortex of primates, and face identification and detection. Experimental Brain Research 101: 473–484. © Springer Nature.)

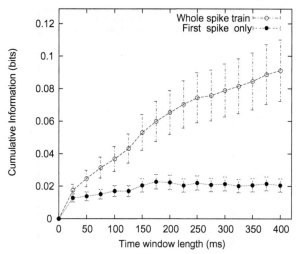

Fig. C.20 Speed of information availability in the inferior temporal visual cortex from single neurons. Cumulative single cell information from all spikes and from the first spike with the analysis starting at 100 ms after stimulus onset. The mean and sem over 21 neurons are shown. (After Rolls, E. T., Franco,L., Aggelopoulos,N.C. and Perez,J.M. (2006) Information in the first spike, the order of spikes, and the number of spikes provided by neurons in the inferior temporal visual cortex. Vision Research 46: 4193–4205. © Elsevier Ltd.)

neurons from which recordings were made, so starting the measure at this time provides the best chance for the single spike measurement to catch a spike that is related to the stimulus. The means and standard errors across the 21 different neurons are shown. The cumulated information from the total number of spikes is larger than that from the first spike, and this is evident and significant within 50 ms of the start of the time epoch. In calculating the information from the first spike, just the first spike in the analysis window starting in this case at 100 ms after stimulus onset was used.

Because any one neuron receiving information from the population being analyzed has multiple inputs, we show in Fig. C.21 the cumulative information that would be available from multiple cells (21) about which of the 20 stimuli was shown, taking both the first spike after the time of stimulus onset (0 ms), and the total number of spikes after 0 ms from each neuron. The cumulative information even from multiple cells is much greater when all the spikes rather than just the first spike are used.

An attractor network might be able to integrate the information arriving over a long time period of several hundred milliseconds (see Section 11.5.1), and might produce the advantage shown in Fig. C.21 for the whole spike train compared to the first spike only. However a single layer pattern association network might only be able to integrate the information over the time constants of its synapses and cell membrane, which might be in the order of 15–30 ms (Panzeri, Rolls, Battaglia and Lavis, 2001; Rolls and Deco, 2002) (see Section B.2). In a hierarchical processing system such as the visual cortical areas, there may only be a short time during which each stage may decode the information from the preceding stage, and then pass on information sufficient to support recognition to the next stage (Rolls and Deco, 2002) (see Chapter 2). We therefore analyzed the information that would be available in short epochs from multiple inputs to a neuron, and show the multiple cell information for the population of 21 neurons in Fig. C.22 (for 20 ms and 50 epochs). We see in this case that the first spike information, because it is being made available from many different neurons (in this case 21 selective neurons discriminating between the stimuli each with $p¡0.001$ in an ANOVA), fares better relative to the information from all the spikes in these short epochs, but is still less than the information from all the spikes (particularly in the 50 ms epoch). In particular, for the epoch starting 100 ms after stimulus onset in Fig. C.23 the information in the 20 ms epoch is

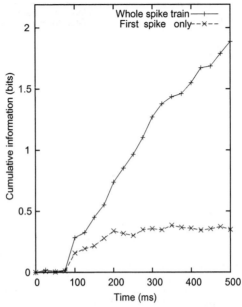

Fig. C.21 Speed of information availability in the inferior temporal visual cortex from a population of neurons. Cumulative multiple cell information from all spikes and first spike starting at the time of stimulus onset (0 ms) for the population of 21 neurons about the set of 20 stimuli. (After Rolls, E. T., Franco,L., Aggelopoulos,N.C. and Perez,J.M. (2006) Information in the first spike, the order of spikes, and the number of spikes provided by neurons in the inferior temporal visual cortex. Vision Research 46: 4193–4205. © Elsevier Ltd.)

0.37 bits, and from the first spike is 0.24 bits. Correspondingly, for a 50 ms epoch, the values in the epoch starting at 100 ms post stimulus were 0.66 bits for the 50 ms epoch, and 0.40 bits for the first spike. Thus with a population of neurons, having just one spike from each can allow considerable information to be read if only a limited period (of e.g. 20 or 50 ms) is available for the readout, though even in these cases, more information was available if all the spikes in the short window are considered (Fig. C.22).

To show how the information increases with the number of neurons in the ensemble in these short epochs, we show in Fig. C.23 the information from different numbers of neurons for a 20 ms epoch starting at time = 100 ms with respect to stimulus onset, for both the first spike condition and the condition with all the spikes in the 20 ms window. The linear increase in the information in both cases indicates that the neurons provide independent information, which could be because there is no redundancy or synergy, or because these cancel (Rolls, Franco, Aggelopoulos and Reece, 2003b,b). It is also clear from Fig. C.23 that even with the population of neurons, and with just a short time epoch of 20 ms, more information is available from the population if all the spikes in 20 ms are considered, and not just the first spike. The 20 ms epoch analyzed for Fig. C.23 is for the post-stimulus time period of 100–120 ms.

To assess whether there is information that is specifically related to the order in which the spikes arrive from the different neurons, Rolls, Franco, Aggelopoulos and Jerez (2006b) computed for every trial the order across the different simultaneously recorded neurons in which the first spike arrived to each stimulus, and used this in the information theoretic analysis. The control condition was to randomly allocate the order values for each trial between the neurons that had any spikes on that trial, thus shuffling or scrambling the order of the spike arrival times in the time window. In both cases, just the first spike in the time window was used in the information analysis. (In both the order and the shuffled control conditions, on some trials some neurons had no spikes, and this itself, in comparison with the fact that

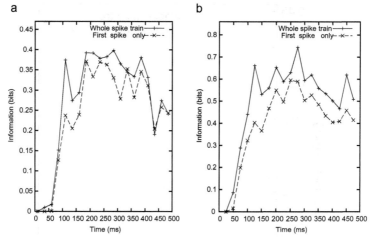

Fig. C.22 Speed of information availability in the inferior temporal visual cortex from a population of neurons. (a) Multiple cell information from all spikes and 1 spike in 20 ms time windows taken at different post-stimulus times starting at time 0. (b) Multiple cell information from all spikes and 1 spike in 50 ms time windows taken at different post-stimulus times starting at time 0. (After Rolls, E. T., Franco,L., Aggelopoulos,N.C. and Perez,J.M. (2006) Information in the first spike, the order of spikes, and the number of spikes provided by neurons in the inferior temporal visual cortex. Vision Research 46: 4193–4205. © Elsevier Ltd.)

some neurons had spiked on that trial, provided some information about which stimulus had been shown. However, by explicitly shuffling in the control condition the order of the spikes for the neurons that had spiked on that trial, comparison of the control with the unshuffled order condition provides a clear measure of whether the order of spike arrival from the different neurons itself carries useful information about which stimulus was shown.) The data set was 36 cells with significantly different ($p¡0.05$) responses to the stimulus set where it was possible to record simultaneously from groups of 3 and 4 cells (so that the order on each trial could be measured) in 11 experiments. Taking a 75 ms time window starting 100 ms after stimulus onset, the information with the order of arrival times of the spikes was 0.142 ± 0.02 bits, and in the control (shuffled order) condition was 0.138 ± 0.02 bits (mean across the 11 experiments $\pm$ sem). Thus the information increase by taking into account the order of spike arrival times relative to the control condition was only $(0.142 - 0.138) = 0.004$ bits per experiment (which was not significant). For comparison, the information calculated for the first spike using the same dot product decoding as described above was 0.136 ± 0.03 bits per experiment. Analogous results were obtained for different time windows. Thus taking the spike order into account compared to a control condition in which the spike order was scrambled made essentially no difference to the amount of information that was available from the populations of neurons about which stimulus was shown.

The results show that although considerable information is present in the first spike, more information is available under the more biologically realistic assumption that neurons integrate spikes over a short time window (depending on their time constants) of for example 20 ms. The results shown in Fig. C.23 are of considerable interest, for they show that even when one increases the number of neurons in the population, the information available from the number of spikes in a 20 ms time window is larger than the information available from just the first spike. Thus although intuitively one might think that one can compensate by taking a population of neurons rather than just a single neuron when using just the first spike instead of the number of spikes available in a fixed time window, this compensation by increasing neuron numbers is insufficient to make the first spike code as efficient as taking the number of spikes.

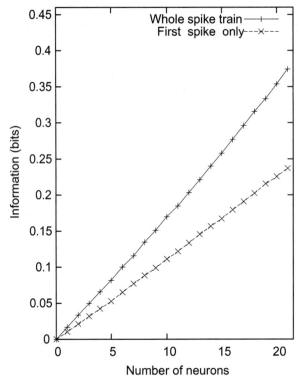

Fig. C.23 Speed of information availability in the inferior temporal visual cortex from populations of neurons. Multiple cell information from all spikes and 1 spike in a 20 ms time window starting at 100 ms after stimulus onset as a function of the number of neurons in the ensemble. (After Rolls, E. T., Franco,L., Aggelopoulos,N.C. and Perez,J.M. (2006) Information in the first spike, the order of spikes, and the number of spikes provided by neurons in the inferior temporal visual cortex. Vision Research 46: 4193–4205. © Elsevier Ltd.)

Further, in this first empirical test of the hypothesis that there is information that is specifically related to the order in which the spikes arrive from the different neurons, which has been proposed by Thorpe et al (Delorme and Thorpe, 2001; Thorpe, Delorme and Van Rullen, 2001; VanRullen, Guyonneau and Thorpe, 2005), we found that in the inferior temporal visual cortex there was no significant evidence that the order of the spike arrival times from different simultaneously recorded neurons is important. Indeed, the evidence found in the experiments was that the number of spikes in the time window is the important property that is related to the amount of information encoded by the spike trains of simultaneously recorded neurons. The fact that there was also more information in the number of spikes in a fixed time window than from the first spike only is also evidence that is not consistent with the spike order hypothesis, for the order between neurons can only be easily read from the first spike, and just using information from the first spike would discard extra information available from further spikes even in short time windows.

The encoding of information that uses the number of spikes in a short time window that is supported by the analyses described by Rolls, Franco, Aggelopoulos and Jerez (2006b) deserves further elaboration. It could be thought of as a rate code, in that the number of spikes in a short time window is relevant, but is not a rate code in the rather artificial sense considered by Thorpe et al. (Delorme and Thorpe, 2001; Thorpe et al., 2001; VanRullen et al., 2005) in which a rate is estimated from the interspike interval. This is not just artificial, but also begs the question of how, once the rate is calculated from the interspike interval, this decoded rate is passed on to the receiving neurons, or how, if the receiving neurons calculate the interspike interval at every synapse, they utilize it. In contrast, the spike count code in a short time window that is considered here is very biologically plausible, in that each spike would inject current into the post-synaptic neuron, and the neuron would integrate all such currents in a dendrite over a time period set by the synaptic and membrane time constants, which will result in an integration time constant in the order of 15–20 ms. Explicit models of exactly this dynamical processing at the integrate-and-fire neuronal level have been described to define precisely these operations (Deco and Rolls, 2003, 2005d; Deco, Rolls and Horwitz, 2004; Deco and Rolls, 2005b; Rolls and Deco, 2002; Rolls, 2016b). Even though the number of spikes in a short time window of e.g. 20 ms is likely to be 0, 1, or 2, it can be 3 or more for effective stimuli (Rolls, Franco, Aggelopoulos and Jerez, 2006b), and this is more efficient than using the first spike.

To add some detail here, a neuron receiving information from a population of inferior temporal cortex neurons of the type described here would have a membrane potential that varied continuously in time reflecting with a time constant in the order of 15–20 ms (resulting from a time constant of order 10 ms for AMPA synapses, 100 ms for NMDA synapses, and 20 ms for the cell membrane) a dot (inner) product over all synapses of each spike count and the synaptic strength. This continuously time varying membrane potential would lead to spikes whenever the results of this integration process produced a depolarization that exceeded the firing threshold. The result is that the spike train of the neuron would reflect continuously with a time constant in the order of 15–20 ms the likelihood that the input spikes it was receiving matched its set of synaptic weights. The spike train would thus indicate in continuous time how closely the stimulus or input matched its most effective stimulus (for a dot product is essentially a correlation). In this sense, no particular starting time is needed for the analysis, and in this respect it is a much better component of a dynamical system than is a decoding that utilizes an order in which the order of the spike arrival times is important and a start time for the analysis must be assumed.

I note that an autoassociation or attractor network implemented by recurrent collateral connections between the neurons can, using its short-term memory, integrate its inputs over much longer periods, for example over 500 ms in a model of how decisions are made (Deco and Rolls, 2006) (see Section 11.5.1), and thus if there is time, the extra information available in more than the first spike or even the first few spikes that is evident in Figs. C.20 and C.21 could be used by the brain.

The conclusions from the single cell information analyses are thus that most of the information is encoded in the spike count; that large parts of this information are available in short temporal epochs of e.g. 20 ms or 50 ms; and that any additional information which appears to be temporally encoded is related to the latency of the neuronal response, and reflects sudden changes in the visual stimuli. Therefore a neuron in the next cortical area would obtain considerable information within 20–50 ms by measuring the firing rate of a single neuron. Moreover, if it took a short sample of the firing rate of many neurons in the preceding area, then very much information is made available in a short time, as shown above and in Section C.3.5.

C.3.5 The information from multiple cells: independent information versus redundancy across cells

The rate at which a single cell provides information translates into an instantaneous information flow across a population (with a simple multiplication by the number of cells) only to the extent that different cells provide different (independent) information. To verify whether this condition holds, one cannot extend to multiple cells the simplified formula for the first time-derivative, because it is made simple precisely by the assumption of independence between spikes, and one cannot even measure directly the full information provided by multiple

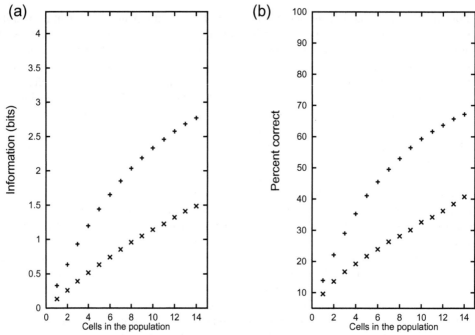

Fig. C.24 The information available from populations of neurons. (a) The information available about which of 20 faces had been seen that is available from the responses measured by the firing rates in a time period of 500 ms (+) or a shorter time period of 50 ms (x) of different numbers of temporal cortex cells. (b) The corresponding percentage correct from different numbers of cells. (From Rolls, E. T., Treves, A. and Tovee, M. J. (1997) The representational capacity of the distributed encoding of information provided by populations of neurons in the primate temporal visual cortex. Experimental Brain Research 114: 149–162. © Springer Nature.)

(more than two to three) cells, because of the limited sampling problem discussed above. Therefore one has to analyze the degree of independence (or conversely of redundancy) either directly among pairs – at most triplets – of cells, or indirectly by using decoding procedures to transform population responses. Obviously, the results of the analysis will vary a great deal with the particular neural system considered and the particular set of stimuli, or in general of neuronal correlates, used. For many systems, before undertaking to quantify the analysis in terms of information measures, it takes only a simple qualitative description of the responses to realize that there is a lot of redundancy and very little diversity in the responses. For example, if one selects pain-responsive cells in the somatosensory system and uses painful electrical stimulation of different intensities, most of the recorded cells are likely to convey pretty much the same information, signalling the intensity of the stimulation with the intensity of their single-cell response. Therefore, an analysis of redundancy makes sense only for a neuronal system that functions to represent, and enable discriminations between, a large variety of stimuli, and only when using a set of stimuli representative, in some sense, of that large variety.

Rolls, Treves and Tovee (1997b) measured the information available from a population of inferior temporal cortex neurons using the decoding method described in Section C.2.3, and found that the information increased approximately linearly, as shown in Fig. 2.18 on page 77, and in Fig. C.24 for a 50 ms interval as well as for a 500 ms measuring period. (It is shown below that the increase is limited only by the information ceiling of 4.32 bits necessary to encode the 20 stimuli. If it were not for this approach to the ceiling, the increase would be approximately linear (Rolls, Treves and Tovee, 1997b).) To the extent that the information increases linearly with the number of neurons, the neurons convey independent information, and there is no redundancy, at least with numbers of neurons in this range. Although these and some of the other results described in this Appendix are for face-selective neurons in the inferior temporal visual cortex, similar results were obtained for neurons responding to objects in the inferior temporal visual cortex (Booth and Rolls, 1998), and for neurons responding to spatial view in the hippocampus (Rolls, Treves, Robertson, Georges-François and Panzeri, 1998b).

Although those neurons were not simultaneously recorded, a similar approximately linear increase in the information from *simultaneously* recorded cells as the number of neurons in the sample increased also occurs (Rolls, Franco, Aggelopoulos and Reece, 2003b; Rolls, Aggelopoulos, Franco and Treves, 2004; Franco, Rolls, Aggelopoulos and Treves, 2004; Aggelopoulos, Franco and Rolls, 2005; Rolls, Franco, Aggelopoulos and Jerez, 2006b). These findings imply little redundancy, and that the number of stimuli that can be encoded increases approximately exponentially with the number of neurons in the population, as illustrated in Figs. 2.19 and C.24.

The issue of redundancy is considered in more detail now. Redundancy can be defined with reference to a multiple channel of capacity $T(C)$ which can be decomposed into C separate channels of capacities $T_i, i = 1, ..., C$:

$$R = 1 - T(C)/\sum_i T_i \tag{C.52}$$

so that when the C channels are multiplexed with maximal efficiency, $T(C) = \sum_i T_i$ and $R = 0$. What is measured more easily, in practice, is the redundancy defined with reference to a specific source (the set of stimuli with their probabilities). Then in terms of mutual information

$$R' = 1 - I(C)/\sum_i I_i. \tag{C.53}$$

Gawne and Richmond (1993) measured the redundancy R' among pairs of nearby primate inferior temporal cortex visual neurons, in their response to a set of 32 Walsh patterns. They found values with a mean $< R' > = 0.1$ (and a mean single-cell transinformation of 0.23 bits). Since to discriminate 32 different patterns takes 5 bits of information, in principle one would need at least 22 cells each providing 0.23 bits of strictly orthogonal information to represent the full entropy of the stimulus set. Gawne and Richmond reasoned, however, that, because of the overlap, y, in the information they provided, more cells would be needed than if the redundancy had been zero. They constructed a simple model based on the notion that the overlap, y, in the information provided by any two cells in the population always corresponds to the average redundancy measured for nearby pairs. A redundancy $R' = 0.1$ corresponds to an overlap $y = 0.2$ in the information provided by the two neurons, since, counting the overlapping information only once, two cells would yield 1.8 times the amount transmitted by one cell alone. If a fraction of $1 - y = 0.8$ of the information provided by a cell is novel with respect to that provided by another cell, a fraction $(1 - y)^2$ of the information provided by a third cell will be novel with respect to what was known from the first pair, and so on, yielding an estimate of $I(C) = I(1) \sum_{i=0}^{C-1} (1-y)^i$ for the total information conveyed by C cells. However such a sum saturates, in the limit of an infinite number of cells, at the level $I(\infty) = I(1)/y$, implying in their case that even with very many cells, no more than $0.23/0.2 = 1.15$ bits could be read off their activity, or less than a quarter of what was available as entropy in the stimulus set! Gawne and Richmond (1993) concluded, therefore, that the average overlap among non-nearby cells must be considerably lower than that measured for cells close to each other.

The model above is simple and attractive, but experimental verification of the actual scaling of redundancy with the number of cells entails collecting the responses of several cells interspersed in a population of interest. Gochin, Colombo, Dorfman, Gerstein and Gross (1994) recorded from up to 58 cells in the primate temporal visual cortex, using sets of two to five visual stimuli, and applied decoding procedures to measure the information content in the population response. The recordings were not simultaneous, but comparison with simultaneous recordings from a smaller number of cells indicated that the effect of recording the individual responses on separate trials was minor. The results were expressed in terms of the *novelty* N in the information provided by C cells, which being defined as the ratio of such information to C times the average single-cell information, can be expressed as

$$N = 1 - R' \tag{C.54}$$

and is thus the complement of the redundancy. An analysis of two different data sets, which included three information measures per data set, indicated a behavior $N(C) \approx 1/\sqrt{C}$, reminiscent of the improvement in the overall noise-to-signal ratio characterizing C independent processes contributing to the same signal. The analysis neglected however to consider limited sampling effects, and more seriously it neglected to consider saturation effects due to the information content approaching its ceiling, given by the entropy of the stimulus set. Since this ceiling was quite low, for 5 stimuli at $\log_2 5 = 2.32$ bits, relative to the mutual information values measured from the population (an average of 0.26 bits, or 1/9 of the ceiling, was provided by single cells), it is conceivable that the novelty would have taken much larger values if larger stimulus sets had been used.

A simple formula describing the approach to the ceiling, and thus the saturation of information values as they come close to the entropy of the stimulus set, can be derived from a natural extension of the Gawne and Richmond (1993) model. In this extension, the information provided by single cells, measured as a fraction of the ceiling, is taken to coincide with the average overlap among pairs of randomly selected, not necessarily nearby, cells from the population. The actual value measured by Gawne and Richmond would have been, again, $1/22 = 0.045$, below the overlap among nearby cells, $y = 0.2$. The assumption that y, measured across any pair of cells, would have been as low as the fraction of information provided by single cells is equivalent to conceiving of single cells as 'covering' a random portion y of information space, and thus of randomly selected pairs of cells as overlapping in a fraction $(y)^2$ of that space, and so on, as postulated by the Gawne and Richmond (1993) model, for higher numbers of cells. The approach to the ceiling is then described by the formula

$$I(C) \approx H\{1 - \exp[C \ln(1 - y)]\} \tag{C.55}$$

that is, a simple exponential saturation to the ceiling. This simple law indeed describes remarkably well the trend in the data analyzed by Rolls, Treves and Tovee (1997b). Although the model has no reason to be exact, and therefore its agreement with the data should not be expected to be accurate, the crucial point it embodies is that deviations from a purely linear increase in information with the number of cells analyzed are due solely to the ceiling effect. Aside from the ceiling, due to the sampling of an information space of finite entropy, the information contents of different cells' responses are independent of each other. Thus, in the model, the observed redundancy (or indeed the overlap) is purely a consequence of the finite size of the stimulus set. If the population were probed with larger and larger sets of stimuli, or more precisely with sets of increasing entropy, and the amount of information conveyed by single cells were to remain approximately the same, then the fraction of space 'covered' by each cell, again y, would get smaller and smaller, tending to eliminate redundancy for very large stimulus entropies (and a fixed number of cells). The actual data were obtained with limited numbers of stimuli, and therefore cannot probe directly the conditions in which redundancy might reduce to zero. The data are consistent, however, with the hypothesis embodied in the simple model, as shown also by the near exponential approach to lower ceilings found for information values calculated with reduced subsets of the original set of stimuli (Rolls, Treves and Tovee, 1997b).

The implication of this set of analyses, some performed towards the end of the ventral visual stream of the monkey, is that the representation of at least some classes of objects in those areas is achieved with minimal redundancy by cells that are allocated each to analyze a different aspect of the visual stimulus. This minimal redundancy is what would be expected of a self-organizing system in which different cells acquired their response selectivities through a random process, with or without local competition among nearby cells (see Section B.4). At the same time, such low redundancy could also very well result in a system that is organized under some strong teaching input, so that the emerging picture is compatible with a simple random process, but could be produced in other ways. The finding that, at least with small numbers of neurons, redundancy may be effectively minimized, is consistent not only with the concept of efficient encoding, but also with the general idea that one of the functions of the early visual system is to progressively minimize redundancy in the representation of visual stimuli (Attneave, 1954; Barlow, 1961). However, the ventral visual system does much more than produce a non-redundant representation of an image, for it transforms the representation from an image to an invariant representation of objects, as described in Chapter 2. Moreover, what is shown in this section is that the information about objects can be read off from just the spike count of a population of neurons, using decoding as simple as the simplest that could be performed by a receiving neuron, dot product decoding. In this sense, the information about objects is made explicit in the firing rate of the neurons in the inferior temporal cortex, in that it can be read off in this way.

We consider in Section C.3.7 whether there is more to it than this. Does the synchronization of neurons (and it would have to be stimulus-dependent synchronization) add significantly to the information that could be encoded by the number of spikes, as has been suggested by some?

Before this, we consider why encoding by a population of neurons is more powerful than the encoding than is possible by single neurons, adding to previous arguments that a distributed representation is much more computationally useful than a local representation, by allowing properties such as generalization, completion, and graceful degradation in associative neuronal networks (see Appendix B).

C.3.6 Should one neuron be as discriminative as the whole organism, in object encoding systems?

In the analysis of random dot motion with a given level of correlation among the moving dots, single neurons in area MT in the dorsal visual system of the primate can be approximately as sensitive or discriminative as the psychophysical performance of the whole animal (Zohary, Shadlen and Newsome, 1994). The arguments and evidence presented here (e.g. in Section C.3.5) suggest that this is not the case for the ventral visual system, concerned with object identification. Why should there be this difference?

Rolls and Treves (1998) suggest that the dimensionality of what is being computed may account for the difference. In the case of visual motion (at least in the study referred to), the problem was effectively one-dimensional, in that the direction of motion of the stimulus along a line in 2D space was extracted from the activity of the neurons. In this low-dimensional stimulus space, the neurons may each perform one of a few similar computations on a particular (local) portion of 2D space, with the side effect that, by averaging over a larger receptive field than in V1, one can extract a signal of a more global nature. Indeed, in the case of more global motion, it is the average of the neuronal activity that can be computed by the larger receptive fields of MT neurons that specifies the average or global direction of motion.

In contrast, in the higher dimensional space of objects, in which there are very many different objects to represent as being different from each other, and in a system that is not concerned with location in visual space but on the contrary tends to be relatively invariant with respect to location, the goal of the representation is to reflect the many aspects of the input information in a way that enables many different objects to be represented, in what is effectively a very high dimensional space. This is achieved by allocating cells, each with an intrinsically limited discriminative power, to sample as thoroughly as possible the many dimensions of the space. Thus the system is geared to use efficiently the parallel computations of all its neurons precisely for tasks such as that of face discrimination, which was used as an experimental probe. Moreover, object representation must be kept higher dimensional, in that it may have to be decoded by dot product decoders in associative memories, in which the input patterns must be in a space that is as high-dimensional as possible (i.e. the activity on different input axons should not be too highly correlated). In this situation, each neuron should act somewhat independently of its neighbours, so that each provides its own separate contribution that adds together with that of the other neurons (in a linear manner, see above and Figs. 2.18, C.24 and 2.19) to provide *in toto* sufficient information to specify which out of perhaps several thousand visual stimuli was seen. The computation involves in this case not an average of neuronal activity (which would be useful for e.g. head direction (Robertson, Rolls, Georges-François and Panzeri, 1999)), but instead comparing the dot product of the activity of the population of neurons with a previously learned vector, stored in, for example, associative memories as the weight vector on a receiving neuron or neurons.

Zohary, Shadlen and Newsome (1994) put forward another argument which suggested to them that the brain could hardly benefit from taking into account the activity of more than a very limited number of neurons. The argument was based on their measurement of a small (0.12) correlation between the activity of simultaneously recorded neurons in area MT. They suggested that there would because of this be decreasing signal-to-noise ratio advantages as more neurons were included in the population, and that this would limit the number of neurons that it would be useful to decode to approximately 100. However, a measure of correlations in the activity of different neurons depends entirely on the way the space of neuronal activity is sampled, that is on the task chosen to probe the system. Among face cells in the temporal cortex, for example, much higher correlations would be observed when the task is a simple two-way discrimination between a face and a non-face, than when the task involves finer identification of several different faces. (It is also entirely possible that some face cells could be found that perform as well in a given particular face / non-face discrimination as the whole animal.) Moreover, their argument depends on the type of decoding of the activity of the population that is envisaged (see further Robertson, Rolls, Georges-François and Panzeri (1999)). It implies that the average of the neuronal activity must be estimated accurately. If a set of neurons uses dot product decoding, and then the activity of the decoding population is scaled or normalized by some negative feedback through inhibitory interneurons, then the effect of such correlated firing in the sending population is reduced, for the decoding effectively measures the relative firing of the different neurons in the population to be decoded. This is equivalent to measuring the angle between the current vector formed by the population of neurons firing, and a previously learned vector, stored in synaptic weights. Thus, with for example this biologically plausible decoding, it is not clear whether the correlation Zohary, Shadlen and Newsome (1994) describe would place a severe limit on the ability of the brain to utilize the information available in a population of neurons.

The main conclusion from this and the preceding Section is that the information available from a set or ensemble of temporal cortex visual neurons increases approximately linearly as more neurons are added to the sample. This is powerful evidence that distributed encoding is used by the brain; and the code can be read just by knowing the firing rates in a short time of the population of neurons. The fact that the code can be read off from the firing rates, and by a principle as simple and neuron-like as dot product decoding, provides strong support for the general approach taken in this book to brain function.

It is possible that more information would be available in the relative time of occurrence of the spikes, either within the spike train of a single neuron, or between the spike trains of different neurons, and it is to this that we now turn.

C.3.7 The information from multiple cells: the effects of cross-correlations between cells

Using the second derivative methods described in Section C.2.5 (see Rolls, Franco, Aggelopoulos and Reece (2003b)), the information available from the number of spikes vs that from the cross-correlations between simultaneously recorded cells has been analyzed for a population of neurons in the inferior temporal visual cortex (Rolls, Aggelopoulos, Franco and Treves, 2004). The stimuli were a set of 20 objects, faces, and scenes presented while the monkey performed a visual discrimination task. If synchronization was being used to bind the parts of each object into the correct spatial relationship to other parts, this might be expected to be revealed by stimulus-dependent cross-correlations in the firing of simultaneously recorded groups of 2–4 cells using multiple single-neuron microelectrodes.

A typical result from the information analysis described in Section C.2.5 on a set of three simultaneously recorded cells from this experiment is shown in Fig. C.25. This shows that most of the information available in a 100 ms time period was available in the rates, and that there was little contribution to the information from stimulus-dependent ('noise') correlations (which would have shown as positive values if for example there was stimulus-dependent synchronization of the neuronal responses); or from stimulus-independent 'noise' correlation effects, which might if present have reflected common input to the different neurons so that their responses tended to be correlated independently of which stimulus was shown.

The results for the 20 experiments with groups of 2–4 simultaneously recorded inferior temporal cortex neurons are shown in Table C.4. (The total information is the total from equations C.43 and C.44 in a 100 ms time window, and is not expected to be the sum of the contributions shown in Table C.4 because only the information from the cross terms (for $i \neq j$) is shown in the table for the contributions related to the stimulus-dependent contributions and the stimulus-independent contributions arising from the 'noise' correlations.) The results show that the greatest contribution to the information is that from the rates, that is from the numbers of spikes from each neuron in the time window of 100 ms. The average value of -0.05 for the cross term of the stimulus independent 'noise' correlation-related contribution is consistent with on average a small amount of common input to neurons in the inferior temporal visual cortex. A positive value for the cross term of the stimulus-dependent 'noise' correlation related contribution would be consistent with on average a small amount of stimulus-dependent synchronization, but the actual value found, 0.04 bits, is so small that for 17 of the 20 experiments it is less than that which can arise by chance statistical fluctuations of the time of arrival of the spikes, as shown by MonteCarlo control rearrangements of the same data. Thus on average there was no significant contribution to the information from stimulus-dependent synchronization effects (Rolls, Aggelopoulos, Franco and Treves, 2004).

Thus, this data set provides evidence for considerable information available from the number of spikes that each cell produces to different stimuli, and evidence for little impact of common input, or of synchronization, on the amount of information provided by

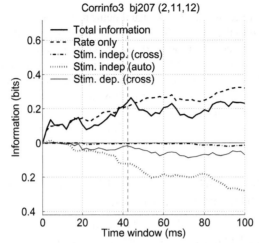

Fig. C.25 Most of the information is present in the firing rates, with little in stimulus-dependent cross-correlations between the spikes of different neurons. A typical result from the information analysis described in Section C.2.5 on a set of 3 simultaneously recorded inferior temporal cortex neurons in an experiment in which 20 complex stimuli effective for IT neurons (objects, faces and scenes) were shown. The graphs show the contributions to the information from the different terms in Equations C.43 and C.44 on page 989, as a function of the length of the time window, which started 100 ms after stimulus onset, which is when IT neurons start to respond. The rate information is the sum of the term in Equation C.43 and the first term of Equation C.44. The contribution of the stimulus-independent noise correlation to the information is the second term of Equation C.44, and is separated into components arising from the correlations between cells (the cross component, for $i \neq j$) and from the autocorrelation within a cell (the auto component, for $i = j$). This term is non-zero if there is some correlation in the variance to a given stimulus, even if it is independent of which stimulus is present. The contribution of the stimulus-dependent noise correlation to the information is the third term of Equation C.44, and only the cross term is shown (for $i \neq j$), as this is the term of interest. (From Rolls, E. T., Aggelopoulos,N.C., Franco,L., and Treves,A. (2004) Information encoding in the inferior temporal cortex: contributions of the firing rates and correlations between the firing of neurons. Biological Cybernetics 90: 19–32. © Springer Nature.)

Table C.4 The average contributions (in bits) of different components of Equations C.43 and C.44 to the information available in a 100 ms time window from 13 sets of simultaneously recorded inferior temporal cortex neurons when shown 20 stimuli effective for the cells.

rate	0.26
stimulus–dependent "noise" correlation-related, cross term	0.04
stimulus–independent "noise" correlation-related, cross term	-0.05
total information	0.31

sets of *simultaneously recorded* inferior temporal cortex neurons. Further supporting data for the inferior temporal visual cortex are provided by Rolls, Franco, Aggelopoulos and Reece (2003b). In that parts as well as whole objects are represented in the inferior temporal cortex (Perrett, Rolls and Caan, 1982), and in that the parts must be bound together in the correct spatial configuration for the inferior temporal cortex neurons to respond (Rolls, Tovee, Purcell, Stewart and Azzopardi, 1994b), we might have expected temporal synchrony, if used to implement feature binding, to have been evident in these experiments.

We have also explored neuronal encoding under natural scene conditions in a task in which top-down attention must be used, a visual search task. We applied the decoding information theoretic method of Section C.2.4 to the responses of neurons in the inferior temporal visual cortex recorded under conditions in which feature binding is likely to be needed, that is when the monkey had to choose to touch one of two simultaneously presented objects, with the stimuli presented in a complex natural background (Aggelopoulos, Franco and Rolls, 2005). The investigation is thus directly relevant to whether stimulus-dependent synchrony

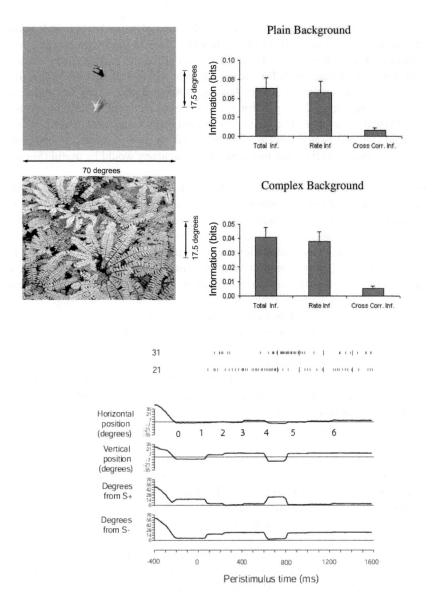

Fig. C.26 Even in complex natural scenes, most of the information is in the firing rates and not in the cross-correlations between the neurons. Left: the objects against the plain background, and in a natural scene. Right: the information available from the firing rates (Rate Inf) or from stimulus-dependent synchrony (Cross-Corr Inf) from populations of simultaneously recorded inferior temporal cortex neurons about which stimulus had been presented in a complex natural scene. The total information (Total Inf) is that available from both the rate and the stimulus-dependent synchrony, which do not necessarily contribute independently. Bottom: eye position recordings and spiking activity from two neurons on a single trial of the task. (Neuron 31 tended to fire more when the macaque looked at one of the stimuli, S−, and neuron 21 tended to fire more when the macaque looked at the other stimulus, S+. Both stimuli were within the receptive field of the neuron.) (After Aggelopoulos,N.C., Franco,L. and Rolls, E. T. (2005) Object perception in natural scenes: encoding by inferior temporal cortex simultaneously recorded neurons. Journal of Neurophysiology 93: 1342–1357. © American Physiological Society.)

contributes to encoding under natural conditions, and when an attentional task was being performed. In the attentional task, the monkey had to find one of two objects and to touch it to obtain reward. This is thus an object-based attentional visual search task, where the top-down bias is for the object that has to be found in the scene (Aggelopoulos, Franco and Rolls,

2005). The objects could be presented against a complex natural scene background. Neurons in the inferior temporal visual cortex respond in some cases to object features or parts, and in other cases to whole objects provided that the parts are in the correct spatial configuration (Perrett, Rolls and Caan, 1982; Desimone, Albright, Gross and Bruce, 1984; Rolls, Tovee, Purcell, Stewart and Azzopardi, 1994b; Tanaka, 1996), and so it is very appropriate to measure whether stimulus-dependent synchrony contributes to information encoding in the inferior temporal visual cortex when two objects are present in the visual field, and when they must be segmented from the background in a natural visual scene, which are the conditions in which it has been postulated that stimulus-dependent synchrony would be useful (Singer, 1999, 2000).

Aggelopoulos, Franco and Rolls (2005) found that between 99% and 94% of the information was present in the firing rates of inferior temporal cortex neurons, and less that 5% in any stimulus-dependent synchrony that was present, as illustrated in Fig. C.26. The implication of these results is that any stimulus-dependent synchrony that is present is not quantitatively important as measured by information theoretic analyses under natural scene conditions. This has been found for the inferior temporal visual cortex, a brain region where features are put together to form representations of objects (Rolls, 2016b) (Chapter 2), where attention has strong effects, at least in scenes with blank backgrounds (Rolls, Aggelopoulos and Zheng, 2003a), and in an object-based attentional search task.

The finding as assessed by information theoretic methods of the importance of firing rates and not stimulus-dependent synchrony is consistent with previous information theoretic approaches (Rolls, Franco, Aggelopoulos and Reece, 2003b; Rolls, Aggelopoulos, Franco and Treves, 2004; Franco, Rolls, Aggelopoulos and Treves, 2004). It would of course also be of interest to test the same hypothesis in earlier visual areas, such as V4, with quantitative, information theoretic, techniques. In connection with rate codes, it should be noted that the findings indicate that the number of spikes that arrive in a given time is what is important for very useful amounts of information to be made available from a population of neurons; and that this time can be very short, as little as 20–50 ms (Tovee and Rolls, 1995; Rolls and Tovee, 1994; Rolls, Tovee and Panzeri, 1999b; Rolls and Deco, 2002; Rolls, Tovee, Purcell, Stewart and Azzopardi, 1994b; Rolls, 2003; Rolls, Franco, Aggelopoulos and Jerez, 2006b). Further, it was shown that there was little redundancy (less than 6%) between the information provided by the spike counts of the simultaneously recorded neurons, making spike counts an efficient population code with a high encoding capacity.

The findings (Aggelopoulos, Franco and Rolls, 2005) are consistent with the hypothesis that feature binding is implemented by neurons that respond to features in the correct relative spatial locations (Rolls and Deco, 2002; Elliffe, Rolls and Stringer, 2002; Rolls, 2016b, 2012d) (Chapter 2), and not by temporal synchrony and attention (Malsburg, 1990; Singer, Gray, Engel, Konig, Artola and Brocher, 1990; Abeles, 1991; Hummel and Biederman, 1992; Singer and Gray, 1995; Singer, 1999, 2000; Rolls, 2016b). In any case, the computational point made in Section 2.8.5.1 is that even if stimulus-dependent synchrony was useful for grouping, it would not without much extra machinery be useful for binding the relative spatial positions of features within an object, or for that matter of the positions of objects in a scene which appears to be encoded in a different way (Aggelopoulos and Rolls, 2005) (see Section 2.8.10).

So far, we know of no analyses that have shown with information theoretic methods that considerable amounts of information are available about the stimulus from the stimulus-dependent correlations between the responses of neurons in the primate ventral visual system. The use of such methods is needed to test quantitatively the hypothesis that stimulus-dependent synchronization contributes substantially to the encoding of information by neurons.

As described in Section C.2.5, one way to measure how the effects of the correlations in the activity of populations of simultaneously recorded neurons influence the total information that can be encoded is to shuffle the data across trials for each neuron in the population (Panzeri et al., 2022). In practice, 'noise' correlations tend to decrease the information that can be decoded from populations of neurons (Panzeri et al., 2022). However, many of these analyses (Panzeri et al., 2022) assume that for example temporal synchrony between the firing of particular pairs of neurons is actually being measured in the brain and taken into account in decoding the information, and that is not at all clear. Overall, 'noise' correlations are not likely to increase the information that is used in the brain, and if anything decrease the information that is being used by the brain (Panzeri et al., 2022).

C.3.8 Conclusions on cortical neuronal encoding

The conclusions emerging from this set of information theoretic analyses, many in cortical areas towards the end of the ventral visual stream of the monkey, and others in the hippocampus for spatial view cells (Rolls, Treves, Robertson, Georges-François and Panzeri, 1998b), in the presubiculum for head direction cells (Robertson, Rolls, Georges-François and Panzeri, 1999), and in the orbitofrontal cortex and related areas for olfactory and taste cells (Rolls, Critchley and Treves, 1996a; Rolls, Critchley, Verhagen and Kadohisa, 2010a) for which subsequent analyses have shown a linear increase in information with the number of cells in the population, are as follows (see also Rolls and Treves (2011)).

The representation of at least some classes of objects in those areas is achieved with minimal redundancy by cells that are allocated each to analyze a different aspect of the visual stimulus (Abbott, Rolls and Tovee, 1996; Rolls, Treves and Tovee, 1997b) (as shown in Sections C.3.5 and C.3.7). This minimal redundancy is what would be expected of a self-organizing system in which different cells acquired their response selectivities through processes that include some randomness in the initial connectivity, and local competition among nearby cells (see Appendix B). Towards the end of the ventral visual stream redundancy may thus be effectively minimized, a finding consistent with the general idea that one of the functions of the early visual system is indeed that of progressively minimizing redundancy in the representation of visual stimuli (Attneave, 1954; Barlow, 1961). Indeed, the evidence described in Sections C.3.5, C.3.7 and C.3.4 shows that the exponential rise in the number of stimuli that can be decoded when the firing rates of different numbers of neurons are analyzed indicates that the encoding of information using firing rates (in practice the number of spikes emitted by each of a large population of neurons in a short time period) is a very powerful coding scheme used by the cerebral cortex, and that the information carried by different neurons is close to independent provided that the number of stimuli being considered is sufficiently large.

Quantitatively, the encoding of information using firing rates (in practice the number of spikes emitted by each of a large population of neurons in a short time period) is likely to be far more important than temporal encoding, in terms of the number of stimuli that can be encoded. Moreover, the information available from an ensemble of cortical neurons when only the firing rates are read, that is with no temporal encoding within or between neurons, is made available very rapidly (see Figs. C.16 and C.17 and Section C.3.4). Further, the neuronal responses in most ventral or 'what' processing streams of behaving monkeys show sustained firing rate differences to different stimuli (see for example Fig. 2.16 for visual representations, for the olfactory pathways Rolls, Critchley and Treves (1996a), for spatial view cells in the hippocampus Rolls, Treves, Robertson, Georges-François and Panzeri (1998b), and for head direction cells in the presubiculum Robertson, Rolls, Georges-François and Panzeri (1999)), so that it may not usually be necessary to invoke temporal encoding for the information about the stimulus. Further, as indicated in Section C.3.7, information theoretic approaches have enabled the information that is available from the firing rate and from the relative time of firing (synchronization) of inferior temporal cortex neurons to be directly compared with the same metric, and most of the information appears to be encoded in the numbers of spikes emitted by a population of cells in a short time period, rather than by the temporal synchronization of the responses of different neurons when certain stimuli appear (see Section C.3.7 and Aggelopoulos, Franco and Rolls (2005)).

Information theoretic approaches have also enabled different types of readout or decoding that could be performed by the brain of the information available in the responses of cell populations to be compared (Rolls, Treves and Tovee, 1997b; Robertson, Rolls, Georges-François and Panzeri, 1999). It has been shown for example that the multiple cell representation of information used by the brain in the inferior temporal visual cortex (Rolls, Treves and Tovee, 1997b; Aggelopoulos, Franco and Rolls, 2005), olfactory cortex (Rolls, Critchley and Treves, 1996a), hippocampus (Rolls, Treves, Robertson, Georges-François and Panzeri, 1998b), and presubiculum (Robertson, Rolls, Georges-François and Panzeri, 1999) can be read fairly efficiently by the neuronally plausible dot product decoding, and that the representation has all the desirable properties of generalization and graceful degradation, as well as exponential coding capacity (see Sections C.3.5 and C.3.7).

Information theoretic approaches have also enabled the information available about different aspects of stimuli to be directly compared. For example, it has been shown that inferior temporal cortex neurons make explicit much more information about what stimulus has been shown rather than where the stimulus is in the visual field (Tovee, Rolls and Azzopardi, 1994), and this is part of the evidence that inferior temporal cortex neurons provide translation invariant representations. In a similar way, information theoretic analysis has provided clear evidence that view invariant representations of objects and faces are present in the inferior temporal visual cortex, in that for example much information is available about what object has been shown from any single trial on which any view of any object is presented (Booth and Rolls, 1998).

Information theory has also helped to elucidate the way in which the inferior temporal visual cortex provides a representation of objects and faces, in which information about which object or face is shown is made explicit in the firing of the neurons in such a way that the information can be read off very simply by memory systems such as the orbitofrontal cortex, amygdala, and perirhinal cortex / hippocampal systems. The information can be read off using dot product decoding, that is by using a synaptically weighted sum of inputs from inferior temporal cortex neurons (see further Section 9.2.7 and Chapter 2). Moreover, information theory has helped to show that for many neurons considerable invariance in the representations of objects and faces are shown by inferior temporal cortex neurons (e.g. Booth and Rolls (1998)). Examples of some of the types of objects and faces that are encoded in this way are shown in Fig. C.7. Information theory has also helped to show that inferior temporal cortex neurons maintain their object selectivity even when the objects are presented in complex natural backgrounds (Aggelopoulos, Franco and Rolls, 2005) (see further Chapter 2 and Section 9.2.7).

Information theory has also enabled the information available in neuronal representations to be compared with that available to the whole animal in its behavior (Zohary, Shadlen and Newsome, 1994) (but see Section C.3.6).

Finally, information theory also provides a metric for directly comparing the information available from neurons in the brain (see Chapter 2 and this Appendix) with that available from single neurons and populations of neurons in simulations of visual information processing (see Chapter 2).

In summary, the evidence from the application of information theoretic and related approaches to how information is encoded in the visual, hippocampal, and olfactory cortical systems described during behavior leads to the following working hypotheses:

1. Much information is available about the stimulus presented in the number of spikes emitted by single neurons in a fixed time period, the firing rate.

2. Much of this firing rate information is available in short periods, with a considerable proportion available in as little as 20 ms. This rapid availability of information enables the next stage of processing to read the information quickly, and thus for multistage processing to operate rapidly. This time is the order of time over which a receiving neuron might be able to utilize the information, given its synaptic and membrane time constants. In this time, a sending neuron is most likely to emit 0, 1, or 2 spikes.

3. This rapid availability of information is confirmed by population analyses, which indicate that across a population on neurons, much information is available in short time periods.

4. More information is available using this rate code in a short period (of e.g. 20 ms) than from just the first spike.

5. Little information is available by time variations within the spike train of individual neurons for static visual stimuli (in periods of several hundred milliseconds), apart from a small amount of information from the onset latency of the neuronal response. A static stimulus encompasses what might be seen in a single visual fixation, what might be tasted with a stimulus in the mouth, what might be smelled in a single sniff, etc. For a time-varying stimulus, clearly the firing rate will vary as a function of time.

6. Across a population of neurons, the firing rate information provided by each neuron tends to be independent; that is, the information increases approximately linearly with the number of neurons. This applies of course only when there is a large amount of information to be encoded, that is with a large number of stimuli. The outcome is that the number of stimuli that can be encoded rises exponentially in the number of neurons in the ensemble. (For a small stimulus set, the information saturates gradually as the amount of information available from the neuronal population approaches that required to code for the stimulus set.) This applies up to the number of neurons tested and the stimulus set sizes used, but as the number of neurons becomes very large, this is likely to hold less well. An implication of the independence is that the response profiles to a set of stimuli of different neurons are uncorrelated.

7. The information in the firing rate across a population of neurons can be read moderately efficiently by a decoding procedure as simple as a dot product. This is the simplest type of processing that might be performed by a neuron, as it involves taking a dot product of the incoming firing rates with the receiving synaptic weights to obtain the activation (e.g. depolarization) of the neuron. This type of information encoding ensures that the simple emergent properties of associative neuronal networks such as generalization, completion, and graceful degradation (see Appendix B) can be realized very naturally and simply.

8. There is little additional information to the great deal available in the firing rates from any stimulus-dependent cross-correlations or synchronization that may be present. Stimulus-dependent synchronization might in any case only be useful for grouping different neuronal populations, and would not easily provide a solution to the binding problem in vision. In-

stead, the binding problem in vision may be solved by the presence of neurons that respond to combinations of features in a given spatial position with respect to each other.

9. There is little information available in the order of the spike arrival times of different neurons for different stimuli that is separate or additional to that provided by a rate code. The presence of spontaneous activity in cortical neurons facilitates rapid neuronal responses, because some neurons are close to threshold at any given time, but this also would make a spike order code difficult to implement.

10. Analysis of the responses of single neurons to measure the sparseness of the representation indicates that the representation is distributed, and not grandmother cell like (or local). Moreover, the nature of the distributed representation, that it can be read by dot product decoding, allows simple emergent properties of associative neuronal networks such as generalization, completion, and graceful degradation (see Appendix B) to be realized very naturally and simply. The evidence becoming available from humans is consistent with this summary (Fried, Rutishauser, Cerf and Kreiman, 2014; Rolls, 2015c, 2017a).

11. The representation is not very sparse in the perceptual systems studied (as shown for example by the values of the single cell sparseness a^s), and this may allow much information to be represented. At the same time, the responses of different neurons to a set of stimuli are decorrelated, in the sense that the correlations between the response profiles of different neurons to a set of stimuli are low. Consistent with this, the neurons convey independent information, at least up to reasonable numbers of neurons. The representation may be more sparse in memory systems such as the hippocampus, and this may help to maximize the number of memories that can be stored in associative networks.

12. The nature of the distributed representation can be understood further by the firing rate probability distribution, which has a long tail with low probabilities of high firing rates. The firing rate probability distributions for some neurons fit an exponential distribution, and for others there are too few very low rates for a good fit to the exponential distribution. An implication of an exponential distribution is that this maximizes the entropy of the neuronal responses for a given mean firing rate under some conditions. It is of interest that in the inferior temporal visual cortex, the firing rate probability distribution is very close to exponential if a large number of neurons are included without scaling of the firing rates of each neuron. An implication is that a receiving neuron would see an exponential firing rate probability distribution.

13. The population sparseness a^p, that is the sparseness of the firing of a population of neurons to a given stimulus (or at one time), is the important measure for setting the capacity of associative neuronal networks. In populations of neurons studied in the inferior temporal cortex, hippocampus, and orbitofrontal cortex, it takes the same value as the single cell sparseness a^s, and this is a situation of weak ergodicity that occurs if the response profiles of the different neurons to a set of stimuli are uncorrelated.

Understanding the neuronal code, the subject of this Appendix, is fundamental for understanding how memory and related perceptual systems in the brain operate, as follows:

Understanding the neuronal code helps to clarify what neuronal operations would be useful in memory and in fact in most mammalian brain systems (e.g. dot product decoding, that is taking a sum in a short time of the incoming firing rates weighted by the synaptic weights).

It clarifies how rapidly memory and perceptual systems in the brain could operate, in terms of how long it takes a receiving neuron to read the code.

It helps to confirm how the properties of those memory systems in terms of generalization, completion, and graceful degradation occur, in that the representation is in the correct form for these properties to be realized.

Understanding the neuronal code also provides evidence essential for understanding the storage capacity of memory systems, and the representational capacity of perceptual systems.

Understanding the neuronal code is also important for interpreting functional neuroimaging, for it shows that functional imaging that reflects incoming firing rates and thus currents injected into neurons, and probably not stimulus-dependent synchronization, is likely to lead to useful interpretations of the underlying neuronal activity and processing. Of course, functional neuroimaging cannot address the details of the representation of information in the brain in the way that is essential for understanding how neuronal networks in the brain could operate, for this level of understanding (in terms of all the properties and working hypotheses described above) comes only from an understanding of how single neurons and populations of neurons encode information.

C.4 Information theory terms – a short glossary

1. The **amount of information**, or **surprise**, in the occurrence of an event (or symbol) s_i of probability $P(s_i)$ is

$$I(s_i) = \log_2(1/P(s_i)) = -\log_2 P(s_i). \tag{C.56}$$

(The measure is in bits if logs to the base 2 are used.) This is also the amount of **uncertainty** removed by the occurrence of the event.

2. The average amount of information per source symbol over the whole alphabet (S) of symbols s_i is the **entropy**,

$$H(S) = -\sum_i P(s_i) \log_2 P(s_i) \tag{C.57}$$

(or *a priori* entropy).

3. The probability of the pair of symbols s and s' is denoted $P(s, s')$, and is $P(s)P(s')$ only when the two symbols are **independent**.

4. Bayes theorem (given the output s', what was the input s ?) states that

$$P(s|s') = \frac{P(s'|s)P(s)}{P(s')} \tag{C.58}$$

where $P(s'|s)$ is the **forward** conditional probability (given the input s, what will be the output s' ?), and $P(s|s')$ is the **backward** (or posterior) conditional probability (given the output s', what was the input s ?). The prior probability is $P(s)$.

5. **Mutual information**. Prior to reception of s', the probability of the input symbol s was $P(s)$. This is the *a priori* probability of s. After reception of s', the probability that the input symbol was s becomes $P(s|s')$, the conditional probability that s was sent given that s' was received. This is the *a posteriori* probability of s. The difference between the *a priori* and

a posteriori uncertainties measures the gain of information due to the reception of s'. Once averaged across the values of both symbols s and s', this is the **mutual information**, or **transinformation**

$$I(S, S') = \sum_{s,s'} P(s, s')\{\log_2[1/P(s)] - \log_2[1/P(s|s')]\} \tag{C.59}$$

$$= \sum_{s,s'} P(s, s') \log_2[P(s|s')/P(s)].$$

Alternatively,
$$I(S, S') = H(S) - H(S|S'). \tag{C.60}$$

$H(S|S')$ is sometimes called the **equivocation** (of S with respect to S').

C.5 Highlights

1. The encoding of information by neuronal responses is described using Shannon information theory.
2. Information is encoded by sparse distributed place coded representations, with almost independent information conveyed by each neuron, up to reasonable numbers of neurons.
3. Place cell encoding conveys much more information than stimulus-dependent synchronicity ('oscillations', coherence) of firing of groups of neurons in the awake behaving animal.
4. Code translated into Matlab that was used for the single neuron information analysis (Rolls, Treves, Tovee and Panzeri, 1997d) and multiple single neuron information analysis Rolls, Treves and Tovee (1997b) is described in Section D.7 and is available at https://www.oxcns.org/software.

Appendix 4 Simulation software for neuronal networks, and information analysis of neuronal encoding

D.1 Introduction

This Appendix of *Brain Computations and Connectivity* (Oxford University Press) (Rolls, 2023a) describes the Matlab software that has been made available with this book to provide simple demonstrations of the operation of some key neuronal networks related to cortical function. Previous versions of some of this software are provided in connection with *Cerebral Cortex: Principles of Operation* (Oxford University Press) (Rolls, 2016b) and *Emotion and Decision-Making Explained* (Oxford University Press) (Rolls, 2014a). The aim of providing the software is to enable those who are learning about these networks to understand how they operate and their properties by running simulations and by providing the programs. The code has been kept simple, but can easily be edited to explore the properties of these networks. The code itself contains comments that help to explain how the code works.

The programs are intended to be used with the descriptions of the networks and their properties provided in Appendix B of this book *Brain Computations and Connectivity* (Rolls, 2023a). Most of the papers cited in this Appendix can be found at https://www.oxcns.org. Exercises are suggested below that will provide insight into the properties of these networks, and will make the software suitable for class use. The code is available at https://www.oxcns.org. The programs are written in Matlab™ (Mathworks Inc). The programs should work in any version of Matlab, whether it is running under Windows, Linux, or Apple software. The programs will also work under GNU Octave, which is available for free download. In addition, for those who use Python, Python versions of these programs are also provided at https://www.oxcns.org.

To get started, copy the Matlab program files PatternAssociationDemo.m, AutoAssociationDemo.m, CompetitiveNetDemo.m and SOMdemo.m, and the function files NormVeclen.m and spars.m, into a directory, and in Matlab cd into that directory.

The corresponding programs for Python are PatternAssociationDemo.py, AutoAssociationDemo.py, CompetitiveNetDemo.py and SOMdemo.py, and the function files NormVeclen.py and spars.py.

Sections D.2–D.4 describe these tutorial neuronal network programs.

In addition, Section D.6 describes tutorial software written in Matlab that illustrates some of the principles of operation of VisNet, the model of invariant visual object recognition described in Section 2.8 of this book (Rolls, 2023a) and by Rolls (2012d). The software is also available at https://www.oxcns.org.

Section D.7 describes code translated into Matlab that was used for the single neuron information analyses described by Rolls, Treves, Tovee and Panzeri (1997d) and the multiple single neuron information analyses described by Rolls, Treves and Tovee (1997b), and in Appendix C. The software is also available at https://www.oxcns.org.

Section D.8 describes Matlab code to illustrate the use of spatial view cells and allocentric bearing to a landmark cells in Navigation described in Section 9.3.15 (Rolls, 2021f). The software is available at https://www.oxcns.org/software.

D.2 Autoassociation or attractor networks

The operation and properties of autoassociation (or attractor) neuronal networks are described in this book (Rolls, 2023a) Appendix B.3.

D.2.1 Running the simulation

In the command window of Matlab, after you have performed a 'cd' into the directory where the source files are, type 'AutoAssociationDemo' (with every command followed by 'Enter' or 'Return'). The program will run for a bit, and then pause so that you can inspect what has been produced so far. A paused state is indicated by the words 'Paused: Press any key' in the bottom of the Matlab window. Press 'Enter' to move to the next stage, until the program finishes and the command prompt reappears. You can edit the code to comment out some of the 'pause' statements if you do not want them, or to add a 'pause' statement if you would like the program to stop at a particular place so that you can inspect the results. To stop the program and exit from it, use 'Ctrl-C'. When at the command prompt, you can access variables by typing the variable name followed by 'Enter'. (Note: if you set '*display = 0*' near the beginning of the program, there will be no pauses, and you will be able to collect data quickly.)

The fully connected autoassociation network has N=100 neurons with the dendrites that receive the synapses shown as vertical columns in the generated figures, and $nSyn = N$ synapses onto each neuron. At the first pause, you will see a figure showing the 10 random binary training patterns with firing rates of 1 or 0, and with a *Sparseness* (referred to as a in the equations below) of 0.5. As these are binary patterns, the *Sparseness* parameter value is the same as the proportion of high firing rates or 1s. At the second pause you will see distorted versions of these patterns to be used as recall cues later. The number of bits that have been flipped $nFlipBits$=14.

Next you will see a figure showing the synaptic matrix being trained with the 10 patterns. Uncomment the pause in the training loop if you wish to see each pattern being presented sequentially. The synaptic weight matrix *SynMat* (the elements of which are referred to as w_{ij} in the equations below) is initialized to zero, and then each pattern is presented as an external input to set the firing rates of the neurons (the postsynaptic term), which because of the recurrent collaterals become also the presynaptic input. Each time a training pattern is presented, the weight change is calculated by a covariance learning rule

$$\delta w_{ij} = \alpha(y_i - a)(y_j - a) \tag{D.1}$$

where α is a learning rate constant, and y_j is the presynaptic firing rate. This learning rule includes (in proportion to y_i the firing rate of the ith postsynaptic neuron) increasing the synaptic weight if $(y_j - a) > 0$ (long-term potentiation), and decreasing the synaptic weight if $(y_j - a) < 0$ (heterosynaptic long-term depression). As these are random binary patterns with sparseness a (the parameter *Sparseness* in AutoassociationDemo.m), a is the average activity $< y_j >$ of an axon across patterns, and a is also the average activity $< y_i >$ of a neuron across patterns. In the exercises, you can try a form of this learning rule that is more biologically plausible, with only heterosynaptic long-term depression. The change of weight is added to the previous synaptic weight. In the figures generated by the code, the maximum weights are shown as white, and the minimum weights are black. Although both these rules lead to some negative synaptic weights, which are not biologically plausible, this limitation can be overcome, as shown in the exercises. In the display of the synaptic weights, remember that each column represents the synaptic weights on a single neuron. The thin row below the synaptic matrix represents the firing rates of the neurons, and the thin column to the left of the synaptic weight matrix the firing rates of the presynaptic input, which are usually the same during training. Rates of 1 are shown as white, and of 0 as black.

Next, testing with the distorted patterns starts, with the output rates allowed to recirculate through the recurrent collateral axons for 9 recall epochs to produce presynaptic inputs that act through the synaptic weight matrix to produce the firing rate for the next recall epoch. The distorted recall cue is presented only on epoch 1 in what is described as the clamped condition, and after that is removed so that the network has a chance to settle into a perfect recall state representing the training pattern without being affected by the distorted recall cue. (In the cortex, this may be facilitated by the greater adaptation of the thalamic inputs than of the recurrent collaterals (Rolls, 2016b)). (Thus on epoch 1 the distorted recall cue is shown as the PreSynaptic Input column on the left of the display, and the Activation row and the Firing Rate row below the synaptic weight matrix are the Activations and Rates produced by the recall cue. On later epochs, the Presynaptic Input column shows the output firing Rate from the preceding epoch, recirculated by the recurrent collateral connections.)

We are interested in how perfect the recall is, that is how correlated the recalled firing rate state is with the original training pattern, with this correlation having a maximum value of 1. Every time you press 'Enter' a new recall epoch is performed, and you will see that over one to several recall epochs the recall usually will become perfect, that is the correlation, which is provided for you in the command window, will become 1. However, on some trials, the network does not converge to perfect recall, and this occurs if by chance the distorted recall cue happened to be much closer to one of the other stored patterns. Do note that with randomly chosen training patterns in relatively small networks this will sometimes occur, and that this 'statistical fluctuation' in how close some of the training patterns are to each other, and how close the distorted test patterns are to individual training patterns, is to be expected. These effects smooth out as the network become larger. (Remember that cortical neurons have in the order of 10,000 recurrent collateral inputs to each neuron, so these statistical fluctuations will be largely smoothed out. Do note also that the performance of the network will be different each time it is run, because the random number generator is set with a different seed on each run.) (Near the beginning of the program, you could uncomment the command that causes the same seed to be used for the random number generator for each run, to help with further program development that you may try.)

After the last test pattern has been presented, the percentage of the patterns that were correctly recalled is shown, using as a criterion that the correlation of the recalled firing rate with the training pattern $r >= 0.98$. For the reasons just described related to the random generation of the training and distorted test patterns, the percentage correct will vary from run to run, so taking the average of several runs is recommended.

Note that the continuing stable firing after the first few recall epochs models the implementation of short-term memory in the cerebral cortex (Rolls, 2008d, 2016b, 2023a).

Note that the retrieval of the correct pattern from a distorted version that includes missing 1s models completion in the cerebral cortex, which is important in episodic memory as implemented in the hippocampus in which the whole of the episodic memory can be retrieved from any part (Rolls, 2008d, 2016b; Kesner and Rolls, 2015) (Chapter 9).

Note that the retrieval of the correct pattern from a distorted version that includes missing 1s or has 1s instead of 0s models correct memory retrieval in the cerebral cortex and hippocampus even if there is some distortion of the recall cue (Rolls, 2016b, 2023a). This also enables generalization to similar patterns or stimuli that have been encountered previously, which is highly behaviorally adaptive (Rolls, 2016b, 2023a). These processes are also important in completion in episodic memory as implemented in the hippocampus in which the whole of the episodic memory can be retrieved from any part (Rolls, 2008d, 2016b; Kesner and Rolls, 2015) (Chapter 9).

D.2.2 Exercises

1. Measure the percent correct as you increase the number of patterns from 10 to 15 with the Sparseness remaining at 0.5. Plot the result. How close is your result to that found by Hopfield (1982), which was $0.14N$ for a sparseness a of 0.5? You could try increasing N by 10 (to 1000) and multiplying the number of training patterns by 10 and increasing $nFlipBits$ to say 100 to see whether your results, with smaller statistical fluctuations, approximate more closely to the theoretical value.

2. Test the effect of reducing the Sparseness (a) to 0.1, which will increase the number of patterns that can be stored and correctly recalled, i.e. the capacity of the network (Treves and Rolls, 1991; Rolls, 2016b, 2023a). (Hint: try a number of patterns in the region of 30.) You could also plot the capacity of the network as a function of the Sparseness (a) with values down to say 0.01 in larger networks, with theoretical results provided by Treves and Rolls (1991) and Rolls (2023a).

3. Test the effect of altering the learning rule, from the covariance rule to the rule with heterosynaptic long term depression (LTD), which is as follows (Rolls, 2023a):

$$\delta w_{ij} = \alpha(y_i)(y_j - a). \tag{D.2}$$

(Hint: in the training loop in the program, at about line 102, comment in the heterosynaptic LTD rule.)

4. Test whether the network operates with positive-only synaptic weights. (Hint: there are two lines (close to 131) just after the training loop that if uncommented will add a constant to all the numbers in the synaptic weight matrix to make all the numbers positive (with the minimum synaptic weight clipped at 0).

5. What happens to the recall if you train more patterns than the critical capacity? (Hint: see Rolls (2023a) Section B.16.)

6. Does it in practice make much difference if you allow self-connections, especially in large networks? (Hint: in the program in the training loop if you comment out the line 'if syn $\sim=$ neuron' and its corresponding 'end', self-connections will be allowed.)

D.3 Pattern association networks

The operation and properties of pattern association networks are described in this book (Rolls, 2023a) Appendix B.2.

D.3.1 Running the simulation

In the command window of Matlab, after you have performed a 'cd' into the directory where the source files are, type 'PatternAssociationDemo'. The program will run for a bit, and then pause so that you can inspect what has been produced so far. A paused state is indicated by the words 'Paused: Press any key'. Press 'Enter' to move to the next stage, until the program finishes and the command prompt reappears. You can edit the code to comment out some of the 'pause' statements if you do not want them, or to add a 'pause' statement if you would like the program to stop at a particular place so that you can inspect the results. To stop the program and exit from it, use 'Ctrl-C'. When at the command prompt, you can access variables by typing the variable name followed by 'Enter'. (Note: if you set 'display = 0' near the beginning of the program, there will be few pauses, and you will be able to collect data quickly.)

The fully connected pattern association network has $N=8$ output neurons with the dendrites that receive the synapses shown as vertical columns in the generated figures, and $nSyn=64$ synapses onto each neuron. At the first pause, you will see the 8 random binary conditioned stimulus (CS) training patterns with firing rates of 1 or 0, and with a sparseness of 0.25 (*InputSparseness*). As these are binary patterns, the sparseness is the same as the proportion of high firing rates or 1s. At the second pause you will see distorted versions of these patterns to be used as recall cues later. The number of bits that have been flipped $nFlipBits=8$.

Next you will see the synaptic matrix being trained with the 8 pattern associations between each conditioned stimulus (CS) and its unconditioned stimulus (US), the output firing. In this simulation, the default is for each US pattern to have one bit on, so that the sparseness of the US, *OutputSparseness* is $1/N$. Uncomment the pause in the training loop if you wish to see each pattern being presented sequentially. The synaptic weight matrix *SynMat* (elements of which are referred to as w_{ij} below) is initialized to zero, and then each pattern pair is presented as a CS and US pair, with the CS specifying the presynaptic input, and the US the firing rate in the N neurons present when the CS is presented. Each time a training pattern pair is presented, the weight change is calculated by an associative learning rule that includes heterosynaptic long term depression

$$\delta w_{ij} = \alpha(y_i)(x_j - a). \tag{D.3}$$

where α is a learning rate constant, and x_j is the presynaptic firing rate. This learning rule includes (in proportion to y_i the firing rate of the ith postsynaptic neuron produced by the US) increasing the synaptic weight if $(y_j - a) > 0$ (long-term potentiation), and decreasing the synaptic weight if $(x_j - a) < 0$ (heterosynaptic long-term depression). As the CS patterns are random binary patterns with sparseness a (the parameter *InputSparseness*), a is the average activity $<x_j>$ of an axon across patterns. The reasons for the use of this learning rule are described in Rolls (2023a) Section B.3.3.6. In the exercises, you can try a Hebbian associative learning rule that does not include this heterosynaptic long-term depression. The change of weight is added to the previous synaptic weight. In the figures generated by the code, the maximum weights are shown as white, and the minimum weights are black. Although both these rules lead to some negative synaptic weights, which are not biologically plausible, this limitation can be overcome, as shown in the exercises. In the display of the synaptic weights, remember that each column represents the synaptic weights on a single neuron. The top thin row below the synaptic matrix represents the activations of the neurons, the bottom thin row the firing rates of the neurons, and the thin column to the left of the synaptic weight matrix the firing rates of the presynaptic input, i.e. the recall (CS) stimulus. Rates of 1 are shown as white, and of 0 as black.

Next, testing with the distorted CS patterns starts. We are interested in how the pattern association network generalizes with distorted inputs to produce the correct US output that should be produced if there were no distortion. The recall performance is measured by how correlated the recalled firing rate state (the Conditioned Response, CR) is with the output that should be produced to the original training CS pattern, with this correlation having a maximum value of 1. Every time you press 'Enter' a new CS is presented. Do note that with randomly chosen distortions of the CS patterns to produce the recall cue, in relatively small networks the distorted CS will sometimes be close of another CS, and that this 'statistical fluctuation' in how close some of the distorted CSs are to the original CSs is to be expected. These effects smooth out as the network become larger. (Remember that cortical neurons have in the order of 10,000 inputs to each neuron (in addition to the recurrent collaterals, Rolls (2023a)), so these statistical fluctuations will be largely smoothed out. Do note also that the performance of the network will be different each time it is run, because the random number generator is set with a different seed on each run. (Near the beginning of the program, you could uncomment the command that causes the same seed to be used for the random number generator for each run, to help with further program development that you may try.)

After the last distorted testing CS pattern has been presented, the percentage of the patterns that were correctly recalled is shown, using a criterion for the correlation of the recalled firing rate with the training pattern $r >= 0.98$. For the reasons just described related to the random generation of the distorted test patterns, the percentage correct will vary from run to run, so taking the average of several runs is recommended.

Note that the retrieval of the correct output (conditioned response, CR) pattern from a distorted CS recall stimulus models generalization in the cerebral cortex, which is highly behaviorally adaptive (Rolls, 2016b, 2023a).

D.3.2 Exercises

1. Test how well the network generalizes to distorted recall cues, by altering $nFlipBits$ to values between 0 and 14. Remember to take the average of several simulation runs.

2. Test the effect of altering the learning rule, from the rule with heterosynaptic long term depression (LTD) as in Eqn. D.3, to a simple associative synaptic modification rule which is as follows (Rolls, 2023a):

$$\delta w_{ij} = \alpha(y_i)(x_j). \tag{D.4}$$

(Hint: in the training loop in the program, at about line 110, comment out the heterosynaptic LTD rule, and uncomment the associative rule.)

If you see little difference, can you suggest conditions under which there may be a difference, such as higher loading? (Hint: check Rolls (2023a) Section B.2.7.)

3. Describe how the threshold non-linearity in the activation function helps to remove interference from other training patterns, and from distortions in the recall cue. (Hint: compare the activations to the firing rates of the output neurons.)

4. In the pattern associator, the conditioned stimulus (CS) retrieves the unconditioned response (UR), that is the effects produced by the unconditioned stimulus (US) with which it has been paired during learning. Can the opposite occur, that is, can the US be used to retrieve the CS? If not, in what type of network is the retrieval symmetrical? (Hint: if you are not sure, read Rolls (2023a) Sections B.2 and B.3.)

5. The network simulated uses local representations for the US, with only one neuron on for each US. If you can program in Matlab, can you write code that would generate distributed representations for the US patterns? Then can you produce new CS patterns with random binary representations and sparsenesses in the range 0.1–0.5, like those used for the

autoassociator, so that you can then investigate the storage capacity of pattern association networks. (Hint: reference to Rolls (2023a) Section B.2.7 and B.2.8 may be useful.)

D.4 Competitive networks and Self-Organizing Maps

The operation and properties of competitive networks are described in this book (Rolls, 2023a) Appendix B.4. This is a self-organizing network, with no teacher. The input patterns are presented in random sequence, and the network learns how to categorise the patterns, placing similar patterns into the same category, and different patterns into different categories. The particular neuron or neurons that represent each category depend on the initial random synaptic weight vectors as well as the learning, so the output neurons are different from simulation run to simulation run. Self-organizing maps are investigated in Exercise 4.

D.4.1 Running the simulation

In the command window of Matlab, after you have performed a 'cd' into the directory where the source files are, type 'CompetitiveNetDemo'. The program will run for a bit, and then pause so that you can inspect what has been produced so far. A paused state is indicated by the words 'Paused: Press any key'. Press 'Enter' to move to the next stage, until the program finishes and the command prompt reappears. You can edit the code to comment out some of the 'pause' statements if you do not want them, or to add a 'pause' statement if you would like the program to stop at a particular place so that you can inspect the results. To stop the program and exit from it, use 'Ctrl-C'. When at the command prompt, you can access variables by typing the variable name followed by 'Enter'. (Note: if you set *display = 0* near the beginning of the program, there will be few pauses, and you will be able to collect data quickly.)

The fully connected competitive network has $N=100$ output neurons with the dendrites that receive the synapses shown as vertical columns, and $nSyn=100$ synapses onto each neuron. With the display on (*display = 1*), at the first pause, you will see the 28 binary input patterns for training with firing rates of 1 or 0. Each pattern is 20 elements long, and each pattern is shifted down 3 elements with respect to the previous pattern, with the parameters supplied. (Each pattern thus overlaps in 17 / 20 locations with its predecessor.)

Next you will see the synaptic matrix being trained with the 28 input patterns, which are presented 20 times each (*nepochs* = 20) in random permuted sequence. Uncomment the pause in the training loop if you wish to see each pattern being presented sequentially. The synaptic weight matrix *SynMat* is initialized so that each neuron has random synaptic weights, with the synaptic weight vector on each neuron normalized to have a length of 1. Normalizing the length of the vector during training is important, for it ensures that no one neuron increases its synaptic strengths to very high values and thus wins for every input pattern. (Biological approximations to this are described by Rolls (2023a) in Section B.4.9.2, and involve a type of heterosynaptic long-term depression of synaptic strength that is large when the postsynaptic term is high, and the presynaptic firing is low.) (In addition, for convenience, each input pattern is normalized to a length of 1, so that when the dot product is computed with a synaptic weight vector on a neuron, the maximum activation of a neuron will be 1.)

The firing rate of each neuron is computed using a binary threshold activation function (which can be changed in the code to threshold linear). The sparseness of the firing rate representation can be set in the code using *OutputSparseness*, and as supplied is set to 0.01 for the first demonstration, which results in one of the $N=100$ output neurons having a high firing rate. Because the (initially random) synaptic weight vectors of each neuron are different, the activations of each of the neurons will be different.

Learning then occurs, using an associative learning rule with synapses increasing between presynaptic neurons with high rates and postsynaptic neurons with high rates. Think of this as moving the synaptic weight vector of a high firing neuron to point closer to the input pattern that is making the neuron fire. At the same time, the other synapses on the same neuron become weaker due to the synaptic weight normalization, so the synaptic weight vector of the neuron moves away from other, different, patterns. In this way, the neurons self-organize so that some neurons point towards some patterns, and other neurons towards other patterns. You can watch these synaptic weight changes during the learning in the figure generated by the code, in which some of the synapses will become stronger (white) on a neuron and correspond to one or several of the patterns, and at the same time the other synapses on the neuron will become weaker (black). In the display of the synaptic weights, remember that each column represents the synaptic weights on a single neuron. The top thin row below the synaptic matrix represents the activations of the neurons, the bottom thin row the firing rates of the neurons, and the thin column to the left of the synaptic weight matrix the firing rates of the presynaptic input, i.e. the pattern currently being presented. Rates of 1 are shown as white, and of 0 as black. Neurons that remain unallocated, and do not respond to any of the input patterns, appear as vertical columns of random synaptic weights onto a neuron. These neurons remain available to potentially categorise different input patterns.

Next, testing with the different patterns starts. We are interested in whether similar input patterns activate the same output neurons; and different input patterns different output neurons. This is described as categorisation (Rolls, 2023a). With the display on (*display* = 1), each time you press 'Enter' the program will step through the patterns in sequence. You will notice in the synaptic matrix that with these initial parameters, only a few neurons have learned. When you step through each testing pattern in sequence, you will observe that one of the neurons responds to several patterns in the sequence, and these patterns are quite closely correlated with each other. Then another neuron becomes active for a further set of close patterns. This is repeated as other patterns are presented, and shows you that similar patterns tend to activate the same output neuron or neurons, and different input patterns tend to activate different output neurons. This illustrates by simulation the categorisation performed by competitive networks.

To illustrate these effects more quantitatively, after the patterns have been presented, you are shown first the correlations between the input patterns, and after that the correlations between the output firing rates produced by each pattern. These results are shown as correlation matrices. You should observe that with the network parameters supplied, the firing rates are grouped into several categories, each corresponding to several input patterns that are highly correlated in the output firing that they produce. The correlation matrix between the output firing rate for the different patterns thus illustrates how a competitive network can categorise similar patterns as similar to each other, and different patterns as different.

D.4.2 Exercises

1. Test the operation of the system with no learning, most easily achieved by setting *nepochs* = 0. This results in the input patterns being mapped to output rates through the random synaptic weight vectors for each neuron. What is your interpretation of what is shown by the correlation matrix between the output firing rates?

(Hint: the randomizing effect of the random synaptic weight vectors on each neuron is to separate out the patterns, with many of the patterns having no correlation with other patterns. In this mode, pattern separation is produced, and not categorisation in that similar inputs are less likely to produce similar outputs, a key property in perception and memory (Rolls, 2023a). Pattern separation is important in its own right as a process (Rolls, 2016f), and is implemented for example by the random non-associatively modifiable connections of the dentate mossy fibre synapses onto the CA3 neurons (Treves and Rolls, 1992; Rolls, 2016b, 2013b; Kesner and Rolls, 2015; Rolls, 2023a).)

2. Investigate and describe the effects of altering the similarity between the patterns on the categorization, by for example altering the value of *shift* in the range 2–20.

3. Investigate and describe the effects of making the output firing rate representation (*OutputSparseness*) less sparse. It is suggested that values in the range 0.01–0.1 are investigated.

4. If there is lateral facilitation of nearby neurons, which might be produced by short-range recurrent collaterals in the cortex, then self-organizing maps can be generated, providing a model of topographic maps in the cerebral cortex (Section B.4.6 and Rolls (2023a) Section B.4.6). Investigate this with the modified competitive network 'SOMdemo'. The map is made clear during the testing, in which the patterns are presented in order, and the neurons activated appear in different mapped positions in the firing rate array. Run the program several times to show that the details of the map are different each time, but that the principles are the same, that nearby neurons tend to respond to similar patterns, and that singularities (discontinuities) in the map can occur, just as are found in the primary visual cortex, V1.

The important change of 'SOMdemo' from 'CompetitiveNetDemo' is a local spatial filter for the firing rate array to simulate the effect of facilitation of the firing rates of nearby neurons by the short-range excitatory recurrent collateral connections between nearby cortical pyramidal cells. This is implemented by the *SpatialFilter* kernel the range of which is set by *FilterRange*. Investigate the effects of altering *FilterRange* from its default value of 11 on the topographic maps that are formed. Other changes to produce 'SOMdemo' include modifying the *OutPutSparseness* of the Firing Rate representation to 0.3. Investigate the effect of modifying this on the maps being formed. Another alteration was to alter the activation function from binary threshold to linear threshold to enable graded firing rate representations to be formed.

What are the advantages of the representations formed when self-organizing maps are present? (Hint: Think of interpolation of untrained input patterns close to those already trained; and check Rolls (2023a) Section B.4.6.)

D.5 Further developments

The neuronal network simulation code supplied and described above may provide a route for readers to develop their own programs. Further examples of Matlab code used to investigate neural systems are available in Anastasio (2010). Matlab itself has a Neural Network Toolbox, with an introduction to its use in modelling simple networks provided in Wallisch et al. (2009).

D.6 Matlab code for a tutorial version of VisNet

Tutorial software written in Matlab that illustrates some of the principles of operation of VisNet, the model of invariant visual object recognition described in Section 2.8 of this book (Rolls, 2023a) and by Rolls (2021d), is available at https://www.oxcns.org/software. This is not the full version of VisNet used for most of the research described in Section 2.8, but it may be useful to illustrate some of the principles of operation of VisNet.

D.7 Matlab code for information analysis of neuronal encoding

Code translated into Matlab that was used for the single neuron information analyses described by Rolls, Treves, Tovee and Panzeri (1997d) and the multiple single neuron information analyses described by Rolls, Treves and Tovee (1997b), and in Appendix C, is also available at https://www.oxcns.org/software.

D.8 Matlab code to illustrate the use of spatial view cells in navigation

Matlab code to illustrate the use of spatial view cells (NavSVC.m), allocentric bearing to a landmark cells (NavABL.m), and combinations of allocentric bearing to a landmark cells using triangulation for navigation (NavTRI.m) described by (Rolls, 2021f) and in Section 9.3.15 is also available at https://www.oxcns.org/software.

D.9 The Automated Anatomical Labelling Atlas 3, AAL3

The Automated Anatomical Labelling Atlas 3, AAL3 (Rolls, Huang, Lin, Feng and Joliot, 2020d), used for some of the research described in this book, is available at https://www.oxcns.org/software.

D.10 The extended Human Connectome Project extended atlas, HCPex

The extended Human Connectome Project Multimodal Parcellation atlas, HCPex (Huang, Rolls, Feng and Lin, 2022), used for some of the research described in this book, is available at https://www.oxcns.org/software.

D.11 Highlights

1. Appendix D describes Matlab software that has been made available with *Brain Computations and Connectivity* (Rolls, 2023a) at https://www.oxcns.org to provide simple demonstrations of the operation of some key neuronal networks related to cortical function.
2. The software demonstrates the operation of pattern association networks, autoassociation / attractor networks, competitive networks, and self-organizing maps.
3. The availability of software to illustrate the operation of VisNet, a model of invariant visual object recognition, has also been described.
4. The availability of software to analyze the encoding of information by single neurons, and by populations of single neurons, has also been described.

Bibliography

Abbott, L. F. (1991). Realistic synaptic inputs for model neural networks, *Network* **2**: 245–258.

Abbott, L. F. and Blum, K. I. (1996). Functional significance of long-term potentiation for sequence learning and prediction, *Cerebral Cortex* **6**: 406–416.

Abbott, L. F. and Nelson, S. B. (2000). Synaptic plasticity: taming the beast, *Nature Neuroscience* **3**: 1178–1183.

Abbott, L. F. and Regehr, W. G. (2004). Synaptic computation, *Nature* **431**: 796–803.

Abbott, L. F., Rolls, E. T. and Tovee, M. J. (1996). Representational capacity of face coding in monkeys, *Cereb Cortex* **6**: 498–505.

Abbott, L. F., Varela, J. A., Sen, K. and Nelson, S. B. (1997). Synaptic depression and cortical gain control, *Science* **275**: 220–224.

Abdallah, C. G., Adams, T. G., Kelmendi, B., Esterlis, I., Sanacora, G. and Krystal, J. H. (2016). Ketamine's mechanism of action: a path to rapid-acting antidepressants, *Depression and Anxiety* **33**: 689–697.

Abeles, M. (1991). *Corticonics: Neural Circuits of the Cerebral Cortex*, Cambridge University Press, Cambridge.

Abramson, N. (1963). *Information Theory and Coding*, McGraw-Hill, New York.

Acharya, L., Aghajan, Z. M., Vuong, C., Moore, J. J. and Mehta, M. R. (2016). Causal influence of visual cues on hippocampal directional selectivity, *Cell* **164**: 197–207.

Ackley, D. H. (1987). *A Connectionist Machine for Genetic Hill-Climbing*, Kluwer Academic Publishers, Dordrecht.

Ackley, D. H., Hinton, G. E. and Sejnowski, T. J. (1985). A learning algorithm for Boltzmann machines, *Cognitive Science* **9**: 147–169.

Ackroff, K. and Sclafani, A. (2014). Rapid post-oral stimulation of intake and flavor conditioning in rats by glucose but not a non-metabolizable glucose analog, *Physiol Behav* **133**: 92–8.

Acsady, L., Kamondi, A., Sik, A., Freund, T. and Buzsaki, G. (1998). GABAergic cells are the major postsynaptic targets of mossy fibers in the rat hippocampus, *J Neurosci* **18**: 3386–403.

Adolphs, R. (2003). Cognitive neuroscience of human social behavior, *Nature Reviews Neuroscience* **4**: 165–178.

Adolphs, R., Tranel, D., Damasio, H. and Damasio, A. (1994). Impaired recognition of emotion in facial expressions following bilateral damage to the human amygdala, *Nature* **372**: 669–672.

Adolphs, R., Baron-Cohen, S. and Tranel, D. (2002a). Impaired recognition of social emotions following amygdala damage, *J Cogn Neurosci* **14**: 1264–74.

Adolphs, R., Tranel, D. and Baron-Cohen, S. (2002b). Amygdala damage impairs recognition of social emotions from facial expressions, *Journal of Cognitive Neuroscience* **14**: 1–11.

Adolphs, R., Gosselin, F., Buchanan, T. W., Tranel, D., Schyns, P. and Damasio, A. R. (2005). A mechanism for impaired fear recognition after amygdala damage, *Nature* **433**: 68–72.

Aertsen, A. M. H. J., Gerstein, G. L., Habib, M. K. and Palm, G. (1989). Dynamics of neuronal firing correlation: modulation of 'effective connectivity', *Journal of Neurophysiology* **61**: 900–917.

Aggelopoulos, N. C. and Rolls, E. T. (2005). Natural scene perception: inferior temporal cortex neurons encode the positions of different objects in the scene, *European Journal of Neuroscience* **22**: 2903–2916.

Aggelopoulos, N. C., Franco, L. and Rolls, E. T. (2005). Object perception in natural scenes: encoding by inferior temporal cortex simultaneously recorded neurons, *Journal of Neurophysiology* **93**: 1342–1357.

Aggleton, J. P. (1992). The functional effects of amygdala lesions in humans: a comparison with findings from monkeys, *in* J. P. Aggleton (ed.), *The Amygdala*, Wiley-Liss, New York, pp. 485–503.

Aggleton, J. P. and Nelson, A. J. D. (2015). Why do lesions in the rodent anterior thalamic nuclei cause such severe spatial deficits?, *Neuroscience & Biobehavioral Reviews* **54**: 108–119.

Aggleton, J. P. and O'Mara, S. M. (2022). The anterior thalamic nuclei: core components of a tripartite episodic memory system, *Nat Rev Neurosci* **23**: 505–516.

Aggleton, J. P., Nelson, A. J. D. and O'Mara, S. M. (2022). Time to retire the serial Papez circuit: Implications for space, memory, and attention, *Neurosci Biobehav Rev* **140**: 104813.

Aguirre, G. K. and D'Esposito, M. (1999). Topographical disorientation: a synthesis and taxonomy, *Brain* **122** (Pt 9): 1613–28.

Ahveninen, J., Huang, S., Nummenmaa, A., Belliveau, J. W., Hung, A. Y., Jaaskelainen, I. P., Rauschecker, J. P., Rossi, S., Tiitinen, H. and Raij, T. (2013). Evidence for distinct human auditory cortex regions for sound location versus identity processing, *Nat Commun* **4**: 2585.

Aigner, T. G., Mitchell, S. J., Aggleton, J. P., DeLong, M. R., Struble, R. G., Price, D. L., Wenk, G. L., Pettigrew, K. D. and Mishkin, M. (1991). Transient impairment of recognition memory following ibotenic acid lesions of the basal forebrain in macaques, *Experimental Brain Research* **86**: 18–26.

Aimone, J. B. and Gage, F. H. (2011). Modeling new neuron function: a history of using computational neuroscience to study adult neurogenesis, *Eur J Neurosci* **33**: 1160–9.

Aimone, J. B., Deng, W. and Gage, F. H. (2010). Adult neurogenesis: integrating theories and separating functions, *Trends Cogn Sci* **14**: 325–37.

Akrami, A., Liu, Y., Treves, A. and Jagadeesh, B. (2009). Converging neuronal activity in inferior temporal cortex during the classification of morphed stimuli, *Cereb Cortex* **19**: 760–76.

Akrami, A., Russo, E. and Treves, A. (2012). Lateral thinking, from the Hopfield model to cortical dynamics, *Brain Res* **1434**: 4–16.

Albus, J. S. (1971). A theory of cerebellar function, *Mathematical Biosciences* **10**: 25–61.

Aleksandrova, L. R., Phillips, A. G. and Wang, Y. T. (2017). Antidepressant effects of ketamine and the roles of AMPA glutamate receptors and other mechanisms beyond NMDA receptor antagonism, *J Psychiatry Neurosci* **42**: 222–229.

Aleman, A. and Kahn, R. S. (2005). Strange feelings: do amygdala abnormalities dysregulate the emotional brain in schizophrenia?, *Progress in Neurobiology* **77**(5): 283–298.

Alexander, A. S. and Nitz, D. A. (2015). Retrosplenial cortex maps the conjunction of internal and external spaces, *Nature Neuroscience* **18**: 1143–1151.

Alexander, A. S., Carstensen, L. C., Hinman, J. R., Raudies, F., Chapman, G. W. and Hasselmo, M. E. (2020). Egocentric boundary vector tuning of the retrosplenial cortex, *Sci Adv* **6**: eaaz2322.

Alexander, L., Clarke, H. F. and Roberts, A. C. (2019). A focus on the functions of area 25, *Brain Sci* **9**: 129.

Alexander, R. D. (1979). *Darwinism and Human Affairs*, University of Washington Press, Seattle.

Alvarez, P. and Squire, L. R. (1994). Memory consolidation and the medial temporal lobe: a simple network model, *Proceedings of the National Academy of Sciences USA* **91**: 7041–7045.

Amaral, D. G. (1986). Amygdalohippocampal and amygdalocortical projections in the primate brain, *in* R. Schwarcz and Y. Ben-Ari (eds), *Excitatory Amino Acids and Epilepsy*, Plenum Press, New York, pp. 3–18.

Amaral, D. G. (1987). Memory: anatomical organization of candidate brain regions, *in* F. Plum and V. Mountcastle (eds), *Higher Functions of the Brain. Handbook of Physiology, Part I*, American Physiological Society, Washington, DC, pp. 211–294.

Amaral, D. G. (1993). Emerging principles of intrinsic hippocampal organization, *Current Opinion in Neurobiology* **3**: 225–229.

Amaral, D. G. (2003). The amygdala, social behavior, and danger detection, *Annals of the New York Academy of Sciences* **1000**: 337–347.

Amaral, D. G. and Price, J. L. (1984). Amygdalo-cortical projections in the monkey (Macaca fascicularis), *Journal of Comparative Neurology* **230**: 465–496.

Amaral, D. G. and Witter, M. P. (1989). The three-dimensional organization of the hippocampal formation: a review of anatomical data, *Neuroscience* **31**: 571–591.

Amaral, D. G. and Witter, M. P. (1995). The hippocampal formation, *in* G. Paxinos (ed.), *The Rat Nervous System*, Academic Press, San Diego, pp. 443–493.

Amaral, D. G., Insausti, R. and Cowan, W. M. (1984). The commissural connections of the monkey hippocampal formation, *J Comp Neurol* **224**: 307–36.

Amaral, D. G., Ishizuka, N. and Claiborne, B. (1990). Neurons, numbers and the hippocampal network, *Progress in Brain Research* **83**: 1–11.

Amaral, D. G., Price, J. L., Pitkanen, A. and Carmichael, S. T. (1992). Anatomical organization of the primate amygdaloid complex, *in* J. P. Aggleton (ed.), *The Amygdala*, Wiley-Liss, New York, chapter 1, pp. 1–66.

Amari, S. (1977). Dynamics of pattern formation in lateral-inhibition type neural fields, *Biological Cybernetics* **27**: 77–87.

Amari, S. (1982). Competitive and cooperative aspects in dynamics of neural excitation and self-organization, *in* S. Amari and M. A. Arbib (eds), *Competition and Cooperation in Neural Nets*, Springer, Berlin, chapter 1, pp. 1–28.

Amari, S., Yoshida, K. and Kanatani, K.-I. (1977). A mathematical foundation for statistical neurodynamics, *SIAM Journal of Applied Mathematics* **33**: 95–126.

Amir, O., Biederman, I. and Hayworth, K. J. (2011). The neural basis for shape preferences, *Vision Res* **51**: 2198–206.

Amit, D. J. (1989). *Modeling Brain Function*, Cambridge University Press, Cambridge.

Amit, D. J. (1995). The Hebbian paradigm reintegrated: local reverberations as internal representations, *Behavioral and Brain Sciences* **18**: 617–657.

Amit, D. J. and Brunel, N. (1997). Model of global spontaneous activity and local structured activity during delay periods in the cerebral cortex, *Cerebral Cortex* **7**: 237–252.
Amit, D. J. and Tsodyks, M. V. (1991). Quantitative study of attractor neural network retrieving at low spike rates. I. Substrate – spikes, rates and neuronal gain, *Network* **2**: 259–273.
Amit, D. J., Gutfreund, H. and Sompolinsky, H. (1985). Spin-glass models of neural networks, **32**: 1007–1018.
Amit, D. J., Gutfreund, H. and Sompolinsky, H. (1987). Statistical mechanics of neural networks near saturation, *Annals of Physics (New York)* **173**: 30–67.
Amunts, K. and Zilles, K. (2012). Architecture and organizational principles of Broca's region, *Trends Cogn Sci* **16**: 418–26.
Anastasio, T. J. (2010). *Tutorial on Neural Systems Modelling*, Sinauer, Sunderland, MA.
Andersen, P., Dingledine, R., Gjerstad, L., Langmoen, I. A. and Laursen, A. M. (1980). Two different responses of hippocampal pyramidal cells to application of gamma-aminobutyric acid, *Journal of Physiology* **307**: 279–296.
Andersen, P., Morris, R., Amaral, D., Bliss, T. and O'Keefe, J. (2007). *The Hippocampus Book*, Oxford University Press, London.
Andersen, R. A. (1989). Visual and eye movement functions of the posterior parietal cortex, *Annu Rev Neurosci* **12**: 377–403.
Andersen, R. A. (1995a). Coordinate transformations and motor planning in the posterior parietal cortex, *in* M. S. Gazzaniga (ed.), *The Cognitive Neurosciences*, MIT Press, Cambridge, MA, chapter 33, pp. 519–532.
Andersen, R. A. (1995b). Encoding of intention and spatial location in the posterior parietal cortex, *Cereb Cortex* **5**: 457–69.
Andersen, R. A. and Cui, H. (2009). Intention, action planning, and decision making in parietal-frontal circuits, *Neuron* **63**: 568–83.
Andersen, R. A. and Mountcastle, V. B. (1983). The influence of the angle of gaze upon the excitability of the light-sensitive neurons of the posterior parietal cortex, *J Neurosci* **3**: 532–48.
Andersen, R. A., Essick, G. K. and Siegel, R. M. (1985). Encoding of spatial location by posterior parietal neurons, *Science* **230**: 456–8.
Andersen, R. A., Batista, A. P., Snyder, L. H., Buneo, C. A. and Cohen, Y. E. (2000). Programming to look and reach in the posterior parietal cortex, *in* M. Gazzaniga (ed.), *The New Cognitive Neurosciences*, 2 edn, MIT Press, Cambridge, MA, chapter 36, pp. 515–524.
Anderson, A. K., Christoff, K., Stappen, I., Panitz, D., Ghahremani, D. G., Glover, G., Gabrieli, J. D. and Sobel, N. (2003). Dissociated neural representations of intensity and valence in human olfaction, *Nature Neuroscience* **6**: 196–202.
Anderson, M. E. (1978). Discharge patterns of basal ganglia neurons during active maintenance of postural stability and adjustment to chair tilt, *Brain Research* **143**: 325–338.
Aparicio, P. L., Issa, E. B. and DiCarlo, J. J. (2016). Neurophysiological organization of the Middle Face Patch in macaque inferior temporal cortex, *J Neurosci* **36**: 12729–12745.
Arbib, M. A. (1964). *Brains, Machines, and Mathematics*, McGraw-Hill, New York (2nd Edn 1987 Springer).
Arcaro, M. J. and Livingstone, M. S. (2021). On the relationship between maps and domains in inferotemporal cortex, *Nat Rev Neurosci* **22**: 573–583.
Archakov, D., DeWitt, I., Kusmierek, P., Ortiz-Rios, M., Cameron, D., Cui, D., Morin, E. L., VanMeter, J. W., Sams, M., Jaaskelainen, I. P. and Rauschecker, J. P. (2020). Auditory representation of learned sound sequences in motor regions of the macaque brain, *Proc Natl Acad Sci U S A* **117**: 15242–15252.
Arcizet, F., Mirpour, K. and Bisley, J. W. (2011). A pure salience response in posterior parietal cortex, *Cerebral Cortex* **21**: 2498–2506.
Armstrong, M. J. and Okun, M. S. (2020). Diagnosis and treatment of Parkinson Disease: a review, *JAMA* **323**: 548–560.
Arnold, P. D., Rosenberg, D. R., Mundo, E., Tharmalingam, S., Kennedy, J. L. and Richter, M. A. (2004). Association of a glutamate (NMDA) subunit receptor gene (GRIN2B) with obsessive-compulsive disorder: a preliminary study, *Psychopharmacology (Berl)* **174**: 530–538.
Arnsten, A. F. and Li, B. M. (2005). Neurobiology of executive functions: catecholamine influences on prefrontal cortical functions, *Biological Psychiatry* **57**: 1377–1384.
Arnsten, A. F. and Wang, M. (2016). Targeting prefrontal cortical systems for drug development: potential therapies for cognitive disorders, *Annu Rev Pharmacol Toxicol* **56**: 339–60.
Aron, A. R., Fletcher, P. C., Bullmore, E. T., Sahakian, B. J. and Robbins, T. W. (2003). Stop-signal inhibition disrupted by damage to inferior frontal gyrus in humans, *Nature Neuroscience* **6**: 115–116.
Aron, A. R., Robbins, T. W. and Poldrack, R. A. (2014). Inhibition and the right inferior frontal cortex: one decade on, *Trends in Cognitive Sciences* **18**: 177–85.
Aronov, D. and Tank, D. W. (2014). Engagement of neural circuits underlying 2D spatial navigation in a rodent virtual reality system, *Neuron* **84**: 442–56.

Aronov, D., Nevers, R. and Tank, D. W. (2017). Mapping of a non-spatial dimension by the hippocampal-entorhinal circuit, *Nature* **543**: 719–722.

Artola, A. and Singer, W. (1993). Long term depression: related mechanisms in cerebellum, neocortex and hippocampus, in M. Baudry, R. F. Thompson and J. L. Davis (eds), *Synaptic Plasticity: Molecular, Cellular and Functional Aspects*, MIT Press, Cambridge, MA, chapter 7, pp. 129–146.

Asaad, W. F., Rainer, G. and Miller, E. K. (2000). Task-specific neural activity in the primate prefrontal cortex, *Journal of Neurophysiology* **84**: 451–459.

Atick, J. J. (1992). Could information theory provide an ecological theory of sensory processing?, *Network* **3**: 213–251.

Atick, J. J. and Redlich, A. N. (1990). Towards a theory of early visual processing, *Neural Computation* **2**: 308–320.

Atick, J. J., Griffin, P. A. and Relich, A. N. (1996). The vocabulary of shape: principal shapes for probing perception and neural response, *Network* **7**: 1–5.

Attneave, F. (1954). Some informational aspects of visual perception, *Psychological Review* **61**: 183–193.

Auger, S. D. and Maguire, E. A. (2013). Assessing the mechanism of response in the retrosplenial cortex of good and poor navigators, *Cortex* **49**: 2904–2913.

Auger, S. D., Mullally, S. L. and Maguire, E. A. (2012). Retrosplenial cortex codes for permanent landmarks, *PLoS One* **7**: e43620.

Averbeck, B. B. (2015). Theory of choice in bandit, information sampling and foraging tasks, *PLoS Comput Biol* **11**: e1004164.

Avila, E., Lakshminarasimhan, K. J., DeAngelis, G. C. and Angelaki, D. E. (2019). Visual and vestibular selectivity for self-motion in macaque Posterior Parietal Area 7a, *Cereb Cortex* **29**: 3932–3947.

Azzi, J. C., Sirigu, A. and Duhamel, J. R. (2012). Modulation of value representation by social context in the primate orbitofrontal cortex, *Proc Natl Acad Sci U S A* **109**: 2126–31.

Bacon-Mace, N., Mace, M. J., Fabre-Thorpe, M. and Thorpe, S. J. (2005). The time course of visual processing: backward masking and natural scene categorisation, *Vision Research* **45**: 1459–1469.

Baddeley, A. (2007). *Working Memory, Thought, and Action*, Oxford University Press, Oxford.

Baddeley, A. (2012). Working memory: theories, models, and controversies, *Annu Rev Psychol* **63**: 1–29.

Baddeley, A. D. (2021). Developing the concept of Working Memory: the role of neuropsychology, *Arch Clin Neuropsychol* **36**: 861–873.

Baddeley, A. D., Hitch, G. J. and Allen, R. J. (2019). From short-term store to multicomponent working memory: The role of the modal model, *Mem Cognit* **47**: 575–588.

Baddeley, R. J., Abbott, L. F., Booth, M. J. A., Sengpiel, F., Freeman, T., Wakeman, E. A. and Rolls, E. T. (1997). Responses of neurons in primary and inferior temporal visual cortices to natural scenes, *Proceedings of the Royal Society B* **264**: 1775–1783.

Bajaj, S., Adhikari, B. M., Friston, K. J. and Dhamala, M. (2016). Bridging the gap: Dynamic Causal Modeling and Granger Causality analysis of resting state functional magnetic resonance imaging, *Brain Connect* **6**: 652–661.

Baker, C. M., Burks, J. D., Briggs, R. G., Conner, A. K., Glenn, C. A., Manohar, K., Milton, C. K., Sali, G., McCoy, T. M., Battiste, J. D., O'Donoghue, D. L. and Sughrue, M. E. (2018). A connectomic atlas of the human cerebrum-Chapter 8: The posterior cingulate cortex, medial parietal lobe, and parieto-occipital sulcus, *Oper Neurosurg (Hagerstown)* **15**: S350–S371.

Baker, K. L., Vasan, G., Gumaste, A., Pieribone, V. A. and Verhagen, J. V. (2019). Spatiotemporal dynamics of odor responses in the lateral and dorsal olfactory bulb, *PLoS Biol* **17**: e3000409.

Bakola, S., Gamberini, M., Passarelli, L., Fattori, P. and Galletti, C. (2010). Cortical connections of parietal field PEc in the macaque: linking vision and somatic sensation for the control of limb action, *Cereb Cortex* **20**: 2592–604.

Baldassano, C., Esteva, A., Fei-Fei, L. and Beck, D. M. (2016). Two distinct scene-processing networks connecting vision and memory, *eNeuro* **3**: e0178–16.2016.

Baldo, J. V., Kacinik, N., Ludy, C., Paulraj, S., Moncrief, A., Piai, V., Curran, B., Turken, A., Herron, T. and Dronkers, N. F. (2018). Voxel-based lesion analysis of brain regions underlying reading and writing, *Neuropsychologia* **115**: 51–59.

Ballard, D. H. (1993). Subsymbolic modelling of hand-eye co-ordination, in D. E. Broadbent (ed.), *The Simulation of Human Intelligence*, Blackwell, Oxford, chapter 3, pp. 71–102.

Balleine, B. W. (2019). The meaning of behavior: discriminating reflex and volition in the brain, *Neuron* **104**: 47–62.

Balleine, B. W. and Dickinson, A. (1998). The role of incentive learning in instrumental outcome revaluation by sensory-specific satiety, *Animal Learning and Behavior* **26**: 46–59.

Balleine, B. W. and O'Doherty, J. P. (2010). Human and rodent homologies in action control: corticostriatal determinants of goal-directed and habitual action, *Neuropsychopharmacology* **35**: 48–69.

Balleine, B. W., Liljeholm, M. and Ostlund, S. B. (2009). The integrative function of the basal ganglia in instrumental conditioning, *Behavioral Brain Research* **199**: 43–52.

Bamford, N. S., Wightman, R. M. and Sulzer, D. (2018). Dopamine's effects on corticostriatal synapses during reward-based behaviors, *Neuron* **97**: 494–510.
Banks, W. P. (1978). Encoding and processing of symbolic information in comparative judgements, *in* G. H. Bower (ed.), *The Psychology of Learning and Motivation: Advances in Theory and Research*, Academic Press, pp. 101–159.
Bannon, S., Gonsalvez, C. J., Croft, R. J. and Boyce, P. M. (2002). Response inhibition deficits in obsessive-compulsive disorder, *Psychiatry Research* **110**: 165–174.
Bannon, S., Gonsalvez, C. J., Croft, R. J. and Boyce, P. M. (2006). Executive functions in obsessive-compulsive disorder: state or trait deficits?, *Aust N Z Journal of Psychiatry* **40**: 1031–1038.
Baraduc, P., Duhamel, J. R. and Wirth, S. (2019). Schema cells in the macaque hippocampus, *Science* **363**: 635–639.
Barat, E., Wirth, S. and Duhamel, J. R. (2018). Face cells in orbitofrontal cortex represent social categories, *Proceedings of the National Academy of Sciences (USA)* **115**: E11158–E11167.
Barbaro, N. and Shackelford, T. K. (2015). Book Review: Nether no more: bringing genital evolution to the forefront, *Evolutionary Psychology* **13**: 262–265.
Barbas, H. (1988). Anatomic organization of basoventral and mediodorsal visual recipient prefrontal regions in the rhesus monkey, *Journal of Comparative Neurology* **276**: 313–342.
Barbas, H. (1993). Organization of cortical afferent input to the orbitofrontal area in the rhesus monkey, *Neuroscience* **56**: 841–864.
Barbas, H. (1995). Anatomic basis of cognitive–emotional interactions in the primate prefrontal cortex, *Neuroscience and Biobehavioral Reviews* **19**: 499–510.
Barbas, H. (2007). Specialized elements of orbitofrontal cortex in primates, *Annals of the New York Academy of Sciences* **1121**: 10–32.
Barbas, H. (2015). General cortical and special prefrontal connections: principles from structure to function, *Annu Rev Neurosci* **38**: 269–89.
Barbas, H. and Pandya, D. N. (1989). Architecture and intrinsic connections of the prefrontal cortex in the rhesus monkey, *Journal of Comparative Neurology* **286**: 353–375.
Barkas, L. J., Henderson, J. L., Hamilton, D. A., Redhead, E. S. and Gray, W. P. (2010). Selective temporal resections and spatial memory impairment: cue dependent lateralization effects, *Behav Brain Res* **208**: 535–44.
Barlow, H. (1995). The neuron doctrine in perception, *in* M. S. Gazzaniga (ed.), *The Cognitive Neurosciences*, MIT Press, Cambridge, MA, chapter 26, pp. 415–435.
Barlow, H. B. (1961). Possible principles underlying the transformation of sensory messages, *in* W. Rosenblith (ed.), *Sensory Communication*, MIT Press, Cambridge, MA.
Barlow, H. B. (1972). Single units and sensation: a neuron doctrine for perceptual psychology, *Perception* **1**: 371–394.
Barlow, H. B. (1985). Cerebral cortex as model builder, *in* D. Rose and V. G. Dobson (eds), *Models of the Visual Cortex*, Wiley, Chichester, pp. 37–46.
Barlow, H. B. (1989). Unsupervised Learning, *Neural Computation* **1**: 295–311.
Barlow, H. B., Kaushal, T. P. and Mitchison, G. J. (1989). Finding minimum entropy codes, *Neural Computation* **1**: 412–423.
Barnes, C. A. (2003). Long-term potentiation and the ageing brain, *Philosophical Transactions of the Royal Society of London B* **358**: 765–772.
Barnes, C. A. (2011). Secrets of aging: What does a normally aging brain look like?, *F1000 Biol Rep* **3**: 22.
Barnes, D. C., Hofacer, R. D., Zaman, A. R., Rennaker, R. L. and Wilson, D. A. (2008). Olfactory perceptual stability and discrimination, *Nat Neurosci* **11**: 1378–80.
Barreiros, I. V., Ishii, H., Walton, M. E. and Panayi, M. C. (2021). Defining an orbitofrontal compass: Functional and anatomical heterogeneity across anterior-posterior and medial-lateral axes, *Behav Neurosci* **135**: 165–173.
Barretto, R. P., Gillis-Smith, S., Chandrashekar, J., Yarmolinsky, D. A., Schnitzer, M. J., Ryba, N. J. and Zuker, C. S. (2015). The neural representation of taste quality at the periphery, *Nature* **517**: 373–6.
Barry, D. N. and Maguire, E. A. (2019). Remote memory and the hippocampus: a constructive critique, *Trends Cogn Sci* **23**: 128–142.
Barry, D. N., Chadwick, M. J. and Maguire, E. A. (2018). Nonmonotonic recruitment of ventromedial prefrontal cortex during remote memory recall, *PLoS Biol* **16**: e2005479.
Barto, A. G. (1985). Learning by statistical cooperation of self-interested neuron-like computing elements, *Human Neurobiology* **4**: 229–256.
Barto, A. G. (1995). Adaptive critics and the basal ganglia, *in* J. C. Houk, J. L. Davis and D. G. Beiser (eds), *Models of Information Processing in the Basal Ganglia*, MIT Press, Cambridge, MA, chapter 11, pp. 215–232.
Barton, J. J. (2011). Disorders of higher visual processing, *Handb Clin Neurol* **102**: 223–61.
Bartus, R. T. (2000). On neurodegenerative diseases, models, and treatment strategies: lessons learned and lessons forgotten a generation following the cholinergic hypothesis, *Experimental Neurology* **163**: 495–529.

Bassett, J. and Taube, J. S. (2005). Head direction signal generation: ascending and descending information streams, *in* S. I. Wiener and J. S. Taube (eds), *Head Direction Cells and the Neural Mechanisms of Spatial Orientation*, MIT Press, Cambridge, MA, chapter 5, pp. 83–109.

Battaglia, F. and Treves, A. (1998a). Stable and rapid recurrent processing in realistic autoassociative memories, *Neural Computation* **10**: 431–450.

Battaglia, F. P. and Treves, A. (1998b). Attractor neural networks storing multiple space representations: a model for hippocampal place fields, *Physical Review E* **58**: 7738–7753.

Battistella, G., Borghesani, V., Henry, M., Shwe, W., Lauricella, M., Miller, Z., Deleon, J., Miller, B. L., Dronkers, N., Brambati, S. M., Seeley, W. W., Mandelli, M. L. and Gorno-Tempini, M. L. (2020). Task-free functional language networks: reproducibility and clinical application, *J Neurosci* **40**: 1311–1320.

Baumann, O. and Mattingley, J. B. (2021). Extrahippocampal contributions to spatial navigation in humans: A review of the neuroimaging evidence, *Hippocampus* **31**: 640–657.

Baumgartner, U., Iannetti, G. D., Zambreanu, L., Stoeter, P., Treede, R. D. and Tracey, I. (2010). Multiple somatotopic representations of heat and mechanical pain in the operculo-insular cortex: a high-resolution fMRI study, *J Neurophysiol* **104**: 2863–72.

Bausch, M., Niediek, J., Reber, T. P., Mackay, S., Bostrom, J., Elger, C. E. and Mormann, F. (2021). Concept neurons in the human medial temporal lobe flexibly represent abstract relations between concepts, *Nat Commun* **12**: 6164.

Baxter, M. G. and Murray, E. A. (2001a). Effects of hippocampal lesions on delayed nonmatching-to-sample in monkeys: a reply to Zola and Squire, *Hippocampus* **11**: 201–203.

Baxter, M. G. and Murray, E. A. (2001b). Opposite relationship of hippocampal and rhinal cortex damage to delayed nonmatching-to-sample deficits in monkeys, *Hippocampus* **11**: 61–71.

Baxter, R. D. and Liddle, P. F. (1998). Neuropsychological deficits associated with schizophrenic syndromes, *Schizophrenia Research* **30**: 239–249.

Baylis, G. C. and Rolls, E. T. (1987). Responses of neurons in the inferior temporal cortex in short term and serial recognition memory tasks, *Experimental Brain Research* **65**: 614–622.

Baylis, G. C., Rolls, E. T. and Leonard, C. M. (1985). Selectivity between faces in the responses of a population of neurons in the cortex in the superior temporal sulcus of the monkey, *Brain Research* **342**: 91–102.

Baylis, G. C., Rolls, E. T. and Leonard, C. M. (1987). Functional subdivisions of the temporal lobe neocortex, *Journal of Neuroscience* **7**: 330–342.

Baylis, L. L. and Rolls, E. T. (1991). Responses of neurons in the primate taste cortex to glutamate, *Physiology and Behavior* **49**: 973–979.

Baylis, L. L., Rolls, E. T. and Baylis, G. C. (1995). Afferent connections of the caudolateral orbitofrontal cortex taste area of the primate, *Neuroscience* **64**: 801–12.

Bazzari, A. H. and Parri, H. R. (2019). Neuromodulators and long-term synaptic plasticity in learning and memory: a steered-glutamatergic perspective, *Brain Sci* **9**: 300.

Bear, M. F. and Singer, W. (1986). Modulation of visual cortical plasticity by acetylcholine and noradrenaline, *Nature* **320**: 172–176.

Beaver, J. D., Lawrence, A. D., Ditzhuijzen, J. v., Davis, M. H., Woods, A. and Calder, A. J. (2006). Individual differences in reward drive predict neural responses to images of food, *Journal of Neuroscience* **26**: 5160–5166.

Bechara, A., Damasio, A. R., Damasio, H. and Anderson, S. W. (1994). Insensitivity to future consequences following damage to human prefrontal cortex, *Cognition* **50**: 7–15.

Bechara, A., Tranel, D., Damasio, H. and Damasio, A. R. (1996). Failure to respond autonomically to anticipated future outcomes following damage to prefrontal cortex, *Cerebral Cortex* **6**: 215–225.

Bechara, A., Damasio, H., Tranel, D. and Damasio, A. R. (1997). Deciding advantageously before knowing the advantageous strategy, *Science* **275**: 1293–1295.

Bechara, A., Damasio, H., Tranel, D. and Damasio, A. R. (2005). The Iowa Gambling Task and the somatic marker hypothesis: some questions and answers, *Trends in Cognitive Sciences* **9**: 159–162.

Beck, A. T. (2008). The evolution of the cognitive model of depression and its neurobiological correlates, *American Journal of Psychiatry* **165**: 969–977.

Beck, D. M. and Kastner, S. (2009). Top-down and bottom-up mechanisms in biasing competition in the human brain, *Vision Research* **49**: 1154–1165.

Becker, N. B., Jesus, S. N., Joao, K., Viseu, J. N. and Martins, R. I. S. (2017). Depression and sleep quality in older adults: a meta-analysis, *Psychol Health Med* **22**: 889–895.

Becker, S. and Hinton, G. E. (1992). Self-organizing neural network that discovers surfaces in random-dot stereograms, *Nature* **355**: 161–163.

Beckstead, R. M. and Norgren, R. (1979). An autoradiographic examination of the central distribution of the trigeminal, facial, glossopharyngeal, and vagal nerves in the monkey, *Journal of Comparative Neurology* **184**: 455–472.

Beckstead, R. M., Morse, J. R. and Norgren, R. (1980). The nucleus of the solitary tract in the monkey: projections to the thalamus and brainstem nuclei, *Journal of Comparative Neurology* **190**: 259–282.

Belin, P. (2019). The vocal brain: core and extended cerebral networks for voice processing, *in* S. Fruhholz and P. Belin (eds), *Oxford Handbook of Voice Perception*, Oxford University Press, Oxford, pp. 37–60.

Bell, A. J. and Sejnowski, T. J. (1995). An information-maximation approach to blind separation and blind deconvolution, *Neural Computation* **7**: 1129–1159.

Bellmund, J. L. S., Gardenfors, P., Moser, E. I. and Doeller, C. F. (2018). Navigating cognition: Spatial codes for human thinking, *Science* **362**: eaat6766.

Bellot, E., Abassi, E. and Papeo, L. (2021). Moving toward versus away from another: how body motion direction changes the representation of bodies and actions in the visual cortex, *Cereb Cortex* **31**: 2670–2685.

Bengio, Y., Goodfellow, I. J. and Courville, A. (2017). *Deep Learning*, MIT Press, Cambridge, MA.

Bennett, A. (1990). Large competitive networks, *Network* **1**: 449–462.

Berg, E. (1948). A simple objective technique for measuring flexibility in thinking, *Journal of General Psychology* **39**: 15–22.

Berlin, H., Rolls, E. T. and Kischka, U. (2004). Impulsivity, time perception, emotion, and reinforcement sensitivity in patients with orbitofrontal cortex lesions, *Brain* **127**: 1108–1126.

Berlin, H., Rolls, E. T. and Iversen, S. D. (2005). Borderline Personality Disorder, impulsivity and the orbitofrontal cortex, *American Journal of Psychiatry* **162**: 2360–2373.

Bermpohl, F., Kahnt, T., Dalanay, U., Hagele, C., Sajonz, B., Wegner, T., Stoy, M., Adli, M., Kruger, S., Wrase, J., Strohle, A., Bauer, M. and Heinz, A. (2010). Altered representation of expected value in the orbitofrontal cortex in mania, *Human Brain Mapping* **31**: 958–969.

Bernard, A., Lubbers, L. S., Tanis, K. Q., Luo, R., Podtelezhnikov, A. A., Finney, E. M., McWhorter, M. M., Serikawa, K., Lemon, T., Morgan, R., Copeland, C., Smith, K., Cullen, V., Davis-Turak, J., Lee, C. K., Sunkin, S. M., Loboda, A. P., Levine, D. M., Stone, D. J., Hawrylycz, M. J., Roberts, C. J., Jones, A. R., Geschwind, D. H. and Lein, E. S. (2012). Transcriptional architecture of the primate neocortex, *Neuron* **73**: 1083–99.

Berners-Lee, A., Feng, T., Silva, D., Wu, X., Ambrose, E. R., Pfeiffer, B. E. and Foster, D. J. (2022). Hippocampal replays appear after a single experience and incorporate greater detail with more experience, *Neuron* **110**: 1829–1842 e5.

Berridge, K. C. and Robinson, T. E. (1998). What is the role of dopamine in reward: hedonic impact, reward learning, or incentive salience?, *Brain Research Reviews* **28**: 309–369.

Berridge, K. C., Robinson, T. E. and Aldridge, J. W. (2009). Dissecting components of reward: 'liking', 'wanting', and learning, *Current Opinion in Pharmacology* **9**: 65–73.

Berthoud, H. R., Morrison, C. D., Ackroff, K. and Sclafani, A. (2021). Learning of food preferences: mechanisms and implications for obesity and metabolic diseases, *Int J Obes (Lond)* **45**: 2156–2168.

Berti, A. and Neppi-Modona, M. (2012). Agnosia (including Prosopagnosia and Anosognosia), *in* V.S.Ramachandran (ed.), *Encyclopedia of Human Behavior*, 2 edn, Vol. 1, Academic Press, pp. 60–67.

Berti, A., Garbarini, F. and Neppi-Modona, M. (2015). Disorders of higher cortical function, *in* M. Zigmond, L. Rowland and J. Coyle (eds), *Neurobiology of Brain Disorders*, Academic Press, pp. 525–541.

Bethlehem, R. A. I., Seidlitz, J. and White, S. R. (2022). Brain charts for the human lifespan, *Nature* **604**: 525–533.

Bhattacharyya, S. and Chakraborty, K. (2007). Glutamatergic dysfunction–newer targets for anti-obsessional drugs, *Recent Patents CNS Drug Discovery* **2**: 47–55.

Bi, G.-Q. and Poo, M.-M. (1998). Activity-induced synaptic modifications in hippocampal culture, dependence on spike timing, synaptic strength and cell type, *Journal of Neuroscience* **18**: 10464–10472.

Bi, G.-Q. and Poo, M.-M. (2001). Synaptic modification by correlated activity: Hebb's postulate revisited, *Annual Review of Neuroscience* **24**: 139–166.

Bialek, W., Rieke, F., de Ruyter van Stevenick, R. R. and Warland, D. (1991). Reading a neural code, *Science* **252**: 1854–1857.

Bicanski, A. and Burgess, N. (2018). A neural-level model of spatial memory and imagery, *Elife* **7**: e33752.

Biederman, I. (1972). Perceiving real-world scenes, *Science* **177**: 77–80.

Biederman, I. (1987). Recognition-by-components: A theory of human image understanding, *Psychological Review* **94**(2): 115–147.

Biederman, I. and Gerhardstein, P. C. (1993). Recognizing depth-rotated objects: Evidence and conditions for 3D viewpoint invariance, *Journal of Experimental Psychology: Human Perception and Performance* **20**(1): 80.

Bienenstock, E. L., Cooper, L. N. and Munro, P. W. (1982). Theory for the development of neuron selectivity: orientation specificity and binocular interaction in visual cortex, *Journal of Neuroscience* **2**: 32–48.

Bierer, L. M., Haroutunian, V., Gabriel, S., Knott, P. J., Carlin, L. S., Purohit, D. P., Perl, D. P., Schmeidler, J., Kanof, P. and Davis, K. L. (1995). Neurochemical correlates of dementia severity in Alzheimer's disease: relative importance of the cholinergic deficits, *Journal of Neurochemistry* **64**: 749–760.

Binder, J. R. (2015). The Wernicke area: Modern evidence and a reinterpretation, *Neurology* **85**: 2170–5.

Binder, J. R. (2017). Current controversies on Wernicke's Area and its role in language, *Curr Neurol Neurosci Rep* **17**: 58.

Binford, T. O. (1981). Inferring surfaces from images, *Artificial Intelligence* **17**: 205–244.
Bishop, C. M. (1995). *Neural Networks for Pattern Recognition*, Clarendon Press, Oxford.
Bisley, J. W. and Goldberg, M. E. (2003). Neuronal activity in the lateral intraparietal area and spatial attention, *Science* **299**: 81–86.
Bisley, J. W. and Goldberg, M. E. (2006). Neural correlates of attention and distractibility in the lateral intraparietal area, *Journal of Neurophysiology* **95**: 1696–1717.
Bisley, J. W. and Goldberg, M. E. (2010). Attention, intention, and priority in the parietal lobe, *Annu Rev Neurosci* **33**: 1–21.
Blair, R. J., Morris, J. S., Frith, C. D., Perrett, D. I. and Dolan, R. J. (1999). Dissociable neural responses to facial expressions of sadness and anger, *Brain* **122**: 883–893.
Blakemore, C., Garey, L. J. and Vital-Durand, F. (1978). The physiological effects of monocular deprivation and their reversal in the monkeys visual cortex, *Journal of Physiology* **283**: 223–262.
Bliss-Moreau, E., Moadab, G., Bauman, M. D. and Amaral, D. G. (2013). The impact of early amygdala damage on juvenile rhesus macaque social behavior, *J Cogn Neurosci* **25**: 2124–40.
Bliss-Moreau, E., Moadab, G., Santistevan, A. and Amaral, D. G. (2017). The effects of neonatal amygdala or hippocampus lesions on adult social behavior, *Behav Brain Res* **322**: 123–137.
Bliss, T. and Collingridge, G. L. (2019). Persistent memories of long-term potentiation and the N-methyl-d-aspartate receptor, *Brain Neurosci Adv* **3**: 2398212819848213.
Bliss, T. V. and Collingridge, G. L. (2013). Expression of NMDA receptor-dependent LTP in the hippocampus: bridging the divide, *Molecular Brain* **6**: 5.
Block, H. D. (1962). The perceptron: a model for brain functioning, *Reviews of Modern Physics* **34**: 123–135.
Bloem, B., Huda, R., Sur, M. and Graybiel, A. M. (2017). Two-photon imaging in mice shows striosomes and matrix have overlapping but differential reinforcement-related responses, *Elife* **6**: 10.7554/eLife.32353.
Blood, A. J. and Zatorre, R. J. (2001). Intensely pleasureable responses to music correlate with activity of brain regions implicated in reward and emotion, *Proceedings of the National Academy of Sciences USA* **98**: 11818–11823.
Blood, A. J., Zatorre, R. J., Bermudez, P. and Evans, A. C. (1999). Emotional responses to pleasant and unpleasant music correlate with activity in paralimbic brain regions, *Nature Neuroscience* **2**: 382–387.
Bloomfield, S. (1974). Arithmetical operations performed by nerve cells, *Brain Research* **69**: 115–124.
Boboeva, V., Brasselet, R. and Treves, A. (2018). The capacity for correlated semantic memories in the cortex, *Entropy (Basel)* **20**: 824.
Boccia, M., Sulpizio, V., Nemmi, F., Guariglia, C. and Galati, G. (2017). Direct and indirect parieto-medial temporal pathways for spatial navigation in humans: evidence from resting-state functional connectivity, *Brain Struct Funct* **222**: 1945–1957.
Bohbot, V. D. and Corkin, S. (2007). Posterior parahippocampal place learning in H.M, *Hippocampus* **17**: 863–72.
Bolles, R. C. and Cain, R. A. (1982). Recognizing and locating partially visible objects: The local-feature-focus method, *International Journal of Robotics Research* **1**: 57–82.
Bonelli, S. B., Powell, R. H., Yogarajah, M., Samson, R. S., Symms, M. R., Thompson, P. J., Koepp, M. J. and Duncan, J. S. (2010). Imaging memory in temporal lobe epilepsy: predicting the effects of temporal lobe resection, *Brain* **133**: 1186–99.
Bonner, M. F. and Price, A. R. (2013). Where is the anterior temporal lobe and what does it do?, *J Neurosci* **33**: 4213–5.
Bonnici, H. M. and Maguire, E. A. (2018). Two years later - Revisiting autobiographical memory representations in vmPFC and hippocampus, *Neuropsychologia* **110**: 159–169.
Booth, D. A. (1985). Food-conditioned eating preferences and aversions with interoceptive elements: learned appetites and satieties, *Annals of the New York Academy of Sciences* **443**: 22–37.
Booth, M. C. A. and Rolls, E. T. (1998). View-invariant representations of familiar objects by neurons in the inferior temporal visual cortex, *Cerebral Cortex* **8**: 510–523.
Bornkessel-Schlesewsky, I., Schlesewsky, M., Small, S. L. and Rauschecker, J. P. (2015). Neurobiological roots of language in primate audition: common computational properties, *Trends Cogn Sci* **19**: 142–50.
Bostan, A. C., Dum, R. P. and Strick, P. L. (2018). Functional anatomy of basal ganglia circuits with the cerebral cortex and the cerebellum, *Prog Neurol Surg* **33**: 50–61.
Botvinick, M., Ritter, S., Wang, J. X., Kurth-Nelson, Z., Blundell, C. and Hassabis, D. (2019). Reinforcement Learning, fast and slow, *Trends Cogn Sci* **23**: 408–422.
Botvinick, M., Wang, J. X., Dabney, W., Miller, K. J. and Kurth-Nelson, Z. (2020). Deep Reinforcement Learning and its neuroscientific implications, *Neuron* **107**: 603–616.
Bouchard, K. E., Mesgarani, N., Johnson, K. and Chang, E. F. (2013). Functional organization of human sensorimotor cortex for speech articulation, *Nature* **495**: 327–32.

Boussaoud, D., Desimone, R. and Ungerleider, L. G. (1991). Visual topography of area TEO in the macaque, *Journal of Computational Neurology* **306**: 554–575.

Bovier, A. and Gayrard, V. (1992). Rigorous bounds on the storage capacity of the dilute Hopfield model, *Journal of Statistical Physics* **69**: 597–627.

Bowers, J. S., Malhotra, G., Dujmovic, M., Montero, M. L., Tsvetkov, C., Biscione, V., Puebla, G., Adolfi, F., Hummel, J. E., Heaton, J. F., Evans, B. D., Mitchell, J. and Blything, R. (2023). Deep problems with neural network models of human vision, *Behavioral and Brain Sciences* p. doi: 10.1017/S0140525X22002813.

Braak, H., Ghebremedhin, E., Rub, U., Bratzke, H. and Del Tredici, K. (2004). Stages in the development of Parkinson's disease-related pathology, *Cell Tissue Res* **318**: 121–34.

Brady, M., Ponce, J., Yuille, A. and Asada, H. (1985). Describing surfaces, *A. I. Memo 882, The Artificial Intelligence* **17**: 285–349.

Braitenberg, V. and Schüz, A. (1991). *Anatomy of the Cortex*, Springer-Verlag, Berlin.

Braitenberg, V. and Schüz, A. (1998). *Cortex: Statistics and Geometry of Neuronal Connectivity*, Springer-Verlag, Berlin.

Bremmer, F., Duhamel, J. R., Ben Hamed, S. and Graf, W. (2000). Stages of self-motion processing in primate posterior parietal cortex, *Int Rev Neurobiol* **44**: 173–98.

Brennan, J. R. (2022). *Language and the Brain: A Slim Guide to Neurolinguistics*, Oxford University Press, Oxford.

Bressler, S. L. and Seth, A. K. (2011). Wiener-Granger Causality: A well established methodology, *Neuroimage* **58**: 323–329.

Bressler, S. L., Tang, W., Sylvester, C. M., Shulman, G. L. and Corbetta, M. (2008). Top-down control of human visual cortex by frontal and parietal cortex in anticipatory visual spatial attention, *Journal of Neuroscience* **28**: 10056–10061.

Bridle, J. S. (1990). Probabilistic interpretation of feedforward classification network outputs, with relationships to statistical pattern recognition, *in* F. Fogelman-Soulie and J. Herault (eds), *Neurocomputing: Algorithms, Architectures and Applications*, Springer-Verlag, New York, pp. 227–236.

Bright, I. M., Meister, M. L. R., Cruzado, N. A., Tiganj, Z., Buffalo, E. A. and Howard, M. W. (2020). A temporal record of the past with a spectrum of time constants in the monkey entorhinal cortex, *Proc Natl Acad Sci U S A* **117**: 20274–20283.

Brincat, S. L. and Miller, E. K. (2015). Frequency-specific hippocampal-prefrontal interactions during associative learning, *Nat Neurosci* **18**: 576–81.

Broca, P. (1878). Anatomie comparée des circonvolutions cérébrales: le grand lobe limbique et la scissure limbique dans la série des mammifères, *Revue Anthropologique* **1**: 385–498.

Brodmann, K. (1909). *Vergleichende Lokalisationslehre der Grosshirnrinde in ihren Prinzipien dargestellt auf Grund des Zellenbaues*, Barth, Leipzig.

Brodmann, K. (1925). *Vergleichende Localisationslehre der Grosshirnrinde. Translated into English by L.J.Garey as Localisation in the Cerebral Cortex 1994 London: Smith-Gordon*, 2 edn, Barth, Leipzig.

Bromberg-Martin, E. S., Matsumoto, M. and Hikosaka, O. (2010a). Dopamine in motivational control: rewarding, aversive, and alerting, *Neuron* **68**: 815–834.

Bromberg-Martin, E. S., Matsumoto, M., Hong, S. and Hikosaka, O. (2010b). A pallidus-habenula-dopamine pathway signals inferred stimulus values, *Journal of Neurophysiology* **104**: 1068–1076.

Brooks, L. R. (1978). Nonanalytic concept formation and memory for instances, *in* E. Rosch and B. B. Lloyd (eds), *Cognition and Categorization*, Erlbaum, Hillsdale, NJ.

Brotchie, P., Andersen, R., Snyder, L. and Goodman, S. (1995). Head position signals used by parietal neurons to encode locations of visual stimuli, *Nature London* **375**: 232–235.

Brothers, L. and Ring, B. (1993). Mesial temporal neurons in the macaque monkey with responses selective for aspects of social stimuli, *Behavioural Brain Research* **57**: 53–61.

Brown, D. A., Gähwiler, B. H., Griffith, W. H. and Halliwell, J. V. (1990a). Membrane currents in hippocampal neurons, *Progress in Brain Research* **83**: 141–160.

Brown, J. M. (2009). Visual streams and shifting attention, *Prog Brain Res* **176**: 47–63.

Brown, M. and Xiang, J. (1998). Recognition memory: neuronal substrates of the judgement of prior occurrence, *Progress in Neurobiology* **55**: 149–189.

Brown, T. H. and Zador, A. (1990). The hippocampus, *in* G. Shepherd (ed.), *The Synaptic Organization of the Brain*, Oxford University Press, New York, pp. 346–388.

Brown, T. H., Kairiss, E. W. and Keenan, C. L. (1990b). Hebbian synapses: biophysical mechanisms and algorithms, *Annual Review of Neuroscience* **13**: 475–511.

Brown, T. H., Ganong, A. H., Kairiss, E. W., Keenan, C. L. and Kelso, S. R. (eds) (1989). *Long-term Potentiation in Two Synaptic Systems of the Hippocampal Brain Slice*, Academic Press, San Diego.

Brown, T. I., Carr, V. A., LaRocque, K. F., Favila, S. E., Gordon, A. M., Bowles, B., Bailenson, J. N. and Wagner, A. D. (2016). Prospective representation of navigational goals in the human hippocampus, *Science* **352**: 1323–6.

Brown, V. J., Desimone, R. and Mishkin, M. (1995). Responses of cells in the tail of the caudate nucleus during visual discrimination learning, *Journal of Neurophysiology* **74**: 1083–1094.

Browning, P. G., Gaffan, D., Croxson, P. L. and Baxter, M. G. (2010). Severe scene learning impairment, but intact recognition memory, after cholinergic depletion of inferotemporal cortex followed by fornix transection, *Cereb Cortex* **20**: 282–93.

Bruce, V. (1988). *Recognising Faces*, Erlbaum, Hillsdale, NJ.

Bruffaerts, R., De Deyne, S., Meersmans, K., Liuzzi, A. G., Storms, G. and Vandenberghe, R. (2019). Redefining the resolution of semantic knowledge in the brain: Advances made by the introduction of models of semantics in neuroimaging, *Neurosci Biobehav Rev* **103**: 3–13.

Brun, V. H., Otnass, M. K., Molden, S., Steffenach, H. A., Witter, M. P., Moser, M. B. and Moser, E. I. (2002). Place cells and place recognition maintained by direct entorhinal–hippocampal circuitry, *Science* **296**: 2243–2246.

Brunel, N. and Wang, X. J. (2001). Effects of neuromodulation in a cortical network model of object working memory dominated by recurrent inhibition, *Journal of Computational Neuroscience* **11**: 63–85.

Brunel, N. and Wang, X. J. (2003). What determines the frequency of fast network oscillations with irregular neural discharges? I. Synaptic dynamics and excitation-inhibition balance, *Journal of Neurophysiology* **90**: 415–430.

Bubb, E. J., Kinnavane, L. and Aggleton, J. P. (2017). Hippocampal - diencephalic - cingulate networks for memory and emotion: An anatomical guide, *Brain Neurosci Adv* **1**: 1–20.

Buck, L. and Axel, R. (1991). A novel multigene family may encode odorant receptors: a molecular basis for odor recognition, *Cell* **65**: 175–187.

Buck, L. and Bargmann, C. I. (2013). Smell and taste: the chemical senses, *in* E. Kandel, J. H. Schwartz, T. H. Jessell, S. A. Siegelbaum and A. J. Hudspeth (eds), *Principles of Neural Science*, 5th edn, McGraw-Hill, New York, chapter 32, pp. 712–742.

Buckley, M. J. and Gaffan, D. (2000). The hippocampus, perirhinal cortex, and memory in the monkey, *in* J. J. Bolhuis (ed.), *Brain, Perception, and Memory: Advances in Cognitive Neuroscience*, Oxford University Press, Oxford, pp. 279–298.

Buckley, M. J. and Gaffan, D. (2006). Perirhinal contributions to object perception, *Trends in Cognitive Sciences* **10**: 100–107.

Buckley, M. J., Booth, M. C. A., Rolls, E. T. and Gaffan, D. (2001). Selective perceptual impairments following perirhinal cortex ablation, *Journal of Neuroscience* **21**: 9824–9836.

Buckner, R. L. and DiNicola, L. M. (2019). The brain's default network: updated anatomy, physiology and evolving insights, *Nat Rev Neurosci* **20**: 593–608.

Buckner, R. L., Krienen, F. M., Castellanos, A., Diaz, J. C. and Yeo, B. T. (2011). The organization of the human cerebellum estimated by intrinsic functional connectivity, *J Neurophysiol* **106**: 2322–45.

Buhl, E. H., Halasy, K. and Somogyi, P. (1994). Diverse sources of hippocampal unitary inhibitory postsynaptic potentials and the number of synaptic release sites, *Nature* **368**: 823–828.

Buhmann, J., Lange, J., von der Malsburg, C., Vorbrüggen, J. C. and Würtz, R. P. (1991). Object recognition in the dynamic link architecture: Parallel implementation of a transputer network, *in* B. Kosko (ed.), *Neural Networks for Signal Processing*, Prentice Hall, Englewood Cliffs, NJ, pp. 121–159.

Bullier, J. and Nowak, L. (1995). Parallel versus serial processing: new vistas on the distributed organization of the visual system, *Current Opinion in Neurobiology* **5**: 497–503.

Bunsey, M. and Eichenbaum, H. (1996). Conservation of hippocampal memory function in rats and humans, *Nature* **379**: 255–257.

Buot, A. and Yelnik, J. (2012). Functional anatomy of the basal ganglia: limbic aspects, *Revue Neurologique (Paris)* **168**: 569–575.

Burgess, N. (2008). Spatial cognition and the brain, *Ann N Y Acad Sci* **1124**: 77–97.

Burgess, N. and O'Keefe, J. (1996). Neuronal computations underlying the firing of place cells and their role in navigation, *Hippocampus* **6**: 749–62.

Burgess, N., Recce, M. and O'Keefe, J. (1994). A model of hippocampal function, *Neural Networks* **7**: 1065–1081.

Burgess, N., Jackson, A., Hartley, T. and O'Keefe, J. (2000). Predictions derived from modelling the hippocampal role in navigation, *Biological Cybernetics* **83**: 301–312.

Burgess, N., Maguire, E. A., Spiers, H. J. and O'Keefe, J. (2001). A temporoparietal and prefrontal network for retrieving the spatial context of lifelike events, *Neuroimage* **14**: 439–53.

Burgess, N., Maguire, E. A. and O'Keefe, J. (2002). The human hippocampus and spatial and episodic memory, *Neuron* **35**: 625–641.

Burke, S. N. and Barnes, C. A. (2006). Neural plasticity in the ageing brain, *Nature Reviews Neuroscience* **7**: 30–40.

Burton, M. J., Rolls, E. T. and Mora, F. (1976). Effects of hunger on the responses of neurones in the lateral hypothalamus to the sight and taste of food, *Experimental Neurology* **51**: 668–677.

Burton, T. J. and Balleine, B. W. (2022). The positive valence system, adaptive behaviour and the origins of reward, *Emerg Top Life Sci* **6**: 501–513.

Burwell, R. D., Witter, M. P. and Amaral, D. G. (1995). Perirhinal and postrhinal cortices of the rat: a review of the neuroanatomical literature and comparison with findings from the monkey brain, *Hippocampus* **5**: 390–408.

Bush, G., Luu, P. and Posner, M. I. (2000). Cognitive and emotional influences in anterior cingulate cortex, *Trends in Cognitive Sciences* **4**: 215–222.

Bush, G., Vogt, B. A., Holmes, J., Dales, A. M., Greve, D., Jenike, M. A. and Rosen, B. R. (2002). Dorsal anterior cingulate cortex: a role in reward-based decision making, *Proceedings of the National Academy of Sciences USA* **99**: 523–528.

Bussey, T. J. and Saksida, L. M. (2005). Object memory and perception in the medial temporal lobe: an alternative approach, *Current Opinion in Neurobiology* **15**: 730–737.

Bussey, T. J., Saksida, L. M. and Murray, E. A. (2002). Perirhinal cortex resolves feature ambiguity in complex visual discriminations, *European Journal of Neuroscience* **15**: 365–374.

Bussey, T. J., Saksida, L. M. and Murray, E. A. (2003). Impairments in visual discrimination after perirhinal cortex lesions: testing "declarative" versus "perceptual-mnemonic" views of perirhinal cortex function, *European Journal of Neuroscience* **17**: 649–660.

Bussey, T. J., Saksida, L. M. and Murray, E. A. (2005). The perceptual-mnemonic / feature conjunction model of perirhinal cortex function, *Quarterly Journal of Experimental Psychology* **58B**: 269–282.

Buzsaki, G. (2015). Hippocampal sharp wave-ripple: A cognitive biomarker for episodic memory and planning, *Hippocampus* **25**: 1073–188.

Buzsaki, G. and Moser, E. I. (2013). Memory, navigation and theta rhythm in the hippocampal-entorhinal system, *Nat Neurosci* **16**: 130–8.

Buzsaki, G. and Tingley, D. (2018). Space and time: the hippocampus as a sequence generator, *Trends Cogn Sci* **22**: 853–869.

Byrne, P., Becker, S. and Burgess, N. (2007). Remembering the past and imagining the future: a neural model of spatial memory and imagery, *Psychol Rev* **114**: 340–75.

Caan, W., Perrett, D. I. and Rolls, E. T. (1984). Responses of striatal neurons in the behaving monkey. 2. Visual processing in the caudal neostriatum, *Brain Research* **290**: 53–65.

Cadieu, C. F., Hong, H., Yamins, D. L., Pinto, N., Ardila, D., Solomon, E. A., Majaj, N. J. and DiCarlo, J. J. (2014). Deep neural networks rival the representation of primate IT cortex for core visual object recognition, *PLoS Comput Biol* **10**: e1003963.

Caffarra, S., Karipidis, I., Yablonski, M. and Yeatman, J. D. (2021). Anatomy and physiology of word-selective visual cortex: from visual features to lexical processing, *Brain Struct Funct* **226**: 3051–3065.

Cahusac, P. M. B., Miyashita, Y. and Rolls, E. T. (1989). Responses of hippocampal formation neurons in the monkey related to delayed spatial response and object-place memory tasks, *Behavioural Brain Research* **33**: 229–240.

Cahusac, P. M. B., Rolls, E. T., Miyashita, Y. and Niki, H. (1993). Modification of the responses of hippocampal neurons in the monkey during the learning of a conditional spatial response task, *Hippocampus* **3**: 29–42.

Cai, X. and Padoa-Schioppa, C. (2012). Neuronal encoding of subjective value in dorsal and ventral anterior cingulate cortex, *Journal of Neuroscience* **32**: 3791–3808.

Cai, X. and Padoa-Schioppa, C. (2019). Neuronal evidence for good-based economic decisions under variable action costs, *Nat Commun* **10**: 393.

Calabresi, P., Maj, R., Pisani, A., Mercuri, N. B. and Bernardi, G. (1992). Long-term synaptic depression in the striatum: physiological and pharmacological characterization, *Journal of Neuroscience* **12**: 4224–4233.

Calder, A. J., Young, A. W., Rowland, D., Perrett, D. I., Hodges, J. R. and Etcoff, N. L. (1996). Facial emotion recognition after bilateral amygdala damage: differentially severe impairment of fear, *Cognitive Neuropsychology* **13**: 699–745.

Caligiore, D., Pezzulo, G., Baldassarre, G., Bostan, A. C., Strick, P. L., Doya, K., Helmich, R. C., Dirkx, M., Houk, J., Jorntell, H., Lago-Rodriguez, A., Galea, J. M., Miall, R. C., Popa, T., Kishore, A., Verschure, P. F., Zucca, R. and Herreros, I. (2017). Consensus paper: towards a systems-level view of cerebellar function: the interplay between cerebellum, basal ganglia, and cortex, *Cerebellum* **16**: 203–229.

Calvert, G. A., Bullmore, E. T., Brammer, M. J., Campbell, R., Williams, S. C. R., McGuire, P. K., Woodruff, P. W. R., Iversen, S. D. and David, A. S. (1997). Activation of auditory cortex during silent lip-reading, *Science* **276**: 593–596.

Camille, N., Tsuchida, A. and Fellows, L. K. (2011). Double dissociation of stimulus-value and action-value learning in humans with orbitofrontal or anterior cingulate cortex damage, *Journal of Neuroscience* **31**: 15048–15052.

Campbell, K. L. and Tyler, L. K. (2018). Language-related domain-specific and domain-general systems in the human brain, *Curr Opin Behav Sci* **21**: 132–137.

Canli, T., Zhao, Z., Desmond, J. E., Kang, E., Gross, J. and Gabrieli, J. D. (2001). An fMRI study of personality influences on brain reactivity to emotional stimuli, *Behavioral Neuroscience* **115**: 33–42.

Canli, T., Sivers, H., Whitfield, S. L., Gotlib, I. H. and Gabrieli, J. D. (2002). Amygdala response to happy faces as a function of extraversion, *Science* **296**: 2191.

Cardinal, N. and Everitt, B. J. (2004). Neural and psychological mechanisms underlying appetitive learning: links to drug addiction, *Current Opinion in Neurobiology* **14**: 156–162.

Cardinal, N., Parkinson, J. A., Hall, J. and Everitt, B. J. (2002). Emotion and motivation: the role of the amygdala, ventral striatum, and prefrontal cortex., *Neuroscience and Biobehavioural Reviews* **26**: 321–52.

Carlson, E. T., Rasquinha, R. J., Zhang, K. and Connor, C. E. (2011). A sparse object coding scheme in area V4, *Curr Biol* **21**: 288–93.

Carmichael, S. T. and Price, J. L. (1994). Architectonic subdivision of the orbital and medial prefrontal cortex in the macaque monkey, *Journal of Comparative Neurology* **346**: 366–402.

Carmichael, S. T. and Price, J. L. (1995a). Limbic connections of the orbital and medial prefrontal cortex in macaque monkeys, *Journal of Comparative Neurology* **363**: 615–641.

Carmichael, S. T. and Price, J. L. (1995b). Sensory and premotor connections of the orbital and medial prefrontal cortex of macaque monkeys, *Journal of Comparative Neurology* **363**: 642–664.

Carmichael, S. T. and Price, J. L. (1996). Connectional networks within the orbital and medial prefrontal cortex of macaque monkeys, *Journal of Comparative Neurology* **371**: 179–207.

Carmichael, S. T., Clugnet, M.-C. and Price, J. L. (1994). Central olfactory connections in the macaque monkey, *Journal of Comparative Neurology* **346**: 403–434.

Carpenter, G. A. (1997). Distributed learning, recognition and prediction by ART and ARTMAP neural networks, *Neural Networks* **10**(8): 1473–1494.

Carruthers, P. (2019). *Human and Animal Minds*, Oxford University Press, Oxford.

Caspers, S. and Zilles, K. (2018). Microarchitecture and connectivity of the parietal lobe, *Handb Clin Neurol* **151**: 53–72.

Caspers, S., Eickhoff, S. B., Geyer, S., Scheperjans, F., Mohlberg, H., Zilles, K. and Amunts, K. (2008). The human inferior parietal lobule in stereotaxic space, *Brain Struct Funct* **212**: 481–95.

Cassaday, H. J. and Rawlins, J. N. (1997). The hippocampus, objects, and their contexts, *Behavioral Neuroscience* **111**: 1228–1244.

Castner, S. A., Williams, G. V. and Goldman-Rakic, P. S. (2000). Reversal of antipsychotic-induced working memory deficits by short-term dopamine D1 receptor stimulation, *Science* **287**: 2020–2022.

Catani, M. and Thiebaut de Schotten, M. (2008). A diffusion tensor imaging tractography atlas for virtual in vivo dissections, *Cortex* **44**: 1105–32.

Cavanna, A. E. and Trimble, M. R. (2006). The precuneus: a review of its functional anatomy and behavioural correlates, *Brain* **129**: 564–83.

Cavina-Pratesi, C., Monaco, S., Fattori, P., Galletti, C., McAdam, T. D., Quinlan, D. J., Goodale, M. A. and Culham, J. C. (2010). Functional magnetic resonance imaging reveals the neural substrates of arm transport and grip formation in reach-to-grasp actions in humans, *J Neurosci* **30**: 10306–23.

Celebrini, S., Thorpe, S., Trotter, Y. and Imbert, M. (1993). Dynamics of orientation coding in area V1 of the awake primate, *Visual Neuroscience* **10**: 811–825.

Cerasti, E. and Treves, A. (2010). How informative are spatial CA3 representations established by the dentate gyrus?, *PLoS Computational Biology* **6**: e1000759.

Cerasti, E. and Treves, A. (2013). The spatial representations acquired in CA3 by self-organizing recurrent connections, *Front Cell Neurosci* **7**: 112.

Cerella, J. (1986). Pigeons and perceptrons, *Pattern Recognition* **19**: 431–438.

Chadwick, M. J., Hassabis, D., Weiskopf, N. and Maguire, E. A. (2010). Decoding individual episodic memory traces in the human hippocampus, *Curr Biol* **20**: 544–7.

Chadwick, M. J., Mullally, S. L. and Maguire, E. A. (2013). The hippocampus extrapolates beyond the view in scenes: an fMRI study of boundary extension, *Cortex* **49**: 2067–79.

Chae, H., Banerjee, A., Dussauze, M. and Albeanu, D. F. (2022). Long-range functional loops in the mouse olfactory system and their roles in computing odor identity, *Neuron* **110**: 3970–3985 e7.

Chakrabarty, K., Bhattacharyya, S., Christopher, R. and Khanna, S. (2005). Glutamatergic dysfunction in OCD, *Neuropsychopharmacology* **30**: 1735–1740.

Chakravarty, I. (1979). A generalized line and junction labeling scheme with applications to scene analysis, *IEEE Transactions PAMI* **1**: 202–205.

Chamberlain, S. R., Fineberg, N. A., Blackwell, A. D., Robbins, T. W. and Sahakian, B. J. (2006). Motor inhibition and cognitive flexibility in obsessive-compulsive disorder and trichotillomania, *American Journal of Psychiatry* **163**: 1282–1284.

Chamberlain, S. R., Fineberg, N. A., Menzies, L. A., Blackwell, A. D., Bullmore, E. T., Robbins, T. W. and Sahakian, B. J. (2007). Impaired cognitive flexibility and motor inhibition in unaffected first-degree relatives of patients with obsessive-compulsive disorder, *American Journal of Psychiatry* **164**: 335–338.

Chamberlain, S. R., Solly, J. E., Hook, R. W., Vaghi, M. M. and Robbins, T. W. (2021). Cognitive Inflexibility in OCD and Related Disorders, *Curr Top Behav Neurosci* **49**: 125–145.

Chang, E. F., Raygor, K. P. and Berger, M. S. (2015). Contemporary model of language organization: an overview for neurosurgeons, *J Neurosurg* **122**: 250–61.

Chang, L. and Tsao, D. Y. (2017). The code for facial identity in the primate brain, *Cell* **169**: 1013–1028 e14.

Chang, L., Egger, B., Vetter, T. and Tsao, D. Y. (2021). Explaining face representation in the primate brain using different computational models, *Curr Biol* **31**: 2785–2795 e4.

Chang, S. W., Gariepy, J. F. and Platt, M. L. (2013). Neuronal reference frames for social decisions in primate frontal cortex, *Nat Neurosci* **16**: 243–50.

Chen, A., Gu, Y., Liu, S., DeAngelis, G. C. and Angelaki, D. E. (2016a). Evidence for a causal contribution of macaque vestibular, but not intraparietal, cortex to heading perception, *J Neurosci* **36**: 3789–98.

Chen, M., Li, B., Guang, J., Wei, L., Wu, S., Liu, Y. and Zhang, M. (2016b). Two subdivisions of macaque LIP process visual-oculomotor information differently, *Proc Natl Acad Sci U S A* **113**: E6263–E6270.

Chen, X., DeAngelis, G. C. and Angelaki, D. E. (2018). Flexible egocentric and allocentric representations of heading signals in parietal cortex, *Proc Natl Acad Sci U S A* **115**: E3305–E3312.

Chen, Y. and Crawford, J. D. (2020). Allocentric representations for target memory and reaching in human cortex, *Ann N Y Acad Sci* **1464**: 142–155.

Chen, Z. and Wilson, M. A. (2017). Deciphering neural codes of memory during sleep, *Trends Neurosci* **40**: 260–275.

Cheney, D. L. and Seyfarth, R. M. (2018). Flexible usage and social function in primate vocalizations, *Proc Natl Acad Sci U S A* **115**: 1974–1979.

Cheng, W., Rolls, E. T., Gu, H., Zhang, J. and Feng, J. (2015). Autism: reduced functional connectivity between cortical areas involved in face expression, theory of mind, and the sense of self, *Brain* **138**: 1382–1393.

Cheng, W., Rolls, E. T., Qiu, J., Liu, W., Tang, Y., Huang, C. C., Wang, X., Zhang, J., Lin, W., Zheng, L., Pu, J., Tsai, S. J., Yang, A. C., Lin, C. P., Wang, F., Xie, P. and Feng, J. (2016a). Medial reward and lateral non-reward orbitofrontal cortex circuits change in opposite directions in depression, *Brain* **139**: 3296–3309.

Cheng, W., Rolls, E. T., Zhang, J., Sheng, W., Ma, L., Wan, L., Luo, Q. and Feng, J. (2016b). Functional connectivity decreases in autism in emotion, self, and face circuits identified by Knowledge-based Enrichment Analysis, *Neuroimage* **148**: 169–178.

Cheng, W., Rolls, E. T., Qiu, J., Xie, X., Lyu, W., Li, Y., Huang, C. C., Yang, A. C., Tsai, S. J., Lyu, F., Zhuang, K., Lin, C. P., Xie, P. and Feng, J. (2018a). Functional connectivity of the human amygdala in health and in depression, *Soc Cogn Affect Neurosci* **13**: 557–568.

Cheng, W., Rolls, E. T., Qiu, J., Xie, X., Wei, D., Huang, C. C., Yang, A. C., Tsai, S. J., Li, Q., Meng, J., Lin, C. P., Xie, P. and Feng, J. (2018b). Increased functional connectivity of the posterior cingulate cortex with the lateral orbitofrontal cortex in depression, *Transl Psychiatry* **8**: 90.

Cheng, W., Rolls, E. T., Qiu, J., Yang, D., Ruan, H., Wei, D., Zhao, L., Meng, J., Xie, P. and Feng, J. (2018c). Functional connectivity of the precuneus in unmedicated patients with depression, *Biol Psychiatry Cogn Neurosci Neuroimaging* **3**: 1040–1049.

Cheng, W., Rolls, E. T., Ruan, H. and Feng, J. (2018d). Functional connectivities in the brain that mediate the association between depressive problems and sleep quality, *JAMA Psychiatry* **75**: 1052–1061.

Cheng, W., Rolls, E. T., Gong, W., Du, J., Zhang, J., Zhang, X. Y., Li, F. and Feng, J. (2021). Sleep duration, brain structure, and psychiatric and cognitive problems in children, *Mol Psychiatry* **26**: 3992–4003.

Cherry, J. A. and Baum, M. J. (2020). Sex differences in main olfactory system pathways involved in psychosexual function, *Genes Brain Behav* **19**: e12618.

Chiba, A. A., Kesner, R. P. and Reynolds, A. M. (1994). Memory for spatial location as a function of temporal lag in rats: role of hippocampus and medial prefrontal cortex, *Behavioral and Neural Biology* **61**: 123–131.

Childress, A. R., Mozley, P. D., McElgin, W., Fitzgerald, J., Reivich, M. and O'Brien, C. P. (1999). Limbic activation during cue-induced cocaine craving, *American Journal of Psychiatry* **156**: 11–18.

Cho, Y. H. and Kesner, R. P. (1995). Relational object association learning in rats with hippocampal lesions, *Behavioural Brain Research* **67**: 91–98.

Cho, Y. K., Li, C. S. and Smith, D. V. (2002). Gustatory projections from the nucleus of the solitary tract to the parabrachial nuclei in the hamster, *Chemical Senses* **27**: 81–90.

Choi, E. Y., Ding, S. L. and Haber, S. N. (2017). Combinatorial inputs to the ventral striatum from the temporal cortex, frontal cortex, and amygdala: implications for segmenting the striatum, *eNeuro* **4**: 6.

Chomsky, N. (1965). *Aspects of the Theory of Syntax*, MIT Press, Cambridge, Massachusetts.

Christie, B. R. (1996). Long-term depression in the hippocampus, *Hippocampus* **6**: 1–2.

Ciaramelli, E. and Treves, A. (2019). A mind free to wander: neural and computational constraints on spontaneous thought, *Front Psychol* **10**: 39.

Ciaramelli, E., De Luca, F., Monk, A. M., McCormick, C. and Maguire, E. A. (2019). What "wins" in VMPFC: Scenes, situations, or schema?, *Neurosci Biobehav Rev* **100**: 208–210.

Cicero, M. T. (55 BC). *De Oratore II*, Vol. II, Cicero, Rome.

Clark, I. A. and Maguire, E. A. (2016). Remembering preservation in hippocampal amnesia, *Annu Rev Psychol* **67**: 51–82.

Clark, I. A., Kim, M. and Maguire, E. A. (2018). Verbal paired associates and the hippocampus: the role of scenes, *J Cogn Neurosci* **30**: 1821–1845.

Clark, I. A., Hotchin, V., Monk, A., Pizzamiglio, G., Liefgreen, A. and Maguire, E. A. (2019). Identifying the cognitive processes underpinning hippocampal-dependent tasks, *J Exp Psychol Gen* **148**: 1861–1881.

Clark, L., Cools, R. and Robbins, T. W. (2004). The neuropsychology of ventral prefrontal cortex: decision-making and reversal learning, *Brain and Cognition* **55**: 41–53.

Clarke, A. and Tyler, L. K. (2014). Object-specific semantic coding in human perirhinal cortex, *J Neurosci* **34**: 4766–75.

Clarke, A. and Tyler, L. K. (2015). Understanding what we see: how we derive meaning from vision, *Trends Cogn Sci* **19**: 677–687.

Clelland, C. D., Choi, M., Romberg, C., Clemenson, G. D., J., Fragniere, A., Tyers, P., Jessberger, S., Saksida, L. M., Barker, R. A., Gage, F. H. and Bussey, T. J. (2009). A functional role for adult hippocampal neurogenesis in spatial pattern separation, *Science* **325**: 210–213.

Clos, M., Amunts, K., Laird, A. R., Fox, P. T. and Eickhoff, S. B. (2013). Tackling the multifunctional nature of Broca's region meta-analytically: co-activation-based parcellation of area 44, *Neuroimage* **83**: 174–88.

Coalson, T. S., Van Essen, D. C. and Glasser, M. F. (2018). The impact of traditional neuroimaging methods on the spatial localization of cortical areas, *Proc Natl Acad Sci U S A* **115**: E6356–E6365.

Colas, J. T., Pauli, W. M., Larsen, T., Tyszka, J. M. and O'Doherty, J. P. (2017). Distinct prediction errors in mesostriatal circuits of the human brain mediate learning about the values of both states and actions: evidence from high-resolution fMRI, *PLoS Comput Biol* **13**: e1005810.

Colby, C. L., Duhamel, J. R. and Goldberg, M. E. (1993). Ventral intraparietal area of the macaque: anatomic location and visual response properties, *J Neurophysiol* **69**: 902–14.

Colby, C. L., Duhamel, J. R. and Goldberg, M. E. (1996). Visual, presaccadic, and cognitive activation of single neurons in monkey lateral intraparietal area, *J Neurophysiol* **76**: 2841–52.

Collins, A. G. E. and Cockburn, J. (2020). Beyond dichotomies in reinforcement learning, *Nat Rev Neurosci* **21**: 576–586.

Collins, J. A. and Olson, I. R. (2014). Beyond the FFA: The role of the ventral anterior temporal lobes in face processing, *Neuropsychologia* **61**: 65–79.

Coltheart, M., Curtis, B., Atkins, P. and Haller, M. (1993). Models of reading aloud: Dual-route and parallel-distributed-processing approaches, *Psychological review* **100**: 589.

Compton, W. M., Wargo, E. M. and Volkow, N. D. (2022). Neuropsychiatric model of addiction simplified, *Psychiatr Clin North Am* **45**: 321–334.

Connolly, J. D., Andersen, R. A. and Goodale, M. A. (2003). FMRI evidence for a 'parietal reach region' in the human brain, *Exp Brain Res* **153**: 140–5.

Constantinescu, A. O., O'Reilly, J. X. and Behrens, T. E. J. (2016). Organizing conceptual knowledge in humans with a gridlike code, *Science* **352**: 1464–1468.

Constantinidis, C., Funahashi, S., Lee, D., Murray, J. D., Qi, X. L., Wang, M. and Arnsten, A. F. T. (2018). Persistent spiking activity underlies working memory, *J Neurosci* **38**: 7020–7028.

Corbetta, M. and Shulman, G. L. (2002). Control of goal-directed and stimulus-driven attention in the brain, *Nature Reviews Neuroscience* **3**: 201–215.

Corcoles-Parada, M., Ubero-Martinez, M., Morris, R. G. M., Insausti, R., Mishkin, M. and Munoz-Lopez, M. (2019). Frontal and insular input to the dorsolateral temporal pole in primates: implications for auditory memory, *Front Neurosci* **13**: 1099.

Corkin, S. (2002). What's new with the amnesic patient H.M.?, *Nat Rev Neurosci* **3**: 153–60.

Cornell, C. E., Rodin, J. and Weingarten, H. (1989). Stimulus-induced eating when satiated, *Physiology and Behavior* **45**: 695–704.

Corrado, G. S., Sugrue, L. P., Seung, H. S. and Newsome, W. T. (2005). Linear-nonlinear-Poisson models of primate choice dynamics, *Journal of the Experimental Analysis of Behavior* **84**: 581–617.

Corrigan, B. W., Gulli, R. A., Doucet, G., Borna, M., Abbass, M., Roussy, M., Rogelio, L. and Martinez-Trujillo, J. C. (2023). View cells in the hippocampus and prefrontal cortex of macaques during virtual navigation, *Hippocampus* **33**: 573–585.

Cortes, C., Jaeckel, L. D., Solla, S. A., Vapnik, V. and Denker, J. S. (1996). Learning curves: asymptotic values and rates of convergence, *Neural Information Processing Systems* **6**: 327–334.

Coslett, H. B. and Schwartz, M. F. (2018). The parietal lobe and language, *Handb Clin Neurol* **151**: 365–375.

Coureaud, G., Thomas-Danguin, T., Sandoz, J. C. and Wilson, D. A. (2022). Biological constraints on configural odour mixture perception, *J Exp Biol* **225**: 242274.

Courtiol, E. and Wilson, D. A. (2017). The olfactory mosaic: bringing an olfactory network together for odor perception, *Perception* **46**: 320–332.

Cover, T. M. (1965). Geometrical and statistical properties of systems of linear inequalities with applications in pattern recognition, *IEEEE Transactions on Electronic Computers* **14**: 326–334.

Cover, T. M. and Thomas, J. A. (1991). *Elements of Information Theory*, Wiley, New York.

Cowell, R. A., Bussey, T. J. and Saksida, L. M. (2006). Why does brain damage impair memory? A connectionist model of object recognition memory in perirhinal cortex, *Journal of Neuroscience* **26**: 12186–12197.

Cowey, A. (1979). Cortical maps and visual perception, *Quarterly Journal of Experimental Psychology* **31**: 1–17.

Cox, J. and Witten, I. B. (2019). Striatal circuits for reward learning and decision-making, *Nat Rev Neurosci* **20**: 482–494.

Coyle, J. T. (2006). Glutamate and schizophrenia: beyond the dopamine hypothesis, *Cellular and Molecular Neurobiology* **26**: 365–384.

Coyle, J. T., Ruzicka, W. B. and Balu, D. T. (2020). Fifty years of research on schizophrenia: the ascendance of the glutamatergic synapse, *Am J Psychiatry* **177**: 1119–1128.

Craig, A. D. (2009). How do you feel–now? The anterior insula and human awareness, *Nat Rev Neurosci* **10**: 59–70.

Craig, A. D. (2011). Significance of the insula for the evolution of human awareness of feelings from the body, *Ann N Y Acad Sci* **1225**: 72–82.

Craig, A. D. (2014). Topographically organized projection to posterior insular cortex from the posterior portion of the ventral medial nucleus in the long-tailed macaque monkey, *J Comp Neurol* **522**: 36–63.

Craik, F. I. M. and Tulving, E. (1975). Depth of processing and the retention of words in episodic memory, *Journal of experimental Psychology: general* **104**: 268.

Crane, J. and Milner, B. (2005). What went where? Impaired object-location learning in patients with right hippocampal lesions, *Hippocampus* **15**: 216–231.

Craver, C. F. and Bechtel, W. (2007). Top-down causation without top-down causes, *Biology and Philosophy* **22**: 547–563.

Creutzfeldt, O. D. (1995). *Cortex Cerebri. Performance, Structural and Functional Organisation of the Cortex*, Oxford University Press, Oxford.

Crick, F. H. C. and Mitchison, G. (1995). REM sleep and neural nets, *Behavioural Brain Research* **69**: 147–155.

Critchley, H. D. and Harrison, N. A. (2013). Visceral influences on brain and behavior, *Neuron* **77**: 624–638.

Critchley, H. D. and Rolls, E. T. (1996a). Hunger and satiety modify the responses of olfactory and visual neurons in the primate orbitofrontal cortex, *J Neurophysiol* **75**: 1673–86.

Critchley, H. D. and Rolls, E. T. (1996b). Olfactory neuronal responses in the primate orbitofrontal cortex: analysis in an olfactory discrimination task, *Journal of Neurophysiology* **75**: 1659–1672.

Critchley, H., Daly, E., Phillips, M., Brammer, M., Bullmore, E., Williams, S., Van Amelsvoort, T., Robertson, D., David, A. and Murphy, D. (2000). Explicit and implicit neural mechanisms for processing of social information from facial expressions: a functional magnetic resonance imaging study, *Hum Brain Mapp* **9**: 93–105.

Cromwell, H. C. and Schultz, W. (2003). Effects of expectations for different reward magntitudes on neuronal activity in primate striatum, *Journal of Neurophysiology* **89**: 2823–2838.

Crooks, B., Stamataki, N. S. and McLaughlin, J. T. (2021). Appetite, the enteroendocrine system, gastrointestinal disease and obesity, *Proc Nutr Soc* **80**: 50–58.

Croxson, P. L., Walton, M. E., O'Reilly, J. X., Behrens, T. E. and Rushworth, M. F. (2009). Effort-based cost-benefit valuation and the human brain, *Journal of Neuroscience* **29**: 4531–4541.

Crutcher, M. D. and DeLong, M. R. (1984a). Single cell studies of the primate putamen. I. Functional organisation, *Experimental Brain Research* **53**: 233–243.

Crutcher, M. D. and DeLong, M. R. (1984b). Single cell studies of the primate putamen. II. Relations to direction of movements and pattern of muscular activity, *Experimental Brain Research* **53**: 244–258.

Culham, J. C., Danckert, S. L., DeSouza, J. F., Gati, J. S., Menon, R. S. and Goodale, M. A. (2003). Visually guided grasping produces fMRI activation in dorsal but not ventral stream brain areas, *Exp Brain Res* **153**: 180–9.

Culham, J. C., Cavina-Pratesi, C. and Singhal, A. (2006). The role of parietal cortex in visuomotor control: what have we learned from neuroimaging?, *Neuropsychologia* **44**: 2668–84.

Cullen, K. E. (2019). Vestibular processing during natural self-motion: implications for perception and action, *Nat Rev Neurosci* **20**: 346–363.

Cullen, K. E. and Taube, J. S. (2017). Our sense of direction: progress, controversies and challenges, *Nat Neurosci* **20**: 1465–1473.

Cummings, D. E. and Overduin, J. (2007). Gastrointestinal regulation of food intake, *J Clin Invest* **117**: 13–23.

da Costa, N. M. and Martin, K. A. (2010). Whose cortical column would that be?, *Frontiers in Neuroanatomy* **4**: 16.

da Costa, N. M. and Martin, K. A. C. (2013). Sparse reconstruction of brain circuits: or, how to survive without a microscopic connectome, *Neuroimage* **80**: 27–36.

Dahan, L., Rampon, C. and Florian, C. (2020). Age-related memory decline, dysfunction of the hippocampus and therapeutic opportunities, *Prog Neuropsychopharmacol Biol Psychiatry* **102**: 109943.

Dalley, J. W. and Robbins, T. W. (2017). Fractionating impulsivity: neuropsychiatric implications, *Nat Rev Neurosci* **18**: 158–171.

Damasio, A., Damasio, H. and Tranel, D. (2013). Persistence of feelings and sentience after bilateral damage of the insula, *Cereb Cortex* **23**: 833–46.

Damasio, A. R. (1994). *Descartes' Error: Emotion, Reason, and the Human Brain*, Grosset/Putnam, New York.

Dan, Y. and Poo, M.-M. (2004). Spike-timing dependent plasticity of neural circuits, *Neuron* **44**: 23–30.

Dan, Y. and Poo, M.-M. (2006). Spike-timing dependent plasticity: from synapse to perception, *Physiological Reviews* **86**: 1033–1048.

Dane, C. and Bajcsy, R. (1982). An object-centred three-dimensional model builder, *Proceedings of the 6th International Conference on Pattern Recognition*, Munich, pp. 348–350.

Darwin, C. (1859). *The Origin of Species*, John Murray [reprinted (1982) by Penguin Books Ltd], London.

Dastgheib, M., Kulanayagam, A. and Dringenberg, H. C. (2022). Is the role of sleep in memory consolidation overrated?, *Neurosci Biobehav Rev* **140**: 104799.

Dastjerdi, M., Foster, B. L., Nasrullah, S., Rauschecker, A. M., Dougherty, R. F., Townsend, J. D., Chang, C., Greicius, M. D., Menon, V., Kennedy, D. P. and Parvizi, J. (2011). Differential electrophysiological response during rest, self-referential, and non-self-referential tasks in human posteromedial cortex, *Proc Natl Acad Sci U S A* **108**: 3023–8.

Daugman, J. (1988). Complete discrete 2D-Gabor transforms by neural networks for image analysis and compression, *IEEE Transactions on Acoustic, Speech, and Signal Processing* **36**: 1169–1179.

Davis, M. (1992). The role of the amygdala in conditioned fear, *in* J. P. Aggleton (ed.), *The Amygdala*, Wiley-Liss, New York, chapter 9, pp. 255–306.

Davis, M. (2000). The role of the amygdala in conditioned and unconditioned fear and anxiety, *in* J. P. Aggleton (ed.), *The Amygdala: a Functional Analysis*, 2nd edn, Oxford University Press, Oxford, chapter 6, pp. 213–287.

Davis, M. (2006). Neural systems involved in fear and anxiety measured with fear-potentiated startle, *American Psychologist* **61**: 741–756.

Davis, M. (2011). NMDA receptors and fear extinction: implications for cognitive behavioral therapy, *Dialogues Clin Neurosci* **13**: 463–74.

Davis, M., Antoniadis, E. A., Amaral, D. G. and Winslow, J. T. (2008). Acoustic startle reflex in rhesus monkeys: a review, *Reviews in Neuroscience* **19**: 171–185.

Davis, S. W., Wing, E. A. and Cabeza, R. (2018). Contributions of the ventral parietal cortex to declarative memory, *Handb Clin Neurol* **151**: 525–553.

Dawkins, M. S. (1986). *Unravelling Animal Behaviour*, 1st edn, Longman, Harlow.

Dawkins, M. S. (1995). *Unravelling Animal Behaviour*, 2nd edn, Longman, Harlow.

Dawkins, M. S. (2021). *The Science of Animal Welfare; Understanding What Animals Want*, Oxford University Press, Oxford.

Dawkins, R. (1976). *The Selfish Gene*, Oxford University Press, Oxford.

Dawkins, R. (1989). *The Selfish Gene*, 2nd edn, Oxford University Press, Oxford.

Day, M., Langston, R. and Morris, R. G. (2003). Glutamate-receptor-mediated encoding and retrieval of paired-associate learning, *Nature* **424**: 205–9.

Dayan, P. and Abbott, L. F. (2001). *Theoretical Neuroscience*, MIT Press, Cambridge, MA.

Dayan, P. and Sejnowski, T. J. (1994). TD(λ) converges with probability 1, *Machine Learning* **14**: 295–301.

De Araujo, I. E. and Rolls, E. T. (2004). Representation in the human brain of food texture and oral fat, *J Neurosci* **24**: 3086–93.

De Araujo, I. E., Rolls, E. T., Kringelbach, M. L., McGlone, F. and Phillips, N. (2003a). Taste-olfactory convergence, and the representation of the pleasantness of flavour, in the human brain, *Eur J Neurosci* **18**: 2059–68.

De Araujo, I. E., Rolls, E. T., Velazco, M. I., Margot, C. and Cayeux, I. (2005). Cognitive modulation of olfactory processing, *Neuron* **46**: 671–9.

De Araujo, I. E., Schatzker, M. and Small, D. M. (2020). Rethinking food reward, *Annu Rev Psychol* **71**: 139–164.

De Araujo, I. E. T., Rolls, E. T. and Stringer, S. M. (2001). A view model which accounts for the spatial fields of hippocampal primate spatial view cells and rat place cells., *Hippocampus* **11**: 699–706.

De Araujo, I. E. T., Kringelbach, M. L., Rolls, E. T. and Hobden, P. (2003b). Representation of umami taste in the human brain, *Journal of Neurophysiology* **90**: 313–319.

De Araujo, I. E. T., Kringelbach, M. L., Rolls, E. T. and McGlone, F. (2003c). Human cortical responses to water in the mouth, and the effects of thirst, *Journal of Neurophysiology* **90**: 1865–1876.

De Falco, E., Ison, M. J., Fried, I. and Quian Quiroga, R. (2016). Long-term coding of personal and universal associations underlying the memory web in the human brain, *Nat Commun* **7**: 13408.

De Gelder, B., Vroomen, J., Pourtois, G. and Weiskrantz, L. (1999). Non-conscious recognition of affect in the absence of striate cortex, *NeuroReport* **10**: 3759–3763.

de Haan, E. H. F. and Dijkerman, H. C. (2020). Somatosensation in the brain: a theoretical re-evaluation and a new model, *Trends Cogn Sci* **24**: 529–541.

de Lafuente, V. and Romo, R. (2005). Neuronal correlates of subjective sensory experience, *Nature Neuroscience* **8**: 1698–1703.

De Luca, F., McCormick, C., Mullally, S. L., Intraub, H., Maguire, E. A. and Ciaramelli, E. (2018). Boundary extension is attenuated in patients with ventromedial prefrontal cortex damage, *Cortex* **108**: 1–12.

De Luca, F., McCormick, C., Ciaramelli, E. and Maguire, E. A. (2019). Scene processing following damage to the ventromedial prefrontal cortex, *Neuroreport* **30**: 828–833.

de Ruyter van Steveninck, R. R. and Laughlin, S. B. (1996). The rates of information transfer at graded-potential synapses, *Nature* **379**: 642–645.

De Sieno, D. (1988). Adding a conscience to competitive learning, *IEEE International Conference on Neural Networks (San Diego 1988)*, Vol. 1, IEEE, New York, pp. 117–124.

De Valois, R. L. and De Valois, K. K. (1988). *Spatial Vision*, Oxford University Press, New York.

Dean, H. L. and Platt, M. L. (2006). Allocentric spatial referencing of neuronal activity in macaque posterior cingulate cortex, *J Neurosci* **26**: 1117–27.

DeAngelis, G. C., Cumming, B. G. and Newsome, W. T. (2000). A new role for cortical area MT: the perception of stereoscopic depth, *in* M. Gazzaniga (ed.), *The New Cognitive Neurosciences, Second Edition*, MIT Press, Cambridge, MA, chapter 21, pp. 305–314.

Debiec, J., LeDoux, J. E. and Nader, K. (2002). Cellular and systems reconsolidation in the hippocampus, *Neuron* **36**: 527–538.

Debiec, J., Doyere, V., Nader, K. and LeDoux, J. E. (2006). Directly reactivated, but not indirectly reactivated, memories undergo reconsolidation in the amygdala, *Proceedings of the National Academy of Sciences USA* **103**: 3428–3433.

deCharms, R. C. and Merzenich, M. M. (1996). Primary cortical representation of sounds by the coordination of action-potential timing, *Nature* **381**: 610–613.

Deco, G. and Rolls, E. T. (2002). Object-based visual neglect: a computational hypothesis, *European Journal of Neuroscience* **16**: 1994–2000.

Deco, G. and Rolls, E. T. (2003). Attention and working memory: a dynamical model of neuronal activity in the prefrontal cortex, *Eur J Neurosci* **18**: 2374–90.

Deco, G. and Rolls, E. T. (2004). A neurodynamical cortical model of visual attention and invariant object recognition, *Vision Res* **44**: 621–42.

Deco, G. and Rolls, E. T. (2005a). Attention, short-term memory, and action selection: a unifying theory, *Progress in Neurobiology* **76**: 236–256.

Deco, G. and Rolls, E. T. (2005b). Neurodynamics of biased competition and co-operation for attention: a model with spiking neurons, *Journal of Neurophysiology* **94**: 295–313.

Deco, G. and Rolls, E. T. (2005c). Sequential memory: a putative neural and synaptic dynamical mechanism, *Journal of Cognitive Neuroscience* **17**: 294–307.

Deco, G. and Rolls, E. T. (2005d). Synaptic and spiking dynamics underlying reward reversal in orbitofrontal cortex, *Cerebral Cortex* **15**: 15–30.

Deco, G. and Rolls, E. T. (2006). A neurophysiological model of decision-making and Weber's law, *European Journal of Neuroscience* **24**: 901–916.

Deco, G., Rolls, E. T. and Horwitz, B. (2004). 'What' and 'where' in visual working memory: a computational neurodynamical perspective for integrating fMRI and single-neuron data, *Journal of Cognitive Neuroscience* **16**: 683–701.

Deco, G., Ledberg, A., Almeida, R. and Fuster, J. (2005). Neural dynamics of cross-modal and cross-temporal associations, *Exp Brain Res* **166**: 325–36.

Deco, G., Scarano, L. and Soto-Faraco, S. (2007). Weber's law in decision making: integrating behavioral data in humans with a neurophysiological model, *Journal of Neuroscience* **27**: 11192–11200.

Deco, G., Rolls, E. T. and Romo, R. (2009). Stochastic dynamics as a principle of brain function, *Progress in Neurobiology* **88**: 1–16.

Deco, G., Rolls, E. T. and Romo, R. (2010). Synaptic dynamics and decision-making, *Proceedings of the National Academy of Sciences* **107**: 7545–7549.

Deco, G., Rolls, E. T., Albantakis, L. and Romo, R. (2013). Brain mechanisms for perceptual and reward-related decision-making, *Prog Neurobiol* **103**: 194–213.

Deco, G., Cabral, J., Woolrich, M. W., Stevner, A. B. A., van Hartevelt, T. J. and Kringelbach, M. L. (2017a). Single or multiple frequency generators in on-going brain activity: A mechanistic whole-brain model of empirical MEG data, *Neuroimage* **152**: 538–550.

Deco, G., Kringelbach, M. L., Jirsa, V. K. and Ritter, P. (2017b). The dynamics of resting fluctuations in the brain: metastability and its dynamical cortical core, *Sci Rep* **7**: 3095.

Deco, G., Cruzat, J., Cabral, J., Tagliazucchi, E., Laufs, H., Logothetis, N. K. and Kringelbach, M. L. (2019). Awakening: Predicting external stimulation to force transitions between different brain states, *Proceedings of the National Academy of Sciences* **116**: 18088–18097.

Deen, B., Koldewyn, K., Kanwisher, N. and Saxe, R. (2015). Functional organization of social perception and cognition in the superior temporal sulcus, *Cereb Cortex* **25**: 4596–4609.

Dehaene, S. (2014). *Consciousness and the Brain*, Penguin, New York.

Dehaene, S. and Cohen, L. (2011). The unique role of the visual word form area in reading, *Trends Cogn Sci* **15**: 254–62.

Dehaene, S., Cohen, L., Sigman, M. and Vinckier, F. (2005). The neural code for written words: a proposal, *Trends Cogn Sci* **9**: 335–41.

Dehaene, S., Lau, H. and Kouider, S. (2017). What is consciousness, and could machines have it?, *Science* **358**: 486–492.

Delatour, B. and Witter, M. P. (2002). Projections from the parahippocampal region to the prefrontal cortex in the rat: evidence of multiple pathways, *European Journal of Neuroscience* **15**: 1400–1407.

Delgado, M. R., Nystrom, L. E., Fissell, C., Noll, D. C. and Fiez, J. A. (2000). Tracking the human hemodynamic responses to reward and punishment in the striatum, *Journal of Neurophysiology* **84**: 3072–3077.

Delgado, M. R., Olsson, A. and Phelps, E. A. (2006). Extending animal models of fear conditioning to humans, *Biol Psychol* **73**: 39–48.

Delgado, M. R., Jou, R. L. and Phelps, E. A. (2011). Neural systems underlying aversive conditioning in humans with primary and secondary reinforcers, *Frontiers in Neuroscience* **5**: 71.

Delhaye, B. P., Long, K. H. and Bensmaia, S. J. (2018). Neural basis of touch and proprioception in primate cortex, *Compr Physiol* **8**: 1575–1602.

Delle Monache, S., Indovina, I., Zago, M., Daprati, E., Lacquaniti, F. and Bosco, G. (2021). Watching the effects of gravity. Vestibular cortex and the neural representation of "visual" gravity, *Front Integr Neurosci* **15**: 793634.

DeLong, M. and Wichmann, T. (2010). Changing views of basal ganglia circuits and circuit disorders, *Clinical EEG and Neuroscience* **41**: 61–67.

DeLong, M. R., Georgopoulos, A. P., Crutcher, M. D., Mitchell, S. J., Richardson, R. T. and Alexander, G. E. (1984). Functional Organization of the Basal ganglia: Contributions of Single-Cell Recording Studies, *Functions of the Basal Ganglia. CIBA Foundation Symposium*, Pitman, London, pp. 64–78.

Delorme, A. and Thorpe, S. J. (2001). Face identification using one spike per neuron: resistance to image degradations, *Neural Networks* **14**: 795–803.

Delorme, R., Gousse, V., Roy, I., Trandafir, A., Mathieu, F., Mouren-Simeoni, M. C., Betancur, C. and Leboyer, M. (2007). Shared executive dysfunctions in unaffected relatives of patients with autism and obsessive-compulsive disorder, *European Psychiatry* **22**: 32–38.

Deming, P., Heilicher, M. and Koenigs, M. (2022). How reliable are amygdala findings in psychopathy? A systematic review of MRI studies, *Neurosci Biobehav Rev* **142**: 104875.

Deng, W. L., Rolls, E. T., Ji, X., Robbins, T. W., Banaschewski, T., Bokde, A., Bromberg, U., Buechel, C., Desrivieres, S., Conrod, P., Flor, H., Frouin, V., Gallinat, J., Garavan, H., Gowland, P., Heinz, A., Ittermann, B., Martinot, J.-L., Lemaitre, H., Nees, F., Papadopoulos Orfanos, D., Poustka, L., Smolka, M. N., Walter, H., Whelan, R., Schumann, G., Feng, J. and the Imagen consortium (2017). Separate neural systems for behavioral change and for emotional responses to failure during behavioral inhibition, *Human Brain Mapping* **38**: 3527–3537.

Depoortere, I. (2014). Taste receptors of the gut: emerging roles in health and disease, *Gut* **63**: 179–90.

Derbyshire, S. W. G., Vogt, B. A. and Jones, A. K. P. (1998). Pain and Stroop interference tasks activate separate processing modules in anterior cingulate cortex, *Experimental Brain Research* **118**: 52–60.

Derdikman, D., Whitlock, J. R., Tsao, A., Fyhn, M., Hafting, T., Moser, M. B. and Moser, E. I. (2009). Fragmentation of grid cell maps in a multicompartment environment, *Nat Neurosci* **12**: 1325–32.

Dere, E., Easton, A., Nadel, L. and Huston, J. (2008). *Handbook of Episodic Memory*, Handbook of Behavioral Neuroscience, Elsevier, Amsterdam.

Descartes, R. (1644). *The Philosophical Writings of Descartes (3 volumes, 1984-1991)*, Cambridge University Press, Cambridge.

Desimone, R. (1996). Neural mechanisms for visual memory and their role in attention, *Proceedings of the National Academy of Sciences USA* **93**: 13494–13499.

Desimone, R. and Duncan, J. (1995). Neural mechanisms of selective visual attention, *Annual Review of Neuroscience* **18**: 193–222.

Desimone, R., Albright, T. D., Gross, C. G. and Bruce, C. (1984). Stimulus-selective properties of inferior temporal neurons in the macaque, *J Neurosci* **4**: 2051–62.

Desrochers, T. M., Amemori, K. and Graybiel, A. M. (2015). Habit learning by naive macaques is marked by response sharpening of striatal neurons representing the cost and outcome of acquired action sequences, *Neuron* **87**: 853–68.

Devereux, B. J., Clarke, A. and Tyler, L. K. (2018). Integrated deep visual and semantic attractor neural networks predict fMRI pattern-information along the ventral object processing pathway, *Sci Rep* **8**: 10636.

DeWeese, M. R. and Meister, M. (1999). How to measure the information gained from one symbol, *Network* **10**: 325–340.

DeWitt, I. and Rauschecker, J. P. (2012). Phoneme and word recognition in the auditory ventral stream, *Proc Natl Acad Sci U S A* **109**: E505–14.

DeWitt, I. and Rauschecker, J. P. (2013). Wernicke's area revisited: parallel streams and word processing, *Brain Lang* **127**: 181–91.

DeWitt, I. and Rauschecker, J. P. (2016). Convergent evidence for the causal involvement of anterior superior temporal gyrus in auditory single-word comprehension, *Cortex* **77**: 164–166.

Di Lorenzo, P. M. (1990). Corticofugal influence on taste responses in the parabrachial pons of the rat, *Brain Research* **530**: 73–84.

Diamanti, E. M., Reddy, C. B., Schroder, S., Muzzu, T., Harris, K. D., Saleem, A. B. and Carandini, M. (2021). Spatial modulation of visual responses arises in cortex with active navigation, *Elife* **10**: e63705.

DiCarlo, J. J. and Maunsell, J. H. R. (2003). Anterior inferotemporal neurons of monkeys engaged in object recognition can be highly sensitive to object retinal position, *Journal of Neurophysiology* **89**: 3264–3278.

DiCarlo, J. J., Zoccolan, D. and Rust, N. C. (2012). How does the brain solve visual object recognition?, *Neuron* **73**: 415–434.

Dickie, E. W., Anticevic, A., Smith, D. E., Coalson, T. S., Manogaran, M., Calarco, N., Viviano, J. D., Glasser, M. F., Van Essen, D. C. and Voineskos, A. N. (2019). Ciftify: A framework for surface-based analysis of legacy MR acquisitions, *Neuroimage* **197**: 818–826.

Diehl, M. M. and Romanski, L. M. (2014). Responses of prefrontal multisensory neurons to mismatching faces and vocalizations, *J Neurosci* **34**: 11233–43.

Dienel, S. J., Schoonover, K. E. and Lewis, D. A. (2022). Cognitive dysfunction and prefrontal cortical circuit alterations in schizophrenia: developmental trajectories, *Biol Psychiatry* **92**: 450–459.

Dillingham, C. M., Frizzati, A., Nelson, A. J. D. and Vann, S. D. (2015). How do mammillary body inputs contribute to anterior thalamic function?, *Neuroscience & Biobehavioral Reviews* **54**: 108–119.

Ding, M., Chen, Y. and Bressler, S. L. (2006). Granger causality: basic theory and application to neuroscience, *in* B. Schelter, M. Winterhalder and J. Timmer (eds), *Handbook of Time Series Analysis*, Wiley, Weinheim, chapter 17, pp. 437–460.

Ding, N., Melloni, L., Zhang, H., Tian, X. and Poeppel, D. (2016). Cortical tracking of hierarchical linguistic structures in connected speech, *Nat Neurosci* **19**: 158–64.

DiNicola, L. M., Braga, R. M. and Buckner, R. L. (2020). Parallel distributed networks dissociate episodic and social functions within the individual, *J Neurophysiol* **123**: 1144–1179.

Divac, I. (1975). Magnocellular nuclei of the basal forebrain project to neocortex, brain stem, and olfactory bulb. Review of some functional correlates, *Brain Research* **93**: 385–398.

Divac, I. and Oberg, R. G. E. (1979). Current conceptions of neostriatal functions, *in* I. Divac and R. G. E. Oberg (eds), *The Neostriatum*, Pergamon, New York, pp. 215–230.

Divac, I., Rosvold, H. E. and Szwarcbart, M. K. (1967). Behavioral effects of selective ablation of the caudate nucleus, *Journal of Comparative and Physiological Psychology* **63**: 184–190.

Dolan, R. J., Fink, G. R., Rolls, E. T., Booth, M., Holmes, A., Frackowiak, R. S. J. and Friston, K. J. (1997). How the brain learns to see objects and faces in an impoverished context, *Nature* **389**: 596–599.

Donahue, C. J., Sotiropoulos, S. N., Jbabdi, S., Hernandez-Fernandez, M., Behrens, T. E., Dyrby, T. B., Coalson, T., Kennedy, H., Knoblauch, K., Van Essen, D. C. and Glasser, M. F. (2016). Using diffusion tractography to predict cortical connection strength and distance: a quantitative comparison with tracers in the monkey, *J Neurosci* **36**: 6758–70.

Donoghue, T., Cao, R., Han, C. Z., Holman, C. M., Brandmeir, N. J., Wang, S. and Jacobs, J. (2023). Single neurons in the human medial temporal lobe flexibly shift representations across spatial and memory tasks, *Hippocampus* **33**: 600–615.

Douglas, R. J. and Martin, K. A. (2004). Neuronal circuits of the neocortex, *Annu Rev Neurosci* **27**: 419–51.

Douglas, R. J. and Martin, K. A. C. (1990). Neocortex, *in* G. M. Shepherd (ed.), *The Synaptic Organization of the Brain*, 3rd edn, Oxford University Press, Oxford, chapter 12, pp. 389–438.

Douglas, R. J., Mahowald, M. A. and Martin, K. A. C. (1996). Microarchitecture of cortical columns, *in* A. Aertsen and V. Braitenberg (eds), *Brain Theory: Biological Basis and Computational Theory of Vision*, Elsevier, Amsterdam.

Douglas, R. J., Markram, H. and Martin, K. A. C. (2004). Neocortex, *in* G. M. Shepherd (ed.), *The Synaptic Organization of the Brain*, 5th edn, Oxford University Press, Oxford, chapter 12, pp. 499–558.

Dow, B. W., Snyder, A. Z., Vautin, R. G. and Bauer, R. (1981). Magnification factor and receptive field size in foveal striate cortex of the monkey, *Experimental Brain Research* **44**: 213–218.

Doya, K. (1999). What are the computations of the cerebellum, the basal ganglia and the cerebral cortex?, *Neural Networks* **12**: 961–974.

Doyere, V., Debiec, J., Monfils, M. H., Schafe, G. E. and LeDoux, J. E. (2007). Synapse-specific reconsolidation of distinct fear memories in the lateral amygdala, *Nature Neuroscience* **10**: 414–416.

Drevets, W. C. (2007). Orbitofrontal cortex function and structure in depression, *Annals of the New York Academy of Sciences* **1121**: 499–527.

Drevets, W. C., Savitz, J. and Trimble, M. (2008). The subgenual anterior cingulate cortex in mood disorders, *CNS Spectr* **13**: 663–81.

Dronkers, N. F., Ivanova, M. V. and Baldo, J. V. (2017). What do language disorders reveal about brain-language relationships? From classic models to network approaches, *J Int Neuropsychol Soc* **23**: 741–754.

Drysdale, A. T., Grosenick, L., Downar, J., Dunlop, K., Mansouri, F., Meng, Y., Fetcho, R. N., Zebley, B., Oathes, D. J., Etkin, A., Schatzberg, A. F., Sudheimer, K., Keller, J., Mayberg, H. S., Gunning, F. M., Alexopoulos, G. S., Fox, M. D., Pascual-Leone, A., Voss, H. U., Casey, B. J., Dubin, M. J. and Liston, C. (2017). Resting-state connectivity biomarkers define neurophysiological subtypes of depression, *Nat Med* **23**: 28–38.

Du, J., Rolls, E. T., Cheng, W., Li, Y., Gong, W., Qiu, J. and Feng, J. (2020). Functional connectivity of the orbitofrontal cortex, anterior cingulate cortex, and inferior frontal gyrus in humans, *Cortex* **123**: 185–199.

Du, J., Rolls, E. T., Gong, W., Cao, M., Vatansever, D., Zhang, J., Kang, J., Cheng, W. and Feng, J. (2022). Association between parental age, brain structure, and behavioral and cognitive problems in children, *Mol Psychiatry* **27**: 967–975.

Dudchenko, P. A., Wood, E. R. and Eichenbaum, H. (2000). Neurotoxic hippocampal lesions have no effect on odor span and little effect on odor recognition memory but produce significant impairments on spatial span, recognition, and alternation, *Journal of Neuroscience* **20**: 2964–2977.

Duff, M. C., Covington, N. V., Hilverman, C. and Cohen, N. J. (2019). Semantic memory and the hippocampus: revisiting, reaffirming, and extending the reach of their critical relationship, *Front Hum Neurosci* **13**: 471.

Duhamel, J. R., Bremmer, F., Ben Hamed, S. and Graf, W. (1997). Spatial invariance of visual receptive fields in parietal cortex neurons, *Nature* **389**: 845–8.

Duman, R. S. and Aghajanian, G. K. (2012). Synaptic dysfunction in depression: potential therapeutic targets, *Science* **338**: 68–72.

Dunbar, R. I. (2017). Group size, vocal grooming and the origins of language, *Psychon Bull Rev* **24**: 209–212.

Dunbar, R. I. M. (2022). Laughter and its role in the evolution of human social bonding, *Philos Trans R Soc Lond B Biol Sci* **377**: 20210176.

Duncan, J. (1996). Cooperating brain systems in selective perception and action, *in* T. Inui and J. L. McClelland (eds), *Attention and Performance XVI*, MIT Press, Cambridge, MA, pp. 549–578.

Duncan, J. and Humphreys, G. (1989). Visual search and stimulus similarity, *Psychological Review* **96**: 433–458.

Dunlop, B. W., Rajendra, J. K., Craighead, W. E., Kelley, M. E., McGrath, C. L., Choi, K. S., Kinkead, B., Nemeroff, C. B. and Mayberg, H. S. (2017). Functional connectivity of the subcallosal cingulate cortex and differential outcomes to treatment with cognitive-behavioral therapy or antidepressant medication for Major Depressive Disorder, *Am J Psychiatry* **174**: 533–545.

Dunnett, S. B. and Iversen, S. D. (1982a). Neurotoxic lesions of ventrolateral but not anteromedial neostriatum impair differential reinforcement of low rates (DRL) performance, *Behavioural Brain Research* **6**: 213–226.

Dunnett, S. B. and Iversen, S. D. (1982b). Sensorimotor impairments following localised kainic acid and 6-hydroxydopamine lesions of the neostriatum, *Brain Research* **248**: 121–127.

Durbin, R. and Mitchison, G. (1990). A dimension reduction framework for understanding cortical maps, *Nature* **343**: 644–647.

D'Urso, G., Dell'Osso, B., Rossi, R., Brunoni, A. R., Bortolomasi, M., Ferrucci, R., Priori, A., de Bartolomeis, A. and Altamura, A. C. (2017). Clinical predictors of acute response to transcranial direct current stimulation (tDCS) in major depression, *J Affect Disord* **219**: 25–30.

Durstewitz, D. and Seamans, J. K. (2002). The computational role of dopamine D1 receptors in working memory, *Neural Networks* **15**: 561–572.

Durstewitz, D., Kelc, M. and Gunturkun, O. (1999). A neurocomputational theory of the dopaminergic modulation of working memory functions, *Journal of Neuroscience* **19**: 2807–2822.

Durstewitz, D., Seamans, J. K. and Sejnowski, T. J. (2000a). Dopamine-mediated stabilization of delay-period activity in a network model of prefrontal cortex, *Journal of Neurophysiology* **83**: 1733–1750.

Durstewitz, D., Seamans, J. K. and Sejnowski, T. J. (2000b). Neurocomputational models of working memory, *Nature Neuroscience* **3 Suppl**: 1184–1191.

Easton, A. and Gaffan, D. (2000). Amygdala and the memory of reward: the importance of fibres of passage from the basal forebrain, *in* J. P. Aggleton (ed.), *The Amygdala: a Functional Analysis*, 2nd edn, Oxford University Press, Oxford, chapter 17, pp. 569–586.

Easton, A., Ridley, R. M., Baker, H. F. and Gaffan, D. (2002). Unilateral lesions of the cholinergic basal forebrain and fornix in one hemisphere and inferior temporal cortex in the opposite hemisphere produce severe learning impairments in rhesus monkeys, *Cerebral Cortex* **12**: 729–736.

Eccles, J. C. (1984). The cerebral neocortex: a theory of its operation, *in* E. G. Jones and A. Peters (eds), *Cerebral Cortex: Functional Properties of Cortical Cells*, Vol. 2, Plenum, New York, chapter 1, pp. 1–36.

Eccles, J. C., Ito, M. and Szentagothai, J. (1967). *The Cerebellum as a Neuronal Machine*, Springer-Verlag, New York.

Eckhorn, R. and Popel, B. (1974). Rigorous and extended application of information theory to the afferent visual system of the cat. I. Basic concepts, *Kybernetik* **16**: 191–200.

Eckhorn, R. and Popel, B. (1975). Rigorous and extended application of information theory to the afferent visual system of the cat. II. Experimental results, *Kybernetik* **17**: 7–17.

Eckhorn, R., Grusser, O. J., Kroller, J., Pellnitz, K. and Popel, B. (1976). Efficiency of different neural codes: information transfer calculations for three different neuronal systems, *Biological Cybernetics* **22**: 49–60.

Edelman, S. (1999). *Representation and Recognition in Vision*, MIT Press, Cambridge, MA.

Edvardsen, V., Bicanski, A. and Burgess, N. (2020). Navigating with grid and place cells in cluttered environments, *Hippocampus* **30**: 220–232.

Eguchi, A., Humphreys, G. W. and Stringer, S. M. (2016). The visually guided development of facial representations in the primate ventral visual pathway: A computer modeling study, *Psychol Rev* **123**: 696–739.

Eichenbaum, H. (1997). Declarative memory: insights from cognitive neurobiology, *Annual Review of Psychology* **48**: 547–572.

Eichenbaum, H. (2014). Time cells in the hippocampus: a new dimension for mapping memories, *Nat Rev Neurosci* **15**: 732–44.

Eichenbaum, H. (2017). On the integration of space, time, and memory, *Neuron* **95**: 1007–1018.

Eichenbaum, H. and Cohen, N. J. (2001). *From Conditioning to Conscious Recollection: Memory Systems of the Brain*, Oxford University Press, New York.

Eichenbaum, H., Otto, T. and Cohen, N. J. (1992). The hippocampus - what does it do?, *Behavioural and Neural Biology* **57**: 2–36.

Eisenberger, N. I. and Lieberman, M. D. (2004). Why rejection hurts: a common neural alarm system for physical and social pain, *Trends in Cognitive Neuroscience* **8**: 294–300.

Ekert, J. O., Gajardo-Vidal, A., Lorca-Puls, D. L., Hope, T. M. H., Dick, F., Crinion, J. T., Green, D. W. and Price, C. J. (2021a). Dissociating the functions of three left posterior superior temporal regions that contribute to speech perception and production, *Neuroimage* **245**: 118764.

Ekert, J. O., Lorca-Puls, D. L., Gajardo-Vidal, A., Crinion, J. T., Hope, T. M. H., Green, D. W. and Price, C. J. (2021b). A functional dissociation of the left frontal regions that contribute to single word production tasks, *Neuroimage* **245**: 118734.

Ekstrom, A. D. and Isham, E. A. (2017). Human spatial navigation: Representations across dimensions and scales, *Curr Opin Behav Sci* **17**: 84–89.

Ekstrom, A. D. and Ranganath, C. (2018). Space, time, and episodic memory: The hippocampus is all over the cognitive map, *Hippocampus* **28**: 680–687.

Ekstrom, A. D., Kahana, M. J., Caplan, J. B., Fields, T. A., Isham, E. A., Newman, E. L. and Fried, I. (2003). Cellular networks underlying human spatial navigation, *Nature* **425**: 184–188.

Ekstrom, A. D., Arnold, A. E. and Iaria, G. (2014). A critical review of the allocentric spatial representation and its neural underpinnings: toward a network-based perspective, *Front Hum Neurosci* **8**: 803.

Ekstrom, A. D., Huffman, D. J. and Starrett, M. (2017). Interacting networks of brain regions underlie human spatial navigation: a review and novel synthesis of the literature, *J Neurophysiol* **118**: 3328–3344.

El Boustani, S., Yger, P., Fregnac, Y. and Destexhe, A. (2012). Stable learning in stochastic network states, *J Neurosci* **32**: 194–214.

Elias, G. J. B., Germann, J., Boutet, A., Loh, A., Li, B., Pancholi, A., Beyn, M. E., Naheed, A., Bennett, N., Pinto, J., Bhat, V., Giacobbe, P., Woodside, D. B., Kennedy, S. H. and Lozano, A. M. (2022a). 3T MRI of rapid brain activity changes driven by subcallosal cingulate deep brain stimulation, *Brain* **145**: 2214–2226.

Elias, G. J. B., Germann, J., Boutet, A., Pancholi, A., Beyn, M. E., Bhatia, K., Neudorfer, C., Loh, A., Rizvi, S. J., Bhat, V., Giacobbe, P., Woodside, D. B., Kennedy, S. H. and Lozano, A. M. (2022b). Structuro-functional surrogates of response to subcallosal cingulate deep brain stimulation for depression, *Brain* **145**: 362–377.

Elliffe, M. C., Rolls, E. T. and Stringer, S. M. (2002). Invariant recognition of feature combinations in the visual system, *Biol Cybern* **86**: 59–71.

Elliffe, M. C. M., Rolls, E. T., Parga, N. and Renart, A. (2000). A recurrent model of transformation invariance by association, *Neural Networks* **13**: 225–237.

Ellis, G. F. R. (2020). The causal closure of physics in real world contexts, *Foundations of physics* **50**: 1057–1097.

Elman, J. A., Rosner, Z. A., Cohn-Sheehy, B. I., Cerreta, A. G. and Shimamura, A. P. (2013). Dynamic changes in parietal activation during encoding: implications for human learning and memory, *Neuroimage* **82**: 44–52.

Elman, J. L. (1990). Finding structure in time, *Cognitive Science* **14**: 179–211.

Elston, G. N. (2007). Specializations in pyramidal cell structure during primate evolution, *in* J. H. Kaas and M. Preuss, T (eds), *Evolution of Nervous Systems*, Academic Press, Oxford, pp. 191–242.

Elston, G. N., Benavides-Piccione, R., Elston, A., Zietsch, B., Defelipe, J., Manger, P., Casagrande, V. and Kaas, J. H. (2006). Specializations of the granular prefrontal cortex of primates: implications for cognitive processing, *Anat Rec A Discov Mol Cell Evol Biol* **288**: 26–35.

Engel, A. K., Konig, P., Kreiter, A. K., Schillen, T. B. and Singer, W. (1992). Temporal coding in the visual system: new vistas on integration in the nervous system, *Trends in Neurosciences* **15**: 218–226.

Epstein, J., Stern, E. and Silbersweig, D. (1999). Mesolimbic activity associated with psychosis in schizophrenia. Symptom-specific PET studies, *Annals of the New York Academy of Sciences* **877**: 562–574.

Epstein, R. (2005). The cortical basis of visual scene processing, *Visual Cognition* **12**: 954–978.

Epstein, R. A. (2008). Parahippocampal and retrosplenial contributions to human spatial navigation, *Trends Cogn Sci* **12**: 388–96.

Epstein, R. A. and Baker, C. I. (2019). Scene perception in the human brain, *Annu Rev Vis Sci* **5**: 373–397.

Epstein, R. A. and Julian, J. B. (2013). Scene areas in humans and macaques, *Neuron* **79**: 615–7.

Epstein, R. and Kanwisher, N. (1998). A cortical representation of the local visual environment, *Nature* **392**: 598–601.

Erickson, L. C., Rauschecker, J. P. and Turkeltaub, P. E. (2017). Meta-analytic connectivity modeling of the human superior temporal sulcus, *Brain Struct Funct* **222**: 267–285.

Eshel, N. and Roiser, J. P. (2010). Reward and punishment processing in depression, *Biological Psychiatry* **68**: 118–124.

Eskandar, E. N., Richmond, B. J. and Optican, L. M. (1992). Role of inferior temporal neurons in visual memory. I. Temporal encoding of information about visual images, recalled images, and behavioural context, *Journal of Neurophysiology* **68**: 1277–1295.

Espinos, A., Fernandez-Ortuno, E., Negri, E. and Borrell, V. (2022). Evolution of genetic mechanisms regulating cortical neurogenesis, *Dev Neurobiol* **82**: 428–453.

Estes, W. K. (1986). Memory for temporal information, *in* J. A. Michon and J. L. Jackson (eds), *Time, Mind and Behavior*, Springer-Verlag, New York, pp. 151–168.

Evans, V. (2014). *The Language Myth: Why Language is Not an Instinct*, Cambridge University Press, Cambridge.

Evarts, E. V. and Wise, S. P. (1984). Basal ganglia outputs and motor control, *Functions of the Basal Ganglia. CIBA Foundation Symposium*, Vol. 107, Pitman, London, pp. 83–96.

Everitt, B. J. and Robbins, T. W. (1992). Amygdala-ventral striatal interactions and reward-related processes, *in* J. P. Aggleton (ed.), *The Amygdala*, Wiley, Chichester, chapter 15, pp. 401–429.

Everitt, B. J. and Robbins, T. W. (2013). From the ventral to the dorsal striatum: devolving views of their roles in drug addiction, *Neurosci Biobehav Rev* **37**: 1946–54.

Everitt, B. J., Belin, D., Economidou, D., Pelloux, Y., Dalley, J. W. and Robbins, T. W. (2008). Review. Neural mechanisms underlying the vulnerability to develop compulsive drug-seeking habits and addiction, *Philos Trans R Soc Lond B Biol Sci* **363**: 3125–35.

Everitt, B. J., Giuliano, C. and Belin, D. (2018). Addictive behaviour in experimental animals: prospects for translation, *Philos Trans R Soc Lond B Biol Sci* **373**: 20170027.

Everling, S., Tinsley, C. J., Gaffan, D. and Duncan, J. (2006). Selective representation of task-relevant objects and locations in the monkey prefrontal cortex, *European Journal of Neuroscience* **23**: 2197–2214.

Fahy, F. L., Riches, I. P. and Brown, M. W. (1993). Neuronal activity related to visual recognition memory and the encoding of recency and familiarity information in the primate anterior and medial inferior temporal and rhinal cortex, *Experimental Brain Research* **96**: 457–492.

Fairhall, S. L. and Caramazza, A. (2013a). Brain regions that represent amodal conceptual knowledge, *J Neurosci* **33**: 10552–8.

Fairhall, S. L. and Caramazza, A. (2013b). Category-selective neural substrates for person- and place-related concepts, *Cortex* **49**: 2748–57.

Faisal, A., Selen, L. and Wolpert, D. (2008). Noise in the nervous system, *Nature Reviews Neuroscience* **9**: 292–303.

Falcone, R., Weintraub, D. B., Setogawa, T., Wittig, J. H., J., Chen, G. and Richmond, B. J. (2019). Temporal coding of reward value in monkey ventral striatal tonically active neurons, *J Neurosci* **39**: 7539–7550.

Farah, M. J. (1990). *Visual Agnosia*, MIT Press, Cambridge, MA.

Farah, M. J. (2000). *The Cognitive Neuroscience of Vision*, Blackwell, Oxford.

Farah, M. J. (2004). *Visual Agnosia*, 2nd edn, MIT Press, Cambridge, MA.

Farah, M. J., Meyer, M. M. and McMullen, P. A. (1996). The living/nonliving dissociation is not an artifact: giving an *a priori* implausible hypothesis a strong test, *Cognitive Neuropsychology* **13**: 137–154.

FarmAnimalWelfare, C. (2009). Farm Animal Welfare in Great Britain: Past, Present and future.

Farooqi, I. S. (2022). Monogenic obesity syndromes provide insights into the hypothalamic regulation of appetite and associated behaviors, *Biol Psychiatry* **91**: 856–859.

Farrow, T. F., Zheng, Y., Wilkinson, I. D., Spence, S. A., Deakin, J. F., Tarrier, N., Griffiths, P. D. and Woodruff, P. W. (2001). Investigating the functional anatomy of empathy and forgiveness, *NeuroReport* **12**: 2433–2438.

Farzanfar, D., Spiers, H. J., Moscovitch, M. and Rosenbaum, R. S. (2023). From cognitive maps to spatial schemas, *Nat Rev Neurosci* **24**: 63–79.

Fatt, P. and Katz, B. (1950). Some observations on biological noise, *Nature* **166**: 597–598.

Fattori, P., Breveglieri, R., Bosco, A., Gamberini, M. and Galletti, C. (2017). Vision for prehension in the medial parietal cortex, *Cereb Cortex* **27**: 1149–1163.

Faugeras, O. D. (1993). *The Representation, Recognition and Location of 3-D Objects*, MIT Press, Cambridge, MA.

Faugeras, O. D. and Hebert, M. (1986). The representation, recognition and location of 3-D objects, *International Journal of Robotics Research* **5**: 27–52.

Fazeli, M. S. and Collingridge, G. L. (eds) (1996). *Cortical Plasticity: LTP and LTD*, Bios, Oxford.

Feffer, K., Fettes, P., Giacobbe, P., Daskalakis, Z. J., Blumberger, D. M. and Downar, J. (2018). 1Hz rTMS of the right orbitofrontal cortex for major depression: Safety, tolerability and clinical outcomes, *Eur Neuropsychopharmacol* **28**: 109–117.

Feigenbaum, J. D. and Rolls, E. T. (1991). Allocentric and egocentric spatial information processing in the hippocampal formation of the behaving primate, *Psychobiology* **19**: 21–40.

Feinstein, J. S., Adolphs, R., Damasio, A. and Tranel, D. (2011). The human amygdala and the induction and experience of fear, *Curr Biol* **21**: 34–8.

Feldman, D. E. (2009). Synaptic mechanisms for plasticity in neocortex, *Annual Reviews of Neuroscience* **32**: 33–55.

Feldman, D. E. (2012). The spike-timing dependence of plasticity, *Neuron* **75**: 556–571.

Feldman, J. A. (1985). Four frames suffice: a provisional model of vision and space, *Behavioural Brain Sciences* **8**: 265–289.

Fellows, L. K. (2007). The role of orbitofrontal cortex in decision making: a component process account, *Annalls of the New York Academy of Sciences* **1121**: 421–430.

Fellows, L. K. (2011). Orbitofrontal contributions to value-based decision making: evidence from humans with frontal lobe damage, *Ann N Y Acad Sci* **1239**: 51–8.

Fellows, L. K. and Farah, M. J. (2003). Ventromedial frontal cortex mediates affective shifting in humans: evidence from a reversal learning paradigm, *Brain* **126**: 1830–1837.

Fellows, L. K. and Farah, M. J. (2005). Different underlying impairments in decision-making after ventromedial and dorsolateral frontal lobe damage in humans, *Cerebral Cortex* **15**: 58–63.

Feng, R., Rolls, E. T., Cheng, W. and Feng, J. (2020). Hypertension is associated with reduced hippocampal connectivity and impaired memory, *EBioMedicine* **61**: 103082.

Ferbinteanu, J., Holsinger, R. M. and McDonald, R. J. (1999). Lesions of the medial or lateral perforant path have different effects on hippocampal contributions to place learning and on fear conditioning to context, *Behavioral Brain Research* **101**: 65–84.

Ferbinteanu, J., Shirvalkar, P. and Shapiro, M. L. (2011). Memory modulates journey-dependent coding in the rat hippocampus, *J Neurosci* **31**: 9135–46.

Ferko, K. M., Blumenthal, A., Martin, C. B., Proklova, D., Minos, A. N., Saksida, L. M., Bussey, T. J., Khan, A. R. and Kohler, S. (2022). Activity in perirhinal and entorhinal cortex predicts perceived visual similarities among category exemplars with highest precision, *Elife* **11**: e66884.

Fernandez-Cabello, S., Kronbichler, M., Van Dijk, K. R. A., Goodman, J. A., Spreng, R. N., Schmitz, T. W. and Alzheimer's Disease Neuroimaging, I. (2020). Basal forebrain volume reliably predicts the cortical spread of Alzheimer's degeneration, *Brain* **143**: 993–1009.

Fernandez, T. V., Leckman, J. F. and Pittenger, C. (2018). Genetic susceptibility in obsessive-compulsive disorder, *Handb Clin Neurol* **148**: 767–781.

Ferre, P., Mamalet, F. and Thorpe, S. J. (2018). Unsupervised feature learning with winner-takes-all based STDP, *Front Comput Neurosci* **12**: 24.

Fettes, P., Schulze, L. and Downar, J. (2017). Cortico-striatal-thalamic loop circuits of the orbitofrontal cortex: promising therapeutic targets in psychiatric illness, *Front Syst Neurosci* **11**: 25.

Fiebelkorn, I. C. and Kastner, S. (2020). Functional specialization in the attention network, *Annu Rev Psychol* **71**: 221–249.

Field, D. J. (1987). Relations between the statistics of natural images and the response properties of cortical cells, *Journal of the Optical Society of America, A* **4**: 2379–2394.

Field, D. J. (1994). What is the goal of sensory coding?, *Neural Computation* **6**: 559–601.

Filimon, F., Nelson, J. D., Huang, R. S. and Sereno, M. I. (2009). Multiple parietal reach regions in humans: cortical representations for visual and proprioceptive feedback during on-line reaching, *J Neurosci* **29**: 2961–71.

Findlay, G., Tononi, G. and Cirelli, C. (2020). The evolving view of replay and its functions in wake and sleep, *Sleep Adv* **1**: zpab002.

Fineberg, N. A. and Robbins, T. W. (2021). *The Neurobiology and Treatment of OCD*, Vol. 49 of *Current Topics in Behavioral Neurosciences*, Springer Nature, Switzerland.

Finkel, L. H. and Edelman, G. M. (1987). Population rules for synapses in networks, *in* G. M. Edelman, W. E. Gall and W. M. Cowan (eds), *Synaptic Function*, John Wiley & Sons, New York, pp. 711–757.

Finzi, D., Gomez, J., Nordt, M., Rezai, A. A., Poltoratski, S. and Grill-Spector, K. (2021). Differential spatial computations in ventral and lateral face-selective regions are scaffolded by structural connections, *Nat Commun* **12**: 2278.

Fiorillo, C. D., Tobler, P. N. and Schultz, W. (2003). Discrete coding of reward probability and uncertainty by dopamine neurons, *Science* **299**: 1898–1902.

Fiske, A. and Holmboe, K. (2019). Neural substrates of early executive function development, *Dev Rev* **52**: 42–62.

Fletcher, P., Shallice, T., Frith, C., Frackowiak, R. and Dolan, R. (1998). The functional roles of prefrontal cortex in episodic memory. II. Retrieval, *Brain* **121**: 1249–1256.

Flinker, A., Korzeniewska, A., Shestyuk, A. Y., Franaszczuk, P. J., Dronkers, N. F., Knight, R. T. and Crone, N. E. (2015). Redefining the role of Broca's area in speech, *Proc Natl Acad Sci U S A* **112**: 2871–5.

Florian, C. and Roullet, P. (2004). Hippocampal CA3-region is crucial for acquisition and memory consolidation in Morris water maze task in mice, *Behavioural Brain Research* **154**: 365–374.

Fodor, J. A. (1994). *The Elm and the Expert: Mentalese and its Semantics*, MIT Press, Cambridge, MA.

Földiák, P. (1991). Learning invariance from transformation sequences, *Neural Computation* **3**: 193–199.

Földiák, P. (2003). Sparse coding in the primate cortex, *in* M. A. Arbib (ed.), *Handbook of Brain Theory and Neural Networks*, 2nd edn, MIT Press, Cambridge, MA, pp. 1064–1608.

Forgeard, M. J., Haigh, E. A., Beck, A. T., Davidson, R. J., Henn, F. A., Maier, S. F., Mayberg, H. S. and Seligman, M. E. (2011). Beyond depression: towards a process-based approach to research, diagnosis, and treatment, *Clinical Psychology (New York)* **18**: 275–299.

Foster, B. L., Dastjerdi, M. and Parvizi, J. (2012). Neural populations in human posteromedial cortex display opposing responses during memory and numerical processing, *Proc Natl Acad Sci U S A* **109**: 15514–9.

Foster, B. L., Kaveh, A., Dastjerdi, M., Miller, K. J. and Parvizi, J. (2013). Human retrosplenial cortex displays transient theta phase locking with medial temporal cortex prior to activation during autobiographical memory retrieval, *J Neurosci* **33**: 10439–46.

Foster, B. L., Koslov, S. R., Aponik-Gremillion, L., Monko, M. E., Hayden, B. Y. and Heilbronner, S. R. (2023). A tripartite view of the posterior cingulate cortex, *Nat Rev Neurosci* **24**: 173–189.

Foster, C., Sheng, W. A., Heed, T. and Ben Hamed, S. (2022). The macaque ventral intraparietal area has expanded into three homologue human parietal areas, *Prog Neurobiol* **209**: 102185.

Foster, D. J. (2017). Replay comes of age, *Annu Rev Neurosci* **40**: 581–602.

Foster, D. J. and Wilson, M. A. (2006). Reverse replay of behavioural sequences in hippocampal place cells during the awake state, *Nature* **440**: 680–3.

Foster, T. C., Castro, C. A. and McNaughton, B. L. (1989). Spatial selectivity of rat hippocampal neurons: dependence on preparedness for movement, *Science* **244**: 1580–1582.

Fox, K. C. R., Foster, B. L., Kucyi, A., Daitch, A. L. and Parvizi, J. (2018). Intracranial electrophysiology of the human Default Network, *Trends Cogn Sci* **22**: 307–324.

Francis, S., Rolls, E. T., Bowtell, R., McGlone, F., O'Doherty, J., Browning, A., Clare, S. and Smith, E. (1999). The representation of pleasant touch in the brain and its relationship with taste and olfactory areas, *NeuroReport* **10**: 453–459.

Franco, L., Rolls, E. T., Aggelopoulos, N. C. and Treves, A. (2004). The use of decoding to analyze the contribution to the information of the correlations between the firing of simultaneously recorded neurons, *Experimental Brain Research* **155**: 370–384.

Franco, L., Rolls, E. T., Aggelopoulos, N. C. and Jerez, J. M. (2007). Neuronal selectivity, population sparseness, and ergodicity in the inferior temporal visual cortex, *Biological Cybernetics* **96**: 547–560.

Frankland, S. M. and Greene, J. D. (2015). An architecture for encoding sentence meaning in left mid-superior temporal cortex, *Proc Natl Acad Sci U S A* **112**: 11732–7.

Franks, K. M., Stevens, C. F. and Sejnowski, T. J. (2003). Independent sources of quantal variability at single glutamatergic synapses, *Journal of Neuroscience* **23**: 3186–3195.

Franzius, M., Sprekeler, H. and Wiskott, L. (2007). Slowness and sparseness lead to place, head-direction, and spatial-view cells, *PLoS Comput Biol* **3**: e166.

Frassle, S., Lomakina, E. I., Razi, A., Friston, K. J., Buhmann, J. M. and Stephan, K. E. (2017). Regression DCM for fMRI, *Neuroimage* **155**: 406–421.

Freedman, D. J. (2015). Learning-dependent plasticity of visual encoding in inferior temporal cortex, *J Vis* **15**: 1420.

Freeman, W. J. and Watts, J. W. (1950). *Psychosurgery in the Treatment of Mental Disorders and Intractable Pain*, 2nd edn, Thomas, Springfield, IL.

Freese, J. L. and Amaral, D. G. (2009). Neuroanatomy of the primate amygdala, *in* P. J. Whalen and E. A. Phelps (eds), *The Human Amygdala*, Guilford, New York, chapter 1, pp. 3–42.

Frégnac, Y. (1996). Dynamics of cortical connectivity in visual cortical networks: an overview, *Journal of Physiology, Paris* **90**: 113–139.

Fregnac, Y., Pananceau, M., Rene, A., Huguet, N., Marre, O., Levy, M. and Shulz, D. E. (2010). A re-examination of Hebbian-covariance rules and spike timing-dependent plasticity in cat visual cortex in vivo, *Frontiers in Synaptic Neuroscience* **2**: 147.

Freiwald, W. A. (2020). The neural mechanisms of face processing: cells, areas, networks, and models, *Curr Opin Neurobiol* **60**: 184–191.

Freiwald, W. A., Tsao, D. Y. and Livingstone, M. S. (2009). A face feature space in the macaque temporal lobe, *Nat Neurosci* **12**: 1187–96.

Fremaux, N. and Gerstner, W. (2015). Neuromodulated spike-timing-dependent plasticity, and theory of three-factor learning rules, *Front Neural Circuits* **9**: 85.

Freton, M., Lemogne, C., Bergouignan, L., Delaveau, P., Lehericy, S. and Fossati, P. (2014). The eye of the self: precuneus volume and visual perspective during autobiographical memory retrieval, *Brain Struct Funct* **219**: 959–68.

Frey, S. and Petrides, M. (2002). Orbitofrontal cortex and memory formation, *Neuron* **36**: 171–176.

Frey, S., Kostopoulos, P. and Petrides, M. (2000). Orbitofrontal involvement in the processing of unpleasant auditory information, *European Journal of Neuroscience* **12**: 3709–3712.

Freyer, F., Roberts, J. A., Becker, R., Robinson, P. A., Ritter, P. and Breakspear, M. (2011). Biophysical mechanisms of multistability in resting-state cortical rhythms, *J Neurosci* **31**: 6353–61.

Freyer, F., Roberts, J. A., Ritter, P. and Breakspear, M. (2012). A canonical model of multistability and scale-invariance in biological systems, *PLOS Computational Biology* **8**: e1002634.

Fried, I., MacDonald, K. A. and Wilson, C. (1997). Single neuron activity in human hippocampus and amygdala during recognition of faces and objects, *Neuron* **18**: 753–765.

Fried, I., Rutishauser, U., Cerf, M. and Kreiman, G. (2014). *Single Neuron Studies of the Human Brain: Probing Cognition*, MIT Press, Cambridge, MA.

Friederici, A. D., Chomsky, N., Berwick, R. C., Moro, A. and Bolhuis, J. J. (2017). Language, mind and brain, *Nat Hum Behav* **1**: 713–722.

Friedman, A., Homma, D., Gibb, L. G., Amemori, K., Rubin, S. J., Hood, A. S., Riad, M. H. and Graybiel, A. M. (2015). A corticostriatal path targeting striosomes controls decision-making under conflict, *Cell* **161**: 1320–33.

Fries, P. (2009). Neuronal gamma-band synchronization as a fundamental process in cortical computation, *Annual Reviews of Neuroscience* **32**: 209–224.

Fries, P. (2015). Rhythms for cognition: communication through coherence, *Neuron* **88**: 220–35.

Friston, K. (2009). Causal modelling and brain connectivity in functional magnetic resonance imaging, *PLoS Biol* **7**: e33.

Friston, K. J. and Frith, C. D. (1995). Schizophrenia: a disconnection syndrome?, *Clin Neurosci* **3**: 89–97.

Friston, K. J., Buechel, C., Fink, G. R., Morris, J., Rolls, E. T. and Dolan, R. J. (1997). Psychophysiological and modulatory interactions in neuroimaging, *Neuroimage* **6**: 218–229.

Friston, K. J., Ashburner, J. T., Kiebel, S. J., Nichols, T. E. and Penny, W. D. (2006). *Statistical Parametric Mapping: the analysis of functional brain images*, Academic Press.

Frith, C. D. and Frith, U. (2012). Mechanisms of social cognition, *Annu Rev Psychol* **63**: 287–313.

Frolov, A. A. and Medvedev, A. V. (1986). Substantiation of the "point approximation" for describing the total electrical activity of the brain with use of a simulation model, *Biophysics* **31**: 332–337.

Fuhrmann, G., Markram, H. and Tsodyks, M. (2002a). Spike frequency adaptation and neocortical rhythms, *Journal of Neurophysiology* **88**: 761–770.

Fuhrmann, G., Segev, I., Markram, H. and Tsodyks, M. (2002b). Coding of temporal information by activity-dependent synapses, *Journal of Neurophysiology* **87**: 140–148.

Fujimichi, R., Naya, Y., Koyano, K. W., Takeda, M., Takeuchi, D. and Miyashita, Y. (2010). Unitized representation of paired objects in area 35 of the macaque perirhinal cortex, *European Journal of Neuroscience* **32**: 659–667.

Fujisawa, T. X. and Cook, N. D. (2011). The perception of harmonic triads: an fMRI study, *Brain Imaging Behav* **5**: 109–125.

Fukushima, K. (1975). Cognitron: a self-organizing neural network, *Biological Cybernetics* **20**: 121–136.

Fukushima, K. (1980). Neocognitron: a self organizing neural network model for a mechanism of pattern recognition unaffected by shift in position, *Biol Cybern* **36**: 193–202.

Fukushima, K. (1988). Neocognitron: a hierarchical neural network capable of visual pattern recognition, *Neural Networks* **1**: 119–130.

Fukushima, K. (1989). Analysis of the process of visual pattern recognition by the neocognitron, *Neural Networks* **2**: 413–420.
Fukushima, K. (1991). Neural networks for visual pattern recognition, *IEEE Transactions E* **74**: 179–190.
Fukushima, K. and Miyake, S. (1982). Neocognitron: A new algorithm for pattern recognition tolerant of deformations and shifts in position, *Pattern Recognition* **15**(6): 455–469.
Fukushima, M., Saunders, R. C., Leopold, D. A., Mishkin, M. and Averbeck, B. B. (2014). Differential coding of conspecific vocalizations in the ventral auditory cortical stream, *J Neurosci* **34**: 4665–76.
Funahashi, S. (2017). Working memory in the prefrontal cortex, *Brain Sci* **7**: 49.
Funahashi, S., Bruce, C. J. and Goldman-Rakic, P. S. (1989). Mnemonic coding of visual space in monkey dorsolateral prefrontal cortex, *Journal of Neurophysiology* **61**: 331–349.
Funahashi, S., Bruce, C. J. and Goldman-Rakic, P. S. (1993). Dorsolateral prefrontal lesions and oculomotor delayed-response performance: evidence for mnemonic "scotomas", *J Neurosci* **13**: 1479–97.
Furuya, Y., Matsumoto, J., Hori, E., Boas, C. V., Tran, A. H., Shimada, Y., Ono, T. and Nishijo, H. (2014). Place-related neuronal activity in the monkey parahippocampal gyrus and hippocampal formation during virtual navigation, *Hippocampus* **24**: 113–30.
Fuster, J. M. (1973). Unit activity in prefrontal cortex during delayed-response performance: neuronal correlates of transient memory, *Joural of Neurophysiology* **36**: 61–78.
Fuster, J. M. (1989). *The Prefrontal Cortex*, 2nd edn, Raven Press, New York.
Fuster, J. M. (1997). *The Prefrontal Cortex*, 3rd edn, Lippincott-Raven, Philadelphia.
Fuster, J. M. (2008). *The Prefrontal Cortex*, 4th edn, Academic Press, London.
Fuster, J. M. (2015). *The Prefrontal Cortex*, 5th edn, Academic Press, London.
Fuster, J. M. and Jervey, J. P. (1982). Neuronal firing in the inferotemporal cortex of the monkey in a visual memory task, *Journal of Neuroscience* **2**: 361–375.
Fuster, J. M., Bauer, R. H. and Jervey, J. P. (1982). Cellular discharge in the dorsolateral prefrontal cortex of the monkey in cognitive tasks, *Experimental Neurology* **77**: 679–694.
Fuster, J. M., Bodner, M. and Kroger, J. K. (2000). Cross-modal and cross-temporal association in neurons of frontal cortex, *Nature* **405**: 347–351.
Fyhn, M., Molden, S., Hollup, S., Moser, M. B. and Moser, E. (2002). Hippocampal neurons responding to first-time dislocation of a target object, *Neuron* **35**: 555–66.
Fyhn, M., Molden, S., Witter, M. P., Moser, E. I. and Moser, M.-B. (2004). Spatial representation in the entorhinal cortex, *Science* **2004**: 1258–1264.
Gabbott, P. L., Warner, T. A., Jays, P. R. and Bacon, S. J. (2003). Areal and synaptic interconnectivity of prelimbic (area 32), infralimbic (area 25) and insular cortices in the rat, *Brain Research* **993**: 59–71.
Gaffan, D. (1993). Additive effects of forgetting and fornix transection in the temporal gradient of retrograde amnesia, *Neuropsychologia* **31**: 1055–1066.
Gaffan, D. (1994). Scene-specific memory for objects: a model of episodic memory impairment in monkeys with fornix transection, *Journal of Cognitive Neuroscience* **6**: 305–320.
Gaffan, D. and Gaffan, E. (1991). Amnesia in man following transection of the fornix. A review, *Brain* **114**: 2611–2618.
Gaffan, D. and Harrison, S. (1989a). A comparison of the effects of fornix section and sulcus principalis ablation upon spatial learning by monkeys, *Behavioural Brain Research* **31**: 207–220.
Gaffan, D. and Harrison, S. (1989b). Place memory and scene memory: effects of fornix transection in the monkey, *Experimental Brain Research* **74**: 202–212.
Gaffan, D. and Saunders, R. C. (1985). Running recognition of configural stimuli by fornix transected monkeys, *Quarterly Journal of Experimental Psychology* **37B**: 61–71.
Gaffan, D., Saunders, R. C., Gaffan, E. A., Harrison, S., Shields, C. and Owen, M. J. (1984). Effects of fornix section upon associative memory in monkeys: role of the hippocampus in learned action, *Quarterly Journal of Experimental Psychology* **36B**: 173–221.
Gajardo-Vidal, A., Lorca-Puls, D. L., Team, P., Warner, H., Pshdary, B., Crinion, J. T., Leff, A. P., Hope, T. M. H., Geva, S., Seghier, M. L., Green, D. W., Bowman, H. and Price, C. J. (2021). Damage to Broca's area does not contribute to long-term speech production outcome after stroke, *Brain* **144**: 817–832.
Galaj, E. and Xi, Z. X. (2021). Progress in opioid reward research: From a canonical two-neuron hypothesis to two neural circuits, *Pharmacol Biochem Behav* **200**: 173072.
Gallagher, M. and Holland, P. C. (1992). Understanding the function of the central nucleus: is simple conditioning enough?, in J. P. Aggleton (ed.), *The Amygdala: Neurobiological Aspects of Emotion, Memory, and Mental Dysfunction*, Wiley-Liss, New York, pp. 307–321.
Gallagher, M. and Holland, P. C. (1994). The amygdala complex: multiple roles in associative learning and attention, *Proceedings of the National Academy of Sciences USA* **91**: 11771–11776.

Gallant, J. L., Connor, C. E. and Van-Essen, D. C. (1998). Neural activity in areas V1, V2 and V4 during free viewing of natural scenes compared to controlled viewing, *NeuroReport* **9**: 85–90.

Galletti, C. and Fattori, P. (2018). The dorsal visual stream revisited: Stable circuits or dynamic pathways?, *Cortex* **98**: 203–217.

Galletti, C., Battaglini, P. P. and Fattori, P. (1993). Parietal neurons encoding spatial locations in craniotopic coordinates, *Exp Brain Res* **96**: 221–9.

Gallivan, J. P. and Goodale, M. A. (2018). The dorsal "action" pathway, *Handb Clin Neurol* **151**: 449–466.

Gallivan, J. P., McLean, A. and Culham, J. C. (2011). Neuroimaging reveals enhanced activation in a reach-selective brain area for objects located within participants' typical hand workspaces, *Neuropsychologia* **49**: 3710–21.

Galvin, V. C., Arnsten, A. F. T. and Wang, M. (2020). Involvement of nicotinic receptors in working memory function, *Curr Top Behav Neurosci* **45**: 89–99.

Gamberini, M., Dal Bo, G., Breveglieri, R., Briganti, S., Passarelli, L., Fattori, P. and Galletti, C. (2018). Sensory properties of the caudal aspect of the macaque's superior parietal lobule, *Brain Struct Funct* **223**: 1863–1879.

Gamberini, M., Passarelli, L., Fattori, P. and Galletti, C. (2020). Structural connectivity and functional properties of the macaque superior parietal lobule, *Brain Struct Funct* **225**: 1349–1367.

Gamberini, M., Passarelli, L., Filippini, M., Fattori, P. and Galletti, C. (2021). Vision for action: thalamic and cortical inputs to the macaque superior parietal lobule, *Brain Struct Funct* **226**: 2951–2966.

Garcia, A. D. and Buffalo, E. A. (2020). Anatomy and function of the primate entorhinal cortex, *Annu Rev Vis Sci* **6**: 411–432.

Garcia-Cabezas, M. A. and Barbas, H. (2017). Anterior cingulate pathways may affect emotions through orbitofrontal cortex, *Cereb Cortex* **27**: 4891–4910.

Gardner, E. (1987). Maximum storage capacity in neural networks, *Europhysics Letters* **4**: 481–485.

Gardner, E. (1988). The space of interactions in neural network models, *Journal of Physics A* **21**: 257–270.

Gardner, E. P. (2008). Dorsal and ventral streams in the sense of touch, *The Senses: A Comprehensive Reference*, Vol. 6, Academic Press, New York, pp. 233–258.

Gardner-Medwin, A. R. (1976). The recall of events through the learning of associations between their parts, *Proceedings of the Royal Society of London, Series B* **194**: 375–402.

Gattass, R., Sousa, A. P. B. and Covey, E. (1985). Cortical visual areas of the macaque: possible substrates for pattern recognition mechanisms, *Experimental Brain Research, Supplement 11, Pattern Recognition Mechanisms* **54**: 1–20.

Gawne, T. J. and Richmond, B. J. (1993). How independent are the messages carried by adjacent inferior temporal cortical neurons?, *Journal of Neuroscience* **13**: 2758–2771.

Gaykema, R. P., van der Kuil, J., Hersh, L. B. and Luiten, P. G. (1991). Patterns of direct projections from the hippocampus to the medial septum-diagonal band complex: anterograde tracing with Phaseolus vulgaris leucoagglutinin combined with immunohistochemistry of choline acetyltransferase, *Neuroscience* **43**: 349–360.

Gazzaniga, M. and LeDoux, J. (1978). *The Integrated Mind*, Plenum, New York.

Gazzaniga, M. S. (1988). Brain modularity: towards a philosophy of conscious experience, *in* A. J. Marcel and E. Bisiach (eds), *Consciousness in Contemporary Science*, Oxford University Press, Oxford, chapter 10, pp. 218–238.

Gazzaniga, M. S. (1995). Consciousness and the cerebral hemispheres, *in* M. S. Gazzaniga (ed.), *The Cognitive Neurosciences*, MIT Press, Cambridge, MA, chapter 92, pp. 1392–1400.

Ge, T., Feng, J., Grabenhorst, F. and Rolls, E. T. (2012). Componential Granger causality, and its application to identifying the source and mechanisms of the top-down biased activation that controls attention to affective vs sensory processing, *Neuroimage* **59**: 1846–1858.

Geesaman, B. J. and Andersen, R. A. (1996). The analysis of complex motion patterns by form/cue invariant MSTd neurons, *Journal of Neuroscience* **16**: 4716–4732.

Georges-François, P., Rolls, E. T. and Robertson, R. G. (1999). Spatial view cells in the primate hippocampus: allocentric view not head direction or eye position or place, *Cerebral Cortex* **9**: 197–212.

Georgopoulos, A. P. (1995). Motor cortex and cognitive processing, *in* M. S. Gazzaniga (ed.), *The Cognitive Neurosciences*, MIT Press, Cambridge, MA, chapter 32, pp. 507–517.

Gerbella, M., Rozzi, S. and Rizzolatti, G. (2017). The extended object-grasping network, *Exp Brain Res* **235**: 2903–2916.

Gerfen, C. R. and Surmeier, D. J. (2011). Modulation of striatal projection systems by dopamine, *Annual Reviews of Neuroscience* **34**: 441–466.

Germann, J. and Petrides, M. (2020a). Area 8A within the posterior Middle Frontal Gyrus underlies cognitive selection between competing visual targets, *eNeuro* **7**: 10.1523/ENEURO.0102–20.2020.

Germann, J. and Petrides, M. (2020b). The ventral part of dorsolateral frontal Area 8A regulates visual attentional selection and the dorsal part auditory attentional selection, *Neuroscience* **441**: 209–216.

Gerstner, W. (1995). Time structure of the activity in neural network models, *Physical Review E* **51**: 738–758.

Gerstner, W. (2000). Population dynamics of spiking neurons: fast transients, asynchronous states, and locking, *Neural Computation* **12**: 43–89.

Gerstner, W. and Kistler, W. (2002). *Spiking Neuron Models: Single Neurons, Populations and Plasticity*, Cambridge University Press, Cambridge.

Gerstner, W., Ritz, R. and Van Hemmen, L. (1993). A biologically motivated and analytically solvable model of collective oscillations in the cortex, *Biological Cybernetics* **68**: 363–374.

Gerstner, W., Kreiter, A. K., Markram, H. and Herz, A. V. (1997). Neural codes: firing rates and beyond, *Proceedings of the National Academy of Sciences USA* **94**: 12740–12741.

Gerstner, W., Kistler, W. M., Naud, R. and Paninski, L. (2014). *Neuronal dynamics: From single neurons to networks and models of cognition*, Cambridge University Press, Cambridge.

Geschwind, N. (1970). The organization of language and the brain, *Science* **170**: 940–4.

Ghasemi, M., Phillips, C., Fahimi, A., McNerney, M. W. and Salehi, A. (2017). Mechanisms of action and clinical efficacy of NMDA receptor modulators in mood disorders, *Neurosci Biobehav Rev* **80**: 555–572.

Ghashghaei, H. T. and Barbas, H. (2002). Pathways for emotion: interactions of prefrontal and anterior temporal pathways in the amygdala of the rhesus monkey, *Neuroscience* **115**: 1261–1279.

Ghosh, V. E. and Gilboa, A. (2014). What is a memory schema? A historical perspective on current neuroscience literature, *Neuropsychologia* **53**: 104–14.

Ghosh, V. E., Moscovitch, M., Melo Colella, B. and Gilboa, A. (2014). Schema representation in patients with ventromedial PFC lesions, *J Neurosci* **34**: 12057–70.

Giarrocco, F. and Averbeck, B. B. (2021). Organization of parietoprefrontal and temporoprefrontal networks in the macaque, *J Neurophysiol* **126**: 1289–1309.

Gibbs, J., Maddison, S. P. and Rolls, E. T. (1981). Satiety role of the small intestine examined in sham-feeding rhesus monkeys, *Journal of Comparative and Physiological Psychology* **95**: 1003–15.

Gibson, J. J. (1950). *The Perception of the Visual World*, Houghton Mifflin, Boston.

Gibson, J. J. (1979). *The Ecological Approach to Visual Perception*, Houghton Mifflin, Boston.

Gilbert, P. E. and Kesner, R. P. (2002). The amygdala but not the hippocampus is involved in pattern separation based on reward value, *Neurobiology of Learning and Memory* **77**: 338–353.

Gilbert, P. E. and Kesner, R. P. (2003). Localization of function within the dorsal hippocampus: the role of the CA3 subregion in paired-associate learning, *Behavioral Neuroscience* **117**: 1385–1394.

Gilbert, P. E. and Kesner, R. P. (2006). The role of dorsal CA3 hippocampal subregion in spatial working memory and pattern separation, *Behavioural Brain Research* **169**: 142–149.

Gilbert, P. E., Kesner, R. P. and DeCoteau, W. E. (1998). Memory for spatial location: role of the hippocampus in mediating spatial pattern separation, *Journal of Neuroscience* **18**: 804–810.

Gilbert, P. E., Kesner, R. P. and Lee, I. (2001). Dissociating hippocampal subregions: double dissociation between dentate gyrus and CA1, *Hippocampus* **11**: 626–636.

Gilbert, S. J. and Burgess, P. W. (2008). Executive function, *Curr Biol* **18**: R110–4.

Gilboa, A. and Marlatte, H. (2017). Neurobiology of schemas and schema-mediated memory, *Trends Cogn Sci* **21**: 618–631.

Gilson, M., Moreno-Bote, R., Ponce-Alvarez, A., Ritter, P. and Deco, G. (2016). Estimation of directed effective connectivity from fMRI functional connectivity hints at asymmetries in the cortical connectome, *PLoS Computational Biology* **12**: e1004762.

Giocomo, L. M. and Hasselmo, M. E. (2007). Neuromodulation by glutamate and acetylcholine can change circuit dynamics by regulating the relative influence of afferent input and excitatory feedback, *Mol Neurobiol* **36**: 184–200.

Giocomo, L. M., Moser, M. B. and Moser, E. I. (2011). Computational models of grid cells, *Neuron* **71**: 589–603.

Glantz, L. A. and Lewis, D. A. (2000). Decreased dendritic spine density on prefrontal cortical pyramidal neurons in schizophrenia, *Arch Gen Psychiatry* **57**: 65–73.

Glascher, J., Adolphs, R., Damasio, H., Bechara, A., Rudrauf, D., Calamia, M., Paul, L. K. and Tranel, D. (2012). Lesion mapping of cognitive control and value-based decision making in the prefrontal cortex, *Proceedings of the National Academy of Sciences U S A* **109**: 14681–14686.

Glasser, M. F., Coalson, T. S., Robinson, E. C., Hacker, C. D., Harwell, J., Yacoub, E., Ugurbil, K., Andersson, J., Beckmann, C. F., Jenkinson, M., Smith, S. M. and Van Essen, D. C. (2016a). A multi-modal parcellation of human cerebral cortex, *Nature* **536**: 171–8.

Glasser, M. F., Smith, S. M., Marcus, D. S., Andersson, J. L., Auerbach, E. J., Behrens, T. E., Coalson, T. S., Harms, M. P., Jenkinson, M., Moeller, S., Robinson, E. C., Sotiropoulos, S. N., Xu, J., Yacoub, E., Ugurbil, K. and Van Essen, D. C. (2016b). The Human Connectome Project's neuroimaging approach, *Nat Neurosci* **19**: 1175–87.

Glausier, J. R. and Lewis, D. A. (2013). Dendritic spine pathology in schizophrenia, *Neuroscience* **251**: 90–107.

Glausier, J. R. and Lewis, D. A. (2018). Mapping pathologic circuitry in schizophrenia, *Handb Clin Neurol* **150**: 389–417.

Glimcher, P. (2005). Indeterminacy in brain and behavior, *Annual Review of Psychology* **56**: 25–56.

Glimcher, P. (2011a). *Foundations of Neuroeconomic Analysis*, Oxford University Press, Oxford.

Glimcher, P. W. (2011b). Understanding dopamine and reinforcement learning: the dopamine reward prediction error hypothesis, *Proceedings of the National Academy of Sciences U S A* **108 Suppl 3**: 15647–15654.

Glimcher, P. W. and Fehr, E. (2013). *Neuroeconomics: Decision-Making and the Brain*, 2nd edn, Academic Press, New York.

Gnadt, J. W. and Andersen, R. A. (1988). Memory related motor planning activity in posterior parietal cortex of macaque, *Exp Brain Res* **70**: 216–20.

Gochin, P. M., Colombo, M., Dorfman, G. A., Gerstein, G. L. and Gross, C. G. (1994). Neural ensemble encoding in inferior temporal cortex, *Journal of Neurophysiology* **71**: 2325–2337.

Gold, A. E. and Kesner, R. P. (2005). The role of the CA3 subregion of the dorsal hippocampus in spatial pattern completion in the rat, *Hippocampus* **15**: 808–814.

Gold, P. W. (2015). The organization of the stress system and its dysregulation in depressive illness, *Molecular Psychiatry* **20**: 32–47.

Goldberg, D. E. (1989). *Genetic Algorithms in Search, Optimization and Machine Learning*, Addison-Wesley Publishing Company, Inc., Boston, MA.

Goldberg, M. E. and Walker, M. F. (2013). The control of gaze, in E. R. Kandel, J. H. Schwartz, T. M. Jessell, S. A. Siegelbaum and A. J. Hudspeth (eds), *Principles of Neural Science*, 5th edn, McGraw-Hill, New York, chapter 40, pp. 894–916.

Goldberg, M. E. and Walker, M. F. (2021). The control of gaze, in E. R. Kandel, J. D. Koester, S. H. Mack and S. A. Siegelbaum (eds), *Principles of Neural Science*, 6 edn, McGraw Hill, New York, chapter 35, pp. 860–882.

Goldberg, M. E., Bisley, J. W., Powell, K. D. and Gottlieb, J. (2006). Saccades, salience and attention: the role of the lateral intraparietal area in visual behavior, *Progress in Brain Research* **155**: 157–175.

Goldman, P. S. and Nauta, W. J. H. (1977). An intricately patterned prefronto-caudate projection in the rhesus monkey, *Journal of Comparative Neurology* **171**: 369–386.

Goldman, P. S., Rosvold, H. E., Vest, B. and Galkin, T. W. (1971). Analysis of the delayed-alternation deficit produced by dorso-lateral pre-frontal lesions in the rhesus monkey, *Journal of Comparative and Physiological Psychology* **77**: 212–220.

Goldman-Rakic, P. (1994). Working memory dysfunction in schizophrenia, *Journal of Neuropsychology and Clinical Neuroscience* **6**: 348–357.

Goldman-Rakic, P. (1996). The prefrontal landscape: implications of functional architecture for understanding human mentation and the central executive, *Philosophical Transactions of the Royal Society B* **351**: 1445–1453.

Goldman-Rakic, P. S. (1987). Circuitry of primate prefrontal cortex and regulation of behavior by representational memory, *Handbook of Physiology, Section 1, The Nervous System*, Vol. V. Higher Functions of the Brain, Part 1, American Physiological Society, Bethesda, MD, pp. 373–417.

Goldman-Rakic, P. S. (1999). The physiological approach: functional architecture of working memory and disordered cognition in schizophrenia, *Biological Psychiatry* **46**: 650–661.

Golomb, D., Kleinfeld, D., Reid, R. C., Shapley, R. M. and Shraiman, B. (1994). On temporal codes and the spatiotemporal response of neurons in the lateral geniculate nucleus, *Journal of Neurophysiology* **72**: 2990–3003.

Golomb, D., Hertz, J. A., Panzeri, S., Treves, A. and Richmond, B. J. (1997). How well can we estimate the information carried in neuronal responses from limited samples?, *Neural Computation* **9**: 649–665.

Gong, W., Rolls, E. T., Du, J., Feng, J. and Cheng, W. (2021). Brain structure is linked to the association between family environment and behavioral problems in children in the ABCD study, *Nature Communications* **12**: 3769.

Gonzalez-Burgos, G. and Lewis, D. A. (2012). NMDA receptor hypofunction, parvalbumin-positive neurons, and cortical gamma oscillations in schizophrenia, *Schizophr Bull* **38**: 950–7.

Gonzalez-Burgos, G., Hashimoto, T. and Lewis, D. A. (2010). Alterations of cortical GABA neurons and network oscillations in schizophrenia, *Curr Psychiatry Rep* **12**: 335–44.

Goodale, M. A. (2004). Perceiving the world and grasping it: dissociations between conscious and unconscious visual processing, in M. S. Gazzaniga (ed.), *The Cognitive Neurosciences III*, MIT Press, Cambridge, MA, pp. 1159–1172.

Goodale, M. A. (2014). How (and why) the visual control of action differs from visual perception, *Proc Biol Sci* **281**: 20140337.

Goodale, M. A. and Milner, A. D. (1992). Separate visual pathways for perception and action, *Trends Neurosci* **15**: 20–5.

Goodrich-Hunsaker, N. J., Hunsaker, M. R. and Kesner, R. P. (2005). Dissociating the role of the parietal cortex and dorsal hippocampus for spatial information processing, *Behavioral Neuroscience* **119**: 1307–1315.

Goodrich-Hunsaker, N. J., Hunsaker, M. R. and Kesner, R. P. (2008). The interactions and dissociations of the dorsal hippocampus subregions: how the dentate gyrus, CA3, and CA1 process spatial information, *Behav Neurosci* **122**: 16–26.

Gothard, K. M., Battaglia, F. P., Erickson, C. A., Spitler, K. M. and Amaral, D. G. (2007). Neural responses to facial expression and face identity in the monkey amygdala, *Journal of Neurophysiology* **97**: 1671–1683.

Gothard, K. M., Mosher, C. P., Zimmerman, P. E., Putnam, P. T., Morrow, J. K. and Fuglevand, A. J. (2018). New perspectives on the neurophysiology of primate amygdala emerging from the study of naturalistic social behaviors, *Wiley Interdiscip Rev Cogn Sci* **9**: 1.

Gotlib, I. H. and Hammen, C. L. (2009). *Handbook of Depression*, Guilford Press, New York.

Gottfried, J. A. (2010). Central mechanisms of odour object perception, *Nature Reviews Neuroscience* **11**: 628–641.

Gottfried, J. A. (2015). Structural and functional imaging of the human olfactory system, *in* R. L. Doty (ed.), *Handbook of Olfaction and Gustation*, 3rd edn, Wiley Liss, New York, chapter 13, pp. 279–304.

Gottfried, J. A., O'Doherty, J. and Dolan, R. J. (2003). Encoding predictive reward value in human amygdala and orbitofrontal cortex, *Science* **301**: 1104–1107.

Gottfried, J. A., Winston, J. S. and Dolan, R. J. (2006). Dissociable codes of odor quality and odorant structure in human piriform cortex, *Neuron* **49**: 467–479.

Goulas, A., Stiers, P., Hutchison, R. M., Everling, S., Petrides, M. and Margulies, D. S. (2017). Intrinsic functional architecture of the macaque dorsal and ventral lateral frontal cortex, *J Neurophysiol* **117**: 1084–1099.

Grabenhorst, F. and Rolls, E. T. (2008). Selective attention to affective value alters how the brain processes taste stimuli, *European Journal of Neuroscience* **27**: 723–729.

Grabenhorst, F. and Rolls, E. T. (2009). Different representations of relative and absolute subjective value in the human brain, *Neuroimage* **48**: 258–268.

Grabenhorst, F. and Rolls, E. T. (2010). Attentional modulation of affective vs sensory processing: functional connectivity and a top down biased activation theory of selective attention, *Journal of Neurophysiology* **104**: 1649–1660.

Grabenhorst, F. and Rolls, E. T. (2011). Value, pleasure, and choice in the ventral prefrontal cortex, *Trends in Cognitive Sciences* **15**: 56–67.

Grabenhorst, F. and Schultz, W. (2021). Functions of primate amygdala neurons in economic decisions and social decision simulation, *Behav Brain Res* **409**: 113318.

Grabenhorst, F., Rolls, E. T., Margot, C., da Silva, M. and Velazco, M. I. (2007). How pleasant and unpleasant stimuli combine in the brain: odor combinations, *Journal of Neuroscience* **27**: 13532–13540.

Grabenhorst, F., Rolls, E. T. and Bilderbeck, A. (2008a). How cognition modulates affective responses to taste and flavor: top down influences on the orbitofrontal and pregenual cingulate cortices, *Cerebral Cortex* **18**: 1549–1559.

Grabenhorst, F., Rolls, E. T. and Parris, B. A. (2008b). From affective value to decision-making in the prefrontal cortex, *European Journal of Neuroscience* **28**: 1930–1939.

Grabenhorst, F., D'Souza, A., Parris, B. A., Rolls, E. T. and Passingham, R. E. (2010a). A common neural scale for the subjective value of different primary rewards, *Neuroimage* **51**: 1265–1274.

Grabenhorst, F., Rolls, E. T., Parris, B. and D'Souza, A. (2010b). How the brain represents the reward value of fat in the mouth, *Cerebral Cortex* **20**: 1082–1091.

Grabenhorst, F., Hernadi, I. and Schultz, W. (2012). Prediction of economic choice by primate amygdala neurons, *Proceedings of the National Academy of Sciences U S A* **109**: 18950–18955.

Grabenhorst, F., Hernadi, I. and Schultz, W. (2016). Primate amygdala neurons evaluate the progress of self-defined economic choice sequences, *Elife* **5**: e18731.

Grabenhorst, F., Baez-Mendoza, R., Genest, W., Deco, G. and Schultz, W. (2019). Primate amygdala neurons simulate decision processes of social partners, *Cell* **177**: 986–998 e15.

Grady, C. L. (2008). Cognitive neuroscience of aging, *Annals of the New York Academy of Sciences* **1124**: 127–144.

Graf, A. B. and Andersen, R. A. (2014). Inferring eye position from populations of lateral intraparietal neurons, *Elife* **3**: e02813.

Granger, C. W. J. (1969). Investigating causal relations by econometric models and cross-spectral methods, *Econometrica* **37**: 414–438.

Grant, J. E. and Chamberlain, S. R. (2019). Obsessive compulsive personality traits: Understanding the chain of pathogenesis from health to disease, *J Psychiatr Res* **116**: 69–73.

Grattan, L. E. and Glimcher, P. W. (2014). Absence of spatial tuning in the orbitofrontal cortex, *PLoS One* **9**: e112750.

Graybiel, A. M. and Grafton, S. T. (2015). The striatum: where skills and habits meet, *Cold Spring Harb Perspect Biol* **7**: a021691.

Graybiel, A. M. and Kimura, M. (1995). Adaptive neural networks in the basal ganglia, *in* J. C. Houk, J. L. Davis and D. G. Beiser (eds), *Models of Information Processing in the Basal Ganglia*, MIT Press, Cambridge, MA, chapter 5, pp. 103–116.

Graziano, M. S. A., Andersen, R. A. and Snowden, R. J. (1994). Tuning of MST neurons to spiral motions, *Journal of Neuroscience* **14**: 54–67.

Green, D. and Swets, J. (1966). *Signal Detection Theory and Psychophysics*, Wiley, New York.

Green, M. F. (1996). What are the functional consequences of neurocognitive deficits in schizophrenia?, *American Journal of Psychiatry* **153**: 321–330.

Greve, D. N. and Fischl, B. (2009). Accurate and robust brain image alignment using boundary-based registration, *Neuroimage* **48**: 63–72.

Grill-Spector, K. and Malach, R. (2004). The human visual cortex, *Annual Review of Neuroscience* **27**: 649–677.

Grill-Spector, K., Sayres, R. and Ress, D. (2006). High-resolution imaging reveals highly selective nonface clusters in the fusiform face area, *Nat Neurosci* **9**: 1177–85.

Grimson, W. E. L. (1990). *Object Recognition by Computer*, MIT Press, Cambridge, MA.

Gross, C. G., Desimone, R., Albright, T. D. and Schwartz, E. L. (1985). Inferior temporal cortex and pattern recognition, *Experimental Brain Research* **11**: 179–201.

Grossberg, S. (1976a). Adaptive pattern classification and universal recoding I: parallel development and coding of neural feature detectors, *Biological Cybernetics* **23**: 121–134.

Grossberg, S. (1976b). Adaptive pattern classification and universal recoding II: feedback, expectation, olfaction, illusions, *Biological Cybernetics* **23**: 1187–202.

Grossberg, S. (1988). Non-linear neural networks: principles, mechanisms, and architectures, *Neural Networks* **1**: 17–61.

Grossberg, S. (2021). *Conscious Mind, Resonant Brain: How Each Brain Makes a Mind*, Oxford University Press, Oxford.

Groves, P. M. (1983). A theory of the functional organization of the neostriatum and the neostriatal control of voluntary movement, *Brain Research Reviews* **5**: 109–132.

Groves, P. M., Garcia-Munoz, M., Linder, J. C., Manley, M. S., Martone, M. E. and Young, S. J. (1995). Elements of the intrinsic organization and information processing in the neostriatum, *in* J. C. Houk, J. L. Davis and D. G. Beiser (eds), *Models of Information Processing in the Basal Ganglia*, MIT Press, Cambridge, MA, chapter 4, pp. 51–96.

Gruber, L. Z., Ullman, S. and Ahissar, E. (2021). Oculo-retinal dynamics can explain the perception of minimal recognizable configurations, *Proc Natl Acad Sci U S A*.

Grusser, O.-J. and Landis, T. (1991). *Visual Agnosias*, MacMillan, London.

Grusser, O. J., Pause, M. and Schreiter, U. (1990). Localization and responses of neurones in the parieto-insular vestibular cortex of awake monkeys (Macaca fascicularis), *J Physiol* **430**: 537–57.

Guell, X. and Schmahmann, J. (2020). Cerebellar functional anatomy: a didactic summary based on human fMRI evidence, *Cerebellum* **19**: 1–5.

Guell, X., Gabrieli, J. D. E. and Schmahmann, J. D. (2018a). Triple representation of language, working memory, social and emotion processing in the cerebellum: convergent evidence from task and seed-based resting-state fMRI analyses in a single large cohort, *Neuroimage* **172**: 437–449.

Guell, X., Schmahmann, J. D., Gabrieli, J. and Ghosh, S. S. (2018b). Functional gradients of the cerebellum, *Elife* **7**: e36652.

Guerguiev, J., Lillicrap, T. P. and Richards, B. A. (2017). Towards deep learning with segregated dendrites, *Elife* **6**: e22901.

Guest, S., Grabenhorst, F., Essick, G., Chen, Y., Young, M., McGlone, F., de Araujo, I. and Rolls, E. T. (2007). Human cortical representation of oral temperature, *Physiology and Behavior* **92**: 975–984.

Gulyas, A. I., Miles, R., Hajos, N. and Freund, T. F. (1993). Precision and variability in postsynaptic target selection of inhibitory cells in the hippocampal CA3 region, *European Journal of Neuroscience* **5**: 1729–1751.

Gurney, K., Prescott, T. J. and Redgrave, P. (2001a). A computational model of action selection in the basal ganglia I: A new functional anatomy, *Biological Cybernetics* **84**: 401–410.

Gurney, K., Prescott, T. J. and Redgrave, P. (2001b). A computational model of action selection in the basal ganglia II: Analysis and simulation of behaviour, *Biological Cybernetics* **84**: 411–423.

Gutig, R. and Sompolinsky, H. (2006). The tempotron: a neuron that learns spike timing-based decisions, *Nature Neuroscience* **9**: 420–428.

Guyenet, S. J. and Schwartz, M. W. (2012). Clinical review: Regulation of food intake, energy balance, and body fat mass: implications for the pathogenesis and treatment of obesity, *Journal of Clinical Endocrinology and Metabolism* **97**: 745–755.

Habas, C. (2021). Functional connectivity of the cognitive cerebellum, *Front Syst Neurosci* **15**: 642225.

Haber, S. N. (2014). The place of dopamine in the cortico-basal ganglia circuit, *Neuroscience* **282**: 248–57.

Haber, S. N. (2016). Corticostriatal circuitry, *Dialogues Clin Neurosci* **18**: 7–21.

Haber, S. N. and Knutson, B. (2009). The reward circuit: linking primate anatomy and human imaging, *Neuropsychopharmacology* **35**: 4–26.

Haberly, L. B. (2001). Parallel-distributed processing in olfactory cortex: new insights from morphological and physiological analysis of neuronal circuitry, *Chemical Senses* **26**: 551–576.

Habib, M. and Sirigu, A. (1987). Pure topographical disorientation: a definition and anatomical basis, *Cortex* **23**: 73–85.

Hafting, T., Fyhn, M., Molden, S., Moser, M. B. and Moser, E. I. (2005). Microstructure of a spatial map in the entorhinal cortex, *Nature* **436**: 801–806.

Hagoort, P. (2017). The core and beyond in the language-ready brain, *Neurosci Biobehav Rev* **81**: 194–204.

Hagoort, P. and Indefrey, P. (2014). The neurobiology of language beyond single words, *Annu Rev Neurosci* **37**: 347–62.

Hale, J. T., Campanelli, L., Li, J., Bhattasali, S., Pallier, C. and Brennan, J. R. (2022). Neurocomputational models of language processing, *Annual Review of Linguistics* **8**: 427–446.

Hamani, C., Mayberg, H., Snyder, B., Giacobbe, P., Kennedy, S. and Lozano, A. M. (2009). Deep brain stimulation of the subcallosal cingulate gyrus for depression: anatomical location of active contacts in clinical responders and a suggested guideline for targeting, *J Neurosurg* **111**: 1209–15.

Hamani, C., Mayberg, H., Stone, S., Laxton, A., Haber, S. and Lozano, A. M. (2011). The subcallosal cingulate gyrus in the context of major depression, *Biol Psychiatry* **69**: 301–8.

Hamilton, J. P., Chen, M. C. and Gotlib, I. H. (2013). Neural systems approaches to understanding major depressive disorder: an intrinsic functional organization perspective, *Neurobiology of Disease* **52**: 4–11.

Hamilton, W. D. (1964). The genetical evolution of social behaviour, *Journal of Theoretical Biology* **7**: 1–52.

Hamilton, W. D. (1996). *Narrow Roads of Gene Land*, W. H. Freeman, New York.

Hamming, R. W. (1990). *Coding and Information Theory*, 2nd edn, Prentice-Hall, Englewood Cliffs, New Jersey.

Hampshire, A. and Owen, A. M. (2006). Fractionating attentional control using event-related fMRI, *Cerebral Cortex* **16**: 1679–1689.

Hampson, R. E., Hedberg, T. and Deadwyler, S. A. (2000). Differential information processing by hippocampal and subicular neurons, *Annals of the New York Academy of Sciences* **911**: 151–165.

Hampton, R. R. (2005). Monkey perirhinal cortex is critical for visual memory, but not for visual perception: reexamination of the behavioural evidence from monkeys, *Quarterly Journal of Experimental Psychology* **58B**: 283–299.

Hampton, R. R., Hampstead, B. M. and Murray, E. A. (2004). Selective hippocampal damage in rhesus monkeys impairs spatial memory in an open-field test, *Hippocampus* **14**: 808–18.

Han, W., Tellez, L. A., Perkins, M. H., Perez, I. O., Qu, T., Ferreira, J., Ferreira, T. L., Quinn, D., Liu, Z. W., Gao, X. B., Kaelberer, M. M., Bohorquez, D. V., Shammah-Lagnado, S. J., de Lartigue, G. and de Araujo, I. E. (2018). A neural circuit for gut-induced reward, *Cell* **175**: 665–678 e23.

Handelmann, G. E. and Olton, D. S. (1981). Spatial memory following damage to hippocampal CA3 pyramidal cells with kainic acid: impairment and recovery with preoperative training, *Brain Research* **217**: 41–58.

Hannagan, T., Agrawal, A., Cohen, L. and Dehaene, S. (2021). Emergence of a compositional neural code for written words: Recycling of a convolutional neural network for reading, *Proc Natl Acad Sci U S A* **118**: e2104779118.

Hannesson, D. K., Howland, G. J. and Phillips, A. G. (2004). Interaction between perirhinal and medial prefrontal cortex is required for temporal order but not recognition memory for objects in rats, *Journal of Neuroscience* **24**: 4596–4604.

Hare, T. A., O'Doherty, J., Camerer, C. F., Schultz, W. and Rangel, A. (2008). Dissociating the role of the orbitofrontal cortex and the striatum in the computation of goal values and prediction errors, *J Neurosci* **28**: 5623–30.

Harel, J., Koch, C. and Perona, P. (2006a). Graph-based visual saliency, *Advances in Neural Information Processing Systems (NIPS)* **19**: 545–552.

Harel, J., Koch, C. and Perona, P. (2006b). A saliency implementation in MATLAB, p. http://www.klab.caltech.edu/ harel/share/gbvs.php.

Hargreaves, E. L., Rao, G., Lee, I. and Knierim, J. J. (2005). Major dissociation between medial and lateral entorhinal input to dorsal hippocampus, *Science* **308**: 1792–1794.

Harmer, C. J. and Cowen, P. J. (2013). 'It's the way that you look at it'–a cognitive neuropsychological account of SSRI action in depression, *Philosophical Transactions of the Royal Society of London B Biological Sciences* **368**: 20120407.

Harris, A. E., Ermentrout, G. B. and Small, S. L. (1997). A model of ocular dominance column development by competition for trophic factor, *Proceedings of the National Academy of Sciences USA* **94**: 9944–9949.

Harris, K. D. and Mrsic-Flogel, T. D. (2013). Cortical connectivity and sensory coding, *Nature* **503**: 51–58.

Harris, K. D. and Shepherd, G. M. (2015). The neocortical circuit: themes and variations, *Nat Neurosci* **18**: 170–81.

Hartley, T., Lever, C., Burgess, N. and O'Keefe, J. (2014). Space in the brain: how the hippocampal formation supports spatial cognition, *Philos Trans R Soc Lond B Biol Sci* **369**: 20120510.

Hartston, H. J. and Swerdlow, N. R. (1999). Visuospatial priming and Stroop performance in patients with obsessive compulsive disorder, *Neuropsychology* **13**: 447–457.

Hassabis, D., Kumaran, D. and Maguire, E. A. (2007). Using imagination to understand the neural basis of episodic memory, *J Neurosci* **27**: 14365–74.

Hassabis, D., Chu, C., Rees, G., Weiskopf, N., Molyneux, P. D. and Maguire, E. A. (2009). Decoding neuronal ensembles in the human hippocampus, *Curr Biol* **19**: 546–54.

Hassanpour, M. S., Simmons, W. K., Feinstein, J. S., Luo, Q., Lapidus, R. C., Bodurka, J., Paulus, M. P. and Khalsa, S. S. (2018). The insular cortex dynamically maps changes in cardiorespiratory interoception, *Neuropsychopharmacology* **43**: 426–434.

Hasselmo, M. E. (1999). Neuromodulation: acetylcholine and memory consolidation, *Trends Cogn Sci* **3**: 351–359.

Hasselmo, M. E. and Bower, J. M. (1993). Acetylcholine and memory, *Trends in Neurosciences* **16**: 218–222.

Hasselmo, M. E. and Giocomo, L. M. (2006). Cholinergic modulation of cortical function, *J Mol Neurosci* **30**: 133–135.

Hasselmo, M. E. and McGaughy, J. (2004). High acetylcholine levels set circuit dynamics for attention and encoding and low acetylcholine levels set dynamics for consolidation, *Prog Brain Res* **145**: 207–31.

Hasselmo, M. E. and Sarter, M. (2011). Modes and models of forebrain cholinergic neuromodulation of cognition, *Neuropsychopharmacology* **36**: 52–73.

Hasselmo, M. E., Rolls, E. T. and Baylis, G. C. (1989a). The role of expression and identity in the face-selective responses of neurons in the temporal visual cortex of the monkey, *Behav Brain Res* **32**: 203–18.

Hasselmo, M. E., Rolls, E. T., Baylis, G. C. and Nalwa, V. (1989b). Object-centred encoding by face-selective neurons in the cortex in the superior temporal sulcus of the monkey, *Experimental Brain Research* **75**: 417–429.

Hasselmo, M. E., Schnell, E. and Barkai, E. (1995). Learning and recall at excitatory recurrent synapses and cholinergic modulation in hippocampal region CA3, *Journal of Neuroscience* **15**: 5249–5262.

Hasselmo, M. E., Giocomo, L. M., Brandon, M. P. and Yoshida, M. (2010). Cellular dynamical mechanisms for encoding the time and place of events along spatiotemporal trajectories in episodic memory, *Behav Brain Res* **215**: 261–74.

Haubrich, J. and Nader, K. (2018). Memory reconsolidation, *Curr Top Behav Neurosci* **37**: 151–176.

Haun, A. M. (2021). What is visible across the visual field?, *Neuroscience of Consciousness* **2021**: niab006.

Hawken, M. J. and Parker, A. J. (1987). Spatial properties of the monkey striate cortex, *Proceedings of the Royal Society, London B* **231**: 251–288.

Haxby, J. V. (2006). Fine structure in representations of faces and objects, *Nature Neuroscience* **9**: 1084–1086.

Haxby, J. V., Gobbini, M. I. and Nastase, S. A. (2020). Naturalistic stimuli reveal a dominant role for agentic action in visual representation, *Neuroimage* **216**: 116561.

Hayden, B. Y., Pearson, J. M. and Platt, M. L. (2011). Neuronal basis of sequential foraging decisions in a patchy environment, *Nature Neuroscience* **14**: 933–939.

Hebb, D. O. (1949). *The Organization of Behavior: a Neuropsychological Theory*, Wiley, New York.

Hegde, J. and Van Essen, D. C. (2000). Selectivity for complex shapes in primate visual area V2, *Journal of Neuroscience* **20**: RC61.

Heilbronner, S. R., Rodriguez-Romaguera, J., Quirk, G. J., Groenewegen, H. J. and Haber, S. N. (2016). Circuit-based corticostriatal homologies between rat and primate, *Biol Psychiatry* **80**: 509–21.

Heilbronner, S. R., Meyer, M. A. A., Choi, E. Y. and Haber, S. N. (2018). How do cortico-striatal projections impact on downstream pallidal circuitry?, *Brain Struct Funct* **223**: 2809–2821.

Hein, G. and Knight, R. T. (2008). Superior temporal sulcus–It's my area: or is it?, *J Cogn Neurosci* **20**: 2125–36.

Heitmann, B. L., Westerterp, K. R., Loos, R. J., Sorensen, T. I., O'Dea, K., McLean, P., Jensen, T. K., Eisenmann, J., Speakman, J. R., Simpson, S. J., Reed, D. R. and Westerterp-Plantenga, M. S. (2012). Obesity: lessons from evolution and the environment, *Obes Rev* **13**: 910–22.

Hellekant, G., Danilova, V. and Ninomiya, Y. (1997). Primate sense of taste: behavioral and single chorda tympani and glossopharyngeal nerve fiber recordings in the rhesus monkey, Macaca mulatta, *J Neurophysiol* **77**: 978–93.

Heller, J., Hertz, J. A., Kjaer, T. W. and Richmond, B. J. (1995). Information flow and temporal coding in primate pattern vision, *Journal of Computational Neuroscience* **2**: 175–193.

Henze, D. A., Wittner, L. and Buzsaki, G. (2002). Single granule cells reliably discharge targets in the hippocampal CA3 network in vivo, *Nat Neurosci* **5**: 790–5.

Hernadi, I., Grabenhorst, F. and Schultz, W. (2015). Planning activity for internally generated reward goals in monkey amygdala neurons, *Nat Neurosci* **18**: 461–9.

Hernandez, A., Zainos, A. and Romo, R. (2002). Temporal evolution of a decision-making process in medial premotor cortex, *Neuron* **33**: 959–972.

Hernandez, M., Fairhall, S. L., Lenci, A., Baroni, M. and Caramazza, A. (2014). Predication drives verb cortical signatures, *J Cogn Neurosci* **26**: 1829–39.

Herrnstein, R. J. (1984). Objects, categories, and discriminative stimuli, *in* H. L. Roitblat, T. G. Bever and H. S. Terrace (eds), *Animal Cognition*, Lawrence Erlbaum and Associates, Hillsdale, NJ, chapter 14, pp. 233–261.

Hertrich, I., Dietrich, S. and Ackermann, H. (2020). The margins of the language network in the brain, *Frontiers in Communication* **5**: 519955.

Hertz, J. A., Krogh, A. and Palmer, R. G. (1991). *Introduction to the Theory of Neural Computation*, Addison-Wesley, Wokingham, UK.

Hertz, J. A., Kjaer, T. W., Eskander, E. N. and Richmond, B. J. (1992). Measuring natural neural processing with artificial neural networks, *International Journal of Neural Systems* **3 (Suppl.)**: 91–103.

Hervig, M. E., Fiddian, L., Piilgaard, L., Bozic, T., Blanco-Pozo, M., Knudsen, C., Olesen, S. F., Alsio, J. and Robbins, T. W. (2020). Dissociable and paradoxical roles of rat medial and lateral orbitofrontal cortex in visual serial reversal learning, *Cereb Cortex* **30**: 1016–1029.

Hesse, J. K. and Tsao, D. Y. (2020). The macaque face patch system: a turtle's underbelly for the brain, *Nat Rev Neurosci* **21**: 695–716.

Hestrin, S., Sah, P. and Nicoll, R. (1990). Mechanisms generating the time course of dual component excitatory synaptic currents recorded in hippocampal slices, *Neuron* **5**: 247–253.

Hickok, G. (2022). The dual stream model of speech and language processing, *Handb Clin Neurol* **185**: 57–69.

Hickok, G. and Poeppel, D. (2007). The cortical organization of speech processing, *Nat Rev Neurosci* **8**: 393–402.

Hickok, G. and Poeppel, D. (2015). Neural basis of speech perception, *Handb Clin Neurol* **129**: 149–60.

Hickok, G., Venezia, J. and Teghipco, A. (2023). Beyond Broca: neural architecture and evolution of a dual motor speech coordination system, *Brain* **146**: 1775–1790.

Hikosaka, K. and Watanabe, M. (2000). Delay activity of orbital and lateral prefrontal neurons of the monkey varying with different rewards, *Cerebral Cortex* **10**: 263–271.

Hikosaka, O., Ghazizadeh, A., Griggs, W. and Amita, H. (2018). Parallel basal ganglia circuits for decision making, *J Neural Transm (Vienna)* **125**: 515–529.

Hill, S. L., Wang, Y., Riachi, I., Schürmann, F. and Markram, H. (2012). Statistical connectivity provides a sufficient foundation for specific functional connectivity in neocortical neural microcircuits, *Proceedings of the National Academy of Sciences* **109**: E2885–E2894.

Hinman, J. R., Brandon, M. P., Climer, J. R., Chapman, G. W. and Hasselmo, M. E. (2016). Multiple running speed signals in medial entorhinal cortex, *Neuron* **91**: 666–79.

Hinton, G. E. (1989). Deterministic Boltzmann learning performs steepest descent in weight-space, *Neural Computation* **1**: 143–150.

Hinton, G. E. and Anderson, J. A. (1981). *Parallel Models of Associative Memory*, Erlbaum, Hillsdale, NJ.

Hinton, G. E. and Ghahramani, Z. (1997). Generative models for discovering sparse distributed representations, *Philosophical Transactions of the Royal Society of London, B* **352**: 1177–1190.

Hinton, G. E. and Salakhutdinov, R. R. (2006). Reducing the dimensionality of data with neural networks, *Science* **313**: 504–507.

Hinton, G. E. and Sejnowski, T. J. (1986). Learning and relearning in Boltzmann machines, *in* D. Rumelhart and J. L. McClelland (eds), *Parallel Distributed Processing*, Vol. 1, MIT Press, Cambridge, MA, chapter 7, pp. 282–317.

Hinton, G. E., Dayan, P., Frey, B. J. and Neal, R. M. (1995). The "wake-sleep" algorithm for unsupervised neural networks, *Science* **268**: 1158–1161.

Hinton, G. E., Osindero, S. and Teh, Y.-W. (2006). A fast learning algorithm for deep belief nets, *Neural computation* **18**: 1527–1554.

Hirabayashi, T., Takeuchi, D., Tamura, K. and Miyashita, Y. (2013). Functional microcircuit recruited during retrieval of object association memory in monkey perirhinal cortex, *Neuron* **77**: 192–203.

Hirshhorn, M., Grady, C., Rosenbaum, R. S., Winocur, G. and Moscovitch, M. (2012). The hippocampus is involved in mental navigation for a recently learned, but not a highly familiar environment: a longitudinal fMRI study, *Hippocampus* **22**: 842–52.

Hodgkin, A. L. and Huxley, A. F. (1952). A quantitative description of membrane current and its application to conduction and excitation in nerve, *Journal of Physiology* **117**: 500–544.

Hoffman, E. A. and Haxby, J. V. (2000). Distinct representations of eye gaze and identity in the distributed neural system for face perception, *Nature Neuroscience* **3**: 80–84.

Hoftman, G. D., Datta, D. and Lewis, D. A. (2017). Layer 3 excitatory and inhibitory circuitry in the prefrontal cortex: developmental trajectories and alterations in schizophrenia, *Biol Psychiatry* **81**: 862–873.

Hoge, J. and Kesner, R. P. (2007). Role of CA3 and CA1 subregions of the dorsal hippocampus on temporal processing of objects, *Neurobiology of Learning and Memory* **88**: 225–231.

Hogeveen, J., Medalla, M., Ainsworth, M., Galeazzi, J. M., Hanlon, C. A., Mansouri, F. A. and Costa, V. D. (2022a). What does the frontopolar cortex contribute to goal-directed cognition and action?, *J Neurosci* **42**: 8508–8513.

Hogeveen, J., Mullins, T. S., Romero, J. D., Eversole, E., Rogge-Obando, K., Mayer, A. R. and Costa, V. D. (2022b). The neurocomputational bases of explore-exploit decision-making, *Neuron* **110**: 1869–1879 e5.

Holland, J. H. (1975). *Adaptation in Natural and Artificial Systems*, The University of Michigan Press, Michigan, USA.

Holland, P. C. and Gallagher, M. (1999). Amygdala circuitry in attentional and representational processes, *Trends in Cognitive Sciences* **3**: 65–73.

Hölscher, C. and Rolls, E. T. (2002). Perirhinal cortex neuronal activity is actively related to working memory in the macaque, *Neural Plasticity* **9**: 41–51.

Hölscher, C., Rolls, E. T. and Xiang, J. Z. (2003). Perirhinal cortex neuronal activity related to long term familiarity memory in the macaque, *European Journal of Neuroscience* **18**: 2037–2046.

Holtzheimer, P. E., Husain, M. M., Lisanby, S. H., Taylor, S. F., Whitworth, L. A., McClintock, S., Slavin, K. V., Berman, J., McKhann, G. M., Patil, P. G., Rittberg, B. R., Abosch, A., Pandurangi, A. K., Holloway, K. L., Lam, R. W., Honey, C. R., Neimat, J. S., Henderson, J. M., DeBattista, C., Rothschild, A. J., Pilitsis, J. G., Espinoza, R. T., Petrides, G., Mogilner, A. Y., Matthews, K., Peichel, D., Gross, R. E., Hamani, C., Lozano, A. M. and Mayberg, H. S. (2017). Subcallosal cingulate deep brain stimulation for treatment-resistant depression: a multisite, randomised, sham-controlled trial, *Lancet Psychiatry* **4**: 839–849.

Holzinger, Y., Ullman, S., Harari, D., Behrmann, M. and Avidan, G. (2019). Minimal recognizable configurations elicit category-selective responses in higher order visual cortex, *J Cogn Neurosci* **31**: 1354–1367.

Hopfield, J. J. (1982). Neural networks and physical systems with emergent collective computational abilities, *Proc Natl Acad Sci U S A* **79**: 2554–8.

Hopfield, J. J. (1984). Neurons with graded response have collective computational properties like those of two-state neurons, *Proceedings of the National Academy of Sciences USA* **81**: 3088–3092.

Hopfield, J. J. and Herz, A. V. (1995). Rapid local synchronization of action potentials: toward computation with coupled integrate-and-fire neurons, *Proceedings of the National Academy of Sciences USA* **92**: 6655–6662.

Hornak, J., Rolls, E. T. and Wade, D. (1996). Face and voice expression identification in patients with emotional and behavioural changes following ventral frontal lobe damage, *Neuropsychologia* **34**: 247–261.

Hornak, J., Bramham, J., Rolls, E. T., Morris, R. G., O'Doherty, J., Bullock, P. R. and Polkey, C. E. (2003). Changes in emotion after circumscribed surgical lesions of the orbitofrontal and cingulate cortices., *Brain* **126**: 1691–1712.

Hornak, J., O'Doherty, J., Bramham, J., Rolls, E. T., Morris, R. G., Bullock, P. R. and Polkey, C. E. (2004). Reward-related reversal learning after surgical excisions in orbitofrontal and dorsolateral prefrontal cortex in humans, *Journal of Cognitive Neuroscience* **16**: 463–478.

Hornykiewicz, O. (1973). Dopamine in the basal ganglia: its role and therapeutic implications including the use of L-Dopa, *British Medical Bulletin* **29**: 172–178.

Horowitz, J. M. and Horwitz, B. A. (2019). Extreme neuroplasticity of hippocampal CA1 pyramidal neurons in hibernating mammalian species, *Front Neuroanat* **13**: 9.

Horowitz, L. F., Saraiva, L. R., Kuang, D., Yoon, K. H. and Buck, L. B. (2014). Olfactory receptor patterning in a higher primate, *J Neurosci* **34**: 12241–52.

Horvitz, J. C. (2000). Mesolimbocortical and nigrostriatal dopamine responses to salient non-reward events, *Neuroscience* **96**: 651–656.

Houk, J. C., Adams, J. L. and Barto, A. C. (1995). A model of how the basal ganglia generates and uses neural signals that predict reinforcement, *in* J. C. Houk, J. L. Davies and D. G. Beiser (eds), *Models of Information Processing in the Basal Ganglia*, MIT Press, Cambridge, MA, chapter 13, pp. 249–270.

Howard, J. D. and Gottfried, J. A. (2014). Configural and elemental coding of natural odor mixture components in the human brain, *Neuron* **84**: 857–69.

Howard, J. D., Gottfried, J. A., Tobler, P. N. and Kahnt, T. (2015). Identity-specific coding of future rewards in the human orbitofrontal cortex, *Proc Natl Acad Sci U S A* **112**: 5195–200.

Howard, J. D., Kahnt, T. and Gottfried, J. A. (2016). Converging prefrontal pathways support associative and perceptual features of conditioned stimuli, *Nat Commun* **7**: 11546.

Howard, M. W. and Eichenbaum, H. (2015). Time and space in the hippocampus, *Brain Res* **1621**: 345–54.

Howard, M. W., MacDonald, C. J., Tiganj, Z., Shankar, K. H., Du, Q., Hasselmo, M. E. and Eichenbaum, H. (2014). A unified mathematical framework for coding time, space, and sequences in the hippocampal region, *J Neurosci* **34**: 4692–707.

Hoydal, O. A., Skytoen, E. R., Andersson, S. O., Moser, M. B. and Moser, E. I. (2019). Object-vector coding in the medial entorhinal cortex, *Nature* **568**: 400–404.

Hsu, C.-C. H., Rolls, E. T., Huang, C.-C., Chong, S. T., Lo, C.-Y. Z., Feng, J. and Lin, C.-P. (2020). Connections of the human orbitofrontal cortex and inferior frontal gyrus, *Cerebral Cortex* **30**: 5830–5843.

Huang, C.-C., Rolls, E. T., Hsu, C.-C., Feng, J. and Lin, C.-P. (2021). Extensive cortical connectivity of the human hippocampal memory system: beyond the "what" and "where" dual-stream model, *Cerebral Cortex* **31**: 4652–4669.

Huang, C. C., Rolls, E. T., Feng, J. and Lin, C. P. (2022). An extended Human Connectome Project multimodal parcellation atlas of the human cortex and subcortical areas, *Brain Struct Funct* **227**: 763–778.

Huang, R. S. and Sereno, M. I. (2018). Multisensory and sensorimotor maps, *Handb Clin Neurol* **151**: 141–161.

Hubel, D. H. and Wiesel, T. N. (1962). Receptive fields, binocular interaction, and functional architecture in the cat's visual cortex, *Journal of Physiology* **160**: 106–154.

Hubel, D. H. and Wiesel, T. N. (1968). Receptive fields and functional architecture of monkey striate cortex, *Journal of Physiology, London* **195**: 215–243.

Hubel, D. H. and Wiesel, T. N. (1977). Functional architecture of the macaque monkey visual cortex, *Proceedings of the Royal Society, London [B]* **198**: 1–59.

Huber, J., Ruehl, M., Flanagin, V. and Zu Eulenburg, P. (2022). Delineating neural responses and functional connectivity changes during vestibular and nociceptive stimulation reveal the uniqueness of cortical vestibular processing, *Brain Struct Funct* **227**: 779–791.

Huerta, P. T., Sun, L. D., Wilson, M. A. and Tonegawa, S. (2000). Formation of temporal memory requires NMDA receptors within CA1 pyramidal neurons, *Neuron* **25**: 473–480.

Hughlings Jackson, J. (1878). *Selected writings of John Hughlings Jackson 2, Edited by J. Taylor, 1932*, Hodder and Staughton, London.

Hull, C. (2020). Prediction signals in the cerebellum: beyond supervised motor learning, *Elife* **9**: e54073.

Hull, C. and Regehr, W. G. (2022). The Cerebellar Cortex, *Annu Rev Neurosci* **45**: 151–175.

Human Genome Sequencing, C. I. (2004). Finishing the euchromatic sequence of the human genome, *Nature* **431**: 931–945.

Hummel, J. E. and Biederman, I. (1992). Dynamic binding in a neural network for shape recognition, *Psychological Review* **99**: 480–517.

Hunsaker, M. R., Rogers, J. L. and Kesner, R. P. (2007). Behavioral characterization of a transection of dorsal CA3 subcortical efferents: comparison with scopolamine and physostigmine infusions into dorsal CA3, *Neurobiol Learn Mem* **88**: 127–36.

Hunsaker, M. R., Lee, B. and Kesner, R. P. (2008). Evaluating the temporal context of episodic memory: the role of CA3 and CA1, *Behav Brain Res* **188**: 310–5.

Hussain, S. S. and Bloom, S. R. (2013). The regulation of food intake by the gut-brain axis: implications for obesity, *Int J Obes (Lond)* **37**: 625–33.

Huth, A. G., de Heer, W. A., Griffiths, T. L., Theunissen, F. E. and Gallant, J. L. (2016). Natural speech reveals the semantic maps that tile human cerebral cortex, *Nature* **532**: 453–458.

Huttenlocher, D. P. and Ullman, S. (1990). Recognizing solid objects by alignment with an image, *International Journal of Computer Vision* **5**: 195–212.

Hölscher, C., Rolls, E. T. and Xiang, J.-Z. (2003). Perirhinal cortex neuronal activity related to long-term familiarity memory in the macaque, *European Journal of Neuroscience* **18**: 2037–2046.

Iadarola, N. D., Niciu, M. J., Richards, E. M., Vande Voort, J. L., Ballard, E. D., Lundin, N. B., Nugent, A. C., Machado-Vieira, R. and Zarate, C. A., J. (2015). Ketamine and other N-methyl-D-aspartate receptor antagonists in the treatment of depression: a perspective review, *Therapeutic Advances in Chronic Disease* **6**: 97–114.

Iadecola, C. and Gottesman, R. F. (2019). Neurovascular and cognitive dysfunction in hypertension, *Circ Res* **124**: 1025–1044.

Imamura, K., Mataga, N. and Mori, K. (1992). Coding of odor molecules by mitral/tufted cells in rabbit olfactory bulb. I. Aliphatic compounds, *Journal of Neurophysiology* **68**: 1986–2002.

Ingvar, D. H. and Franzen, G. (1974). Abnormalities of cerebral blood flow distribution in patients with chronic schizophrenia, *Acta Psychiatrica Scandinavica* **50**: 425–462.

Insabato, A., Pannunzi, M., Rolls, E. T. and Deco, G. (2010). Confidence-related decision-making, *Journal of Neurophysiology* **104**: 539–547.

Ishai, A., Ungerleider, L. G., Martin, A., Schouten, J. L. and Haxby, J. V. (1999). Distributed representation of objects in the human ventral visual pathway, *Proceedings of the National Academy of Sciences USA* **96**: 9379–9384.

Ishizuka, N., Weber, J. and Amaral, D. G. (1990). Organization of intrahippocampal projections originating from CA3 pyramidal cells in the rat, *Journal of Comparative Neurology* **295**: 580–623.

Ison, M. J., Quian Quiroga, R. and Fried, I. (2015). Rapid encoding of new memories by individual neurons in the human brain, *Neuron* **87**: 220–30.

Issa, E. B. and DiCarlo, J. J. (2012). Precedence of the eye region in neural processing of faces, *The Journal of Neuroscience* **32**: 16666–16682.

Ito, M. (1984). *The Cerebellum and Neural Control*, Raven Press, New York.

Ito, M. (1989). Long-term depression, *Annual Review of Neuroscience* **12**: 85–102.

Ito, M. (1993a). Cerebellar mechanisms of long-term depression, *in* M. Baudry, R. F. Thompson and J. L. Davis (eds), *Synaptic Plasticity: Molecular, Cellular and Functional Aspects*, MIT Press, Cambridge, MA, chapter 6, pp. 117–128.

Ito, M. (1993b). Synaptic plasticity in the cerebellar cortex and its role in motor learning, *Canadian Journal of Neurological Science* **Suppl. 3**: S70–S74.

Ito, M. (2006). Cerebellar circuitry as a neuronal machine, *Progress in Neurobiology* **78**: 272–303.

Ito, M. (2010). Cerebellar cortex, *in* G. M. Shepherd and S. Grillner (eds), *Handbook of Brain Microcircuits*, Oxford University Press, Oxford, chapter 28, pp. 293–300.

Ito, M. (2013). Error detection and representation in the olivo-cerebellar system, *Frontiers in Neural Circuits* **7**: 1.

Ito, M. and Komatsu, H. (2004). Representation of angles embedded within contour stimuli in area V2 of macaque monkeys, *Journal of Neuroscience* **24**: 3313–3324.

Ito, M., Yamaguchi, K., Nagao, S. and Yamazaki, T. (2014). Long-term depression as a model of cerebellar plasticity, *Progress in Brain Research* **210**: 1–30.

Itskov, P. M., Vinnik, E. and Diamond, M. E. (2011). Hippocampal representation of touch-guided behavior in rats: persistent and independent traces of stimulus and reward location, *PLoS One* **6**: e16462.

Itti, L. and Koch, C. (2000). A saliency-based search mechanism for overt and covert shifts of visual attention, *Vision Research* **40**: 1489–1506.

Iversen, S. D. (1979). Behaviour after neostriatal lesions in animals, *in* I. Divac (ed.), *The Neostriatum*, Pergamon, Oxford, pp. 195–210.

Iversen, S. D. (1984). Behavioural effects of manipulation of basal ganglia neurotransmitters, *Functions of the Basal Ganglia. CIBA Foundation Symposium*, Vol. 107, Pitman, London, pp. 183–195.

Izquierdo, A. (2017). Functional heterogeneity within rat orbitofrontal cortex in reward learning and decision making, *J Neurosci* **37**: 10529–10540.

Jackendoff, R. (2002). *Foundations of Language. Brain, Meaning, Grammar, Evolution*, Oxford University Press, Oxford.

Jackendoff, R. (2003). Precis of Foundations of language: brain, meaning, grammar, evolution, *Behav Brain Sci* **26**: 651–65; discussion 666–707.

Jackendoff, R. (2007). A Parallel Architecture perspective on language processing, *Brain Res* **1146**: 2–22.

Jackson, B. S. (2004). Including long-range dependence in integrate-and-fire models of the high interspike-interval variability of cortical neurons, *Neural Computation* **16**: 2125–2195.

Jackson, M. B. (2013). Recall of spatial patterns stored in a hippocampal slice by long-term potentiation, *Journal of Neurophysiology* **110**: 2511–2519.

Jacobs, J., Weidemann, C. T., Miller, J. F., Solway, A., Burke, J. F., Wei, X. X., Suthana, N., Sperling, M. R., Sharan, A. D., Fried, I. and Kahana, M. J. (2013). Direct recordings of grid-like neuronal activity in human spatial navigation, *Nat Neurosci* **16**: 1188–90.

Jacoby, L. L. (1983a). Perceptual enhancement: persistent effects of an experience, *Journal of Experimental Psychology: Learning, Memory, and Cognition* **9**: 21–38.

Jacoby, L. L. (1983b). Remembering the data: analyzing interaction processes in reading, *Journal of Verbal Learning and Verbal Behavior* **22**: 485–508.

Jahr, C. and Stevens, C. (1990). Voltage dependence of NMDA-activated macroscopic conductances predicted by single-channel kinetics, *Journal of Neuroscience* **10**: 3178–3182.

Jakab, R. L. and Leranth, C. (1995). Septum, *in* G. Paxinos (ed.), *The Rat Nervous System*, Academic Press, San Diego.

Janssen, P., Vogels, R. and Orban, G. A. (1999). Macaque inferior temporal neurons are selective for disparity-defined three-dimensional shapes, *Proceedings of the National Academy of Sciences* **96**: 8217–8222.

Janssen, P., Vogels, R. and Orban, G. A. (2000). Selectivity for 3D shape that reveals distinct areas within macaque inferior temporal cortex, *Science* **288**: 2054–2056.

Janssen, P., Vogels, R., Liu, Y. and Orban, G. A. (2003). At least at the level of inferior temporal cortex, the stereo correspondence problem is solved, *Neuron* **37**: 693–701.

Jarrard, L. E. (1993). On the role of the hippocampus in learning and memory in the rat, *Behavioral and Neural Biology* **60**: 9–26.

Jarrard, L. E. and Davidson, T. L. (1990). Acquisition of concurrent conditional discriminations in rats with ibotenate lesions of hippocampus and subiculum, *Psychobiology* **18**: 68–73.

Jarrett, K., Kavukcuoglu, K., Ranzato, M. and LeCun, Y. (2009). What is the Best Multi-Stage Architecture for Object Recognition?, *2009 IEEE 12th International Conference on Computer Vision (ICCV)* pp. 2146–2153.

Jay, T. M. and Witter, M. P. (1991). Distribution of hippocampal CA1 and subicular efferents in the prefrontal cortex of the rat studied by means of anterograde transport of Phaseolus vulgaris–leucoagglutinin, *Journal of Comparative Neurology* **313**: 574–586.

Jeffery, K. J. and Hayman, R. (2004). Plasticity of the hippocampal place cell representation, *Reviews in the Neurosciences* **15**: 309–331.

Jeffery, K. J., Anderson, M. I., Hayman, R. and Chakraborty, S. (2004). A proposed architecture for the neural representation of spatial context, *Neuroscience and Biobehavioral Reviews* **28**: 201–218.

Jenkinson, M., Beckmann, C. F., Behrens, T. E., Woolrich, M. W. and Smith, S. M. (2012). FSL, *Neuroimage* **62**: 782–90.

Jerman, T., Kesner, R. P. and Hunsaker, M. R. (2006). Disconnection analysis of CA3 and DG in mediating encoding but not retrieval in a spatial maze learning task, *Learning and Memory* **13**: 458–464.

Jeurissen, B., Descoteaux, M., Mori, S. and Leemans, A. (2019). Diffusion MRI fiber tractography of the brain, *NMR Biomed* **32**: e3785.

Jezek, K., Henriksen, E. J., Treves, A., Moser, E. I. and Moser, M.-B. (2011). Theta-paced flickering between place-cell maps in the hippocampus, *Nature* **278**: 246–249.

Jia, X., Hong, H. and DiCarlo, J. J. (2021). Unsupervised changes in core object recognition behavior are predicted by neural plasticity in inferior temporal cortex, *Elife* **10**: 60830.

Jiang, R., Andolina, I. M., Li, M. and Tang, S. (2021). Clustered functional domains for curves and corners in cortical area V4, *Elife* **10**: e63798.

Jiao, Z., Lai, Y., Kang, J., Gong, W., Ma, L., Jia, T., Xie, C., Xiang, S., Cheng, W., Heinz, A., Desrivieres, S., Schumann, G., Consortium, I., Sun, F. and Feng, J. (2022). A model-based approach to assess reproducibility for large-scale high-throughput MRI-based studies, *Neuroimage* **255**: 119166.

Jobard, G., Crivello, F. and Tzourio-Mazoyer, N. (2003). Evaluation of the dual route theory of reading: a metanalysis of 35 neuroimaging studies, *Neuroimage* **20**: 693–712.

Johansen-Berg, H., Gutman, D. A., Behrens, T. E., Matthews, P. M., Rushworth, M. F., Katz, E., Lozano, A. M. and Mayberg, H. S. (2008). Anatomical connectivity of the subgenual cingulate region targeted with deep brain stimulation for treatment-resistant depression, *Cereb Cortex* **18**: 1374–83.

Johansen, J. P., Tarpley, J. W., LeDoux, J. E. and Blair, H. T. (2010). Neural substrates for expectation-modulated fear learning in the amygdala and periaqueductal gray, *Nat Neurosci* **13**: 979–86.

Johns, D. J., Hartmann-Boyce, J., Jebb, S. A., Aveyard, P. and Behavioural Weight Management Review, G. (2014). Diet or exercise interventions vs combined behavioral weight management programs: a systematic review and meta-analysis of direct comparisons, *J Acad Nutr Diet* **114**: 1557–68.

Johnson, S. C., Baxter, L. C., Wilder, L. S., Pipe, J. G., Heiserman, J. E. and Prigatano, G. P. (2002). Neural correlates of self-reflection, *Brain* **125**: 1808–14.

Johnston, D. and Amaral, D. (2004). Hippocampus, *in* G. M. Shepherd (ed.), *The Synaptic Organization of the Brain*, 5th edn, Oxford University Press, Oxford, chapter 11, pp. 455–498.

Johnston, S. T., Shtrahman, M., Parylak, S., Goncalves, J. T. and Gage, F. H. (2016). Paradox of pattern separation and adult neurogenesis: A dual role for new neurons balancing memory resolution and robustness, *Neurobiol Learn Mem* **129**: 60–8.

Johnstone, S. and Rolls, E. T. (1990). Delay, discriminatory, and modality specific neurons in striatum and pallidum during short-term memory tasks, *Brain Research* **522**: 147–151.

Jonas, E. A. and Kaczmarek, L. K. (1999). The inside story: subcellular mechanisms of neuromodulation, *in* P. S. Katz (ed.), *Beyond Neurotransmission*, Oxford University Press, New York, chapter 3, pp. 83–120.

Jones, E. G. and Peters, A. (eds) (1984). *Cerebral Cortex, Functional Properties of Cortical Cells*, Vol. 2, Plenum, New York.

Jones, E. G. and Powell, T. P. S. (1970). An anatomical study of converging sensory pathways within the cerebral cortex of the monkey, *Brain* **93**: 793–820.

Julian, J. B., Keinath, A. T., Frazzetta, G. and Epstein, R. A. (2018). Human entorhinal cortex represents visual space using a boundary-anchored grid, *Nat Neurosci* **21**: 191–194.

Jung, M. W. and McNaughton, B. L. (1993). Spatial selectivity of unit activity in the hippocampal granular layer, *Hippocampus* **3**: 165–182.

Kaas, J. H. and Hackett, T. A. (2000). Subdivisions of auditory cortex and processing streams in primates, *Proc Natl Acad Sci U S A* **97**: 11793–9.

Kacelnik, A. and Brito e Abreu, F. (1998). Risky choice and Weber's Law, *Journal of Theoretical Biology* **194**: 289–298.

Kadohisa, M. (2015). Beyond flavour to the gut and back, *Flavour* **4**: 1–11.

Kadohisa, M. and Wilson, D. A. (2006). Separate encoding of identity and similarity of complex familiar odors in piriform cortex, *Proceedings of the National Academy of Sciences U S A* **103**: 15206–15211.

Kadohisa, M., Rolls, E. T. and Verhagen, J. V. (2004). Orbitofrontal cortex neuronal representation of temperature and capsaicin in the mouth, *Neuroscience* **127**: 207–221.

Kadohisa, M., Rolls, E. T. and Verhagen, J. V. (2005a). Neuronal representations of stimuli in the mouth: the primate insular taste cortex, orbitofrontal cortex, and amygdala, *Chemical Senses* **30**: 401–419.

Kadohisa, M., Rolls, E. T. and Verhagen, J. V. (2005b). The primate amygdala: neuronal representations of the viscosity, fat texture, grittiness and taste of foods, *Neuroscience* **132**: 33–48.

Kadohisa, M., Kusunoki, M., Mitchell, D. J., Bhatia, C., Buckley, M. J. and Duncan, J. (2023). Frontal and temporal coding dynamics in successive steps of complex behavior, *Neuron* **111**: 430–443 e3.

Kagel, J. H., Battalio, R. C. and Green, L. (1995). *Economic Choice Theory: An Experimental Analysis of Animal Behaviour*, Cambridge University Press, Cambridge.

Kamps, F. S., Julian, J. B., Kubilius, J., Kanwisher, N. and Dilks, D. D. (2016). The occipital place area represents the local elements of scenes, *Neuroimage* **132**: 417–424.

Kandel, E. R., Koester, J. D., Mack, S. H. and Siegelbaum, S. A. (2021). *Principles of Neural Science*, 6 edn, McGraw-Hill, New York.

Kanske, P., Bockler, A. and Singer, T. (2017). Models, mechanisms and moderators dissociating empathy and theory of mind, *Curr Top Behav Neurosci* **30**: 193–206.

Kanter, I. and Sompolinsky, H. (1987). Associative recall of memories without errors, *Physical Review A* **35**: 380–392.

Kanwisher, N., McDermott, J. and Chun, M. M. (1997). The fusiform face area: A module in human extrastriate cortex specialized for face perception, *Journal Of Neuroscience* **17**: 4302–4311.

Karabanov, A. N., Paine, R., Chao, C. C., Schulze, K., Scott, B., Hallett, M. and Mishkin, M. (2015). Participation of the classical speech areas in auditory long-term memory, *PLoS One* **10**: e0119472.

Karno, M., Golding, J. M., Sorenson, S. B. and Burnam, M. A. (1988). The epidemiology of obsessive-compulsive disorder in five US communities, *Archives of General Psychiatry* **45**: 1094–1099.

Karthik, S., Sharma, L. P. and Narayanaswamy, J. C. (2020). Investigating the role of glutamate in obsessive-compulsive disorder: current perspectives, *Neuropsychiatr Dis Treat* **16**: 1003–1013.

Kastner, S., Chen, Q., Jeong, S. K. and Mruczek, R. E. B. (2017). A brief comparative review of primate posterior parietal cortex: A novel hypothesis on the human toolmaker, *Neuropsychologia* **105**: 123–134.

Kato, T. (2019). Current understanding of bipolar disorder: Toward integration of biological basis and treatment strategies, *Psychiatry Clin Neurosci* **73**: 526–540.

Kayaert, G., Biederman, I. and Vogels, R. (2005a). Representation of regular and irregular shapes in macaque inferotemporal cortex, *Cerebral Cortex* **15**: 1308–1321.

Kayaert, G., Biederman, I., Op de Beeck, H. P. and Vogels, R. (2005b). Tuning for shape dimensions in macaque inferior temporal cortex, *Eur J Neurosci* **22**: 212–24.

Kelley, A. E. (2004). Ventral striatal control of appetitive motivation: role in ingestive behaviour and reward-related learning, *Neuroscience and Biobehavioral Reviews* **27**: 765–776.

Kelley, A. E. and Berridge, K. C. (2002). The neuroscience of natural rewards: relevance to addictive drugs, *Journal of Neuroscience* **22**: 3306–3311.

Kelly, C., Uddin, L. Q., Shehzad, Z., Margulies, D. S., Castellanos, F. X., Milham, M. P. and Petrides, M. (2010). Broca's region: linking human brain functional connectivity data and non-human primate tracing anatomy studies, *Eur J Neurosci* **32**: 383–98.

Kelly, K. M., Nadon, N. L., Morrison, J. H., Thibault, O., Barnes, C. A. and Blalock, E. M. (2006). The neurobiology of aging, *Epilepsy Research* **68, Supplement 1**: S5–S20.

Kemmerer, D. (2015). *Cognitive Neuroscience of Language*, Psychology Press, New York.

Kemmerer, D. (2019). Grammatical categories, *in* G. I. d. Zubicaray and N. O. Schiller (eds), *The Oxford Handbook of Neurolinguistics*, Oxford University Press, Oxford, pp. 1–33.

Kemp, J. M. and Powell, T. P. S. (1970). The cortico-striate projections in the monkey, *Brain* **93**: 525–546.

Kennedy, D. P. and Adolphs, R. (2011). Reprint of: Impaired fixation to eyes following amygdala damage arises from abnormal bottom-up attention, *Neuropsychologia* **49**: 589–95.

Kennerley, S. W. and Wallis, J. D. (2009). Encoding of reward and space during a working memory task in the orbitofrontal cortex and anterior cingulate sulcus, *Journal of Neurophysiology* **102**: 3352–3364.

Kennerley, S. W., Walton, M. E., Behrens, T. E., Buckley, M. J. and Rushworth, M. F. (2006). Optimal decision making and the anterior cingulate cortex, *Nature Neuroscience* **9**: 940–947.

Kennerley, S. W., Behrens, T. E. and Wallis, J. D. (2011). Double dissociation of value computations in orbitofrontal and anterior cingulate neurons, *Nature Neuroscience* **14**: 1581–1589.

Kennis, M., Rademaker, A. R. and Geuze, E. (2013). Neural correlates of personality: an integrative review, *Neuroscience and Biobehavioural Reviews* **37**: 73–95.

Kesner, R. P. (1998). Neural mediation of memory for time: role of hippocampus and medial prefrontal cortex, *Psychological Bulletin Reviews* **5**: 585–596.

Kesner, R. P. (2018). An analysis of dentate gyrus function (an update), *Behav Brain Res* **354**: 84–91.

Kesner, R. P. and Gilbert, P. E. (2006). The role of the medial caudate nucleus, but not the hippocampus, in a delayed-matching-to sample task for motor response, *European Journal of Neuroscience* **23**: 1888–1894.

Kesner, R. P. and Rolls, E. T. (2001). Role of long term synaptic modification in short term memory, *Hippocampus* **11**: 240–250.

Kesner, R. P. and Rolls, E. T. (2015). A computational theory of hippocampal function, and tests of the theory: new developments, *Neuroscience and Biobehavioral Reviews* **48**: 92–147.

Kesner, R. P. and Warthen, D. K. (2010). Implications of CA3 NMDA and opiate receptors for spatial pattern completion in rats, *Hippocampus* **20**: 550–7.

Kesner, R. P., Gilbert, P. E. and Barua, L. A. (2002). The role of the hippocampus in memory for the temporal order of a sequence of odors, *Behavioral Neuroscience* **116**: 286–290.

Kesner, R. P., Lee, I. and Gilbert, P. (2004). A behavioral assessment of hippocampal function based on a subregional analysis, *Reviews in the Neurosciences* **15**: 333–351.

Kesner, R. P., Hunsaker, M. R. and Gilbert, P. E. (2005). The role of CA1 in the acquisition of an object-trace-odor paired associate task, *Behavioral Neuroscience* **119**: 781–786.

Kesner, R. P., Hunsaker, M. R. and Warthen, M. W. (2008). The CA3 subregion of the hippocampus is critical for episodic memory processing by means of relational encoding in rats, *Behavioral Neuroscience* **122**: 1217–1225.

Kesner, R. P., Hunsaker, M. R. and Ziegler, W. (2011). The role of the dorsal and ventral hippocampus in olfactory working memory, *Neurobiol Learn Mem* **96**: 361–6.

Kesner, R. P., Hui, X., Sommer, T., Wright, C., Barrera, V. R. and Fanselow, M. S. (2014). The role of postnatal neurogenesis in supporting remote memory and spatial metric processing, *Hippocampus* **24**: 1663–71.

Keysers, C. and Perrett, D. I. (2002). Visual masking and RSVP reveal neural competition, *Trends in Cognitive Sciences* **6**: 120–125.

Keysers, C. and Perrett, D. I. (2004). Demystifying social cognition: a Hebbian perspective, *Trends in Cognitive Sciences* **8**: 501–507.

Keysers, C., Xiao, D., Foldiak, P. and Perrett, D. (2001). The speed of sight, *Journal of Cognitive Neuroscience* **13**: 90–101.

Khalil, H. (1996). *Nonlinear Systems*, Prentice Hall, Upper Saddle River, NJ.

Khandhadia, A. P., Murphy, A. P., Romanski, L. M., Bizley, J. K. and Leopold, D. A. (2021). Audiovisual integration in macaque face patch neurons, *Curr Biol* **31**: 1826–1835 e3.

Kheradpisheh, S. R., Ganjtabesh, M., Thorpe, S. J. and Masquelier, T. (2018). STDP-based spiking deep convolutional neural networks for object recognition, *Neural Netw* **99**: 56–67.

Kievit, J. and Kuypers, H. G. J. M. (1975). Subcortical afferents to the frontal lobe in the rhesus monkey studied by means of retrograde horseradish peroxidase transport, *Brain Research* **85**: 261–266.

Kikuchi, Y., Horwitz, B., Mishkin, M. and Rauschecker, J. P. (2014). Processing of harmonics in the lateral belt of macaque auditory cortex, *Front Neurosci* **8**: 204.

Killcross, S. and Coutureau, E. (2003). Coordination of actions and habits in the medial prefrontal cortex of rats, *Cerebral Cortex* **13**: 400–408.

Killcross, S., Robbins, T. and Everitt, B. (1997). Different types of fear-conditioned behaviour mediated by separate nuclei within amygdala, *Nature* **388**: 377–380.

Killian, N. J., Jutras, M. J. and Buffalo, E. A. (2012). A map of visual space in the primate entorhinal cortex, *Nature* **491**: 761–4.

Kim, H., Shimojo, S. and O'Doherty, J. P. (2006). Is avoiding an aversive outcome rewarding? Neural substrates of avoidance learning in the human brain, *PLoS Biol* **4**: e233.

Kim, H. F. and Hikosaka, O. (2015). Parallel basal ganglia circuits for voluntary and automatic behaviour to reach rewards, *Brain* **138**: 1776–800.

Kim, H. F., Ghazizadeh, A. and Hikosaka, O. (2015a). Dopamine neurons encoding long-term memory of object value for habitual behavior, *Cell* **163**: 1165–1175.

Kim, J. (2011). *Philosophy of Mind*, 3 edn, Westview Press, Boulder, CO, USA.

Kim, J., Delcasso, S. and Lee, I. (2011). Neural correlates of object-in-place learning in hippocampus and prefrontal cortex, *J Neurosci* **31**: 16991–7006.

Kim, J. G. and Biederman, I. (2012). Greater sensitivity to nonaccidental than metric changes in the relations between simple shapes in the lateral occipital cortex, *Neuroimage* **63**: 1818–26.

Kim, J. G., Aminoff, E. M., Kastner, S. and Behrmann, M. (2015b). A neural basis for developmental topographic disorientation, *J Neurosci* **35**: 12954–69.

Kim, T., Bair, W. and Pasupathy, A. (2019). Neural coding for shape and texture in macaque area V4, *J Neurosci* **39**: 4760–4774.

Kircher, T. T. and Thienel, R. (2005). Functional brain imaging of symptoms and cognition in schizophrenia, *Progress in Brain Research* **150**: 299–308.

Kircher, T. T., Senior, C., Phillips, M. L., Benson, P. J., Bullmore, E. T., Brammer, M., Simmons, A., Williams, S. C., Bartels, M. and David, A. S. (2000). Towards a functional neuroanatomy of self processing: effects of faces and words, *Brain Res Cogn Brain Res* **10**: 133–44.

Kircher, T. T., Brammer, M., Bullmore, E., Simmons, A., Bartels, M. and David, A. S. (2002). The neural correlates of intentional and incidental self processing, *Neuropsychologia* **40**: 683–92.

Kirkwood, A., Dudek, S. M., Gold, J. T., Aizenman, C. D. and Bear, M. F. (1993). Common forms of synaptic plasticity in the hippocampus and neocortex "in vitro", *Science* **260**: 1518–1521.

Kjaer, T. W., Hertz, J. A. and Richmond, B. J. (1994). Decoding cortical neuronal signals: network models, information estimation and spatial tuning, *Journal of Computational Neuroscience* **1**: 109–139.

Klam, F. and Graf, W. (2003). Vestibular response kinematics in posterior parietal cortex neurons of macaque monkeys, *Eur J Neurosci* **18**: 995–1010.

Kleckner, I. R., Zhang, J., Touroutoglou, A., Chanes, L., Xia, C., Simmons, W. K., Quigley, K. S., Dickerson, B. C. and Barrett, L. F. (2017). Evidence for a large-scale brain system supporting allostasis and interoception in humans, *Nat Hum Behav* **1**: 0069.

Klein-Flugge, M. C., Bongioanni, A. and Rushworth, M. F. S. (2022a). Medial and orbital frontal cortex in decision-making and flexible behavior, *Neuron* **110**: 2743–2770.

Klein-Flugge, M. C., Jensen, D. E. A., Takagi, Y., Priestley, L., Verhagen, L., Smith, S. M. and Rushworth, M. F. S. (2022b). Relationship between nuclei-specific amygdala connectivity and mental health dimensions in humans, *Nat Hum Behav* **6**: 1705–1722.

Kleinfeld, D. (1986). Sequential state generation by model neural networks, *Proceedings of the National Academy of Sciences of the USA* **83**: 9469–9473.

Klingner, C. M. and Witte, O. W. (2018). Somatosensory deficits, *Handb Clin Neurol* **151**: 185–206.

Kluver, H. and Bucy, P. C. (1939). Preliminary analysis of functions of the temporal lobe in monkeys, *Archives of Neurology and Psychiatry* **42**: 979–1000.

Knierim, J. J. and Neunuebel, J. P. (2016). Tracking the flow of hippocampal computation: Pattern separation, pattern completion, and attractor dynamics, *Neurobiology of Learning and Memory* **129**: 38–49.

Knierim, J. J. and Rao, G. (2003). Distal landmarks and hippocampal place cells: effects of relative translation versus rotation, *Hippocampus* **13**: 604–17.

Knierim, J. J., Neunuebel, J. P. and Deshmukh, S. S. (2014). Functional correlates of the lateral and medial entorhinal cortex: objects, path integration and local-global reference frames, *Philosophical Transactions of the Royal Society London B Biological Sciences* **369**: 20130369.

Knudsen, E. I. (2011). Control from below: the role of a midbrain network in spatial attention, *European Journal of Neuroscience* **33**: 1961–1972.

Knutson, B., Adams, C. M., Fong, G. W. and Hommer, D. (2001). Anticipation of increasing monetary reward selectively recruits nucleus accumbens, *Journal of Neuroscience* **21**: 1–5.

Knutson, B., Delgado, M. R. and Phillips, E. M. (2009). Representation of subjective value in the striatum, *in* P. W. Glimcher, C. F. Camerer, E. Fehr and R. A. Poldrack (eds), *Neuroeconomics. Decision Making and the Brain*, Academic Press, London, chapter 25, pp. 389–406.

Kobayashi, Y. and Amaral, D. G. (2007). Macaque monkey retrosplenial cortex: III. Cortical efferents, *J Comp Neurol* **502**: 810–33.

Kocagoncu, E., Clarke, A., Devereux, B. J. and Tyler, L. K. (2017). Decoding the cortical dynamics of sound-meaning mapping, *J Neurosci* **37**: 1312–1319.

Koch, C. (1999). *Biophysics of Computation*, Oxford University Press, Oxford.

Koch, K. W. and Fuster, J. M. (1989). Unit activity in monkey parietal cortex related to haptic perception and temporary memory, *Experimental Brain Research* **76**: 292–306.

Koenderink, J. J. (1990). *Solid Shape*, MIT Press, Cambridge, MA.

Koenderink, J. J. and Van Doorn, A. J. (1979). The internal representation of solid shape with respect to vision, *Biological Cybernetics* **32**: 211–217.

Koenderink, J. J. and van Doorn, A. J. (1991). Affine structure from motion, *Journal of the Optical Society of America, A* **8**: 377–385.

Kohonen, T. (1977). *Associative Memory: A System Theoretical Approach*, Springer, New York.

Kohonen, T. (1982). Clustering, taxonomy, and topological maps of patterns, *in* M. Lang (ed.), *Proceedings of the Sixth International Conference on Pattern Recognition*, IEEE Computer Society Press, Silver Spring, MD, pp. 114–125.

Kohonen, T. (1988). *Self-Organization and Associative Memory*, 2nd edn, Springer-Verlag, New York.

Kohonen, T. (1989). *Self-Organization and Associative Memory*, 3rd (1984, 1st edn; 1988, 2nd edn) edn, Springer-Verlag, Berlin.

Kohonen, T. (1995). *Self-Organizing Maps*, Springer-Verlag, Berlin.

Kohonen, T., Oja, E. and Lehtio, P. (1981). Storage and processing of information in distributed memory systems, *in* G. E. Hinton and J. A. Anderson (eds), *Parallel Models of Associative Memory*, Erlbaum, Hillsdale, NJ, chapter 4, pp. 105–143.

Kokrashvili, Z., Mosinger, B. and Margolskee, R. F. (2009a). T1r3 and alpha-gustducin in gut regulate secretion of glucagon-like peptide-1, *Ann N Y Acad Sci* **1170**: 91–4.

Kokrashvili, Z., Mosinger, B. and Margolskee, R. F. (2009b). Taste signaling elements expressed in gut enteroendocrine cells regulate nutrient-responsive secretion of gut hormones, *Am J Clin Nutr* **90**: 822S–825S.

Kolb, B. and Whishaw, I. Q. (2021). *Fundamentals of Human Neuropsychology*, 8th edn, MacMillan, New York.

Kolling, N., Wittmann, M. K., Behrens, T. E., Boorman, E. D., Mars, R. B. and Rushworth, M. F. (2016). Value, search, persistence and model updating in anterior cingulate cortex, *Nat Neurosci* **19**: 1280–5.

Kolster, H., Peeters, R. and Orban, G. A. (2010). The retinotopic organization of the human middle temporal area MT/V5 and its cortical neighbors, *J Neurosci* **30**: 9801–20.

Komorowski, R. W., Manns, J. R. and Eichenbaum, H. (2009). Robust conjunctive item-place coding by hippocampal neurons parallels learning what happens where, *J Neurosci* **29**: 9918–29.

Kondo, H., Saleem, K. S. and Price, J. L. (2003). Differential connections of the temporal pole with the orbital and medial prefrontal networks in macaque monkeys, *J Comp Neurol* **465**: 499–523.

Kondo, H., Lavenex, P. and Amaral, D. G. (2009). Intrinsic connections of the macaque monkey hippocampal formation: II. CA3 connections, *Journal of Comparative Neurology* **515**: 349–377.

Konopaske, G. T., Lange, N., Coyle, J. T. and Benes, F. M. (2014). Prefrontal cortical dendritic spine pathology in schizophrenia and bipolar disorder, *JAMA Psychiatry* **71**: 1323–31.

Koob, G. F. and Volkow, N. D. (2016). Neurobiology of addiction: a neurocircuitry analysis, *Lancet Psychiatry* **3**: 760–73.

Kornblith, S., Cheng, X., Ohayon, S. and Tsao, D. Y. (2013). A network for scene processing in the macaque temporal lobe, *Neuron* **79**: 766–81.

Kosar, E., Grill, H. J. and Norgren, R. (1986). Gustatory cortex in the rat. II. Thalamocortical projections, *Brain Research* **379**: 342–352.

Koski, L. and Paus, T. (2000). Functional connectivity of anterior cingulate cortex within human frontal lobe: a brain mapping meta-analysis, *Experimental Brain Research* **133**: 55–65.

Kostadinov, D. and Hausser, M. (2022). Reward signals in the cerebellum: Origins, targets, and functional implications, *Neuron* **110**: 1290–1303.

Kourtzi, Z. and Connor, C. E. (2011). Neural representations for object perception: structure, category, and adaptive coding, *Annu Rev Neurosci* **34**: 45–67.

Kovacs, G., Vogels, R. and Orban, G. A. (1995). Cortical correlate of pattern backward masking, *Proceedings of the National Academy of Sciences USA* **92**: 5587–5591.

Kraus, B. J., Robinson, R. J., White, J. A., Eichenbaum, H. and Hasselmo, M. E. (2013). Hippocampal "time cells": time versus path integration, *Neuron* **78**: 1090–1101.

Kraus, B. J., Brandon, M. P., Robinson, R. J., Connerney, M. A., Hasselmo, M. E. and Eichenbaum, H. (2015). During running in place, grid cells integrate elapsed time and distance run, *Neuron* **88**: 578–89.

Kravitz, D. J., Saleem, K. S., Baker, C. I. and Mishkin, M. (2011). A new neural framework for visuospatial processing, *Nat Rev Neurosci* **12**: 217–30.

Kravitz, D. J., Saleem, K. S., Baker, C. I., Ungerleider, L. G. and Mishkin, M. (2013). The ventral visual pathway: an expanded neural framework for the processing of object quality, *Trends Cogn Sci* **17**: 26–49.

Krebs, J. R. and Davies, N. B. (1991). *Behavioural Ecology*, 3rd edn, Blackwell, Oxford.

Kreiman, G., Koch, C. and Fried, I. (2000). Category-specific visual responses of single neurons in the human medial temporal lobe, *Nat Neurosci* **3**: 946–53.

Kringelbach, M. L. and Deco, G. (2020). Brain states and transitions: insights from computational neuroscience, *Cell Rep* **32**: 108128.

Kringelbach, M. L. and Rolls, E. T. (2003). Neural correlates of rapid reversal learning in a simple model of human social interaction, *Neuroimage* **20**: 1371–1383.

Kringelbach, M. L. and Rolls, E. T. (2004). The functional neuroanatomy of the human orbitofrontal cortex: evidence from neuroimaging and neuropsychology, *Progress in Neurobiology* **72**: 341–372.

Kringelbach, M. L., O'Doherty, J., Rolls, E. T. and Andrews, C. (2003). Activation of the human orbitofrontal cortex to a liquid food stimulus is correlated with its subjective pleasantness., *Cerebral Cortex* **13**: 1064–1071.

Kringelbach, M. L., McIntosh, A. R., Ritter, P., Jirsa, V. K. and Deco, G. (2015). The rediscovery of slowness: exploring the timing of cognition, *Trends Cogn Sci* **19**: 616–628.

Kroes, M. C., Schiller, D., LeDoux, J. E. and Phelps, E. A. (2016). Translational approaches targeting reconsolidation, *Curr Top Behav Neurosci* **28**: 197–230.

Kropff, E. and Treves, A. (2005). The storage capacity of Potts models for semantic memory retrieval, *Journal of Statistical Mechanics: Theory and Experiment* **2005**: P08010.

Kropff, E. and Treves, A. (2008). The emergence of grid cells: Intelligent design or just adaptation?, *Hippocampus* **18**: 1256–69.

Kropff, E., Carmichael, J. E., Moser, M. B. and Moser, E. I. (2015). Speed cells in the medial entorhinal cortex, *Nature* **523**: 419–24.

Kubota, Y. (2014). Untangling GABAergic wiring in the cortical microcircuit, *Current Opinion in Neurobiology* **26**: 7–14.

Kuhn, R. (1990). Statistical mechanics of neural networks near saturation, *in* L. Garrido (ed.), *Statistical Mechanics of Neural Networks*, Springer-Verlag, Berlin.

Kuhn, R., Bos, S. and van Hemmen, J. L. (1991). Statistical mechanics for networks of graded response neurons, *Physical Review A* **243**: 2084–2087.

Kuwabara, M., Kang, N., Holy, T. E. and Padoa-Schioppa, C. (2020). Neural mechanisms of economic choices in mice, *Elife* **9**: e49669.

Kuznetsov, Y. A. (2013). *Elements of applied bifurcation theory*, Vol. 112, Springer Science and Business Media, New York.

Lai, M. C., Lombardo, M. V. and Baron-Cohen, S. (2014). Autism, *Lancet* **383**: 896–910.

Lally, N., Nugent, A. C., Luckenbaugh, D. A., Niciu, M. J., Roiser, J. P. and Zarate, C. A., J. (2015). Neural correlates of change in major depressive disorder anhedonia following open-label ketamine, *Journal of Psychopharmacology* **29**: 596–607.

Land, M. F. (1999). Motion and vision: why animals move their eyes, *Journal of Comparative Physiology A* **185**: 341–352.

Land, M. F. and Collett, T. S. (1997). A survey of active vision in invertebrates, *in* M. V. Srinivasan and S. Venkatesh (eds), *From Living Eyes to Seeing Machines*, Oxford University Press, Oxford, pp. 16–36.

Lane, R. D., Reiman, E. M., Ahern, G. L., Schwartz, G. E. and Davidson, R. J. (1997a). Neuroanatomical correlates of happiness, sadness, and disgust, *American Journal of Psychiatry* **154**: 926–933.

Lane, R. D., Reiman, E. M., Bradley, M. M., Lang, P. J., Ahern, G. L., Davidson, R. J. and Schwartz, G. E. (1997b). Neuroanatomical correlates of pleasant and unpleasant emotion, *Neuropsychologia* **35**: 1437–1444.

Lane, R. D., Reiman, E., Axelrod, B., Yun, L.-S., Holmes, A. H. and Schwartz, G. (1998). Neural correlates of levels of emotional awareness. Evidence of an interaction between emotion and attention in the anterior cingulate cortex, *Journal of Cognitive Neuroscience* **10**: 525–535.

Lanthorn, T., Storm, J. and Andersen, P. (1984). Current-to-frequency transduction in CA1 hippocampal pyramidal cells: slow prepotentials dominate the primary range firing, *Experimental Brain Research* **53**: 431–443.

Lassalle, J. M., Bataille, T. and Halley, H. (2000). Reversible inactivation of the hippocampal mossy fiber synapses in mice impairs spatial learning, but neither consolidation nor memory retrieval, in the Morris navigation task, *Neurobiology of Learning and Memory* **73**: 243–257.

Lau, H. (2022). *In Consciousness We Trust: the cognitive neuroscience of conscious experience*, Oxford University Press, Oxford.

Lau, H. and Rosenthal, D. (2011). Empirical support for higher-order theories of conscious awareness, *Trends Cogn Sci* **15**: 365–73.

Lavenex, P. and Amaral, D. G. (2000). Hippocampal-neocortical interaction: a hierarchy of associativity, *Hippocampus* **10**: 420–430.

Lavenex, P. B., Amaral, D. G. and Lavenex, P. (2006). Hippocampal lesion prevents spatial relational learning in adult macaque monkeys, *J Neurosci* **26**: 4546–58.

Lavenex, P., Suzuki, W. A. and Amaral, D. G. (2004). Perirhinal and parahippocampal cortices of the macaque monkey: Intrinsic projections and interconnections, *Journal of Comparative Neurology* **472**: 371–394.

Laxton, A. W., Neimat, J. S., Davis, K. D., Womelsdorf, T., Hutchison, W. D., Dostrovsky, J. O., Hamani, C., Mayberg, H. S. and Lozano, A. M. (2013). Neuronal coding of implicit emotion categories in the subcallosal cortex in patients with depression, *Biological Psychiatry* **74**: 714–719.

Leaver, A. M. and Rauschecker, J. P. (2016). Functional topography of human auditory cortex, *J Neurosci* **36**: 1416–28.

LeCun, Y., Kavukcuoglu, K. and Farabet, C. (2010). Convolutional networks and applications in vision, *2010 IEEE International Symposium on Circuits and Systems* pp. 253–256.

LeCun, Y., Bengio, Y. and Hinton, G. (2015). Deep learning, *Nature* **521**: 436–444.

LeDoux, J. (1994). Emotion, memory and the brain, *Scientific American* **270**: 32–39.

LeDoux, J. (1996). *The Emotional Brain*, Simon and Schuster, New York.

LeDoux, J. (2012a). Rethinking the emotional brain, *Neuron* **73**: 653–76.

LeDoux, J. E. (1992). Emotion and the amygdala, *in* J. P. Aggleton (ed.), *The Amygdala*, Wiley-Liss, New York, chapter 12, pp. 339–351.

LeDoux, J. E. (1995). Emotion: clues from the brain, *Annu Rev Psychol* **46**: 209–35.

LeDoux, J. E. (2000). Emotion circuits in the brain, *Annual Review of Neuroscience* **23**: 155–184.

LeDoux, J. E. (2008). Emotional coloration of consciousness: how feelings come about, *in* L. Weiskrantz and M. Davies (eds), *Frontiers of Consciousness*, Oxford University Press, Oxford, pp. 69–130.

LeDoux, J. E. (2012b). Rethinking the emotional brain, *Neuron* **73**: 653–676.

LeDoux, J. E. (2017). Semantics, surplus meaning, and the science of fear, *Trends Cogn Sci* **21**: 303–306.

LeDoux, J. E. (2020). Thoughtful feelings, *Curr Biol* **30**: R619–R623.

LeDoux, J. E. and Daw, N. D. (2018). Surviving threats: neural circuit and computational implications of a new taxonomy of defensive behaviour, *Nat Rev Neurosci* **19**: 269–282.

LeDoux, J. E. and Pine, D. S. (2016). Using neuroscience to help understand fear and anxiety: a two-system framework, *Am J Psychiatry* **173**: 1083–1093.

LeDoux, J., Brown, R., Pine, D. and Hofmann, S. (2018). Know thyself: well-being and subjective experience, *Cerebrum* **2018**: https://www.ncbi.nlm.nih.gov/pmc/articles/PMC6353121/.

Lee, H., Grosse, R., Ranganath, R. and Ng, A. Y. (2011). Unsupervised learning of hierarchical representations with convolutional deep belief networks, *Communications of the ACM* **54**: 95–103.

Lee, I. and Kesner, R. P. (2002). Differential contribution of NMDA receptors in hippocampal subregions to spatial working memory, *Nature Neuroscience* **5**: 162–168.

Lee, I. and Kesner, R. P. (2003a). Differential roles of dorsal hippocampal subregions in spatial working memory with short versus intermediate delay, *Behavioral Neuroscience* **117**: 1044–1053.

Lee, I. and Kesner, R. P. (2003b). Time-dependent relationship between the dorsal hippocampus and the prefrontal cortex in spatial memory, *Journal of Neuroscience* **23**: 1517–1523.

Lee, I. and Kesner, R. P. (2004a). Differential contributions of dorsal hippocampal subregions to memory acquisition and retrieval in contextual fear-conditioning, *Hippocampus* **14**: 301–310.

Lee, I. and Kesner, R. P. (2004b). Encoding versus retrieval of spatial memory: double dissociation between the dentate gyrus and the perforant path inputs into CA3 in the dorsal hippocampus, *Hippocampus* **14**: 66–76.

Lee, I., Rao, G. and Knierim, J. J. (2004). A double dissociation between hippocampal subfields: differential time course of CA3 and CA1 place cells for processing changed environments, *Neuron* **42**: 803–815.

Lee, I., Jerman, T. S. and Kesner, R. P. (2005). Disruption of delayed memory for a sequence of spatial locations following CA1 or CA3 lesions of the dorsal hippocampus, *Neurobiology of Learning and Memory* **84**: 138–147.

Lee, T. S. (1996). Image representation using 2D Gabor wavelets, *IEEE Transactions on Pattern Analysis and Machine Intelligence* **18,10**: 959–971.

Leech, R. and Sharp, D. J. (2014). The role of the posterior cingulate cortex in cognition and disease, *Brain* **137**: 12–32.

Leech, R. and Smallwood, J. (2019). The posterior cingulate cortex: Insights from structure and function, *Handb Clin Neurol* **166**: 73–85.

Lehky, S. R. and Tanaka, K. (2016). Neural representation for object recognition in inferotemporal cortex, *Curr Opin Neurobiol* **37**: 23–35.

Lehky, S. R., Sejnowski, T. J. and Desimone, R. (2005). Selectivity and sparseness in the responses of striate complex cells, *Vision Research* **45**: 57–73.

Lehn, H., Steffenach, H. A., van Strien, N. M., Veltman, D. J., Witter, M. P. and Haberg, A. K. (2009). A specific role of the human hippocampus in recall of temporal sequences, *Journal of Neuroscience* **29**: 3475–3484.

Leibo, J. Z., Liao, Q., Anselmi, F., Freiwald, W. A. and Poggio, T. (2017). View-tolerant face recognition and Hebbian learning imply mirror-symmetric neural tuning to head orientation, *Curr Biol* **27**: 62–67.

Leonard, C. M., Rolls, E. T., Wilson, F. A. W. and Baylis, G. C. (1985). Neurons in the amygdala of the monkey with responses selective for faces, *Behavioural Brain Research* **15**: 159–176.

Lerch, J. P., van der Kouwe, A. J., Raznahan, A., Paus, T., Johansen-Berg, H., Miller, K. L., Smith, S. M., Fischl, B. and Sotiropoulos, S. N. (2017). Studying neuroanatomy using MRI, *Nat Neurosci* **20**: 314–326.

Leung, H., Gore, J. and Goldman-Rakic, P. (2002). Sustained mnemonic response in the human middle frontal gyrus during on-line storage of spatial memoranda, *Journal of Cognitive Neuroscience* **14**: 659–671.

Leutgeb, J. K., Leutgeb, S., Moser, M. B. and Moser, E. I. (2007). Pattern separation in the dentate gyrus and CA3 of the hippocampus, *Science* **315**: 961–966.

Leutgeb, S. and Leutgeb, J. K. (2007). Pattern separation, pattern completion, and new neuronal codes within a continuous CA3 map, *Learn Mem* **14**: 745–57.

Leutgeb, S., Leutgeb, J. K., Treves, A., Moser, M. B. and Moser, E. I. (2004). Distinct ensemble codes in hippocampal areas CA3 and CA1, *Science* **305**: 1295–1298.

Leutgeb, S., Leutgeb, J. K., Barnes, C. A., Moser, E. I., McNaughton, B. L. and Moser, M. B. (2005a). Independent codes for spatial and episodic memory in hippocampal neuronal ensembles, *Science* **309**: 619–23.

Leutgeb, S., Leutgeb, J. K., Treves, A., Meyer, R., Barnes, C. A., McNaughton, B. L., Moser, M.-B. and Moser, E. I. (2005b). Progressive transformation of hippocampal neuronal representations in "morphed" environments, *Neuron* **48**: 345–358.

Leutgeb, S., Leutgeb, J. K., Moser, E. I. and Moser, M. B. (2006). Fast rate coding in hippocampal CA3 cell ensembles, *Hippocampus* **16**: 765–74.

LeVay, S., Wiesel, T. N. and Hubel, D. H. (1980). The development of ocular dominance columns in normal and visually deprived monkeys, *Journal of Comparative Neurology* **191**: 1–51.

Lever, C., Burton, S., Jeewajee, A., O'Keefe, J. and Burgess, N. (2009). Boundary vector cells in the subiculum of the hippocampal formation, *J Neurosci* **29**: 9771–7.

Levitt, J. B., Lund, J. S. and Yoshioka, T. (1996). Anatomical substrates for early stages in cortical processing of visual information in the macaque monkey, *Behavioural Brain Research* **76**: 5–19.

Levy, W. B. (1985). Associative changes in the synapse: LTP in the hippocampus, *in* W. B. Levy, J. A. Anderson and S. Lehmkuhle (eds), *Synaptic Modification, Neuron Selectivity, and Nervous System Organization*, Erlbaum, Hillsdale, NJ, chapter 1, pp. 5–33.

Levy, W. B. (1989). A computational approach to hippocampal function, *in* R. D. Hawkins and G. H. Bower (eds), *Computational Models of Learning in Simple Neural Systems*, Academic Press, San Diego, pp. 243–305.

Levy, W. B. and Baxter, R. A. (1996). Energy efficient neural codes, *Neural Computation* **8**: 531–543.

Levy, W. B. and Desmond, N. L. (1985). The rules of elemental synaptic plasticity, *in* W. B. Levy, J. A. Anderson and S. Lehmkuhle (eds), *Synaptic Modification, Neuron Selectivity, and Nervous System Organization*, Erlbaum, Hillsdale, NJ, chapter 6, pp. 105–121.

Levy, W. B., Colbert, C. M. and Desmond, N. L. (1990). Elemental adaptive processes of neurons and synapses: a statistical/computational perspective, *in* M. Gluck and D. Rumelhart (eds), *Neuroscience and Connectionist Theory*, Erlbaum, Hillsdale, NJ, chapter 5, pp. 187–235.

Levy, W. B., Wu, X. and Baxter, R. A. (1995). Unification of hippocampal function via computational/encoding considerations, *International Journal of Neural Systems* **6, Suppl.**: 71–80.

Lewis, D. A. (2014). Inhibitory neurons in human cortical circuits: substrate for cognitive dysfunction in schizophrenia, *Curr Opin Neurobiol* **26**: 22–6.

Li, C. S. and Cho, Y. K. (2006). Efferent projection from the bed nucleus of the stria terminalis suppresses activity of taste-responsive neurons in the hamster parabrachial nuclei, *American Journal of Physiology Regul Integr Comp Physiol* **291**: R914–R926.

Li, C. S., Cho, Y. K. and Smith, D. V. (2002). Taste responses of neurons in the hamster solitary nucleus are modulated by the central nucleus of the amygdala, *Journal of Neurophysiology* **88**: 2979–2992.

Li, H., Matsumoto, K. and Watanabe, H. (1999). Different effects of unilateral and bilateral hippocampal lesions in rats on the performance of radial maze and odor-paired associate tasks, *Brain Research Bulletin* **48**: 113–119.

Li, N. and DiCarlo, J. J. (2010). Unsupervised natural visual experience rapidly reshapes size-invariant object representation in inferior temporal cortex, *Neuron* **67**: 1062–75.

Li, N. and DiCarlo, J. J. (2012). Neuronal learning of invariant object representation in the ventral visual stream is not dependent on reward, *J Neurosci* **32**: 6611–20.

Li, Y. and Dulac, C. (2018). Neural coding of sex-specific social information in the mouse brain, *Curr Opin Neurobiol* **53**: 120–130.

Liddle, P. F. (1987). The symptoms of chronic schizophrenia: a re-examination of the positive-negative dichotomy, *British Journal of Psychiatry* **151**: 145–151.

Lillicrap, T. P., Santoro, A., Marris, L., Akerman, C. J. and Hinton, G. (2020). Backpropagation and the brain, *Nat Rev Neurosci* **21**: 335–346.

Lim, J. J. and Poppitt, S. D. (2019). How satiating are the 'satiety' peptides: a problem of pharmacology versus physiology in the development of novel foods for regulation of food intake, *Nutrients* **11**: doi: 10.3390/nu11071517.

Lisberger, S. G. and Thach, W. T. (2013). The cerebellum, *in* E. Kandel, J. H. Schwartz, T. M. Jessell, S. A. Siegelbaum and A. J. Hudspeth (eds), *Principles of Neural Science*, 5th edn, McGraw-Hill, New York, chapter 24, pp. 960–981.

Lisman, J. E., Fellous, J. M. and Wang, X. J. (1998). A role for NMDA-receptor channels in working memory, *Nature Neuroscience* **1**: 273–275.

Little, S. and Brown, P. (2020). Debugging adaptive deep brain stimulation for Parkinson's Disease, *Mov Disord* **35**: 555–561.

Little, W. A. (1974). The existence of persistent states in the brain, *Mathematical Bioscience* **19**: 101–120.

Liu, B., Tian, Q. and Gu, Y. (2021). Robust vestibular self-motion signals in macaque posterior cingulate region, *Elife* **10**: e64569.

Liu, Y. and Wang, X.-J. (2001). Spike-frequency adaptation of a generalized leaky integrate-and-fire model neuron, *Journal of Computational Neuroscience* **10**: 25–45.

Liuzzi, A. G., Bruffaerts, R. and Vandenberghe, R. (2019). The medial temporal written word processing system, *Cortex* **119**: 287–300.

Logothetis, N. K. and Sheinberg, D. L. (1996). Visual object recognition, *Annual Review of Neuroscience* **19**: 577–621.

Logothetis, N. K., Pauls, J., Bulthoff, H. H. and Poggio, T. (1994). View-dependent object recognition by monkeys, *Current Biology* **4**: 401–414.

Logothetis, N. K., Pauls, J. and Poggio, T. (1995). Shape representation in the inferior temporal cortex of monkeys, *Current Biology* **5**: 552–563.

Loh, M., Rolls, E. T. and Deco, G. (2007a). A dynamical systems hypothesis of schizophrenia, *PLoS Computational Biology* **3**: e228. doi:10.1371/journal.pcbi.0030228.

Loh, M., Rolls, E. T. and Deco, G. (2007b). Statistical fluctuations in attractor networks related to schizophrenia, *Pharmacopsychiatry* **40**: S78–84.

Long, M. A., Katlowitz, K. A., Svirsky, M. A., Clary, R. C., Byun, T. M., Majaj, N., Oya, H., Howard, M. A., r. and Greenlee, J. D. W. (2016). Functional segregation of cortical regions underlying speech timing and articulation, *Neuron* **89**: 1187–1193.

Loonen, A. J. and Ivanova, S. A. (2016). Circuits regulating pleasure and happiness: the evolution of the amygdalar-hippocampal-habenular connectivity in vertebrates, *Front Neurosci* **10**: 539.
Lowe, D. (1985). *Perceptual Organization and Visual Recognition*, Kluwer, Boston.
Lozano, A. M., Giacobbe, P., Hamani, C., Rizvi, S. J., Kennedy, S. H., Kolivakis, T. T., Debonnel, G., Sadikot, A. F., Lam, R. W., Howard, A. K., Ilcewicz-Klimek, M., Honey, C. R. and Mayberg, H. S. (2012). A multicenter pilot study of subcallosal cingulate area deep brain stimulation for treatment-resistant depression, *J Neurosurg* **116**: 315–22.
Lujan, J. L., Chaturvedi, A., Choi, K. S., Holtzheimer, P. E., Gross, R. E., Mayberg, H. S. and McIntyre, C. C. (2013). Tractography-activation models applied to subcallosal cingulate deep brain stimulation, *Brain Stimul* **6**: 737–9.
Luk, C. H. and Wallis, J. D. (2009). Dynamic encoding of responses and outcomes by neurons in medial prefrontal cortex, *Journal of Neuroscience* **29**: 7526–7539.
Luk, C. H. and Wallis, J. D. (2013). Choice coding in frontal cortex during stimulus-guided or action-guided decision-making, *Journal of Neuroscience* **33**: 1864–1871.
Lund, J. S. (1984). Spiny stellate neurons, *in* A. Peters and E. Jones (eds), *Cerebral Cortex, Vol. 1, Cellular Components of the Cerebral Cortex*, Plenum, New York, chapter 7, pp. 255–308.
Lundy, R. F., J. and Norgren, R. (2004). Activity in the hypothalamus, amygdala, and cortex generates bilateral and convergent modulation of pontine gustatory neurons, *Journal of Neurophysiology* **91**: 1143–1157.
Luo, Q., Ge, T., Grabenhorst, F., Feng, J. and Rolls, E. T. (2013). Attention-dependent modulation of cortical taste circuits revealed by Granger causality with signal-dependent noise, *PLoS Computational Biology* **9**: e1003265.
Luscher, C., Robbins, T. W. and Everitt, B. J. (2020). The transition to compulsion in addiction, *Nat Rev Neurosci* **21**: 247–263.
Luskin, M. B. and Price, J. L. (1983). The topographic organization of associational fibers of the olfactory system in the rat, including centrifugal fibers to the olfactory bulb, *Journal of Comparative Neurology* **216**: 264–291.
Lynch, G. and Gall, C. M. (2006). AMPAkines and the threefold path to cognitive enhancement, *Trends in Neuroscience* **29**: 554–562.
Lynch, M. A. (2004). Long-term potentiation and memory, *Physiological Reviews* **84**: 87–136.
Ma, Q., Rolls, E. T., Huang, C.-C., Cheng, W. and Feng, J. (2022a). Extensive cortical functional connectivity of the human hippocampal memory system, *Cortex* **147**: 83–101.
Ma, Q., Wang, H., Rolls, E. T., Xiang, S., Li, J., Li, Y., Zhou, Q., Cheng, W. and Li, F. (2022b). Lower gestational age is associated with lower cortical volume and cognitive and educational performance in adolescence, *BMC Med* **20**: 424.
Ma, Y. (2015). Neuropsychological mechanism underlying antidepressant effect: a systematic meta-analysis, *Molecular Psychiatry* **20**: 311–319.
Maaswinkel, H., Jarrard, L. E. and Whishaw, I. Q. (1999). Hippocampectomized rats are impaired in homing by path integration, *Hippocampus* **9**: 553–561.
Macdonald, C. J., Lepage, K. Q., Eden, U. T. and Eichenbaum, H. (2011). Hippocampal "time cells" bridge the gap in memory for discontiguous events, *Neuron* **71**: 737–749.
MacDonald, M. L., Alhassan, J., Newman, J. T., Richard, M., Gu, H., Kelly, R. M., Sampson, A. R., Fish, K. N., Penzes, P., Wills, Z. P., Lewis, D. A. and Sweet, R. A. (2017). Selective loss of smaller spines in schizophrenia, *Am J Psychiatry* **174**: 586–594.
MacGregor, R. J. (1987). *Neural and Brain Modelling*, Academic Press, San Diego, CA.
MacKay, D. M. and McCulloch, W. S. (1952). The limiting information capacity of a neuronal link, *Bulletin of Mathematical Biophysics* **14**: 127–135.
Maddison, S., Wood, R. J., Rolls, E. T., Rolls, B. J. and Gibbs, J. (1980). Drinking in the rhesus monkey: peripheral factors, *J Comp Physiol Psychol* **94**: 365–74.
Madsen, J. and Kesner, R. P. (1995). The temporal-distance effect in subjects with dementia of the Alzheimer type, *Alzheimer's Disease and Associated Disorders* **9**: 94–100.
Maguire, E. A. (2001). The retrosplenial contribution to human navigation: a review of lesion and neuroimaging findings, *Scand J Psychol* **42**: 225–38.
Maguire, E. A. (2014). Memory consolidation in humans: new evidence and opportunities, *Exp Physiol* **99**: 471–86.
Maguire, E. A., Intraub, H. and Mullally, S. L. (2016). Scenes, spaces, and memory traces: what does the hippocampus do?, *Neuroscientist* **22**: 432–9.
Maier-Hein, K. H., Neher, P. F., Houde, J. C., Cote, M. A., Garyfallidis, E., Zhong, J., Chamberland, M., Yeh, F. C., Lin, Y. C., Ji, Q., Reddick, W. E., Glass, J. O., Chen, D. Q., Feng, Y., Gao, C., Wu, Y., Ma, J., He, R., Li, Q., Westin, C. F., Deslauriers-Gauthier, S., Gonzalez, J. O. O., Paquette, M., St-Jean, S., Girard, G., Rheault, F., Sidhu, J., Tax, C. M. W., Guo, F., Mesri, H. Y., David, S., Froeling, M., Heemskerk, A. M., Leemans, A., Bore, A., Pinsard, B., Bedetti, C., Desrosiers, M., Brambati, S., Doyon, J., Sarica, A., Vasta, R., Cerasa, A., Quattrone, A., Yeatman, J., Khan, A. R., Hodges, W., Alexander, S., Romascano, D., Barakovic, M., Auria, A., Esteban, O., Lemkaddem, A., Thiran, J. P., Cetingul, H. E., Odry, B. L., Mailhe, B., Nadar, M. S., Pizzagalli, F., Prasad, G., Villalon-Reina, J. E., Galvis, J., Thompson, P. M., Requejo, F. S., Laguna, P. L., Lacerda, L. M., Barrett, R.,

Dell'Acqua, F., Catani, M., Petit, L., Caruyer, E., Daducci, A., Dyrby, T. B., Holland-Letz, T., Hilgetag, C. C., Stieltjes, B. and Descoteaux, M. (2017). The challenge of mapping the human connectome based on diffusion tractography, *Nat Commun* **8**: 1349.

Maier, S. F. and Seligman, M. E. (2016). Learned helplessness at fifty: Insights from neuroscience, *Psychol Rev* **123**: 349–67.

Majaj, N. J., Hong, H., Solomon, E. A. and DiCarlo, J. J. (2015). Simple learned weighted sums of inferior temporal neuronal firing rates accurately predict human core object recognition performance, *J Neurosci* **35**: 13402–18.

Malkova, L. and Mishkin, M. (2003). One-trial memory for object-place associations after separate lesions of hippocampus and posterior parahippocampal region in the monkey, *Journal of Neuroscience* **23**: 1956–1965.

Malkova, L., Bachevalier, J., Mishkin, M. and Saunders, R. C. (2001). Neurotoxic lesions of perirhinal cortex impair visual recognition memory in rhesus monkeys, *Neuroreport* **12**: 1913–1917.

Malsburg, C. v. d. (1973). Self-organization of orientation-sensitive columns in the striate cortex, *Kybernetik* **14**: 85–100.

Malsburg, C. v. d. (1990). A neural architecture for the representation of scenes, in J. L. McGaugh, N. M. Weinburger and G. Lynch (eds), *Brain Organization and Memory: Cells, Systems and Circuits*, Oxford University Press, Oxford, chapter 18, pp. 356–372.

Maltbie, E. A., Kaundinya, G. S. and Howell, L. L. (2017). Ketamine and pharmacological imaging: use of functional magnetic resonance imaging to evaluate mechanisms of action, *Behav Pharmacol* **28**: 610–622.

Manohar, S. G. (2022). Computational neuroscience: a grand unifying theory?, *Brain* **145**: 1189–1190.

Mansouri, F. A., Egner, T. and Buckley, M. J. (2017a). Monitoring demands for executive control: shared functions between human and nonhuman primates, *Trends Neurosci* **40**: 15–27.

Mansouri, F. A., Koechlin, E., Rosa, M. G. P. and Buckley, M. J. (2017b). Managing competing goals - a key role for the frontopolar cortex, *Nat Rev Neurosci* **18**: 645–657.

Manwani, A. and Koch, C. (2001). Detecting and estimating signals over noisy and unreliable synapses: information-theoretic analysis, *Neural Computation* **13**: 1–33.

Mao, D., Avila, E., Caziot, B., Laurens, J., Dickman, J. D. and Angelaki, D. E. (2021). Spatial modulation of hippocampal activity in freely moving macaques, *Neuron* **109**: 3521–3534 e6.

Maravita, A. and Romano, D. (2018). The parietal lobe and tool use, *Handb Clin Neurol* **151**: 481–498.

Margolskee, R. F., Dyer, J., Kokrashvili, Z., Salmon, K. S., Ilegems, E., Daly, K., Maillet, E. L., Ninomiya, Y., Mosinger, B. and Shirazi-Beechey, S. P. (2007). T1R3 and gustducin in gut sense sugars to regulate expression of Na+-glucose cotransporter 1, *Proc Natl Acad Sci U S A* **104**: 15075–80.

Markov, N. T., Ercsey-Ravasz, M., Lamy, C., Ribeiro Gomes, A. R., Magrou, L., Misery, P., Giroud, P., Barone, P., Dehay, C., Toroczkai, Z., Knoblauch, K., Van Essen, D. C. and Kennedy, H. (2013). The role of long-range connections on the specificity of the macaque interareal cortical network, *Proceedings of the National Academy of Sciences USA* **110**: 5187–5192.

Markov, N. T., Ercsey-Ravasz, M. M., Ribeiro Gomes, A. R., Lamy, C., Magrou, L., Vezoli, J., Misery, P., Falchier, A., Quilodran, R., Gariel, M. A., Sallet, J., Gamanut, R., Huissoud, C., Clavagnier, S., Giroud, P., Sappey-Marinier, D., Barone, P., Dehay, C., Toroczkai, Z., Knoblauch, K., Van Essen, D. C. and Kennedy, H. (2014a). A weighted and directed interareal connectivity matrix for macaque cerebral cortex, *Cereb Cortex* **24**: 17–36.

Markov, N. T., Vezoli, J., Chameau, P., Falchier, A., Quilodran, R., Huissoud, C., Lamy, C., Misery, P., Giroud, P., Ullman, S., Barone, P., Dehay, C., Knoblauch, K. and Kennedy, H. (2014b). Anatomy of hierarchy: Feedforward and feedback pathways in macaque visual cortex, *Journal of Comparative Neurology* **522**: 225–259.

Markram, H. and Segal, M. (1992). The inositol 1,4,5-triphosphate pathway mediates cholinergic potentiation of rat hippocampal neuronal responses to NMDA, *Journal of Physiology* **447**: 513–533.

Markram, H. and Tsodyks, M. (1996). Redistribution of synaptic efficacy between neocortical pyramidal neurons, *Nature* **382**: 807–810.

Markram, H., Lübke, J., Frotscher, M. and Sakmann, B. (1997). Regulation of synaptic efficacy by coincidence of postsynaptic APs and EPSPs, *Science* **275**: 213–215.

Markram, H., Pikus, D., Gupta, A. and Tsodyks, M. (1998). Information processing with frequency-dependent synaptic connections, *Neuropharmacology* **37**: 489–500.

Markram, H., Gerstner, W. and Sjöström, P. J. (2012). Spike-timing-dependent plasticity: a comprehensive overview, *Frontiers in Synaptic Neuroscience* **4**: 2.

Markram, H., Muller, E., Ramaswamy, S., Reimann, M. W., Abdellah, M., Sanchez, C. A., Ailamaki, A., Alonso-Nanclares, L., Antille, N., Arsever, S., Kahou, G. A., Berger, T. K., Bilgili, A., Buncic, N., Chalimourda, A., Chindemi, G., Courcol, J. D., Delalondre, F., Delattre, V., Druckmann, S., Dumusc, R., Dynes, J., Eilemann, S., Gal, E., Gevaert, M. E., Ghobril, J. P., Gidon, A., Graham, J. W., Gupta, A., Haenel, V., Hay, E., Heinis, T., Hernando, J. B., Hines, M., Kanari, L., Keller, D., Kenyon, J., Khazen, G., Kim, Y., King, J. G., Kisvarday, Z., Kumbhar, P., Lasserre, S., Le Be, J. V., Magalhaes, B. R., Merchan-Perez, A., Meystre, J., Morrice, B. R., Muller, J., Munoz-Cespedes, A., Muralidhar, S., Muthurasa, K., Nachbaur, D., Newton, T. H., Nolte, M., Ovcharenko, A., Palacios, J., Pastor, L., Perin, R., Ranjan, R., Riachi, I., Rodriguez, J. R., Riquelme, J. L., Rossert, C., Sfyrakis,

K., Shi, Y., Shillcock, J. C., Silberberg, G., Silva, R., Tauheed, F., Telefont, M., Toledo-Rodriguez, M., Trankler, T., Van Geit, W., Diaz, J. V., Walker, R., Wang, Y., Zaninetta, S. M., DeFelipe, J., Hill, S. L., Segev, I. and Schurmann, F. (2015). Reconstruction and simulation of neocortical microcircuitry, *Cell* **163**: 456–92.

Markus, E. J., Qin, Y. L., Leonard, B., Skaggs, W., McNaughton, B. L. and Barnes, C. A. (1995). Interactions between location and task affect the spatial and directional firing of hippocampal neurons, *Journal of Neuroscience* **15**: 7079–7094.

Marr, D. (1969). A theory of cerebellar cortex, *Journal of Physiology* **202**: 437–470.

Marr, D. (1970). A theory for cerebral cortex, *Proceedings of The Royal Society of London, Series B* **176**: 161–234.

Marr, D. (1971). Simple memory: a theory for archicortex, *Philosophical Transactions of The Royal Society of London, Series B* **262**: 23–81.

Marr, D. (1982). *Vision*, Freeman, San Francisco.

Marr, D. and Nishihara, H. K. (1978). Representation and recognition of the spatial organization of three dimensional structure, *Proceedings of the Royal Society of London B* **200**: 269–294.

Marreiros, A. C., Kiebel, S. J. and Friston, K. J. (2008). Dynamic causal modelling for fMRI: a two-state model, *Neuroimage* **39**: 269–78.

Marshall, J. (1951). Sensory disturbances in cortical wounds with special reference to pain, *Journal of Neurology, Neurosurgery and Psychiatry* **14**: 187–204.

Marslen-Wilson, W. D. and Welsh, A. (1978). Processing interactions and lexical access during word recognition in continuous speech, *Cognitive psychology* **10**: 29–63.

Marti, D., Deco, G., Mattia, M., Gigante, G. and Del Giudice, P. (2008). A fluctuation-driven mechanism for slow decision processes in reverberant networks, *PLoS ONE* **3**: e2534. doi:10.1371/journal.pone.0002534.

Martin, K. A. C. (1984). Neuronal circuits in cat striate cortex, *in* E. Jones and A. Peters (eds), *Cerebral Cortex, Vol. 2, Functional Properties of Cortical Cells*, Plenum, New York, chapter 9, pp. 241–284.

Martin, S. J., Grimwood, P. D. and Morris, R. G. (2000). Synaptic plasticity and memory: an evaluation of the hypothesis, *Annual Review of Neuroscience* **23**: 649–711.

Martinez, C. O., Do, V. H., Martinez, J. L. J. and Derrick, B. E. (2002). Associative long-term potentiation (LTP) among extrinsic afferents of the hippocampal CA3 region in vivo, *Brain Research* **940**: 86–94.

Martinez-Garcia, M., Rolls, E. T., Deco, G. and Romo, R. (2011). Neural and computational mechanisms of postponed decisions, *Proc Natl Acad Sci U S A* **108**: 11626–31.

Mascaro, M. and Amit, D. J. (1999). Effective neural response function for collective population states, *Network* **10**: 351–373.

Mason, A. and Larkman, A. (1990). Correlations between morphology and electrophysiology of pyramidal neurones in slices of rat visual cortex. I. Electrophysiology, *Journal of Neuroscience* **10**: 1415–1428.

Masuda, N. and Aihara, K. (2003). Ergodicity of spike trains: when does trial averaging make sense?, *Neural Computation* **15**: 1341–1372.

Matchin, W. and Hickok, G. (2020). The cortical organization of syntax, *Cereb Cortex* **30**: 1481–1498.

Matchin, W., Basilakos, A., Ouden, D. D., Stark, B. C., Hickok, G. and Fridriksson, J. (2022). Functional differentiation in the language network revealed by lesion-symptom mapping, *Neuroimage* **247**: 118778.

Mathiasen, M. L., O'Mara, S. M. and Aggleton, J. P. (2020). The anterior thalamic nuclei and nucleus reuniens: So similar but so different, *Neurosci Biobehav Rev* **119**: 268–280.

Matsumoto, K., Suzuki, W. and Tanaka, K. (2003). Neuronal correlates of goal-based motor selection in the prefrontal cortex, *Science* **301**: 229–232.

Matsumoto, M. and Hikosaka, O. (2009). Two types of dopamine neuron distinctly convey positive and negative motivational signals, *Nature* **459**: 837–841.

Matsumoto, M., Matsumoto, K., Abe, H. and Tanaka, K. (2007). Medial prefrontal selectivity signalling prediction errors of action values, *Nature Neuroscience* **10**: 647–656.

Matsumura, N., Nishijo, H., Tamura, R., Eifuku, S., Endo, S. and Ono, T. (1999). Spatial- and task-dependent neuronal responses during real and virtual translocation in the monkey hippocampal formation, *Journal of Neuroscience* **19**: 2318–2393.

Mattia, M. and Del Giudice, P. (2002). Population dynamics of interacting spiking neurons, *Physical Review E* **66**: 051917.

Mattia, M. and Del Giudice, P. (2004). Finite-size dynamics of inhibitory and excitatory interacting spiking neurons, *Physical Review E* **70**: 052903.

Mayberg, H. S. (2003). Positron emission tomography imaging in depression: a neural systems perspective, *Neuroimaging Clin N Am* **13**: 805–15.

Maynard Smith, J. (1982). *Evolution and the Theory of Games*, Cambridge University Press, Cambridge.

Maynard Smith, J. (1984). Game theory and the evolution of behaviour, *Behavioral and Brain Sciences* **7**: 95–125.

McAdams, C. and Maunsell, J. H. R. (1999). Effects of attention on orientation-tuning functions of single neurons in macaque cortical area V4, *Journal of Neuroscience* **19**: 431–441.

McCabe, C. and Rolls, E. T. (2007). Umami: a delicious flavor formed by convergence of taste and olfactory pathways in the human brain, *European Journal of Neuroscience* **25**: 1855–1864.

McCabe, C., Rolls, E. T., Bilderbeck, A. and McGlone, F. (2008). Cognitive influences on the affective representation of touch and the sight of touch in the human brain, *Social, Cognitive and Affective Neuroscience* **3**: 97–108.

McClelland, J. L. (1981). Retrieving general and specific information from stored knowledge of specifics, *Proceedings of the third annual meeting of the Cognitive Science Society*, Citeseer.

McClelland, J. L. and Rumelhart, D. E. (1986). A distributed model of human learning and memory, *in* J. L. McClelland and D. E. Rumelhart (eds), *Parallel Distributed Processing*, Vol. 2, MIT Press, Cambridge, MA, chapter 17, pp. 170–215.

McClelland, J. L. and Rumelhart, D. E. (1989). *Explorations in parallel distributed processing: A handbook of models, programs, and exercises*, MIT Press, Cambridge, MA.

McClelland, J. L., Rumelhart, D. E. and Hinton, G. E. (1986). The appeal of parallel distributed processing, *MIT Press, Cambridge MA* pp. 3–44.

McClelland, J. L., McNaughton, B. L. and O'Reilly, R. C. (1995). Why there are complementary learning systems in the hippocampus and neocortex: insights from the successes and failures of connectionist models of learning and memory, *Psychological Review* **102**: 419–457.

McClelland, J. L., McNaughton, B. L. and Lampinen, A. K. (2020). Integration of new information in memory: new insights from a complementary learning systems perspective, *Philos Trans R Soc Lond B Biol Sci* **375**: 20190637.

McClure, S. M., Berns, G. S. and Montague, P. R. (2003). Temporal prediction errors in a passive learning task activate human striatum, *Neuron* **38**: 339–346.

McClure, S. M., Laibson, D. I., Loewenstein, G. and Cohen, J. D. (2004). Separate neural systems value immediate and delayed monetary rewards, *Science* **306**: 503–507.

McCormick, C. and Maguire, E. A. (2021). The distinct and overlapping brain networks supporting semantic and spatial constructive scene processing, *Neuropsychologia* **158**: 107912.

McCormick, C., Ciaramelli, E., De Luca, F. and Maguire, E. A. (2018). Comparing and contrasting the cognitive effects of hippocampal and ventromedial prefrontal cortex damage: a review of human lesion studies, *Neuroscience* **374**: 295–318.

McCormick, C., Barry, D. N., Jafarian, A., Barnes, G. R. and Maguire, E. A. (2020). vmPFC drives hippocampal processing during autobiographical memory recall regardless of remoteness, *Cereb Cortex* **30**: 5972–5987.

McGaugh, J. L. (2000). Memory - a century of consolidation, *Science* **287**: 248–251.

McGurk, H. and MacDonald, J. (1976). Hearing lips and seeing voices, *Nature* **264**: 746–748.

McLeod, P., Plunkett, K. and Rolls, E. T. (1998). *Introduction to Connectionist Modelling of Cognitive Processes*, Oxford University Press, Oxford.

McNaughton, B. L. (1991). Associative pattern completion in hippocampal circuits: new evidence and new questions, *Brain Research Reviews* **16**: 193–220.

McNaughton, B. L. and Morris, R. G. M. (1987). Hippocampal synaptic enhancement and information storage within a distributed memory system, *Trends in Neuroscience* **10**: 408–415.

McNaughton, B. L. and Nadel, L. (1990). Hebb-Marr networks and the neurobiological representation of action in space, *in* M. A. Gluck and D. E. Rumelhart (eds), *Neuroscience and Connectionist Theory*, Erlbaum, Hillsdale, NJ, pp. 1–64.

McNaughton, B. L., Barnes, C. A. and O'Keefe, J. (1983). The contributions of position, direction, and velocity to single unit activity in the hippocampus of freely-moving rats, *Experimental Brain Research* **52**: 41–49.

McNaughton, B. L., Barnes, C. A., Meltzer, J. and Sutherland, R. J. (1989). Hippocampal granule cells are necessary for normal spatial learning but not for spatially selective pyramidal cell discharge, *Experimental Brain Research* **76**: 485–496.

McNaughton, B. L., Chen, L. L. and Markus, E. J. (1991). "Dead reckoning", landmark learning, and the sense of direction: a neurophysiological and computational hypothesis, *Journal of Cognitive Neuroscience* **3**: 190–202.

McNaughton, B. L., Barnes, C. A., Gerrard, J. L., Gothard, K., Jung, M. W., Knierim, J. J., Kudrimoti, H., Qin, Y., Skaggs, W. E., Suster, M. and Weaver, K. L. (1996). Deciphering the hippocampal polyglot: the hippocampus as a path integration system, *Journal of Experimental Biology* **199**: 173–185.

McNaughton, B. L., Battaglia, F. P., Jensen, O., Moser, E. I. and Moser, M. (2006). Path integration and the neural basis of the 'cognitive map', *Nature Reviews Neuroscience* **7**: 663–678.

Medalla, M. and Barbas, H. (2010). Anterior cingulate synapses in prefrontal areas 10 and 46 suggest differential influence in cognitive control, *J Neurosci* **30**: 16068–81.

Medalla, M. and Barbas, H. (2014). Specialized prefrontal "auditory fields": organization of primate prefrontal-temporal pathways, *Front Neurosci* **8**: 77.

Medin, D. L. and Schaffer, M. M. (1978). Context theory of classification learning, *Psychological Review* **85**: 207–238.

Mehta, M. R., Quirk, M. C. and Wilson, M. A. (2000). Experience-dependent asymmetric shape of hippocampal receptive fields, *Neuron* **25**: 707–15.

Meister, M. L. R. and Buffalo, E. A. (2018). Neurons in primate entorhinal cortex represent gaze position in multiple spatial reference frames, *J Neurosci* **38**: 2430–2441.

Mel, B. W. (1997). SEEMORE: Combining color, shape, and texture histogramming in a neurally-inspired approach to visual object recognition, *Neural Computation* **9**: 777–804.

Mel, B. W. and Fiser, J. (2000). Minimizing binding errors using learned conjunctive features, *Neural Computation* **12**: 731–762.

Mel, B. W., Ruderman, D. L. and Archie, K. A. (1998). Translation-invariant orientation tuning in visual "complex" cells could derive from intradendritic computations, *Journal of Neuroscience* **18**(11): 4325–4334.

Mel, B. W., Schiller, J. and Poirazi, P. (2017). Synaptic plasticity in dendrites: complications and coping strategies, *Curr Opin Neurobiol* **43**: 177–186.

Melzack, R. and Wall, P. D. (1996). *The Challenge of Pain*, Penguin, Harmondsworth, UK.

Menon, V. and Uddin, L. Q. (2010). Saliency, switching, attention and control: a network model of insula function, *Brain Struct Funct* **214**: 655–67.

Menzies, L., Chamberlain, S. R., Laird, A. R., Thelen, S. M., Sahakian, B. J. and Bullmore, E. T. (2008). Integrating evidence from neuroimaging and neuropsychological studies of obsessive-compulsive disorder: The orbitofronto-striatal model revisited, *Neuroscience and Biobehavioral Reviews* **32**: 525–549.

Meredith, M. (2001). Human vomeronasal organ function: a critical review of best and worst cases, *Chemical Senses* **26**: 433–445.

Meshulam, L., Gauthier, J. L., Brody, C. D., Tank, D. W. and Bialek, W. (2017). Collective behavior of place and non-place neurons in the hippocampal network, *Neuron* **96**: 1178–1191 e4.

Mesulam, M. M. (1990). Human brain cholinergic pathways, *Prog Brain Res* **84**: 231–41.

Mesulam, M. M. (2023). Temporopolar regions of the human brain, *Brain* **146**: 20–41.

Mesulam, M.-M. and Mufson, E. J. (1982a). Insula of the Old World monkey. I: Architectonics in the insulo-orbito-temporal component of the paralimbic brain, *Journal of Comparative Neurology* **212**: 1–22.

Mesulam, M.-M. and Mufson, E. J. (1982b). Insula of the Old World monkey. III. Efferent cortical output and comments on function, *Journal of Comparative Neurology* **212**: 38–52.

Middleton, F. A. and Strick, P. L. (1996a). New concepts about the organization of the basal ganglia., *in* J. A. Obeso (ed.), *Advances in Neurology: The Basal Ganglia and the Surgical Treatment for Parkinson's Disease*, Raven, New York.

Middleton, F. A. and Strick, P. L. (1996b). The temporal lobe is a target of output from the basal ganglia, *Proceedings of the National Academy of Sciences of the USA* **93**: 8683–8687.

Mikami, A., Nakamura, K. and Kubota, K. (1994). Neuronal responses to photographs in the superior temporal sulcus of the rhesus monkey, *Behavioural Brain Research* **60**: 1–13.

Miller, E. K. and Buschman, T. J. (2013). Cortical circuits for the control of attention, *Current Opinion in Neurobiology* **23**: 216–222.

Miller, E. K. and Desimone, R. (1994). Parallel neuronal mechanisms for short-term memory, *Science* **263**: 520–522.

Miller, E. K., Li, L. and Desimone, R. (1993). Activity of neurons in anterior inferior temporal cortex during a short-term memory task, *Journal of Neuroscience* **13**: 1460–1478.

Miller, E. K., Erickson, C. and Desimone, R. (1996). Neural mechanisms of visual working memory in prefrontal cortex of the macaque, *Journal of Neuroscience* **16**: 5154–5167.

Miller, E. K., Nieder, A., Freedman, D. J. and Wallis, J. D. (2003). Neural correlates of categories and concepts, *Current Opinion in Neurobiology* **13**: 198–203.

Miller, E. K., Lundqvist, M. and Bastos, A. M. (2018). Working Memory 2.0, *Neuron* **100**: 463–475.

Miller, G. A. (1955). Note on the bias of information estimates, *Information Theory in Psychology; Problems and Methods II-B* pp. 95–100.

Miller, G. F. (2000). *The Mating Mind*, Heinemann, London.

Miller, J. F., Neufang, M., Solway, A., Brandt, A., Trippel, M., Mader, I., Hefft, S., Merkow, M., Polyn, S. M., Jacobs, J., Kahana, M. J. and Schulze-Bonhage, A. (2013). Neural activity in human hippocampal formation reveals the spatial context of retrieved memories, *Science* **342**: 1111–4.

Miller, K. D. (1994). Models of activity-dependent neural development, *Progress in Brain Research* **102**: 303–308.

Miller, K. D. (2016). Canonical computations of cerebral cortex, *Curr Opin Neurobiol* **37**: 75–84.

Miller, P. and Wang, X.-J. (2006). Power-law neuronal fluctuations in a recurrent network model of parametric working memory, *Journal of Neurophysiology* **95**: 1099–1114.

Millhouse, O. and DeOlmos, J. (1983). Neuronal configuration in lateral and basolateral amygdala, *Neuroscience* **10**: 1269–1300.

Milner, A. (2008). Conscious and unconscious visual processing in the human brain, *in* L. Weiskrantz and M. Davies (eds), *Frontiers of Consciousness*, Oxford University Press, Oxford, chapter 5, pp. 169–214.

Milner, A. and Goodale, M. (1995). *The Visual Brain in Action*, Oxford University Press, Oxford.

Milner, P. (1974). A model for visual shape recognition, *Psychological Review* **81**: 521–535.

Milton, A. L., Lee, J. L., Butler, V. J., Gardner, R. and Everitt, B. J. (2008). Intra-amygdala and systemic antagonism of NMDA receptors prevents the reconsolidation of drug-associated memory and impairs subsequently both novel and previously acquired drug-seeking behaviors, *Journal of Neuroscience* **28**: 8230–8237.

Milton, C. K., Dhanaraj, V., Young, I. M., Taylor, H. M., Nicholas, P. J., Briggs, R. G., Bai, M. Y., Fonseka, R. D., Hormovas, J., Lin, Y. H., Tanglay, O., Conner, A. K., Glenn, C. A., Teo, C., Doyen, S. and Sughrue, M. E. (2021). Parcellation-based anatomic model of the semantic network, *Brain Behav* **11**: e02065.

Minai, A. A. and Levy, W. B. (1993). Sequence learning in a single trial, *International Neural Network Society World Congress of Neural Networks* **2**: 505–508.

Mineault, P. J., Khawaja, F. A., Butts, D. A. and Pack, C. C. (2012). Hierarchical processing of complex motion along the primate dorsal visual pathway, *Proc Natl Acad Sci U S A* **109**: E972–80.

Minsky, M. L. and Papert, S. A. (1969). *Perceptrons*, expanded 1988 edn, MIT Press, Cambridge, MA.

Mirenowicz, J. and Schultz, W. (1996). Preferential activation of midbrain dopamine neurons by appetitive rather than aversive stimuli, *Nature* **279**: 449–451.

Mishkin, M. (1979). Analogous neural models for tactual and visual learning, *Neuropsychologia* **17**: 139–51.

Miyashita, Y. (1988). Neuronal correlate of visual associative long-term memory in the primate temporal cortex, *Nature* **335**: 817–820.

Miyashita, Y. (1993). Inferior temporal cortex: where visual perception meets memory, *Annual Review of Neuroscience* **16**: 245–263.

Miyashita, Y. (2019). Perirhinal circuits for memory processing, *Nat Rev Neurosci* **20**: 577–592.

Miyashita, Y. and Chang, H. S. (1988). Neuronal correlate of pictorial short-term memory in the primate temporal cortex, *Nature* **331**: 68–70.

Miyashita, Y., Rolls, E. T., Cahusac, P. M. B., Niki, H. and Feigenbaum, J. D. (1989). Activity of hippocampal neurons in the monkey related to a conditional spatial response task, *Journal of Neurophysiology* **61**: 669–678.

Miyashita, Y., Okuno, H., Tokuyama, W., Ihara, T. and Nakajima, K. (1996). Feedback signal from medial temporal lobe mediates visual associative mnemonic codes of inferotemporal neurons, *Cognitive Brain Research* **5**: 81–86.

Miyashita, Y., Kameyama, M., Hasegawa, I. and Fukushima, T. (1998). Consolidation of visual associative long-term memory in the temporal cortex of primates, *Neurobiology of Learning and Memory* **1**: 197–211.

Mizumori, S. J. and Tryon, V. L. (2015). Integrative hippocampal and decision-making neurocircuitry during goal-relevant predictions and encoding, *Progress in Brain Research* **219**: 217–242.

Mkrtchian, A., Evans, J. W., Kraus, C., Yuan, P., Kadriu, B., Nugent, A. C., Roiser, J. P. and Zarate, C. A., J. (2021). Ketamine modulates fronto-striatal circuitry in depressed and healthy individuals, *Mol Psychiatry* **26**: 3292–3301.

Mobbs, D., Adolphs, R., Fanselow, M. S., Barrett, L. F., LeDoux, J. E., Ressler, K. and Tye, K. M. (2019). Viewpoints: Approaches to defining and investigating fear, *Nat Neurosci* **22**: 1205–1216.

Moerel, M., De Martino, F. and Formisano, E. (2014). An anatomical and functional topography of human auditory cortical areas, *Front Neurosci* **8**: 225.

Molnar, Z., Kaas, J. H., de Carlos, J. A., Hevner, R. F., Lein, E. and Nemec, P. (2014). Evolution and development of the mammalian cerebral cortex, *Brain Behav Evol* **83**: 126–39.

Mombaerts, P. (2006). Axonal wiring in the mouse olfactory system, *Annual Review of Cell and Developmental Biology* **22**: 713–737.

Monaco, S., Cavina-Pratesi, C., Sedda, A., Fattori, P., Galletti, C. and Culham, J. C. (2011). Functional magnetic resonance adaptation reveals the involvement of the dorsomedial stream in hand orientation for grasping, *J Neurophysiol* **106**: 2248–63.

Monaghan, D. T. and Cotman, C. W. (1985). Distribution of N-methyl-D-aspartate-sensitive L-[3H]glutamate-binding sites in the rat brain, *Journal of Neuroscience* **5**: 2909–2919.

Montague, P. R., Gally, J. A. and Edelman, G. M. (1991). Spatial signalling in the development and function of neural connections, *Cerebral Cortex* **1**: 199–220.

Montague, P. R., King-Casas, B. and Cohen, J. D. (2006). Imaging valuation models in human choice, *Annual Review of Neuroscience* **29**: 417–448.

Montaldi, D., Spencer, T. J., Roberts, N. and Mayes, A. R. (2006). The neural system that mediates familiarity memory, *Hippocampus* **16**: 504–20.

Moore, D. B., Lee, P., Paiva, M., Walker, D. W. and Heaton, M. B. (1998). Effects of neonatal ethanol exposure on cholinergic neurons of the rat medial septum, *Alcohol* **15**: 219–226.

Mora, F., Rolls, E. T. and Burton, M. J. (1976). Modulation during learning of the responses of neurones in the lateral hypothalamus to the sight of food, *Experimental Neurology* **53**: 508–519.

Mora, F., Mogenson, G. J. and Rolls, E. T. (1977). Activity of neurones in the region of the substantia nigra during feeding, *Brain Research* **133**: 267–276.

Morecraft, R. J. and Tanji, J. (2009). Cingulofrontal interactions and the cingulate motor areas, *in* B. Vogt (ed.), *Cingulate Neurobiology and Disease*, Oxford University Press, Oxford, chapter 5, pp. 113–144.

Morecraft, R. J., Geula, C. and Mesulam, M.-M. (1992). Cytoarchitecture and neural afferents of orbitofrontal cortex in the brain of the monkey, *Journal of Comparative Neurology* **323**: 341–358.

Morel, A., Garraghty, P. E. and Kaas, J. H. (1993). Tonotopic organization, architectonic fields, and connections of auditory cortex in macaque monkeys, *J Comp Neurol* **335**: 437–59.

Moreno-Bote, R., Rinzel, J. and Rubin, N. (2007). Noise-induced alternations in an attractor network model of perceptual bistability, *Journal of Neurophysiology* **98**: 1125–1139.

Mori, K. and Sakano, H. (2011). How is the olfactory map formed and interpreted in the mammalian brain?, *Annual Reviews of Neuroscience* **34**: 467–499.

Mori, K., Mataga, N. and Imamura, K. (1992). Differential specificities of single mitral cells in rabbit olfactory bulb for a homologous series of fatty acid odor molecules, *Journal of Neurophysiology* **67**: 786–789.

Mori, K., Nagao, H. and Yoshihara, Y. (1999). The olfactory bulb: coding and processing of odor molecule information, *Science* **286**: 711–715.

Morin, E. L., Hadj-Bouziane, F., Stokes, M., Ungerleider, L. G. and Bell, A. H. (2015). Hierarchical encoding of social cues in primate inferior temporal cortex, *Cereb Cortex* **25**: 3036–45.

Mormann, F., Kornblith, S., Cerf, M., Ison, M. J., Kraskov, A., Tran, M., Knieling, S., Quian Quiroga, R., Koch, C. and Fried, I. (2017). Scene-selective coding by single neurons in the human parahippocampal cortex, *Proc Natl Acad Sci U S A* **114**: 1153–1158.

Morris, A. M., Churchwell, J. C., Kesner, R. P. and Gilbert, P. E. (2012). Selective lesions of the dentate gyrus produce disruptions in place learning for adjacent spatial locations, *Neurobiol Learn Mem* **97**: 326–31.

Morris, J. S., Fritch, C. D., Perrett, D. I., Rowland, D., Young, A. W., Calder, A. J. and Dolan, R. J. (1996). A differential neural response in the human amygdala to fearful and happy face expressions, *Nature* **383**: 812–815.

Morris, L. S., Kundu, P., Dowell, N., Mechelmans, D. J., Favre, P., Irvine, M. A., Robbins, T. W., Daw, N., Bullmore, E. T., Harrison, N. A. and Voon, V. (2016). Fronto-striatal organization: Defining functional and microstructural substrates of behavioural flexibility, *Cortex* **74**: 118–33.

Morris, R. G., Garrud, P., Rawlins, J. N. and O'Keefe, J. (1982). Place navigation impaired in rats with hippocampal lesions, *Nature* **297**: 681–3.

Morris, R. G., Moser, E. I., Riedel, G., Martin, S. J., Sandin, J., Day, M. and O'Carroll, C. (2003). Elements of a neurobiological theory of the hippocampus: the role of activity-dependent synaptic plasticity in memory, *Philosophical Transactions of the Royal Society of London B* **358**: 773–786.

Morris, R. G. M. (1989). Does synaptic plasticity play a role in information storage in the vertebrate brain?, in R. G. M. Morris (ed.), *Parallel Distributed Processing: Implications for Psychology and Neurobiology*, Oxford University Press, Oxford, chapter 11, pp. 248–285.

Morris, R. G. M. (2003). Long-term potentiation and memory, *Philosophical Transactions of the Royal Society of London B* **358**: 643–647.

Morris, R. W., Dezfouli, A., Griffiths, K. R., Le Pelley, M. E. and Balleine, B. W. (2022). The neural bases of action-outcome learning in humans, *J Neurosci* **42**: 3636–3647.

Morrison, S. E., Saez, A., Lau, B. and Salzman, C. D. (2011). Different time courses for learning-related changes in amygdala and orbitofrontal cortex, *Neuron* **71**: 1127–40.

Morton, G. J., Meek, T. H. and Schwartz, M. W. (2014). Neurobiology of food intake in health and disease, *Nature Reviews Neuroscience* **15**: 367–378.

Morton, N. W. and Preston, A. R. (2021). Concept formation as a computational cognitive process, *Curr Opin Behav Sci* **38**: 83–89.

Moscovitch, M., Rosenbaum, R. S., Gilboa, A., Addis, D. R., Westmacott, R., Grady, C., McAndrews, M. P., Levine, B., Black, S., Winocur, G. and Nadel, L. (2005). Functional neuroanatomy of remote episodic, semantic and spatial memory: a unified account based on multiple trace theory, *Journal of Anatomy* **207**: 35–66.

Moscovitch, M., Cabeza, R., Winocur, G. and Nadel, L. (2016). Episodic memory and beyond: the hippocampus and neocortex in transformation, *Annu Rev Psychol* **67**: 105–34.

Moser, E. I., Moser, M. B. and Roudi, Y. (2014a). Network mechanisms of grid cells, *Philosophical Transactions of the Royal Society of London B Biological Science* **369**: 20120511.

Moser, E. I., Roudi, Y., Witter, M. P., Kentros, C., Bonhoeffer, T. and Moser, M. B. (2014b). Grid cells and cortical representation, *Nature Reviews Neuroscience* **15**: 466–481.

Moser, E. I., Moser, M. B. and McNaughton, B. L. (2017). Spatial representation in the hippocampal formation: a history, *Nat Neurosci* **20**: 1448–1464.

Moser, E. I., Moser, M.-B. and Siegelbaum, S. A. (2021). The hippocampus and the neural basis of explicit memory storage, in E. R. Kandel, J. D. Koester, S. H. Mack and S. A. Siegelbaum (eds), *Principles of Neural Science*, 6 edn, McGraw-Hill, New York, chapter 54, pp. 1339–1369.

Moser, M. B., Rowland, D. C. and Moser, E. I. (2015). Place cells, grid cells, and memory, *Cold Spring Harb Perspect Biol* **7**: a021808.

Mountcastle, V. B. (1957). Modality and topographic properties of single neurons of cat's somatosensory cortex, *Journal of Neurophysiology* **20**: 408–434.

Mountcastle, V. B. (1984). Central nervous mechanisms in mechanoreceptive sensibility, *in* I. Darian-Smith (ed.), *Handbook of Physiology, Section 1: The Nervous System, Vol III, Sensory Processes, Part 2*, American Physiological Society, Bethesda, MD, pp. 789–878.

Mountcastle, V. B., Lynch, J. C., Georgopoulos, A., Sakata, H. and Acuna, C. (1975). Posterior parietal association cortex of the monkey: command functions for operations within extrapersonal space, *J Neurophysiol* **38**: 871–908.

Movshon, J. A., Adelson, E. H., Gizzi, M. S. and Newsome, W. T. (1985). The analysis of moving visual patterns, *in* C. Chagas, R. Gattass and C. G. Gross (eds), *Pattern Recognition Mechanisms*, Springer-Verlag, New York, pp. 117–151.

Moyer, J. R. J., Deyo, R. A. and Disterhoft, J. F. (1990). Hippocampectomy disrupts trace eye-blink conditioning in rabbits, *Behavioral Neuroscience* **104**: 243–252.

Mozer, M. C. (1991). *The Perception of Multiple Objects: A Connectionist Approach*, MIT Press, Cambridge, MA.

Mrsic-Flogel, T. D., King, A. J. and Schnupp, J. W. (2005). Encoding of virtual acoustic space stimuli by neurons in ferret primary auditory cortex, *J Neurophysiol* **93**: 3489–503.

Mueser, K. T. and McGurk, S. R. (2004). Schizophrenia, *Lancet* **363**: 2063–2072.

Muir, J. L., Everitt, B. J. and Robbins, T. W. (1994). AMPA-induced excitotoxic lesions of the basal forebrain: a significant role for the cortical cholinergic system in attentional function, *Journal of Neuroscience* **14**: 2313–2326.

Muller, R. U., Kubie, J. L., Bostock, E. M., Taube, J. S. and Quirk, G. J. (1991). Spatial firing correlates of neurons in the hippocampal formation of freely moving rats, *in* J. Paillard (ed.), *Brain and Space*, Oxford University Press, Oxford, pp. 296–333.

Muller, R. U., Ranck, J. B. and Taube, J. S. (1996). Head direction cells: properties and functional significance, *Current Opinion in Neurobiology* **6**: 196–206.

Mundy, J. and Zisserman, A. (1992). Introduction – towards a new framework for vision, *in* J. Mundy and A. Zisserman (eds), *Geometric Invariance in Computer Vision*, MIT Press, Cambridge, MA, pp. 1–39.

Munoz-Lopez, M., Insausti, R., Mohedano-Moriano, A., Mishkin, M. and Saunders, R. C. (2015). Anatomical pathways for auditory memory II: information from rostral superior temporal gyrus to dorsolateral temporal pole and medial temporal cortex, *Front Neurosci* **9**: 158.

Munuera, J. and Duhamel, J. R. (2020). The role of the posterior parietal cortex in saccadic error processing, *Brain Struct Funct* **225**: 763–784.

Munuera, J., Rigotti, M. and Salzman, C. D. (2018). Shared neural coding for social hierarchy and reward value in primate amygdala, *Nat Neurosci* **21**: 415–423.

Murata, A., Fadiga, L., Fogassi, L., Gallese, V., Raos, V. and Rizzolatti, G. (1997). Object representation in the ventral premotor cortex (area F5) of the monkey, *J Neurophysiol* **78**: 2226–30.

Murray, E. A. and Fellows, L. K. (2022). Prefrontal cortex interactions with the amygdala in primates, *Neuropsychopharmacology* **47**: 163–179.

Murray, E. A. and Izquierdo, A. (2007). Orbitofrontal cortex and amygdala contributions to affect and action in primates, *Annals of the New York Academy of Sciences* **1121**: 273–296.

Murray, E. A. and Rudebeck, P. H. (2018). Specializations for reward-guided decision-making in the primate ventral prefrontal cortex, *Nat Rev Neurosci* **19**: 404–417.

Murray, E. A., Gaffan, D. and Mishkin, M. (1993). Neural substrates of visual stimulus–stimulus association in rhesus monkeys, *Journal of Neuroscience* **13**: 4549–4561.

Murray, E. A., Baxter, M. G. and Gaffan, D. (1998). Monkeys with rhinal cortex damage or neurotoxic hippocampal lesions are impaired on spatial scene learning and object reversals, *Behavioral Neuroscience* **112**: 1291–1303.

Mutch, J. and Lowe, D. G. (2008). Object class recognition and localization using sparse features with limited receptive fields, *International Journal of Computer Vision* **80**: 45–57.

Myers, M. G., J., Affinati, A. H., Richardson, N. and Schwartz, M. W. (2021). Central nervous system regulation of organismal energy and glucose homeostasis, *Nat Metab* **3**: 737–750.

Naber, P. A., Lopes da Silva, F. H. and Witter, M. P. (2001). Reciprocal connections between the entorhinal cortex and hippocampal fields CA1 and the subiculum are in register with the projections from CA1 to the subiculum, *Hippocampus* **11**: 99–104.

Nadal, J. P., Toulouse, G., Changeux, J. P. and Dehaene, S. (1986). Networks of formal neurons and memory palimpsests, *Europhysics Letters* **1**: 535–542.

Nadasdy, Z., Nguyen, T. P., Torok, A., Shen, J. Y., Briggs, D. E., Modur, P. N. and Buchanan, R. J. (2017). Context-dependent spatially periodic activity in the human entorhinal cortex, *Proc Natl Acad Sci U S A* **114**: E3516–E3525.

Nagahama, Y., Okada, T., Katsumi, Y., Hayashi, T., Yamauchi, H., Oyanagi, C., Konishi, J., Fukuyama, H. and Shibasaki, H. (2001). Dissociable mechanisms of attentional control within the human prefrontal cortex, *Cerebral Cortex* **11**: 85–92.

Nagai, Y., Critchley, H. D., Featherstone, E., Trimble, M. R. and Dolan, R. J. (2004). Activity in ventromedial prefrontal cortex covaries with sympathetic skin conductance level: a physiological account of a "default mode" of brain function, *Neuroimage* **22**: 243–251.

Nakahara, H., Amari, S. and Hikosaka, O. (2002). Self-organisation in the basal ganglia with modulation of reinforcement signals, *Neural Computation* **14**: 819–844.

Nakazawa, K., Quirk, M. C., Chitwood, R. A., Watanabe, M., Yeckel, M. F., Sun, L. D., Kato, A., Carr, C. A., Johnston, D., Wilson, M. A. and Tonegawa, S. (2002). Requirement for hippocampal CA3 NMDA receptors in associative memory recall, *Science* **297**: 211–218.

Nakazawa, K., Sun, L. D., Quirk, M. C., Rondi-Reig, L., Wilson, M. A. and Tonegawa, S. (2003). Hippocampal CA3 NMDA receptors are crucial for memory acquisition of one-time experience, *Neuron* **38**: 305–315.

Nakazawa, K., McHugh, T. J., Wilson, M. A. and Tonegawa, S. (2004). NMDA receptors, place cells and hippocampal spatial memory, *Nature Reviews Neuroscience* **5**: 361–372.

Nam, Y., Sato, T., Uchida, G., Malakhova, E., Ullman, S. and Tanifuji, M. (2021). View-tuned and view-invariant face encoding in IT cortex is explained by selected natural image fragments, *Sci Rep* **11**: 7827.

Nandy, A. S., Sharpee, T. O., Reynolds, J. H. and Mitchell, J. F. (2013). The fine structure of shape tuning in area V4, *Neuron* **78**: 1102–15.

Nanry, K. P., Mundy, W. R. and Tilson, H. A. (1989). Colchicine-induced alterations of reference memory in rats: role of spatial versus non-spatial task components, *Behavioral Brain Research* **35**: 45–53.

Nasr, S., Liu, N., Devaney, K. J., Yue, X., Rajimehr, R., Ungerleider, L. G. and Tootell, R. B. (2011). Scene-selective cortical regions in human and nonhuman primates, *J Neurosci* **31**: 13771–85.

Natu, V. S., Arcaro, M. J., Barnett, M. A., Gomez, J., Livingstone, M., Grill-Spector, K. and Weiner, K. S. (2021). Sulcal depth in the medial ventral temporal cortex predicts the location of a place-selective region in macaques, children, and adults, *Cereb Cortex* **31**: 48–61.

Nau, M., Julian, J. B. and Doeller, C. F. (2018a). How the brain's navigation system shapes our visual experience, *Trends Cogn Sci* **22**: 810–825.

Nau, M., Navarro Schroder, T., Bellmund, J. L. S. and Doeller, C. F. (2018b). Hexadirectional coding of visual space in human entorhinal cortex, *Nat Neurosci* **21**: 188–190.

Naya, Y., Chen, H., Yang, C. and Suzuki, W. A. (2017). Contributions of primate prefrontal cortex and medial temporal lobe to temporal-order memory, *Proc Natl Acad Sci U S A* **114**: 13555–13560.

Nelken, I., Prut, Y., Vaadia, E. and Abeles, M. (1994). Population responses to multifrequency sounds in the cat auditory cortex: one- and two-parameter families of sounds, *Hearing Research* **72**: 206–222.

Nesse, R. M. and Lloyd, A. T. (1992). The evolution of psychodynamic mechanisms, *in* J. H. Barkow, L. Cosmides and J. Tooby (eds), *The Adapted Mind*, Oxford University Press, New York, pp. 601–624.

Newman, E. L., Gupta, K., Climer, J. R., Monaghan, C. K. and Hasselmo, M. E. (2012). Cholinergic modulation of cognitive processing: insights drawn from computational models, *Front Behav Neurosci* **6**: 24.

Newsome, W. T., Britten, K. H. and Movshon, J. A. (1989). Neuronal correlates of a perceptual decision, *Nature* **341**: 52–54.

Nicolaidis, S. and Rowland, N. (1977). Intravenous self-feeding: long-term regulation of energy balance in rats, *Science* **195**: 589–591.

Nicoll, R. A. (1988). The coupling of neurotransmitter receptors to ion channels in the brain, *Science* **241**: 545–551.

Niemiro, G. M., Rewane, A. and Algotar, A. M. (2022). Exercise and fitness effect on obesity, *StatPearls*, StatPearls, Treasure Island (FL), p. https://www.ncbi.nlm.nih.gov/pubmed/30969715.

Niki, H. and Watanabe, M. (1979). Prefrontal and cingulate unit activity during timing behavior in the monkey, *Brain Research* **171**: 213–224.

Niv, Y., Duff, M. O. and Dayan, P. (2005). Dopamine, uncertainty, and TD learning, *Behavioral and Brain Functions* **1**: 6.

Noonan, M. P., Mars, R. B. and Rushworth, M. F. (2011). Distinct roles of three frontal cortical areas in reward-guided behavior, *J Neurosci* **31**: 14399–412.

Norgren, R. (1974). Gustatory afferents to ventral forebrain, *Brain Research* **81**: 285–295.

Norgren, R. (1976). Taste pathways to hypothalamus and amygdala, *Journal of Comparative Neurology* **166**: 17–30.

Norgren, R. (1990). Gustatory system, *in* G. Paxinos (ed.), *The Human Nervous System*, Academic, San Diego, pp. 845–861.

Norgren, R. and Leonard, C. M. (1971). Taste pathways in rat brainstem, *Science* **173**: 1136–1139.

Norman, Y., Yeagle, E. M., Khuvis, S., Harel, M., Mehta, A. D. and Malach, R. (2019). Hippocampal sharp-wave ripples linked to visual episodic recollection in humans, *Science* **365**: eaax1030.

Nowak, L. and Bullier, J. (1997). The timing of information transfer in the visual system, *in* K. Rockland, J. Kaas and A. Peters (eds), *Cerebral Cortex: Extrastriate Cortex in Primate*, Plenum, New York, p. 870.

Nugent, A. C., Milham, M. P., Bain, E. E., Mah, L., Cannon, D. M., Marrett, S., Zarate, C. A., Pine, D. S., Price, J. L. and Drevets, W. C. (2006). Cortical abnormalities in bipolar disorder investigated with MRI and voxel-based morphometry, *Neuroimage* **30**: 485–497.

Nusslock, R., Young, C. B. and Damme, K. S. (2014). Elevated reward-related neural activation as a unique biological marker of bipolar disorder: assessment and treatment implications, *Behaviour Research and Therapy* **62**: 74–87.

Oberg, R. G. E. and Divac, I. (1979). "Cognitive" functions of the striatum, *in* I. Divac and R. G. E. Oberg (eds), *The Neostriatum*, Pergamon, New York, pp. 291–314.

Oberhuber, M., Hope, T. M. H., Seghier, M. L., Parker Jones, O., Prejawa, S., Green, D. W. and Price, C. J. (2016). Four Functionally Distinct Regions in the Left Supramarginal Gyrus Support Word Processing, *Cereb Cortex* **26**: 4212–4226.

O'Connor, D. H., Krubitzer, L. and Bensmaia, S. (2021). Of mice and monkeys: Somatosensory processing in two prominent animal models, *Prog Neurobiol* **201**: 102008.

O'Doherty, J., Rolls, E. T., Francis, S., Bowtell, R., McGlone, F., Kobal, G., Renner, B. and Ahne, G. (2000). Sensory-specific satiety related olfactory activation of the human orbitofrontal cortex, *NeuroReport* **11**: 893–897.

O'Doherty, J., Kringelbach, M. L., Rolls, E. T., Hornak, J. and Andrews, C. (2001a). Abstract reward and punishment representations in the human orbitofrontal cortex., *Nature Neuroscience* **4**: 95–102.

O'Doherty, J., Rolls, E. T., Francis, S., Bowtell, R. and McGlone, F. (2001b). The representation of pleasant and aversive taste in the human brain, *Journal of Neurophysiology* **85**: 1315–1321.

O'Doherty, J., Deichmann, R., Critchley, H. D. and Dolan, R. J. (2002). Neural response during anticipation of a primary taste reward, *Neuron* **33**: 815–826.

O'Doherty, J., Dayan, P., Friston, K. J., Critchley, H. D. and Dolan, R. J. (2003a). Temporal difference models and reward-related learning in the human brain, *Neuron* **38**: 329–337.

O'Doherty, J., Winston, J., Critchley, H., Perrett, D., Burt, D. M. and Dolan, R. J. (2003b). Beauty in a smile: the role of medial orbitofrontal cortex in facial attractiveness, *Neuropsychologia* **41**: 147–55.

O'Doherty, J., Dayan, P., Schultz, J., Deichmann, R., Friston, K. and Dolan, R. J. (2004). Dissociable roles of ventral and dorsal striatum in instrumental conditioning, *Science* **304**: 452–454.

O'Doherty, J. P., Cockburn, J. and Pauli, W. M. (2017). Learning, reward, and decision making, *Annu Rev Psychol* **68**: 73–100.

Oemisch, M., Westendorff, S., Azimi, M., Hassani, S. A., Ardid, S., Tiesinga, P. and Womelsdorf, T. (2019). Feature-specific prediction errors and surprise across macaque fronto-striatal circuits, *Nat Commun* **10**: 176.

Oertel, D. and Doupe, A. J. (2013). The auditory central nervous system, *in* E. R. Kandel, J. H. Schwartz, T. M. Jessell, S. A. Siegelbaum and A. J. Hudspeth (eds), *Principles of Neuroscience*, 5th edn, McGraw-Hill, New York, chapter 31, pp. 682–711.

Oertel, D. and Wang, X. (2021). Auditory processing by the central nervous system, *in* E. R. Kandel, J. D. Koester, S. H. Mack and S. A. Siegelbaum (eds), *Principles of Neural Science*, 6 edn, McGraw-Hill, New York, chapter 28, pp. 651–679.

Ohashi, H. and Ostry, D. J. (2021). Neural development of speech sensorimotor learning, *J Neurosci* **41**: 4023–4035.

Oja, E. (1982). A simplified neuron model as a principal component analyzer, *Journal of Mathematical Biology* **15**: 267–273.

O'Kane, D. and Treves, A. (1992). Why the simplest notion of neocortex as an autoassociative memory would not work, *Network* **3**: 379–384.

O'Keefe, J. (1979). A review of the hippocampal place cells, *Progress in Neurobiology* **13**: 419–439.

O'Keefe, J. (1984). Spatial memory within and without the hippocampal system, *in* W. Seifert (ed.), *Neurobiology of the Hippocampus*, Academic Press, London, pp. 375–403.

O'Keefe, J. (1990). A computational theory of the hippocampal cognitive map, *Progress in Brain Research* **83**: 301–312.

O'Keefe, J. (1991). The hippocampal cognitive map and navigational strategies, *in* J. Paillard (ed.), *Brain and Space*, Oxford University Press, Oxford, pp. 273–295.

O'Keefe, J. and Dostrovsky, J. (1971). The hippocampus as a spatial map: preliminary evidence from unit activity in the freely moving rat, *Brain Research* **34**: 171–175.

O'Keefe, J. and Krupic, J. (2021). Do hippocampal pyramidal cells respond to nonspatial stimuli?, *Physiol Rev* **101**: 1427–1456.

O'Keefe, J. and Nadel, L. (1978). *The Hippocampus as a Cognitive Map*, Clarendon Press, Oxford.

O'Keefe, J. and Speakman, A. (1987). Single unit activity in the rat hippocampus during a spatial memory task, *Experimental Brain Research* **68**(1): 1–27.

O'Keefe, J., Burgess, N., Donnett, J. G., Jeffery, K. J. and Maguire, E. A. (1998). Place cells, navigational accuracy, and the human hippocampus, *Philosophical Transactions of the Royal Society B* **353**: 1333–40.

Olausson, H., Lamarre, Y., Backlund, H., Morin, C., Wallin, B. G., Starck, G., Ekholm, S., Strigo, I., Worsley, K., Vallbo, A. B. and Bushnell, M. C. (2002). Unmyelinated tactile afferents signal touch and project to insular cortex, *Nature Neuroscience* **5**: 900–904.

Olausson, H., Wessberg, J., Morrison, I., McGlone, F. and Vallbo, A. (2010). The neurophysiology of unmyelinated tactile afferents, *Neurosci Biobehav Rev* **34**: 185–91.

Olausson, H., Wessberg, J. and McGlone, F. (2016). *Affective touch and the neurophysiology of CT afferents*, Springer.

Oliva, A. (2022). CA2 physiology underlying social memory, *Curr Opin Neurobiol* **77**: 102642.

Olshausen, B. A. and Field, D. J. (1997). Sparse coding with an incomplete basis set: a strategy employed by V1, *Vision Research* **37**: 3311–3325.

Olshausen, B. A. and Field, D. J. (2004). Sparse coding of sensory inputs, *Current Opinion in Neurobiology* **14**: 481–487.

Olshausen, B. A., Anderson, C. H. and Van Essen, D. C. (1993). A neurobiological model of visual attention and invariant pattern recognition based on dynamic routing of information, *Journal of Neuroscience* **13**: 4700–4719.

Olshausen, B. A., Anderson, C. H. and Van Essen, D. C. (1995). A multiscale dynamic routing circuit for forming size- and position-invariant object representations, *Journal of Computational Neuroscience* **2**: 45–62.

O'Mara, S. M. and Aggleton, J. P. (2019). Space and memory (far) beyond the hippocampus: many subcortical structures also support cognitive mapping and mnemonic processing, *Front Neural Circuits* **13**: 52.

O'Mara, S. M., Rolls, E. T., Berthoz, A. and Kesner, R. P. (1994). Neurons responding to whole-body motion in the primate hippocampus, *Journal of Neuroscience* **14**: 6511–6523.

O'Neill, M. J. and Dix, S. (2007). AMPA receptor potentiators as cognitive enhancers, *IDrugs* **10**: 185–192.

Ongur, D. and Price, J. L. (2000). The organisation of networks within the orbital and medial prefrontal cortex of rats, monkeys and humans, *Cerebral Cortex* **10**: 206–219.

Ongur, D., Ferry, A. T. and Price, J. L. (2003). Architectonic subdivision of the human orbital and medial prefrontal cortex, *Journal of Comparative Neurology* **460**: 425–449.

Optican, L. M. and Richmond, B. J. (1987). Temporal encoding of two-dimensional patterns by single units in primate inferior temporal cortex: III. Information theoretic analysis, *Journal of Neurophysiology* **57**: 162–178.

Optican, L. M., Gawne, T. J., Richmond, B. J. and Joseph, P. J. (1991). Unbiased measures of transmitted information and channel capacity from multivariate neuronal data, *Biological Cybernetics* **65**: 305–310.

O'Rahilly, S. (2009). Human genetics illuminates the paths to metabolic disease, *Nature* **462**: 307–14.

Oram, M. W. and Perrett, D. I. (1994). Modeling visual recognition from neurophysiological constraints, *Neural Networks* **7**: 945–972.

Orban, G. A., Lanzilotto, M. and Bonini, L. (2021a). From observed action identity to social affordances, *Trends Cogn Sci* **25**: 493–505.

Orban, G. A., Sepe, A. and Bonini, L. (2021b). Parietal maps of visual signals for bodily action planning, *Brain Struct Funct* **226**: 2967–2988.

O'Regan, J. K., Rensink, R. A. and Clark, J. J. (1999). Change-blindness as a result of 'mudsplashes', *Nature* **398**: 1736–1753.

O'Reilly, R. C. and Munakata, Y. (2000). *Computational Explorations in Cognitive Neuroscience*, MIT Press, Cambridge, MA.

O'Reilly, R. C. and Rudy, J. W. (2001). Conjunctive representations in learning and memory: principles of cortical and hippocampal function, *Psychological Review* **108**: 311–345.

Orzylowski, M., Fujiwara, E., Mousseau, D. D. and Baker, G. B. (2021). An overview of the involvement of D-serine in cognitive impairment in normal aging and dementia, *Front Psychiatry* **12**: 754032.

O'Scalaidhe, S. P., Wilson, F. A. and Goldman-Rakic, P. S. (1997). Areal segregation of face-processing neurons in prefrontal cortex, *Science* **278**: 1135–1138.

Otto, T. and Eichenbaum, H. (1992). Neuronal activity in the hippocampus during delayed non-match to sample performance in rats: evidence for hippocampal processing in recognition memory, *Hippocampus* **2**: 323–334.

Owen, M. J., Sawa, A. and Mortensen, P. B. (2016). Schizophrenia, *Lancet* **388**: 86–97.

Padoa-Schioppa, C. (2007). Orbitofrontal cortex and the computation of economic value, *Ann N Y Acad Sci* **1121**: 232–53.

Padoa-Schioppa, C. (2011). Neurobiology of economic choice: a good-based model, *Annual Review of Neuroscience* **34**: 333–359.

Padoa-Schioppa, C. and Assad, J. A. (2006). Neurons in the orbitofrontal cortex encode economic value, *Nature* **441**: 223–6.

Padoa-Schioppa, C. and Assad, J. A. (2008). The representation of economic value in the orbitofrontal cortex is invariant for changes of menu, *Nat Neurosci* **11**: 95–102.

Padoa-Schioppa, C. and Cai, X. (2011). The orbitofrontal cortex and the computation of subjective value: consolidated concepts and new perspectives, *Ann N Y Acad Sci* **1239**: 130–7.

Padoa-Schioppa, C. and Conen, K. E. (2017). Orbitofrontal cortex: A neural circuit for economic decisions, *Neuron* **96**: 736–754.

Pager, J., Giachetti, I., Holley, A. and LeMagnen, J. (1972). A selective control of olfactory bulb electrical activity in relation to food deprivation and satiety in rats, *Physiology and Behavior* **9**: 573–580.

Palomero-Gallagher, N. and Zilles, K. (2004). Isocortex, *in* G. Paxinos (ed.), *The Rat Nervous System*, Elsevier Academic Press, San Diego, pp. 729–757.

Pandya, D. N., Seltzer, B., Petrides, M. and Cipolloni, P. B. (2015). *Cerebral Cortex: Architecture, Connections, and the Dual Origin Concept*, Oxford University Press, New York.

Pantelis, C., Barber, F. Z., Barnes, T. R., Nelson, H. E., Owen, A. M. and Robbins, T. W. (1999). Comparison of set-shifting ability in patients with chronic schizophrenia and frontal lobe damage, *Schizophrenia Research* **37**: 251–270.

Panzeri, S. and Treves, A. (1996). Analytical estimates of limited sampling biases in different information measures, *Network* **7**: 87–107.

Panzeri, S., Biella, G., Rolls, E. T., Skaggs, W. E. and Treves, A. (1996). Speed, noise, information and the graded nature of neuronal responses, *Network* **7**: 365–370.

Panzeri, S., Schultz, S. R., Treves, A. and Rolls, E. T. (1999a). Correlations and the encoding of information in the nervous system, *Proceedings of the Royal Society B* **266**: 1001–1012.

Panzeri, S., Treves, A., Schultz, S. and Rolls, E. T. (1999b). On decoding the responses of a population of neurons from short time windows, *Neural Computation* **11**: 1553–1577.

Panzeri, S., Rolls, E. T., Battaglia, F. and Lavis, R. (2001). Speed of feedforward and recurrent processing in multilayer networks of integrate-and-fire neurons, *Network: Computation in Neural Systems* **12**: 423–440.

Panzeri, S., Moroni, M., Safaai, H. and Harvey, C. D. (2022). The structures and functions of correlations in neural population codes, *Nat Rev Neurosci* **23**: 551–567.

Papagno, C. (2018). Memory deficits, *Handbook of Clinical Neurology, Parietal Cortex* **151**: 377–393.

Papp, G. and Treves, A. (2008). Network analysis of the significance of hippocampal subfields, *in* S. J. Y. Mizumori (ed.), *Hippocampal Place Fields: Relevance to Learning and Memory.*, Oxford University Press, New York, chapter 20, pp. 328–342.

Parga, N. and Rolls, E. T. (1998). Transform invariant recognition by association in a recurrent network, *Neural Computation* **10**: 1507–1525.

Parisi, G. (1986). A memory which forgets, *Journal of Physics A* **19**: L617–L619.

Parker, A. J. (2007). Binocular depth perception and the cerebral cortex, *Nature Reviews Neuroscience* **8**: 379–391.

Parker, A. J., Cumming, B. G. and Dodd, J. V. (2000). Binocular neurons and the perception of depth, *in* M. Gazzaniga (ed.), *The New Cognitive Neurosciences, Second Edition*, MIT Press, Cambridge, MA, chapter 18, pp. 263–277.

Parker, H. E., Gribble, F. M. and Reimann, F. (2014). The role of gut endocrine cells in control of metabolism and appetite, *Exp Physiol* **99**: 1116–20.

Parkinson, J. K., Murray, E. A. and Mishkin, M. (1988). A selective mnemonic role for the hippocampus in monkeys: memory for the location of objects, *Journal of Neuroscience* **8**: 4059–4167.

Passarelli, L., Gamberini, M. and Fattori, P. (2021). The superior parietal lobule of primates: a sensory-motor hub for interaction with the environment, *J Integr Neurosci* **20**: 157–171.

Passingham, R. E. (2021). *Understanding the Prefrontal Cortex: selective advantage, connectivity and neural operations*, Oxford University Press, Oxford.

Passingham, R. E. P. and Wise, S. P. (2012). *The Neurobiology of the Prefrontal Cortex*, Oxford University Press, Oxford.

Pasupathy, A., Kim, T. and Popovkina, D. V. (2019). Object shape and surface properties are jointly encoded in mid-level ventral visual cortex, *Curr Opin Neurobiol* **58**: 199–208.

Patel, G. H., Sestieri, C. and Corbetta, M. (2019). The evolution of the temporoparietal junction and posterior superior temporal sulcus, *Cortex* **118**: 38–50.

Paton, J. J., Belova, M. A., Morrison, S. E. and Salzman, C. D. (2006). The primate amygdala represents the positive and negative value of visual stimuli during learning, *Nature* **439**: 865–870.

Patterson, K., Nestor, P. J. and Rogers, T. T. (2007). Where do you know what you know? The representation of semantic knowledge in the human brain, *Nat Rev Neurosci* **8**: 976–87.

Paul, S. (2009). Binaural recording technology: a historical review and possible future developments, *Acta Acustica united with Acustica* **95**: 767–788.

Pauls, D. L., Abramovitch, A., Rauch, S. L. and Geller, D. A. (2014). Obsessive-compulsive disorder: an integrative genetic and neurobiological perspective, *Nat Rev Neurosci* **15**: 410–24.

Penades, R., Catalan, R., Andres, S., Salamero, M. and Gasto, C. (2005). Executive function and nonverbal memory in obsessive-compulsive disorder, *Psychiatry Research* **133**: 81–90.

Penades, R., Catalan, R., Rubia, K., Andres, S., Salamero, M. and Gasto, C. (2007). Impaired response inhibition in obsessive compulsive disorder, *European Psychiatry* **22**: 404–410.

Peng, H. C., Sha, L. F., Gan, Q. and Wei, Y. (1998). Energy function for learning invariance in multilayer perceptron, *Electronics Letters* **34**(3): 292–294.

Pennartz, C. M., Ameerun, R. F., Groenewegen, H. J. and Lopes da Silva, F. H. (1993). Synaptic plasticity in an in vitro slice preparation of the rat nucleus accumbens, *European Journal of Neuroscience* **5**: 107–117.

Percheron, G., Yelnik, J. and François, C. (1984a). The primate striato-pallido-nigral system: an integrative system for cortical information, *in* J. S. McKenzie, R. E. Kemm and L. N. Wilcox (eds), *The Basal Ganglia: Structure and Function*, Plenum, New York, pp. 87–105.

Percheron, G., Yelnik, J. and François, C. (1984b). A Golgi analysis of the primate globus pallidus. III. Spatial organization of the striato-pallidal complex, *Journal of Comparative Neurology* **227**: 214–227.

Percheron, G., Yelnik, J., François, C., Fenelon, G. and Talbi, B. (1994). Informational neurology of the basal ganglia related system, *Revue Neurologique (Paris)* **150**: 614–626.

Perez Castillo, I. and Skantzos, N. S. (2004). The Little-Hopfield model on a sparse random graph, *Journal of Physics A: Math Gen* **37**: 9087–9099.

Perrett, D., Mistlin, A. and Chitty, A. (1987). Visual neurons responsive to faces, *Trends in Neurosciences* **10**: 358–364.

Perrett, D. I., Rolls, E. T. and Caan, W. (1979). Temporal lobe cells of the monkey with visual responses selective for faces, *Neuroscience Letters* **S3**: S358.

Perrett, D. I., Rolls, E. T. and Caan, W. (1982). Visual neurons responsive to faces in the monkey temporal cortex, *Experimental Brain Research* **47**: 329–342.

Perrett, D. I., Smith, P. A. J., Mistlin, A. J., Chitty, A. J., Head, A. S., Potter, D. D., Broennimann, R., Milner, A. D. and Jeeves, M. A. (1985a). Visual analysis of body movements by neurons in the temporal cortex of the macaque monkey: a preliminary report, *Behavioural Brain Research* **16**: 153–170.

Perrett, D. I., Smith, P. A. J., Potter, D. D., Mistlin, A. J., Head, A. S., Milner, D. and Jeeves, M. A. (1985b). Visual cells in temporal cortex sensitive to face view and gaze direction, *Proceedings of the Royal Society of London, Series B* **223**: 293–317.

Perry, C. J. and Fallah, M. (2014). Feature integration and object representations along the dorsal stream visual hierarchy, *Front Comput Neurosci* **8**: 84.

Perry, G., Rolls, E. T. and Stringer, S. M. (2006). Spatial vs temporal continuity in view invariant visual object recognition learning, *Vision Res* **46**: 3994–4006.

Perry, G., Rolls, E. T. and Stringer, S. M. (2010). Continuous transformation learning of translation invariant representations, *Experimental Brain Research* **204**: 255–270.

Persichetti, A. S. and Dilks, D. D. (2019). Distinct representations of spatial and categorical relationships across human scene-selective cortex, *Proc Natl Acad Sci U S A* **116**: 21312–21317.

Personnaz, L., Guyon, I. and Dreyfus, G. (1985). Information storage and retrieval in spin-glass-like neural networks, *Journal de Physique Lettres (Paris)* **46**: 359–365.

Pessoa, L. (2009). How do emotion and motivation direct executive control?, *Trends in Cognitive Sciences* **13**: 160–166.

Pessoa, L. and Adolphs, R. (2010). Emotion processing and the amygdala: from a 'low road' to 'many roads' of evaluating biological significance, *Nature Reviews Neuroscience* **11**: 773–783.

Pessoa, L. and Hof, P. R. (2015). From Paul Broca's great limbic lobe to the limbic system, *J Comp Neurol* **523**: 2495–500.

Peters, A. (1984a). Bipolar cells, *in* A. Peters and E. G. Jones (eds), *Cerebral Cortex, Vol. 1, Cellular Components of the Cerebral Cortex*, Plenum, New York, chapter 11, pp. 381–407.

Peters, A. (1984b). Chandelier cells, *in* A. Peters and E. G. Jones (eds), *Cerebral Cortex, Vol. 1, Cellular Components of the Cerebral Cortex*, Plenum, New York, chapter 10, pp. 361–380.

Peters, A. and Jones, E. G. (eds) (1984). *Cerebral Cortex, Vol. 1, Cellular Components of the Cerebral Cortex*, Plenum, New York.

Peters, A. and Regidor, J. (1981). A reassessment of the forms of nonpyramidal neurons in area 17 of the cat visual cortex, *Journal of Comparative Neurology* **203**: 685–716.

Peters, A. and Saint Marie, R. L. (1984). Smooth and sparsely spinous nonpyramidal cells forming local axonal plexuses, *in* A. Peters and E. G. Jones (eds), *Cerebral Cortex, Vol. 1, Cellular Components of the Cerebral Cortex*, New York, Plenum, chapter 13, pp. 419–445.

Peterson, C. and Anderson, J. R. (1987). A mean field theory learning algorithm for neural networks, *Complex Systems* **1**: 995–1015.

Petkov, C. I., Kikuchi, Y., Milne, A. E., Mishkin, M., Rauschecker, J. P. and Logothetis, N. K. (2015). Different forms of effective connectivity in primate frontotemporal pathways, *Nat Commun* **6**: 6000.

Petri, H. L. and Mishkin, M. (1994). Behaviorism, cognitivism, and the neuropsychology of memory, *American Scientist* **82**: 30–37.

Petrides, M. (1985). Deficits on conditional associative-learning tasks after frontal- and temporal-lobe lesions in man, *Neuropsychologia* **23**: 601–614.

Petrides, M. (1996). Specialized systems for the processing of mnemonic information within the primate frontal cortex, *Philosophical Transactions of the Royal Society of London B* **351**: 1455–1462.

Petrides, M. (2014). *Neuroanatomy of Language Regions of the Human Brain*, Academic Press, New York.

Petrides, M. and Pandya, D. N. (1988). Association fiber pathways to the frontal cortex from the superior temporal region in the rhesus monkey, *Journal of Comparative Neurology* **273**: 52–66.

Petrides, M. and Pandya, D. N. (1999). Dorsolateral prefrontal cortex: comparative cytoarchitectonic analysis in the human and the macaque brain and corticocortical connection patterns, *Eur J Neurosci* **11**: 1011–36.

Petrides, M. and Pandya, D. N. (2002). Comparative cytoarchitectonic analysis of the human and the macaque ventrolateral prefrontal cortex and corticocortical connection patterns in the monkey, *Eur J Neurosci* **16**: 291–310.

Petrides, M., Tomaiuolo, F., Yeterian, E. H. and Pandya, D. N. (2012). The prefrontal cortex: comparative architectonic organization in the human and the macaque monkey brains, *Cortex* **48**: 46–57.

Phelps, E. A. (2004). Human emotion and memory: interactions of the amygdala and hippocampal complex, *Curr Opin Neurobiol* **14**: 198–202.

Phelps, E. A. (2006). Emotion and cognition: insights from studies of the human amygdala, *Annu Rev Psychol* **57**: 27–53.

Phelps, E. A. and LeDoux, J. E. (2005). Contributions of the amygdala to emotion processing: from animal models to human behavior, *Neuron* **48**: 175–87.

Phelps, E., O'Connor, K. J., Gatenby, J. C., Gore, J. C., Grillon, C. and Davis, M. (2001). Activation of the left amygdala to a cognitive representation of fear, *Nature Neuroscience* **4**: 437–441.

Phillips, A. G., Mora, F. and Rolls, E. T. (1981). Intra-cerebral self-administration of amphetamine by rhesus monkeys, *Neuroscience Letters* **24**: 81–86.

Phillips, M. L., Drevets, W. C., Rauch, S. L. and Lane, R. (2003). Neurobiology of emotion perception II: Implications for major psychiatric disorders, *Biological Psychiatry* **54**: 515–528.

Phillips, R. R., Malamut, B. L., Bachevalier, J. and Mishkin, M. (1988). Dissociation of the effects of inferior temporal and limbic lesions on object discrimination learning with 24-h intertrial intervals, *Behavioural Brain Research* **27**: 99–107.

Phillips, W. A., Kay, J. and Smyth, D. (1995). The discovery of structure by multi-stream networks of local processors with contextual guidance, *Network* **6**: 225–246.

Pinker, S. (1995). *The Language Instinct: The New Science of Language and Mind*, Vol. 7529, Penguin UK.

Pinto, N., Cox, D. D. and DiCarlo, J. J. (2008). Why is real-world visual object recognition hard?, *PLoS Computational Biology* **4**: e27.

Pinto, N., Doukhan, D., DiCarlo, J. J. and Cox, D. D. (2009). A high-throughput screening approach to discovering good forms of biologically inspired visual representation, *PLoS Computational Biology* **5**: e1000579.

Piray, P., Dezfouli, A., Heskes, T., Frank, M. J. and Daw, N. D. (2019). Hierarchical Bayesian inference for concurrent model fitting and comparison for group studies, *PLoS Comput Biol* **15**: e1007043.

Pirmoradian, S. and Treves, A. (2013). Encoding words into a Potts attractor network, *in* J. Mayor and P. Gomez (eds), *Computational Models of Cognitive Processes: Proceedings of the 13th Neural Computation and Psychology Workshop (NCPW13)*, World Scientific Press, Singapore, pp. 29–42.

Pitcher, D. and Ungerleider, L. G. (2021). Evidence for a third visual pathway specialized for social perception, *Trends Cogn Sci* **25**: 100–110.

Pitcher, D., Ianni, G. and Ungerleider, L. G. (2019). A functional dissociation of face-, body- and scene-selective brain areas based on their response to moving and static stimuli, *Sci Rep* **9**: 8242.

Pitkanen, A., Kelly, J. L. and Amaral, D. G. (2002). Projections from the lateral, basal, and accessory basal nuclei of the amygdala to the entorhinal cortex in the macaque monkey, *Hippocampus* **12**: 186–205.

Pittenger, C. (2015). Glutamatergic agents for OCD and related disorders, *Curr Treat Options Psychiatry* **2**: 271–283.

Pittenger, C. (2021). Pharmacotherapeutic strategies and new targets in OCD, *Curr Top Behav Neurosci* **49**: 331–384.

Pittenger, C., Krystal, J. H. and Coric, V. (2006). Glutamate-modulating drugs as novel pharmacotherapeutic agents in the treatment of obsessive-compulsive disorder, *NeuroRx* **3**(1): 69–81.

Pittenger, C., Bloch, M. H. and Williams, K. (2011). Glutamate abnormalities in obsessive compulsive disorder: Neurobiology, pathophysiology, and treatment, *Pharmacology and Therapeutics* **132**: 314–332.

Pitzalis, S., Sereno, M. I., Committeri, G., Fattori, P., Galati, G., Tosoni, A. and Galletti, C. (2013). The human homologue of macaque area V6A, *Neuroimage* **82**: 517–30.

Pitzalis, S., Fattori, P. and Galletti, C. (2015). The human cortical areas V6 and V6A, *Vis Neurosci* **32**: E007.

Pitzalis, S., Serra, C., Sulpizio, V., Di Marco, S., Fattori, P., Galati, G. and Galletti, C. (2019). A putative human homologue of the macaque area PEc, *Neuroimage* **202**: 116092.

Plakke, B. and Romanski, L. M. (2014). Auditory connections and functions of prefrontal cortex, *Front Neurosci* **8**: 199.

Plakke, B. and Romanski, L. M. (2016). Neural circuits in auditory and audiovisual memory, *Brain Res* **1640**: 278–88.

Plakke, B., Diltz, M. D. and Romanski, L. M. (2013). Coding of vocalizations by single neurons in ventrolateral prefrontal cortex, *Hear Res* **305**: 135–43.

Platt, M. L. and Glimcher, P. W. (1999). Neural correlates of decision variables in parietal cortex, *Nature* **400**: 233–238.

Platt, M. L., Seyfarth, R. M. and Cheney, D. L. (2016). Adaptations for social cognition in the primate brain, *Philos Trans R Soc Lond B Biol Sci* **371**: 20150096.

Plebe, A. and Grasso, G. (2019). The unbearable shallow understanding of deep learning, *Minds and Machines* **29**: 515–553.

Ploux, E., Freret, T. and Billard, J. M. (2020). d-serine in physiological and pathological brain aging, *Biochim Biophys Acta Proteins Proteom* **1869**: 140542.

Poggio, T. and Edelman, S. (1990). A network that learns to recognize three-dimensional objects, *Nature* **343**: 263–266.

Poggio, T. and Girosi, F. (1990a). Networks for approximation and learning, *Proceedings of the IEEE* **78**: 1481–1497.

Poggio, T. and Girosi, F. (1990b). Regularization algorithms for learning that are equivalent to multilayer networks, *Science* **247**: 978–982.

Pollen, D. and Ronner, S. (1981). Phase relationship between adjacent simple cells in the visual cortex, *Science* **212**: 1409–1411.

Poremba, A., Saunders, R. C., Crane, A. M., Cook, M., Sokoloff, L. and Mishkin, M. (2003). Functional mapping of the primate auditory system, *Science* **299**: 568–572.

Posner, M. I. and Keele, S. W. (1968). On the genesis of abstract ideas, *Journal of Experimental Psychology* **77**: 353–363.

Postle, B. R. and D'Esposito, M. (1999). "What" – then – "Where" in visual working memory: An event-related fMRI study, *Journal of Cognitive Neuroscience* **11**: 585–597.

Postle, B. R. and D'Esposito, M. (2000). Evaluating models of the topographical organization of working memory function in frontal cortex with event-related fMRI, *Psychobiology* **28**: 132–145.

Poucet, B. (1989). Object exploration, habituation, and response to a spatial change in rats following septal or medial frontal cortical damage, *Behavioral Neuroscience* **103**: 1009–1016.

Poulter, S., Hartley, T. and Lever, C. (2018). The neurobiology of mammalian navigation, *Curr Biol* **28**: R1023–R1042.

Powell, T. P. S. (1981). Certain aspects of the intrinsic organisation of the cerebral cortex, *in* O. Pompeiano and C. Ajmone Marsan (eds), *Brain Mechanisms and Perceptual Awareness*, Raven Press, New York, pp. 1–19.

Power, J. M. and Sah, P. (2008). Competition between calcium-activated K+ channels determines cholinergic action on firing properties of basolateral amygdala projection neurons, *Journal of Neuroscience* **28**: 3209–3220.

Prado, J., Clavagnier, S., Otzenberger, H., Scheiber, C., Kennedy, H. and Perenin, M. T. (2005). Two cortical systems for reaching in central and peripheral vision, *Neuron* **48**: 849–58.

Preston, A. R. and Eichenbaum, H. (2013). Interplay of hippocampus and prefrontal cortex in memory, *Curr Biol* **23**: R764–73.

Preuss, T. M. (1995). Do rats have prefrontal cortex? The Rose-Woolsey-Akert program reconsidered, *Journal of Cognitive Neuroscience* **7**: 1–24.

Preuss, T. M. and Goldman-Rakic, P. S. (1989). Connections of the ventral granular frontal cortex of macaques with perisylvian premotor and somatosensory areas: anatomical evidence for somatic representation in primate frontal association cortex, *Journal of Comparative Neurology* **282**: 293–316.

Price, A. R., Bonner, M. F., Peelle, J. E. and Grossman, M. (2015). Converging evidence for the neuroanatomic basis of combinatorial semantics in the angular gyrus, *J Neurosci* **35**: 3276–84.

Price, J. L. (2006). Connections of orbital cortex, *in* D. H. Zald and S. L. Rauch (eds), *The Orbitofrontal Cortex*, Oxford University Press, Oxford, chapter 3, pp. 39–55.

Price, J. L. and Drevets, W. C. (2010). Neurocircuitry of mood disorders, *Neuropsychopharmacology* **35**: 192–216.

Price, J. L. and Drevets, W. C. (2012). Neural circuits underlying the pathophysiology of mood disorders, *Trends Cogn Sci* **16**: 61–71.

Price, J. L., Carmichael, S. T., Carnes, K. M., Clugnet, M.-C. and Kuroda, M. (1991). Olfactory input to the prefrontal cortex, *in* J. L. Davis and H. Eichenbaum (eds), *Olfaction: A Model System for Computational Neuroscience*, MIT Press, Cambridge, MA, pp. 101–120.

Price, S. L. and Bloom, S. R. (2014). Protein PYY and its role in metabolism, *Front Horm Res* **42**: 147–54.

Pritchard, S. C., Coltheart, M., Marinus, E. and Castles, A. (2018). A computational model of the self-teaching hypothesis based on the dual-route cascaded model of reading, *Cogn Sci* **42**: 722–770.

Pritchard, T. C., Hamilton, R. B. and Norgren, R. (1989). Neural coding of gustatory information in the thalamus of Macaca mulatta, *Journal of Neurophysiology* **61**: 1–14.

Pritchard, T., Hamilton, R., Morse, J. and Norgren, R. (1986). Projections of thalamic gustatory and lingual areas in the monkey, Macaca fascicularis, *Journal of Comparative Neurology* **244**: 213–228.

Procyk, E., Wilson, C. R., Stoll, F. M., Faraut, M. C., Petrides, M. and Amiez, C. (2016). Midcingulate motor map and feedback detection: converging data from humans and monkeys, *Cereb Cortex* **26**: 467–76.

Proulx, C. D., Hikosaka, O. and Malinow, R. (2014). Reward processing by the lateral habenula in normal and depressive behaviors, *Nat Neurosci* **17**: 1146–52.

Prusky, G. T., West, P. W. and Douglas, R. M. (2000). Behavioral assessment of visual acuity in mice and rats, *Vision Res* **40**: 2201–9.

Pryce, C. R., Azzinnari, D., Spinelli, S., Seifritz, E., Tegethoff, M. and Meinlschmidt, G. (2011). Helplessness: a systematic translational review of theory and evidence for its relevance to understanding and treating depression, *Pharmacol Ther* **132**: 242–267.

Quesque, F. and Brass, M. (2019). The role of the TemporoParietal Junction in self-other distinction, *Brain Topogr* **32**: 943–955.

Quian Quiroga, R. (2012). Concept cells: the building blocks of declarative memory functions, *Nat Rev Neurosci* **13**: 587–97.

Quian Quiroga, R. (2013). Gnostic cells in the 21st century, *Acta Neurobiol Exp (Wars)* **73**: 463–71.

Quian Quiroga, R. (2023). An integrative view of human hippocampal function: differences with other species and capacity considerations, *Hippocampus* **33**: 616–634.

Quian Quiroga, R., Reddy, L., Kreiman, G., Koch, C. and Fried, I. (2005). Invariant visual representation by single neurons in the human brain, *Nature* **435**: 1102–7.

Quirk, G. J., Armony, J. L., Repa, J. C., Li, X. F. and LeDoux, J. E. (1996). Emotional memory: a search for sites of plasticity, *Cold Spring Harb Symp Quant Biol* **61**: 247–57.

Rachlin, H. (1989). *Judgement, Decision, and Choice: A Cognitive/Behavioural Synthesis*, Freeman, New York.

Raffi, M., Maioli, M. G. and Squatrito, S. (2011). Optic flow direction coding in area PEc of the behaving monkey, *Neuroscience* **194**: 136–49.

Rajalingham, R., Issa, E. B., Bashivan, P., Kar, K., Schmidt, K. and DiCarlo, J. J. (2018). Large-scale, high-resolution comparison of the core visual object recognition behavior of humans, monkeys, and state-of-the-art deep artificial neural networks, *J Neurosci* **38**: 7255–7269.

Rajalingham, R., Kar, K., Sanghavi, S., Dehaene, S. and DiCarlo, J. J. (2020). The inferior temporal cortex is a potential cortical precursor of orthographic processing in untrained monkeys, *Nat Commun* **11**: 3886.

Ranck, Jr., J. B. (1985). Head direction cells in the deep cell layer of dorsolateral presubiculum in freely moving rats, in G. Buzsáki and C. H. Vanderwolf (eds), *Electrical Activity of the Archicortex*, Akadémiai Kiadó, Budapest.

Rao, S. C., Rainer, G. and Miller, E. K. (1997). Integration of what and where in the primate prefrontal cortex, *Science* **276**: 821–824.

Rao, V. R., Sellers, K. K., Wallace, D. L., Lee, M. B., Bijanzadeh, M., Sani, O. G., Yang, Y., Shanechi, M. M., Dawes, H. E. and Chang, E. F. (2018). Direct electrical stimulation of lateral orbitofrontal cortex acutely improves mood in individuals with symptoms of depression, *Curr Biol* **28**: 3893–3902 e4.

Rauschecker, J. P. (1998a). Cortical processing of complex sounds, *Curr Opin Neurobiol* **8**: 516–21.

Rauschecker, J. P. (1998b). Parallel processing in the auditory cortex of primates, *Audiol Neurootol* **3**: 86–103.

Rauschecker, J. P. (2011). An expanded role for the dorsal auditory pathway in sensorimotor control and integration, *Hear Res* **271**: 16–25.

Rauschecker, J. P. (2012). Ventral and dorsal streams in the evolution of speech and language, *Front Evol Neurosci* **4**: 7.

Rauschecker, J. P. (2015). Auditory cortex, *Reference Module in Neuroscience and Biobehavioral Psychology. Brain Mapping* **2**: 299–304.

Rauschecker, J. P. (2018a). Where did language come from? Precursor mechanisms in nonhuman primates, *Curr Opin Behav Sci* **21**: 195–204.

Rauschecker, J. P. (2018b). Where, When, and How: Are they all sensorimotor? Towards a unified view of the dorsal pathway in vision and audition, *Cortex* **98**: 262–268.

Rauschecker, J. P. and Scott, S. K. (2009). Maps and streams in the auditory cortex: nonhuman primates illuminate human speech processing, *Nat Neurosci* **12**: 718–24.

Rauschecker, J. P. and Tian, B. (2000). Mechanisms and streams for processing of "what" and "where" in auditory cortex, *Proc Natl Acad Sci U S A* **97**: 11800–6.

Rauschecker, J. P., Tian, B. and Hauser, M. (1995). Processing of complex sounds in the macaque nonprimary auditory cortex, *Science* **268**: 111–4.

Rawlins, J. N. P. (1985). Associations across time: the hippocampus as a temporary memory store, *Behavioral Brain Science* **8**: 479–496.

Razi, A., Seghier, M. L., Zhou, Y., McColgan, P., Zeidman, P., Park, H. J., Sporns, O., Rees, G. and Friston, K. J. (2017). Large-scale DCMs for resting-state fMRI, *Netw Neurosci* **1**: 222–241.

Reber, J., Feinstein, J. S., O'Doherty, J. P., Liljeholm, M., Adolphs, R. and Tranel, D. (2017). Selective impairment of goal-directed decision-making following lesions to the human ventromedial prefrontal cortex, *Brain* **140**: 1743–1756.

Redgrave, P., Prescott, T. J. and Gurney, K. (1999). Is the short-latency dopamine response too short to signal reward error?, *Trends in Neuroscience* **22**: 146–151.

Reichle, E. D. (2021). *Computational Models of Reading: A Handbook*, Oxford University Press, Oxford.

Rempel-Clower, N. L. and Barbas, H. (1998). Topographic organization of connections between the hypothalamus and prefrontal cortex in the rhesus monkey, *Journal of Comparative Neurology* **398**: 393–419.

Renart, A., Parga, N. and Rolls, E. T. (1999a). Associative memory properties of multiple cortical modules, *Network* **10**: 237–255.

Renart, A., Parga, N. and Rolls, E. T. (1999b). Backprojections in the cerebral cortex: implications for memory storage, *Neural Computation* **11**: 1349–1388.

Renart, A., Parga, N. and Rolls, E. T. (2000). A recurrent model of the interaction between the prefrontal cortex and inferior temporal cortex in delay memory tasks, *in* S. Solla, T. Leen and K.-R. Mueller (eds), *Advances in Neural Information Processing Systems*, Vol. 12, MIT Press, Cambridge, MA, pp. 171–177.

Renart, A., Moreno, R., Rocha, J., Parga, N. and Rolls, E. T. (2001). A model of the IT–PF network in object working memory which includes balanced persistent activity and tuned inhibition, *Neurocomputing* **38–40**: 1525–1531.

Rensink, R. A. (2000). Seeing, sensing, and scrutinizing, *Vision Research* **40**: 1469–1487.

Rensink, R. A. (2014). Limits to the usability of iconic memory, *Front Psychol* **5**: 971.

Rensink, R. A. (2018). To have seen or not to have seen: a look at Rensink, O'Regan, and Clark (1997), *Perspect Psychol Sci* **13**: 230–235.

Rescorla, R. A. and Wagner, A. R. (1972). A theory of Pavlovian conditioning: the effectiveness of reinforcement and non-reinforcement, *Classical Conditioning II: Current Research and Theory*, Appleton-Century-Crofts, New York, pp. 64–69.

Rey, H. G., Ison, M. J., Pedreira, C., Valentin, A., Alarcon, G., Selway, R., Richardson, M. P. and Quian Quiroga, R. (2015). Single-cell recordings in the human medial temporal lobe, *J Anat* **227**: 394–408.

Reynolds, J. N. and Wickens, J. R. (2002). Dopamine-dependent plasticity of corticostriatal synapses, *Neural Networks* **15**: 507–521.

Rhee, T. G., Shim, S. R., Forester, B. P., Nierenberg, A. A., McIntyre, R. S., Papakostas, G. I., Krystal, J. H., Sanacora, G. and Wilkinson, S. T. (2022). Efficacy and safety of ketamine vs electroconvulsive therapy among patients with Major Depressive Episode: A systematic review and meta-analysis, *JAMA Psychiatry* **79**: 1162–1172.

Rhodes, P. (1992). The open time of the NMDA channel facilitates the self-organisation of invariant object responses in cortex, *Society for Neuroscience Abstracts* **18**: 740.

Ridley, M. (1993). *The Red Queen: Sex and the Evolution of Human Nature*, Penguin, London.

Rieke, F., Warland, D. and Bialek, W. (1993). Coding efficiency and information rates in sensory neurons, *Europhysics Letters* **22**: 151–156.

Rieke, F., Warland, D., de Ruyter van Steveninck, R. R. and Bialek, W. (1997). *Spikes: Exploring the Neural Code*, MIT Press, Cambridge, MA.

Riesenhuber, M. and Poggio, T. (1998). Just one view: Invariances in inferotemporal cell tuning, *in* M. I. Jordan, M. J. Kearns and S. A. Solla (eds), *Advances in Neural Information Processing Systems*, Vol. 10, MIT Press, Cambridge, MA, pp. 215–221.

Riesenhuber, M. and Poggio, T. (1999a). Are cortical models really bound by the "binding problem"?, *Neuron* **24**: 87–93.

Riesenhuber, M. and Poggio, T. (1999b). Hierarchical models of object recognition in cortex, *Nature Neuroscience* **2**: 1019–1025.

Riesenhuber, M. and Poggio, T. (2000). Models of object recognition, *Nature Neuroscience Supplement* **3**: 1199–1204.

Risold, P. Y. and Swanson, L. W. (1997). Connections of the rat lateral septal complex, *Brain Research Reviews* **24**: 115–195.

Riva-Posse, P., Choi, K. S., Holtzheimer, P. E., Crowell, A. L., Garlow, S. J., Rajendra, J. K., McIntyre, C. C., Gross, R. E. and Mayberg, H. S. (2018). A connectomic approach for subcallosal cingulate deep brain stimulation surgery: prospective targeting in treatment-resistant depression, *Mol Psychiatry* **23**: 843–849.

Rivard, B., Li, Y., Lenck-Santini, P. P., Poucet, B. and Muller, R. U. (2004). Representation of objects in space by two classes of hippocampal pyramidal cells, *J Gen Physiol* **124**: 9–25.

Rizzolatti, G. and Craighero, L. (2004). The mirror-neuron system, *Annual Review of Neuroscience* **27**: 169–192.

Rizzolatti, G. and Kalaska, J. F. (2013). Voluntary movement: the parietal and premotor cortex, *in* E. R. Kandel, J. H. Schwartz, T. M. Jessell, S. A. Siegelbaum and A. J. Hudspeth (eds), *Principles of neural science*, Vol. 5, McGraw-Hill, New York, pp. 865–893.

Rizzolatti, G. and Rozzi, S. (2018). The mirror mechanism in the parietal lobe, *Handb Clin Neurol* **151**: 555–573.

Rizzolatti, G. and Sinigaglia, C. (2016). The mirror mechanism: a basic principle of brain function, *Nat Rev Neurosci* **17**: 757–765.

Robbins, T. W. and Costa, R. M. (2017). Habits, *Curr Biol* **27**: R1200–R1206.

Robbins, T. W., Cador, M., Taylor, J. R. and Everitt, B. J. (1989). Limbic-striatal interactions in reward-related processes, *Neuroscience and Biobehavioral Reviews* **13**: 155–162.

Robbins, T. W., Vaghi, M. M. and Banca, P. (2019). Obsessive-Compulsive Disorder: puzzles and prospects, *Neuron* **102**: 27–47.

Robertson, R. G., Rolls, E. T. and Georges-François, P. (1998). Spatial view cells in the primate hippocampus: Effects of removal of view details, *Journal of Neurophysiology* **79**: 1145–1156.

Robertson, R. G., Rolls, E. T., Georges-François, P. and Panzeri, S. (1999). Head direction cells in the primate pre-subiculum, *Hippocampus* **9**: 206–219.

Robin, J., Hirshhorn, M., Rosenbaum, R. S., Winocur, G., Moscovitch, M. and Grady, C. L. (2015). Functional connectivity of hippocampal and prefrontal networks during episodic and spatial memory based on real-world environments, *Hippocampus* **25**: 81–93.

Robinson, L. and Rolls, E. T. (2015). Invariant visual object recognition: biologically plausibile approaches, *Biological Cybernetics* **109**: 505–535.

Rockland, K. S., Saleem, K. S. and Tanaka, K. (1994). Divergent Feedback Connections From Areas V4 and Teo In the Macaque, *Visual Neuroscience* **11**: 579–600.

Rodin, J. (1976). The role of perception of internal and external signals in the regulation of feeding in overweight and non-obese individuals, *Dahlem Konferenzen, Life Sciences Research Report* **2**: 265–281.

Roe, A. W., Chelazzi, L., Connor, C. E., Conway, B. R., Fujita, I., Gallant, J. L., Lu, H. and Vanduffel, W. (2012). Toward a unified theory of visual area V4, *Neuron* **74**: 12–29.

Rogan, M. T., Staubli, U. V. and LeDoux, J. E. (1997). Fear conditioning induces associative long-term potentiation in the amygdala, *Nature* **390**: 604–607.

Rogers Flattery, C. N., Rosen, R. F., Farberg, A. S., Dooyema, J. M., Hof, P. R., Sherwood, C. C., Walker, L. C. and Preuss, T. M. (2020). Quantification of neurons in the hippocampal formation of chimpanzees: comparison to rhesus monkeys and humans, *Brain Struct Funct* **225**: 2521–2531.

Rogers, J. L. and Kesner, R. P. (2003). Cholinergic modulation of the hippocampus during encoding and retrieval, *Neurobiology of Learning and Memory* **80**: 332–342.

Rogers, J. L. and Kesner, R. P. (2004). Cholinergic modulation of the hippocampus during encoding and retrieval of tone/shock-induced fear conditioning, *Learning and Memory* **11**: 102–107.

Rogers, J. L., Hunsaker, M. R. and Kesner, R. P. (2006). Effects of ventral and dorsal CA1 subregional lesions on trace fear conditioning, *Neurobiology of Learning and Memory* **86**: 72–81.

Rogers, R. D., Andrews, T. C., Grasby, P. M., Brooks, D. J. and Robbins, T. W. (2000). Contrasting cortical and subcortical activations produced by attentional-set shifting and reversal learning in humans, *Journal of Cognitive Neuroscience* **12**: 142–162.

Rolls, B. J. (2012a). Dietary strategies for weight management, *Nestle Nutrition Institute Workshop Series* **73**: 37–48.

Rolls, B. J., Rolls, E. T. and Rowe, E. A. (1980a). Sensory specific satiety and its influences on feeding, *Appetite* **1**: 85–86.

Rolls, B. J., Rolls, E. T., Rowe, E. A. and Sweeney, K. (1981a). How sensory properties of foods affect human feeding behaviour, *Physiology and Behavior* **29**: 409–417.

Rolls, B. J., Rolls, E. T., Rowe, E. A. and Sweeney, K. (1981b). Sensory specific satiety in man, *Physiology and Behavior* **27**: 137–142.

Rolls, B. J., Rowe, E. A., Rolls, E. T., Kingston, B., Megson, A. and Gunary, R. (1981c). Variety in a meal enhances food intake in man, *Physiology and Behavior* **26**: 215–221.

Rolls, B. J., Rolls, E. T. and Rowe, E. A. (1982a). The influence of variety on human food selection, *in* L. Barker (ed.), *Psychobiology of Human Food Selection*, AVI Publishing Company, Westport, Connecticut, pp. 101–122.

Rolls, B. J., Rowe, E. A. and Rolls, E. T. (1982b). How flavour and appearance affect human feeding, *Proceedings of the Nutrition Society,* **41**: 109–117.

Rolls, B. J., Rowe, E. A. and Rolls, E. T. (1982c). How sensory properties of foods affect human feeding behavior, *Physiology and Behavior* **29**: 409–417.

Rolls, E. T. (1973). Polar frequency response of the human ear, *Journal of Physiology* **134**: 18–19P.

Rolls, E. T. (1975). *The Brain and Reward*, Pergamon Press, Oxford.

Rolls, E. T. (1981a). Central nervous mechanisms related to feeding and appetite, *British Medical Bulletin* **37**: 131–134.

Rolls, E. T. (1981b). Processing beyond the inferior temporal visual cortex related to feeding, learning, and striatal function, *in* Y. Katsuki, R. Norgren and M. Sato (eds), *Brain Mechanisms of Sensation*, Wiley, New York, chapter 16, pp. 241–269.

Rolls, E. T. (1981c). Responses of amygdaloid neurons in the primate, *in* Y. Ben-Ari (ed.), *The Amygdaloid Complex*, Elsevier, Amsterdam, pp. 383–393.

Rolls, E. T. (1982). Neuronal mechanisms underlying the formation and disconnection of associations between visual stimuli and reinforcement in primates, *in* C. D. Woody (ed.), *Conditioning: Representation of Involved Neural Functions*, Plenum, New York, pp. 363–373.

Rolls, E. T. (1984). Neurons in the cortex of the temporal lobe and in the amygdala of the monkey with responses selective for faces, *Human Neurobiology* **3**: 209–222.

Rolls, E. T. (1986a). Neural systems involved in emotion in primates, *in* R. Plutchik and H. Kellerman (eds), *Emotion: Theory, Research, and Experience*, Vol. 3: Biological Foundations of Emotion, Academic Press, New York, chapter 5, pp. 125–143.

Rolls, E. T. (1986b). Neuronal activity related to the control of feeding, *in* R. Ritter, S. Ritter and C. Barnes (eds), *Feeding Behavior: Neural and Humoral Controls*, Academic Press, New York, chapter 6, pp. 163–190.

Rolls, E. T. (1986c). A theory of emotion, and its application to understanding the neural basis of emotion, *in* Y. Oomura (ed.), *Emotions. Neural and Chemical Control*, Japan Scientific Societies Press; and Karger, Tokyo; and Basel, pp. 325–344.

Rolls, E. T. (1987). Information representation, processing and storage in the brain: analysis at the single neuron level, *in* J.-P. Changeux and M. Konishi (eds), *The Neural and Molecular Bases of Learning*, Wiley, Chichester, pp. 503–540.

Rolls, E. T. (1989a). Functions of neuronal networks in the hippocampus and cerebral cortex in memory, *in* R. Cotterill (ed.), *Models of Brain Function*, Cambridge University Press, Cambridge, pp. 15–33.

Rolls, E. T. (1989b). Functions of neuronal networks in the hippocampus and neocortex in memory, *in* J. H. Byrne and W. O. Berry (eds), *Neural Models of Plasticity: Experimental and Theoretical Approaches*, Academic Press, San Diego, pp. 240–265.

Rolls, E. T. (1989c). Information processing and basal ganglia function, *in* C. Kennard and M. Swash (eds), *Hierarchies in Neurology*, Springer-Verlag, London, chapter 15, pp. 123–142.

Rolls, E. T. (1989d). Information processing in the taste system of primates, *Journal of Experimental Biology* **146**: 141–164.

Rolls, E. T. (1989e). Parallel distributed processing in the brain: implications of the functional architecture of neuronal networks in the hippocampus, *in* R. G. M. Morris (ed.), *Parallel Distributed Processing: Implications for Psychology and Neurobiology*, Oxford University Press, Oxford, chapter 12, pp. 286–308.

Rolls, E. T. (1989f). The representation and storage of information in neuronal networks in the primate cerebral cortex and hippocampus, *in* R. Durbin, C. Miall and G. Mitchison (eds), *The Computing Neuron*, Addison-Wesley, Wokingham, England, chapter 8, pp. 125–159.

Rolls, E. T. (1990a). Functions of the primate hippocampus in spatial processing and memory, *in* D. S. Olton and R. P. Kesner (eds), *Neurobiology of Comparative Cognition*, L. Erlbaum, Hillsdale, NJ, chapter 12, pp. 339–362.

Rolls, E. T. (1990b). Theoretical and neurophysiological analysis of the functions of the primate hippocampus in memory, *Cold Spring Harbor Symposia in Quantitative Biology* **55**: 995–1006.

Rolls, E. T. (1990c). A theory of emotion, and its application to understanding the neural basis of emotion, *Cognition and Emotion* **4**: 161–190.

Rolls, E. T. (1992a). Neurophysiological mechanisms underlying face processing within and beyond the temporal cortical visual areas, *Philosophical Transactions of the Royal Society of London B* **335**: 11–21.

Rolls, E. T. (1992b). Neurophysiology and functions of the primate amygdala, *in* J. P. Aggleton (ed.), *The Amygdala*, Wiley-Liss, New York, chapter 5, pp. 143–165.

Rolls, E. T. (1993). The neural control of feeding in primates, *in* D. Booth (ed.), *Neurophysiology of Ingestion*, Pergamon, Oxford, chapter 9, pp. 137–169.

Rolls, E. T. (1994a). Brain mechanisms for invariant visual recognition and learning, *Behavioural Processes* **33**: 113–138.

Rolls, E. T. (1994b). Neurophysiological and neuronal network analysis of how the primate hippocampus functions in memory, *in* J. Delacour (ed.), *The Memory System of the Brain*, World Scientific, London, pp. 713–744.

Rolls, E. T. (1994c). Neurophysiology and cognitive functions of the striatum, *Revue Neurologique (Paris)* **150**: 648–660.

Rolls, E. T. (1995a). Learning mechanisms in the temporal lobe visual cortex, *Behavioural Brain Research* **66**: 177–185.

Rolls, E. T. (1995b). A model of the operation of the hippocampus and entorhinal cortex in memory, *International Journal of Neural Systems* **6**: 51–70.

Rolls, E. T. (1996a). The orbitofrontal cortex, *Philosophical Transactions of the Royal Society B* **351**: 1433–1444.

Rolls, E. T. (1996b). The representation of space in the primate hippocampus, and its relation to memory, *in* K. Ishikawa, J. L. McGaugh and H. Sakata (eds), *Brain Processes and Memory*, Elsevier, Amsterdam, pp. 203–227.

Rolls, E. T. (1996c). Roles of Long Term Potentiation and Long Term Depression in neuronal network operations in the brain, *in* M. S. Fazeli and G. L. Collingridge (eds), *Cortical Plasticity: LTP and LTD*, Bios, Oxford, chapter 11, pp. 223–250.

Rolls, E. T. (1996d). A theory of hippocampal function in memory, *Hippocampus* **6**: 601–620.

Rolls, E. T. (1997a). Brain mechanisms of vision, memory, and consciousness, *in* M. Ito, Y. Miyashita and E. Rolls (eds), *Cognition, Computation, and Consciousness*, Oxford University Press, Oxford, pp. 81–120.

Rolls, E. T. (1997b). Consciousness in neural networks?, *Neural Networks* **10**: 1227–1240.

Rolls, E. T. (1997c). A neurophysiological and computational approach to the functions of the temporal lobe cortical visual areas in invariant object recognition, *in* M. Jenkin and L. Harris (eds), *Computational and Psychophysical Mechanisms of Visual Coding*, Cambridge University Press, Cambridge, chapter 9, pp. 184–220.

Rolls, E. T. (1999a). *The Brain and Emotion*, Oxford University Press, Oxford.

Rolls, E. T. (1999b). The functions of the orbitofrontal cortex, *Neurocase* **5**: 301–312.

Rolls, E. T. (1999c). Spatial view cells and the representation of place in the primate hippocampus, *Hippocampus* **9**: 467–480.

Rolls, E. T. (2000a). Functions of the primate temporal lobe cortical visual areas in invariant visual object and face recognition, *Neuron* **27**: 205–18.

Rolls, E. T. (2000b). Memory systems in the brain, *Annual Review of Psychology* **51**: 599–630.

Rolls, E. T. (2000c). Neurophysiology and functions of the primate amygdala, and the neural basis of emotion, *in* J. P. Aggleton (ed.), *The Amygdala: Second Edition. A Functional Analysis*, Oxford University Press, Oxford, chapter 13, pp. 447–478.

Rolls, E. T. (2000d). The orbitofrontal cortex and reward, *Cerebral Cortex* **10**: 284–294.

Rolls, E. T. (2000e). Precis of The Brain and Emotion, *Behav Brain Sci* **23**: 177–91; discussion 192–233.

Rolls, E. T. (2001). The rules of formation of the olfactory representations found in the orbitofrontal cortex olfactory areas in primates, *Chemical Senses* **26**: 595–604.

Rolls, E. T. (2003). Consciousness absent and present: a neurophysiological exploration, *Progress in Brain Research* **144**: 95–106.

Rolls, E. T. (2004a). The functions of the orbitofrontal cortex, *Brain and Cognition* **55**: 11–29.

Rolls, E. T. (2004b). A higher order syntactic thought (HOST) theory of consciousness, *in* R. J. Gennaro (ed.), *Higher-Order Theories of Consciousness: An Anthology*, John Benjamins, Amsterdam, pp. 137–172.

Rolls, E. T. (2005a). *Emotion Explained*, Oxford University Press, Oxford.

Rolls, E. T. (2005b). Head direction and spatial view cells in primates, and brain mechanisms for path integration and episodic memory, *in* S. I. Wiener and J. S. Taube (eds), *Head Direction Cells and the Neural Mechanisms of Spatial Orientation*, MIT Press, Cambridge, MA, pp. 299–318, Chapter 14.

Rolls, E. T. (2006a). Consciousness absent and present: a neurophysiological exploration of masking, *in* H. Ogmen and B. G. Breitmeyer (eds), *The First Half Second*, MIT Press, Cambridge, MA, chapter 6, pp. 89–108.

Rolls, E. T. (2006b). The neurophysiology and functions of the orbitofrontal cortex, *in* D. H. Zald and S. L. Rauch (eds), *The Orbitofrontal Cortex*, Oxford University Press, Oxford, chapter 5, pp. 95–124.

Rolls, E. T. (2007a). The affective neuroscience of consciousness: higher order linguistic thoughts, dual routes to emotion and action, and consciousness, *in* P. Zelazo, M. Moscovitch and E. Thompson (eds), *Cambridge Handbook of Consciousness*, Cambridge University Press, Cambridge, chapter 29, pp. 831–859.

Rolls, E. T. (2007b). A computational neuroscience approach to consciousness, *Neural Networks* **20**: 962–82.

Rolls, E. T. (2007c). Invariant representations of objects in natural scenes in the temporal cortex visual areas, *in* S. Funahashi (ed.), *Representation and Brain*, Springer, Tokyo, chapter 3, pp. 47–102.

Rolls, E. T. (2007d). Memory systems: multiple systems in the brain and their interactions, *in* H. L. Roediger, Y. Dudai and S. M. Fitzpatrick (eds), *Science of Memory: Concepts*, Oxford University Press, New York, chapter 59, pp. 345–351.

Rolls, E. T. (2007e). The representation of information about faces in the temporal and frontal lobes of primates including humans, *Neuropsychologia* **45**: 124–143.

Rolls, E. T. (2007f). Sensory processing in the brain related to the control of food intake, *Proceedings of the Nutrition Society* **66**: 96–112.

Rolls, E. T. (2007g). Understanding the mechanisms of food intake and obesity, *Obesity Reviews* **8**: 67–72.

Rolls, E. T. (2008a). Emotion, higher order syntactic thoughts, and consciousness, *in* L. Weiskrantz and M. K. Davies (eds), *Frontiers of Consciousness*, Oxford University Press, Oxford, chapter 4, pp. 131–167.

Rolls, E. T. (2008b). Face representations in different brain areas, and critical band masking, *Journal of Neuropsychology* **2**: 325–360.

Rolls, E. T. (2008c). Functions of the orbitofrontal and pregenual cingulate cortex in taste, olfaction, appetite and emotion, *Acta Physiologica Hungarica* **95**: 131–164.

Rolls, E. T. (2008d). *Memory, Attention, and Decision-Making. A Unifying Computational Neuroscience Approach*, Oxford University Press, Oxford.

Rolls, E. T. (2008e). The primate hippocampus and episodic memory, *in* E. Dere, A. Easton, L. Nadel and J. P. Huston (eds), *Handbook of Episodic Memory*, Elsevier, Amsterdam, chapter 4.2, pp. 417–438.

Rolls, E. T. (2008f). Top-down control of visual perception: attention in natural vision, *Perception* **37**: 333–354.

Rolls, E. T. (2009a). The anterior and midcingulate cortices and reward, *in* B. Vogt (ed.), *Cingulate Neurobiology and Disease*, Oxford University Press, Oxford, chapter 8, pp. 191–206.

Rolls, E. T. (2009b). Functional neuroimaging of umami taste: what makes umami pleasant, *American Journal of Clinical Nutrition* **90**: 803S–814S.

Rolls, E. T. (2010a). The affective and cognitive processing of touch, oral texture, and temperature in the brain, *Neuroscience and Biobehavioral Reviews* **34**: 237–245.

Rolls, E. T. (2010b). A computational theory of episodic memory formation in the hippocampus, *Behavioural Brain Research* **215**: 180–196.

Rolls, E. T. (2010c). Noise in the brain, decision-making, determinism, free will, and consciousness, *in* E.Perry, D.Collerton, F.Lebeau and H. Ashton (eds), *New Horizons in the Neuroscience of Consciousness*, John Benjamins, Amsterdam, pp. 113–120.

Rolls, E. T. (2011a). Chemosensory learning in the cortex, *Frontiers in Systems Neuroscience* **5**: 78 (1–13).

Rolls, E. T. (2011b). Consciousness, decision-making, and neural computation, *in* V.Cutsuridis, A.Hussain and J.G.Taylor (eds), *Perception-Action Cycle: Models, Algorithms and Systems*, Springer, Berlin, chapter 9, pp. 287–333.

Rolls, E. T. (2011c). David Marr's Vision: floreat computational neuroscience, *Brain* **134**: 913–916.

Rolls, E. T. (2011d). Face neurons, *in* A. J. Calder, G. Rhodes, M. H. Johnson and J. V. Haxby (eds), *The Oxford Handbook of Face Perception*, Oxford University Press, Oxford, chapter 4, pp. 51–75.

Rolls, E. T. (2011e). The neural representation of oral texture including fat texture, *Journal of Texture Studies* **42**: 137–156.

Rolls, E. T. (2011f). Taste, olfactory, and food texture reward processing in the brain and obesity, *International Journal of Obesity* **35**: 550–561.

Rolls, E. T. (2012b). Advantages of dilution in the connectivity of attractor networks in the brain, *Biologically Inspired Cognitive Architectures* **1**: 44–54.

Rolls, E. T. (2012c). Glutamate, obsessive-compulsive disorder, schizophrenia, and the stability of cortical attractor neuronal networks, *Pharmacology, Biochemistry and Behavior* **100**: 736–751.

Rolls, E. T. (2012d). Invariant visual object and face recognition: neural and computational bases, and a model, VisNet, *Frontiers in Computational Neuroscience* **6**(35): 1–70.

Rolls, E. T. (2012e). *Neuroculture: On the Implications of Brain Science*, Oxford University Press, Oxford.

Rolls, E. T. (2012f). Taste, olfactory, and food texture reward processing in the brain and the control of appetite, *Proceedings of the Nutrition Society* **71**: 488–501.

Rolls, E. T. (2013a). A biased activation theory of the cognitive and attentional modulation of emotion, *Frontiers in Human Neuroscience* **7**: 74.

Rolls, E. T. (2013b). The mechanisms for pattern completion and pattern separation in the hippocampus, *Frontiers in Systems Neuroscience* **7**: 74.

Rolls, E. T. (2013c). A quantitative theory of the functions of the hippocampal CA3 network in memory, *Frontiers in Cellular Neuroscience* **7**: 98.

Rolls, E. T. (2013d). What are emotional states, and why do we have them?, *Emotion Review* **5**: 241–247.

Rolls, E. T. (2014a). *Emotion and Decision-Making Explained*, Oxford University Press, Oxford.

Rolls, E. T. (2014b). Emotion and Decision-Making Explained: Precis, *Cortex* **59**: 185–193.

Rolls, E. T. (2015a). Diluted connectivity in pattern association networks facilitates the recall of information from the hippocampus to the neocortex, *Progress in Brain Research* **219**: 21–43.

Rolls, E. T. (2015b). Limbic systems for emotion and for memory, but no single limbic system, *Cortex* **62**: 119–157.

Rolls, E. T. (2015c). The neuronal representation of information in the human brain. Review, *Brain* **138**: 3459–3462.

Rolls, E. T. (2015d). Taste, olfactory, and food reward value processing in the brain, *Progress in Neurobiology* **127-128**: 64–90.

Rolls, E. T. (2016a). Brain processing of reward for touch, temperature, and oral texture, *in* H. Olausson, J. Wessberg, I. Morrison and F. McGlone (eds), *Affective Touch and the Neurophysiology of CT Afferents*, Springer, Berlin, chapter 13, pp. 209–225.

Rolls, E. T. (2016b). *Cerebral Cortex: Principles of Operation*, Oxford University Press, Oxford.

Rolls, E. T. (2016c). Functions of the anterior insula in taste, autonomic, and related functions, *Brain and Cognition* **110**: 4–19.

Rolls, E. T. (2016d). Motivation Explained: Ultimate and proximate accounts of hunger and appetite, *Advances in Motivation Science* **3**: 187–249.

Rolls, E. T. (2016e). A non-reward attractor theory of depression, *Neurosci Biobehav Rev* **68**: 47–58.

Rolls, E. T. (2016f). Pattern separation, completion, and categorisation in the hippocampus and neocortex, *Neurobiology of Learning and Memory* **129**: 4–28.

Rolls, E. T. (2016g). Reward systems in the brain and nutrition, *Annual Review of Nutrition* **36**: 435–470.

Rolls, E. T. (2017a). Cortical coding, *Language, Cognition and Neuroscience* **32**: 316–329.

Rolls, E. T. (2017b). Evolution of the emotional brain, *in* S. Watanabe, M. A. Hofman and T. Shimizu (eds), *Evolution of Brain, Cognition, and Emotion in Vertebrates*, Springer, Tokyo, chapter 12, pp. 251–272.

Rolls, E. T. (2017c). The roles of the orbitofrontal cortex via the habenula in non-reward and depression, and in the responses of serotonin and dopamine neurons, *Neurosci Biobehav Rev* **75**: 331–334.

Rolls, E. T. (2017d). A scientific theory of *ars memoriae*: spatial view cells in a continuous attractor network with linked items, *Hippocampus* **27**: 570–579.

Rolls, E. T. (2018a). *The Brain, Emotion, and Depression*, Oxford University Press, Oxford.

Rolls, E. T. (2018b). The storage and recall of memories in the hippocampo-cortical system, *Cell and Tissue Research* **373**: 577–604.

Rolls, E. T. (2019a). Attractor network dynamics, transmitters, and the memory and cognitive changes in aging, *in* K. M. Heilman and S. E. Nadeau (eds), *Cognitive Changes and the Aging Brain*, Cambridge University Press, Cambridge, chapter 14, pp. 203–225.

Rolls, E. T. (2019b). The cingulate cortex and limbic systems for action, emotion, and memory, *in* B. A. Vogt (ed.), *Handbook of Clinical Neurology: Cingulate Cortex*, Vol. 166, Elsevier, Oxford, chapter 2, pp. 23–37.

Rolls, E. T. (2019c). The cingulate cortex and limbic systems for emotion, action, and memory, *Brain Struct Funct* **224**: 3001–3018.

Rolls, E. T. (2019d). Emotion and reasoning in human decision-making, *Economics: The Open-Access, Open-Assessment E-Journal* **13**: http://dx.doi.org/10.5018/economics–ejournal.ja.2019–39.

Rolls, E. T. (2019e). *The Orbitofrontal Cortex*, Oxford University Press, Oxford.

Rolls, E. T. (2019f). The orbitofrontal cortex and emotion in health and disease, including depression, *Neuropsychologia* **128**: 14–43.

Rolls, E. T. (2019g). Taste and smell processing in the brain, *in* R. L. Doty (ed.), *Handbook of Clinical Neurology Vol 164 (3rd series): Smell and Taste*, Vol. 164, Elsevier, Oxford, chapter 7, pp. 97–118.

Rolls, E. T. (2020a). Neural computations underlying phenomenal consciousness: a Higher Order Syntactic Thought theory, *Frontiers in Psychology (Consciousness Research)* **11**: 655.

Rolls, E. T. (2020b). Spatial coordinate transforms linking the allocentric hippocampal and egocentric parietal primate brain systems for memory, action in space, and navigation, *Hippocampus* **30**: 332–353.

Rolls, E. T. (2020c). The texture and taste of food in the brain, *Journal of Texture Studies* **51**: 23–44.

Rolls, E. T. (2021a). Attractor cortical neurodynamics, schizophrenia, and depression, *Translational Psychiatry* **11**: 215.

Rolls, E. T. (2021b). *Brain Computations: What and How*, Oxford University Press, Oxford.

Rolls, E. T. (2021c). The connections of neocortical pyramidal cells can implement the learning of new categories, attractor memory, and top-down recall and attention, *Brain Structure and Function* **226**: 2523–2536.

Rolls, E. T. (2021d). Learning invariant object and spatial view representations in the brain using slow unsupervised learning, *Frontiers in Computational Neuroscience* **15**: 686239.

Rolls, E. T. (2021e). Mind causality: a computational neuroscience approach, *Frontiers in Computational Neuroscience* **15**: 70505.

Rolls, E. T. (2021f). Neurons including hippocampal spatial view cells, and navigation in primates including humans, *Hippocampus* **31**: 593–611.

Rolls, E. T. (2021g). A neuroscience levels of explanation approach to the mind and the brain, *Frontiers in Computational Neuroscience* **15**: 649679.

Rolls, E. T. (2021h). The neuroscience of emotional disorders, *in* K. M. Heilman and S. E. Nadeau (eds), *Handbook of Clinical Neurology: Disorders of Emotion in Neurologic Disease*, Vol. 183, Elsevier, Oxford, chapter 1, pp. 1–26.

Rolls, E. T. (2021i). On pattern separation in the primate including human hippocampus, *Trends in Cognitive Sciences* **25**: 920–922.

Rolls, E. T. (2022a). *The Brain, Emotion, and Depression*, chinese edn, East China Normal University Press, Shanghai, China.

Rolls, E. T. (2022b). The hippocampus, ventromedial prefrontal cortex, and episodic and semantic memory, *Prog Neurobiol* **217**: 102334.

Rolls, E. T. (2023a). *Brain Computations and Connectivity*, Oxford University Press, Oxford.

Rolls, E. T. (2023b). Emotion, motivation, decision-making, the orbitofrontal cortex, anterior cingulate cortex, and the amygdala, *Brain Structure and Function* pp. doi: 10.1007/s00429-023-02644-9.

Rolls, E. T. (2023c). Hippocampal spatial view cells for memory and navigation, and their underlying connectivity in humans, *Hippocampus* **33**: 533–572.

Rolls, E. T. (2023d). Hippocampal spatial view cells, place cells, and concept cells: view representations, *Hippocampus* **33**: 667–687.

Rolls, E. T. (2023e). Hippocampal storage and recall of neocortical 'what'-'where' representations.

Rolls, E. T. (2023f). The orbitofrontal cortex, food reward, body weight and obesity, *Soc Cogn Affect Neurosci* **18**: nsab044.

Rolls, E. T. and Baylis, G. C. (1986). Size and contrast have only small effects on the responses to faces of neurons in the cortex of the superior temporal sulcus of the monkey, *Experimental Brain Research* **65**: 38–48.

Rolls, E. T. and Baylis, L. L. (1994). Gustatory, olfactory and visual convergence within the primate orbitofrontal cortex, *Journal of Neuroscience* **14**: 5437–5452.

Rolls, E. T. and Cowey, A. (1970). Topography of the retina and striate cortex and its relationship to visual acuity in rhesus monkeys and squirrel monkeys, *Exp Brain Res* **10**: 298–310.

Rolls, E. T. and de Waal, A. W. L. (1985). Long-term sensory-specific satiety: evidence from an Ethiopian refugee camp, *Physiology and Behavior* **34**: 1017–1020.

Rolls, E. T. and Deco, G. (2002). *Computational Neuroscience of Vision*, Oxford University Press, Oxford.

Rolls, E. T. and Deco, G. (2006). Attention in natural scenes: neurophysiological and computational bases, *Neural Networks* **19**: 1383–1394.

Rolls, E. T. and Deco, G. (2010). *The Noisy Brain: Stochastic Dynamics as a Principle of Brain Function*, Oxford University Press, Oxford.

Rolls, E. T. and Deco, G. (2011a). A computational neuroscience approach to schizophrenia and its onset, *Neuroscience and Biobehavioral Reviews* **35**: 1644–1653.

Rolls, E. T. and Deco, G. (2011b). Prediction of decisions from noise in the brain before the evidence is provided, *Frontiers in Neuroscience* **5**: 33.

Rolls, E. T. and Deco, G. (2015a). Networks for memory, perception, and decision-making, and beyond to how the syntax for language might be implemented in the brain, *Brain Research* **1621**: 316–334.

Rolls, E. T. and Deco, G. (2015b). Stochastic cortical neurodynamics underlying the memory and cognitive changes in aging, *Neurobiol Learn Mem* **118**: 150–61.

Rolls, E. T. and Deco, G. (2016). Non-reward neural mechanisms in the orbitofrontal cortex, *Cortex* **83**: 27–38.

Rolls, E. T. and Grabenhorst, F. (2008). The orbitofrontal cortex and beyond: from affect to decision-making, *Prog Neurobiol* **86**: 216–44.

Rolls, E. T. and Johnstone, S. (1992). Neurophysiological analysis of striatal function, *in* G. Vallar, S. Cappa and C. Wallesch (eds), *Neuropsychological Disorders Associated with Subcortical Lesions*, Oxford University Press, Oxford, chapter 3, pp. 61–97.

Rolls, E. T. and Kesner, R. P. (2006a). A computational theory of hippocampal function, and empirical tests of the theory, *Progress in Neurobiology* **79**: 1–48.

Rolls, E. T. and Kesner, R. P. (2006b). A theory of hippocampal function, and tests of the theory, *Progress in Neurobiology* **79**: 1–48.

Rolls, E. T. and Kesner, R. P. (2016). Pattern separation and pattern completion in the hippocampal system, *Neurobiology of Learning and Memory* **129**: 1–3.

Rolls, E. T. and McCabe, C. (2007). Enhanced affective brain representations of chocolate in cravers vs non-cravers, *European Journal of Neuroscience* **26**: 1067–1076.

Rolls, E. T. and Mills, P. (2019). The generation of time in the hippocampal memory system, *Cell Rep* **28**: 1649–1658 e6.

Rolls, E. T. and Mills, W. P. C. (2017). Computations in the deep vs superficial layers of the cerebral cortex, *Neurobiol Learn Mem* **145**: 205–221.

Rolls, E. T. and Mills, W. P. C. (2018). Non-accidental properties, metric invariance, and encoding by neurons in a model of ventral stream visual object recognition, VisNet, *Neurobiology of Learning and Memory* **152**: 20–31.

Rolls, E. T. and Milward, T. (2000). A model of invariant object recognition in the visual system: learning rules, activation functions, lateral inhibition, and information-based performance measures, *Neural Computation* **12**: 2547–2572.

Rolls, E. T. and O'Mara, S. (1993). Neurophysiological and theoretical analysis of how the hippocampus functions in memory, *in* T. Ono, L. Squire, M. Raichle, D. Perrett and M. Fukuda (eds), *Brain Mechanisms of Perception and Memory: From Neuron to Behavior*, Oxford University Press, New York, chapter 17, pp. 276–300.

Rolls, E. T. and O'Mara, S. M. (1995). View-responsive neurons in the primate hippocampal complex, *Hippocampus* **5**: 409–24.

Rolls, E. T. and Rolls, B. J. (1982). Brain mechanisms involved in feeding, *in* L. Barker (ed.), *Psychobiology of Human Food Selection*, AVI Publishing Company, Westport, Connecticut, chapter 3, pp. 33–62.

Rolls, E. T. and Rolls, J. H. (1997). Olfactory sensory-specific satiety in humans, *Physiology and Behavior* **61**: 461–473.

Rolls, E. T. and Scott, T. R. (2003). Central taste anatomy and neurophysiology, *in* R. Doty (ed.), *Handbook of Olfaction and Gustation*, 2nd edn, Dekker, New York, chapter 33, pp. 679–705.

Rolls, E. T. and Stringer, S. M. (2000). On the design of neural networks in the brain by genetic evolution, *Prog Neurobiol* **61**: 557–79.

Rolls, E. T. and Stringer, S. M. (2001a). Invariant object recognition in the visual system with error correction and temporal difference learning, *Network: Computation in Neural Systems* **12**: 111–129.

Rolls, E. T. and Stringer, S. M. (2001b). A model of the interaction between mood and memory, *Network: Computation in Neural Systems* **12**: 89–109.

Rolls, E. T. and Stringer, S. M. (2005). Spatial view cells in the hippocampus, and their idiothetic update based on place and head direction, *Neural Networks* **18**: 1229–1241.

Rolls, E. T. and Stringer, S. M. (2006a). Invariant global motion recognition in the dorsal visual system: a unifying theory, *Neural Computation* **19**: 139–169.

Rolls, E. T. and Stringer, S. M. (2006b). Invariant visual object recognition: a model, with lighting invariance, *Journal of Physiology – Paris* **100**: 43–62.

Rolls, E. T. and Tovee, M. J. (1994). Processing speed in the cerebral cortex and the neurophysiology of visual masking, *Proceedings of the Royal Society, B* **257**: 9–15.

Rolls, E. T. and Tovee, M. J. (1995a). The responses of single neurons in the temporal visual cortical areas of the macaque when more than one stimulus is present in the visual field, *Experimental Brain Research* **103**: 409–420.

Rolls, E. T. and Tovee, M. J. (1995b). Sparseness of the neuronal representation of stimuli in the primate temporal visual cortex, *Journal of Neurophysiology* **73**: 713–726.

Rolls, E. T. and Treves, A. (1990). The relative advantages of sparse versus distributed encoding for associative neuronal networks in the brain, *Network* **1**: 407–421.

Rolls, E. T. and Treves, A. (1994). Neural networks in the brain involved in memory and recall, *Prog Brain Res* **102**: 335–41.

Rolls, E. T. and Treves, A. (1998). *Neural Networks and Brain Function*, Oxford University Press, Oxford.

Rolls, E. T. and Treves, A. (2011). The neuronal encoding of information in the brain, *Progress in Neurobiology* **95**: 448–490.

Rolls, E. T. and Webb, T. J. (2012). Cortical attractor network dynamics with diluted connectivity, *Brain Research* **1434**: 212–225.

Rolls, E. T. and Webb, T. J. (2014). Finding and recognising objects in natural scenes: complementary computations in the dorsal and ventral visual systems, *Frontiers in Computational Neuroscience* **8**: 85.

Rolls, E. T. and Williams, G. V. (1987a). Neuronal activity in the ventral striatum of the primate, *in* M. B. Carpenter and A. Jayamaran (eds), *The Basal Ganglia II – Structure and Function – Current Concepts*, Plenum, New York, pp. 349–356.

Rolls, E. T. and Williams, G. V. (1987b). Sensory and movement-related neuronal activity in different regions of the primate striatum, *in* J. S. Schneider and T. I. Lidsky (eds), *Basal Ganglia and Behavior: Sensory Aspects and Motor Functioning*, Hans Huber, Bern, pp. 37–59.

Rolls, E. T. and Wirth, S. (2018). Spatial representations in the primate hippocampus, and their functions in memory and navigation, *Prog Neurobiol* **171**: 90–113.

Rolls, E. T. and Wirth, S. (2023). Hippocampal system neurons encoding views in different species: Introduction to the Special Issue of Hippocampus 2023, *Hippocampus* **33**: 445–447.

Rolls, E. T. and Xiang, J.-Z. (2005). Reward-spatial view representations and learning in the hippocampus, *Journal of Neuroscience* **25**: 6167–6174.

Rolls, E. T. and Xiang, J.-Z. (2006). Spatial view cells in the primate hippocampus, and memory recall, *Reviews in the Neurosciences* **17**: 175–200.

Rolls, E. T., Burton, M. J. and Mora, F. (1976). Hypothalamic neuronal responses associated with the sight of food, *Brain Research* **111**: 53–66.

Rolls, E. T., Judge, S. J. and Sanghera, M. (1977). Activity of neurones in the inferotemporal cortex of the alert monkey, *Brain Research* **130**: 229–238.

Rolls, E. T., Perrett, D., Thorpe, S. J., Puerto, A., Roper-Hall, A. and Maddison, S. (1979a). Responses of neurons in area 7 of the parietal cortex to objects of different significance, *Brain Research* **169**: 194–198.

Rolls, E. T., Sanghera, M. K. and Roper-Hall, A. (1979b). The latency of activation of neurons in the lateral hypothalamus and substantia innominata during feeding in the monkey, *Brain Research* **164**: 121–135.

Rolls, E. T., Thorpe, S. J., Maddison, S., Roper-Hall, A., Puerto, A. and Perrett, D. (1979c). Activity of neurones in the neostriatum and related structures in the alert animal, *in* I. Divac and R. Oberg (eds), *The Neostriatum*, Pergamon Press, Oxford, pp. 163–182.

Rolls, E. T., Burton, M. J. and Mora, F. (1980b). Neurophysiological analysis of brain-stimulation reward in the monkey, *Brain Research* **194**: 339–357.

Rolls, E. T., Perrett, D. I. and Thorpe, S. J. (1980c). The influence of motivation on the responses of neurons in the posterior parietal association cortex, *The Behavioral and Brain Sciences* **3**: 514–515.

Rolls, E. T., Perrett, D. I., Caan, A. W. and Wilson, F. A. W. (1982d). Neuronal responses related to visual recognition, *Brain* **105**: 611–646.

Rolls, E. T., Rolls, B. J. and Rowe, E. A. (1983a). Sensory-specific and motivation-specific satiety for the sight and taste of food and water in man, *Physiology and Behavior* **30**: 185–192.

Rolls, E. T., Thorpe, S. J. and Maddison, S. P. (1983b). Responses of striatal neurons in the behaving monkey. 1. Head of the caudate nucleus, *Behavioural Brain Research* **7**: 179–210.

Rolls, E. T., Thorpe, S. J., Boytim, M., Szabo, I. and Perrett, D. I. (1984). Responses of striatal neurons in the behaving monkey. 3. Effects of iontophoretically applied dopamine on normal responsiveness, *Neuroscience* **12**: 1201–1212.

Rolls, E. T., Baylis, G. C. and Leonard, C. M. (1985). Role of low and high spatial frequencies in the face-selective responses of neurons in the cortex in the superior temporal sulcus in the monkey, *Vision Research* **25**: 1021–35.

Rolls, E. T., Murzi, E., Yaxley, S., Thorpe, S. J. and Simpson, S. J. (1986). Sensory-specific satiety: food-specific reduction in responsiveness of ventral forebrain neurons after feeding in the monkey, *Brain Res* **368**: 79–86.

Rolls, E. T., Baylis, G. C. and Hasselmo, M. E. (1987). The responses of neurons in the cortex in the superior temporal sulcus of the monkey to band-pass spatial frequency filtered faces, *Vision Research* **27**: 311–326.

Rolls, E. T., Scott, T. R., Sienkiewicz, Z. J. and Yaxley, S. (1988). The responsiveness of neurones in the frontal opercular gustatory cortex of the macaque monkey is independent of hunger, *Journal of Physiology* **397**: 1–12.

Rolls, E. T., Baylis, G. C., Hasselmo, M. and Nalwa, V. (1989a). The representation of information in the temporal lobe visual cortical areas of macaque monkeys, *in* J. Kulikowski, C. Dickinson and I. Murray (eds), *Seeing Contour and Colour*, Pergamon, Oxford.

Rolls, E. T., Baylis, G. C., Hasselmo, M. E. and Nalwa, V. (1989b). The effect of learning on the face-selective responses of neurons in the cortex in the superior temporal sulcus of the monkey, *Experimental Brain Research* **76**: 153–164.

Rolls, E. T., Miyashita, Y., Cahusac, P. M. B., Kesner, R. P., Niki, H., Feigenbaum, J. and Bach, L. (1989c). Hippocampal neurons in the monkey with activity related to the place in which a stimulus is shown, *Journal of Neuroscience* **9**: 1835–1845.

Rolls, E. T., Sienkiewicz, Z. J. and Yaxley, S. (1989d). Hunger modulates the responses to gustatory stimuli of single neurons in the caudolateral orbitofrontal cortex of the macaque monkey, *Eur J Neurosci* **1**: 53–60.

Rolls, E. T., Yaxley, S. and Sienkiewicz, Z. J. (1990). Gustatory responses of single neurons in the caudolateral orbitofrontal cortex of the macaque monkey, *J Neurophysiol* **64**: 1055–66.

Rolls, E. T., Cahusac, P. M. B., Feigenbaum, J. D. and Miyashita, Y. (1993). Responses of single neurons in the hippocampus of the macaque related to recognition memory, *Experimental Brain Research* **93**: 299–306.

Rolls, E. T., Hornak, J., Wade, D. and McGrath, J. (1994a). Emotion-related learning in patients with social and emotional changes associated with frontal lobe damage, *Journal of Neurology, Neurosurgery and Psychiatry* **57**: 1518–1524.

Rolls, E. T., Tovee, M. J., Purcell, D. G., Stewart, A. L. and Azzopardi, P. (1994b). The responses of neurons in the temporal cortex of primates, and face identification and detection, *Experimental Brain Research* **101**: 474–484.

Rolls, E. T., Critchley, H. D. and Treves, A. (1996a). The representation of olfactory information in the primate orbitofrontal cortex, *Journal of Neurophysiology* **75**: 1982–1996.

Rolls, E. T., Critchley, H. D., Mason, R. and Wakeman, E. A. (1996b). Orbitofrontal cortex neurons: role in olfactory and visual association learning, *Journal of Neurophysiology* **75**: 1970–1981.

Rolls, E. T., Critchley, H., Wakeman, E. A. and Mason, R. (1996c). Responses of neurons in the primate taste cortex to the glutamate ion and to inosine 5'-monophosphate, *Physiology and Behavior* **59**: 991–1000.

Rolls, E. T., Robertson, R. G. and Georges-François, P. (1997a). Spatial view cells in the primate hippocampus, *European Journal of Neuroscience* **9**: 1789–1794.

Rolls, E. T., Treves, A. and Tovee, M. J. (1997b). The representational capacity of the distributed encoding of information provided by populations of neurons in the primate temporal visual cortex, *Experimental Brain Research* **114**: 177–185.

Rolls, E. T., Treves, A., Foster, D. and Perez-Vicente, C. (1997c). Simulation studies of the CA3 hippocampal subfield modelled as an attractor neural network, *Neural Networks* **10**: 1559–1569.

Rolls, E. T., Treves, A., Tovee, M. J. and Panzeri, S. (1997d). Information in the neuronal representation of individual stimuli in the primate temporal visual cortex, *Journal of Computational Neuroscience* **4**: 309–333.

Rolls, E. T., Critchley, H. D., Browning, A. and Hernadi, I. (1998a). The neurophysiology of taste and olfaction in primates, and umami flavor, *Annals of the New York Academy of Sciences* **855**: 426–437.

Rolls, E. T., Treves, A., Robertson, R. G., Georges-François, P. and Panzeri, S. (1998b). Information about spatial view in an ensemble of primate hippocampal cells, *Journal of Neurophysiology* **79**: 1797–1813.

Rolls, E. T., Critchley, H. D., Browning, A. S., Hernadi, A. and Lenard, L. (1999a). Responses to the sensory properties of fat of neurons in the primate orbitofrontal cortex, *Journal of Neuroscience* **19**: 1532–1540.

Rolls, E. T., Tovee, M. J. and Panzeri, S. (1999b). The neurophysiology of backward visual masking: information analysis, *Journal of Cognitive Neuroscience* **11**: 335–346.

Rolls, E. T., Stringer, S. M. and Trappenberg, T. P. (2002). A unified model of spatial and episodic memory, *Proceedings of The Royal Society B* **269**: 1087–1093.

Rolls, E. T., Aggelopoulos, N. C. and Zheng, F. (2003a). The receptive fields of inferior temporal cortex neurons in natural scenes., *Journal of Neuroscience* **23**: 339–348.

Rolls, E. T., Franco, L., Aggelopoulos, N. C. and Reece, S. (2003b). An information theoretic approach to the contributions of the firing rates and the correlations between the firing of neurons, *Journal of Neurophysiology* **89**: 2810–2822.

Rolls, E. T., Kringelbach, M. L. and De Araujo, I. E. T. (2003c). Different representations of pleasant and unpleasant odors in the human brain, *European Journal of Neuroscience* **18**: 695–703.

Rolls, E. T., O'Doherty, J., Kringelbach, M. L., Francis, S., Bowtell, R. and McGlone, F. (2003d). Representations of pleasant and painful touch in the human orbitofrontal and cingulate cortices, *Cereb Cortex* **13**: 308–17.

Rolls, E. T., Verhagen, J. V. and Kadohisa, M. (2003e). Representations of the texture of food in the primate orbitofrontal cortex: neurons responding to viscosity, grittiness, and capsaicin, *Journal of Neurophysiology* **90**: 3711–3724.

Rolls, E. T., Aggelopoulos, N. C., Franco, L. and Treves, A. (2004). Information encoding in the inferior temporal visual cortex: contributions of the firing rates and the correlations between the firing of neurons, *Biological Cybernetics* **90**: 19–32.

Rolls, E. T., Browning, A. S., Inoue, K. and Hernadi, S. (2005a). Novel visual stimuli activate a population of neurons in the primate orbitofrontal cortex., *Neurobiology of Learning and Memory* **84**: 111–123.

Rolls, E. T., Franco, L. and Stringer, S. M. (2005b). The perirhinal cortex and long-term familiarity memory, *Q J Exp Psychol B* **58**: 234–45.

Rolls, E. T., Xiang, J.-Z. and Franco, L. (2005c). Object, space and object-space representations in the primate hippocampus, *Journal of Neurophysiology* **94**: 833–844.

Rolls, E. T., Critchley, H. D., Browning, A. S. and Inoue, K. (2006a). Face-selective and auditory neurons in the primate orbitofrontal cortex, *Experimental Brain Research* **170**: 74–87.

Rolls, E. T., Franco, L., Aggelopoulos, N. C. and Jerez, J. M. (2006b). Information in the first spike, the order of spikes, and the number of spikes provided by neurons in the inferior temporal visual cortex, *Vision Research* **46**: 4193–4205.

Rolls, E. T., Stringer, S. M. and Elliot, T. (2006c). Entorhinal cortex grid cells can map to hippocampal place cells by competitive learning, *Network: Computation in Neural Systems* **17**: 447–465.

Rolls, E. T., Grabenhorst, F. and Parris, B. (2008a). Warm pleasant feelings in the brain, *Neuroimage* **41**: 1504–1513.

Rolls, E. T., Grabenhorst, F., Margot, C., da Silva, M. and Velazco, M. I. (2008b). Selective attention to affective value alters how the brain processes olfactory stimuli, *Journal of Cognitive Neuroscience* **20**: 1815–1826.

Rolls, E. T., Loh, M. and Deco, G. (2008c). An attractor hypothesis of obsessive-compulsive disorder, *European Journal of Neuroscience* **28**: 782–793.

Rolls, E. T., Loh, M., Deco, G. and Winterer, G. (2008d). Computational models of schizophrenia and dopamine modulation in the prefrontal cortex, *Nature Reviews Neuroscience* **9**: 696–709.

Rolls, E. T., McCabe, C. and Redoute, J. (2008e). Expected value, reward outcome, and temporal difference error representations in a probabilistic decision task, *Cerebral Cortex* **18**: 652–663.

Rolls, E. T., Tromans, J. M. and Stringer, S. M. (2008f). Spatial scene representations formed by self-organizing learning in a hippocampal extension of the ventral visual system, *Eur J Neurosci* **28**: 2116–27.

Rolls, E. T., Grabenhorst, F. and Franco, L. (2009). Prediction of subjective affective state from brain activations, *Journal of Neurophysiology* **101**: 1294–1308.

Rolls, E. T., Critchley, H. D., Verhagen, J. V. and Kadohisa, M. (2010a). The representation of information about taste and odor in the orbitofrontal cortex, *Chemosensory Perception* **3**: 16–33.

Rolls, E. T., Grabenhorst, F. and Deco, G. (2010b). Choice, difficulty, and confidence in the brain, *Neuroimage* **53**: 694–706.

Rolls, E. T., Grabenhorst, F. and Deco, G. (2010c). Decision-making, errors, and confidence in the brain, *Journal of Neurophysiology* **104**: 2359–2374.

Rolls, E. T., Grabenhorst, F. and Parris, B. A. (2010d). Neural systems underlying decisions about affective odors, *Journal of Cognitive Neuroscience* **10**: 1068–1082.

Rolls, E. T., Webb, T. J. and Deco, G. (2012). Communication before coherence, *European Journal of Neuroscience* **36**: 2689–2709.

Rolls, E. T., Dempere-Marco, L. and Deco, G. (2013). Holding multiple items in short term memory: a neural mechanism, *PLoS One* **8**: e61078.

Rolls, E. T., Joliot, M. and Tzourio-Mazoyer, N. (2015a). Implementation of a new parcellation of the orbitofrontal cortex in the automated anatomical labeling atlas, *Neuroimage* **122**: 1–5.

Rolls, E. T., Kellerhals, M. B. and Nichols, T. E. (2015b). Age differences in the brain mechanisms of good taste, *Neuroimage* **113**: 298–309.

Rolls, E. T., Lu, W., Wan, L., Yan, H., Wang, C., Yang, F., Tan, Y.-L., Li, L., Chinese-Schizophrenia-Collaboration, G., Yu, H., Liddle, P. F., Palaniyappan, L., Zhang, D., Yue, W. and Feng, J. (2017). Individual differences in schizophrenia, *British Journal of Psychiatry Open* **3**: 265–273.

Rolls, E. T., Cheng, W., Gilson, M., Qiu, J., Hu, Z., Ruan, H., Li, Y., Huang, C. C., Yang, A. C., Tsai, S. J., Zhang, X., Zhuang, K., Lin, C. P., Deco, G., Xie, P. and Feng, J. (2018a). Effective connectivity in depression, *Biol Psychiatry Cogn Neurosci Neuroimaging* **3**: 187–197.

Rolls, E. T., Mills, T., Norton, A., Lazidis, A. and Norton, I. T. (2018b). Neuronal encoding of fat using the coefficient of sliding friction in the cerebral cortex and amygdala, *Cerebral Cortex* **28**: 4080–4089.

Rolls, E. T., Cheng, W., Gong, W., Qiu, J., Zhou, C., Zhang, J., Lv, W., Ruan, H., Wei, D., Cheng, K., Meng, J., Xie, P. and Feng, J. (2019). Functional connectivity of the anterior cingulate cortex in depression and in health, *Cereb Cortex* **29**: 3617–3630.

Rolls, E. T., Cheng, W. and Feng, J. (2020a). The orbitofrontal cortex: reward, emotion, and depression, *Brain Communications* **2**: fcaa196.

Rolls, E. T., Cheng, W., Du, J., Wei, D., Qiu, J., Dai, D., Zhou, Q., Xie, P. and Feng, J. (2020b). Functional connectivity of the right inferior frontal gyrus and orbitofrontal cortex in depression, *Soc Cogn Affect Neurosci* **15**: 75–86.

Rolls, E. T., Cheng, W., Gilson, M., Gong, W., Deco, G., Lo, C. Z., Yang, A. C., Tsai, S. J., Liu, M. E., Lin, C. P. and Feng, J. (2020c). Beyond the disconnectivity hypothesis of schizophrenia, *Cerebral Cortex* **30**: 1213–1233.

Rolls, E. T., Huang, C. C., Lin, C. P., Feng, J. and Joliot, M. (2020d). Automated anatomical labelling atlas 3, *Neuroimage* **206**: 116189.

Rolls, E. T., Vatansever, D., Li, Y., Cheng, W. and Feng, J. (2020e). Rapid rule-based reward reversal and the lateral orbitofrontal cortex, *Cerebral Cortex Communications* **1**: tgaa087 doi: 10.1093/texcom/tgaa087.

Rolls, E. T., Zhou, Y., Cheng, W., Gilson, M., Deco, G. and Feng, J. (2020f). Effective connectivity in autism, *Autism Research* **13**: 32–44.

Rolls, E. T., Cheng, W. and Feng, J. (2021a). Brain dynamics: Synchronous peaks, functional connectivity, and its temporal variability, *Human Brain Mapping* **42**: 2790–2801.

Rolls, E. T., Cheng, W. and Feng, J. (2021b). Brain dynamics: the temporal variability of connectivity, and differences in schizophrenia and ADHD, *Translational Psychiatry* **11**: 70.

Rolls, E. T., Deco, G., Huang, C. C. and Feng, J. (2022a). The effective connectivity of the human hippocampal memory system, *Cereb Cortex* **32**: 3706–3725.

Rolls, E. T., Deco, G., Huang, C.-C. and Feng, J. (2022b). The human language effective connectome, *Neuroimage* **258**: 119352.

Rolls, E. T., Wan, Z., Cheng, W. and Feng, J. (2022c). Risk-taking in humans and the medial orbitofrontal cortex reward system, *Neuroimage* **249**: 118893.

Rolls, E. T., Deco, G., Huang, C.-C. and Feng, J. (2023a). The connectivity of the human frontal pole cortex, and a theory of its involvement in exploit vs explore.

Rolls, E. T., Deco, G., Huang, C.-C. and Feng, J. (2023b). Human amygdala compared to orbitofrontal cortex connectivity, and emotion, *Progress in Neurobiology* **220**: 102385.

Rolls, E. T., Deco, G., Huang, C. C. and Feng, J. (2023c). The human orbitofrontal cortex, vmPFC, and anterior cingulate cortex effective connectome: emotion, memory, and action, *Cereb Cortex* **33**: 330–359.

Rolls, E. T., Deco, G., Huang, C. C. and Feng, J. (2023d). The human posterior parietal cortex: effective connectome, and its relation to function, *Cereb Cortex* **33**: 3142–3170.

Rolls, E. T., Deco, G., Huang, C.-C. and Feng, J. (2023e). Multiple cortical visual streams in humans, *Cerebral Cortex* **33**: 3319–3349.

Rolls, E. T., Deco, G., Huang, C. C. and Feng, J. (2023f). Prefrontal and somatosensory-motor cortex effective connectivity in humans, *Cereb Cortex* **33**: 4939–4963.

Rolls, E. T., Feng, R., Cheng, W. and Feng, J. (2023g). Orbitofrontal cortex connectivity is associated with food reward and body weight in humans, *Soc Cogn Affect Neurosci* **18**: nsab083.

Rolls, E. T., Rauschecker, J. P., Deco, G., Huang, C. C. and Feng, J. (2023h). Auditory cortical connectivity in humans, *Cereb Cortex* **33**: 6207–6227.

Rolls, E. T., Wirth, S., Deco, G., Huang, C.-C. and Feng, J. (2023i). The human posterior cingulate, retrosplenial and medial parietal cortex effective connectome, and implications for memory and navigation, *Human Brain Mapping* **44**: 629–655.

Romanski, L. M. and Diehl, M. M. (2011). Neurons responsive to face-view in the primate ventrolateral prefrontal cortex, *Neuroscience* **189**: 223–35.

Romanski, L. M., Tian, B., Fritz, J., Mishkin, M., Goldman-Rakic, P. S. and Rauschecker, J. P. (1999). Dual streams of auditory afferents target multiple domains in the primate orbitofrontal cortex, *Nature Neuroscience* **2**: 1131–1136.

Romanski, L. M., Averbeck, B. B. and Diltz, M. (2005). Neural representation of vocalizations in the primate ventrolateral prefrontal cortex, *Journal of Neurophysiology* **93**: 734–747.

Romo, R. and Salinas, E. (2001). Touch and Go: Decision-making mechanisms in Somatosensation, *Annual Review of Neuroscience* **24**: 107–137.

Romo, R. and Salinas, E. (2003). Flutter discrimination: Neural codes, perception, memory and decision making, *Nature Reviews Neuroscience* **4**: 203–218.

Romo, R., Hernandez, A., Zainos, A., Lemus, L. and Brody, C. (2002). Neural correlates of decision-making in secondary somatosensory cortex, *Nature Neuroscience* **5**: 1217–1225.

Romo, R., Hernandez, A., Zainos, A. and Salinas, E. (2003). Correlated neuronal discharges that increase coding efficiency during perceptual discrimination, *Neuron* **38**: 649–657.

Romo, R., Hernandez, A. and Zainos, A. (2004). Neuronal correlates of a perceptual decision in ventral premotor cortex, *Neuron* **41**: 165–173.

Ronchi, R., Park, H. D. and Blanke, O. (2018). Bodily self-consciousness and its disorders, *Handb Clin Neurol* **151**: 313–330.

Rondi-Reig, L., Libbey, M., Eichenbaum, H. and Tonegawa, S. (2001). CA1-specific N-methyl-D-aspartate receptor knockout mice are deficient in solving a nonspatial transverse patterning task, *Proc Natl Acad Sci U S A* **98**: 3543–8.

Roper, S. D. and Chaudhari, N. (2017). Taste buds: cells, signals and synapses, *Nat Rev Neurosci* **18**: 485–497.

Rosati, A. G. (2017). The evolution of primate executive function: from response control to strategic decision-making, *in* J. H. Kaas (ed.), *Evolution of Nervous Systems, 2nd edition, Volume 3*, 2nd edn, Vol. 3, Elsevier, Amsterdam, chapter 23, pp. 423–437.

Rosch, E. (1975). Cognitive representations of semantic categories, *Journal of Experimental Psychology: General* **104**: 192–233.

Rosenbaum, R. S., Gilboa, A. and Moscovitch, M. (2014). Case studies continue to illuminate the cognitive neuroscience of memory, *Ann N Y Acad Sci* **1316**: 105–33.

Rosenberg, D. R., MacMaster, F. P., Keshavan, M. S., Fitzgerald, K. D., Stewart, C. M. and Moore, G. J. (2000). Decrease in caudate glutamatergic concentrations in pediatric obsessive-compulsive disorder patients taking paroxetine, *Journal of the American Academy of Child and Adolescent Psychiatry* **39**: 1096–1103.

Rosenberg, D. R., MacMillan, S. N. and Moore, G. J. (2001). Brain anatomy and chemistry may predict treatment response in paediatric obsessive–compulsive disorder, *International Journal of Neuropsychopharmacology* **4**: 179–190.

Rosenberg, D. R., Mirza, Y., Russell, A., Tang, J., Smith, J. M., Banerjee, S. P., Bhandari, R., Rose, M., Ivey, J., Boyd, C. and Moore, G. J. (2004). Reduced anterior cingulate glutamatergic concentrations in childhood OCD and major depression versus healthy controls, *Journal of the American Academy of Child and Adolescent Psychiatry* **43**: 1146–1153.

Rosenblatt, F. (1961). *Principles of Neurodynamics: Perceptrons and the Theory of Brain Mechanisms*, Spartan, Washington, DC.

Rosenkilde, C. E., Bauer, R. H. and Fuster, J. M. (1981). Single unit activity in ventral prefrontal cortex in behaving monkeys, *Brain Research* **209**: 375–394.

Rosenthal, D. (2012). Higher-order awareness, misrepresentation and function, *Philos Trans R Soc Lond B Biol Sci* **367**: 1424–38.

Rosenthal, D. M. (2005). *Consciousness and Mind*, Oxford University Press, Oxford.

Rosenthal-von der Putten, A. M., Kramer, N. C., Maderwald, S., Brand, M. and Grabenhorst, F. (2019). Neural mechanisms for accepting and rejecting artificial social partners in the Uncanny Valley, *J Neurosci* **39**: 6555–6570.

Rossi, A. F., Pessoa, L., Desimone, R. and Ungerleider, L. G. (2009). The prefrontal cortex and the executive control of attention, *Experimental Brain Research* **192**: 489–497.

Rottschy, C., Langner, R., Dogan, I., Reetz, K., Laird, A. R., Schulz, J. B., Fox, P. T. and Eickhoff, S. B. (2012). Modelling neural correlates of working memory: a coordinate-based meta-analysis, *Neuroimage* **60**: 830–846.

Roudi, Y. and Treves, A. (2006). Localized activity profiles and storage capacity of rate-based autoassociative networks, *Physical Review E* **73**: 061904.

Roudi, Y. and Treves, A. (2008). Representing where along with what information in a model of a cortical patch, *PLoS Computational Biology* **4**(3): e1000012.

Roux, F. E., Miskin, K., Durand, J. B., Sacko, O., Rehault, E., Tanova, R. and Demonet, J. F. (2015). Electrostimulation mapping of comprehension of auditory and visual words, *Cortex* **71**: 398–408.

Royet, J. P., Zald, D., Versace, R., Costes, N., Lavenne, F., Koenig, O. and Gervais, R. (2000). Emotional responses to pleasant and unpleasant olfactory, visual, and auditory stimuli: a positron emission tomography study, *J Neurosci* **20**: 7752–9.

Rubinov, M. and Sporns, O. (2010). Complex network measures of brain connectivity: uses and interpretations, *Neuroimage* **52**: 1059–69.

Rudebeck, P. H., Behrens, T. E., Kennerley, S. W., Baxter, M. G., Buckley, M. J., Walton, M. E. and Rushworth, M. F. (2008). Frontal cortex subregions play distinct roles in choices between actions and stimuli, *Journal of Neuroscience* **28**: 13775–13785.

Rudebeck, P. H., Saunders, R. C., Lundgren, D. A. and Murray, E. A. (2017). Specialized representations of value in the orbital and ventrolateral prefrontal cortex: desirability versus availability of outcomes, *Neuron* **95**: 1208–1220 e5.

Rueckemann, J. W. and Buffalo, E. A. (2017). Spatial responses, immediate experience, and memory in the monkey hippocampus, *Current Opinion in Behavioral Sciences* **17**: 155–160.

Rumelhart, D. E. and McClelland, J. L. (1986). *Parallel Distributed Processing*, Vol. 1: Foundations, MIT Press, Cambridge, MA.

Rumelhart, D. E. and Zipser, D. (1985). Feature discovery by competitive learning, *Cognitive Science* **9**: 75–112.

Rumelhart, D. E., Hinton, G. E. and Williams, R. J. (1986a). Learning internal representations by error propagation, in D. E. Rumelhart, J. L. McClelland and the PDP Research Group (eds), *Parallel Distributed Processing: Explorations in the Microstructure of Cognition*, Vol. 1, MIT Press, Cambridge, MA, chapter 8, pp. 318–362.

Rumelhart, D. E., Hinton, G. E. and Williams, R. J. (1986b). Learning representations by back-propagating errors, *Nature* **323**: 533–536.

Rupniak, N. M. J. and Gaffan, D. (1987). Monkey hippocampus and learning about spatially directed movements, *Journal of Neuroscience* **7**: 2331–2337.

Rushworth, M. F., Noonan, M. P., Boorman, E. D., Walton, M. E. and Behrens, T. E. (2011). Frontal cortex and reward-guided learning and decision-making, *Neuron* **70**: 1054–69.

Rushworth, M. F., Kolling, N., Sallet, J. and Mars, R. B. (2012). Valuation and decision-making in frontal cortex: one or many serial or parallel systems?, *Curr Opin Neurobiol* **22**: 946–55.

Rushworth, M. F. S., Hadland, K. A., Paus, T. and Sipila, P. K. (2002). Role of the human medial frontal cortex in task-switching: a combined fMRI and TMS study, *Journal of Neurophysiology* **87**: 2577–2592.

Rushworth, M. F. S., Walton, M. E., Kennerley, S. W. and Bannerman, D. M. (2004). Action sets and decisions in the medial frontal cortex, *Trends in Cognitive Sciences* **8**: 410–417.

Rushworth, M. F. S., Behrens, T. E., Rudebeck, P. H. and Walton, M. E. (2007a). Contrasting roles for cingulate and orbitofrontal cortex in decisions and social behaviour, *Trends in Cognitive Sciences* **11**: 168–176.

Rushworth, M. F. S., Buckley, M. J., Behrens, T. E., Walton, M. E. and Bannerman, D. M. (2007b). Functional organization of the medial frontal cortex, *Current Opinion in Neurobiology* **17**: 220–227.

Russchen, F. T., Amaral, D. G. and Price, J. L. (1985). The afferent connections of the substantia innominata in the monkey, Macaca fascicularis, *Journal of Comparative Neurology* **242**: 1–27.

Rust, N. C. and DiCarlo, J. J. (2010). Selectivity and tolerance ("invariance") both increase as visual information propagates from cortical area V4 to IT, *J Neurosci* **30**: 12978–95.

Rutishauser, U. (2019). Testing models of human declarative memory at the single-neuron level, *Trends Cogn Sci* **23**: 510–524.

Rutishauser, U., Tudusciuc, O., Neumann, D., Mamelak, A. N., Heller, A. C., Ross, I. B., Philpott, L., Sutherling, W. W. and Adolphs, R. (2011). Single-unit responses selective for whole faces in the human amygdala, *Current Biology* **21**: 1654–1660.

Rutishauser, U., Mamelak, A. N. and Adolphs, R. (2015). The primate amygdala in social perception - insights from electrophysiological recordings and stimulation, *Trends Neurosci* **38**: 295–306.

Rutishauser, U., Reddy, L., Mormann, F. and Sarnthein, J. (2021). The architecture of human memory: insights from human single-neuron recordings, *J Neurosci* **41**: 883–890.

Ryali, S., Supekar, K., Chen, T., Kochalka, J., Cai, W., Nicholas, J., Padmanabhan, A. and Menon, V. (2016). Temporal dynamics and developmental maturation of salience, default and central-executive network interactions revealed by variational Bayes Hidden Markov modeling, *PLoS Comput Biol* **12**: e1005138.

Ryom, K. I., Stendardi, D., Ciaramelli, E. and Treves, A. (2023). Computational constraints on the associative recall of spatial scenes, *Hippocampus* **33**: 635–645.

Saez, R. A., Saez, A., Paton, J. J., Lau, B. and Salzman, C. D. (2017). Distinct roles for the amygdala and orbitofrontal cortex in representing the relative amount of expected reward, *Neuron* **95**: 70–77 e3.

Sah, P. (1996). Ca^{2+}-activated K^+ currents in neurones: types, physiological roles and modulation, *Trends in Neuroscience* **19**: 150–154.

Sah, P. and Faber, E. S. (2002). Channels underlying neuronal calcium-activated potassium currents, *Progress in Neurobiology* **66**: 345–353.

Saint-Cyr, J. A., Ungerleider, L. G. and Desimone, R. (1990). Organization of visual cortical inputs to the striatum and subsequent outputs to the pallido-nigral complex in the monkey, *Journal of Comparative Neurology* **298**: 129–156.

Salakhutdinov, R. and Larochelle, H. (2010). Efficient learning of deep Boltzmann machines, *International Conference on Artificial Intelligence and Statistics*, pp. 693–700.

Saleem, K. S., Kondo, H. and Price, J. L. (2008). Complementary circuits connecting the orbital and medial prefrontal networks with the temporal, insular, and opercular cortex in the macaque monkey, *Journal of Comparative Neurology* **506**: 659–693.

Saleem, K. S., Miller, B. and Price, J. L. (2014). Subdivisions and connectional networks of the lateral prefrontal cortex in the macaque monkey, *Journal of Comparative Neurology* **522**: 1641–1690.

Salinas, E. and Abbott, L. F. (1995). Transfer of coded information from sensory to motor networks, *J Neurosci* **15**: 6461–74.

Salinas, E. and Abbott, L. F. (1996). A model of multiplicative neural responses in parietal cortex, *Proc Natl Acad Sci U S A* **93**: 11956–61.

Salinas, E. and Abbott, L. F. (1997). Invariant visual responses from attentional gain fields, *Journal of Neurophysiology* **77**: 3267–3272.

Salinas, E. and Abbott, L. F. (2001). Coordinate transformations in the visual system: how to generate gain fields and what to compute with them, *Prog Brain Res* **130**: 175–90.

Salinas, E. and Sejnowski, T. J. (2001). Gain modulation in the central nervous system: where behavior, neurophysiology, and computation meet, *Neuroscientist* **7**: 430–40.

Sallet, J., Mars, R. B., Noonan, M. P., Neubert, F. X., Jbabdi, S., O'Reilly, J. X., Filippini, N., Thomas, A. G. and Rushworth, M. F. (2013). The organization of dorsal frontal cortex in humans and macaques, *J Neurosci* **33**: 12255–74.

Sallet, J., Noonan, M. P., Thomas, A., O'Reilly, J. X., Anderson, J., Papageorgiou, G. K., Neubert, F. X., Ahmed, B., Smith, J., Bell, A. H., Buckley, M. J., Roumazeilles, L., Cuell, S., Walton, M. E., Krug, K., Mars, R. B. and Rushworth, M. F. S. (2020). Behavioral flexibility is associated with changes in structure and function distributed across a frontal cortical network in macaques, *PLoS Biol* **18**: e3000605.

Salz, D. M., Tiganj, Z., Khasnabish, S., Kohley, A., Sheehan, D., Howard, M. W. and Eichenbaum, H. (2016). Time cells in hippocampal area CA3, *J Neurosci* **36**: 7476–84.

Samsonovich, A. and McNaughton, B. L. (1997). Path integration and cognitive mapping in a continuous attractor neural network model, *Journal of Neuroscience* **17**: 5900–5920.

Sanghera, M. K., Rolls, E. T. and Roper-Hall, A. (1979). Visual responses of neurons in the dorsolateral amygdala of the alert monkey, *Experimental Neurology* **63**: 610–626.

Saper, C. B., Swanson, L. W. and Cowan, W. M. (1979). An autoradiographic study of the efferent connections of the lateral hypothalamic area in the rat, *Journal of Comparative Neurology* **183**: 689–706.

Sargolini, F., Fyhn, M., Hafting, T., McNaughton, B. L., Witter, M. P., Moser, M. B. and Moser, E. I. (2006). Conjunctive representation of position, direction, and velocity in entorhinal cortex, *Science* **312**: 758–762.

Sawaguchi, T. and Goldman-Rakic, P. S. (1991). D1 dopamine receptors in prefrontal cortex: Involvement in working memory, *Science* **251**: 947–950.

Sawaguchi, T. and Goldman-Rakic, P. S. (1994). The role of D1-dopamine receptor in working memory: local injections of dopamine antagonists into the prefrontal cortex of rhesus monkeys performing an oculomotor delayed-response task, *Journal of Neurophysiology* **71**: 515–528.

Saxe, A. M., McClelland, J. L. and Ganguli, S. (2019). A mathematical theory of semantic development in deep neural networks, *Proc Natl Acad Sci U S A* **116**: 11537–11546.

Schachter, S. (1971). Importance of cognitive control in obesity, *American Psychologist* **26**: 129–144.

Schacter, G. B., Yang, C. R., Innis, N. K. and Mogenson, G. J. (1989). The role of the hippocampal–nucleus accumbens pathway in radial-arm maze performance, *Brain Research* **494**: 339–349.

Scheuerecker, J., Ufer, S., Zipse, M., Frodl, T., Koutsouleris, N., Zetzsche, T., Wiesmann, M., Albrecht, J., Bruckmann, H., Schmitt, G., Moller, H. J. and Meisenzahl, E. M. (2008). Cerebral changes and cognitive dysfunctions in medication-free schizophrenia – An fMRI study, *Journal of Psychiatric Research* **42**: 469–476.

Schiller, D., Monfils, M. H., Raio, C. M., Johnson, D. C., LeDoux, J. E. and Phelps, E. A. (2010). Preventing the return of fear in humans using reconsolidation update mechanisms, *Nature* **463**: 49–53.

Schlesiger, M. I., Boublil, B. L., Hales, J. B., Leutgeb, J. K. and Leutgeb, S. (2018). Hippocampal global remapping can occur without input from the medial entorhinal cortex, *Cell Rep* **22**: 3152–3159.

Schliebs, R. and Arendt, T. (2006). The significance of the cholinergic system in the brain during aging and in Alzheimer's disease, *Journal of Neural Transmission* **113**: 1625–1644.

Schliebs, R. and Arendt, T. (2011). The cholinergic system in aging and neuronal degeneration, *Behav Brain Res* **221**: 555–63.

Schmaal, L., Hibar, D. P., Samann, P. G., Hall, G. B., Baune, B. T., Jahanshad, N., Cheung, J. W., van Erp, T. G. M., Bos, D., Ikram, M. A., Vernooij, M. W., Niessen, W. J., Tiemeier, H., Hofman, A., Wittfeld, K., Grabe, H. J., Janowitz, D., Bulow, R., Selonke, M., Volzke, H., Grotegerd, D., Dannlowski, U., Arolt, V., Opel, N., Heindel, W., Kugel, H., Hoehn, D., Czisch, M., Couvy-Duchesne, B., Renteria, M. E., Strike, L. T., Wright, M. J., Mills, N. T., de Zubicaray, G. I., McMahon, K. L., Medland, S. E., Martin, N. G., Gillespie, N. A., Goya-Maldonado, R., Gruber, O., Kramer, B., Hatton, S. N., Lagopoulos, J., Hickie, I. B., Frodl, T., Carballedo, A., Frey, E. M., van Velzen, L. S., Penninx, B., van Tol, M. J., van der Wee, N. J., Davey, C. G., Harrison, B. J., Mwangi, B., Cao, B., Soares, J. C., Veer, I. M., Walter, H., Schoepf, D., Zurowski, B., Konrad, C., Schramm, E., Normann, C., Schnell, K., Sacchet, M. D., Gotlib, I. H., MacQueen, G. M., Godlewska, B. R., Nickson, T., McIntosh, A. M., Papmeyer, M., Whalley, H. C., Hall, J., Sussmann, J. E., Li, M., Walter, M., Aftanas, L., Brack, I., Bokhan, N. A., Thompson, P. M. and Veltman, D. J. (2017). Cortical abnormalities in adults and adolescents with major depression based on brain scans from 20 cohorts worldwide in the ENIGMA Major Depressive Disorder Working Group, *Mol Psychiatry* **22**: 900–909.

Schmahmann, J. D. (2021). Emotional disorders and the cerebellum: Neurobiological substrates, neuropsychiatry, and therapeutic implications, *Handb Clin Neurol* **183**: 109–154.

Schmahmann, J. D., Guell, X., Stoodley, C. J. and Halko, M. A. (2019). The theory and neuroscience of cerebellar cognition, *Annu Rev Neurosci* **42**: 337–364.

Schmidt, E. R. E. and Polleux, F. (2021). Genetic mechanisms underlying the evolution of connectivity in the human cortex, *Front Neural Circuits* **15**: 787164.

Schmolesky, M., Wang, Y., Hanes, D., Thompson, K., Leutgeb, S., Schall, J. and Leventhal, A. (1998). Signal timing across the macaque visual system, *Journal of Neurophysiology* **79**: 3272–3277.

Schoenbaum, G., Roesch, M. R., Stalnaker, T. A. and Takahashi, Y. K. (2009). A new perspective on the role of the orbitofrontal cortex in adaptive behaviour, *Nature Reviews Neuroscience* **10**: 885–892.

Schonfeld, F. and Wiskott, L. (2015). Modeling place field activity with hierarchical slow feature analysis, *Front Comput Neurosci* **9**: 51.

Schonsberg, F., Roudi, Y. and Treves, A. (2021). Efficiency of local learning rules in threshold-linear associative networks, *Phys Rev Lett* **126**: 018301.

Schultz, S. and Rolls, E. T. (1999). Analysis of information transmission in the Schaffer collaterals, *Hippocampus* **9**: 582–598.

Schultz, W. (1998). Predictive reward signal of dopamine neurons, *Journal of Neurophysiology* **80**: 1–27.

Schultz, W. (2004). Neural coding of basic reward terms of animal learning theory, game theory, microeconomics and behavioural ecology, *Current Opinion in Neurobiology* **14**: 139–147.

Schultz, W. (2006). Behavioral theories and the neurophysiology of reward, *Annual Review of Psychology* **57**: 87–115.

Schultz, W. (2013). Updating dopamine reward signals, *Current Opinion in Neurobiology* **23**: 229–238.

Schultz, W. (2016a). Dopamine reward prediction error coding, *Dialogues Clin Neurosci* **18**: 23–32.

Schultz, W. (2016b). Dopamine reward prediction-error signalling: a two-component response, *Nat Rev Neurosci* **17**: 183–95.

Schultz, W. (2016c). Reward functions of the basal ganglia, *J Neural Transm (Vienna)* **123**: 679–693.

Schultz, W. (2017). Reward prediction error, *Curr Biol* **27**: R369–R371.

Schultz, W. (2019). Recent advances in understanding the role of phasic dopamine activity, *F1000Res* **8**: 1680.

Schultz, W., Apicella, P., Scarnati, E. and Ljungberg, T. (1992). Neuronal activity in the ventral striatum related to the expectation of reward, *Journal of Neuroscience* **12**: 4595–4610.

Schultz, W., Apicella, P., Romo, R. and Scarnati, E. (1995a). Context-dependent activity in primate striatum reflecting past and future behavioral events, in J. C. Houk, J. L. Davis and D. G. Beiser (eds), *Models of Information Processing in the Basal Ganglia*, MIT Press, Cambridge, MA, chapter 2, pp. 11–27.

Schultz, W., Romo, R., Ljunberg, T., Mirenowicz, J., Hollerman, J. R. and Dickinson, A. (1995b). Reward-related signals carried by dopamine neurons, in J. C. Houk, J. L. Davis and D. G. Beiser (eds), *Models of Information Processing in the Basal Ganglia*, MIT Press, Cambridge, MA, chapter 12, pp. 233–248.

Schultz, W., Dayan, P. and Montague, P. R. (1997). A neural substrate of prediction and reward, *Science* **275**: 1593–1599.

Schultz, W., Tremblay, L. and Hollerman, J. R. (2000). Reward processing in primate orbitofrontal cortex and basal ganglia, *Cereb Cortex* **10**: 272–84.

Schultz, W., Tremblay, L. and Hollerman, J. R. (2003). Changes in behavior-related neuronal activity in the striatum during learning, *Trends in Neurosciences* **26**: 312–328.

Schurz, M., Tholen, M. G., Perner, J., Mars, R. B. and Sallet, J. (2017). Specifying the brain anatomy underlying temporo-parietal junction activations for theory of mind: A review using probabilistic atlases from different imaging modalities, *Hum Brain Mapp* **38**: 4788–4805.

Schwindel, C. D. and McNaughton, B. L. (2011). Hippocampal-cortical interactions and the dynamics of memory trace reactivation, *Progress in Brain Research* **193**: 163–177.

Sclafani, A. (2013). Gut-brain nutrient signaling. Appetition vs. satiation, *Appetite* **71**: 454–8.

Sclafani, A., Ackroff, K. and Schwartz, G. J. (2003). Selective effects of vagal deafferentation and celiac-superior mesenteric ganglionectomy on the reinforcing and satiating action of intestinal nutrients, *Physiology and Behavior* **78**: 285–294.

Scott, B. H. and Mishkin, M. (2016). Auditory short-term memory in the primate auditory cortex, *Brain Res* **1640**: 264–77.

Scott, B. H., Mishkin, M. and Yin, P. (2014). Neural correlates of auditory short-term memory in rostral superior temporal cortex, *Curr Biol* **24**: 2767–75.

Scott, B. H., Leccese, P. A., Saleem, K. S., Kikuchi, Y., Mullarkey, M. P., Fukushima, M., Mishkin, M. and Saunders, R. C. (2017). Intrinsic connections of the Core Auditory Cortical regions and rostral supratemporal plane in the macaque monkey, *Cereb Cortex* **27**: 809–840.

Scott, S. H. and Kalaska, J. F. (2021). Voluntary movement: motor cortices, *in* E. R. Kandel, J. D. Koester, S. H. Mack and S. A. Siegelbaum (eds), *Principles of Neural Science*, McGraw-Hill, New York, chapter 34, pp. 815–859.

Scott, S. K., Young, A. W., Calder, A. J., Hellawell, D. J., Aggleton, J. P. and Johnson, M. (1997). Impaired auditory recognition of fear and anger following bilateral amygdala lesions, *Nature* **385**: 254–7.

Scott, T. R. (2011). Learning through the taste system, *Front Syst Neurosci* **5**: 87.

Scott, T. R. and Small, D. M. (2009). The role of the parabrachial nucleus in taste processing and feeding, *Annals of the New York Academy of Sciences* **1170**: 372–377.

Scott, T. R., Yaxley, S., Sienkiewicz, Z. J. and Rolls, E. T. (1986a). Gustatory responses in the frontal opercular cortex of the alert cynomolgus monkey, *Journal of Neurophysiology* **56**: 876–890.

Scott, T. R., Yaxley, S., Sienkiewicz, Z. J. and Rolls, E. T. (1986b). Taste responses in the nucleus tractus solitarius of the behaving monkey, *Journal of Neurophysiology* **55**: 182–200.

Scott, T. R., Messersmith, A. R., McCrary, W. J., Herlong, J. L. and Burgess, S. C. (2005). Hematopoietic prostaglandin D2 synthase in the chicken Harderian gland, *Vet Immunol Immunopathol* **108**: 295–306.

Scoville, W. and Milner, B. (1957). Loss of recent memory after bilateral hippocampal lesions, *J. Neurol. Neurosurg. Psychiatry* **20**: 11–21.

Seamans, J. K. and Yang, C. R. (2004). The principal features and mechanisms of dopamine modulation in the prefrontal cortex, *Progress in Neurobiology* **74**: 1–58.

Seeley, R. J., Kaplan, J. M. and Grill, H. J. (1995). Effect of occluding the pylorus on intraoral intake: a test of the gastric hypothesis of meal termination, *Physiol Behav* **58**: 245–9.

Segerdahl, A. R., Mezue, M., Okell, T. W., Farrar, J. T. and Tracey, I. (2015). The dorsal posterior insula subserves a fundamental role in human pain, *Nat Neurosci* **18**: 499–500.

Seghier, M. L. (2013). The angular gyrus: multiple functions and multiple subdivisions, *Neuroscientist* **19**: 43–61.

Seghier, M. L., Fagan, E. and Price, C. J. (2010). Functional subdivisions in the left angular gyrus where the semantic system meets and diverges from the default network, *J Neurosci* **30**: 16809–17.

Seigel, M. and Auerbach, J. M. (1996). Neuromodulators of synaptic strength, *in* M. S. Fazeli and G. L. Collingridge (eds), *Cortical Plasticity*, Bios, Oxford, chapter 7, pp. 137–148.

Sejnowski, T. J. (2020). The unreasonable effectiveness of deep learning in artificial intelligence, *Proc Natl Acad Sci U S A*.

Seleman, L. D. and Goldman-Rakic, P. S. (1985). Longitudinal topography and interdigitation of corticostriatal projections in the rhesus monkey, *Journal of Neuroscience* **5**: 776–794.

Selfridge, O. G. (1959). Pandemonium: A paradigm for learning, *in* D. Blake and A.Uttley (eds), *The Mechanization of Thought Processes*, H. M. Stationery Office, London, pp. 511–529.

Seltzer, B. and Pandya, D. N. (1978). Afferent cortical connections and architectonics of the superior temporal sulcus and surrounding cortex in the rhesus monkey, *Brain Research* **149**: 1–24.

Seltzer, B. and Pandya, D. N. (1989). Frontal lobe connections of the superior temporal sulcus in the rhesus monkey, *Journal of Comparative Neurology* **281**: 97–113.

Semework, M., Steenrod, S. C. and Goldberg, M. E. (2018). A spatial memory signal shows that the parietal cortex has access to a craniotopic representation of space, *Elife* **7**: e30762.

Sendhilnathan, N., Basu, D., Goldberg, M. E., Schall, J. D. and Murthy, A. (2021). Neural correlates of goal-directed and non-goal-directed movements, *Proc Natl Acad Sci U S A* **118**: e2006372118.

Senn, W., Markram, H. and Tsodyks, M. (2001). An algorithm for modifying neurotransmitter release probability based on pre- and postsynaptic spike timing, *Neural Computation* **13**: 35–67.

Serre, T., Kreiman, G., Kouh, M., Cadieu, C., Knoblich, U. and Poggio, T. (2007a). A quantitative theory of immediate visual recognition, *Progress in Brain Research* **165**: 33–56.

Serre, T., Oliva, A. and Poggio, T. (2007b). A feedforward architecture accounts for rapid categorization, *Proceedings of the National Academy of Sciences* **104**: 6424–6429.

Serre, T., Wolf, L., Bileschi, S., Riesenhuber, M. and Poggio, T. (2007c). Robust object recognition with cortex-like mechanisms, *IEEE Transactions on Pattern Analysis and Machine Intelligence* **29**: 411–426.

Seyfarth, R. M. and Cheney, D. L. (2010). Production, usage, and comprehension in animal vocalizations, *Brain Lang* **115**: 92–100.

Seymour, B., O'Doherty, J., Dayan, P., Koltzenburg, M., Jones, A. K., Dolan, R. J., Friston, K. J. and Frackowiak, R. S. (2004). Temporal difference models describe higher-order learning in humans, *Nature* **429**: 664–667.

Shadlen, M. and Newsome, W. (1995). Is there a signal in the noise?, *Current Opinion in Neurobiology* **5**: 248–250.

Shadlen, M. and Newsome, W. (1998). The variable discharge of cortical neurons: implications for connectivity, computation and coding, *Journal of Neuroscience* **18**: 3870–3896.

Shadlen, M. N. and Movshon, J. A. (1999). Synchrony unbound: A critical evaluation of the temporal binding hypothesis, *Neuron* **24**: 67–77.

Shallice, T. and Burgess, P. (1996). The domain of supervisory processes and temporal organization of behaviour, *Philos Trans R Soc Lond B Biol Sci* **351**: 1405–11.

Shallice, T. and Burgess, P. W. (1991). Deficits in strategy application following frontal lobe damage in man, *Brain* **114 (Pt 2)**: 727–41.

Shallice, T. and Cipolotti, L. (2018). The prefrontal cortex and neurological impairments of active thought, *Annu Rev Psychol* **69**: 157–180.

Shannon, C. E. (1948). A mathematical theory of communication, *AT&T Bell Laboratories Technical Journal* **27**: 379–423.

Shapiro, M. L., Tanila, H. and Eichenbaum, H. (1997). Cues that hippocampal place cells encode: dynamic and hierarchical representation of local and distal stimuli, *Hippocampus* **7**: 624–42.

Sharp, P. E. (1996). Multiple spatial-behavioral correlates for cells in the rat postsubiculum: multiple regression analysis and comparison to other hippocampal areas, *Cerebral Cortex* **6**: 238–259.

Sharpe, M. J., Stalnaker, T., Schuck, N. W., Killcross, S., Schoenbaum, G. and Niv, Y. (2019). An integrated model of action selection: distinct modes of cortical control of striatal decision making, *Annu Rev Psychol* **70**: 53–76.

Shashua, A. (1995). Algebraic functions for recognition, *IEEE Transactions on Pattern Analysis and Machine Intelligence* **17**: 779–789.

Sheinberg, D. L. and Logothetis, N. K. (2001). Noticing familiar objects in real world scenes: the role of temporal cortical neurons in natural vision, *J Neurosci* **21**: 1340–50.

Shepherd, G. M. (2004). *The Synaptic Organisation of the Brain*, 5th edn, Oxford University Press, Oxford.

Shepherd, G. M. and Grillner, S. (eds) (2010). *Handbook of Brain Microcircuits*, Oxford University Press, Oxford.

Shepherd, G. M. and Rowe, T. B. (2017). Neocortical lamination: insights from neuron types and evolutionary precursors, *Front Neuroanat* **11**: 100.

Shepherd, G. M. G. and Yamawaki, N. (2021). Untangling the cortico-thalamo-cortical loop: cellular pieces of a knotty circuit puzzle, *Nat Rev Neurosci* **22**: 389–406.

Shergill, S. S., Brammer, M. J., Williams, S. C., Murray, R. M. and McGuire, P. K. (2000). Mapping auditory hallucinations in schizophrenia using functional magnetic resonance imaging, *Archives of General Psychiatry* **57**: 1033–1038.

Sherrill, K. R., Chrastil, E. R., Ross, R. S., Erdem, U. M., Hasselmo, M. E. and Stern, C. E. (2015). Functional connections between optic flow areas and navigationally responsive brain regions during goal-directed navigation, *Neuroimage* **118**: 386–96.

Shevelev, I. A., Novikova, R. V., Lazareva, N. A., Tikhomirov, A. S. and Sharaev, G. A. (1995). Sensitivity to cross-like figures in cat striate neurons, *Neuroscience* **69**: 51–57.

Shiino, M. and Fukai, T. (1990). Replica-symmetric theory of the nonlinear analogue neural networks, *Journal of Physics A: Mathematical and General* **23**: L1009–L1017.

Shima, K. and Tanji, J. (1998). Role for cingulate motor area cells in voluntary movement selection based on reward, *Science* **13**: 1335–1338.

Shizgal, P. and Arvanitogiannis, A. (2003). Gambling on dopamine, *Science* **299**: 1856–1858.

Si, B. and Treves, A. (2009). The role of competitive learning in the generation of DG fields from EC inputs, *Cogn Neurodyn* **3**: 177–87.

Sidhu, M. K., Stretton, J., Winston, G. P., Bonelli, S., Centeno, M., Vollmar, C., Symms, M., Thompson, P. J., Koepp, M. J. and Duncan, J. S. (2013). A functional magnetic resonance imaging study mapping the episodic memory encoding network in temporal lobe epilepsy, *Brain* **136**: 1868–1888.

Siegelbaum, S. A. and Kandel, E. R. (2013). Prefrontal cortex, hippocampus, and the biology of memory storage, in E. R. Kandel, J. H. Schwartz, T. M. Jessell, S. A. Siegelbaum and A. J. Hudspeth (eds), *Principles of Neural Science*, 5 edn, McGraw Hill, New York, chapter 67, pp. 1487–1521.

Sigala, N. and Logothetis, N. K. (2002). Visual categorisation shapes feature selectivity in the primate temporal cortex, *Nature* **415**: 318–320.

Sikström, S. (2007). Computational perspectives on neuromodulation of aging, *Acta Neurochirurgica, Supplement* **97**: 513–518.

Sillito, A. M. (1984). Functional considerations of the operation of GABAergic inhibitory processes in the visual cortex, *in* E. G. Jones and A. Peters (eds), *Cerebral Cortex, Vol. 2, Functional Properties of Cortical Cells*, Plenum, New York, chapter 4, pp. 91–117.

Sillito, A. M., Grieve, K. L., Jones, H. E., Cudeiro, J. and Davis, J. (1995). Visual cortical mechanisms detecting focal orientation discontinuities, *Nature* **378**: 492–496.

Silson, E. H., Steel, A. D. and Baker, C. I. (2016). Scene-selectivity and retinotopy in medial parietal cortex, *Front Hum Neurosci* **10**: 412.

Silson, E. H., Steel, A., Kidder, A., Gilmore, A. W. and Baker, C. I. (2019). Distinct subdivisions of human medial parietal cortex support recollection of people and places, *Elife* **8**: e47391.

Silventoinen, K., Magnusson, P. K., Tynelius, P., Kaprio, J. and Rasmussen, F. (2008). Heritability of body size and muscle strength in young adulthood: a study of one million Swedish men, *Genet Epidemiol* **32**: 341–9.

Simmen, M. W., Rolls, E. T. and Treves, A. (1996a). On the dynamics of a network of spiking neurons, *in* F. Eekman and J. Bower (eds), *Computations and Neuronal Systems: Proceedings of CNS95*, Kluwer, Boston.

Simmen, M. W., Treves, A. and Rolls, E. T. (1996b). Pattern retrieval in threshold-linear associative nets, *Network* **7**: 109–122.

Simmons, J. M., Ravel, S., Shidara, M. and Richmond, B. J. (2007). A comparison of reward-contingent neuronal activity in monkey orbitofrontal cortex and ventral striatum: guiding actions toward rewards, *Annals of the New York Academy of Sciences* **1121**: 376–394.

Singer, A. C. and Frank, L. M. (2009). Rewarded outcomes enhance reactivation of experience in the hippocampus, *Neuron* **64**: 910–21.

Singer, W. (1987). Activity-dependent self-organization of synaptic connections as a substrate for learning, *in* J.-P. Changeux and M. Konishi (eds), *The Neural and Molecular Bases of Learning*, Wiley, Chichester, pp. 301–335.

Singer, W. (1995). Development and plasticity of cortical processing architectures, *Science* **270**: 758–764.

Singer, W. (1999). Neuronal synchrony: A versatile code for the definition of relations?, *Neuron* **24**: 49–65.

Singer, W. (2000). Response synchronisation: A universal coding strategy for the definition of relations, *in* M. Gazzaniga (ed.), *The New Cognitive Neurosciences*, 2nd edn, MIT Press, Cambridge, MA, chapter 23, pp. 325–338.

Singer, W. and Gray, C. M. (1995). Visual Feature Integration and the Temporal Correlation Hypothesis, *Annual Review of Neuroscience* **18**: 555–586.

Singer, W., Gray, C., Engel, A., Konig, P., Artola, A. and Brocher, S. (1990). Formation of Cortical Cell Assemblies, *Cold Spring Harbor Symposium on Quantitative Biology* **55**: 939–952.

Singer, W., Sejnowski, T. J. and Rakic, P. (2019). *The Neocortex*, MIT Press, Cambridge, MA.

Sjöström, P. J., Turrigiano, G. G. and Nelson, S. B. (2001). Rate, timing, and cooperativity jointly determine cortical synaptic plasticity, *Neuron* **32**: 1149–1164.

Skaggs, W. E. and McNaughton, B. L. (1992). Quantification of what it is that hippocampal cell firing encodes, *Society for Neuroscience Abstracts* **18**: 1216.

Skaggs, W. E., McNaughton, B. L., Gothard, K. and Markus, E. (1993). An information theoretic approach to deciphering the hippocampal code, *in* S. Hanson, J. D. Cowan and C. L. Giles (eds), *Advances in Neural Information Processing Systems*, Vol. 5, Morgan Kaufmann, San Mateo, CA, pp. 1030–1037.

Skaggs, W. E., Knierim, J. J., Kudrimoti, H. S. and McNaughton, B. L. (1995). A model of the neural basis of the rat's sense of direction, *in* G. Tesauro, D. S. Touretzky and T. K. Leen (eds), *Advances in Neural Information Processing Systems*, Vol. 7, MIT Press, Cambridge, MA, pp. 173–180.

Sloper, J. J. and Powell, T. P. S. (1979a). An experimental electron microscopic study of afferent connections to the primate motor and somatic sensory cortices, *Philosophical Transactions of the Royal Society of London, Series B* **285**: 199–226.

Sloper, J. J. and Powell, T. P. S. (1979b). A study of the axon initial segment and proximal axon of neurons in the primate motor and somatic sensory cortices, *Philosophical Transactions of the Royal Society of London, Series B* **285**: 173–197.

Small, D. M. (2010). Taste representation in the human insula, *Brain Structre and Function* **214**: 551–561.

Small, D. M. and Scott, T. R. (2009). Symposium overview: What happens to the pontine processing? Repercussions of interspecies differences in pontine taste representation for tasting and feeding, *Annals of the New York Academy of Science* **1170**: 343–346.

Small, D. M., Zald, D. H., Jones-Gotman, M., Zatorre, R. J., Petrides, M. and Evans, A. C. (1999). Human cortical gustatory areas: a review of functional neuroimaing data, *NeuroReport* **8**: 3913–3917.

Small, D. M., Bender, G., Veldhuizen, M. G., Rudenga, K., Nachtigal, D. and Felsted, J. (2007). The role of the human orbitofrontal cortex in taste and flavor processing, *Annals of the New York Academy of Sciences* **1121**: 136–151.

Smerieri, A., Rolls, E. T. and Feng, J. (2010). Decision time, slow inhibition, and theta rhythm, *Journal of Neuroscience* **30**: 14173–14181.

Smith, A. T., Beer, A. L., Furlan, M. and Mars, R. B. (2018). Connectivity of the cingulate sulcus visual area (CSv) in the human cerebral cortex, *Cereb Cortex* **28**: 713–725.

Smith, M. L. and Milner, B. (1981). The role of the right hippocampus in the recall of spatial location, *Neuropsychologia* **19**: 781–793.

Smith, S. M., Jenkinson, M., Woolrich, M. W., Beckmann, C. F., Behrens, T. E., Johansen-Berg, H., Bannister, P. R., De Luca, M., Drobnjak, I., Flitney, D. E., Niazy, R. K., Saunders, J., Vickers, J., Zhang, Y., De Stefano, N., Brady, J. M. and Matthews, P. M. (2004). Advances in functional and structural MR image analysis and implementation as FSL, *Neuroimage* **23 Suppl 1**: S208–19.

Smucny, J., Dienel, S. J., Lewis, D. A. and Carter, C. S. (2022). Mechanisms underlying dorsolateral prefrontal cortex contributions to cognitive dysfunction in schizophrenia, *Neuropsychopharmacology* **47**: 292–308.

Snyder, L. H., Grieve, K. L., Brotchie, P. and Andersen, R. A. (1998). Separate body- and world-referenced representations of visual space in parietal cortex, *Nature* **394**: 887–91.

Sokolov, A. A., Miall, R. C. and Ivry, R. B. (2017). The cerebellum: adaptive prediction for movement and cognition, *Trends Cogn Sci* **21**: 313–332.

Solari, N. and Hangya, B. (2018). Cholinergic modulation of spatial learning, memory and navigation, *Eur J Neurosci* **48**: 2199–2230.

Soldatkina, O., Schonsberg, F. and Treves, A. (2022). Challenges for place and grid cell models, *Adv Exp Med Biol* **1359**: 285–312.

Solstad, T., Boccara, C. N., Kropff, E., Moser, M. B. and Moser, E. I. (2008). Representation of geometric borders in the entorhinal cortex, *Science* **322**: 1865–8.

Soltani, A. and Koch, C. (2010). Visual saliency computations: mechanisms, constraints, and the effect of feedback, *Journal of Neuroscience* **30**: 12831–12843.

Somogyi, P. (2010). Hippocampus: intrinsic organisation, *in* G. M. Shepherd and S. Grillner (eds), *Handbook of Brain Microcircuits*, Oxford University Press, Oxford, chapter 15, pp. 148–164.

Somogyi, P. and Cowey, A. C. (1984). Double bouquet cells, *in* A. Peters and E. G. Jones (eds), *Cerebral Cortex, Vol. 1, Cellular Components of the Cerebral Cortex*, Plenum, New York, chapter 9, pp. 337–360.

Somogyi, P., Kisvarday, Z. F., Martin, K. A. C. and Whitteridge, D. (1983). Synaptic connections of morphologically identified and physiologically characterized large basket cells in the striate cortex of the cat, *Neuroscience* **10**: 261–294.

Somogyi, P., Tamas, G., Lujan, R. and Buhl, E. H. (1998). Salient features of synaptic organisation in the cerebral cortex, *Brain Research Reviews* **26**: 113–135.

Sompolinsky, H. (1987). The theory of neural networks: the Hebb rule and beyond, *in* L. van Hemmen and I. Morgenstern (eds), *Heidelberg Colloquium on Glassy Dynamics*, Vol. 275, Springer, New York, pp. 485–527.

Sompolinsky, H. and Kanter, I. I. (1986). Temporal association in asymmetric neural networks, *Physical Review Letters* **57**: 2861–2864.

Song, S., Yao, H. and Treves, A. (2014). A modular latching chain, *Cognitive neurodynamics* **8**: 37–46.

Spalla, D., Cornacchia, I. M. and Treves, A. (2021). Continuous attractors for dynamic memories, *Elife*.

Spalla, D., Treves, A. and Boccara, C. N. (2022). Angular and linear speed cells in the parahippocampal circuits, *Nat Commun* **13**: 1907.

Spezio, M. L., Huang, P. Y., Castelli, F. and Adolphs, R. (2007). Amygdala damage impairs eye contact during conversations with real people, *J Neurosci* **27**: 3994–7.

Spiers, H. J. and Gilbert, S. J. (2015). Solving the detour problem in navigation: a model of prefrontal and hippocampal interactions, *Front Hum Neurosci* **9**: 125.

Spiers, H. J. and Maguire, E. A. (2006). Thoughts, behaviour, and brain dynamics during navigation in the real world, *Neuroimage* **31**: 1826–40.

Spiridon, M., Fischl, B. and Kanwisher, N. (2006). Location and spatial profile of category-specific regions in human extrastriate cortex, *Human Brain Mapping* **27**: 77–89.

Spoerer, C. J., Eguchi, A. and Stringer, S. M. (2016). A computational exploration of complementary learning mechanisms in the primate ventral visual pathway, *Vision Research* **119**: 16–28.

Sprung-Much, T., Eichert, N., Nolan, E. and Petrides, M. (2022). Broca's area and the search for anatomical asymmetry: commentary and perspectives, *Brain Struct Funct* **227**: 441–449.

Spruston, N., Jonas, P. and Sakmann, B. (1995). Dendritic glutamate receptor channel in rat hippocampal CA3 and CA1 pyramidal neurons, *Journal of Physiology* **482**: 325–352.

Squire, L. (1992). Memory and the hippocampus: A synthesis from findings with rats, monkeys and humans, *Psychological Review* **99**: 195–231.

Squire, L. R. and Wixted, J. T. (2011). The cognitive neuroscience of human memory since H.M, *Annu Rev Neurosci* **34**: 259–88.

Squire, L. R. and Zola, S. M. (1996). Structure and function of declarative and nondeclarative memory systems, *Proceedings of the National Academy of Sciences U S A* **93**: 13515–22.

Squire, L. R., Genzel, L., Wixted, J. T. and Morris, R. G. (2015). Memory consolidation, *Cold Spring Harb Perspect Biol* **7**: a021766.

Srinivasan, S., Carlo, C. N. and Stevens, C. F. (2015). Predicting visual acuity from the structure of visual cortex, *Proc Natl Acad Sci U S A* **112**: 7815–20.

Stankiewicz, B. and Hummel, J. (1994). MetriCat: A representation for basic and subordinate-level classification, *in* G. W. Cottrell (ed.), *Proceedings of the 18th Annual Conference of the Cognitive Science Society*, Erlbaum, San Diego, pp. 254–259.

Staresina, B. P., Reber, T. P., Niediek, J., Bostrom, J., Elger, C. E. and Mormann, F. (2019). Recollection in the human hippocampal-entorhinal cell circuitry, *Nat Commun* **10**: 1503.

Stefanacci, L., Suzuki, W. A. and Amaral, D. G. (1996). Organization of connections between the amygdaloid complex and the perirhinal and parahippocampal cortices in macaque monkeys, *Journal of Comparative Neurology* **375**: 552–582.

Stein, D. J., Kogan, C. S., Atmaca, M., Fineberg, N. A., Fontenelle, L. F., Grant, J. E., Matsunaga, H., Reddy, Y. C., Simpson, H. B., Thomsen, P. H., van den Heuvel, O. A., Veale, D., Woods, D. W. and Reed, G. M. (2016). The classification of Obsessive-Compulsive and Related Disorders in the ICD-11, *J Affect Disord* **190**: 663–74.

Stella, F., Cerasti, E. and Treves, A. (2013). Unveiling the metric structure of internal representations of space, *Frontiers in Neural Circuits* **7**: 81.

Stent, G. S. (1973). A psychological mechanism for Hebb's postulate of learning, *Proceedings of the National Academy of Sciences USA* **70**: 997–1001.

Stephan, K. E. and Roebroeck, A. (2012). A short history of causal modeling of fMRI data, *Neuroimage* **62**: 856–863.

Stephan, K. E., Weiskopf, N., Drysdale, P. M., Robinson, P. A. and Friston, K. J. (2007). Comparing hemodynamic models with DCM, *Neuroimage* **38**: 387–401.

Stephan, K. E., Penny, W. D., Moran, R. J., den Ouden, H. E., Daunizeau, J. and Friston, K. J. (2010). Ten simple rules for dynamic causal modeling, *Neuroimage* **49**: 3099–109.

Stern, C. E. and Passingham, R. E. (1995). The nucleus accumbens in monkeys (Macaca fascicularis): III. Reversal learning, *Experimental Brain Research* **106**: 239–247.

Stern, C. E. and Passingham, R. E. (1996). The nucleus accumbens in monkeys (Macaca fascicularis): II. Emotion and motivation, *Behavioural Brain Research* **75**: 179–193.

Sternson, S. M. (2013). Hypothalamic survival circuits: blueprints for purposive behaviors, *Neuron* **77**: 810–24.

Sterpenich, V., Vidal, S., Hofmeister, J., Michalopoulos, G., Bancila, V., Warrot, D., Dayer, A., Desseilles, M., Aubry, J. M., Kosel, M., Schwartz, S. and Vutskits, L. (2019). Increased reactivity of the mesolimbic reward system after ketamine injection in patients with Treatment-Resistant Major Depressive Disorder, *Anesthesiology* **130**: 923–935.

Stewart, S. E., Fagerness, J. A., Platko, J., Smoller, J. W., Scharf, J. M., Illmann, C., Jenike, E., Chabane, N., Leboyer, M., Delorme, R., Jenike, M. A. and Pauls, D. L. (2007). Association of the SLC1A1 glutamate transporter gene and obsessive-compulsive disorder, *American Journal of Medical Genetics B: Neuropsychiatric Genetics* **144**: 1027–1033.

Stockhausen, K. (1972). Four Criteria of Electronic Music, pp. https://www.youtube.com/watch?v=ZzDhg–MoHlo.

Stoodley, C. J. and Tsai, P. T. (2021). Adaptive prediction for social contexts: the cerebellar contribution to typical and atypical social behaviors, *Annu Rev Neurosci* **44**: 475–493.

Stoodley, C. J., Valera, E. M. and Schmahmann, J. D. (2010). An fMRI study of intra-individual functional topography in the human cerebellum, *Behav Neurol* **23**: 65–79.

Stoodley, C. J., Valera, E. M. and Schmahmann, J. D. (2012). Functional topography of the cerebellum for motor and cognitive tasks: an fMRI study, *Neuroimage* **59**: 1560–70.

Stoodley, C. J., MacMore, J. P., Makris, N., Sherman, J. C. and Schmahmann, J. D. (2016). Location of lesion determines motor vs. cognitive consequences in patients with cerebellar stroke, *Neuroimage Clin* **12**: 765–775.

Storm-Mathiesen, J., Zimmer, J. and Ottersen, O. P. (1990). Understanding the brain through the hippocampus, *Progress in Brain Research* **83**: 1–.

Strait, C. E., Blanchard, T. C. and Hayden, B. Y. (2014). Reward value comparison via mutual inhibition in ventromedial prefrontal cortex, *Neuron* **82**: 1357–66.

Strigo, I. A. and Craig, A. D. (2016). Interoception, homeostatic emotions and sympathovagal balance, *Philos Trans R Soc Lond B Biol Sci* **371**: 20160010.

Stringer, S. M. and Rolls, E. T. (2000). Position invariant recognition in the visual system with cluttered environments, *Neural Networks* **13**: 305–315.

Stringer, S. M. and Rolls, E. T. (2002). Invariant object recognition in the visual system with novel views of 3D objects, *Neural Comput* **14**: 2585–96.

Stringer, S. M. and Rolls, E. T. (2006). Self-organizing path integration using a linked continuous attractor and competitive network: path integration of head direction, *Network: Computation in Neural Systems* **17**: 419–445.

Stringer, S. M. and Rolls, E. T. (2007). Hierarchical dynamical models of motor function, *Neurocomputing* **70**: 975–990.
Stringer, S. M. and Rolls, E. T. (2008). Learning transform invariant object recognition in the visual system with multiple stimuli present during training, *Neural Networks* **21**: 888–903.
Stringer, S. M., Rolls, E. T., Trappenberg, T. P. and De Araujo, I. E. (2002a). Self-organizing continuous attractor networks and path integration: two-dimensional models of place cells, *Network* **13**: 429–46.
Stringer, S. M., Trappenberg, T. P., Rolls, E. T. and De Araujo, I. E. (2002b). Self-organizing continuous attractor networks and path integration: one-dimensional models of head direction cells, *Network* **13**: 217–42.
Stringer, S. M., Rolls, E. T. and Trappenberg, T. P. (2004). Self-organising continuous attractor networks with multiple activity packets, and the representation of space, *Neural Networks* **17**: 5–27.
Stringer, S. M., Rolls, E. T. and Trappenberg, T. P. (2005). Self-organizing continuous attractor network models of hippocampal spatial view cells, *Neurobiol Learn Mem* **83**: 79–92.
Stringer, S. M., Perry, G., Rolls, E. T. and Proske, J. H. (2006). Learning invariant object recognition in the visual system with continuous transformations, *Biological Cybernetics* **94**: 128–142.
Stringer, S. M., Rolls, E. T. and Taylor, P. (2007a). Learning movement sequences with a delayed reward signal in a hierarchical model of motor function, *Neural Networks* **29**: 172–181.
Stringer, S. M., Rolls, E. T. and Tromans, J. M. (2007b). Invariant object recognition with trace learning and multiple stimuli present during training, *Network* **18**: 161–87.
Strong, S. P., Koberle, R., de Ruyter van Steveninck, R. R. and Bialek, W. (1998). Entropy and information in neural spike trains, *Physical Review Letters* **80**: 197–200.
Sugase, Y., Yamane, S., Ueno, S. and Kawano, K. (1999). Global and fine information coded by single neurons in the temporal visual cortex, *Nature* **400**: 869–873.
Sugiura, M., Watanabe, J., Maeda, Y., Matsue, Y., Fukuda, H. and Kawashima, R. (2005). Cortical mechanisms of visual self-recognition, *Neuroimage* **24**: 143–9.
Sugrue, L. P., Corrado, G. S. and Newsome, W. T. (2005). Choosing the greater of two goods: neural currencies for valuation and decision making, *Nature Reviews Neuroscience* **6**: 363–375.
Sulpizio, V., Galati, G., Fattori, P., Galletti, C. and Pitzalis, S. (2020). A common neural substrate for processing scenes and egomotion-compatible visual motion, *Brain Struct Funct* **225**: 2091–2110.
Sun, C., Tang, K., Wu, J., Xu, H., Zhang, W., Cao, T., Zhou, Y., Yu, T. and Li, A. (2019a). Leptin modulates olfactory discrimination and neural activity in the olfactory bulb, *Acta Physiol (Oxf)* **227**: e13319.
Sun, J., Liu, Z., Rolls, E. T., Chen, Q., Yao, Y., Yang, W., Wei, D., Zhang, Q., Zhang, J., Feng, J. and Qiu, J. (2019b). Verbal creativity correlates with the temporal variability of brain networks during the resting state, *Cereb Cortex* **29**: 1047–1058.
Suri, R. E. and Schultz, W. (1998). Learning of sequential movements by neural network model with dopamine-like reinforcement signal, *Experimental Brain Research* **121**: 350–354.
Sutherland, N. S. (1968). Outline of a theory of visual pattern recognition in animal and man, *Proceedings of the Royal Society, B* **171**: 297–317.
Sutherland, R. J. and Rudy, J. W. (1991). Exceptions to the rule of space, *Hippocampus* **1**: 250–252.
Sutherland, R. J., Whishaw, I. Q. and Kolb, B. (1983). A behavioural analysis of spatial localization following electrolytic, kainate- or colchicine-induced damage to the hippocampal formation in the rat, *Behavioral Brain Research* **7**: 133–153.
Sutton, R. S. (1988). Learning to predict by the methods of temporal differences, *Machine Learning* **3**: 9–44.
Sutton, R. S. and Barto, A. G. (1981). Towards a modern theory of adaptive networks: expectation and prediction, *Psychological Review* **88**: 135–170.
Sutton, R. S. and Barto, A. G. (1990). Time-derivative models of Pavlovian reinforcement, *in* M. Gabriel and J. Moore (eds), *Learning and Computational Neuroscience*, MIT Press, Cambridge, MA, pp. 497–537.
Sutton, R. S. and Barto, A. G. (1998). *Reinforcement Learning*, MIT Press, Cambridge, MA.
Sutton, R. S. and Barto, A. G. (2018). *Reinforcement Learning: An Introduction*, MIT Press, Cambridge, MA.
Suzuki, W. A. and Amaral, D. G. (1994a). Perirhinal and parahippocampal cortices of the macaque monkey – cortical afferents, *Journal of Comparative Neurology* **350**: 497–533.
Suzuki, W. A. and Amaral, D. G. (1994b). Topographic organization of the reciprocal connections between the monkey entorhinal cortex and the perirhinal and parahippocampal cortices, *Journal of Neuroscience* **14**: 1856–1877.
Suzuki, W. A., Miller, E. K. and Desimone, R. (1997). Object and place memory in the macaque entorhinal cortex, *Journal of Neurophysiology* **78**: 1062–1081.
Swann, A. C. (2009). Impulsivity in mania, *Current Psychiatry Reports* **11**: 481–487.
Swanson, L. W. and Cowan, W. M. (1977). An autoradiographic study of the organization of the efferent connections of the hippocampal formation in the rat, *Journal of Comparative Neurology* **172**: 49–84.

Swanson, S. J., Conant, L. L., Humphries, C. J., LeDoux, M., Raghavan, M., Mueller, W. M., Allen, L., Gross, W. L., Anderson, C. T., Carlson, C. E., Busch, R. M., Lowe, M., Tivarus, M. E., Drane, D. L., Loring, D. W., Jacobs, M., Morgan, V. L., Szaflarski, J., Bonilha, L., Bookheimer, S., Grabowski, T., Phatak, V., Vannest, J., Binder, J. R. and study, F. i. A. T. E. S. (2020). Changes in description naming for common and proper nouns after left anterior temporal lobectomy, *Epilepsy Behav* **106**: 106912.

Swash, M. (1989). John Hughlings Jackson: a historical introduction, *in* C. Kennard and M. Swash (eds), *Hierarchies in Neurology*, Springer, London, chapter 1, pp. 3–10.

Szabo, M., Almeida, R., Deco, G. and Stetter, M. (2004). Cooperation and biased competition model can explain attentional filtering in the prefrontal cortex, *European Journal of Neuroscience* **19**: 1969–1977.

Szabo, M., Deco, G., Fusi, S., Del Giudice, P., Mattia, M. and Stetter, M. (2006). Learning to attend: Modeling the shaping of selectivity in infero-temporal cortex in a categorization task, *Biological Cybernetics* **94**: 351–365.

Szentagothai, J. (1978). The neuron network model of the cerebral cortex: a functional interpretation, *Proceedings of the Royal Society of London, Series B* **201**: 219–248.

Szpunar, K. K., Chan, J. C. and McDermott, K. B. (2009). Contextual processing in episodic future thought, *Cereb Cortex* **19**: 1539–48.

Tabuchi, E., Mulder, A. B. and Wiener, S. I. (2003). Reward value invariant place responses and reward site associated activity in hippocampal neurons of behaving rats, *Hippocampus* **13**: 117–132.

Taira, K. and Rolls, E. T. (1996). Receiving grooming as a reinforcer for the monkey, *Physiology and Behavior* **59**: 1189–1192.

Takahashi, N., Kawamura, M., Shiota, J., Kasahata, N. and Hirayama, K. (1997). Pure topographic disorientation due to right retrosplenial lesion, *Neurology* **49**: 464–9.

Takashima, A., Petersson, K. M., Rutters, F., Tendolkar, I., Jensen, O., Zwarts, M. J., McNaughton, B. L. and Fernandez, G. (2006). Declarative memory consolidation in humans: a prospective functional magnetic resonance imaging study, *Proc Natl Acad Sci U S A* **103**: 756–61.

Takeuchi, T., Duszkiewicz, A. J. and Morris, R. G. (2014). The synaptic plasticity and memory hypothesis: encoding, storage and persistence, *Philos Trans R Soc Lond B Biol Sci* **369**: 20130288.

Tan, H., Ng, T. P. Y., Owens, C., Libedinsky, C. and Yen, S.-C. (2021). Independent influences of place and view in the hippocampus of the non-human primate, *Society for Neuroscience Abstracts* p. P869.08.

Tanaka, H., Ishikawa, T., Lee, J. and Kakei, S. (2020). The cerebro-cerebellum as a locus of forward model: a review, *Front Syst Neurosci* **14**: 19.

Tanaka, K. (1993). Neuronal mechanisms of object recognition, *Science* **262**: 685–688.

Tanaka, K. (1996). Inferotemporal cortex and object vision, *Annual Review of Neuroscience* **19**: 109–139.

Tanaka, K., Saito, C., Fukada, Y. and Moriya, M. (1990). Integration of form, texture, and color information in the inferotemporal cortex of the macaque, *in* E. Iwai and M. Mishkin (eds), *Vision, Memory and the Temporal Lobe*, Elsevier, New York, chapter 10, pp. 101–109.

Tanaka, K., Saito, H., Fukada, Y. and Moriya, M. (1991). Coding visual images of objects in the inferotemporal cortex of the macaque monkey, *Journal of Neurophysiology* **66**: 170–189.

Tanaka, S. C., Doya, K., Okada, G., Ueda, K., Okamoto, Y. and Yamawaki, S. (2004). Prediction of immediate and future rewards differentially recruits cortico-basal ganglia loops, *Nature Neuroscience* **7**: 887–893.

Tanila, H. (1999). Hippocampal place cells can develop distinct representations of two visually identical environments, *Hippocampus* **9**: 235–246.

Taschereau-Dumouchel, V., Michel, M., Lau, H., Hofmann, S. G. and LeDoux, J. E. (2022). Putting the "mental" back in "mental disorders": a perspective from research on fear and anxiety, *Mol Psychiatry* **27**: 1322–1330.

Taube, J. S., Muller, R. U. and Ranck, J. B., J. (1990a). Head-direction cells recorded from the postsubiculum in freely moving rats. I. Description and quantitative analysis, *J Neurosci* **10**: 420–35.

Taube, J. S., Muller, R. U. and Ranck, Jr., J. B. (1990b). Head-direction cells recorded from the postsubiculum in freely moving rats. II. Effects of environmental manipulations, *Journal of Neuroscience* **10**: 436–447.

Taube, J. S., Goodridge, J. P., Golob, E. J., Dudchenko, P. A. and Stackman, R. W. (1996). Processing the head direction signal: A review and commentary., *Brain Res. Bull.* **40**: 477–486.

Taylor, J. G. (1999). Neural 'bubble' dynamics in two dimensions: foundations, *Biological Cybernetics* **80**: 393–409.

Teghil, A., Bonavita, A., Guariglia, C. and Boccia, M. (2021). Commonalities and specificities between environmental navigation and autobiographical memory: A synthesis and a theoretical perspective, *Neurosci Biobehav Rev* **127**: 928–945.

Temido-Ferreira, M., Coelho, J. E., Pousinha, P. A. and Lopes, L. V. (2019). Novel players in the aging synapse: impact on cognition, *J Caffeine Adenosine Res* **9**: 104–127.

Teng, E. and Squire, L. R. (1999). Memory for places learned long ago is intact after hippocampal damage, *Nature* **400**: 675–7.

Terrazas, A., Krause, M., Lipa, P., Gothard, K. M., Barnes, C. A. and McNaughton, B. L. (2005). Self-motion and the hippocampal spatial metric, *J Neurosci* **25**: 8085–96.

Teyler, T. J. and DiScenna, P. (1986). The hippocampal memory indexing theory, *Behavioral Neuroscience* **100**: 147–154.

Thapar, A., Eyre, O., Patel, V. and Brent, D. (2022). Depression in young people, *Lancet* **400**: 617–631.

Thomson, A. M. and Deuchars, J. (1994). Temporal and spatial properties of local circuits in neocortex, *Trends in Neurosciences* **17**: 119–126.

Thorpe, S. J. and Imbert, M. (1989). Biological constraints on connectionist models, *in* R. Pfeifer, Z. Schreter and F. Fogelman-Soulie (eds), *Connectionism in Perspective*, Elsevier, Amsterdam, pp. 63–92.

Thorpe, S. J., Maddison, S. and Rolls, E. T. (1979). Single unit activity in the orbitofrontal cortex of the behaving monkey, *Neuroscience Letters* **S3**: S77.

Thorpe, S. J., Rolls, E. T. and Maddison, S. (1983). The orbitofrontal cortex: neuronal activity in the behaving monkey, *Exp Brain Res* **49**: 93–115.

Thorpe, S. J., O'Regan, J. K. and Pouget, A. (1989). Humans fail on XOR pattern classification problems, *in* L. Personnaz and G. Dreyfus (eds), *Neural Networks: From Models to Applications*, I.D.S.E.T., Paris, pp. 12–25.

Thorpe, S. J., Fize, D. and Marlot, C. (1996). Speed of processing in the human visual system, *Nature* **381**: 520–522.

Thorpe, S. J., Delorme, A. and Van Rullen, R. (2001). Spike-based strategies for rapid processing, *Neural Networks* **14**: 715–725.

Tian, B., Reser, D., Durham, A., Kustov, A. and Rauschecker, J. P. (2001). Functional specialization in rhesus monkey auditory cortex, *Science* **292**: 290–3.

Tiganj, Z., Cromer, J. A., Roy, J. E., Miller, E. K. and Howard, M. W. (2018). Compressed timeline of recent experience in monkey lateral prefrontal cortex, *J Cogn Neurosci* **30**: 935–950.

Timbie, C., Garcia-Cabezas, M. A., Zikopoulos, B. and Barbas, H. (2020). Organization of primate amygdalar-thalamic pathways for emotions, *PLoS Biol* **18**: e3000639.

Tirko, N. N., Eyring, K. W., Carcea, I., Mitre, M., Chao, M. V., Froemke, R. C. and Tsien, R. W. (2018). Oxytocin transforms firing mode of CA2 hippocampal neurons, *Neuron* **100**: 593–608 e3.

Tobler, P. N., Dickinson, A. and Schultz, W. (2003). Coding of predicted reward omission by dopamine neurons in a conditioned inhibition paradigm, *Journal of Neuroscience* **23**: 10402–10410.

Toda, T., Parylak, S. L., Linker, S. B. and Gage, F. H. (2019). The role of adult hippocampal neurogenesis in brain health and disease, *Mol Psychiatry* **24**: 67–87.

Tonegawa, S., Nakazawa, K. and Wilson, M. A. (2003). Genetic neuroscience of mammalian learning and memory, *Philosophical Transactions of the Royal Society of London B Biological Sciences* **358**: 787–795.

Tosoni, A., Pitzalis, S., Committeri, G., Fattori, P., Galletti, C. and Galati, G. (2015). Resting-state connectivity and functional specialization in human medial parieto-occipital cortex, *Brain Struct Funct* **220**: 3307–21.

Tou, J. T. and Gonzalez, A. G. (1974). *Pattern Recognition Principles*, Addison-Wesley, Reading, MA.

Tovee, M. J. and Rolls, E. T. (1995). Information encoding in short firing rate epochs by single neurons in the primate temporal visual cortex, *Visual Cognition* **2**: 35–58.

Tovee, M. J., Rolls, E. T., Treves, A. and Bellis, R. P. (1993). Information encoding and the responses of single neurons in the primate temporal visual cortex, *Journal of Neurophysiology* **70**: 640–654.

Tovee, M. J., Rolls, E. T. and Azzopardi, P. (1994). Translation invariance in the responses to faces of single neurons in the temporal visual cortical areas of the alert macaque, *J Neurophysiol* **72**: 1049–60.

Tovee, M. J., Rolls, E. T. and Ramachandran, V. S. (1996). Rapid visual learning in neurones of the primate temporal visual cortex, *NeuroReport* **7**: 2757–2760.

Tracey, I. (2017). Neuroimaging mechanisms in pain: from discovery to translation, *Pain* **158 Suppl 1**: S115–S122.

Trappenberg, T. P., Rolls, E. T. and Stringer, S. M. (2002). Effective size of receptive fields of inferior temporal visual cortex neurons in natural scenes, *in* T. G. Dietterich, S. Becker and Z. Gharamani (eds), *Advances in Neural Information Processing Systems*, Vol. 14, MIT Press, Cambridge, MA, pp. 293–300.

Tremblay, L. and Schultz, W. (1998). Modifications of reward expectation-related neuronal activity during learning in primate striatum, *Journal of Neurophysiology* **80**: 964–977.

Tremblay, L. and Schultz, W. (1999). Relative reward preference in primate orbitofrontal cortex, *Nature* **398**: 704–708.

Tremblay, L. and Schultz, W. (2000). Modifications of reward expectation-related neuronal activity during learning in primate orbitofrontal cortex, *Journal of Neurophysiology* **83**: 1877–1885.

Treves, A. (1990). Graded-response neurons and information encodings in autoassociative memories, *Physical Review A* **42**: 2418–2430.

Treves, A. (1991a). Are spin-glass effects relevant to understanding realistic auto-associative networks?, *Journal of Physics A* **24**: 2645–2654.

Treves, A. (1991b). Dilution and sparse coding in threshold-linear nets, *Journal of Physics A* **24**: 327–335.

Treves, A. (1993). Mean-field analysis of neuronal spike dynamics, *Network* **4**: 259–284.

Treves, A. (1995). Quantitative estimate of the information relayed by the Schaffer collaterals, *Journal of Computational Neuroscience* **2**: 259–272.

Treves, A. (1997). On the perceptual structure of face space, *Biosystems* **40**: 189–196.

Treves, A. (2005). Frontal latching networks: a possible neural basis for infinite recursion, *Cognitive Neuropsychology* **22**: 276–291.

Treves, A. (2016). The dentate gyrus, defining a new memory of David Marr, *in* L. M. Vaina and R. E. Passingham (eds), *Computational Theories and their Implementation in the Brain: The Legacy of David Marr*, Oxford University Press, Oxford.

Treves, A. and Panzeri, S. (1995). The upward bias in measures of information derived from limited data samples, *Neural Computation* **7**: 399–407.

Treves, A. and Rolls, E. T. (1991). What determines the capacity of autoassociative memories in the brain?, *Network* **2**: 371–397.

Treves, A. and Rolls, E. T. (1992). Computational constraints suggest the need for two distinct input systems to the hippocampal CA3 network, *Hippocampus* **2**: 189–99.

Treves, A. and Rolls, E. T. (1994). A computational analysis of the role of the hippocampus in memory, *Hippocampus* **4**: 374–391.

Treves, A., Rolls, E. T. and Simmen, M. (1997). Time for retrieval in recurrent associative memories, *Physica D* **107**: 392–400.

Treves, A., Panzeri, S., Rolls, E. T., Booth, M. and Wakeman, E. A. (1999). Firing rate distributions and efficiency of information transmission of inferior temporal cortex neurons to natural visual stimuli, *Neural Computation* **11**: 601–631.

Trivers, R. L. (1985). *Social Evolution*, Benjamin, Cummings, CA.

Troiani, V., Stigliani, A., Smith, M. E. and Epstein, R. A. (2014). Multiple object properties drive scene-selective regions, *Cereb Cortex* **24**: 883–97.

Tsao, A., Sugar, J., Lu, L., Wang, C., Knierim, J. J., Moser, M. B. and Moser, E. I. (2018). Integrating time from experience in the lateral entorhinal cortex, *Nature* **561**: 57–62.

Tsao, D. (2014). The macaque face patch system: a window into object representation, *Cold Spring Harb Symp Quant Biol* **79**: 109–14.

Tsao, D. Y., Freiwald, W. A., Tootell, R. B. and Livingstone, M. S. (2006). A cortical region consisting entirely of face-selective cells, *Science* **311**: 617–618.

Tschacher, W., Giersch, A. and Friston, K. (2017). Embodiment and schizophrenia: a review of implications and applications, *Schizophr Bull* **43**: 745–753.

Tsitsiklis, M., Miller, J., Qasim, S. E., Inman, C. S., Gross, R. E., Willie, J. T., Smith, E. H., Sheth, S. A., Schevon, C. A., Sperling, M. R., Sharan, A., Stein, J. M. and Jacobs, J. (2020). Single-neuron representations of spatial targets in humans, *Curr Biol* **30**: 245–253 e4.

Tsuchida, A. and Fellows, L. K. (2012). Are you upset? Distinct roles for orbitofrontal and lateral prefrontal cortex in detecting and distinguishing facial expressions of emotion, *Cereb Cortex* **22**: 2904–12.

Tuckwell, H. (1988). *Introduction to Theoretical Neurobiology*, Cambridge University Press, Cambridge.

Turken, A. U. and Dronkers, N. F. (2011). The neural architecture of the language comprehension network: converging evidence from lesion and connectivity analyses, *Front Syst Neurosci* **5**: 1.

Turova, T. and Rolls, E. T. (2019). Analysis of biased competition and cooperation for attention in the cerebral cortex, *Front Comput Neurosci* **13**: 51.

Tyler, L. K., Randall, B. and Stamatakis, E. A. (2008). Cortical differentiation for nouns and verbs depends on grammatical markers, *J Cogn Neurosci* **20**: 1381–9.

Ullman, S. (1996). *High-Level Vision. Object Recognition and Visual Cognition*, Bradford/MIT Press, Cambridge, MA.

Ullman, S., Assif, L., Fetaya, E. and Harari, D. (2016). Atoms of recognition in human and computer vision, *Proc Natl Acad Sci U S A* **113**: 2744–9.

Ullsperger, M. and von Cramon, D. Y. (2001). Subprocesses of performance monitoring: a dissociation of error processing and response competition revealed by event-related fMRI and ERPs, *Neuroimage* **14**: 1387–1401.

Umbach, G., Kantak, P., Jacobs, J., Kahana, M., Pfeiffer, B. E., Sperling, M. and Lega, B. (2020). Time cells in the human hippocampus and entorhinal cortex support episodic memory, *Proc Natl Acad Sci U S A* **117**: 28463–28474.

Underwood, A. G., Guynn, M. J. and Cohen, A. L. (2015). The future orientation of past memory: the role of BA 10 in prospective and retrospective retrieval modes, *Front Hum Neurosci* **9**: 668.

Ungerleider, L. G. (1995). Functional brain imaging studies of cortical mechanisms for memory, *Science* **270**: 769–775.

Ungerleider, L. G. and Haxby, J. V. (1994). 'What' and 'where' in the human brain, *Curr Opin Neurobiol* **4**: 157–65.

Ungerleider, L. G. and Mishkin, M. (1982). Two cortical visual systems, *in* D. J. Ingle, M. A. Goodale and R. J. W. Mansfield (eds), *Analysis of Visual Behavior*, MIT Press, Cambridge, MA, pp. 549–586.

Uno, Y. and Coyle, J. T. (2019). Glutamate hypothesis in schizophrenia, *Psychiatry Clin Neurosci* **73**: 204–215.

Uran, C., Peter, A., Lazar, A., Barnes, W., Klon-Lipok, J., Shapcott, K. A., Roese, R., Fries, P., Singer, W. and Vinck, M. (2022). Predictive coding of natural images by V1 firing rates and rhythmic synchronization, *Neuron* **110**: 2886–2887.

Urgen, B. A. and Orban, G. A. (2021). The unique role of parietal cortex in action observation: Functional organization for communicative and manipulative actions, *Neuroimage* **237**: 118220.

Usher, M. and Niebur, E. (1996). Modelling the temporal dynamics of IT neurons in visual search: A mechanism for top-down selective attention, *Journal of Cognitive Neuroscience* **8**: 311–327.

Valdes-Sosa, P. A., Roebroeck, A., Daunizeau, J. and Friston, K. (2011). Effective connectivity: influence, causality and biophysical modeling, *Neuroimage* **58**: 339–61.

van Assche, M., Kebets, V., Vuilleumier, P. and Assal, F. (2016). Functional dissociations within posterior parietal cortex during scene integration and viewpoint changes, *Cereb Cortex* **26**: 586–598.

van Beest, E. H., Mukherjee, S., Kirchberger, L., Schnabel, U. H., van der Togt, C., Teeuwen, R. R. M., Barsegyan, A., Meyer, A. F., Poort, J., Roelfsema, P. R. and Self, M. W. (2021). Mouse visual cortex contains a region of enhanced spatial resolution, *Nat Commun* **12**: 4029.

van den Heuvel, M. P., de Reus, M. A., Feldman Barrett, L., Scholtens, L. H., Coopmans, F. M., Schmidt, R., Preuss, T. M., Rilling, J. K. and Li, L. (2015). Comparison of diffusion tractography and tract-tracing measures of connectivity strength in rhesus macaque connectome, *Hum Brain Mapp* **36**: 3064–75.

van den Heuvel, O. A., Veltman, D. J., Groenewegen, H. J., Cath, D. C., van Balkom, A. J., van Hartskamp, J., Barkhof, F. and van Dyck, R. (2005). Frontal-striatal dysfunction during planning in obsessive-compulsive disorder, *Archives of General Psychiatry* **62**: 301–309.

van den Heuvel, O. A., van Wingen, G., Soriano-Mas, C., Alonso, P., Chamberlain, S. R., Nakamae, T., Denys, D., Goudriaan, A. E. and Veltman, D. J. (2016). Brain circuitry of compulsivity, *Eur Neuropsychopharmacol* **26**: 810–27.

van der Heijden, K., Rauschecker, J. P., de Gelder, B. and Formisano, E. (2019). Cortical mechanisms of spatial hearing, *Nat Rev Neurosci* **20**: 609–623.

van der Klaauw, A. A. and Farooqi, I. S. (2015). The hunger genes: pathways to obesity, *Cell* **161**: 119–32.

van der Linden, M., Berkers, R. M. W. J., Morris, R. G. M. and Fernandez, G. (2017). Angular gyrus involvement at encoding and retrieval Is associated with durable but less specific memories, *J Neurosci* **37**: 9474–9485.

Van Essen, D. C. and Glasser, M. F. (2018). Parcellating cerebral cortex: how invasive animal studies inform noninvasive mapmaking in humans, *Neuron* **99**: 640–663.

Van Essen, D., Anderson, C. H. and Felleman, D. J. (1992). Information processing in the primate visual system: an integrated systems perspective, *Science* **255**: 419–423.

van Haeften, T., Baks-te Bulte, L., Goede, P. H., Wouterlood, F. G. and Witter, M. P. (2003). Morphological and numerical analysis of synaptic interactions between neurons in deep and superficial layers of the entorhinal cortex of the rat, *Hippocampus* **13**: 943–952.

Van Hoesen, G. W. (1981). The differential distribution, diversity and sprouting of cortical projections to the amygdala in the rhesus monkey, in Y. Ben-Ari (ed.), *The Amygdaloid Complex*, Elsevier, Amsterdam, pp. 77–90.

Van Hoesen, G. W. (1982). The parahippocampal gyrus. New observations regarding its cortical connections in the monkey, *Trends in Neurosciences* **5**: 345–350.

Van Hoesen, G. W., Yeterian, E. H. and Lavizzo-Mourey, R. (1981). Widespread corticostriate projections from temporal cortex of the rhesus monkey, *Journal of Comparative Neurology* **199**: 205–219.

Van Overwalle, F., Manto, M., Cattaneo, Z., Clausi, S., Ferrari, C., Gabrieli, J. D. E., Guell, X., Heleven, E., Lupo, M., Ma, Q., Michelutti, M., Olivito, G., Pu, M., Rice, L. C., Schmahmann, J. D., Siciliano, L., Sokolov, A. A., Stoodley, C. J., van Dun, K., Vandervert, L. and Leggio, M. (2020). Consensus paper: cerebellum and social cognition, *Cerebellum* **19**: 833–868.

van Strien, N. M., Cappaert, N. L. and Witter, M. P. (2009). The anatomy of memory: an interactive overview of the parahippocampal-hippocampal network, *Nature Reviews Neuroscience* **10**: 272–282.

van Veen, V., Cohen, J. D., Botvinick, M. M., Stenger, A. V. and Carter, C. S. (2001). Anterior cingulate cortex, conflict monitoring, and levels of processing, *Neuroimage* **14**: 1302–1308.

van Vugt, B., Dagnino, B., Vartak, D., Safaai, H., Panzeri, S., Dehaene, S. and Roelfsema, P. R. (2018). The threshold for conscious report: Signal loss and response bias in visual and frontal cortex, *Science* **360**: 537–542.

Vann, S. D. and Aggleton, J. P. (2004). The mammillary bodies: two memory systems in one?, *Nature Reviews Neuroscience* **5**: 35–44.

Vann, S. D., Aggleton, J. P. and Maguire, E. A. (2009). What does the retrosplenial cortex do?, *Nat Rev Neurosci* **10**: 792–802.

Vanni, S., Hokkanen, H., Werner, F. and Angelucci, A. (2020). Anatomy and physiology of macaque visual cortical areas V1, V2, and V5/MT: bases for biologically realistic models, *Cereb Cortex* **30**: 3483–3517.

VanRullen, R., Guyonneau, R. and Thorpe, S. J. (2005). Spike times make sense, *Trends in Neuroscience* **28**: 1–4.

Veale, D. M., Sahakian, B. J., Owen, A. M. and Marks, I. M. (1996). Specific cognitive deficits in tests sensitive to frontal lobe dysfunction in obsessive-compulsive disorder, *Psychological Medicine* **26**: 1261–1269.

Vedder, L. C., Miller, A. M. P., Harrison, M. B. and Smith, D. M. (2017). Retrosplenial cortical neurons encode navigational cues, trajectories and reward locations during goal directed navigation, *Cereb Cortex* **27**: 3713–3723.

Ventre-Dominey, J. (2014). Vestibular function in the temporal and parietal cortex: distinct velocity and inertial processing pathways, *Front Integr Neurosci* **8**: 53.

Verhagen, J. V., Rolls, E. T. and Kadohisa, M. (2003). Neurons in the primate orbitofrontal cortex respond to fat texture independently of viscosity, *J Neurophysiol* **90**: 1514–25.

Verhagen, J. V., Kadohisa, M. and Rolls, E. T. (2004). The primate insular/opercular taste cortex: neuronal representations of the viscosity, fat texture, grittiness, temperature and taste of foods, *Journal of Neurophysiology* **92**: 1685–1699.

Verhagen, J. V., Baker, K. L., Vasan, G., Pieribone, V. A. and Rolls, E. T. (2023). Odor encoding by signals in the olfactory bulb, *J Neurophysiol* **129**: 431–444.

Vigliocco, G., Vinson, D. P., Druks, J., Barber, H. and Cappa, S. F. (2011). Nouns and verbs in the brain: a review of behavioural, electrophysiological, neuropsychological and imaging studies, *Neuroscience and Biobehavioral Reviews* **35**: 407–426.

Vinckier, F., Dehaene, S., Jobert, A., Dubus, J. P., Sigman, M. and Cohen, L. (2007). Hierarchical coding of letter strings in the ventral stream: dissecting the inner organization of the visual word-form system, *Neuron* **55**: 143–56.

Vinje, W. E. and Gallant, J. L. (2000). Sparse coding and decorrelation in primary visual cortex during natural vision, *Science* **287**: 1273–1276.

Virasoro, M. A. (1989). Categorization in neural networks and prosopagnosia, *Physics Reports* **184**: 301–306.

Vogels, R. (2022). More than the face: representations of bodies in the inferior temporal cortex, *Annu Rev Vis Sci* **8**: 383–405.

Vogels, R. and Biederman, I. (2002). Effects of illumination intensity and direction on object coding in macaque inferior temporal cortex, *Cerebral Cortex* **12**: 756–766.

Vogels, R., Biederman, I., Bar, M. and Lorincz, A. (2001). Inferior temporal neurons show greater sensitivity to nonaccidental than to metric shape differences, *J Cogn Neurosci* **13**: 444–53.

Vogt, B. A. (2009). *Cingulate Neurobiology and Disease*, Oxford University Press, Oxford.

Vogt, B. A. (2016). Midcingulate cortex: Structure, connections, homologies, functions and diseases, *J Chem Neuroanat* **74**: 28–46.

Vogt, B. A. (2019a). The cingulate cortex in neurologic diseases: History, Structure, Overview, *Handb Clin Neurol* **166**: 3–21.

Vogt, B. A. (2019b). *Handbook of Clinical Neurology: Cingulate Cortex*, Vol. 166 of *Handbook of Clinical Neurology*, 3 edn, Elsevier, Oxford.

Vogt, B. A. and Pandya, D. N. (1987). Cingulate cortex of the rhesus monkey: II. Cortical afferents, *Journal of Comparative Neurology* **262**: 271–289.

Vogt, B. A. and Sikes, R. W. (2000). The medial pain system, cingulate cortex, and parallel processing of nociceptive information, *Progress in Brain Research* **122**: 223–235.

Vogt, B. A., Nimchinsky, E. A., Vogt, L. J. and Hof, P. R. (1995). Human cingulate cortex: surface features, flat maps, and cytoarchitecture, *J Comp Neurol* **359**: 490–506.

Vogt, B. A., Derbyshire, S. and Jones, A. K. P. (1996). Pain processing in four regions of human cingulate cortex localized with co-registered PET and MR imaging, *European Journal of Neuroscience* **8**: 1461–1473.

Vogt, B. A., Berger, G. R. and Derbyshire, S. W. G. (2003). Structural and functional dichotomy of human midcingulate cortex, *European Journal of Neuroscience* **18**: 3134–3144.

Volkow, N. D., Wang, G. J., Tomasi, D. and Baler, R. D. (2013). Obesity and addiction: neurobiological overlaps, *Obes Rev* **14**: 2–18.

Volkow, N. D., Wise, R. A. and Baler, R. (2017). The dopamine motive system: implications for drug and food addiction, *Nat Rev Neurosci* **18**: 741–752.

Völlm, B. A., De Araujo, I. E. T., Cowen, P. J., Rolls, E. T., Kringelbach, M. L., Smith, K. A., Jezzard, P., Heal, R. J. and Matthews, P. M. (2004). Methamphetamine activates reward circuitry in drug naive human subjects, *Neuropsychopharmacology* **29**: 1715–1722.

Waelti, P., Dickinson, A. and Schultz, W. (2001). Dopamine responses comply with basic assumptions of formal learning theory, *Nature* **412**: 43–48.

Walker, M. P. and Stickgold, R. (2006). Sleep, memory, and plasticity, *Annual Review of Psychology* **57**: 139–166.

Wallace, D. G. and Whishaw, I. Q. (2003). NMDA lesions of Ammon's horn and the dentate gyrus disrupt the direct and temporally paced homing displayed by rats exploring a novel environment: evidence for a role of the hippocampus in dead reckoning, *European Journal of Neuroscience* **18**: 513–523.

Wallis, G. and Baddeley, R. (1997). Optimal unsupervised learning in invariant object recognition, *Neural Computation* **9**: 883–894.

Wallis, G. and Bülthoff, H. (1999). Learning to recognize objects, *Trends in Cognitive Sciences* **3**: 22–31.

Wallis, G. and Rolls, E. T. (1997). Invariant face and object recognition in the visual system, *Prog Neurobiol* **51**: 167–94.

Wallis, G., Rolls, E. T. and Földiák, P. (1993). Learning invariant responses to the natural transformations of objects, *International Joint Conference on Neural Networks* **2**: 1087–1090.

Wallis, J. D. and Miller, E. K. (2003). Neuronal activity in primate dorsolateral and orbital prefrontal cortex during performance of a reward preference task, *European Journal of Neuroscience* **18**: 2069–2081.

Wallis, J. D., Anderson, K. C. and Miller, E. K. (2001). Single neurons in prefrontal cortex encode abstract rules, *Nature* **411**: 953–956.

Wallisch, P., Lusignan, M., Benayoun, M., Baker, T. L., Dickey, A. S. and Hatsoupoulos, N. G. (2009). *MATLAB for Neuroscientists*, Academic Press, Burlington, MA.

Walton, M. E., Bannerman, D. M. and Rushworth, M. F. S. (2002). The role of rat medial frontal cortex in effort-based decision making, *Journal of Neuroscience* **22**: 10996–11003.

Walton, M. E., Bannerman, D. M., Alterescu, K. and Rushworth, M. F. S. (2003). Functional Specialization within Medial Frontal Cortex of the Anterior Cingulate for Evaluating Effort-Related Decisions, *Journal of Neuroscience* **23**: 6475–6479.

Walton, M. E., Devlin, J. T. and Rushworth, M. F. (2004). Interactions between decision making and performance monitoring within prefrontal cortex, *Nature Neuroscience* **7**: 1259–1265.

Wan, Z., Rolls, E. T., Cheng, W. and Feng, J. (2020). Sensation-seeking is related to functional connectivities of the medial orbitofrontal cortex with the anterior cingulate cortex, *Neuroimage* **215**: 116845.

Wan, Z., Rolls, E. T., Cheng, W. and Feng, J. (2022). Brain functional connectivities that mediate the association between childhood traumatic events and adult mental health and cognition, *EBioMedicine* **79**: 104002.

Wang, C., Chen, X. and Knierim, J. J. (2020a). Egocentric and allocentric representations of space in the rodent brain, *Curr Opin Neurobiol* **60**: 12–20.

Wang, C. H., Monaco, J. D. and Knierim, J. J. (2020b). Hippocampal place cells encode local surface-texture boundaries, *Curr Biol* **30**: 1397–1409 e7.

Wang, H., Rolls, E. T., Du, X., Du, J., Yang, D., Li, J. ., Li, F., Cheng, W. and Feng, J. (2020c). Severe nausea and vomiting in pregnancy: psychiatric and cognitive problems, and brain structure in children, *BMC Medicine* **18**: 228.

Wang, L., Cheng, W., Rolls, E. T., Dai, F., Gong, W., Du, J., Zhang, W., Wang, S., Liu, F., Wang, J., Brown, P. and Feng, J. (2020d). Association of specific biotypes in patients with Parkinson disease and disease progression, *Neurology* **95**: e1445–e1460.

Wang, P. Y., Boboila, C., Chin, M., Higashi-Howard, A., Shamash, P., Wu, Z., Stein, N. P., Abbott, L. F. and Axel, R. (2020e). Transient and persistent representations of odor value in prefrontal cortex, *Neuron* **108**: 209–224 e6.

Wang, S., Yu, R., Tyszka, J. M., Zhen, S., Kovach, C., Sun, S., Huang, Y., Hurlemann, R., Ross, I. B., Chung, J. M., Mamelak, A. N., Adolphs, R. and Rutishauser, U. (2017). The human amygdala parametrically encodes the intensity of specific facial emotions and their categorical ambiguity, *Nat Commun* **8**: 14821.

Wang, S.-H. and Morris, R. G. M. (2010). Hippocampal-neocortical interactions in memory formation, consolidation, and reconsolidation, *Annual Review of Psychology* **61**: 49–79.

Wang, X. J. (1999). Synaptic basis of cortical persistent activity: the importance of NMDA receptors to working memory, *Journal of Neuroscience* **19**: 9587–9603.

Wang, X. J. (2001). Synaptic reverberation underlying mnemonic persistent activity, *Trends in Neurosciences* **24**: 455–463.

Wang, X. J. (2002). Probabilistic decision making by slow reverberation in cortical circuits, *Neuron* **36**: 955–968.

Wang, X.-J. (2008). Decision making in recurrent neuronal circuits, *Neuron* **60**: 215–234.

Wang, X. J. (2010). Neurophysiological and computational principles of cortical rhythms in cognition, *Physiological Reviews* **90**: 1195–1268.

Warrington, E. K. and Weiskrantz, L. (1973). An analysis of short-term and long-term memory defects in man, *in* J. A. Deutsch (ed.), *The Physiological Basis of Memory*, Academic Press, New York, chapter 10, pp. 365–395.

Wasserman, E., Kirkpatrick-Steger, A. and Biederman, I. (1998). Effects of geon deletion, scrambling, and movement on picture identification in pigeons, *Journal of Experimental Psychology – Animal Behavior Processes* **24**: 34–46.

Watanabe, K., Lauwereyns, J. and Hikosaka, O. (2003). Neural correlates of rewarded and unrewarded eye movements in the primate caudate nucleus, *Journal of Neuroscience* **23**: 10052–10057.

Watanabe, S., Lea, S. E. G. and Dittrich, W. H. (1993). What can we learn from experiments on pigeon discrimination?, *in* H. P. Zeigler and H.-J. Bischof (eds), *Vision, Brain, and Behavior in Birds*, MIT Press, Cambridge, MA, pp. 351–376.

Waters, S. J., Basile, B. M. and Murray, E. A. (2023). Reevaluating the role of the hippocampus in memory: A meta-analysis of neurotoxic lesion studies in nonhuman primates, *Hippocampus* p. doi: 10.1002/hipo.23499.

Watkins, L. H., Sahakian, B. J., Robertson, M. M., Veale, D. M., Rogers, R. D., Pickard, K. M., Aitken, M. R. and Robbins, T. W. (2005). Executive function in Tourette's syndrome and obsessive-compulsive disorder, *Psychological Medicine* **35**: 571–582.

Webb, T. J. and Rolls, E. T. (2014). Deformation-specific and deformation-invariant visual object recognition: pose vs identity recognition of people and deforming objects, *Frontiers in Computational Neuroscience* **8**: 37.

Webb, T. J., Rolls, E. T., Deco, G. and Feng, J. (2011). Noise in attractor networks in the brain produced by graded firing rate representations, *PLoS One* **6**: e23620.

Weghenkel, B. and Wiskott, L. (2018). Slowness as a proxy for temporal predictability: an empirical comparison, *Neural Comput* **30**: 1151–1179.

Wegrzyn, D., Juckel, G. and Faissner, A. (2022). Structural and functional deviations of the hippocampus in schizophrenia and schizophrenia animal models, *Int J Mol Sci* **23**: 5482.

Weiller, C., Reisert, M., Peto, I., Hennig, J., Makris, N., Petrides, M., Rijntjes, M. and Egger, K. (2021). The ventral pathway of the human brain: A continuous association tract system, *Neuroimage* **234**: 117977.

Weiner, K. S. and Grill-Spector, K. (2015). The evolution of face processing networks, *Trends Cogn Sci* **19**: 240–1.

Weiner, K. S., Barnett, M. A., Lorenz, S., Caspers, J., Stigliani, A., Amunts, K., Zilles, K., Fischl, B. and Grill-Spector, K. (2017). The cytoarchitecture of domain-specific regions in human high-level visual cortex, *Cereb Cortex* **27**: 146–161.

Weiskrantz, L. (1956). Behavioral changes associated with ablation of the amygdaloid complex in monkeys, *Journal of Comparative and Physiological Psychology* **49**: 381–391.

Weiskrantz, L. (1997). *Consciousness Lost and Found*, Oxford University Press, Oxford.

Weiskrantz, L. (1998). *Blindsight*, 2nd edn, Oxford University Press, Oxford.

Weiskrantz, L. (2009). Is blindsight just degraded normal vision?, *Experimental Brain Research* **192**: 413–416.

Weiss, A. P. and Heckers, S. (1999). Neuroimaging of hallucinations: a review of the literature, *Psychiatry Research* **92**: 61–74.

Weiss, C., Bouwmeester, H., Power, J. M. and Disterhoft, J. F. (1999). Hippocampal lesions prevent trace eyeblink conditioning in the freely moving rat, *Behavioural Brain Research* **99**: 123–132.

Weissman, M. M., Bland, R. C., Canino, G. J., Greenwald, S., Hwu, H. G., Lee, C. K., Newman, S. C., Oakley-Browne, M. A., Rubio-Stipec, M., Wickramaratne, P. J. et al. (1994). The cross national epidemiology of obsessive compulsive disorder. The Cross National Collaborative Group, *Journal of Clinical Psychiatry* **55 Suppl**: 5–10.

Wessa, M., Kanske, P. and Linke, J. (2014). Bipolar disorder: a neural network perspective on a disorder of emotion and motivation, *Restorative Neurology and Neuroscience* **32**: 51–62.

Whalen, P. J. and Phelps, E. A. (2009). *The Human Amygdala*, Guilford, New York.

Wheeler, E. Z. and Fellows, L. K. (2008). The human ventromedial frontal lobe is critical for learning from negative feedback, *Brain* **131**: 1323–1331.

Whishaw, I. Q., Hines, D. J. and Wallace, D. G. (2001). Dead reckoning (path integration) requires the hippocampal formation: evidence from spontaneous exploration and spatial learning tasks in light (allothetic) and dark (idiothetic) tests, *Behavioral Brain Research* **127**: 49–69.

Whitehouse, P., Price, D., Struble, R., Clarke, A., Coyle, J. and Delong, M. (1982). Alzheimer's disease in senile dementia: loss of neurones in the basal forebrain, *Science* **215**: 1237–1239.

Whitsel, B. L., Vierck, C. J., Waters, R. S., Tommerdahl, M. and Favorov, O. V. (2019). Contributions of Nociresponsive Area 3a to Normal and Abnormal Somatosensory Perception, *J Pain* **20**: 405–419.

Whittlesea, B. W. A. (1983). *Representation and Generalization of Concepts: the Abstractive and Episodic Perspectives Evaluated*, Unpublished doctoral dissertation, MacMaster University.

WHO, . (2017). World Health Organization: Depression and other common mental disorders: global health estimates, p. https://www.who.int/mental_health/management/depression/prevalence_global_health_estimates/en/.

Wickens, J. and Kotter, R. (1995). Cellular models of reinforcement, *in* J. C. Houk, J. L. Davis and D. G. Beiser (eds), *Models of Information Processing in the Basal Ganglia*, MIT Press, Cambridge, MA, chapter 10, pp. 187–214.

Wickens, J. R., Begg, A. J. and Arbuthnott, G. W. (1996). Dopamine reverses the depression of rat corticostriatal synapses which normally follows high-frequency stimulation of cortex in vitro, *Neuroscience* **70**: 1–5.

Widrow, B. and Hoff, M. E. (1960). Adaptive switching circuits, *1960 IRE WESCON Convention Record, Part 4 (Reprinted in Anderson and Rosenfeld, 1988)*, IRE, New York, pp. 96–104.

Widrow, B. and Stearns, S. D. (1985). *Adaptive Signal Processing*, Prentice-Hall, Englewood Cliffs, NJ.

Wiech, K., Jbabdi, S., Lin, C. S., Andersson, J. and Tracey, I. (2014). Differential structural and resting state connectivity between insular subdivisions and other pain-related brain regions, *Pain* **155**: 2047–55.

Wiener, N. (1956). The theory of prediction, *in* E. Beckenbach (ed.), *Modern Mathematics for Engineers*, McGraw-Hill, New York, chapter 8, pp. 165–190.

Wiener, S. I. and Taube, J. (eds) (2005). *Head Direction Cells and the Neural Mechanisms Underlying Directional Orientation*, MIT Press, Cambridge, MA.

Wilber, A. A., Clark, B. J., Forster, T. C., Tatsuno, M. and McNaughton, B. L. (2014). Interaction of egocentric and world-centered reference frames in the rat posterior parietal cortex, *J Neurosci* **34**: 5431–46.

Wilber, A. A., Skelin, I., Wu, W. and McNaughton, B. L. (2017). Laminar organization of encoding and memory reactivation in the parietal cortex, *Neuron* **95**: 1406–1419 e5.

Wild, B. and Treue, S. (2021). Primate extrastriate cortical area MST: a gateway between sensation and cognition, *J Neurophysiol* **125**: 1851–1882.

Wilkinson, S. T., Katz, R. B., Toprak, M., Webler, R., Ostroff, R. B. and Sanacora, G. (2018). Acute and longer-term outcomes using ketamine as a clinical treatment at the Yale Psychiatric Hospital, *J Clin Psychiatry* **79**: doi: 10.4088/JCP.17m11731.

Wilks, D. C., Besson, H., Lindroos, A. K. and Ekelund, U. (2011). Objectively measured physical activity and obesity prevention in children, adolescents and adults: a systematic review of prospective studies, *Obes Rev* **12**: e119–29.

Williams, G. V., Rolls, E. T., Leonard, C. M. and Stern, C. (1993). Neuronal responses in the ventral striatum of the behaving macaque, *Behav Brain Res* **55**: 243–52.

Wills, T. J., Lever, C., Cacucci, F., Burgess, N. and O'Keefe, J. (2005). Attractor dynamics in the hippocampal representation of the local environment, *Science* **308**: 873–876.

Willshaw, D. J. (1981). Holography, associative memory, and inductive generalization, *in* G. E. Hinton and J. A. Anderson (eds), *Parallel Models of Associative Memory*, Erlbaum, Hillsdale, NJ, chapter 3, pp. 83–104.

Willshaw, D. J. and Buckingham, J. T. (1990). An assessment of Marr's theory of the hippocampus as a temporary memory store, *Philosophical Transactions of The Royal Society of London, Series B* **329**: 205–215.

Willshaw, D. J. and Longuet-Higgins, H. C. (1969). The holophone – recent developments, *in* D. Mitchie (ed.), *Machine Intelligence*, Vol. 4, Edinburgh University Press, Edinburgh.

Willshaw, D. J. and von der Malsburg, C. (1976). How patterned neural connections can be set up by self-organization, *Proceedings of The Royal Society of London, Series B* **194**: 431–445.

Willshaw, D. J., Dayan, P. and Morris, R. G. (2015). Memory, modelling and Marr: a commentary on Marr (1971) 'Simple memory: a theory of archicortex', *Philos Trans R Soc Lond B Biol Sci* **370**: 20140383.

Wilson, C. J. (1995). The contribution of cortical neurons to the firing pattern of striatal spiny neurons, *in* J. C. Houk, J. L. Davis and D. G. Beiser (eds), *Models of Information Processing in the Basal Ganglia*, MIT Press, Cambridge, MA, chapter 3, pp. 29–50.

Wilson, D. A. and Sullivan, R. M. (2011). Cortical processing of odor objects, *Neuron* **72**: 506–519.

Wilson, D. A., Xu, W., Sadrian, B., Courtiol, E., Cohen, Y. and Barnes, D. C. (2014a). Cortical odor processing in health and disease, *Progress in Brain Research* **208**: 275–305.

Wilson, F. A., O'Scalaidhe, S. P. and Goldman-Rakic, P. S. (1994a). Functional synergism between putative gamma-aminobutyrate-containing neurons and pyramidal neurons in prefrontal cortex, *Proceedings of the Natlional Academy of Sciences U S A* **91**: 4009–4013.

Wilson, F. A. W. and Rolls, E. T. (1990a). Learning and memory are reflected in the responses of reinforcement-related neurons in the primate basal forebrain, *Journal of Neuroscience* **10**: 1254–1267.

Wilson, F. A. W. and Rolls, E. T. (1990b). Neuronal responses related to reinforcement in the primate basal forebrain, *Brain Research* **509**: 213–231.

Wilson, F. A. W. and Rolls, E. T. (1990c). Neuronal responses related to the novelty and familiarity of visual stimuli in the substantia innominata, diagonal band of Broca and periventricular region of the primate, *Experimental Brain Research* **80**: 104–120.

Wilson, F. A. W. and Rolls, E. T. (1993). The effects of stimulus novelty and familiarity on neuronal activity in the amygdala of monkeys performing recognition memory tasks, *Experimental Brain Research* **93**: 367–382.

Wilson, F. A. W. and Rolls, E. T. (2005). The primate amygdala and reinforcement: a dissociation between rule-based and associatively-mediated memory revealed in amygdala neuronal activity., *Neuroscience* **133**: 1061–1072.

Wilson, F. A. W., Riches, I. P. and Brown, M. W. (1990). Hippocampus and medial temporal cortex: neuronal responses related to behavioural responses during the performance of memory tasks by primates, *Behavioral Brain Research* **40**: 7–28.

Wilson, F. A. W., Scalaidhe, S. P. and Goldman-Rakic, P. S. (1993). Dissociation of object and spatial processing domains in primate prefrontal cortex, *Science* **260**: 1955–8.

Wilson, F. A. W., O'Scalaidhe, S. P. and Goldman-Rakic, P. (1994b). Functional synergism between putative gamma-aminobutyrate-containing neurons and pyramidal neurons in prefrontal cortex, *Proceedings of the National Academy of Science* **91**: 4009–4013.

Wilson, H. R. (1999). *Spikes, Decisions and Actions: Dynamical Foundations of Neuroscience*, Oxford University Press, Oxford.

Wilson, H. R. and Cowan, J. D. (1972). Excitatory and inhibitory interactions in localised populations of model neurons, *Biophysics Journal* **12**: 1–24.

Wilson, M. A. (2002). Hippocampal memory formation, plasticity, and the role of sleep, *Neurobiology of Learning and Memory* **78**: 565–569.

Wilson, M. A. and McNaughton, B. L. (1993). Dynamics of the hippocampal ensemble code for space, *Science* **261**: 1055–8.

Wilson, M. A. and McNaughton, B. L. (1994). Reactivation of hippocampal ensemble memories during sleep, *Science* **265**: 676–679.

Wilson, R. C., Takahashi, Y. K., Schoenbaum, G. and Niv, Y. (2014b). Orbitofrontal cortex as a cognitive map of task space, *Neuron* **81**: 267–279.

Winocur, G. and Moscovitch, M. (2011). Memory transformation and systems consolidation, *J Int Neuropsychol Soc* **17**: 766–80.

Winston, P. H. (1975). Learning structural descriptions from examples, *in* P. H. Winston (ed.), *The Psychology of Computer Vision*, McGraw-Hill, New York, pp. 157–210.

Winterer, G., Ziller, M., Dorn, H., Frick, K., Mulert, C., Wuebben, Y., Herrmann, W. M. and Coppola, R. (2000). Schizophrenia: reduced signal-to-noise ratio and impaired phase-locking during information processing, *Clinical Neurophysiology* **111**: 837–849.

Winterer, G., Coppola, R., Goldberg, T. E., Egan, M. F., Jones, D. W., Sanchez, C. E. and Weinberger, D. R. (2004). Prefrontal broadband noise, working memory, and genetic risk for schizophrenia, *American Journal of Psychiatry* **161**: 490–500.

Winterer, G., Musso, F., Beckmann, C., Mattay, V., Egan, M. F., Jones, D. W., Callicott, J. H., Coppola, R. and Weinberger, D. R. (2006). Instability of prefrontal signal processing in schizophrenia, *American Journal of Psychiatry* **163**: 1960–1968.

Wirth, S. (2023). A place with a view: a first-person perspective in the hippocampal memory space, *Hippocampus* **33**: 658–666.

Wirth, S., Yanike, M., Frank, L. M., Smith, A. C., Brown, E. N. and Suzuki, W. A. (2003). Single neurons in the monkey hippocampus and learning of new associations, *Science* **300**: 1578–1581.

Wirth, S., Avsar, E., Chiu, C. C., Sharma, V., Smith, A. C., Brown, E. and Suzuki, W. A. (2009). Trial outcome and associative learning signals in the monkey hippocampus, *Neuron* **61**: 930–40.

Wirth, S., Baraduc, P., Plante, A., Pinede, S. and Duhamel, J. R. (2017). Gaze-informed, task-situated representation of space in primate hippocampus during virtual navigation, *PLoS Biol* **15**: e2001045.

Wirth, S., Soumier, A., Eliava, M., Derdikman, D., Wagner, S., Grinevich, V. and Sirigu, A. (2021). Territorial blueprint in the hippocampal system, *Trends Cogn Sci* **25**: 831–842.

Wise, R. A. and Jordan, C. J. (2021). Dopamine, behavior, and addiction, *J Biomed Sci* **28**: 83.

Wise, S. P. (2008). Forward frontal fields: phylogeny and fundamental function, *Trends in Neuroscience* **31**: 599–608.

Wiskott, L. (2003). Slow feature analysis: A theoretical analysis of optimal free responses, *Neural Computation* **15**: 2147–2177.

Wiskott, L. and Sejnowski, T. J. (2002). Slow feature analysis: unsupervised learning of invariances, *Neural Comput* **14**: 715–70.

Witter, M. P. (1993). Organization of the entorhinal–hippocampal system: a review of current anatomical data, *Hippocampus* **3**: 33–44.

Witter, M. P. (2007). Intrinsic and extrinsic wiring of CA3: indications for connectional heterogeneity, *Learning and Memory* **14**: 705–713.

Witter, M. P. and Amaral, D. G. (2021). The entorhinal cortex of the monkey: VI. Organization of projections from the hippocampus, subiculum, presubiculum, and parasubiculum, *J Comp Neurol* **529**: 828–852.

Witter, M. P., Groenewegen, H. J., Lopes da Silva, F. H. and Lohman, A. H. M. (1989a). Functional organization of the extrinsic and intrinsic circuitry of the parahippocampal region, *Progress in Neurobiology* **33**: 161–254.

Witter, M. P., Van Hoesen, G. W. and Amaral, D. G. (1989b). Topographical organisation of the entorhinal projection to the dentate gyrus of the monkey, *Journal of Neuroscience* **9**: 216–228.

Witter, M. P., Naber, P. A., van Haeften, T., Machielsen, W. C., Rombouts, S. A., Barkhof, F., Scheltens, P. and Lopes da Silva, F. H. (2000a). Cortico-hippocampal communication by way of parallel parahippocampal-subicular pathways, *Hippocampus* **10**: 398–410.

Witter, M. P., Wouterlood, F. G., Naber, P. A. and Van Haeften, T. (2000b). Anatomical organization of the parahippocampal-hippocampal network, *Annals of the New York Academcy of Sciences* **911**: 1–24.

Wolkin, A., Sanfilipo, M., Wolf, A. P., Angrist, B., Brodie, J. D. and Rotrosen, J. (1992). Negative symptoms and hypofrontality in chronic schizophrenia, *Archives of General Psychiatry* **49**: 959–965.

Wood, E. R., Dudchenko, P. A. and Eichenbaum, H. (1999). The global record of memory in hippocampal neuronal activity, *Nature* **397**: 613–6.

Wood, E. R., Dudchenko, P. A., Robitsek, R. J. and Eichenbaum, H. (2000). Hippocampal neurons encode information about different types of memory episodes occurring in the same location, *Neuron* **27**: 623–33.

Wood, E. R., Agster, K. M. and Eichenbaum, H. (2004). One-trial odor–reward association: a form of event memory not dependent on hippocampal function, *Behavioral Neuroscience* **118**: 526–539.

Woodward, J. (2005). *Making things happen: A theory of causal explanation*, Oxford University Press.

Woodward, J. (2015). Interventionism and causal exclusion, *Philosophy and Phenomenological Research* **91**: 303–347.

Woodward, J. (2020). Levels: What are they and what are they good for?, *in* K. S. Kendler, J. Parnas and P. Zachar (eds), *Levels of Analysis in Psychopathology: Cross Disciplinary Perspectives*, Cambridge University Press, Cambridge, pp. 424–449.

Woodward, J. (2021a). Downward causation and levels, *in* D. S. Brooks, J. DiFrisco and W. C. Wimsatt (eds), *Levels of Organization in the Biological Sciences*, MIT Press, Cambridge, MA, pp. http://philsci-archive.pitt.edu/id/eprint/18004.

Woodward, J. (2021b). Downward causation defended, *in* J. Voosholz and M. Gabriel (eds), *Top-Down Causation and Emergence*, Springer, pp. 217–251.

Wu, A., Dvoryanchikov, G., Pereira, E., Chaudhari, N. and Roper, S. D. (2015). Breadth of tuning in taste afferent neurons varies with stimulus strength, *Nat Commun* **6**: 8171.

Wu, C. C., Sacchet, M. D. and Knutson, B. (2012). Toward an affective neuroscience account of financial risk taking, *Frontiers in Neuroscience* **6**: 159.

Wu, X., Baxter, R. A. and Levy, W. B. (1996). Context codes and the effect of noisy learning on a simplified hippocampal CA3 model, *Biological Cybernetics* **74**: 159–165.

Wurm, M. F. and Caramazza, A. (2019). Distinct roles of temporal and frontoparietal cortex in representing actions across vision and language, *Nat Commun* **10**: 289.

Wurtz, R. H. and Duffy, C. J. (1992). Neuronal correlates of optic flow stimulation, *Ann N Y Acad Sci* **656**: 205–19.

Wyatt, T. D. (2014). *Pheromones and Animal Behaviour*, 2nd edn, Cambridge University Press, Cambridge.

Wyatt, T. D. (2020). Reproducible research into human chemical communication by cues and pheromones: learning from psychology's renaissance, *Philos Trans R Soc Lond B Biol Sci* **375**: 20190262.

Wyss, R., Konig, P. and Verschure, P. F. (2006). A model of the ventral visual system based on temporal stability and local memory, *PLoS Biol* **4**: e120.

Xavier, G. F., Oliveira-Filho, F. J. and Santos, A. M. (1999). Dentate gyrus-selective colchicine lesion and disruption of performance in spatial tasks: difficulties in "place strategy" because of a lack of flexibility in the use of environmental cues?, *Hippocampus* **9**: 668–681.

Xiang, J. Z. and Brown, M. W. (1998). Differential neuronal encoding of novelty, familiarity and recency in regions of the anterior temporal lobe, *Neuropharmacology* **37**: 657–676.

Xiang, J. Z. and Brown, M. W. (2004). Neuronal responses related to long-term recognition memory processes in prefrontal cortex, *Neuron* **42**: 817–829.

Xie, C., Jia, T., Rolls, E. T., Robbins, T. W., Sahakian, B. J., Zhang, J., Liu, Z., Cheng, W., Luo, Q., Zac Lo, C.-Y., Wang, H., Banaschewski, T., Barker, G., Bodke, A., Buchel, C., Quinlan, E. B., Desrivieres, S., Flor, H., Grigis, A., Garavan, H., Gowland, P., Heinz, A., Hohmann, S., Ittermann, B., Martinot, J.-L., Martinot, M.-L. P., Nees, F., Papadopoulos Orfanos, D., Paus, T., Poustka, L., Frohner, J. H., Smolka, M. N., Walter, H., Whelan, R., Schumann, G., Feng, J. and IMAGEN, C. (2021). Reward vs non-reward sensitivity of the medial vs lateral orbitofrontal cortex relates to the severity of depressive symptoms, *Biological Psychiatry: Cognitive Neuroscience and Neuroimaging* **6**: 259–269.

Xue, G. (2018). The neural representations underlying human episodic memory, *Trends Cogn Sci* **22**: 544–561.

Yamada, H., Louie, K., Tymula, A. and Glimcher, P. W. (2018). Free choice shapes normalized value signals in medial orbitofrontal cortex, *Nat Commun* **9**: 162.

Yamamoto, S., Kim, H. F. and Hikosaka, O. (2013). Reward value-contingent changes of visual responses in the primate caudate tail associated with a visuomotor skill, *Journal of Neuroscience* **33**: 11227–11238.

Yamane, S., Kaji, S. and Kawano, K. (1988). What facial features activate face neurons in the inferotemporal cortex of the monkey?, *Experimental Brain Research* **73**: 209–214.

Yamins, D. L. and DiCarlo, J. J. (2016). Using goal-driven deep learning models to understand sensory cortex, *Nat Neurosci* **19**: 356–65.

Yamins, D. L., Hong, H., Cadieu, C. F., Solomon, E. A., Seibert, D. and DiCarlo, J. J. (2014). Performance-optimized hierarchical models predict neural responses in higher visual cortex, *Proc Natl Acad Sci U S A* **111**: 8619–24.

Yan, J. and Scott, T. R. (1996). The effect of satiety on responses of gustatory neurons in the amygdala of alert cynomolgus macaques, *Brain Research* **740**: 193–200.

Yang, A. C., Rolls, E. T., Dong, G., Du, J., Li, Y., Feng, J., Cheng, W. and Zhao, X.-M. (2022). Longer screen time utilization is associated with the polygenic risk for Attention-deficit/hyperactivity disorder with mediation by brain white matter microstructure, *EBioMedicine* **80**: 104039.

Yang, C., Chen, H. and Naya, Y. (2023). Allocentric information represented by self-referenced spatial coding in the primate medial temporal lobe, *Hippocampus* **33**: 522–532.

Yates, F. A. (1992). *The Art of Memory*, University of Chicago Press, Chicago, Ill.

Yaxley, S., Rolls, E. T., Sienkiewicz, Z. J. and Scott, T. R. (1985). Satiety does not affect gustatory activity in the nucleus of the solitary tract of the alert monkey, *Brain Research* **347**: 85–93.

Yaxley, S., Rolls, E. T. and Sienkiewicz, Z. J. (1988). The responsiveness of neurons in the insular gustatory cortex of the macaque monkey is independent of hunger, *Physiology and Behavior* **42**: 223–229.

Yaxley, S., Rolls, E. T. and Sienkiewicz, Z. J. (1990). Gustatory responses of single neurons in the insula of the macaque monkey, *Journal of Neurophysiology* **63**: 689–700.

Yeatman, J. D. and White, A. L. (2021). Reading: The Confluence of Vision and Language, *Annu Rev Vis Sci* **7**: 487–517.

Yelnik, J. (2002). Functional anatomy of the basal ganglia, *Movement Disorders* **17 Suppl 3**: S15–S21.

Yeterian, E. H., Pandya, D. N., Tomaiuolo, F. and Petrides, M. (2012). The cortical connectivity of the prefrontal cortex in the monkey brain, *Cortex* **48**: 58–81.

Yoganarasimha, D., Yu, X. and Knierim, J. J. (2006). Head direction cell representations maintain internal coherence during conflicting proximal and distal cue rotations: comparison with hippocampal place cells, *Journal of Neuroscience* **26**: 622–631.

Yokoyama, C., Autio, J. A., Ikeda, T., Sallet, J., Mars, R. B., Van Essen, D. C., Glasser, M. F., Sadato, N. and Hayashi, T. (2021). Comparative connectomics of the primate social brain, *Neuroimage* **245**: 118693.

Young, A. W., Aggleton, J. P., Hellawell, D. J., Johnson, M., Broks, P. and Hanley, J. R. (1995). Face processing impairments after amygdalotomy, *Brain* **118**: 15–24.

Young, A. W., Hellawell, D. J., Van De Wal, C. and Johnson, M. (1996). Facial expression processing after amygdalotomy, *Neuropsychologia* **34**: 31–9.

Zaborszky, L., Hoemke, L., Mohlberg, H., Schleicher, A., Amunts, K. and Zilles, K. (2008). Stereotaxic probabilistic maps of the magnocellular cell groups in human basal forebrain, *Neuroimage* **42**: 1127–41.

Zaborszky, L., Gombkoto, P., Varsanyi, P., Gielow, M. R., Poe, G., Role, L. W., Ananth, M., Rajebhosale, P., Talmage, D. A., Hasselmo, M. E., Dannenberg, H., Minces, V. H. and Chiba, A. A. (2018). Specific basal forebrain-cortical cholinergic circuits coordinate cognitive operations, *J Neurosci* **38**: 9446–9458.

Zaharia, A. D., Goris, R. L. T., Movshon, J. A. and Simoncelli, E. P. (2019). Compound stimuli reveal the structure of visual motion selectivity in macaque MT neurons, *eNeuro* **6**: ENEURO.0258–19.2019.

Zangemeister, L., Grabenhorst, F. and Schultz, W. (2016). Neural basis for economic saving strategies in human amygdala-prefrontal reward circuits, *Curr Biol* **26**: 3004–3013.

Zanos, P. and Gould, T. D. (2018). Mechanisms of ketamine action as an antidepressant, *Mol Psychiatry* **23**: 801–811.

Zanos, P., Moaddel, R., Morris, P. J., Georgiou, P., Fischell, J., Elmer, G. I., Alkondon, M., Yuan, P., Pribut, H. J., Singh, N. S., Dossou, K. S., Fang, Y., Huang, X. P., Mayo, C. L., Wainer, I. W., Albuquerque, E. X., Thompson, S. M., Thomas, C. J., Zarate, C. A., J. and Gould, T. D. (2016). NMDAR inhibition-independent antidepressant actions of ketamine metabolites, *Nature* **533**: 481–6.

Zapiec, B. and Mombaerts, P. (2015). Multiplex assessment of the positions of odorant receptor-specific glomeruli in the mouse olfactory bulb by serial two-photon tomography, *Proc Natl Acad Sci U S A* **112**: E5873–82.

Zatorre, R. J., Jones-Gotman, M., Evans, A. C. and Meyer, E. (1992). Functional localization of human olfactory cortex, *Nature* **360**: 339–340.

Zatorre, R. J., Jones-Gotman, M. and Rouby, C. (2000). Neural mechanisms involved in odor pleasantness and intensity judgments, *NeuroReport* **11**: 2711–2716.

Zeidman, P. and Maguire, E. A. (2016). Anterior hippocampus: the anatomy of perception, imagination and episodic memory, *Nat Rev Neurosci* **17**: 173–82.

Zeidman, P., Mullally, S. L. and Maguire, E. A. (2015). Constructing, perceiving, and maintaining scenes: hippocampal activity and connectivity, *Cereb Cortex* **25**: 3836–55.

Zeisel, A., Hochgerner, H., Lonnerberg, P., Johnsson, A., Memic, F., van der Zwan, J., Haring, M., Braun, E., Borm, L. E., La Manno, G., Codeluppi, S., Furlan, A., Lee, K., Skene, N., Harris, K. D., Hjerling-Leffler, J., Arenas, E., Ernfors, P., Marklund, U. and Linnarsson, S. (2018). Molecular architecture of the mouse nervous system, *Cell* **174**: 999–1014 e22.

Zhang, B., Rolls, E. T., Wang, X., Xie, C., Cheng, W. and Feng, J. (2023a). Roles of the medial and lateral orbitofrontal cortex in major depression and its treatment.

Zhang, H., Japee, S., Stacy, A., Flessert, M. and Ungerleider, L. G. (2020). Anterior superior temporal sulcus is specialized for non-rigid facial motion in both monkeys and humans, *Neuroimage* **218**: 116878.

Zhang, K. (1996). Representation of spatial orientation by the intrinsic dynamics of the head-direction cell ensemble: A theory, *Journal of Neuroscience* **16**: 2112–2126.

Zhang, R., Rolls, E. T., Cheng, W. and Feng, J. (2023b). Different cortical connectivities in human females and males relate to differences in strength and body composition, reward and emotional systems, and memory, p. in review.

Zhao, D., Si, B. and Tang, F. (2019). Unsupervised feature learning for visual place recognition in changing environments, *2019 International Joint Conference on Neural Networks (IJCNN)* **IEEE**: 1–8.

Zhao, X., Wang, Y., Spruston, N. and Magee, J. C. (2020). Membrane potential dynamics underlying context-dependent sensory responses in the hippocampus, *Nat Neurosci* **23**: 881–891.

Zhao, X., Hsu, C. L. and Spruston, N. (2022). Rapid synaptic plasticity contributes to a learned conjunctive code of position and choice-related information in the hippocampus, *Neuron* **110**: 96–108 e4.

Zhu, S. L., Lakshminarasimhan, K. J. and Angelaki, D. E. (2023). Computational cross-species views of the hippocampal formation, *Hippocampus* **33**: 586–599.

Zhuang, C., Yan, S., Nayebi, A., Schrimpf, M., Frank, M. C., DiCarlo, J. J. and Yamins, D. L. K. (2021). Unsupervised neural network models of the ventral visual stream, *Proc Natl Acad Sci U S A* **118**: e2014196118.

Zihl, J., Von Cramon, D. and Mai, N. (1983). Selective disturbance of movement vision after bilateral brain damage, *Brain* **106**: 313–340.

Zilli, E. A. (2012). Models of grid cell spatial firing published 2005–2011, *Frontiers in Neural Circuits* **6**: 16.

Zink, C. F., Pagnoni, G., Martin, M. E., Dhamala, M. and Berns, G. S. (2003). Human striatal responses to salient nonrewarding stimuli, *Journal of Neuroscience* **23**: 8092–8097.

Zink, C. F., Pagnoni, G., Martin-Skurski, M. E., Chappelow, J. C. and Berns, G. S. (2004). Human striatal responses to monetary reward depend on saliency, *Neuron* **42**: 509–517.

Zohary, E., Shadlen, M. N. and Newsome, W. T. (1994). Correlated neuronal discharge rate and its implications for psychophysical performance, *Nature* **370**: 140–143.

Zola-Morgan, S., Squire, L. R., Amaral, D. G. and Suzuki, W. A. (1989). Lesions of perirhinal and parahippocampal cortex that spare the amygdala and hippocampal formation produce severe memory impairment, *Journal of Neuroscience* **9**: 4355–4370.

Zola-Morgan, S., Squire, L. R. and Ramus, S. J. (1994). Severity of memory impairment in monkeys as a function of locus and extent of damage within the medial temporal lobe memory system, *Hippocampus* **4**: 483–494.

Zorumski, C. F., Izumi, Y. and Mennerick, S. (2016). Ketamine: NMDA receptors and beyond, *J Neurosci* **36**: 11158–11164.

Zucker, S. W., Dobbins, A. and Iverson, L. (1989). Two stages of curve detection suggest two styles of visual computation, *Neural Computation* **1**: 68–81.

Zwir, I., Del-Val, C., Hintsanen, M., Cloninger, K. M., Romero-Zaliz, R., Mesa, A., Arnedo, J., Salas, R., Poblete, G. F., Raitoharju, E., Raitakari, O., Keltikangas-Jarvinen, L., de Erausquin, G. A., Tattersall, I., Lehtimaki, T. and Cloninger, C. R. (2022). Evolution of genetic networks for human creativity, *Mol Psychiatry* **27**: 354–376.

Index

ΔI, 549–554
3D model, 94–96
3D object recognition, 153–159
5HT, 482–483

accessory olfactory system, 252
accumulation of evidence, 719
acetylcholine, 13, 347, 395, 527, 761–765, 943, 1011
acetylcholine and memory, 442
action in space, 201–220
action-outcome learning, 527, 588–590, 778–780
actions
    cost, 488
activation, 7
activation function, 7, 834, 844
active vision, 97
adaptation, 7, 347, 651, 762, 764, 843, 891–892, 915, 941, 1011
addiction, 518–520, 692
ADHD, 760, 793
adolescents, 766
advantages of cortical architecture, 692
ageing, 836, 943
aging, 758–765
agnosia
    associative, 303
AIP, 219, 464
alignment approach to object recognition, 96–97
allocentric, 208, 451
allocentric auditory space, 293
allocentric bearing to a landmark cells, 425–427
allocentric coordinates, 592
allocentric coordinates definition, 206
allocentric representation, 420
allocentric scene representation, 452
allocentric sound location cells, 293
Alzheimer's disease, 348, 761–765
ambiguity, 490
ambiguous figures, 192
amnesia, 346–353, 382, 456
    retrograde, 324, 382
amphetamine, 518
amygdala, 529–544, 1001
    and reversal, 558
    connections, 531
    lesions, 532
    not involved in conscious feelings, 538
amygdala lesions
    macaques, 533
amygdala neuronal responses, 535–537
analysis by synthesis, 190
AND, 809
angular gyrus, 631
animal welfare, 517
anterior cingulate cortex, 359–363, 527

anterior thalamic nuclei, 346, 347
    and memory, 505
anterior thalamus, 350
aperture problem, 202
aphasia, 303
ars memoriae, 418
art of memory, 418
artificial intelligence, 728
associative learning, 172, 613, 815–855
associative processes, 530–531
associative reward–penalty algorithm, 933–934
asymmetric receptive fields, 170
attention, 162–172, 609–622
    biased activation theory of, 247–250
    binding, 195
    feature integration theory, 195
    top-down, 195
attention and emotion, 238–239
attention deficit hyperactivity disorder, ADHD, 760
attractor network, 19, 159–162, 544–554, 832–887, 911–915
attractor network dynamics, 711–767, 892–900
attractor network simulations, 1036–1038
attractor networks
    diluted connectivity, 843–854
    discrete and continuous, 887
    hierarchically organized, 620
    obsessive-compulsive disorder, 739–742
auditory cortex in humans, 293–298
auditory cortical streams, 291, 293
auditory feature hierarchy, 292
auditory localization, 287–290
auditory processing, 286–298
auditory representation in the orbitofrontal cortex, 292
auditory representation in the prefrontal cortex, 292
autism, 80
autoassociation network, 19, 159–162, 832–855
autoassociation network simulations, 1036–1038
autocorrelation memory, 835
autonomic responses, 531, 535, 581
autonomic system, 589
avoidance, 530–531

backprojections, 107, 192, 266, 403, 405–412, 555, 854, 864–866
    quantitative analysis, 409–412
backpropagation learning and vision, 88
backpropagation of error network, 18, 922–928
backpropagation of error networks, 98, 775
basal forebrain, 761–765
basal forebrain cholingeric nucleus, 527
basal forebrain neurons, 442
basal ganglia, 665–694, 703, 778–780
basal ganglia and reward, 528

basal ganglia computation, 669–694
basal magnocellular cholinergic neurons, 763–765
basal magnocellular forebrain nuclei of Meynert, 762
Bayes' theorem, 1033
bearing, 208
bearing to a landmark cells, 425–427
biased activation hypothesis of attention, 247–250
biased activation theory of attention, 247–250
biased competition, 162–172, 908–909
biased competition hypothesis of attention, 195–198
binding, 65, 95–96, 106, 134–147, 195, 624–659, 1028
binocular rivalry, 192
biologically plausible computation, 787–791
biologically plausible models of object recognition, 183–188
biologically plausible networks, 18, 775–778
bipolar disorder, 756–758
bits per spike and sparseness, 1009
blindsight, 510
blood pressure, 766
body motion cells, 336, 586
body movements, 84
body parts, 84
BOLD signal, 231
Boltzmann machine, 930–931
brain development, 766
brain vs digital computers, 769–775
Brain-Inspired Intelligence, 769, 791
Brain-Inspired Medicine, 792
breadth of tuning, 226
Broca's area, 604, 637
Brodmann areas, 22–27

CA1 neurons, 400–405
CA2, 367
CA3 neurons, 378–400
capacity, 809
    autoassociator, 839–840
    competitive network, 859
    pattern associator, 827–829, 831
catastrophic changes in the qualitative shape descriptors, 154
categorisation, 303
categorization, 855, 858
category formation, 938
caudate nucleus
    head, 667, 669, 676–681
    tail, 674–675
causality, 780, 782
Central Executive Network, 786
central tendency, 825, 837
cerebellar cortex, 695–708
cerebellar Purkinje cell, 700
cerebellum and cognition, 702
change blindness, 192–194
chart, 388
cholinergic neurons, 761–765
cholinergic system, 359–363
cingulate cortex, 238–241, 564–595
    midcingulate, 588
    posterior, 581
    subgenual, 581
cingulate cortex and hippocampus, 592
cingulate motor area, 588
clamped inputs, 835
classical conditioning, 535, 672, 934
classification, 855
climbing fibres in the cerebellum, 698
cluster analysis, 862
cluttered environment, 147–153
coarse coding, 16
cocaine, 518
Code for information theoretic analysis of neuronal activity, 1044
Code for VisNet, 1043
coding, 17, 74–79, 771, 824, 831, 966–1034
coefficient of sliding friction, 234
cognition and olfaction, 260
cognitive map, 388
Cognitron, 103–104
coherence, 136
cold, 272
columnar organization, 84
combinatorial explosion, 107, 147
command neurons, 270, 664
common scale of value, 576
communication before coherence, 136
communication through coherence, 136
competitive network, 19, 104, 397, 855–876
competitive network simulations, 1041–1043
competitive networks
    diluted connectivity, 858
completion, 438, 442, 834, 836
computation
    by the whole brain, 769
computation of non-reward, 559
computational neurology, 792
computational psychiatry, 792
computers, 769–778
concept cells, 302, 322, 323, 629
    in humans, 302
    in macaques, 322
    in monkeys, 302
conditional expected value neurons, 486
conditional reward neurons, 486, 556
conditioned response, 530, 531
conditioned stimulus, 530, 531
conditioning, 530–531, 815–831
conductances, 889–892
confabulation, 515, 727
confidence, 549–554
configural learning, 399
conflict, 514
connectionism, 18
connectionist networks, 311
connectivity
    modifiable, 773
    ventral visual streams, 85–92
consciousness, 726, 780, 784, 785, 1011
consolidation, 405, 457
    memory, 359–363
content addressability, 769, 832
context, 840

continuous attractor networks, 178, 193, 345, 384–389, 418, 441, 876–887
continuous attractors, 384
continuous spatial transformation learning, 172–173
contrastive Hebbian learning, 97, 930–931
convergence, 104
convolution networks, 98, 189, 775, 928–930
convolutional neural network, 189
coordinate transforms, 420, 471
correlation, 805
cortex, 544
   decision-making, 709–765
   noisy operation, 709–765
   stability, 709–765
   stochastic dynamics, 711–767
cortical
   backprojections, 405–412
cortical architecture
   advantages, 692
   design and evolution, 266
   disadvantages, 692
   quantitative aspects, 44–52
cortical circuits, 46–52
cortical computations, 695–708
cortical design, 39–52, 84, 945–965
cortical structure, 39–52
cost of actions, 488
cost–benefit analysis, 514
costs, 490
coupled attractor networks, 911–915
creative thought, 728
creativity, 728
credit assignment, 927
critical band masking, 67
critical period, 943
cross-correlation, 1025–1029
cross-correlations
   between neuronal spike trains, 982–990
crossmodal association, 620
curves, 61

deception, 514, 515
decision
   under ambiguity, 490
   under risk, 490
decision time, 717–721
decision times, 552–553
decision-making
   medial prefrontal cortex, 549–554
decision-making in the somatosensory system, 276
decoding, 74, 978–982
Deep Belief Networks, 931
deep learning, 98, 189, 311, 928–930
deep learning and vision, 88
deep lerning, 928
deep networks, 775
Default Mode Network, 786
deformation-invariant object recognition, 175–176
delayed match to sample, 559, 675, 762
delta rule, 917
delta rule learning, 934–938
dementia, 303

dentate granule cells, 393–400, 432
depression, 576, 742–758, 793
   ketamine, 753
   theory of, 742–758
desire vs pleasure, 535
determinism, 727
deterministic behavior, 727
devaluation, 487, 567, 576
difference of Gaussian (DOG) filtering, 113–115
difficult vs easy decisions, 549–552
diffusion tractography, 37
digital computers vs brain computation, 769–775
diluted connectivity, 390–392, 412
   competitive networks, 858
dilution of the connectivity, 829
discoveries
   properties of inferior temporal visual cortex neurons, 52–200
   theories of schizophrenia, obsessive-compulsive disorder, depression, and normal aging, 709–765
   theory of hippocampal operation, 313–458
   theory of invariant visual object recognition, 52–200
distributed computation, 772
distributed encoding, 107
distributed representation, 15–18, 74–79, 824, 831, 991–1002, 1023–1025
   advantages, 17–18
divisive inhibition, 42
dopamine, 13, 482–483, 518, 528, 760, 778–780, 790
   and reward, 688
   and reward prediction error, 688, 937
   reward prediction error hypothesis, 680
dopamine and schizophrenia, 729–738
dopamine neurons
   error signal, 688–694
   reward, 688–694
dorsal cortical auditory stream, 293
dorsal visual cortical stream in humans, 217–220
dorsal visual pathway, 22
dorsal visual system, 178, 201–220, 869
dorsolateral prefrontal cortex, 606
dot product, 92, 803–806, 812
   neuronal operation, 821
dot product decoding, 981–982
downward causality, 782
dual stream model of language comprehension, 627
dynamical systems properties, 774
dynamics, 887–915

effective connectivity, 37
egocentric, 208, 451
egocentric coordinates, 592
egocentric coordinates definition, 206
egocentric representation, 420
emotion, 589
   and attention, 238–239
   and memory, 761–765
   definition, 506
emotion-related learning, 530–531
empathy, 517

encoding, 15, 74, 966–1034
energy
  in an autoassociator, 835
energy landscape, 384, 552, 714–721, 731–765, 835, 848–854
entorhinal cortex, 337, 369, 372, 386–387, 398–399, 403
epilepsy, 692, 774
episodic memory, 313–458, 854, 887
  'where', 177
ergodicity, 903, 998, 1000–1001
error correction, 915–928
error correction and invariance learning, 126
error correction learning, 125–134, 934–938
error correction network, 915
error learning, 934–938
error neurons, 495–500, 555, 559, 688–694, 743, 937
error signal, 934
error signals, 590
escape, 530–531
escaping time, 717–721
evolution, 945–965
evolution of cortex, 945–965
evolution of emotion, 515
evolutionary history of the orbitofrontal cortex, 562
evolutionary utility, 725
excitatory cortical neurons, 40–41
executive function, 511, 596
exocentric coordinates definition, 206
expansion recoding, 698, 830, 863
expected reward value, 487, 934–938
expected utility, 672–674
expected value, 237, 257, 484, 680, 934
experienced reward value and emotion, 225
explicit processing, 726
exploit, 577
exploit vs explore, 564
explore, 577
exponential firing rate distribution, 994–1005
expression, 80–85
  face, 80, 492, 496, 536, 538–539
extinction, 495–500, 934
extraversion, 539
eye position, 206

face attractiveness, 492, 494
face expression, 80–85, 299, 492, 496
  amygdala, 538–539
face gesture, 299
face identity, 62–85, 492
face patch, 190
face processing
  neuroimaging, 83
false binding errors, 146–147
familiarity, 350
Fano factor, 712
fat, 234, 535, 571, 669
fat texture, 234
fault tolerance, 770, 823, 836
fear, 538
feature
  binding, 106

  combinations, 106
feature analysis, 857
feature analyzer, 862
feature analyzers, 20, 102, 106, 234
feature binding, 134–147, 1028
feature binding in a hierarchical network, 139
feature combinations, 61, 67, 98, 118, 134–147
feature hierarchies, 98–200
  introduction, 98–103
feature hierarchy, 98, 107–200
feature integration theory, 195
feature spaces, 93–94
feature subsets and supersets, 134–139
features, 98
feedback inhibition, 44
feedback processing, 892–900
feedforward processing, 897–900
finite size noise, 713
firing rate distribution, 840, 991–1002
  exponential, 991–1002
firing rate encoding, 392
flavor, 236, 257
flow, 714–721
fMRI, 231
food reward, 241, 793
food texture, 234–236, 502, 535, 571
foraging, 564, 577, 726
forgetting, 323, 382, 940–945
fornix, 505
forward replay, 376
free will, 726, 727
frontal lobes, 22
frontal pole cortex, 612
FST, 218
functional connectivity, 37

GABA, 683
GABA, gamma-amino-butyric acid, 41–44, 834
Gabor filters, 113, 115
gambling, 502
gamma oscillations, 548
gamma rhythm, 136
gene-defined goal, 506–509
generalization, 144–147, 822, 836
generic view, 154
genes, 945
genetic algorithm, 869, 951
genetic algorithms, 945
genetic specification
  of brain connectivity, 773, 945–965
global motion, 202, 204–206, 269
global workspace hypothesis of consciousness, 784
glomerulus, 253, 262
glucose, 535
Go/NoGo task, 535, 556, 677
goal for action, 506–509
goal-related action, 589
graceful degradation, 770, 823, 836
gradient of retrograde amnesia, 383
grammar, 624–659
grandmother cell, 16, 74, 105
grandmother cell encoding, 15

Granger causality, 611, 781
granule cells, 366–400, 697–708
granule cells in the cerebellum, 698
grid cells, 337, 386–387, 398–399

habenula, 482–483
habit learning, 535, 589, 679, 688, 790
hairpin maze, 333
HCNN, 189
HCP MMP atlas, 27–36
head direction cells, 344–346, 386, 455, 878–884
Hebb rule, 8–14, 816, 817, 826, 833, 838
Hebbian associative learning, 159
hedonic assessment, 535
hidden units, 927
hierarchical convolutional neural networks, 189
hierarchical feature analysis networks for object recognition, 98–200
hierarchical networks, 20, 102, 106, 234
hierarchical processing, 774, 866, 897–900
hierarchy, 104, 515
    feature, 107–200
higher order syntactic thought theory of consciousness, 784
higher order thought theory of consciousness, 784
hippocampal chart, 388
hippocampal design, 266
hippocampal function
    rodents, 445–450
hippocampal simulation, 413
hippocampal theory
    evaluation, 454–458
hippocampus, 313–458, 527, 592, 707, 763, 863, 1001
    anatomy, 316–319
    backprojections, 403, 405–412
    CA1, 442–445
    CA3, 435–442
    CA3 neurons, 378–397
    completion, 438
    lesions, 319–321
    memory, 450
    navigation, 450
    neurophysiology, 324–344
    object–spatial view neurons, 337
    recall, 403
    reward–spatial view neurons, 339
    Rolls' theory of, 313–458
    speed cells, 336
    summary, 450
    tests of the theory, 432–445
    theory, 364–414
hippocampus and memory, 313–458
hippocampus and parahippocampal cortex in navigation, 431
hippocampus, blood pressure, and memory, 766
hippocampus: random allocation of CA3 neurons to new memories, 395
hippocmpal spatial view cells, 353–356
HMAX, 183–188
Hodgkin-Huxley equations, 889–890
Hopfield, 835
human auditory cortex, 293–298

human brains compared to rodent brains, 796–802
human cortical coding, 1032
human lateral orbitofrontal cortex, 523
human medial orbitofrontal cortex, 521
human navigation, 429, 431
human somatosensory cortex, 278–283
human STS semantic cortex, 305–311
hypertension and memory, 766
hypothalamus
    lateral, 761–765
hypotheses, invariant object recognition, 104–107

idiothetic (self-motion) inputs, 882–884
idiothetic navigation, 427–432
idiothetic update, 334, 471
imaging, 83
implicit processing, 726
implicit responses, 516
impulsiveness, 497
incentive motivation, 518
indexing theory of hippocampal memory recall, 409
inferior frontal gyrus, 497, 604
inferior parietal cortex, 467
inferior temporal cortex
    models, 52–200
    subdivisions, 80–85
    topology, 867
inferior temporal visual cortex, 190
    learning, 71
information
    bits per spike and sparseness, 1009
    continuous variables, 974–976
    in the cross-correlation, 1025–1029
    in the rate, 1025–1029
    limited sampling problem, 976–982
    multiple cell, 978–990, 1019–1033
    mutual, 971, 1033
    neuronal, 976–1033
    neuronal synchronization, 982–990, 1025–1029
    odor, 1007
    single neuron, 971–974
    speed of transfer, 1007–1019
    temporal, 1007
    temporal encoding within a spike train, 991–1007
information encoding, 966–1033
information encoding software, 1044
information from multiple neurons, 1019–1029
information theoretic analysis of neuronal responses, 990–1033
information theory, 77, 966–1034
inhibitory cortical neurons, 41–44
inhibitory neurons, 502, 555, 686, 834
inner product, 803, 821
instrumental learning, 531, 589
instrumental reinforcers, 530–531, 535, 554
insula, 272, 589
insular taste cortex, 1001
integrate-and-fire model, 196
integrate-and-fire neuronal networks, 713–725, 887–900
interacting attractor networks, 911–915
interests, 512

gene-defined, 512
of the individual defined by the reasoning system, 512
interference, 829
intraparietal cortex, 219
introversion, 539
invariance, 53–200
　dendritic computation, 190
　rotation, 105
　scale, 105
　size, 105
　spatial frequency, 105
　translation, 105, 144–147
　view, 106, 153–159
invariance learning, 870–871
invariant object recognition, 774
　approaches, 92–103
　hypotheses, 104–107
　models, 52–200
invariant representations, 62–71, 92
invariant visual object recognition, 1043
invertebrate neural systems, 961
invertible networks, 97–98
Iowa Gambling Task, 502
IP1, 219

Jennifer Aniston neuron, 322

ketamine and depression, 753
Kohonen map, 866–870

labelled line encoding, 15
language, 292, 301–312, 624–659, 773
lateral hypothalamus, 535, 761–765
lateral inhibition, 41, 42, 266, 856, 866
lateral intraparietal cortex, LIP, 178
lateralization of function, 320
learning, 760
　action–outcome, 588–589
　associative, 484–489, 530–531, 815–831
　habit, 589, 688
　in a cluttered environment, 151–152
　instrumental, 530–531, 554, 589, 680
　of emotional responses, 530
　of emotional states, 530–531
　stimulus–response, 589, 688
learning in IT, 71
learning in the neocortex, 938
learning rule
　local, 826, 838
learning set, 554–559
least mean squares rule, 917
levels of explanation, 780, 785
levels of investigation, 785
lighting invariance, 173–174
linear algebra, 803–814
linear separability, 807–813, 860
linearity, 807
linearly independent vectors, 807–813
LIP, 206, 219, 464
local learning rule, 10, 18, 826, 838
local representation, 16, 831

logical operations, 774
long-term depression, 700
long-term depression (LTD), 10–15, 554, 558, 940
long-term familiarity memory, 350
long-term memory, 346–353
long-term potentiation (LTP), 10–15, 817
low order feature combinations, 20, 102, 106, 234
LTD, 10–15, 700, 940
LTP, 10–15

macaque brains, 796–802
Machiavellian intelligence, 515
machine learning, 20, 928
magnetoencephalography, MEG, 38
mammillary bodies, 346, 350, 505
mammillothalamic tract, 505
mania, 756–758
map, 84, 866–870
mapping in short-term memory, 620
Marr, 409
masking, 1011–1012
McGurk effect, 866, 913–914
mean field neurodynamics, 901–911
medial prefrontal cortex, 549–554, 576
memory, 313–458, 511, 527, 544, 559, 675, 761–765, 815
　anterior thalamic nuclei, 505
　for sequences, 389
　hippocampus, 313–458
　object recognition, 52–200
　perirhinal cortex, 346–353
　recognition, 346–353
　subcortical paths, 505
memory and hypertension, 766
memory and the ventromedial prefrontal cortex, 504
memory capacity, 85
memory consolidation, 359–363, 457, 527
memory reconsolidation, 942–943
mice, 796–802
middle temporal gyrus, 299
mind–body problem, 780
mind–brain problem, 780
mind–brain relationship, 780–785
minimal recognizable configurations, 188
MIP, 219, 464
mirror neurons, 274, 662–664
mixture states, 841
model of reversal learning, 554–559
modular organization, 868
modularity, 45–52, 774
monetary reward, 499–501, 571, 672–674, 680
monitoring, 649
mood, 571
mossy fibres, 393–396
motion, 201–206
motor control, 665–708, 887
motor cortex, 283
motor cortical areas, 660–664
MST, 218
MT, 218, 869
multicompartment neurons, 897
multilayer perceptron, 922–928

multimodal representations, 865
multimodular dynamics, 909–915
multiple cell information, 1019–1033
multiple cell information analysis, 1044
multiple decision-making systems, 515
multiple memory systems, 67
multiple objects, 146, 162–172
multiple objects in a scene, 170
multiplicative interactions, 910
multistability, 719–721
music, 495, 517
mutual information, 1033

natural scene, 147–153
natural scene object recognition, 178–181
natural scenes, 64–66, 135, 162–172
Navigation, 419–432, 473–474
navigation, 333, 335, 450, 586
   goals for, 359
   idiothetic, 427–432
navigation in primates, 423
navigation using spatial view cells, 423
navigation with allocentric bearing to a landmark cells, 425–427
navigation: hippocampus and parahippocampal cortex, 431
navigational strategy in primates including humans, 425, 800
navigational strategy in rodents, 425, 800
negative reward prediction error, 559
Neocognitron, 103–104
neocortex, 22–52, 703, 707, 938
neocortex cerebellum comparison, 703
neocortex model, 407
neocortical computation, 787–791
neocortical design, 266
neocortical learning, 395
neocortical model, 789
net value, 490
neural encoding, 74–79, 824
neural networks
   effects of damage, 303
neuroeconomics, 490–492
neurogenesis, 400, 434
neuroimaging, 72, 83, 553
neuromodulation, 13
neuronal encoding, 966–1034
neuronal network simulation software, 1035–1044
neuronal networks, 19–21, 815–966
neuronal regeneration, 262
neurons, 5–18, 39–52
neuroticism, 539
NMDA receptors, 10–15, 534, 558, 758, 829, 874, 885
noise, 719–767, 772
   definition, 713
   finite size, 713
   measurement, 713
noise and diluted connectivity, 391
noise in the brain
   source, 711–713
noise reduction, 825, 837

noisy cortex, 711–767
non-accidental properties of object transforms, 181
non-linear networks, 812–814
non-linearity, 807
   in the learning rule, 874
non-reward, 500, 507, 577, 680
non-reward and depression, 743–756
non-reward computation, 559
non-reward neurons, 495–500, 555, 589, 742–743
noradrenaline, 760
norepinephrine, 760
normalization
   of neuronal activity, 42
   of synaptic weights, 873
nucleus accumbens, 669–674

obesity, 243, 793
object identification, 84, 194
object motion, 204–206
object recognition, 52–200
   biologically plausible models, 183–188
   Rolls' theory of, 52–200
object recognition in natural scenes, 178–181
object representations, 79, 352, 990–1033
object vs spatial view representations, 176, 342
object-based encoding, 69–71
object-based motion, 206
obsessive-compulsive disorder, 738–742
occipital place area, 353–356
occlusion, 70, 152–153
odor, 238–239, 251–267
Oja learning rule, 159, 874
olfaction, 571
   orbitofrontal cortex, 256
   attentional influences, 238–239
   modulation by cognition, 260
olfaction and orbitofrontal cortex, 267
olfaction and taste, 257
olfactory bulb, 253, 262
olfactory bulb information, 1007
olfactory cortex, 255
olfactory epithelium, 253, 262
olfactory receptor gene, 253, 262
olfactory reversal learning, 257
olfactory reward, 259
olfactory system, 251–267
olfactory with taste convergence, 257
opiates, 535
optic flow, 206
orbitofrontal cortex, 80, 292, 359–363, 669, 778–780, 1001
   anatomy, 479–483
   auditory responses, 495
   behavioral problems, 528
   connections, 479–483
   emotional problems, 528
   evolutionary history, 562
   face representations, 492–495
   influences of attention, 238–239
   olfaction, 256
   relative preference, 502
   reward, 259

topology, 500–502
visual inputs, 484–495
orbitofrontal cortex and emotion, 506
orbitofrontal cortex and memory, 527
orbitofrontal cortex and olfaction, 257
orbitofrontal cortex connectivity in humans, 521
orbitofrontal cortex lesions
macaques, 498, 533
orthogonalization, 397, 858, 863
oscillations, 136
outcome, 934
output systems for emotion, 535, 581–589
ownership, 350
oxytocin, 367

pain, 272–276, 284, 569–589, 672
palimpsest, 940
parahippocampal gyrus, 353–356
parahippocampal scene area, 177, 353–356
parallel computation, 772
parallel distributed computation, 771, 772
parallel fibres in the cerebellum, 697
parietal cortex, 631
parietal cortex, area 7, 466
parietal cortex, intraparietal regions, 464
parietal visual cortex, 467
Parkinson's disease, 760
path integration, 345, 386–387, 441, 882–887
pattern association, 412
pattern association memory, 815–831
pattern association network, 19
pattern association network simulations, 1038–1041
pattern separation, 393–400, 432–434, 707, 860
Pavlovian conditioning, 530, 672, 934
percent correct, 552
perceptron, 701, 809, 915–928
perceptual learning, 71
perforant path, 396
perirhinal cortex, 301, 346–353
perirhinal cortex and territoriality, 350
personality, 497, 539, 793
PFm, 470
PGp, 471
PGs, 470
pheromone, 252
phonemes, 292
phonological processing, 631
place cells, 324–344, 416, 450
place cells vs spatial view cells, 414–416
place code, 642
place coding, 15
planning, 596, 623, 692
pleasant touch, 272–276, 284, 571
pleasure map, 501
pleasure scaling, 576
pointer theory of hippocampal memory recall, 409
Poisson firing, 772
Poisson process, 712
population sparseness, 998–1002
posterior cingulate cortex, 581
Potts attractor network, 657
Potts attractor networks, 854

predicted reward value, 673, 934–938
prediction error, 482
prediction error hypothesis, 672–674, 680, 688–694, 937
preference
relative, 484, 502
prefrontal cortex, 22, 596–623, 784
computational necessity for, 616–623
medial, 549–554, 576
premotor cortex, 283
primary reinforcers, 507, 530, 535
primate brains compared to rodent brains, 796–802
principal component analysis (PCA), 862
prospective memory, 693
prototype extraction, 825, 837
psychiatric problems, 766
psychiatric states, 709–765
pyriform cortex, 238, 255
pyriform cortex connectivity in humans, 255
pyriform cortex design, 266

Q-learning, 938

radial basis function (RBF) networks, 871–872
rational choice, 515
rational, reasoning, 508
rationality, 512
rats, 796–802
reaction time, 717–721
reaction times, 552–553
reading, 627
reasoning, 512
recall, 321, 405–412, 816, 818, 833
in autoassociation memories, 834
semantic, 405
recall of semantic representation, 405
recency effect in short-term memory, 602
receptive field size, 104
receptive fields
asymmetric, 170
recognition
of objects, 52–200
recognition memory, 346–353
reconsolidation, 534, 942–943
recurrent collateral connections, 544
redundancy, 857, 863, 1019–1025
regeneration, 262
reinforcement learning, 590, 692, 703, 778–780, 790, 928, 932–938
reinforcers, 507–509, 514, 530–531, 535, 554
secondary, 484–500
relative preference, 484, 502
remapping, 333, 388
replay, 376, 457
representation
semantic, 405
representations
of objects, 79, 352, 990–1033
retrograde amnesia, 321–324, 382, 383
retrospective memory, 693
retrosplenial cortex, 592
retrosplenial place area, 353–356

retrosplenial scene area, 586, 587
reversal, 577
reversal learning, 484–500, 778–780
reversal learning set, 554–559
reversal learning, model of, 554–559
reverse replay, 376
reward, 241, 688–694
reward devaluation, 487
reward in the cerebellum, 702
reward magnitude, 934
reward outcome, 934
reward outcome value, 231
reward predicting neuron, 484, 677
reward prediction error, 495–500, 555, 589, 672, 680, 934–935
reward prediction error does not produce emotion, 780
reward systems, 793
reward value, 230, 259, 270, 664, 688–694
reward value and the hippocampal memory system, 358
rhythms in the brain, 136
Riesenhuber and Poggio model of invariant recognition, 183–188
ripples, 457
risk, 490
rodent hippocampal function, 445–450
rodents, 796–802
Rolls'
  biased activation theory of attention, 247–250
  discoveries on neuronal encoding, 966–1034
  discovery of hippocampal spatial view cells, 324–344
  discovery of olfactory reward neurons, 257–258
  discovery of sensory-specific satiety, 230–233
  hypotheses about the implementation of syntax in the cortex, 624–659
  hypotheses of how the cortex is specified and evolves, 945–965
  theory of depression, 742–758
  theory of hippocampal function, 313–458
  theory of invariant global motion recognition in the dorsal visual system, 204–206
  theory of normal aging, 758–765
  theory of obsessive-compulsive disorder, 738–742
  theory of schizophrenia, 729–738
  theory of visual object recognition, 52–200
Rolls' model of invariant recognition, 98–200
Rolls' theory of invariant object recognition, 774
routes to action, 508

saccade generation, 206
salience, 535, 671, 676–681
Saliency Network, 786
salted nut phenomenon, 518
satiety, 230–233, 241
scene representation, 176–178
schema, 388
schizophrenia, 729–738, 793
secondary reinforcers, 534
segregation of processing streams, 869
segregation of visual pathways

principles, 870
selection of action, 683
self-motion, 206
self-motion update, 334
self-organization, 857
self-organizing map, 84
selfish gene, 512–513
selfish individual, 512–513
selfish phene, 512–513
selfish phenotype, 512–513
semantic cell, 322
semantic memory, 301–312, 324, 854
semantic representation, 322, 405
semantic representations, 301–312, 629
semantics, 631, 640
  learning, 640
sensation-seeking, 497
sensory-specific satiety, 230–233, 487, 795
septal nuclei, 359–363
sequence memory, 389, 401, 403, 623, 841, 915
serotonin, 482–483
sexual behavior, 534
sharp wave ripples, 457
shift invariance, 105
short-term memory, 73, 195–198, 555, 596–623, 675, 692, 693, 762, 815, 832, 854, 911
  for visual stimuli, 73
  stability, 721–725
  stimulus-response mapping, 620
  visual, 192
shunting inhibition, 42
Sigma-Pi neurons, 9, 136, 190, 813–814
signal-detection theory, 712
signal-to-noise ratio, 713
simulation software, 1035–1044
simulations: attractor networks, 1036–1038
simulations: autoassociation networks, 1036–1038
simulations: competitive networks, 1041–1043
simulations: pattern association networks, 1038–1041
simultanagnosia, 192–194
single cell information analysis, 1044
size constancy, 67
size invariance, 67
sleep, 323
sleep and memory, 944–945
slow learning, 183
smell, 238–239, 251–267
social behavior, 367
social group, 350
soft competition, 874–875
soft max, 874
software, 1035–1044
somatosensory cortex in humans, 278–283
somatosensory insula, 272
somatosensory system, 268–285
sparseness, 16, 76, 226, 824, 829, 831, 859, 991–1002
sparseness and bits per spike, 1009
sparseness, population, 998–1002
sparsification, 863
spatial continuity, 172–173
spatial frequency, 67

spatial pattern separation, 432
spatial scene formation, 177
spatial scene learning, 418
spatial view cells, 176, 177, 324–344, 416, 423, 450
    anticipation of a scene, 334
spatial view cells and foveal vision, 342
spatial view cells and navigation, 423–432
spatial view cells and scene memory, 426
spatial view vs object representations, 176, 342
speed cells, 336, 586
speed of computation, 771
speed of operation of memory systems, 389
speed of processing, 45, 825, 837, 887–900
spike response model, 900–901
spike timing-dependent plasticity (STDP), 14
spin glass, 835
spontaneous firing
    principles, 711–714, 837
spontaneous firing of neurons, 711
spontaneous firing rate, 45
stability
    short-term memory, 721–725
stability of attractor networks in the cortex, 709–765
statistical mechanics, 835
STDP, 14
stimulus–reinforcer association learning, 484–489, 495–500, 532–536, 815–831
stimulus–reinforcer reversal learning, model of, 554–559
stimulus–response habits, 688
stimulus-response learning, 778–780, 790
stimulus-response mapping in short-term memory, 620
stochastc gradient descent, 928
stochastic dynamics, 772
stochastic resonance, 726
stop-signal task, 497
striatal neuronal activity, 670–682
striatum, 665–694
    ventral, 482–483
structural description, 94
structural differences in the brain, 766
structural shape descriptions, 94–96
STS, 80
STS semantic cortex in humans, 305–311
STS visual stream, 89, 632
subgenual anterior cingulate area 25, 574
subgenual cingulate cortex, 564, 569, 576, 581
subjective value, 680
substantia innominata, 347
substantia nigra, 528
superior temporal sulcus, 80
superior temporal sulcus visual stream, 89, 632
supervised learning, 21
supramarginal gyrus, 631
symmetric synaptic weights, 833
synaptic modifiability, 773
synaptic modification, 8–15, 554–555, 558, 760
synaptic weight vector, 816–831
synchronization, 135–136, 1025–1029
synchrony, 641
syntactic binding, 135–136

syntactic pattern recognition, 94–96
syntax, 301–312, 624–659, 773, 784

taste, 535, 571
taste cortex in humans, 281
TD learning, 938
temperature, 272
template matching, 96–97
temporal difference (TD) error, 672, 935–938
temporal difference (TD) learning, 125–134, 672–674, 935–938
temporal difference learning, 129–134, 935–938
temporal encoding within a spike train, 991–1007
temporal information, 1007
temporal lobe, 299–312
temporal order memory, 623
temporal pole, 303
temporal synchronization, 135, 1025–1029
territory, 301, 322–323, 350
territory cell, 322
texture, 234–236, 535, 571
    fat, 234
thalamus, 267
    functions of, 267
theories of hippocampal function, 454–458
theory of mind, 511, 517
third visual stream, 80
time cells, 372–378, 403, 623
top-down attention, 195
topographic map, 866–870, 1041–1043
touch, 268–285, 501, 531, 571
trace learning rule, 105, 109–110, 125–134
trace rule value η, 121, 124–125
tractography, 37
translation invariance, 105, 144–147
triangulation, 426

uncertainty, 688–694, 937
unclamped inputs, 835
unconditioned response, 530
unconditioned stimulus, 530, 554, 815–824
unconscious processing, 726
unifying approach, 787–791
unifying principles, 176, 198, 206, 416, 458
unpredictable behavior, 726, 729
unsupervised learning, 20, 107
unsupervised networks, 855–876
upward causality, 782

V2, 61, 106
V3A, 217
V4, 61, 106, 869
V6, 217
V6A, 217
valence, 670, 671, 676–681
value, 680
vector, 803, 816–831
    angle, 805
    correlation, 805
    dot product, 803
    length, 804
    linear combination, 807–813

linear independence, 807–813
linear separability, 807–813
normalization, 805
normalized dot product, 805
outer product, 806
vector quantization, 858
vector similarity computation, 770–774
ventral cortical auditory stream, 291
ventral forebrain nuclei of Meynert, 347
ventral striatum, 80, 534, 535, 669–674
ventral visual pathway, 22, 52–200
   principles, 870
ventral visual stream, 869
ventral visual system, 178
ventrolateral visual stream, 86
ventromedial cortical visual stream, 353–356
ventromedial prefrontal cortex, 347, 359–363, 549–554, 568, 576
ventromedial prefrontal cortex and memory, 504
vestibular inputs, 336
view invariance, 106, 122–124, 153–159
view-based object recognition, 98–200
view-based scene representation, 452
view-invariant representation, 69–71
viewpoint-dependent representations, 452
VIP, 206, 219, 464
virtual environment, 333
viscosity, 234, 535, 571
vision, 52–200
   association learning, 484–495
   deep learning, 88, 189
   princioal dimensions, 190
VisNet, 107–200, 416, 774, 1043
   3D transforms, 153–159
   and spatial view cells, 176, 416
   architecture, 108–115
   attention, 162–172
   attractor version, 159–162
   capacity, 159–162
   cluttered environment, 147–153
   continuous spatial transformation learning, 172
   feature binding, 134–147
   generalization, 144–147
   lighting invariance, 173
   motion, 204
   multiple objects, 162–172
   natural scenes, 162–172
   object motion, 204
   occlusion, 152–153
   performance measures, 115–117
   receptive field size, 162–172
   simulation code, 1043
   trace learning rule, 109–110
   trace rule, 125–134
   trace rule value η, 121, 124–125
   translation invariance, 121–122
   view invariance, 122–124
visual parietal cortex, 467
visual scene representations, 353–356
visual system connectivity, 85–92
Visual Word Form Area, 627
visuo-spatial scratchpad, 192–194

VMPFC, 504, 549–554, 568
vmPFC, 359–363
voluntary action, 596

wake-sleep algorithm, 930
warmth, 272
weight normalization, 873
welfare, 517
Wernicke's area, 635
what visual stream, 22, 52–200
where visual stream, 22
where visual system, 201–220
whole body motion cells, 336, 586
whole brain computation, 769
Widrow–Hoff rule, 917
winner-take-all, 105, 857
wiring length, 84, 868
word, 405
words, 292
working memory, 596, 623

XOR, 809